Contemporary Obstetrics and Gynecology for Developing Countries

Friday Okonofua • Joseph A. Balogun
Kunle Odunsi • Victor N. Chilaka
Editors

Contemporary Obstetrics and Gynecology for Developing Countries

Second Edition

Springer

Editors
Friday Okonofua
Centre of Excellence in Reproductive
Health Innovation
Department of Obstetrics and
Gynaecology, University of Benin
Benin City
Nigeria

Women's Health and Action Research Centre
Benin City
Nigeria

University of Medical Sciences
Ondo City, Ondo State
Nigeria

Kunle Odunsi
Roswell Park Cancer Institute
Buffalo, NY
USA

Joseph A. Balogun
College of Health Sciences
Chicago State University
Chicago, IL
USA

Victor N. Chilaka
Clinical Obstetrics and Gynaecology
Weil Cornell Medicine
Doha
Qatar

1st edition: © Women's Health and Action Research Centre (WHARC)2005
ISBN 978-3-030-75384-9 ISBN 978-3-030-75385-6 (eBook)
https://doi.org/10.1007/978-3-030-75385-6

This Springer imprint is published by the registered company Springer Nature Switzerland AG
The registered company address is: Gewerbestrasse 11, 6330 Cham, Switzerland

This book is dedicated to:

1. **Dr Natalia Kanem** – *Executive director of the United Nations Fund for Population Activities (UNFPA), a global champion for women's health and human rights, and a mentor to many health practitioners and civil society organizations in developing countries.*
2. **Dr Nahid Toubia** – *Sudanese medical doctor who has worked tirelessly for the abolishment of female genital mutilation, now officially prohibited in Sudan.*
3. **Professor Kelsey Harrison** – *Nigerian obstetrician and gynaecologist, whose publications in the mid-1980s on the adverse circumstances under which women in developing countries give birth led to the safe motherhood initiative and several international conferences that provided renewed commitments on maternal health.*
4. **Professor Mahmoud Fathalla** – *An Egyptian, past president of the International Federation of Gynaecology and Obstetrics (FIGO) provided and continues to provide a strong compelling voice for international programming and research on women's health.*
5. **Late Professor Fred Sai** – *A Ghanaian chaired the 1994 International Conference on Population and Development (ICPD) in Cairo, Egypt, a milestone event that provided great ascendancy for the field of sexual and reproductive health and rights.*
6. **Late Professor Allan Rosenfield** – *An international human rights advocate who wrote strongly on the importance of improving maternal health especially in developing countries from human rights and social justice perspectives.*
7. **Late Professor Olikoye Ransome-Kuti** – *A past minister of Health of Nigeria, whose legacies in promoting primary health care as the instrument for achieving universal health coverage in developing countries remain unsurpassed.*
8. **Late John Bateman Lawson** – *A Briton, the Foundation Professor of Obstetrics and Gynaecology at the University of Ibadan. A teacher of teachers, he excelled in the surgery of vesico-vaginal surgery and provided needed expertise and skills that remain legendary.*

They inspired and continue to inspire us.

Foreword

The invitation to pen a foreword to this magnificent book was accepted with alacrity, the major reason being that I was gripped by the sheer scale of its coverage, and that there was enough well-structured information in it to make it appeal to its diverse target readership. However, this assessment brought back a piece of history. I have already come across many curious readers who asked to be told whether or not there were earlier textbooks in living memory with broadly similar aims and objectives as this. The answer was a resounding yes (Table 1). The first that I knew was published in 1967. Edited by two Britons, JB Lawson of Ibadan University and DB Stewart of University of West Indies at Jamaica, it was titled *Obstetrics and Gynaecology in the Tropics and Developing Countries.* The next, edited by JB Lawson, KA Harrison, and S Bergstrom of Karolinska University Sweden, was titled *Maternity Care in Developing Countries.* The timing of its publication in 2001 was greatly influenced by the safe motherhood initiative, one important result being the cutting out of the whole section on gynaecology, which by all accounts was considered a mistake – and I wholeheartedly agreed. The same criticism could not be levelled on what came next in 2004, which was the first edition of *Contemporary Obstetrics and Gynaecology in Developing Countries.* The latest effort – the second edition – edited by F Okonofua, K Odunsi, JA Balogun and VN Chilaka and ably assisted by 80 seasoned and committed professionals has now landed us in a different territory as it were. Take section six for example. Its contents throw up so many other salient lessons worth learning. Such lessons correctly applied should help to bring about positive changes in the lives of the generality of women in developing countries.

Finally, I congratulate Professor Friday Okonofua and his entire team for putting this work together so well. It has been a pleasure, a privilege, and indeed an honor to live to see all these remarkable changes in one's lifetime.

Tuusula, Finland

Kelsey A. Harrison

Table 1 The evolution of some important textbooks on women's health in developing countries 1967–2020

S/N	Book Title	Editors	Number of Contributors	Year of Publication	Publisher
1	Obstetrics And Gynaecology in Tropics and Developing Countries	JB Lawson DB Stewart	12	1967	Edward Arnold English Language Book Societies
2	Maternity Care in Developing Countries	JB Lawson KA Harrison S Bergstrom	22	2001	RCOG Press
3.	Contemporary Obstetrics and Gynaecology in Developing Countries First Edition	F Okonofua K Odunsi	43	2004	Women's Health and Action Research Centre
4	Contemporary Obstetrics and Gynaecology for Developing Countries Second Edition	F Okonofua JA Balogun K Odunsi VN Chilaka	80	2020	Springer

Preface

The first edition of *Contemporary Obstetrics and Gynaecology for Developing Countries* was published in 2005. Since then, several groundbreaking discoveries and innovations have taken place in the discipline, including within the context of developing countries. The widespread enthusiasm with which the first edition was received, and the opportunity to incorporate the suggestions of numerous readers and stakeholders, justify the publication of this second edition. Many countries in the developing world continue to witness some of the most daunting clinical scenarios relating to reproductive health, obstetrics and gynaecology, and women's health. It is beyond doubt that these challenges and scenarios require specific and novel methods differing from those applied in other parts of the world. It is, therefore, necessary and appropriate to devote a specific textbook and enable the development of approaches and methodologies to address these challenges.

The editors of this textbook possess rich scientific backgrounds, with years of clinical practice, research, and service delivery in many parts of the developing world. As such, we are conversant with some of the drawbacks in educational delivery and pedagogy which continue to feature in the curricula of many undergraduate and postgraduate programs. In particular, there remains a deficit of skills, clinical orientation, and broad-based practices that limit the ability of graduates to deal with contemporary challenges connected to women's health and its related components in the region. Some of these deficits include poor linkage of science to service delivery, misalignment of competencies to patient and population needs, poor interprofessional teamwork, narrow technical focus without broader contextual understanding of a practitioner's role in the health system, the predominance of a hospital-based orientation at the expense of public health (especially with respect to reproductive health and primary health care), and weak understanding of the importance of leadership and business in firmly positioning the discipline within societal infrastructure.

The need to address these deficits has guided the development of this second edition of the textbook. The volume now comprises 70 chapters written by a multidisciplinary team of 81 authors. Apart from updating information on specific topics in obstetrics and gynaecology, we have expanded the sections on sexual and reproductive health, and gynaecological oncology. These are two key areas that currently generate intense interest in most of the developing world. We have also incorporated chapters that were missing in the first edition, especially those related to research methodology, epidemiology, biostatistics, physical therapy, health management, human rights, and the legal context of obstetrics and gynaecology. We believe that these additional topics will provide readers with a single integrated resource which contextualizes the interconnections between different concepts and principles that underpin the practice of the discipline in the region.

In summary, this second edition of *Contemporary Obstetrics and Gynaecology for Developing Countries* will be an exciting and essential textbook for undergraduate and postgraduate students in obstetrics and gynaecology, public health, health economics, nursing, physical therapy, reproductive health, demography, medical sociology, gender studies, and related fields in many parts of the developing world, especially sub-Saharan Africa. To the best of our knowledge, this textbook is currently the most comprehensive, detailed, and multidisciplinary of its kind in the region. It will be of use for researchers, programmers, development workers, and women's advocates in the developed world who have research interests or conduct health promotion activities in the developing world.

We conclude by opining that, in themselves, good textbooks are no more than useful guides to good clinical practices. The fundamental element remains the determination of those who read this book to be passionate and unwavering in offering the best clinical practices in line with their professional principles and oaths of practice. We are happy and firmly believe that this second edition of the textbook meets the laudable goals set out in the first edition.

Benin City, Nigeria — Friday Okonofua
Buffalo, NY, USA — Kunle Odunsi
Chicago, IL, USA — Joseph A. Balogun
Doha, Qatar — Victor N. Chilaka
August 2019

Reviewers

Prof. Jacob A. Unuigbe
Prof. Kelson A. Harrison
Dr. Barbara Crane
Prof. Joseph A. Balogun
Barr. Oludamilola Adejumo
Prof. Friday Okonofua
Dr. Tony Marinho
Prof. Hakeem Fawehinmi
Dr. Uche Menakaya
Prof. Shittu Oladapo
Prof. Nimi Briggs
Prof. Olaitan Soyannwo
Dr. Lindsay Edouard
Prof. Odunayo Oluwatosin
Prof. Adesuyi Ajayi
Dr. Victor N. Chilaka
Prof. O.A. Olatunbosun
Prof. A.A. Fasumade
Prof. Fola Esan
Prof. Durosimi M.
Prof. Kunle Odunsi
Prof. Nkoli Aniekwu

Acknowledgements

We dedicate this book to all mothers who labor hard to bring forth Africa's new generation of women and men, and pray for the repose of the souls of women worldwide who die through childbirth. We are grateful to all staff of the Women's Health and Action Research Centre (WHARC) and the *African Journal of Reproductive Health* (AJRH) in Nigeria, who supported the editing and publication of this book.

We are particularly grateful to Mr. Karl Eromosele Eimuhi, Managing Editor at the AJRH, who served in finalizing the typesetting and collation of the chapters in the book. Ms. MaryJane Emiowele, Secretary at WHARC, also provided secretarial assistance during the compilation of the book.

Contents

About the Editors

Friday Okonofua, MB CHB, PhD, FWACS, FRCOG, FAS is a Fellow of the Nigerian Academy of Science and the African Academy of Science. He is a professor of Obstetrics and Gynaecology, and the pioneer Vice-Chancellor of the University of Medical Sciences in Ondo State, Nigeria. He is also the Centre Leader of the World Bank–funded Africa Centre of Excellence in Reproductive Health Innovation at the University of Benin, Nigeria. He is a global champion of women's health, an area in which he has published 294 articles. He has served as Honorary Adviser on Health to President Olusegun Obasanjo of Nigeria, the Executive Director of the International Federation of Gynaecology and Obstetrics, and member of the International Advisory Board of the MacArthur Foundation, among several other positions.

Joseph A. Balogun, PhD, FACSM, FNSP, FAS, FAcadMS is Distinguished University Professor at Chicago State University, USA. He is also Emeritus Professor of Physiotherapy and Associate Director of Research Development and Innovation at the University of Medical Sciences, Ondo City, Nigeria. He is the founder and President/CEO of Joseph Rehabilitation Centre; a social service organization at Tinley Park, Illinois, that provides community-integrated living arrangement services for adults with disabilities. He has authored six books, eighteen book chapters, technical compendia, 170 articles, and 24 peer-reviewed conference abstracts and proceedings. He is a Fellow of the Academy of Medicine Specialties (FAcadMedS), Fellow of the Royal Society for Public Health, Fellow of the Academy of Science, Fellow of the Nigeria Society of Physiotherapy, and Fellow of the American College of Sports Medicine.

Kunle Odunsi, MD, PhD, FRCOG, FACOG is the Cancer Centre Deputy Director at Roswell Park Comprehensive Cancer Centre, USA, and a Fellow of the Nigerian Academy of Science. In 2018, he was elected to the United States National Academy of Medicine. He maintains an active independent laboratory research program that focuses on understanding the mechanisms of immune recognition and tolerance in human ovarian cancer, and translation of the findings to clinical immunotherapy trials. He has authored or coauthored more than 340 journal publications or book chapters, including papers in the *Proceedings of the National Academy of Sciences USA, Nature Genetics, Immunity, and New England Journal of Medicine*. He is also principal investigator of a multimillion dollar grant from NYSTEM to pioneer a novel strategy of re-programming human hematopoietic stem cells to become a life-long supply of anti-tumour immune cells in patients.

Victor N. Chilaka, MBBS, FRCOG, FWACS is Assistant Professor of Clinical Obstetrics and Gynaecology at the Hamad Medical Corporation, Weill Cornell Medical College, Qatar. He is also a senior consultant in Obstetrics and Gynaecology with special interest in urogynaecology and pelvic floor reconstruction at the Women's Wellness and Research Centre in Doha, Qatar. In 2003, he was appointed at the University Teaching Hospital of Derby, where he is the lead consultant for women with female genital mutilation and blood-borne viral infections in pregnancy, including HIV. He was awarded Fellowship of the Royal College of Obstetricians and Gynaecologists in 2006, and the West African College of Surgeons in 1994, in recognition of his contribution to the specialty.

Contributors

Peter Adefuye, MBBS, FWACS, FICS Department of Obstetrics and Gynaecology, Olabisi Onabanjo University Teaching Hospital, Sagamu, Nigeria

Adedokun Isaac Adegoke, MBBS, FWACS Department of Obstetrics and Gynaecology, University of Medical Sciences Teaching Hospital, Ondo, Nigeria

Oluwadamilola A. Adejumo, LLM, BL, ACIArb (UK) Faculty of Law, Obafemi Awolowo University, Ile-Ife, Ife, Nigeria

Olusegun Adeoye, MBBS, MScPH, LMIH Society of Gynaecology and Obstetrics of Nigeria (SOGON), Kaura District Abuja, Nigeria

Clement A. Adepiti, MBChB, FWACS, FMCOG Department of Obstetrics, Gynaecology and Perinatology, Faculty of Clinical Sciences, College of Health Sciences, Obafemi Awolowo University, Ile-Ife, Nigeria

Olalekan O. Adetoro, FWACS, FICS Department of Obstetrics and Gynaecology, Olabisi Onabanjo University, Sagamu, Nigeria

Olubukola Adesina Adewole, MBBS, MSc, FWACS College of Medicine, University of Ibadan, University College Hospital, Ibadan, Nigeria

Joseph Ifeanyi Brian-D Adinma, BM, BCh, FWACS, FICS, FISS College of Health Sciences, Nnamdi Azikiwe University and Teaching Hospital, Nnewi, Nigeria

Ekwueme Centre for Multidisciplinary Research/Centre for Health and Allied Legal Demographical Development, Research and Training (CHALADDRAT), Nnamdi Azikiwe University, Awka, Nigeria

Chris Ovoroyeguono Agboghoroma, MBBS, MA, MPH, FWACS, FMCOG Reproductive Medicine and Endocrinology Unit, Department of Obstetrics & Gynaecology, National Hospital, Abuja, Nigeria

Kingsley N. Agholor, MBBS, FWACS, FMCOG Central Hospital, Warri, Nigeria

Christopher O. Aimakhu, MBBS, FWACS, FMCOG, FICS College of Medicine, University of Ibadan and University College Hospital, Ibadan, Nigeria

Society of Gynaecology and Obstetrics of Nigeria (SOGON), Kaura District Abuja, Nigeria

Aderemi O. Aisien, MBBS, FMCOG, FICS University of Benin, Benin City, Nigeria

Olukunle Ajayi, MD York Teaching Hospital NHS, East Riding Hospital, and Scarborough Hospital, York, UK

Olusegun Kayode Ajenifuja, MD, FWACS, MPH, FMCOG College of Health Sciences, Obafemi Awolowo University, Ile-Ife, Nigeria

Obafemi Awolowo University Teaching Hospitals, Ile-Ife, Nigeria

Oluwole Akande, OON, DPhil (Oxford), FRCOG (UK)s College of Medicine, University College Hospital, Ibadan, Nigeria

Dilly O. C. Anumba, MBBS, MD, LLM (Medical Law) Faculty of Medicine, Dentistry and Health, University of Sheffield, Sheffield, UK

The Jessop Wing, Sheffield Teaching Hospitals NHS Foundation Trust, Sheffield, UK

Obasohan Austine, MBBS, FWACP, FMCP, FACC, FRCP College of Medicine Science, University of Benin, Benin City, Nigeria

University of Benin Teaching Hospital, Benin City, Nigeria

Aderonke F. Awe, MBBS, MRCOG Shrewsbury and Telford Hospitals NHS Trust, Shropshire, Shrewsbury, UK

Plymouth University, Plymouth, UK

Omolade Awodu, MbChB, FMCPath University of Benin/University of Benin Teaching Hospital, Benin City, Nigeria

Olusegun Badejoko, MBChB, FWACS, FMCOG, FMAS Department of Obstetrics, Gynaecology and Perinatology, Obafemi Awolowo University, Ile-Ife, Nigeria

Abdulmalik Bako, MBBS, MA, MMeD, FMCOG, FWACS Women's Wellness and Research Centre, Hamad Medical Corporation, Doha, Qatar

Weill Cornell Medicine-Qatar, Doha, Qatar

Joseph A. Balogun, PT, PhD, FACSM, FNSP, FAS, FRSPH Chicago State University, Chicago, IL, USA

University of Medical Sciences, Ondo City, Nigeria

Centre of Excellence in Reproductive Health Innovation, University of Benin, Benin City, Nigeria

Sophia Bornstein, MD, PhD Department of Radiation Medicine, Oregon Health and Science University, Portland, OR, USA

Chioma Uchenna Chilaka Specialty Registrar, East Midlands, UK

Victor N. Chilaka, MBBS, FWACS, FRCOG Women's Wellness and Research Centre, Hamad Medical Corporation, Doha, Qatar

Stephen C. Collins, MD, PhD, FACOG Yale University School of Medicine, New Haven, CT, USA

Lynette Denny, MD, PhD Obstetrics and Gynaecology, University of Cape Town, Cape Town, South Africa

Gynaecological Cancer Research Centre, Cape Town, South Africa

Lindsay Edouard, MBBS, MSc, FFPHM, FFSRH, FRCOG Department of Obstetrics and Gynaecology, College of Medicine, University of Saskatchewan, Saskatoon, SK, Canada

Tarek Elshamy, MBBCH, MSc, MRCOG West Middlesex University Hospital, London, UK

Ehigha Enabudoso, MBBS, FWACS, FMCOG, MPH Department of Obstetrics & Gynaecology, University of Benin Teaching Hospital, Benin City, Nigeria

Nosakhare O. Enaruna, MBBS, FWACS, FMCOG University of Benin, Benin City, Nigeria

University of Benin Teaching Hospital, Benin City, Nigeria

Mathew Ebose Enosolease, MBBS, FMCPath Department of Haematology, University of Benin, Benin City, Nigeria

University of Benin Teaching Hospital, Benin City, Nigeria

Michael Chudi Ezeanochie, MBBS, FWACS University of Benin Teaching Hospital, Benin City, Nigeria

Department of Obstetrics & Gynaecology, University of Benin, Benin City, Nigeria

Yomi Finnih, MBBS, FRCOG Society of Gynaecology and Obstetrics of Nigeria (SOGON), Finnih Medical Centre, Lagos, Nigeria

Aisha Amal Galadanci, MBBS, FMCPath Aminu Kano Teaching Hospital, Bayero University, Kano, Nigeria

Hadiza Shehu Galadanci, MBBS, MSc, FWACS, FRCOG College of Health Sciences, Africa Centre of Excellence for Population Health and Policy, Bayero University, Kano, Nigeria

Michael Olumide Gbala, MBBS, FWACS, FICS University of Medical Sciences (UNIMED) Teaching Hospital, Ondo, Nigeria

UNIMED, Ondo, Nigeria

Etedafe P. Gharoro, MBBS, FMCOG, FWACS, FICS Faculty of Obstetrics & Gynaecology, Liberian College of Physicians and Surgeons, JFK Liberian-Japanese Friendship Maternity Hospital, Monrovia, Liberia

University of Benin Teaching Hospital, Benin City, Nigeria

Aiwuyo O. Henry, MBBS, FWACP, Cert AHA Instructor Delog Nigerian Limited, Lagos, Nigeria

Okechukwu A. Ibeanu, MD, FWACS Gynaecologic Oncology, John Hopkins University, Baltimore, MD, USA

Alvin & Lois Lapidus Cancer Institute, Sinai and Northwest Hospital, Baltimore, MD, USA

Abiodun O. Ilesanmi, JP, PMP®, FNIM, NPOM, OON College of Medicine, University of Ibadan and University College Hospital, Ibadan, Nigeria

Charles Imarengiaye, MBBS, FWACS, FMCA School of Medicine, University of Benin, University of Benin Teaching Hospital, Benin City, Nigeria

Pius E. Iribhogbe, MBBS, FWACS, Cert. T. RACS, FICS University of Benin, Benin City, Nigeria

Jerry J. Jaboin, MD, PhD Department of Radiation Medicine, Oregon Health and Science University, Portland, OR, USA

Rotimi A. K. Jaiyesimi, MBBS, MBA, FRSPH, FWACS, FRCOG Mid and South Essex University Hospitals NHS Foundation Trust, Basildon, UK

Faculty of Law, University of Ibadan, Ibadan, Nigeria

Toby Kenneth Maduako, MBBS, MSc, FWACS University of Benin Teaching Hospital, Benin City, Nigeria

J. Ryan Martin, MD, FACOG Shady Grove Fertility, Warrington, PA, USA

Uche A. Menakaya, MBBS (Benin), MCE (Monash) JUNIC Specialist Imaging and Women's Centre, Coombs, ACT, Australia

Calvary Public Hospital, Bruce, ACT, Australia

Calvary Private Hospital, Bruce, ACT, Australia

Francis Githae Muriithi, MBChB, MMed, MSc, MRCOG East Midlands North Deanery, Queen's Medical Centre, Nottingham University Hospitals NHS Foundation Trust, Nottingham, UK

Osric Banfegha Navti, MBBS, FRCOG Al Wakra Hospital, Hamad Medical Corporation, Doha, Qatar

Kunle Odunsi, MD, PhD, FRCOG, FACOG Roswell Park Comprehensive Cancer Centre (Roswell Park), Buffalo, NY, USA

Department of Gynaecologic Oncology, Centre for Immunotherapy, Roswell Park, Buffalo, NY, USA

University of Buffalo, Buffalo, NY, USA

Olatoye Ogunbode, MBBS, FWACS, FRCOG Department of Obstetrics and Gynaecology, University of Ibadan, Ibadan, Nigeria

Olayinka Ogunbode, MBBS, FWACS Department of Obstetrics & Gynaecology, University of Ibadan, Ibadan, Nigeria

University College Hospital, Ibadan, Nigeria

Tinuade A. Ogunlesi, MB ChB, MPH, FWACP(Paed) Department of Paediatrics, Olabisi Onabanjo University, Sagamu, Nigeria

Department of Paediatrics, Olabisi Onabanjo University Teaching Hospital, Sagamu, Nigeria

Rosemary N. Ogu, MBBS, MSc(RH), FWACS, FMCOG University of Port Harcourt Teaching Hospital, University of Port Harcourt, Port Harcourt, Nigeria

Gestational DM Study Group, WHARC WHO FMOH MNCH Study Team, Abuja, Nigeria

Adegbola Ojo, PhD School of Geography and Lincoln Centre for Water and Planetary Health, University of Lincoln, Lincolnshire, UK

Oluropo Ebenezer Ojo, MBBS, FRCOG, FNCOG, FFFP Cedarpark Healthcare Lincoln, Lincolnshire East CCG, Lincoln, UK

Elizade University Healthcare Centre, Ilara Mokin, Nigeria

Friday Okonofua, MB CHB, PhD, FWACS, FRCOG, FAS Centre of Excellence in Reproductive Health Innovation, Department of Obstetrics and Gynaecology, University of Benin, Benin City, Nigeria

Women's Health and Action Research Centre, Benin City, Nigeria

University of Medical Sciences, Ondo City, Ondo State, Nigeria

Biodun Olagbuji, MBBS, MPH, FWACS Ekiti State University Teaching Hospital, Ado-Ekiti, Nigeria

Adeola Olaitan, MBBS, MD, FRCOG UCLH Gynaecological Cancer Centre, London, UK

North London Gynaecological Cancer Network, London, UK

Olufemi A. Olatunbosun, MD, FRCSC, FACOG Department of Obstetrics and Gynaecology, College of Medicine, University of Saskatchewan, Saskatoon, SK, Canada

Alex Olawaiye, MBBS, FWACS, FRCOG Gynaecologic Cancer Research, Mage Women's Hospital, University of Pittsburgh Medical Centre, Pittsburgh, PA, USA

Gynaecologic Oncology, University of Pittsburgh Cancer Institute, Pittsburgh, PA, USA

Joseph Onakewhor, MBBS, MSc (Anatomy), FMCOG University of Benin, Benin City, Nigeria

University of Benin Teaching Hospital, Benin City, Nigeria

Uchenna Onwudiegwu Department of Obstetrics, Gynaecology and Perinatology, Obafemi Awolowo University, Ile-Ife, Nigeria

Foluso J. Owotade, BChD, PhD, FWACS Department of Oral & Maxillofacial Surgery and Oral Pathology, Faculty of Dentistry, Obafemi Awolowo University, Ile-Ife, Nigeria

Lubna Pal, MBBS, MS, FACOG, FRCOG (UK) Division of Reproductive Endocrinology & Infertility, Department of Obstetrics, Gynaecology and Reproductive Sciences, Yale School of Medicine, New Haven, CT, USA

Tanja Pejovic, MD, PhD Oregon Health and Science University, Portland, OR, USA

Shushan Rana, MD Department of Radiation Medicine, Oregon Health and Science University, Portland, OR, USA

Rakiya Saidu, MBBS, MPH College of Health Sciences, University of Ilorin, Ilorin, Nigeria

University of Cape Town, Cape Town, South Africa

Dan O. Selo-Ojeme, MBBS, MBA, FWACS, FMCOG Urogynaecological Services, Barnet and Chase Farm Hospital, The Royal Free London NHS Foundation Trust, London, UK

Jedidiah Dase Kingsley Sodje, FWACS, MBBS Department of Obstetrics & Gynaecology, University of Benin and University of Benin Teaching Hospital, Benin City, Nigeria

Nasreen M. N. Soliman, MBBS, MD, MRCOG, DFSRH Shrewsbury & Telford Hospitals NHS Trust, Shrewsbury, UK

Morounfolu Olaleye Thompson, MBBS, FWACS, FRCOG, DMFM Fetal Medicine, Queens University Hospital, Romford, UK

Institute of Health Sciences, Barts and The London School of Medicine and Dentistry, Queen Mary University of London, London, UK

Kingsley Ufuoma Tobi, MBBS, PGDA, FMCA, FWACS Department of Surgery and Anaesthesiology, University of Namibia, Windhoek, Namibia

University of Benin Teaching Hospital, Benin City, Nigeria

Jacob A. Unuigbe, MBBS, (Ibadan), FWACS, FICS College of Health Sciences, Igbinedion University, Okada, Nigeria

Part I

Women's Reproductive Health

Sexual and Reproductive Health and Rights: An Overview

1

Ebenezer Oluwole Akande

Learning Objectives

At the conclusion of this chapter, the reader will:

- Know the definition and components of sexual and reproductive health and rights (SRHR)
- Understand why sexual and reproductive health and rights are central to the practice of obstetrics and gynaecology
- Recognise the role of obstetricians and gynaecologists in promoting and advancing sexual and reproductive health and rights
- Understand the international dimensions of sexual and reproductive health and rights

Sexual and reproductive health (SRH) and rights encompass efforts to eliminate preventable maternal and neonatal mortality and morbidity, to ensure quality sexual and reproductive health services, including contraceptive services, and to address sexually transmitted infections and cervical cancer, violence against women and girls, and the sexual and reproductive health needs of adolescents [1]. Women's reproductive health needs have not always been respected as basic human rights. On the contrary, the neglect of women's reproductive health, perpetuated by law, is part of a larger, systematic discrimination against women [2].

The second half of the twentieth century witnessed a vast expansion of health technologies and of health care services related to reproduction and sexual health. These services were, however, fragmented and not oriented to respond to the needs of women and men in a holistic fashion. This fragmentation of services and their lack of orientation resulted in the recent emergence of the concept of sexual and reproductive health that offers a comprehensive and integrated approach to health needs related to reproduction and sexual health. The concept puts women at the centre of the process, and recognises, respects and responds to the needs of women throughout their reproductive career, and not only to those of mothers.

The concept of reproductive health received great attention in the United Nations International Conference on Population and Development (ICPD), held in Cairo in 1994 [1]. It was endorsed as showing the way forward, as a preferable alternative to narrowly focusing on family planning programmes.

1.1 What Is Reproductive Health?

Reproductive health, according to the consensus definition agreed on at the ICPD in 1994, is a 'state of complete physical, mental and social well-being, and not merely the absence of disease or infirmity, in all matters relating to the reproductive system and to its functions and processes'. This definition was drawn up within the context of the positive definition of health in the constitution of the World Health Organization (WHO) as a 'state of complete physical, mental and social well-being and not merely the absence of disease or infirmity' [3].

1.2 Sexual Health

The ICPD in Cairo also expanded the definition of reproductive health to include 'a satisfying and safe sex life', a theme that was further elaborated at the 1995 World Conference on Women in Beijing [4]. The ICPD Programme of Action stated that 'reproductive health implies that people are able to have a satisfying and safe sex life, and that they have the capability to reproduce and the freedom to decide if, when

E. O. Akande (✉)
College of Medicine, University College Hospital, Ibadan, Nigeria

F. Okonofua et al. (eds.), *Contemporary Obstetrics and Gynecology for Developing Countries*,
https://doi.org/10.1007/978-3-030-75385-6_1

and how often to do so' [1]. Reproductive and sexual health, therefore, encompasses freedom from fear of unwanted pregnancy, disease and abuse, and from the shame and guilt that surrounds sexuality in many cultures [5].

Sexual health is, therefore, part of reproductive health and includes healthy sexual development; equitable and responsible relationships, and sexual fulfilment; and freedom from illness, disease, disability, violence and other harmful practices related to sexuality [6].

Sexual and reproductive health also implies that people have the ability to reproduce, to regulate their fertility, and to practice and enjoy sexual relationships. It further implies that reproduction is carried to a successful outcome through infant and child survival, growth and healthy development. It finally implies that women can go safely through pregnancy and childbirth, that fertility regulation can be achieved without health hazards, that women are safe while participating in sex [3, 6], and enjoy the freedom to decide if, when and how often to do so [7].

1.3 Components of Sexual and Reproductive Health

The following constitute the basic components of sexual and reproductive health:

- Fertility regulation
- Infertility: prevention and treatment
- Safe motherhood
- Infant and child survival, growth and development
- Sexually transmitted disease including HIV/AIDS
- Unsafe abortion: prevention and management
- Reproductive system cancers

To these should be added the following other important considerations:

- Gender equity
- Sexual behaviour
- Adolescent reproductive health and sexuality
- Harmful traditional practices and violence against women
- Reproductive health of older women and men

1.4 What Is New About the Concept of Sexual and Reproductive Health?

The comprehensive approach to sexual and reproductive health described in the ICPD Programme of Action seeks to build upon the strengths of existing service delivery systems and the gains that have been made in providing family planning, maternal and child health (MCH), and other vertical (stand-alone) programmes.

At the same time, the ICPD approach aims to improve service quality and broaden existing programmes to offer clients a full range of sexual and reproductive health services, through integration of services or strong links between components of care. Such an approach recognises that providing care for one aspect of sexual and reproductive health (e.g. prevention of sexually transmitted diseases) can have a positive impact on other aspects (e.g. healthy pregnancy and delivery, as well as the prevention of infertility) and help prevent future ill health. In addition to improving health status, this integrated approach to service provision can also reduce duplication of efforts, promote the efficient use of existing human resources, and improve client satisfaction and the use of available services.

Sexual and reproductive health, therefore, does not start out from a list of diseases or problems – such as sexually transmitted diseases (STD), maternal mortality – or from a list of programmes – such as maternal and child health, safe motherhood, family planning and so on. Instead, reproductive health must be understood in the context of relationship: such as fulfilment and risk, and the opportunity to have a desired child, or alternatively to avoid unwanted pregnancy. Reproductive health contributes enormously to physical and physiological comfort and closeness, and to personal and social maturation – poor reproductive health is frequently associated with disease, abuse, exploitation, unwanted pregnancy and even death.

Programmes dealing with various components of reproductive health exist in some form almost everywhere. But they have been delivered in disparate and separate ways, unconnected to programmes dealing with closely interdependent topics. For example, the objectives, design and evaluation of family planning programmes were largely driven by demographic imperatives, without due consideration to related health issues such as a maternal health or STD prevention and management. Evaluation was largely in terms of quantity rather than quality – such as numbers of contraceptive acceptors, as opposed to the ability and opportunity to make informed decisions about health issues. In general, such programmes exclusively targeted women, taking little account of the social, cultural and intimate realities of their reproductive lives and decision-making powers. They tended to serve only married people, excluding, in particular, young people. Services were rarely designed to serve men even though they have reproductive health concerns of their own. Moreover, the involvement of men in reproductive health is important because they have a role to play as family decision-makers with regard to family size, family planning and the use of health services.

A reproductive health approach would differ from a narrow family planning approach in several ways. It would aim to build on what exists and at the same time to modify current narrow, vertical programmes to ones in which every opportunity is taken to offer women and men a full range of reproductive health services in a linked way. The underlying assumption is that people with needs in one particular area – say treatment of STDs – also have needs in other areas – such as family planning or antenatal and postpartum care. Such programmes would recognise that dealing with one aspect of reproductive health could have synergistic effects in dealing with others. For example, management of infertility is difficult and expensive but it can be largely prevented through appropriate care during and after delivery and prevention and management of STDs. Promotion of breast-feeding has an impact on reproductive health in many ways – it helps prevent certain postpartum problems, delays the return to fertility, may prevent ovarian and breast cancer, and improves neonatal health.

Another important difference between the existing programmes and those developed to respond to the new concept of reproductive health is the way in which people – particularly women and young people who are the most affected by reproductive health concerns – are involved in programme development, implementation and evaluation. When women are more involved in programmes, it becomes clearer to them that they have concerns beyond motherhood. Also, dealing with reproductive health leads to a profound rethinking of the behavioural, social, gender and cultural dimensions of decision-making that affect women's reproductive lives.

1.5 The Role of Men in Sexual and Reproductive Health

Men too have reproductive health concerns and needs, though their general health is affected by reproductive health to a lesser extent than women. Not only do men have reproductive health concerns of their own, but their health status and behaviours also affect women's reproductive health. Men's reproductive health needs include sexuality, protection against sexually transmitted diseases, infertility prevention and management, and fertility regulation. Protection against prostatic hypertrophy and prostatic cancer is another concern. Men can play a positive role in promoting women's reproductive health by sharing responsibility of family planning using a male method, by supporting their partners in using female contraception and deciding on appropriate family size, and by responsible sexual behaviour. Young men need to be educated to respect women and treat them as equals, to support efforts to enhance the status of women, and to prevent gender-based violence.

Because of men's central roles, it is imperative that men join women in sharing the responsibility for sexual and reproductive health and achieving gender equity and equality.

At each stage of life, individual needs differ. However, there is a cumulative effect across the life course – events at each phase having important implications for future well-being. Failure to deal with problems at any stage in life sets the tone for later health and developmental problems.

1.6 The Concept of Sexual and Reproductive Health and Rights: A Paradigm Shift in Population Activities

Sexual and reproductive health and rights (SRHR) is the concept of human rights applied to sexuality and reproduction [8]. The International Conference on Population and Development (ICPD) held in Cairo in 1994 represented a significant shift in the world's perception of population dynamics. For the first time, the conference not only focused on population but also on development. The ICPD represented a paradigm shift in population activities. Pre-Cairo, the emphasis was on population size versus resources as well as population growth versus economic development. Post-Cairo, the emphasis shifted to human rights, reproductive health and individual choice. Pre-Cairo, the major players were economists and development planners, whilst post-Cairo, the identities of the major players shifted to health professionals and human right activists.

The concept of sexual and reproductive health and rights was firmly put in place at the Cairo conference. Significantly, it also placed sexual and reproductive health at the centre of development efforts, making it clear that the aim of the interventions is to enhance reproductive health and promote reproductive rights, rather than population policies and fertility control. This implies the empowerment of women (including through better access to education): the involvement of women and young people in the development and implementation of programmes and services; reaching out to the poor, the marginalised and the excluded and assuming responsibility for reproductive health on the part of men.

SRHR encompass the right of all individuals to make decisions about their sexual activity and reproduction free from discrimination, coercion and violence, and to achieve the highest attainable standard of sexual health. Specifically, access to SRH services allows individuals to choose whether, when and with whom to engage in sexual activity; to choose whether and when to have children and to have access to the information and means to make those choices.

To maintain one's sexual and reproductive health, people need access to accurate information and the safe, effective, affordable and acceptable contraception method of their choice. They must be informed and empowered to protect themselves from STDs. And when they decide to have children, women must have access to services that facilitate successful pregnancy, safe delivery and a healthy baby.

Comprehensive sexual and reproductive health (SRH) services include [9, 10]:

- Contraceptive information and services, including emergency contraception and a range of modern contraceptive methods
- Maternity care, including antenatal and postnatal care, and delivery care, particularly skilled attendance and emergency obstetric care
- Prevention and appropriate treatment of infertility
- Safe abortion and post-abortion care
- Prevention, care and treatment of STDs, HIV/AIDS, reproductive tract infections and reproductive cancers
- Information, education and counselling
- Prevention and surveillance of violence against women (VAW), care for survivors of violence
- Actions to eliminate harmful traditional practices such as Female Genital Mutilation (FGM) and early and forced marriage

1.7 Why Is Sexual and Reproductive Health Important?

Sexual and reproductive health, probably more than any other health field, has an impact that extends beyond the individual and family, to the society at large and even to the world as a whole. This impact involves crucial areas of global concern such as health, population development, status of women and the environment. Reproductive health is a crucial part of general health and a central feature of development. It is a reflection of health during childhood, and it is crucial during adolescence and adulthood. It sets the stage for health beyond the reproductive years for both women and men, and affects the health of the next generation. The health of the newborn is largely a function of the mother's health and nutrition status, and her access to health care.

SRH is a universal concern, but it is of particular importance for women during the reproductive years. Although most reproductive health problems arise during the reproductive years, in old age general health continues to reflect earlier reproductive health life events. Healthy sexual and reproductive behaviour sets the stage for good health before, during and beyond the reproductive years for both women and men, and has a significant impact on the health of the next generation. Women bear by far the greatest burden of sexual and reproductive health problems, due to their physiology, their ability to give birth and the limited power many women have over sexual decisions [6]. Women are at risk of complications from pregnancy and childbirth, suffer the complications of unsafe abortion and bear most of the burden of contraception.

Sexual and reproductive ill health accounts for more than a third of the global burden of disease for women of childbearing age and one-fifth of the burden for the whole population [1].

> Because reproductive health is such an important component of general health, it is a prerequisite for social, economic and human development. The highest attainable level of health is not only a fundamental human right for all; it is also a social and economic imperative, because human energy and creativity are the driving force of development [11, 12]. Every effort should be made towards the goal of universal access to sexual and reproductive health and rights, including family planning.

References

1. UN, Population and Development, i. Programme of action adopted at the international conference on population and development (ICPD), Cairo, 5–13 September 1994. New York: United Nations, Department for Economic and Social Information and Policy Analysis; 1994.
2. Cook RJ. International human rights and women's reproductive health. Stud Fam Plan. 1993;24(2):73–86.
3. Fathalla MF. Promotion of research in human reproduction: global needs and perspectives. Hum Reprod. 1988;3:7–10.
4. UN, Department of Public Information. Platform for action and Beijing declaration. Fourth world conference on women, Beijing, China, 4–15 September 1995. New York: UN; 1995.
5. Barnett J, Stein J. Women's voices, Women's lives: a synthesis of findings from the Women's studies project. Research Triangle Park: Family Health International; 1998.
6. Fathalla MF. From obstetrics and gynaecology to women's health: the road ahead. New York and London: Parthenon; 1997. p. 33–48.
7. Cook R, Dickens BM, Fathalla MF. Reproductive health and human rights. Oxford University Press; 2003.
8. Cook RJ, Fathalla MF. Advancing reproductive rights beyond Cairo and Beijing. Int Fam Plann Persp. 1996;22(3):115–21.
9. Framework of actions of the follow-up to the programme of action of international conference on population and development (ICPD) Beyond 2014. ICPD Beyond 2014; 2014 Jan 20.
10. International Planned Parenthood Federation. Charter on sexual and reproductive rights. London: International Planned Parenthood Federation; 1996.
11. Family Care International (FCI). Millennium development goals & sexual & reproductive health. New York: Family Care International; 2005.
12. Family Health Care International. Meeting the Cairo challenge: progress in sexual and reproductive health – implementing the ICPD programme of action. New York; 1999.

Clinical Diagnosis in Obstetrics and Gynaecology

2

Yomi Finnih

Learning Objectives

At the conclusion of this chapter, the reader will:

- Understand the clinical approach to history taking and physical examination in obstetrics and gynaecology
- Be knowledgeable about the basic investigations in women with obstetrics and gynaecological disorders
- Appreciate the importance of compassionate care and counselling of women with obstetrics and gynaecological disorders
- Understand the connection between obstetrics and gynaecology and sexual and reproductive health

Women's health is a recognised sub-specialty in reproductive health, which has been defined as "a state of physical, mental and social wellbeing in all matters relating to the reproductive system", at all stages of life. It encompasses the ability of women to have fulfilling and safe sex lives, as well as the capability to reproduce, and the liberty to make decisions if, when and how often to do so. It provides that men and women should be informed about reproduction and have access to safe, effective, affordable and acceptable methods of family planning of their choice, and the right to appropriate health care services that enable them to go safely through pregnancy and childbirth.
Obstetrics and gynaecology is the medical specialty that deals specifically with the reproductive health challenges of women [1]. It is critical that medical students and resident doctors should master the clinical approach to women, and the special art and skills of obstetrics and gynaecological practice. The purpose of taking history is to arrive at a diagnosis so that proper management can be offered to the patient. The questions asked must therefore be comprehensive and be relevant to how the patient should be managed. The handling and the examination of the patient can only be properly taught and learnt in the consulting room and at the bedside, and there are several ways of doing this adequately.

Y. Finnih (✉)
Society of Gynaecology and Obstetrics of Nigeria (SOGON), Finnih Medical Centre, Lagos, Nigeria

2.1 Gynaecological History Taking

Gynaecological history taking involves methodological questioning of a woman with the aim of developing a diagnosis, or a differential diagnosis, on which the further management of the patient may be organised. The treatment plan may involve examination of the patient, further investigative testing and treatment of a diagnosed condition.

There is a basic structure for eliciting gynaecological histories from women, but this can differ slightly depending on the nature of the presenting complaint [2].

2.1.1 Introduction

This includes the introduction of the clinician to the woman, and the elicitation of general information including name, age and address, level of education, religion and marital status.

2.1.2 History of Presenting Complaint

It is important to ask an open-ended question in this part of the history. This will enable the woman to state her problem in the most explanatory way and in the language she understands. The history of the complaint will differ depending on the nature of the complaint, but it is advised that as much as possible, a value-free and non-judgmental approach is used.

If pain is involved, the site and characteristics of the pain should be ascertained. The onset, periodicity, duration and recurrence should also be noted. The history of aggravating

F. Okonofua et al. (eds.), *Contemporary Obstetrics and Gynecology for Developing Countries*,
https://doi.org/10.1007/978-3-030-75385-6_2

and relieving factors, as well as severity, is taken. Information about the nature and severity of any associated bleeding should also be obtained.

2.1.3 Menstrual History

The age of menarche or menopause, first day of the last menstrual period (LMP), duration of menstrual bleeding, frequency and regularity, bleeding between periods and bleeding after intercourse should be noted. History of any post-menopausal bleeding is taken. The nature of the menstrual periods is noted in terms of heaviness, passage of clots or flooding.

2.1.4 Past Gynaecological History

The clinician should also ask about any previous gynaecological diagnoses, surgery, contraception and date and results of previous cervical smears.

2.1.5 Past Obstetric History

This includes information on gravidity and parity, as well as dates of deliveries, duration of pregnancies, whether labour was spontaneous or induced, type of delivery, weight and sex of babies, as well as complications before, during and after delivery.

2.1.6 Past Medical and Surgical History

The history of current or past illnesses, hospital admissions and past surgeries should be taken. It is important to ask about prescribed and non-prescribed medications, herbal drugs, as well as drug allergies. Medical conditions in the family should be noted, as well as family history of medical conditions such as diabetes and hypertension, as well as malignancies.

The social history will include information pertaining to smoking habits and alcohol use.

2.2 The Gynaecological Examination

Women are often apprehensive about undergoing a pelvic examination [3]. They feel vulnerable and exposed during this examination. The positioning for the examination creates a significant imbalance of power in the patient/provider interaction and carries sexual connotations for many women. If the provider explains what is going on, maintains eye contact as much as possible and comments on findings, the patient is more likely to feel relaxed and safe.

The complete gynaecological examination comprises a general physical examination, examinations of the breasts and abdomen, as well as a pelvic examination.

2.2.1 General Physical Examination

This should be carried out in a comfortable, private area under a good light source. The patient is examined for pallor, jaundice, dehydration, pedal oedema, varicosities and enlarged lymph nodes. The respiratory system is examined, while the pulse and blood pressure are recorded. The neck is examined for evidence of enlargement, tenderness or lumps. The breasts are examined for symmetry, visible lumps and galactorrhoea.

2.2.2 Examination of the Abdomen

The urinary bladder should be empty during abdominal examination. There should be adequate exposure of the abdomen between the xiphisternum and just below the pubic hair line. The abdomen is first inspected for shape and contour. It should be noted whether the abdomen is symmetrical, hollow, flat or distended. The umbilicus could be inverted, flat or everted. The presence of scarification marks and surgical scars should also be noted.

A superficial palpation of the abdomen is then carried out, essentially to elicit areas of tenderness. It is traditionally carried out in the nine regions of the abdomen. Thereafter, deep palpation is carried out to detect any enlargement of the liver and the spleen, as well as the ability to ballot the kidneys.

2.2.3 Pelvic Examination

After explaining the procedure, the patient is positioned on a couch. The external genitalia are inspected for normalcy of appearance and hair distribution. Any lesions or developmental abnormalities are noted. The Bartholin's and Skene's glands are visualised. The patient is asked to cough or bear down, with the labia separated by the left middle and index fingers. The Cusco's speculum is inserted into the vagina until the cervix is brought into view. The vaginal walls are examined, as well as the cervix, for colour, position, surface characteristics, bleeding and discharge. A cervical smear will be taken if required.

To conduct the bimanual examination, the two gloved fingers are inserted in the vagina; the cervix is palpated noting the position, shape, consistency, regularity, mobility and tenderness. The fornices are palpated. The uterus is palpated, noting the size, shape, consistency, mobility, any tenderness or masses. Each ovary is palpated, as well as the adnexae.

After careful history taking and physical examination, a presumptive diagnosis is often possible. Further confirmation of the diagnosis and management will depend on the outcome of the general and specific investigations.

2.3 Investigations in Gynaecology

The common investigations carried out in gynaecological practice include the following:

1. Blood values
2. Urine examination
3. Urethral, vaginal and endocervical swabs
4. Colposcopy
5. Imaging techniques
6. Endometrial sampling
7. Biopsy
8. Endoscopy
9. Hormonal assays

Routine Blood Investigations:

(a) Haemoglobin estimations – useful in cases of excessive bleeding
(b) Total and differential counts – useful in cases of pelvic inflammatory disease
(c) Erythrocyte sedimentation rate
(d) Platelet count
(e) Serology (Venereal Disease Research Laboratory (VDRL) test, HIV, Hepatitis B and C)

Urine Analysis:

(a) Urine microscopy, culture and sensitivity
(b) Urine pregnancy test

The collection of urine from gynaecological patients may be by midstream, catheter or suprapubic bladder puncture.

2.3.1 Urethral, Vaginal and Endocervical Swabs

Swabs can be collected from the urethra, the posterior fornix of the vagina and the endocervix for microscopy, culture and sensitivity studies.

2.3.2 Papanicolaou Test or Pap Smear

This can be used to screen for cervical cancer, identify local viral infections like herpes and condylomata acuminata and for cytohormonal studies. An endocervical sampling can be done by scraping the endocervix with a cytobrush and adding to the slide.

This is carried out by exfoliative cytology. It is a non-invasive study of the epithelium for hormonal status. It is based on the principle that the vaginal epithelium is sensitive to oestrogen and progesterone. Oestrogen leads to superficial maturation, while progesterone leads to intermediate cell maturation. Scrapings are taken from the lateral wall of the upper third of the vagina.

2.3.3 Uterine Aspiration Cytology

This is the screening test for endometrial cancer by endometrial sampling. The sample is obtained by endometrial pipette, or by uterine aspiration syringe or brush.

2.3.4 Cold Cone Biopsy

This involves excising a large area of tissue for examination in suspected cases of Cervical Intraepithelial Neoplasia (CIN).

2.3.5 Culdocentesis

This involves the trans-vaginal aspiration of peritoneal fluid from the Pouch of Douglas. It is sometimes useful as a diagnostic procedure in cases of pelvic abscess and ruptured ectopic pregnancy and to detect malignant cells in cases of ascites associated with ovarian tumours.

2.3.6 Hormone Assay

The usual hormones assayed in gynaecological practice are follicle stimulating hormone (FSH), luteinising hormone (LH), prolactin, progesterone, oestradiol, testosterone, aldosterone, cortisol, human chorionic gonadotropin (HCG), dehydroepiandrosterone sulphate (DHEAS) and androstenedione. They are useful in the diagnosis of menopause, polycystic ovarian disease, anovulation and hyperprolactinaemia, as well as in monitoring the treatment regimes in ovulation induction and assisted reproductive techniques.

2.3.7 Imaging Techniques

1. Plain abdominal X rays
2. Hysterosalpingography (HSG)
3. Sonohysterosalpingography
4. Transabdominal ultrasound
5. Transvaginal sonography (TVS)

TVS is useful in infertility workup to carry out the folliculometric measurement of ovarian follicles and measurement of endometrial thickness and to provide evidence of ovulation internal echoes and free fluid in the Pouch of Douglas. It is also used for sonographic-guided oocyte retrieval during in vitro fertilisation. It is also able to view a tubal ring in the adnexa with an empty uterine cavity in cases of ectopic pregnancy, as well as the evaluation of a pelvic mass.

In oncology, TVS can be used to assess the vascularity of tumours. It can also be used for endometrial thickness studies in dysfunctional uterine bleeding. It can locate a misplaced Intrauterine Contraceptive Device (IUCD) and is useful in falloposcopy to study the medial end of the fallopian tube. It may be able to diagnose endometriosis as well as to study ovarian pathologies such as PCOD, ovarian cysts and tumours. It is useful in the diagnosis of congenital abnormalities of the uterus as well as adnexal masses.

6. Transvaginal colour Doppler sonography

   This gives information regarding blood flow to, from or within the uterus or adnexa.
7. Computerised tomography (CT)

   This investigation supplements information from ultrasonography. It is accurate in assessing local tumour invasion and enables accurate localisation of a directed biopsy. It can diagnose pelvic vein thrombophlebitis, intra-abdominal abscess and other extra genital abnormalities. It is, however, contraindicated in pregnancy.
8. Magnetic resonance imaging (MRI)

   It is indicated when a sonogram or CT fails to detect a lesion, or to differentiate post-treatment fibrosis or tumour. It is, however, limited by cost, time and availability.
9. Positron emission tomography (PET)

2.3.8 Diagnostic Endoscopy

This includes laparoscopy and hysteroscopy.

2.4 Obstetric History Taking

Pregnancy is not a disease but should be regarded as a significant biological event. Sensitivity and tactful questioning concerning this event are important [4].

For the antenatal patient, it is critical during history taking to capture as much information as possible, in order to be able to accurately categorise the patient as no risk or high risk. Risk factors will emerge from asking questions pertaining to the following:

2.4.1 Biodata

Name, age, occupation, gravidity, parity, last normal menstrual period and gestational age should be noted.

2.4.2 History of Current Pregnancy

The history of the current pregnancy is noted. It should be determined whether the pregnancy was desired and planned, and whether it occurred spontaneously or by means of assisted conception technique. The date of the last menstrual period (LMP) should be elicited, in order to enable the calculation of the estimated date of delivery (EDD).

A history of when and how the pregnancy was confirmed should be taken. Exaggerated early pregnancy symptoms or any other complaint should be noted. The first sonogram carried out should be examined. The results of routine antenatal investigations should be elicited. These include packed cell volume (PCV), human immunodeficiency virus (HIV) status, genotype, blood group, urinalysis and hepatitis B and C tests. A history of tetanus toxoid commencement or completion is elicited, as well as intermittent preventive therapy (IPT). The routine antenatal drugs being taken should be noted.

2.4.3 Past Obstetric History

Each previous pregnancy should be detailed chronologically. The month and year, the health institution where the pregnancy was registered, the gestational age and the history of the antenatal period should be elicited. The gestational age at delivery, the nature of onset of labour, whether spontaneous or induced, intranatal events, type of delivery and any complications in the third stage of labour should be elicited. The condition of the baby at birth, the birth weight and need for intensive neonatal care should also be elicited. History of the type of infant feeding, routine immunisations and developmental milestones should be obtained. Finally, the current condition of the baby should be ascertained.

2.4.4 Gynaecological History

A history is taken of the regularity of the menstrual periods, including cycle length and duration. The presence of menorrhagia and dysmenorrhoea is noted. Use of contraception is elicited, including the type used and the duration. Any previous gynaecological surgery is noted. Any history of spontaneous miscarriages or induced abortions is also elicited, including associated complications.

2.4.5 Past Medical and Surgical History

The patient is asked about any ongoing or previous major medical conditions, including diabetes mellitus and hypertension. Any hospital admissions apart from confinements are also documented. Any previous surgery is documented.

2.4.6 Drug History and Allergy

A history of past or current drug use is taken as well as any allergy to any particular drug.

2.4.7 Family and Social History

Details regarding the woman's home setting are obtained, including husband's occupation, whether it is a monogamous or polygamous matrimony and the kind of accommodation they reside in. The history of first-degree family members with hypertension, diabetes mellitus or sickle cell disease should also be sought.

2.4.8 Systemic Review

The patient is asked specific questions related to each of the systems in the body including the central nervous, respiratory, cardiovascular, gastrointestinal, reproductive and musculoskeletal systems.

2.5 Obstetric Examination

The obstetric examination comprises general and systemic examinations.

2.5.1 General Examination

A brief description of the patient's appearance is given. The patient is then examined for conjunctival pallor, jaundice, fever, palmar pallor, capillary refill and oedema on the feet, sacrum and fingers. The neck is examined for enlargement, tenderness and lumps suggestive of thyroid mass. The breasts are examined next. This may indeed be the first time a pregnant woman will have her breasts examined professionally. Particular attention is paid to the size, shape, symmetry, as well as dimpling and retraction. On palpation, tenderness and masses are checked for.

2.5.2 Abdominal Examination

An inspection of the abdomen is carried out with particular attention to the shape, whether scaphoid, flat or distended. It is then examined for linea nigra, striae gravidarum, scarification marks, scars and foetal movements. The nine regions of the abdomen are palpated for any area of tenderness, after which the liver and spleen are checked for enlargement. The kidneys are checked to determine if they are ballotable. Thereafter, the symphysio-fundal height is measured in centimetres.

The lie, presentation, position, foetal head engagement and the presence of foetal heart tones are determined using the 4-step Leopold's manoeuvres.

2.6 Conclusion

Detailed history taking and examination will usually point to possible diagnosis in the majority of cases in gynaecological practice. Appropriate investigations need to be requested with careful consideration in view of the high cost, especially in the developing world countries.

References

1. King's College London School of Medicine. Reproductive and sexual Health Book. Curriculum Guidelines.
2. Ibrahim A, Mahmoud NM, Othman MS. Gynaecological history taking. In: Ibrahim A, editor. Wikiversity. History taking and clinical examination for obstetrics and gynaecology patients. 1st ed. Kota Bhanu Egypt; 2009.
3. Finnih OA. Clinical diagnosis in obstetrics and gynaecology. In: Okonofua F, Odunsi K, editors. Contemporary obstetrics and gynaecology for developing countries. Benin City: Women's Health and Action Research Centre; 2003. p. 3–11.
4. Abedi HO, Ebeigbe PN. Examination of the obstetric patient. In: Ebeigbe PN, editor. Foundations of clinical obstetrics in the tropics. Fodah Global Ultimate Limited. Abraka, Delta state, Nigeria; 2012. p. 10–7.

Maternal Mortality in Developing Countries

3

Friday Okonofua

Learning Objectives

At the conclusion of this chapter, the reader will:

- Understand the causes and social determinants of maternal mortality in developing countries.
- Come to terms with the prevention of maternal mortality, including recent advances in primary prevention, secondary prevention and emergency obstetrics care.
- Be able to relate maternal mortality as an essential challenge to be addressed to achieve the sustainable development goals in the developing countries.
- Be able to identify the research gaps and interventions needed to reduce maternal mortality in the developing countries.

The World Health Organization defines maternal mortality as the death of a woman during pregnancy or in the 42 days (6 weeks) following delivery regardless of the gestational age and site of the pregnancy. The death of a woman during pregnancy is a very distressing experience to the immediate and extended family of the woman, her friends and associates, providers of health care, and her immediate community at large. While maternal deaths occur in all countries and in all societies, sub-Saharan Africa is the region of the world with the highest numbers and rates of deaths, largely due to preventable causes including poverty and the low socio-economic status of women. With the growing knowledge that maternal mortality is highly associated with under-development and social marginalisation, the estimation and comparisons of the rate of maternal death are now regarded as one of the best indices for measuring societal development globally.

Three categories of maternal deaths have been identified. These include *direct maternal death*, which includes a maternal death occurring as a complication of a pregnancy. This implies that such a death (e.g. from postpartum haemorrhage) would not have occurred if the woman was not pregnant. An *indirect maternal death* is a death occurring from a medical condition that was present before the woman became pregnant, but which was made worse as a result of pregnancy. An example is a woman who had sickle cell disease prior to pregnancy, but who died as a result of a severe complication of sickle cell disease occurring in pregnancy. By contrast, an *associated maternal death* refers to an accidental death, not related to the pregnancy or its complications. Examples of associated indirect maternal deaths include deaths from suicide, severe trauma from any cause, and homicidal deaths. Thus, it is clear that all forms of death in a pregnant woman within 42 days after delivery can be included in the definition of a maternal death.

The prevention of maternal mortality is now one of the most important functions of health systems around the world. The safe motherhood initiative was a global effort in the late 1980s to galvanise political will and mobilise resources to reduce the rate of maternal mortality. However, to date, the problem remains a relentless and discomforting human experience. Indeed and unfortunately, maternal mortality remains one of the most important unmet needs for human development. This chapter reviews the epidemiology and causes of maternal mortality, especially within the context of developing countries, and deal extensively with current and past efforts being made to prevent maternal mortality in these countries.

F. Okonofua (✉)
Centre of Excellence in Reproductive Health Innovation, Department of Obstetrics and Gynaecology, University of Benin, Benin City, Nigeria

Women's Health and Action Research Centre, Benin City, Nigeria

University of Medical Sciences, Ondo City, Ondo State, Nigeria

F. Okonofua et al. (eds.), *Contemporary Obstetrics and Gynecology for Developing Countries*, https://doi.org/10.1007/978-3-030-75385-6_3

3.1 Definitions and Measurements of Maternal Deaths

To enable the development of clear benchmarks and the comparison of maternal deaths around the world, some basic definitions of terminologies are frequently in use. The *maternal mortality ratio*, defined as the number of maternal deaths per 100,000 live births, is used to measure the number of maternal deaths in a health facility at any level. When measured accurately, it enables the comparison of maternal deaths in a single institution over time, as well as the comparison of deaths between institutions of similar status. With the estimation of the maternal mortality ratios, it is possible to determine whether interventions to prevent or reduce maternal mortality are working within or between health facilities.

By contrast, the *maternal mortality rate (MMR)* is defined as the number of maternal deaths per 100,000 women of reproductive age (15–49 years). While the maternal mortality ratio takes account of deaths in single institutions, the maternal mortality rate measures the proportion of maternal deaths that occur in communities and within health systems. Apart from institutional deaths, the maternal mortality rate also takes into consideration deaths that occur outside the health care system – including deaths occurring at home, in the homes of traditional and faith-based attendants, and deaths from unattended deliveries. Thus, the maternal mortality rate refers to the comprehensive experience of maternal mortality at sub-national, national and regional levels, and allows for the comparison of maternal mortality between countries and regions, and between communities and states within countries. The estimation of the maternal mortality rate is used to assess the effectiveness of maternal health interventions and the performance of health care systems in improving women's health.

Although simplistic in their definitions, the measurement of the maternal mortality ratio and rates are often difficult, especially within developing countries. This is primarily due to the lack of vital registration systems and the difficulty in documenting births and deaths in many developing countries. Data in health institutions to accurately document the numbers of maternal deaths and births are often lacking, even in big referral hospitals. When the lack of information on deliveries that take place at home and in informal health facilities is added, it shows a complex system of inadequate data gathering relating to maternal mortality that has remained unsolved in many developing countries over time.

Despite the difficulty, maternal mortality ratios and rates have been assessed in different parts of the developing world, albeit with different degrees of accuracy. The available methods include the following:

Civil registration and vital statistics (CRVS) This is the civil registration of births and deaths that allows for the calculation of crude birth rates, death rates and maternal mortality rates. Such systems are usually put in place by governments as part of efforts to monitor social systems and the growth of populations. Unfortunately, CRVS has not worked in many developing countries, especially in sub-Saharan Africa, while it is reliable in developed countries. Although the UN has recommended CRVS to be 'universal, continuous, compulsory and confidential', many sub-Saharan African countries have yet to pass legislations to put it into practice. The UN further estimates that 72 (out of 193) member states have complete (≥90%) recording of deaths. Of these, only one (Mauritius) is in sub-Saharan Africa. Indeed, according to Professor Kelsey Harrison (personal communication), 'the initiation of civil registration and vital statistics is the most important single intervention that can improve the delivery of maternal health care in sub-Saharan Africa'.

Household surveys These are conducted with the intention of obtaining estimates of maternal mortality rates from representative random samples. This would better represent target communities or regions, and normally allows for external generalisation of the results. Household surveys simply ask the time of death relative to pregnancy and measure pregnancy-related deaths. The methods have been well summarised and described by Kenneth Hill, 2010 [1]. They include the use of the original sisterhood method, the sibling-history-based method and the identification of all female deaths in the household in some reference period.

The major advantage of household surveys is that they provide all information required to estimate pregnancy-related mortality, including fertility. They are also relatively inexpensive to carry out, especially if done in the context of national demographic surveys. On the downside, they are extremely demanding in terms of data processing requirements. Large sample sizes are also required, including complex designs and sampling procedures. More importantly, they tend to underestimate overall mortality, including pregnancy-related mortality.

Facility-based studies These are studies of maternal mortality obtained from health facilities with existing records. Such studies have the potential for gold standard care, and for assessment of standards of maternal health care in health facilities. They are especially useful for identifying areas for improved care, in particular when confidential enquiry procedures are used. However, the quality of such studies is often difficult to evaluate, since facility-based deaths (and births) may be selected on the basis of characteristics that may (not?) be fully disclosed. Also, the results are often not generalisable to national maternal mortality estimates unless selection probabilities are known and well defined.

National population censuses The 2010 Principles and Recommendations for Population and Housing Censuses recommended that countries that lack complete vital registration systems can include questions on deaths in households in defined reference periods in population censuses. However, the reported deaths of women of reproductive age often trigger additional questions about the timing of death relative to pregnancy. This can make census reporting much more complex.

The major concern relating to including questions on maternal death in censuses is that such deaths can be missed in single-person households. Also, the death of a leading household figure may result in the break-up of the household, leading to missing information. Repeated experiences suggest that there is always under-reporting of maternal deaths with the use of census statistics.

Reproductive Age Mortality Studies (RAMOS) This was initially thought to be the gold standard for measuring maternal deaths. However, the method has recently been questioned as a method at all due to its unreliability. It relies on multiple sources of data to identify adult female deaths. These sources include vital registration, medical records, undertaker records, records from traditional birth attendants and faith-based healers, mothers' groups, women's associations, markets, newspaper and related publications, and verbal autopsy. However, such data are difficult to collect in countries with no culture of data keeping or reasonable vital registration base. Once adult female deaths are identified, a verbal autopsy or medical records, or a combination of both, will then be used to determine the cause of death.

The main advantage of RAMOS is that it provides a more complete method of identifying maternal deaths, due to the multiple sources of data collection. It also allows for important data collection on avoidable causes of death both in health facilities and at home, and therefore enables the assessment of care-seeking behaviour as a determinant of maternal death. However, the method is expensive and labour intensive, and can only be considered in settings with greater than 60% completeness of reporting of adult female deaths in vital registration. It also does not provide for the number of births, and without a denominator, maternal mortality rates or ratios cannot be determined.

National Demographic and Health Surveys (NDHS) Questions about the death of sisters have tended to be incorporated into National Demographic and Health Surveys that have been conducted in many developing countries since the beginning of the millennium. Respondents, who are typically women of reproductive age, are asked questions about each of their sisters' current age or, if applicable, age at death, when death occurred, and whether it occurred during a pregnancy, childbirth or within 6 weeks of the end of the pregnancy.

In NDHS, maternal deaths are identified on the basis of the time of death. Such deaths are pregnancy associated rather than being true maternal deaths. Thus, a major drawback of NDHS as a means of estimating maternal deaths is that non-maternal deaths may be counted, while many maternal deaths may be left uncounted because the respondent may not have complete information about the pregnancy status of the woman at the time of her death. In many parts of Africa because of cultural sensitivity, even when the respondents know the causes of death, they may not be willing to disclose such information. This is particularly so when the cause of death may be an abortion or HIV/AIDS.

Statistical models Without reliable data, especially in developing countries, organisations such as the UNICEF, UNFPA, WHO and the World Bank have relied on statistical modelling to estimate global trends in maternal mortality rates. Such estimates have been published over several years, but it has to be recognised that they are only estimates and not true rates based on accurate data. Due to the difficulty in obtaining relevant data, the true accuracy of statistical modelling has never been tested, which makes interpretation a real problem in development planning.

3.2 Global Trends in Maternal Mortality Rates

Data on the high rates of maternal mortality in Nigeria were first published in the mid-1980s by Professor Kelsey Harrison [2]. Since then, periodic reports have been published as single reports from health facilities, countries or regions from across the world. The most recent estimates confirm the continuing higher rates of maternal mortality in the developing world as compared to high-income countries. The most recent report [3] (summarised in Fig. 3.1), jointly published by the WHO, UNICEF. , UNFPA, the World Bank Group and the United Nations Population Division, suggests that between 1990 and 2015, maternal mortality rates (MMR) fell globally by 44%. The results showed that MMR fell from a mean of 385 per 100,000 in 1990 to a mean of 216 per 100,000 in 2015. The actual annual numbers of maternal deaths were estimated to have fallen from 532,000 in 1990 to 303,000 in 2015. The global lifetime risk of a maternal death also fell from 1 in 73 to 1 in 180 during the period.

The report also showed that developing countries still accounted for 99% (302,000) of the global maternal deaths in 2015. Sub-Saharan Africa alone account for 66% (201,000) of the annual maternal deaths, followed by Southern Asia (66,000). At the national level, Nigeria and India together accounted for over 33% of all maternal deaths worldwide in 2015, with approximately 58,000 deaths occurring in India and 45,000 deaths recorded in Nigeria. Indeed, Nigeria

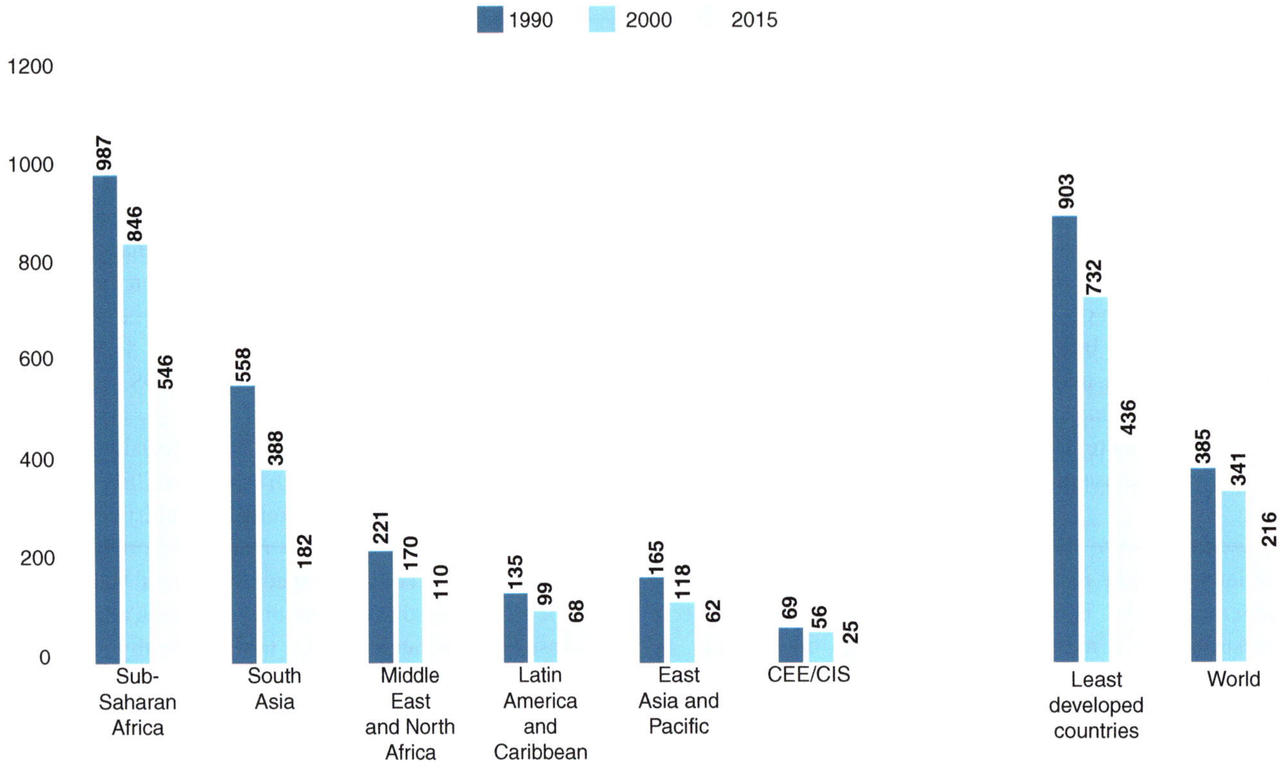

Fig. 3.1 Global rates of maternal mortality between 1990 and 2015: Data from the WHO, UNICEF. UNFPA, the World Bank Group and the United Nations Population Division Report

accounted for 15% of global maternal deaths in 2015, whereas it accounted for 10% in 2000. This implies a worsening maternal mortality scenario in Africa's most populous country. In 2015, sub-Saharan African countries had the highest MMR in the world, with Sierra Leone leading with a rate of 1360 per 100,000. Nigeria had an MMR of 814 per 100,000.

Thus, it is evident that despite the inclusion of maternal mortality reduction in the Millennium Declaration with an MDG-5 premised on reducing maternal mortality by 75% between 1990 and 2015, many developing countries, especially in sub-Saharan Africa, failed to achieve the benchmark. Cape Verde and Rwanda were the only two sub-Saharan African countries that achieved the MDG-5 target. Now that the Sustainable Development Goals (SDGs) have focused in Goal 3.1 on reducing MMR below 70 per 100,000 by 2030, it will require accelerated action by all governments and nations to achieve the target.

3.3 Medical and Direct Causes of Maternal Mortality

The medical and obstetric causes of maternal mortality have been published from various parts of the world. In 2014, the WHO undertook a systematic analysis of the causes of maternal deaths that summarised the results of nearly 23 eligible studies published between 2003 and 2012, and that included 417 datasets from 115 countries and 60,799 maternal deaths [4]. The results showed that about 73% of the maternal deaths worldwide between 2003 and 2009 were attributable to direct obstetric cases, while indirect causes accounted for 27.5% of the maternal deaths.

Obstetric haemorrhage topped the list of direct causes of maternal deaths, accounting for 27.1%, while hypertensive disorders of pregnancy contributed 14% of deaths. Other causes were sepsis (10.7%), unsafe abortion (7.9%), embolism (3.2%), and other direct causes (9.6%). Indirect causes include conditions that existed before pregnancy but that were made worse by pregnancy, examples being sickle cell disease and HIV/AIDS.

Evidently there were regional variations, with causes such as obstructed labour and uterine rupture featuring more in sub-Saharan African countries. These were broadly categorised under infections and haemorrhage, and did not feature as separate entities. Whereas haemorrhage, hypertensive diseases and infections featured as causes of maternal death in developing countries, deaths in developed countries were more likely to be due to embolism and to indirect causes. Despite the prevalence of severe obstetric complications in all countries, mortality from these complications tended to occur more in developing countries as compared to developed countries. It is now recognised that part of the reasons for the higher rate of maternal mortality in developing countries is the adverse social circumstances under which women become pregnant and give birth, and the inadequate response of health systems to maternal health care.

3.4 Social Context of Maternal Mortality

Most maternal deaths occur as a result of poorly managed severe pregnancy complications. Delay in health seeking and in the management of pregnancy complications is now known to be the most important single factor that leads to maternal deaths in developing countries. If a pregnancy complication is promptly recognised, and promptly reported and managed in an adequately equipped and staffed maternal health facility, it is unlikely that such a complication would lead to a maternal death. Such is the situation in many developed countries, and is the reason for the low rate of maternal mortality in those countries. By contrast, in many developing countries, delay in the management of pregnancy complications due to adverse personal social factors, and health systems' underperformance has been identified as the major intermediate determinant of maternal death.

In an elegant paper, Thaddeus and Maine [5] identified three types of delays that are associated with maternal deaths, and also pinpointed some of the social factors that may lead to such delays. According to the model, *type 1 delay* is the failure of a woman to seek care when she experiences a complication during pregnancy. To this, we would add the failure of a woman to seek antenatal or delivery care at the right time during pregnancy or onset of labour. Type 1 delay is largely due to ignorance and illiteracy, and possibly to cultural preference for traditional methods of pregnancy and delivery care. Also, there is now abundant evidence that Type 1 delay may be due to women's perceptions relating to high costs of services and poor or abusive services in health facilities [6].

Type 2 delay is when women delay in receiving treatment for pregnancy complications as a result of difficulty with transportation. This could be due to the fact that health facilities are located far away from places where women live, or to the inability to obtain actual means of transportation at the time the complications occur.

By contrast, type 3 delays are those due to delays in treatment after the woman has arrived in hospital. Experience suggests that there are multiple scenarios with type 3 delays, including failure to start treatment in time as immediate emergencies in health facilities; women presenting themselves in poorly equipped health facilities, with the facilities delaying in referring such women to higher-level facilities; the lack of treatment tools such as blood, infusions and antibiotics when women with complications arrive in health facilities; women with complications arriving in health facilities at the time of lock-outs by health workers; and poor staff attitudes and skills resulting in delays and inadequate or incorrect treatment or treatment errors [7, 8]. The results of our most recent publications suggest that many of these occurrences are associated with poor staff attitudes and skills, inadequate staffing of health facilities with consequent heavy workloads and low staff motivation, inadequate information given to patients and the poor organisation of maternal health services [9–13].

The results of a careful analytical and qualitative study we conducted in Ile-Ife, Nigeria [14] revealed that up to 40% of delays that led to maternal death at a leading teaching hospital were due to type 1 delay and 20% of maternal deaths occurred as a result of type 2 delay, while 40% were attributable to type 3 delays. Major efforts to eliminate delays in care-giving for pregnancy and delivery would significantly reduce the incidence and prevalence of maternal deaths in many developing countries.

3.5 Risk Factors for Maternal Mortality

Some identified risk factors for maternal mortality include the following:

Poverty Maternal mortality is higher among women of lower social economic status, and among unemployed women, as well as women in poorer households and those in the lower wealth quintiles. According to the UNFPA [15], 'maternal mortality rates reflect disparities between rich and poor countries more than any other measure of health'. Within countries, it measures the huge gap between poor and rich citizens more than any other social indicator.

Education Results from several studies [2, 16] indicate that maternal mortality is higher among women with lower education as compared to women with higher levels of education. Indeed, Kelsey Harrison has repeatedly shown this relationship in his many studies and publications of the effects of social determinants on maternal mortality [2, 17–20], and showed that more than 90% of maternal deaths in Nigeria occurred among women with no education or with primary-level education. By contrast, among Nigerian women with tertiary-level education, the maternal mortality ratio was similar to those of women in the UK.

Place of residence Research evidence suggests that maternal deaths are twice as likely to occur in rural areas as compared to urban areas [21]. Even within urban areas, maternal deaths are significantly more common in sub-urban areas as compared to more urbanised communities, even after controlling for socio-economic factors such as poverty and education. This is likely to be due to the fact that maternal health facilities are often located in urban areas in many developing countries as compared to rural communities. Therefore, women in rural communities may have poorer access to emergency obstetric care due to distance, poor roads and difficulties with transportation.

Maternal Age Initial studies showed that teenagers and adolescents had higher rates of maternal mortality due to higher prevalence of anaemia, eclampsia and obstructed labour [2, 22, 23]. Additionally, young mothers are likely not to be experienced and supported in pregnancy, and so less likely to receive antenatal care and skilled delivery care, which predisposes them to higher rates of unmanaged complications and consequently higher risk of death. However, recent evidence also suggests that older maternal age (age >35 years) exposes women to greater risks of maternal death during pregnancy and childbirth, essentially due to higher rates of pregnancy complications (postpartum haemorrhage, ruptured uterus and pregnancy hypertension) that lead to maternal death.

Past obstetric experiences Past obstetric experiences that lead to increased risks of maternal mortality in developing countries include grand multi-parity (Para ≥5), short pregnancy intervals (less than 2 years), previous caesarean section, and past pregnancy complications (such as past obstetric haemorrhage). By contrast, although death often occurs as a result of caesarean delivery, no systematic research has yet been undertaken to investigate the effect of caesarean delivery on the likelihood of maternal mortality in developing countries. While our recent study showed that caesarean delivery reduces the likelihood of still-births in eight referral hospitals in Nigeria [24], it is not clear if this association also lies with maternal deaths. Caesarean delivery carries inherent risks especially in poorly resourced settings. Therefore, it would be critical to prospectively investigate the practice and safety of caesarean section within the context of developing countries.

Non-use of contraceptives by women not desiring pregnancies Unwanted pregnancy due to non-use of contraceptives by sexually active women is one of the most important risk factors for maternal mortality. Indeed, data from the WHO indicate that up to 50% of the decline in maternal mortality that occurred between 1911 and 2016 was predominantly due to increases in contraceptive prevalence rates. Low contraceptive prevalence rates prevail in many developing countries with high rates of maternal mortality. These low rates account for high rates of adolescent and teenager pregnancies, and unwanted and unplanned pregnancies, which lead to unsafe abortions with higher risks of maternal mortality. Unwanted term pregnancies are also likely to be unsupported and to be associated with inappropriate health-seeking behaviour, with limited access to skilled pregnancy care.

Unmet need for contraception (defined as sexually active women who do not wish to become pregnant but are not using contraceptives) is high in many developing countries with high rates of maternal mortality. Nigeria, with the second-highest global numbers of maternal deaths, had a contraceptive prevalence rate (proportion of women using modern methods of contraceptives) of less 10%, and an unmet need of about 16% in 2013 [25]. By contrast, the global unmet need declined to 12.3% in the same period. Absolute numbers for unmet need for contraception are expected to rise to 214 million in developing countries in 2017, with most of the increase occurring in developing countries.

Some of the most common reasons for low use of contraceptives and unmet need in developing countries have been well documented [26]. These include lack of choice and access to contraceptives; non-evidence-based medical rules (e.g. not giving contraceptives to women unless they are menstruating; high costs of family planning commodities and services; providers' bias and misinformation; and women's fear and inaccurate perceptions of the side-effects of contraceptives). Efforts to address these challenges are needed to increase the use of family planning and reduce maternal mortality in many developing countries.

Restrictive abortion policies and laws Data from the WHO indicate that countries with restrictive abortion laws not only have higher rates of unwanted pregnancy but also have higher rates of unsafe abortion and abortion-related deaths. About 25% of countries globally have highly restrictive abortion laws. These are countries mostly in sub-Saharan Africa, Asia and Latin America. Women living in these countries, especially in sub-Saharan Africa, experience higher rates of abortion-related deaths and maternal mortality, as compared to countries (mostly high-income countries) with less restrictive and more liberal abortion laws.

Low use of antenatal care The proportion of pregnant women using evidence-based antenatal care is a good predictor of the likelihood of maternal deaths. Published data indicate that 'unbooked women', who have not received antenatal care during pregnancy and who present as complicated emergencies in referral facilities, have substantially increased chances of dying in pregnancy as compared to 'booked' women [2, 27]. The WHO recommends clinical standards for provision of antenatal care for positive pregnancy experience and to save lives [28]. However, evidence abounds to indicate that essential components of antenatal care are not followed in many developing countries, mainly because pregnant women in developing countries (especially in sub-Saharan Africa) do not present themselves for antenatal care in health facilities. By contrast, many pregnant women either do not receive antenatal care at all, or receive care in the homes of unskilled birth attendants or traditional providers.

Data from UNICEF show that in 2016 [29], while about 86% of women globally received antenatal care with a skilled health provider at least once during pregnancy, only 62% received at least four antenatal visits, as recommended by the WHO. In regions and countries with the highest rates of maternal mortality, an even lower proportion of pregnant women received at least four antenatal visits. This amounted to only 52% in sub-Saharan Africa overall and only 64% in Nigeria. As expected, urban women, better-educated women and women in the richest quintiles were more likely to receive antenatal care as compared to rural women, women with no education and those in the poorest quintiles. Efforts to address these bottlenecks would greatly increase antenatal attendance and reduce maternal mortality in developing countries.

Unskilled birth attendance In our experience, of all the risks associated with maternal mortality in developing countries, the non-use of a skilled birth attendant (doctor or midwife) at the time of delivery is one of the most dangerous risks to which women are exposed, which has the highest proclivity to lead (likelihood of leading) to maternal death. Even when all risks are aggregated, if women have access to a skilled attendant to manage delivery and possible complications, the chances of maternal mortality will be substantially reduced.

The current reality is that sadly, only a low proportion of pregnant women in developing countries have access to a skilled birth attendant at the time of delivery. Skilled birth attendance was one of the indicators for measuring access to maternal health care in the Millennium Development Goals (MDGs). It remains a universal indicator for measuring the success of maternal health interventions. Countries with the lowest maternal mortality rates, such as Sweden, have nearly 100% skilled birth attendance, whereas countries with high maternal rates have substantially lower rates. Nigeria has a skilled birth attendance rate of only 33%. The 2011 MDG report showed that many countries made progress in increasing the skilled birth attendance rate, from 55% in 1990 to 65% in 2009 [30], but substantial progress still needs to be made.

3.6 Prevention of Maternal Mortality

Prevention of maternal mortality can conveniently be divided into three categories as follows:

- Primary prevention: Family planning to prevent unwanted and mistimed pregnancies
- Secondary prevention: Safe termination of a pregnancy when not wanted, or the continuation of a wanted pregnancy to term through quality antenatal and delivery care; and
- Tertiary prevention: The management of complications of pregnancy that lead to maternal deaths.

However, these three prevention components must be based on a strong health system that ensures the over-arching coordination of activities related to prevention. Essential to the prevention of maternal deaths (also called safe motherhood) is the recognition that no single intervention can prevent a maternal death without the inputs of the other components. Indeed, prevention of maternal death is one of the most important indicators that all components of societal development are working within a geo-political entity. Thus, governance has to work to coordinate the delivery of basic health care, based on the development of basic health services, rested on the principles of universal access to services for all citizens, equity and social justice. It is the lack of performance of health systems, based on poorly performing governance, that is the under-pinning reason that all types of prevention activities do not work for maternal mortality prevention in many parts of Africa.

However, there is rising evidence [31] and hope that the political will and commitment to provide essential maternal and reproductive health services to prevent maternal deaths may be rising in parts of Africa. Our earlier report not only confirmed this observation [31], but there is evidence that some governments have recently taken specific steps to tackle high rates of maternal mortality in their communities. A good example is Ondo State, one of the 36 federal states in Nigeria, located in the southwest region of the country. In 2007, Ondo State experienced the highest rate of maternal mortality in southwest Nigeria. Between 2009 and 2016, the government of the state under Dr. Olusegun Mimiko launched an aggressive safe motherhood programme tagged the *Abiye project* [32], which provided free delivery and caesarean sections to women, and coordinated the referral of pregnant women from the homes of traditional birth attendants to adequately funded referral facilities. The programme witnessed a nearly 70% decline in maternal mortality within a short period, such that the state now has the lowest maternal mortality in Nigeria and was the only state in the country that achieved the MDG-5. This confirms that regardless of the work non-governmental organisations and international agencies may be doing in preventing maternal deaths in developing countries, advocacy to increase the political commitment of governments to scale up best practices can work [33], and are an important and critical intervention.

3.6.1 Primary Prevention of Maternal Mortality

Improving family planning is one of the most effective measures to decrease the rates of unwanted and mistimed pregnancies, and to reduce maternal mortality rates worldwide. The United Nations Sustainable Development Goals (SDGs) [34] –Goal 3 recommends that 'by 2030, (governments) should ensure universal access to sexual and reproductive health care services, including family planning information and education, and the integration of reproductive health into national strategies and programs'. In order to ensure that this is achieved, national governments must work in partnership with civil society organisations, communities and health providers, as well as international partners, to strengthen reproductive health and family planning programmes, ensuring increased accessed to the most at-risk men, women and families in the coming two decades.

Comprehensive and multi-sectorial methods for family planning delivery that need to be used include the following:

- Clinic-based methods.
- Mobile clinics to ensure that family planning reaches men and women in places where they work or reside.
- Community-based distribution – such approaches must include delivery methods that are acceptable to community members.
- Social marketing – influencing social behaviours that benefit the target audience and the general society on issues related to family planning.
- Targeting of special groups – postpartum, post-abortion, adolescents, workplace.

Integrating family planning into primary health care now offers the best opportunity to reach the most vulnerable men and women in the most remote areas, especially rural and suburban locations. The WHO [35] recommends that this approach be used more widely in efforts to scale up family planning delivery and use, especially in developing countries.

3.6.2 Secondary Prevention of Maternal Mortality

When women experience unwanted and mistimed pregnancies and desire to terminate such pregnancies, experiences have shown that they will do so regardless of the law. Due to legal restrictions, many women with unwanted pregnancies in developing countries resort to the use of dangerous methods of abortion that cause them harm, disability and death. Evidence abounds to show that restrictive abortion laws do not prevent induced abortions; they merely make such abortions unsafe and dangerous [36]. On the basis of this, promoting women's access to safe abortion care is now one of the most important secondary prevention methods for maternal mortality.

The World Health Organization has provided guidelines on safe abortion care [37] for integration into policies and programmes of health care delivery systems in various countries. A proper use of these guidelines will considerably improve safe abortion policy and practice, and result in significant reduction in abortion-related deaths and maternal mortality.

The most important consideration for secondary prevention is the use of antenatal care by women desiring continuation of their pregnancies. Antenatal care refers to the care given to a pregnant woman from time of conception until the beginning of labour. It is a preventative and cost-effective service. The goals of antenatal care are fourfold: (1) to ensure a mother's health; (2) to ensure delivery of a healthy infant; (3) to anticipate problems; and (4) to diagnose and manage problems early.

The World Health Organization has provided guidelines for the delivery of antenatal care [28]. Countries are encouraged to follow these guidelines for the effective delivery of antenatal care. Both demand and supply factors that hinder the use of antenatal care by pregnant women should be addressed to encourage increased access for women. In particular, as primary health care promises easier entry to the most vulnerable women in rural and hard-to-reach areas, the use of the primary health care approach needs to be better promoted for the delivery of antenatal care in developing countries in order to achieve universal coverage, especially for disadvantaged rural women.

3.6.3 Tertiary Prevention of Maternal Mortality

Tertiary prevention of maternal mortality is rested on the provision of quality emergency care to promptly manage women who present with obstetric complications in health facilities. Less than 50% of pregnant women presently have access to emergency obstetric care in sub-Saharan African countries. To achieve universal access to emergency obstetric care, the UNFPA recommends Basic Emergency Obstetrics Care (BEOC) in primary healthcare settings. This includes skilled delivery care, administration of antibiotics, manual removal of the placenta, removal of retained products of conception, assisted vaginal delivery possibly with a vacuum extractor, and basic neonatal care, including neonatal resuscitation. By contrast, Comprehensive Emergency Obstetrics Care (CEOC) will provide all BEOC services in addition to caesarean section and safe blood transfusion services, and make provisions for the treatment of the sick baby.

Unfortunately, the health systems in many developing countries are not properly structured to provide such services. Many are characterised by the lack of facilities, inadequate coordination, poor training and motivation of staff, and inadequate funding. Improving the demand and supply of BEOC and CEOC is currently one of the most important strategies that can help reduce high rates of maternal mortality in many developing countries.

3.7 Recommendations and Conclusion

The global community has given attention to the prevention of maternal mortality over the past two decades. Despite these efforts, a lot still remains to be done. Some priority areas requiring urgent global action include the following:

- As payment for maternal health services considerably hurts the poor, the removal of financial barriers will greatly boost maternal health service utilisation in many parts of the developing world. Efforts should be made to provide subsidies, remove financial barriers and even incentives (such as conditional cash transfers) to enable the most vulnerable pregnant women to gain access to evidence-based maternal health services.
- Re-training programmes for traditional and faith-based birth attendants have repeatedly been shown not to be effective in preventing maternal deaths [39–41]. Therefore, such training programmes should no longer be encouraged in developing countries. By contrast, efforts should be concentrated on increasing women's access to skilled pregnancy and delivery care.
- The absence of vital registration systems is currently one of the most critical bottlenecks besetting (impacting) the accurate determination of the rates and causes of maternal deaths in many developing countries. Going forward, and with the aim of achieving SDG-3, efforts should be made in every developing country to improve vital registration systems for the accurate recording of births and deaths, as recommended by the World Health Organization. Additionally, confidential enquiries into maternal deaths, which have proven useful in developed countries for identifying and rectifying the medical and social causes of maternal mortality, should be put in place in the health and governance systems of developing countries. This would engender systems-wide accountability to ensure that all components of development are pulled together to prevent maternal deaths and improve the well-being of citizens.
- A new era of strategic thinking must be cultivated in all developing countries to ensure that care during pregnancy for all women is prioritised. All women should be able to deliver in health centres, with midwives working in teams, while poor and rural women in greatest need should be targeted.
- Policy-makers must make strategic human resource decisions to ensure 100% coverage of maternal health services with health professionals. Plans for the training and deployment of sufficient numbers of health professionals to the most rural communities must be developed and implemented. Quality counts, and so it is important to ensure that skills and competencies to provide evidence-based care are strengthened in maternal health facilities. And investments must be made to retain existing and competent staff.
- Great financial resources are needed to protect the poorest families from the catastrophic consequences of unaffordable emergency care. Maternal mortality reduction requires a consistent and significant effort over the next 10 years and beyond, and so national governments need to invest greater resources. Donors also need to increase financial contributions in low-income countries to fill the resource gap.
- Finally, political commitment is necessary to ensure the new era of strategic thinking on promoting maternal health is translated into programmes. Governments, donors and civil society need to work in concert to ensure that this happens.

In conclusion, the prevention of maternal mortality is one of the most important indicators of improved social attainment in developing countries in years to come. Efforts put in place at the present time will be rewarding for developing countries now and in the future.

References

1. Hill K. Methods for measuring maternal mortality. Presentation prepared for workshop on improving national capacity to track maternal mortality towards the attainment of the MDG5. Nairobi, Kenya. December, 2010.
2. Harrison K. Childbearing, health and social priorities: a survey of 22,774 consecutive hospital births in Zaria, northern Nigeria. BJOG. 1985;92(Supplement 5):1–119.
3. WHO, UNICEF, UNFPA, World Bank, the United Nations Population Group. Trends in maternal mortality: 1990 to 2015. WHO, 2015. ISBN 978 92 41565141. NLM Classification: WQ 16.
4. Say L, Chou D, Gemmil A, et al. Global causes of maternal deaths: a WHO systematic analysis. Lancet Glob Health. 2014;2(6): e323–33. https://doi.org/10.1016/S2214-109X(14)70227-X.
5. Thaddeus S, Maine D. Too far to walk – maternal mortality in context. Soc Sci Med. 1994;38:1091–110.
6. Okonofua FE, Ntoimo LF, Ogu RN. Women's perceptions on reasons for Maternal Deaths: Implications for policies and programs in

low-income countries. Health Care for Women International. 2018; 39:1, 95–109. https://doi.org/10.1080/07399332.2017. 1365868. PMID 28829240
7. Hussein J, Hirose A, Owolabi O, Imamura M, Kanguru L, Okonofua F. Maternal death and obstetric audits in Nigeria: a systematic review of barriers and enabling factors in the provision of emergency care. Reprod Health. 2016;13:47.
8. Bregje de Kok, Imamura M, Kanguru L, Owolabi O, Okonofua F, Hussein J. Achieving accountability through maternal death reviews in Nigeria: A process analysis. Health Policy and Planning 2017:1–9. https://doi.org/10.1093/healop/c2x012.
9. Okonofua F, Agholor K, Ogu R, Okike O, Abdus-salam A, Gana M, et al. Qualitative assessment of women's satisfaction with maternal health care in referral hospitals in Nigeria. BMC Reprod Health. 2017;14:44. https://doi.org/10.1186/s12978-017-0305-6. REPH-D-16-00234.
10. Okonofua F, Randawa A, Ogu R, Agholor K, Okike O, Abdus-salam A, Galadanci H. Views of senior health personnel about quality of emergency obstetric care: a qualitative study in Nigeria. PLoS One. 2017;12(3):e01734. https://doi.org/10.1371/journalPONE-D-16-41470.
11. Hirose A, Owolabi O, Imamura M, Okonofua FE, Hussein J. Systematic review of obstetric care from a women-centred perspective in Nigeria. Int J Gynaecol Obstet. 2017;136(1):13–8.
12. Okonofua FE, Ogu RN, Ntoimo LF. Opinion of women on workloads in maternity hospitals and its effect on quality of maternal health care. Midwifery. 2017;56:1–6. https://doi.org/100.1016/jmidw2017.08.008.
13. Okonofua FE, Ogu RN, Ntoimo LF, Gana M, Okike O, Durodola A, et al. Where do delays occur when women receive antenatal care in referral hospitals in Nigeria? A client flow multi-site study. Ghana Medical Journal 2017;51(3).
14. Okonofua FE, Abejide OR, Makanjuola RO. Maternal mortality in Ile-Ife, Nigeria: a study of risk factors. Stud Fam Plan. 1992;23(5):319–24.
15. UNFPA. The social determinants of maternal death and disability. UNFPA – EN_SRH facts sheet; 2012.
16. Bhalotra S, Clarke D. Educational attainment and maternal mortality. Background paper prepared for the education for all global monitoring report. 2013/4. Teaching and learning: achieving quality education for all. UNESCO, 2013. 2014/ED/EFA/MRT/P1/14.
17. Harrison KA. The struggle to reduce maternal mortality in Nigeria. Afr J Reprod Health. 2009;13(3):9–20.
18. Harrison KA. Reproductive health struggles in Nigeria. Lancet. 2003;362:582.
19. Harrison KA, Bergstrom S. Poverty, deprivation and unsafe motherhood. In: Lawson JB, Harrison KA, Bergstrom S, editors. Maternity care in developing countries. London: RCOG Press. 2001 page 1.
20. Harrison KA. We reap what we sow. Lecture delivered at the 1st distinguished guest lecture. Ondo City: University of Medical Sciences; May 2016.
21. Banda R, Fylkesnes K, Sandoy IF. Rural-urban differentials in pregnancy-related mortality in Zambia: estimates using data collected in a census. Popul Health Metrics. 2015;12:32. https://doi.org/10.1186/s12963-015-0066-9.
22. Gibbs CM, Wendt A, Peters S, Hogue CJ. The impact of early age at first childbirth on maternal and infant health. Paediatr Perinat Epidemiol. 2012;26(01):259–84.
23. Benli AR, Benli NC, Usla AT, et al. Effect of maternal age on pregnancy outcome and cesarean delivery rate. J Clin Med Res. 2015;7(2):97–102.
24. Okonofua FE, Ntoimo LFC, Ogu R, Galadanci H, Mohammed G, Adetoye D, Abe E, Okike O, Agholor K, Abdus-Salam R, Randawa A. Prevalence and risk factors for stillbirths in Nigerian referral hospitals: A multi-centre study. BMC Pregnancy and Childbirth. 2019;19(1):533. https://doi.org/10.1186/s/12884-019-2682-2.
25. Alkema L, et al. National, regional and global rates and trends in contraceptive prevalence and unmet need for family planning between 1990 and 2015: a systematic and comprehensive analysis. Lancet. 2013;381(9878):1642–52.
26. Campbell A, et al. Barriers to fertility regulation. Stud Fam Plan. 2006;37:87–98.
27. Ntiomo L, Okonofua FE, Gana M, Ogu R., Abdus-salam A, Galadanci H., Durodola A, Randawa A. Prevalence and risk factors for maternal mortality in Nigerian referral hospitals. Int J Women's Health 2018;10:69–76. https://doi.org/10.2147/IFWH.S151784. PMID 29440934.
28. WHO. New guidelines on antenatal care for a positive pregnancy experience. WHO, Geneva 2016. Accessed from: www.who.int/reproductivehealth/publications/maternal_perinatal_health/anc.../en/. 22 Dec 2017.
29. UNICEF. Monitoring the situation of children and women – Global databases 2017 based on MICS and DHS. Accessed from: https://data.unicef.org/topic/maternal-health/antenatal-care/#. 23 Dec 2017.
30. United Nations. The Millennium Development Goals Report 2011. UN, 2011. Accessed from http://www.un.org/millenniumgoals/pdf/ 23 Dec 2017.
31. Shiffman J, Okonofua FE. The state of political priority for safe motherhood in Nigeria. Br J Obstet Gynaecol. 2007;114:127–33.
32. Olusegun M. Experiences with universal health coverage of maternal health care in Ondo State, Nigeria, 2009-2017. Afr J Reprod Health. 2017;20:3, 1–18.
33. Okonofua FE, Lambo E. Advocacy for free maternal and child health care in Nigeria – results and outcomes. J Health Policy. 2011;99:131–8.
34. United Nations: Transforming our world: the 2030 Agenda for sustainable development. Accessed from: https://sustainabledevelopment.un.org/?menu=1300. 24 Dec 2017.
35. World Health Organization. Primary health care now more than ever. World health report 2008. Geneva: WHO; 2008. p. 65. http://www.who.int/whr/2008/whr08en.df
36. Berer M. Abortion law and policy around the world. Health Hum Rights. 2017;19(1):13–27.
37. World Health Organization. Safe abortion: technical and policy guidance for health systems. Geneva: WHO; 2012.
38. UNFPA. Setting standards for emergency obstetric and neonatal care – basic and comprehensive care. UNFPA. Accessed from: http://www.unfpa.org/resources/setting-standards-emergency-obstetric-and-newborn-care/. 24 Dec 2017.
39. Head to Head. Are traditional birth attendants good for improving maternal and perinatal health? BMJ. 2011;342(d3308):1340–12341.
40. Bergstrom S, Goodburn E. The role of traditional birth attendants in the reduction of maternal mortality. Accessed from http://citeseerx.ist.psu.edu/viewdoc/download?doi=10.1.1.576.6630&rep=rep1&type=pdf. 24 Dec 2017.
41. Staffan B. Enhancing maternal survival in Africa. In: Okonofua F, editor. Reproductive health challenges in Africa – a textbook for students and development practitioners. Irvine: Women's Health and Action Research Centre (WHARC) and Brown Walker Press; 2014 . ISBN = 1-62734-508-6. p. 57–90.

Preventing Perinatal Mortality in the Developing Countries

4

Tinuade A. Ogunlesi and Olalekan O. Adetoro

Learning Objectives

At the conclusion of this chapter, the reader will be able to:

- Define perinatal mortality and perinatal mortality rate.
- Describe the epidemiology of stillbirths and early neonatal mortality across continents and across parts of the developing world.
- Itemise the predisposing factors in perinatal mortality.
- List the common causes of perinatal mortality (maternal and foetal) in the developing world.
- Describe specific effective preventive measures for perinatal mortality in the developing world.
- Identify key global interventions targeted at preventing perinatal and neonatal mortality in the developing world.

4.1 Introduction

Perinatal death remains a common pregnancy outcome in developing countries. The developing parts of the world, presently re-classified into low-income and lower middle-income countries, are characterised by large population, poor socio-economic indices and low expenditure on health. The proportion of the population living on less than $1 per day, as at 2013, was 43.6% for low-income countries, compared to less than 2.0% for high-income countries [1]. Similarly, the expenditure on health as a percentage of Gross Domestic Product (as at 2012) was 2.9% for low-income countries, compared with 9.6% for high-income countries [1]. It is not surprising, therefore, that the perinatal mortality rate in the developing world is close to 50 per 1000 births, compared to about 10 per 1000 births in the developed world [2].

The perinatal mortality rate is a sensitive index of socio-economic development and quality of prenatal, delivery and early infant care practices available in a community. In addition, perinatal mortality is a major contributor to overall childhood mortality [3]. Recent estimates suggest that 75% of all neonatal deaths occur during the first week of life and perinatal mortality accounts for about 45% of under-five mortality globally [4]. According to the World Health Organization (WHO), the perinatal period extends from the 22nd week of pregnancy till the end of the first week of life [5], and this is the most vulnerable period in life when the foetus may have difficulty transiting to independent extra-uterine life. Perinatal deaths encompass foetal deaths (still births) and early neonatal deaths (neonatal deaths in the first 7 days of life). Each year, close to 7 million perinatal deaths occur worldwide (3 to 4 million stillbirths and 3 million early neonatal deaths), with close to 99% of these deaths occurring in the low- and middle-income parts of the world [6].

The demographic picture of most developing countries provides a background to poor reproductive health indices and the unusually high perinatal mortality. For example, Nigeria has a current population of over 190 million people (2017) (ref), with a woman having an average of six births during her reproductive years. Adolescents account for 22% of the population with an adolescent fertility rate of 122 per 1000. The current contraceptive prevalence rate in Nigeria is only 15% (ref). In spite of the fact that 46% of the population reside in the urban parts of Nigeria, over 60% of babies are delivered outside health facilities with 38% skilled attendance at birth [7]. This implies that the lack of quality repro-

T. A. Ogunlesi (✉)
Department of Paediatrics, Olabisi Onabanjo University, Sagamu, Nigeria

Department of Paediatrics, Olabisi Onabanjo University Teaching Hospital, Sagamu, Nigeria

O. O. Adetoro
Department of Obstetrics and Gynaecology, Olabisi Onabanjo University, Sagamu, Nigeria

F. Okonofua et al. (eds.), *Contemporary Obstetrics and Gynecology for Developing Countries*,
https://doi.org/10.1007/978-3-030-75385-6_4

ductive health care services and the unfavourable socio-economic environment contribute to the high perinatal mortality. The need to reduce this alarmingly high perinatal death rate is a critical concern in the developing world [8, 9].

This chapter aims to highlight the pattern of perinatal mortality in low- and middle-income countries with emphasis on the common risk factors and known etiological factors for perinatal deaths. Evidence-based preventive measures and interventions which are applicable to the developing world situation will be discussed.

4.2 Definitions

Perinatal mortality is the combination of foetal deaths (or still births) and early neonatal deaths. The stillbirth rate (SBR) is defined as the number of foetal deaths prior to or during labour per 1000 total births, while the early neonatal death rate (ENDR) refers to the number of deaths occurring within the first week of life per 1000 live births. Therefore, the perinatal mortality rate (PNMR) is defined as the total number of stillbirths and early neonatal deaths per 1000 total births. Foetal death refers to death of a product of human conception occurring after 20 weeks of gestation but prior to the complete expulsion or extraction from the mother. According to the 10th Edition of the International Classification of Diseases (ICD-10), foetal deaths are subdivided into early (22 to 27 weeks gestation, weight > 500 g, crown-rump-length ≥ 25 cm) or late (≥28 weeks of gestation, weight ≥ 1000 g, crown-rump-length ≥ 35 cm). Therefore, foetal deaths at 22 weeks gestation or more defines stillbirth while the foetal deaths before 22 weeks gestation or weight less than 500 g define miscarriages [10, 11]. However, the definition of stillbirth using the gestational age and foetal weight at birth varies in different regions of the world, and this contributes to the variation of perinatal mortality rates recorded in the different regions of the world. For instance, whilst foetal viability is defined by 20 weeks of gestation or 500 g birth weight in the developed world, 28 weeks of gestation and above or birth weight of 700 g and above is used in developing countries. The definition accepted in various parts of the world depends on cultural disposition to foetal losses, definitions of foetal viability and availability of vital health statistics such as birth rates and death rates. Therefore, to facilitate international comparability of data, the World Health Organization uses the definition spanning 28 weeks of gestation to the first 7 days of life for perinatal deaths [10].

4.3 Incidence of Perinatal Mortality

Perinatal mortality rates vary from place to place in all regions of the world. In addition to the accepted definition of terms, the difference in PNMR is related to the socio-economic conditions and availability of acceptable qualitative medical services. According to the World Health Organization, PNMR was highest in the poorest parts of the world (Africa, Asia and Oceania), where it varied between 42/1000 and 56/1000 births, compared with richer parts of the world (Latin America, Europe and North Americas), where PNMR varied between 7/1000 births and 20/1000 births [12].

The pattern of PNMR in some African countries is shown in Table 4.1. The more developed countries in northern and southern Africa have relatively lower perinatal mortality rates when compared with countries in the eastern and western parts of the continent.

Table 4.1 Pattern of perinatal mortality rates (PNMR), stillbirth rates (SBR) and neonatal mortality rates (NMR) in some African countries

Countries	PNMR/1000 births	SBR/1000 births (2009)	NMR/1000 live births (2012)
Egypt	28 (2008)	13	12
Ethiopia	46 (2011)	26	29
Ghana	39 (2008)	22	28
Kenya	37 (2009)	22	27
Lesotho	54 (2009)	25	45
Malawi	40 (2010)	24	24
Mali	47 (2006)	23	42
Mozambique	38 (2011)	28	30
Niger	33 (2012)	23	28
Nigeria	39 (2008)	42	39
Senegal	38 (2011)	34	24
Tanzania	36 (2010)	26	21
Zambia	38 (2007)	26	29

Adapted from: www.who.int/maternal_child_adolescent/epidemiology/profiles/maternal/en/

Table 4.2 Pattern of perinatal mortality rates (PNMR) reported from health facilities in parts of Nigeria

City	Year of publication	PNMR/1000 births
Ibadan [13]	1982	86.9
Sagamu [14]	1994	119.9
Ilesha [15]	2003	77
Enugu [16]	2007	133.9
Lagos [17]	2011	84.6
Abakaliki/Port Harcourt [18]	2011	62.7
Lagos/Abuja/Katsina [19]	2011	78
Ilorin [20]	2012	81
Abuja [21]	2014	60.4
Katsina [22]	2014	130
Eku, Delta [23]	2014	94.1

The 2013 Demographic and Health Survey in Nigeria showed that the regional PNMR for the southwest, southeast, south-south, northwest, northeast and north-central zones were 42/1000, 36/1000, 37/1000, 44/1000, 45/1000 and 34/1000, respectively. In addition, hospital-based perinatal mortality rates recorded from different parts of Nigeria, as shown in Table 4.2, showed that most perinatal mortality rates varied between 60/1000 births and 134/1000 births over the years. These are not remarkably different from the range of rates reported from other parts of the developing world. A multi-centre study conducted in Burkina Faso, Cote d'Ivoire, Mali, Mauritania, Niger and Senegal reported a mean perinatal mortality rate of 42/1000 [24] and 118/1000 from Kenya [25]. Interestingly, the current trend of PNMR reported from countries in Africa (Table 4.1) shows no consistent pattern across the board.

While there is no strong evidence on which to base these observations, it is plausible that there had been deliberate efforts at tackling the problem of high perinatal mortality in most places, but the degree of success recorded in countries varies. Unfortunately, recent investigations suggest that the perinatal mortality rate in some parts of Nigeria may be rising. PNMR recorded in Ilesha, southwest Nigeria, rose from 57.8/1000 in 1995 to 77.03/1000 in 2003 [15, 26]. Similarly, the rate has not changed remarkably in Lagos, from 84.4/1000 in 2004 to 84.6/1000 in 2011 [17, 27]. These observations underscore the persistently high perinatal mortality rates in parts of Nigeria.

4.4 Epidemiology of Perinatal Deaths

Globally, about 2.6 million children die in the first 28 days of life, and a similar number are stillborn [28]. Over 98% of these perinatal deaths occur in low- and middle-income countries. Unfortunately, most of these deaths are unrecorded because they occur in parts of the world where vital statistics are poorly kept, and notifications of perinatal deaths are rarely made for socio-cultural reasons [29]. This implies that the figures presently used for local and international epidemiology, and for planning interventions, may indeed be under-estimations.

In 2015, for every 1000 total births, 18.4 babies were delivered stillborn and two-thirds of these stillbirths occurred following intrapartum complications. Although the bulk of these stillbirths occur in low- and middle-income countries, for example 28/1000 in sub-Saharan Africa, high-income countries are not spared as the stillbirth rates vary between 1.3/1000 and 8/1000 births [30]. This implies that stillbirth is a global problem and that there is a need for global attention to reduce the scourge of this important perinatal health issue. The global stillbirth rate declined from 22.1/1000 births in 1995 to 18.9/1000 births in 2009, representing a 14% decline.

Table 4.3 Changes in Stillbirth rates between 1995 and 2009 in different regions of the world

Regions	Stillbirth rates (per 1000 total births) 1995	Stillbirth rates (per 1000 total births) 2009
Africa	31.0	28.1
Americas	9.8	7.0
East Mediterranean	29.7	27.2
Europe	8.1	6.3
South East Asia	25.9	22.0
Western Pacific	17.4	10.2

Table 4.3 shows the rate of decline in stillbirth rates in different parts of the world. In low- and middle-income countries, the greatest rate of decline in stillbirth rates occurred in South East Asia and the Western Pacific regions, compared to Africa and the Americas. The stillbirth rates appear to remain high in parts of the world where access to quality perinatal health care is poor, with inequity in the distribution of the available health resources, poor maternal health indices such as fertility rates, contraceptive use and skilled attendance at birth. Therefore, it is not surprising that more recent literature shows that more than three-quarters of global stillbirths occur in sub-Saharan Africa (40.5%) and South Asia (36.9%), while the remaining one-quarter was spread across the other regions of the world [11].

A lot still needs to be done to further reduce neonatal deaths to 12/1000 live births by the year 2030, according to the tenets of the Sustainable Development Goals [4]. In 2013, the neonatal mortality rates were highest in Africa (30.5/1000), South East Asia (25.9/1000) and the Eastern Mediterranean (25.8/1000). On the other hand, the Western Pacific, the Americas and Europe recorded significantly lower neonatal mortality rates (8.4/1000, 7.6/1000 and 6.1/1000, respectively) during the same period. Although significant progress has been made from the 1990 neonatal mortality rates, the bulk of the countries with a neonatal mortality rate above 30/1000 births in 2013 are in the African region [1]. Apart from prematurity and its complications, severe intrapartum events are the next leading causes of neonatal deaths, constituting 11% of childhood deaths. These severe intrapartum events unarguably comprise foetal hypoxia, perinatal asphyxia and birth injuries. The slowest progress in the reduction of neonatal deaths was made with regard to prematurity and sepsis [31, 32]. This implies that with more efforts directed at severe intrapartum events, both stillbirths and early neonatal deaths will be further reduced. With the advent of the Sustainable Development Goals, the 2030 target is to achieve national neonatal mortality rates of 20/1000 live births or fewer. While a hundred countries globally had already met the stated target, 29 countries, which are in the low-income countries category, will have to double their rates of progress in order to meet that target. The national stillbirth rate is also targeted at 12/1000 total births or fewer. This translates into reducing stillbirths from 2.6 million to 1.1 million and this feat requires 56 countries to at least double their rate of progress [33, 34].

4.5 Factors Predisposing to Perinatal Mortality

Perinatal deaths, world over, occur as a result of poor health care during pregnancy, during labour and delivery, and immediately after child birth. Factors contributing to poor maternity and early neonatal care are similar across the globe, although with varying frequencies and relative import. These factors can be classified as follows:

4.5.1 Environmental Factors

Rural or urban slum residence is characterised by poor housing with poor environmental hygiene as a result of poor refuse and sewage disposal and poor supply of safe water. All these factors predispose to infections in pregnancy, which may adversely affect the foetus in utero or the baby soon after birth. Getting prompt and adequate health care in rural or urban slum settings may also be impaired by poor transportation (caused by bad roads or difficult water ways), lack of electricity and water supply, lack of facilities for emergency obstetric and neonatal care, as well as personnel with adequate expertise [35]. Other important factors which may predispose to perinatal death include poverty, ignorance, harmful cultural practices and religious beliefs, all of which ultimately affect health care-seeking practices. Poor nutrition also contributes remarkably to morbidities in pregnancy, resulting in perinatal losses [36]. The effect of unfavourable health-related policy reforms has been documented to adversely influence human behaviour, particularly with regard to accessing health care, and this worsens perinatal loss in a developing economy [26].

4.5.2 Biosocial Factors

Extremes of reproductive age (less than 20 and greater than 35 years) are known to be associated with poor perinatal outcomes arising from complications such as hypertensive diseases, malnutrition, malaria and anaemia. These complications may explain the higher frequencies of perinatal loss among women in those age groups [37]. Indeed, the best perinatal outcome is obtained among mothers aged between 20 and 24 years. Similarly, high parity (i.e. greater than four deliveries), elderly primigravida and very young primigravida are at increased risk of pregnancy and labour complications, which, in turn, increase their risk of perinatal mortality [38, 39]. Pregnant women in the lower social classes are most at risk of perinatal deaths compared with the other social classes due to factors such as poverty, ignorance and poor access to helpful health information. The overall effects of these factors include increased risk of poor nutrition, anaemia, infections and poor utilisation of available health resources. Neonatal tetanus is a good example of a leading cause of perinatal mortality in low-income and lower-middle-income countries, which is closely related to low socioeconomic status of families. Tetanus is a major contributor to perinatal deaths in Nigeria and other developing countries [40, 41]. Mothers of newborn infants with tetanus in various parts of Nigeria have been repeatedly shown to be poor with no record of quality prenatal care, lack of adequate immunisation against tetanus during pregnancy and childbirth in unhygienic environments [42–44]. Similarly, mothers who did not register for facility-based prenatal care (unbooked) are more vulnerable to perinatal mortality compared with booked mothers [45]. In addition, both maternal obesity and short stature predispose to perinatal deaths through difficult labour and the various associated mechanical and hypoxic injuries in the baby [46, 47]. Birth weight and intra-uterine growth status also contribute to perinatal deaths. Babies with extremes of abnormal birth weight (low birth weight and macrosomic babies) and extremes of abnormal intra-uterine growth (small for gestational age or large for gestational age babies) have higher risks of complications, which frequently result in perinatal mortality [48].

4.5.3 Obstetric and Gynaecological Factors

Poor utilisation of family planning services, antenatal care services and quality delivery services characterise low- and middle-income countries, where economic indices are poor and fertility rate per woman is high, as shown in Table 4.4.

Previous abortion increases the risk of perinatal death in subsequent pregnancies [49]. Other important obstetric and gynaecological determinants of perinatal death include pregnancy complications, such as antepartum haemorrhage, abnormal labour and assisted deliveries. Assisted deliveries contribute to high perinatal mortality through higher risk of

Table 4.4 Socio-economic and obstetric care indices in different areas of the world

Countries	Total Fertility Rate per woman (2013)	Population living on < $1 per Day (2013)	Population living in urbanised areas (%) (2013)	Unmet need for Family planning (%) (2014)	Contraceptive prevalence (%) (2013)	Antenatal Care coverage – at least 4 visits (%) (2014)	Births attended by skilled personnel (%) (2014)	Births by Caesarean Section (%) (2014)
Africa	4.9	47.0	38	24	28	48	51	4
Americas	2.1	2.7	80	9	74	90	96	38
South East Asia	2.4	23.9	35	13	60	70	68	10
Europe	1.7	<2.0	71	10	68	–	98	25
East Mediterranean	3.1	8.9	51	18	48	48	67	22
West Pacific	1.8	6.4	56	6	80	–	96	25

Adapted from the World Health Statistics 2015 [1]

mechanical injuries to viscera and concealed haemorrhages. Other obstetric and gynaecological disorders predisposing to perinatal mortality include severe maternal or intrauterine infection, malposition, malpresentation and abnormal labour, which predispose to preterm birth and low birth weight with various complications such as perinatal asphyxia, intraventricular haemorrhage, idiopathic respiratory distress, hypothermia, hypoglycaemia, recurrent apnoea and septicaemia [50, 51].

4.6 Causes of Perinatal Mortality

The causes of perinatal mortality may be broadly classified into direct and indirect: the former are mainly medical disorders in the mother, foetus or baby, which may cause foetal or early neonatal death. The indirect causes are biological, cultural, socio-economic and anthropological problems, which enhance the occurrence and effects of the direct causes of perinatal death. The two classes of causes of perinatal deaths are usually interwoven, such that it is difficult in the developing world to ascribe perinatal death to a single factor. Unfortunately, most cases of foetal or neonatal death occur outside the hospital; thus, the exact causes of the foetal death may not be known.

4.6.1 Direct Causes

4.6.1.1 Prolonged Obstructed Labour

This is common in developing countries for reasons such as poor attendance of antenatal care and poor utilisation of quality delivery services [52]. The obstruction to foetal passage frequently follows cephalopelvic disproportion, either from contracted pelvis or a relatively big baby. The strong uterine contractions over a long period of time impair placental functions and cause intrapartum foetal hypoxic-ischaemic injury and perinatal asphyxia.

4.6.1.2 Anaemia and Malnutrition

Malaria, iron and folate deficiency, and haemoglobinopathies are common causes of anaemia and malnutrition in pregnancy. These factors cause placental dysfunction, impair nutrient supply to the foetus and cause restriction of foetal growth, thus predisposing to poor pregnancy outcomes [36]. The leading and synergistic roles of malaria, malnutrition and anaemia in the aetiology of intrauterine growth restriction and preterm delivery are well known [53]. Added to this burden is HIV infection, which further enhances the susceptibility of the placenta to the effects of malaria in pregnancy [54]. In addition, perinatal death from maternal anaemia in pregnancy is associated with foetal anaemia, premature labour, low birth weight and intrapartum hypoxia, causing stillbirth or early neonatal death [55]. Obesity is also becoming a matter of concern in the developing world despite widespread under-nutrition, due to westernisation of life styles and increasing consumption of unhealthy foods. Maternal obesity is associated with higher risk of hypertensive disorders in pregnancy, shoulder dystocia, foetal distress, stillbirth and early neonatal death from severe perinatal asphyxia [47].

4.6.1.3 Hypertensive Diseases of Pregnancy

Pre-eclampsia, eclampsia and pre-gestational essential hypertension are associated with higher rates of perinatal mortality. Eclampsia has been shown to cause more stillbirths than early neonatal deaths in Nigeria [56]. Perinatal death rate increases with the severity of the disease, and inversely with the gestational age at the onset of the disease [57, 58]. High perinatal loss in hypertensive diseases is related to macro-vascular damage, impaired placental blood flow or premature placental separation. These factors cause intrauterine hypoxia, intrauterine growth restriction and preterm delivery [59].

4.6.1.4 Antepartum Haemorrhage

Bleeding in pregnancy predisposes to perinatal death [60] from compromised foetal circulation, anaemia and intrauterine hypoxia. Placental abruption, in particular, causes premature delivery in settings equipped for emergency obstetric practice, or intra-uterine death where such facilities are lacking. Other associated complications of haemorrhage which may contribute to perinatal deaths include congenital malformations (where bleeding occurs early in pregnancy), intra-uterine hypoxia resulting in perinatal asphyxia, neonatal anaemia and early-onset sepsis. The latter conditions may cause perinatal deaths from shock, congestive cardiac failure or multiple organ failure.

4.6.1.5 Diabetes Mellitus in Pregnancy

Sudden and unexplained foetal and early neonatal death occurs in about 30% of pregnancies complicated by diabetes mellitus [61]. However, improved hospital-based care for diabetes in pregnancy has drastically reduced the risk of associated adverse perinatal outcome. Although gestational diabetes increases the risk of preterm delivery [62], the perinatal mortality rate is higher among women with pre-gestational diabetes mellitus, especially when it is poorly controlled, compared with the gestational type [63]. In addition to the known co-existence of diabetes in pregnancy and hypertensive disorders [64], the common complications of diabetes mellitus in pregnancy which contribute to perinatal death include hydramnios, hydrops fetalis, congenital malformations, particularly of the intestine and heart, foetal macrosomia, intrauterine growth restriction and preterm birth with respiratory distress syndrome. Perinatal asphyxia and other forms of birth injury may be caused by difficulty delivery as a result of foetal macrosomia. However, foetal macrosomia is not universal in diabetes during pregnancy, as foetal size depends on the degree of glycaemic control and integrity of utero-placental circulation. With poor glycaemic control of diabetes in pregnancy, microvascular damage results in poor placental blood flow and secondary intrauterine growth restriction. Both macrosomia and small-for-gestational age predispose to intrapartum stillbirth, and increased risk of early neonatal death from the complications of asphyxia.

4.6.1.6 Birth Trauma

Birth trauma contributes remarkably to perinatal loss, as factors predisposing babies to birth trauma such as macrosomia, cephalopelvic disproportion, shoulder dystocia, prolonged or difficult labour, precipitous delivery, abnormal presentations and instrumental delivery are frequent obstetric occurrences in parts of the developing world [65]. Soft tissue injuries are more frequently associated with perinatal deaths compared to bony or neuronal injuries. Soft tissue injuries such as intraventricular, cephalohaematoma, subgaleal haemorrhage and visceral rupture, particularly adrenal gland rupture, may also cause life-threatening complications.

4.6.1.7 Infections

Apart from causing systemic inflammatory response, which may be harmful to the mother and the foetus through circulatory failure and multi-organ failure, systemic bacterial sepsis in pregnancy may cause perinatal death through anaemia and intra-uterine hypoxia. Localised infections in the gastrointestinal and genitourinary tract are also known to precipitate preterm delivery [66]. Prolonged rupture of foetal membranes or preterm premature rupture of membranes cause ascending intra-uterine infections, which predispose to perinatal deaths [67]. Intra-uterine infection with TORCHES organisms (Rubella, Toxoplasma gondi, Treponema pallidum, Herpes simplex and Epstein-Barr virus) are common in the developing world due to poor hygiene and poverty. These organisms are capable of causing perinatal deaths through severe congenital malformations, intrauterine growth restriction and preterm delivery. Perinatal HIV infection is important because it causes embryopathy and congenital malformations, with remarkably higher risk of perinatal mortality from intrauterine growth restriction and preterm delivery. Pregnant women who are sero-positive for HIV have been shown to be more likely to have preterm delivery, low-birth-weight babies, intrauterine growth restriction and perinatal mortality [68].

4.6.1.8 Prematurity

Perinatal death is jointly influenced by birth weight and gestational age. Perinatal mortality has an inverse relationship with gestational age and birth weight. Indeed, perinatal mortality increases in very preterm (less than 34 weeks) and very-low-birth-weight babies (less than 1500 g). Preterm delivery has been shown to be the leading single cause of perinatal deaths in the developing world, with contribution as high as 40% in India [69]. These babies are most at risk of severe conditions such as asphyxia, respiratory distress syndrome, septicaemia, hyperbilirubinaemia, hypothermia, hypoglycaemia, intraventricular haemorrhage, apnoea, anaemia, congenital cardiac malformations and serious gastrointestinal disorders such as necrotising enterocolitis [48, 50, 51]. These complications often require highly specialised expertise, huge infrastructural support and intensive care facilities, which are almost non-existent in the parts of the world where the incidence of preterm birth is paradoxically high. Therefore, preterm birth is associated with a high rate of perinatal death in the developing countries.

4.6.1.9 Intrauterine Growth Restriction

Intrauterine growth restriction is an important cause of perinatal mortality [6, 70]. Many maternal diseases in pregnancy which affect the utero-placental circulation cause intrauterine growth restriction. Other causes include specific intrinsic foetal disorders such as chromosomal anomalies, particularly the trisomies. High perinatal loss associated with IUGR is usually due to intrapartum asphyxia, hypoglycaemia, hypothermia, hyperviscosity syndrome from polycythaemia, hyperbilirubinaemia and congenital malformations, particularly, of the heart.

4.6.1.10 Malpresentation

Breech presentation is the commonest abnormal presentation and, like others such as shoulder, face, brow, transverse and cord presentation, accounts for high perinatal loss. Malpresentation may be a cause of prolonged or obstructed labour with a significant risk of intrapartum hypoxia, asphyxia and mechanical birth injuries. Inappropriate mode of delivery may contribute to high perinatal loss associated with malpresentation. This is because babies with abnormal presentations are usually risky to deliver, and experienced and well-trained obstetricians are required. The lack of the required equipment, and scarcity of highly skilled specialists, increase perinatal mortality in babies with malpresentation.

4.6.1.11 Perinatal Asphyxia

Most cases of stillbirth are caused by severe intrapartum events. Foetal loss in labour usually occurs as a result of intrapartum hypoxia due to sudden oxygen deprivation to the foetus, usually from severe compromise of the utero-placental circuit. Therefore, complications of pregnancy and labour such as hypoxic maternal conditions, post-maturity, intrapartum bleeding from placenta praevia, prolonged obstructed labour and malpresentation, particularly breech delivery, which are associated with intrapartum hypoxia, cause foetal death, and consequently, increased perinatal mortality.

Undue stress of labour associated with trial of labour or abnormal uterine action, and difficult assisted delivery, may be associated with stillbirth. In early neonatal life, the effects of perinatal asphyxia, which increase the chances of perinatal death, include hypoxic-ischaemic encephalopathy, apnoea, intracranial haemorrhage, pulmonary haemorrhage, cardiac failure, consumptive coagulopathy, hypothermia and hypoglycaemia [71].

4.6.1.12 Post Maturity

Perinatal loss in pregnancies prolonged beyond 42 weeks is three times higher than in pregnancies ending between 38 and 42 weeks. The decline in placental function, in some cases of macrosomic foetus, coupled with the stress of labour, makes post-term foetuses more susceptible to perinatal death.

4.6.2 Indirect Causes

Studies have shown that low socio-economic status is associated with increased risk of poor perinatal outcome [72]. Some of the reasons why the poor tend to have poorer pregnancy outcomes include poor access to health services, either in terms of physical location and transportation difficulties or in terms of cost, in the absence of social supports. Other factors include ignorance from poor access to helpful health information, poor feeding, poor hygiene, higher likelihood of pregnancy complications bordering on the state of maternal health and poor health care-seeking behaviours [73]. In the developing countries where adult literacy level averages 60% [1], it is commonplace for pregnant women to decline operative deliveries in the face of complicated labour. The rates of caesarean delivery in different parts of the world are depicted in Table 4.4, and the poor parts of the world (Africa and South East Asia) have the lowest rates of caesarean delivery compared to the more advanced countries. Studies in Nigeria have also shown the poor acceptability of caesarean section by pregnant women across various parts of the country [74–76]. The poor acceptability of caesarean section cannot be separated from low maternal education and sociocultural disapproval by the family. The poor acceptability of caesarean section has implications for perinatal survival.

The socio-economic status of the inhabitants of any country influences perinatal mortality. For instance, perinatal mortality is seven times higher amongst the low socioeconomic group in India than in the higher social class [77]. Malnutrition and poverty serve as major factors predisposing to poor perinatal outcome. Maternal malnutrition may arise from poverty, or from food insecurity in the form of drought and famine during natural disasters, or occurring in situations of war, civil strife, displacement and refuge, all of which are common in low-income and lower-middle-income countries compared to upper middle- and high-income countries. Poor maternal nutrition impairs foetal nutrition, retards intrauterine growth and causes low birth weight. It also worsens the depressed immunity of pregnancy, thus, predisposing to infections, which may either precipitate preterm delivery or cause foetal death. Chronic malnutrition, especially in the form of hypovitaminosis D, predisposes to maternal short stature, deformed pelvic bones and contracted pelvis, which will ultimately predispose to obstructed labour. Inequity in the distribution of health resources in the poor parts of the world contributes to the burden of high perinatal mortality in such places. Compared to urban areas, rural areas where the larger proportion of the population reside, usually lack personnel and equipment required to manage emergency obstetric services. Due to poor planning and inefficient health policies, most skilled personnel are located in urban areas, particularly in the secondary and tertiary levels of care, where they are less needed. This pattern of distribution further reduces the chances of survival of a large number of babies delivered in rural and less developed areas.

Appropriate health care-seeking behaviour is strongly influenced by socio-economic and cultural factors, culminating in delays in receiving appropriate care. Prominent among these factors is the patriarchal family system in most parts of Africa and Asia, by which the power to take decisions on when to seek care, where to seek care and what type of care to seek rests squarely on the male head of the family [78]. Therefore, the pregnant woman is deprived of the right to take decisions concerning her health and the pregnancy. The decision of the family head on when to seek medical help may be inappropriate, or may come too late, thus predisposing to poor perinatal outcomes. Even when the decision to seek appropriate obstetric care is eventually taken, there may be other confounding challenges such as transportation difficulties and lack of funds to contend with. These factors further worsen the delay in seeking quality care, and increase the risk of perinatal death. In addition, certain cultures in some developing countries permit teenage pregnancy, and make facility-delivery culturally unattractive for primigravida women. Teenage girls, who are immature in height and pelvic size, are exposed to complications of pregnancy and delivery with an overall increase in perinatal loss [37]. Other non-specific variables indirectly contributing to perinatal deaths include extremes of maternal age (<18 years and >35 years), high parity, multiple gestation and poor utilisation of antenatal care services. Women aged 35 years or more have been shown to have higher risk of perinatal mortality from obstructed labour compared to those aged 20 to 34 years [79]. Similarly, expectant mothers who did not receive antenatal care have been shown to be at higher risk of preterm birth, small-for-gestational babies and perinatal mortality, compared with mothers who were booked for antenatal care [45]. In addition, birth interval between 18 and 23 months is associated with the lowest risk of adverse perinatal outcome [79]. Female genital mutilation is a strong cultural practice in most parts of the developing world. This practice increases the risk of obstructed labour due to the restrictive effect of the scarred vulva, and also predisposes to perinatal loss in poor settings in the absence of highly skilled obstetric care. High perinatal mortality is associated with multiple gestations as a result of higher likelihood of preterm delivery and low birth weight in the babies. The second twin has been shown to be more susceptible to severe intrapartum events and mortality, possibly from partial placental separation and cord accidents following the delivery of the first twin [80]. Therefore, efforts must be made to identify these indirect causes of perinatal loss during antenatal care, and the delivery must be supervised to minimise perinatal losses.

4.7 Prevention

4.7.1 Primary Prevention

The general population in the low- and middle-income countries needs to be educated about the burden of perinatal deaths and the methods available to tackle the problem. This intervention should be community based and client focused, using mass media methods of health campaigns. This intervention is meant to improve the utilisation of the available health services, improve health during pregnancy and childbirth, accept life-saving delivery methods including caesarean section and stop harmful cultural practices, and to enhance maternal and neonatal outcomes of pregnancies. Such a community approach to perinatal health has been shown to reduce maternal morbidity, neonatal mortality, stillbirth rate and perinatal mortality, and to increase referrals to health facilities [81]. Similarly, educational interventions have been shown to improve child care practices in Tanzania [82]. Family planning and birth control interventions are helpful with adequate child spacing, enhanced maternal health, better family preparedness for pregnancy and child birth, and better pregnancy outcomes. This requires outreach programmes on maternal and child health that will incorporate family planning services as suggested [83]. Family planning services should be targeted at teenagers, the elderly, the excessively multiparous and those with short birth intervals, who are most at risk of poor perinatal outcome [84]. Nutritional interventions should start very early in childhood through adolescence, without sex discrimination, in order to prevent short maternal stature and small-for-gestational age babies, and to improve perinatal survival. Improved personal and environmental hygiene practices, both at home and in health facilities, are essential in the prevention of infections and infestations which may threaten perinatal survival [85]. The practice of clean birthing would reduce the risk of early-onset sepsis, which is a major contributor to perinatal mortality in the developing world.

The combination of poverty, ignorance and harmful cultural practices represents a major risk factor for perinatal mortality. Therefore, educational qualification, social status and the financial empowerment of mothers should be enhanced to improve their health status and to reduce the risk of perinatal mortality. Specially packaged interventions to improve perinatal survival should be targeted at the socially disadvantaged parts of the community, using good road networks, and affordable and safe means of transportation.

Furthermore, in order to effectively reduce perinatal mortality, efforts should be concentrated on three levels of participants. The first level is the health team, whose members must receive adequate training relevant to the health needs of the community, and be trained to deliver health education interventions. An additional task of collecting data and disseminating information on perinatal deaths should be routinely performed by the health team. Second, the government agencies and health policy makers must formulate appropriate policies to allow and encourage universal formal education. Finally, the community must be mobilised and sensitised to use quality and safe health services, invest in their own health, and raise resources to facilitate safe pregnancy and childbirth.

4.7.2 Secondary Prevention

Secondary prevention involves the prevention of perinatal loss through the establishment of properly organised and efficient antenatal care services. The early identification of high-risk pregnancies through an effective screening system and timely community-to-facility referral or inter-facility referral is essential. A major step towards the secondary prevention of perinatal deaths is the provision of skilled health workers to serve hard-to-reach areas where poverty, ignorance and social disadvantage make accessibility of quality maternity services difficult. Community health workers have been shown to have roles in providing pregnancy and childbirth care, mobilising communities to embrace life-saving interventions for care during labour and delivery, and changing some of the long-standing harmful practices on newborn care, especially for poor families [86, 87]. Successful actualisation of these roles requires innovative community based strategies and health system strengthening. The Midwives Service Scheme was introduced by the Nigerian government to increase accessibility to quality and safe obstetric care in the rural and socially disadvantaged parts of the country [88]. This scheme addresses the twin problem of inequity in the distribution of health resources, and poor obstetric and perinatal outcomes [89]. In addition, efforts should be made to engage traditional birth attendants in frequent training programmes, preferably, with incentives attached. The training of this group of care providers on safe clean delivery and newborn resuscitation has been shown to reduce neonatal mortality by almost half, though more efforts are required with respect to stillbirth and perinatal death rates [90]. With the introduction of the Focused Antenatal Care system, emphasis includes Birth Preparedness and Complications Readiness (BP/CP). This entails important decision-making before the onset of labour. The components include the identification of danger signs in pregnancy, identifying a health worker to attend labour and take safe decisions, saving money in preparation for delivery, arranging transport system in case referral becomes inevitable, and obtaining the support of the family and relations ahead of confinement [91]. Where home delivery is preferred, this can be planned ahead with the appropriate arrangements for prompt referral in case of emergencies. Efforts should be made to ensure that every delivery is supervised and attended by people skilled in basic live-saving skills, including neonatal resuscitation. It is desirable that every health worker should be skilled in neonatal resuscitation, particularly with bag and mask ventilation. This would reduce the number of babies lost to intrapartum hypoxia through stillbirth or early neonatal death. In Nigeria, some professional bodies now organise neonatal resuscitation training programme for nurse-midwives and physicians on a national scale and Help the Baby Breathe training programmes at the lower tiers of healthcare [92]. These efforts have been shown to be helpful and should be entrenched in national health policy.

For pregnancies at risk of preterm delivery, the current emphasis is on the prevention of preterm labour, and improved quality care for prematurely delivered babies. Tocolysis using magnesium sulphate is recommended by the WHO for prolonging pregnancies and protecting the immature foetal brain [93]. It has the advantage of reducing the risk of cerebral palsy among infants delivered preterm [94]. The other components of the management of preterm labour as recommended by the WHO include the use of antenatal corticosteroid therapy to improve lung maturity of the foetus and prevent idiopathic respiratory distress syndrome, as well as erythromycin therapy for foetuses at risk of sepsis [93]. Antenatal corticosteroids therapy is most useful when administered within 7 days of preterm delivery [95]. Other important components of care for the preterm infant, which have been found to reduce mortality by half among babies weighing less than 2 kg, include rapid and effective resuscitation, thermoregulation using the Kangaroo Mother Care Technique and feeding supports [96]. These measures cannot be separated from *Essential Newborn Care*, which is a key component of Every Newborn Action Plan. The plan includes the strategies of care at birth (to prevent intrapartum hypoxia), and care of small and sick newborn babies (to prevent deaths from prematurity, infections, jaundice) [97]. The focus of *Essential Newborn Care* includes basic preventive newborn care (support to breathe at birth, clean delivery, temperature maintenance, immediate exclusive breastfeeding, and eye and cord care), early detection of danger signs in the newborn, and treatment of key morbidities in early neonatal life, with emphasis on sepsis and asphyxia [98].

4.7.3 Tertiary Prevention

Cardiopulmonary supports are crucial to the survival of preterm and other critically ill babies. The facilities required for mechanical ventilation, including exogenous or synthetic surfactant, are usually expensive and may not be affordable for poor families. This strongly calls for the establishment of a special government funding system for such specialised care, at least on a regional basis, with an efficient referral system attached to it. In addition, community-based health insurance systems, which would subsidise the cost of specialised care like neonatal intensive care, may also be instituted to alleviate the cost of care of high-risk infants, to encourage presentation at well-equipped facilities for the desired care, and to minimise perinatal deaths.

The WHO estimated that 1.1 million stillbirths could be prevented using interventions such as comprehensive emergency obstetric and neonatal care, syphilis detection and treatment, detection and management of hypertension during pregnancy, detection and management of foetal growth restriction, identification and induction for mothers >41 weeks gestation, malaria prevention, including treated bed-nets and intermittent preventive treatment for malaria in pregnancy, folic acid fortification before conception, and detection and management of diabetes in pregnancy [6].

One of the major challenges in planning the reduction of stillbirths is inadequate data from the poor registration of births and deaths in low- and middle-income countries [10, 99]. Even in settings where data are available, the use of several classification systems, and multiple definitions of foetal death and stillbirth makes the comparison of the available data with other international datasets challenging. Therefore, international health agencies concerned with obstetric and perinatal health need to agree on a harmonised system of definitions and classifications, possibly including investigations such as post-mortem examinations and histologic studies [99]. In addition, the existing health systems need to be strengthened for more efficient delivery of perinatal services using the deployment of highly skilled personnel and task-shifting in hard-to-reach areas. Community-to-facility referral should be strengthened to save many foetuses with intrapartum hypoxia. Clinical genetics and paediatric surgical services should be made available to supplement obstetric and neonatal care services, particularly for babies with congenital malformations. This networking between specialties should be supported in ways that babies with congenital malformations may still be helped to survive with good quality of life.

4.8 Conclusion

The bulk of perinatal deaths occur in the poorer parts of the world – the low- and middle-income countries. Early neonatal deaths also form about a quarter of under-five deaths and most cases occur in the perinatal period. These facts reflect the relationship between economic realities and access to good health and development. Therefore, global attention is shifting towards addressing these health-related socio-economic inadequacies. Although several evidence-based interventions and action plans are coming up to strengthen the existing weak health system in the resource-poor part of the world, and to improve the outcome of pregnancies, reduce stillbirth rates and increase the survival of newborn babies, improved literacy through formal education of women, and women empowerment through better employment and better rights of decision-making, are also essential. With improved education, the standard of living will equally improve and so will the access to health services. Government policies should aim at improved funding of health services through participatory local health insurance schemes. More importantly, interventions which had caused a sharp decline in perinatal mortality rates in high-income countries should be replicated in low- and middle-income countries.

References

1. WHO. World Health Statistics 2015. World Health Organization; 2015.
2. WHO. Neonatal and perinatal mortality: Country, Regional and Global Estimates. World Health Organization; 2006.
3. WHO. The World Health Report 2005: make every mother and child count. Geneva: World Health Organization; 2005.
4. WHO. Media Centre. Children: reducing mortality. Fact sheet. Updated January 2016.
5. Wikipedia. Perinatal mortality. Available at https://en.m.wikipedia.org/wiki/Perinatal_mortality.
6. WHO. 2.6 million babies stillborn in 2009. WHO News release 2011. Available at http://www.who.int/mediacentre/news/release/2011/stillbirths_20110414/en/.
7. UNICEF. State of the World's Children 2015.
8. Liu L, Johnson HL, Cousens S, Perin J, Scott S, Lawn JE, Rudan I, Campbell H, et al. Global, regional and national causes of child mortality: an updated systematic analysis for 2010 with time trends since 2000. Lancet. 2012;379(9832):151–61.
9. Lawn JE, Kerber K, Enweronu-Laryea C, Cousens S. 3.6 million neonatal deaths – What is progressing and what is not? Semin Perinatol. 2010;34(6):371–86.
10. Barfield WD. Committee on Foetus and Newborn. Clinical reports – Standard Terminology for fetal, infant and perinatal deaths. Pediatrics. 2011;128(1):177–81.
11. Blencowe H, Cousens S, Jassir FB, Say L, Chou D, Mathers C, Hogan D, et al. National, regional and worldwide estimates of Stillbirth Rate in 2015, with trends from 2000: a systematic review. Lancet Glob Health. 2016;4:e98–108.
12. WHO. Perinatal mortality: country, regional and global estimates. World Health Organization 2007.
13. Adeleye JA. A two-year study of caesarean section and perinatal mortality at the University College Hospital, Ibadan, Nigeria. East Afr Med J. 1982;59(6):383–9.
14. Njokanma OF, Sule-Odu OA, Akesode FA. Perinatal mortality at the Ogun State University Teaching Hospital, Sagamu, Nigeria. J Trop Paediatr. 1994;40:78–81.
15. Kuti O, Orji EO, Ogunlola IO. Analysis of perinatal mortality in a Nigerian Teaching Hospital. J Obst Gynaecol. 2003;23(5):512–4.
16. Adimora GN, Odetunde IO. Perinatal mortality in University of Nigeria Teaching Hospital (UNTH), Enugu at the end of the last millennium. Niger J Clin Pract. 2007;10(1):19–23.
17. Ekure EN, Ezeaka VC, Iroha E, Egri-Okwaji MTC. Prospective audit of perinatal mortality among inborn babies in a tertiary health centre in Lagos, Nigeria. Niger J Clin Pract. 2011;14(1):88–94.

18. Ibekwe P, Ugboma H, Onyire N, Muoneke U. perinatal mortality in southern Nigeria: less than half a decade to the MDG. Ann Med Health Sci Res. 2011;1(2):215–22.
19. Fawole AO, Shah A, Tongo O, Dara K, El-Ladan AM, Umezulike AU, et al. determinants of perinatal mortality in Nigeria. Int J Gynecol Obstet. 2011;114(1):37–42.
20. Suleiman BM, Mokuolu OA, Adesiyun OO. Pattern of perinatal mortality in babies delivered at the University of Ilorin Teaching Hospital, Ilorin, Nigeria. West Afr J Med. 2012;31(2):102–8.
21. Mairami AB, Audu LI, Aikhionbare HA. Risk factors for perinatal deaths in Abuja, Nigeria. Peak J Med Med Res. 2014;2(3): 23–32.
22. Suleiman MB, Mokuolu OA. Perinatal mortality in a Northwestern Nigerian City: a wake-up call. Front Pediatr. 2014;2:105.
23. Igberase GO. Perinatal mortality in a rural referral hospital in the Niger Delta, Nigeria. Afr J Med Health Sci. 2014;13(1):47–50.
24. Chalumeau M, Salanave B, Bouvier-Colle MH, de Bernis L, Prua A, Breart G. Risk factors for perinatal mortality in West Africa: a population-based study of 20326 pregnancies. Acta Paediatr. 2000;89(9):1115–21.
25. Weiner R, Ronsmans C, Dorman E, Jilo H, Muhoro A, Shulman C. Labour complications remains the most important risk factors for perinatal mortality in rural Kenya. Bull World Health Org. 2003;81(7):1–6.
26. Owa JA, Osinaike AI, Makinde O. Trends in utilisation of obstetric care at Wesley Guild Hospital, Ilesa, Nigeria. Effects of a depressed economy. Trop Geogr Med. 1995;47(2):86–8.
27. Ekure EN, Iroha EO, Egri-Okwaji MTC, Ogedengbe OK. Perinatal mortality at the close of the 20th century in Lagos University Teaching Hospital. Niger J Paediatr. 2004;31(1):14–8.
28. Richardus JH, Graafmans WC, Verloove-Vanhorick SP, Mackenbach JP. The perinatal mortality rate as an indicator of quality of care in international comparisons. Med Care. 1998;36(1):54.
29. UNICEF. Levels and trends in child mortality report. UNICEF, 2010.
30. WHO. Sexual and reproductive health. The Neglected tragedy of stillbirths. World Health Organization. Available at http://www.who.int/reproductivehealth/topics/maternal_perinatal/stillbirth/en/.
31. Lawn J. Millennium Development Goals to Sustainable Development Goals: What next for women and children health? Available at www.imperial.ac.uk/media/imperial-college/centre-for-international-child-health/public/Joy_CICH_Jan2016-keynote.pdf Accessed on 22 Dec 2018.
32. Liu L, Oza S, Hogan D, Perin J, Rudan I, Lawn J, et al. Global, regional and national causes of child mortality in 2000-2013 with projections to inform post-2015 priorities: an updated systematic analysis. Lancet. 2015;385(9966):430–40.
33. De Bernis L, Kinney MV, Stones W, Hoope-Bender P, Vivio D, Leishner SH. Stillbirths: ending preventable deaths by 2030. Lancet. 2016;387(10019):703–16.
34. WHO/UNICEF. Every newborn action plan. 2014.
35. Harrison KA, Briggs ND, Oruamabo RS. Technology free obstetrics. Letter to Editor. Lancet. 1991;358:383.
36. Abu-Saad K, Fraser D. Maternal nutrition and birth outcomes. Epidemiol Rev. 2010;32(1):5–25.
37. Ogunlesi TA, Ayeni VA, Jagun OE, Ogunfowora OB. Socio-clinical factors related to the perinatal outcome of teenage pregnancies in a Nigerian Teaching Hospital. Niger J Paediatr. 2013;40(3): 290–4.
38. Kwast BE. Reduction of maternal and perinatal mortality in rural and pre-urban settings. What works? Eur J Obst Gynaecol Reprod Biol. 1996;69(1):47–53.
39. Adedoyin MA, Adetoro OO. Pregnancy and its outcome among teenage mothers in Ilorin. Nigeria East Afr Med J. 1989;66(7): 448–52.
40. Oruamabo RS. Neonatal tetanus in Nigeria: does it still pose a major threat to neonatal survival? Arch Dis Child. 2007;92(1):9–10.
41. Ibinda F, Bauni E, Kariuki SM, Fegan G, Lewa J, Mwikamba M, Boga M, et al. incidence and risk factors for neonatal tetanus in admission to Kilifi County Hospital, Kenya. PLoS One. 2015;10(4):e0122606.
42. Ogunlesi TA, Okeniyi JAO, Owa JA, Oyedeji GA. Neonatal tetanus at the close of the 20th century in Ilesa, Nigeria. Trop Doct. 2007;37:165–7.
43. Fetuga MB, Ogunlesi TA, Adekanmbi AF, Runsewe-Abiodun TI, Ogunfowora OB. Neonatal Tetanus in Sagamu, Nigeria during the Expanded Programme on Immunisation and National Programme on Immunisation eras: a comparative analysis. Int J Pediatr Neonatol. 2010;12:1. Available at http://www.ispub.com/ijpn/.
44. Alhaji MA, Bello MA, Elechi HA, Akuhwa RT, Bukar FL, Ibrahim HA. A review of neonatal tetanus in University of Maiduguri Teaching Hospital, Northeastern Nigeria. Niger Med J. 2013;54(6):398–401.
45. Owolabi AT, Fatusi AO, Kuti O, Adeyemi A, Faturoti SO, Obianjunwa PO. Maternal complications and perinatal outcomes in booked and unbooked Nigerian mothers. Singap Med J. 2008;49(7):526.
46. Ozumba BC, Ucheagbu H. Incidence and management of obstructed labour in eastern Nigeria. Aust New Zealand J Obst Gynaecol. 1991;31(3):213–6.
47. Cedergren MI. Maternal morbid obesity and the risk of adverse pregnancy outcome. Obstet Gynecol. 2004;103(2):219–24.
48. KhoshnoodShariati M, Karmi Z, Rezaienejad M, Basiri A, Torkestani F, SalehGargari S. Perinatal complications associated with preterm deliveries at 24 to 33 weeks and 6 days gestation (2011-2012): a hospital-based retrospective study. Iran J Reprod Med. 2015;13(11):697–702.
49. Okonofua FE, Onwudiegwu U, Odutayo R. Pregnancy outcome after illegal induced abortion in Nigeria, a retrospective controlled historical study. Afr J Med Med Sci. 1994;23(2):165–9.
50. Ogunlesi TA, Ogunfowora OB. Predictors of mortality in neonatal septicaemia in an under-resourced setting. J Natl Med Assoc. 2010;102(10):915–21.
51. Adegoke SA, Ayoola AO, Bankole KP, Ogunlesi TA. Intravenous haemorrhage in newborns weighing <1500g: Epidemiology and short-term outcome in a resource-poor setting. Ann Trop Med Pub Health. 2014;7(1):48–54.
52. Ali AA, Adam I. Maternal and perinatal outcome of obstructed labour in Kassala Hospital, Sudan. J Obst Gynecol. 2010;30(4): 376–7.
53. Uneke CJ. Impact of placental Plasmodium falciparum malaria on pregnancy and perinatal outcome in sub-Saharan Africa. Yale J Biol Med. 2007;80(2):39–50.
54. Ticconi C, Mapfuno M, Dorrucci M, Naha N, Tarira E, Pietropolli A, Rezza G. Effect of maternal HIV and malaria infection on pregnancy and perinatal outcome in Zimbabwe. J AIDS. 2003;34(3):289–94.
55. Adam I, Babiker S, Mohammed AA, Salih MM, Prins MH, Zaki ZM. Low body mass index, anaemia and poor perinatal outcome in a rural hospital in Eastern Sudan. J Trop Pediatr. 2008;54(3):202–4.
56. Adamu AN, Ekele BA, Ahmed Y, Mohammed BA, Isezuo SA, Abdullahi AA. Pregnancy outcome in women with eclampsia at a tertiary centre in northern Nigeria. Afr J Med Med Sci. 2012;41(2):211–9.
57. Gaugler-Senden IPM, Huijsson AG, Visser W, Stugers EAP, de Groot CJM. Maternal and perinatal outcome of pre-eclampsia with an onset before 24 weeks gestation. Eur J Obstet Gynaecol Reprod Biol. 2006;128(1):216–21.
58. Lisonkova S, Joseph KS. Incidence of pre-eclampsia: risk factors and outcomes associated with early versus late-onset disease. Am J Obstet Gynecol. 2013;209(6):544e1–e12.
59. Njokanma OF, Olanrewaju DM. A study of neonatal deaths at the Ogun State University Teaching Hospital, Sagamu, Nigeria. J Trop Med Hyg. 1995;98(3):155–60.
60. Kalter HD, Khazen RR, Barghouthi M, Odeh M. Prospective community-based cluster census and case-control study of still-

births and neonatal deaths in the West Bank and Gaza Strip. Paediatr Perinat Epidemiol. 2008;22(4):321–33.
61. Maouris P. Reducing perinatal mortality in Vila Central Hospital, Vanuatu. Papau New Guinea Med J. 1994;35(5):495–501.
62. Gashim TI. Gestational diabetes mellitus: maternal and perinatal outcomes in 220 Saudi women. Oman Med J. 2012;27(2):140–4.
63. Abu-Heija AT, Al-Bash M, Mathew M. Gestational and pre-gestational diabetes mellitus in Omani Women: Comparison of obstetric and perinatal outcomes. Sultan Qaboos Univ Med J. 2015;15(4):e496–500.
64. Ozumba BC, Obi SN, Oli JM. Diabetes mellitus in pregnancy in an African population. Int J Gynecol Obstet. 2004;84(2): 114–9.
65. Njokanma OF, Kehinde OA. Mechanical birth trauma – an evaluation of predisposing factors at the Ogun State University Teaching Hospital, Sagamu. Niger J Paediatr. 2002;29:61–5.
66. Ananya D, Subrat P, Ahanthem SS, Sourah GD, BhanuPratap SG. Preterm birth: analysis of risk factors and neonatal outcome. Gynecol Obstet Case Rep. 2015;1:1. Available at www.gynaecology-obstetrics.imedpub.com.
67. Yu H, Wang X, Gao H, You Y, Xing A. Perinatal outcome outcomes of pregnancies complicated by preterm premature rupture of the membranes before 34 weeks of gestation in a tertiary centre in China: a retrospective review. Biosci Trends. 2015;9(1):35–41.
68. Ellis J, Williams H, Graves W, Lindsay MK. Human immunodeficiency virus infection is a risk factor for adverse perinatal outcomes. Am J Obstet Gynaecol. 2002;186(5):903–6.
69. Viswanath K, Ps R, Charkaborty A, Prasad JH, Minz S, George K. A community-based case-control study on determination of perinatal mortality in a tribal population of southern India. Rural Remote Health. 2015;15(3):3388.
70. Simchen MJ, Beiner ME, Strauss-Liviathan N, Dulitzky M, Kuint J, Mashiach S, Schiff E. Neonatal outcome in growth-restricted versus appropriately grown preterm infants. Am J Perinatol. 2000;17(4):187–92.
71. Ogunfowora OB, Ogunlesi TA, Fetuga MB, Oyinlade AO. Clinical manifestations and outcome of hospitalised babies with birth asphyxia in Sagamu. Niger J Paediatr. 2009;35:12–8.
72. Dubay L, Joyce T, Kaestner R, et al. Changes in prenatal care timing and low birth weight by race and socioeconomic status: implications for the Medicaid expansion for pregnant women. Health Serv Res. 2001;36(2):399–403.
73. Kramer MS, Seguin L, Lydon J, et al. Socioeconomic disparities in pregnancy outcome: why do the poor fare so poorly? Paediatr Perinat Epidemiol. 2000;14(3):194–210.
74. Orji EO, Ogunniyi SO, Onwudiegwu U. Beliefs and perceptions of pregnant women at Ilesha about Caesarean section. Trop J Obstet Gynaecol. 2003;20:141–3.
75. Sunday-Adeoye I, Kalu CA. Pregnant Nigerian women's view of Caesarean section. Niger J Clin Pract. 2011;14(3):276–9.
76. Aziken M, Omo-Aghoja I, Okonofua F. Perceptions and attitudes of pregnant women towards caesarean section in urban Nigeria. Acta Obstet Gynecol. 2007;86(1):42–7.
77. Kwast BE. Building a community based maternal program. Int J Gynaecol Obstet. 1995;48(Suppl 1):567–82.
78. Magoma M, Requejo J, Campbell OM, Cousens S, Filippi V. High ANC coverage and low skilled attendance in a rural Tanzanian district: a case for implementing a birth plan intervention. BMC Pregnancy Childbirth. 2010;10:13.
79. Zhu B-P, Rolfs RT, Nangle BE, Horan JM. Effect of the interval between pregnancy on perinatal outcomes. N Engl J Med. 1999;340:589–94.
80. Armson BA, O'Connell C, Persad V, Joseph KS, Young DC, Baskett T. Determinants of perinatal mortality and serious neonatal morbidity in the second twin. Obstet Gynecol. 2006;108(3):556–64.
81. Lassi ZS, Haider BA, Bhutta ZA. Community-based intervention packages for reducing maternal and neonatal morbidity and mortality and improving neonatal outcomes. Cochrane Database Syst Rev. 2010;11:CD007754.
82. Penfold S, Manzi F, Mkumbo E, Temu S, Jaribu J, Shamba DD, et al. Effect of home-based counselling on newborn care practices in southern Tanzania, one year after implementation: a cluster randomised controlled trial. BMC Pediatr. 2014;14:187.
83. Alan Guttmacher Institute. Facts on investing on family planning and maternal and newborn health. Issues in Brief 2010. Available at www.guttmacher.org.
84. Kozuki N, Katz J, Lee AC, Vogel JP, Silveira MF, Sania A, Stevens GA. Short maternal stature increases the risk of small-for-gestational age and preterm births in low-and middle-income countries; individual participants data meta-analysis and population attributable fraction. J Nutr. 2015;14(11):2542–50.
85. Jehan I, Harris H, Salat S, Zeb A, Mobeen N, Pasha O, et al. Neonatal mortality, risk factors and causes: a prospective population-based cohort study in urban Pakistan. Bull World Health Org. 2009;87:130–8.
86. Darmstadt GL, Lee AC, Cousens S, Sibley L, Bhutta ZA, Donney F, et al. 60 million non-facility births: who can deliver in community settings to reduce intrapartum related deaths? Int J Gynecol Obstet. 2009;107(Suppl 1):S89–S112.
87. Walswa P, Pariyo G, Kallander K, Akuze J, Namazzi G, Ekirapa-Kiracho E, Kerber K, et al. Effect of the Ugandan Newborn Study on care seeking and care practices; a cluster randomised controlled trial. Glob Health Action. 2015;8:24584.
88. National Primary Health Development Agency, Nigeria. Nigerian Midwives Service Scheme. Available at www.who.int/workforcealliance/forum/2011/hrhawardscs26/en/.
89. Enweronu-Larygea C, Dickson KE, Moxon SG, Simen-Kapen A, Nyange C, Niermeyer S, et al. Basic newborn care and neonatal resuscitation: a multi-country analysis of health system bottlenecks and potential solutions. BMC Pregnancy Childbirth. 2015;15 Suppl 2:S4.
90. Sibley LM, Sipe TA, Barry D. Traditional birth attendants training for improving health behaviours and pregnancy outcomes. Cochrane Database Syst Rev. 2012;8:CD005460.
91. JHPIEGO Trainer News. Focused antenatal care: planning and providing care during pregnancy – A Maternal and Neonatal Health Programme Best Practices. 2003.
92. Disu EA, Ferguson IC, Njokanma OF, Anga LA, Solarin AU, Olutekunbi AO, Ekure EU, Ezeaka CV, Esangbedo DO, Ogunlesi TA. National Neonatal Resuscitation Training in Nigeria (2008-2012): a preliminary report. Niger J Clin Pract. 2015;18(1): 102–9.
93. WHO. WHO recommendations on interventions to improve preterm birth outcomes. Geneva; 2015.
94. Magee L, Sawchuck D, Synnes A, von Dadelszen P. SOGC Clinical Practice Guidelines: Magnesium sulphate for fetal neuroprotection. J Obstet Gynaecol Can. 2011;33(5):516–29.
95. Melamed N, Shah J, Soraishan A, Yoon EW, Lee SK, Shah PS, Murphy KE. Association between antenatal corticosteroid administration-to-birth interval and outcomes of preterm neonates. Obstet Gynecol. 2015;125(6):1377–84.
96. Lawn JE, Davidge R, Paul VK, von Xylander S, de Graft JJ, Costello A, et al. Born too soon: care for the preterm baby. Reprod Health. 2013;10(Suppl 1):55.
97. Akseer N, Lawn JE, Keenan W, Koustantopoulous A, Cooper P, Ismail Z, et al. Ending preventable newborn deaths in a generation. Int J Gynaecol Obstet. 2015;131(Suppl 1):S43–8.
98. Narayanan I, Rose M, Cordero D, Faillace S, Sanghvi T. The components of essential newborn care. Basics support for institutionalizing child survival project (BASICS II) for the United States Agency for International Development, 2004.
99. Maeda K. Global statistics of perinatal medicine. J Health Med Informt. 2013;S11:1.

Abortion

5

Friday Okonofua

Learning Objectives

At the conclusion of this chapter, the reader will be able to:

- Differentiate between spontaneous and induced abortion.
- Discuss the aetiology, risk factors and clinical presentation of spontaneous abortion.
- Describe the differential diagnosis, management and prevention of spontaneous abortion.
- Discuss the risk factors, consequences, primary, secondary and tertiary prevention of induced abortion.
- Enumerate the prevalence, management and prevention of induced abortion.
- Discuss the human rights, gender, legal and policy contexts for induced abortion.

5.1 Introduction

Abortion is defined as the voluntary or involuntary loss of a pregnancy before the age of viability. The age of viability of a pregnancy is traditionally set at 28 weeks, but with increasing technology, babies born at much lesser age now have significant chances of survival. Consequently, the World Health Organization now defines abortion as the loss of a pregnancy before 20 weeks of gestation or a foetus weighing less than 500 g. Despite this, the definition of abortion often varies according to the laws of individual countries.

F. Okonofua (✉)
Centre of Excellence in Reproductive Health Innovation, Department of Obstetrics and Gynaecology, University of Benin, Benin City, Nigeria

Women's Health and Action Research Centre, Benin City, Nigeria

University of Medical Sciences, Ondo City, Ondo State, Nigeria

Abortion may be spontaneous or induced. Spontaneous abortion is the involuntary loss of pregnancy when the couple intended to continue the pregnancy to term. By contrast, induced abortion is the deliberate act of termination of a pregnancy, often because it is not wanted, it is mistimed or because it would endanger the woman's physical, psychological or emotional health and social well-being. Both types of abortion have implications for women's reproductive health and are significant causes of maternal morbidity and mortality. In this chapter, we describe the types of abortion, and explain how they can be prevented or managed to improve women's health and social well-being.

5.2 Spontaneous Abortion

Also called 'miscarriage', spontaneous abortion is the natural loss of a pregnancy before 20 weeks. It is the most common early complication of pregnancy and is frequently not recognised by women. Among women who know they are pregnant, spontaneous abortion complicates between 10% and 20% of pregnancies, while it may be as high as 30–50% in women who may not even know they have been pregnant. Repeat spontaneous abortion occurs in about 5% of women. Although there have been limited recent reports and publications on spontaneous abortion, it is evident that the rates do not differ significantly between the different regions of the world. However, we conjecture that regions or individuals at highest risk of congenital malformations may also have higher rates of spontaneous abortion.

5.2.1 Aetiology

With respect to aetiology, spontaneous abortion can be divided into those occurring in the first trimester or those that occur in the second trimester. First trimester spontaneous abortions are most often due to congenital foetal malformations, the most

F. Okonofua et al. (eds.), *Contemporary Obstetrics and Gynecology for Developing Countries*,
https://doi.org/10.1007/978-3-030-75385-6_5

important of which are chromosomal anomalies, especially trisomies, monosomies and triploidies. However, some cases of spontaneous abortion in the second trimester may also be due to congenital malformations of the foetus. Published data [1] indicate that up to 90% of spontaneous abortions occurring within 6 weeks of pregnancy (so-called anembryonic conceptions) are due to abnormal foetal karyotypes, compared to 50% in abortions occurring at 8–11 weeks gestation, with 30% occurring at 16–19 weeks of pregnancy.

The frequencies of congenital malformations as causes of first trimester spontaneous abortion have been categorised as follows:

Autosomal trisomies – 52%
Monosomy X – 19%
Polyploidies/triploidies – 22%
Others – 7%

Trisomy 16 is by far the most common and the most lethal autosomal trisomy. Most of these abnormalities arise de novo, but many may be inherited from parental karyotypic abnormalities, such as balanced translocations. By contrast, most second trimester spontaneous abortions are due to host factor problems – the inability of the host to continue with the pregnancy due to inherent defects. These include the following:

- Acquired or congenital uterine abnormalities, for example, uterine septal defects, uterine leiomyomata, uterine synechiae and cervical incompetence. Cervical incompetence deserves a special mention because of its high prevalence in developing countries. Previous damage to the cervix because of forceful dilatations, difficult deliveries associated with un-repaired tears of the cervix and perhaps congenital defects may result in the laxity of the cervical tissues and its inability to contain a growing pregnancy.
- Acute maternal infections, such as listeria monocytogenes, toxoplasmosis, parvovirus B19, rubella, cytomegalovirus inclusion disease, maternal malaria and herpes simplex.
- Maternal endocrinopathies – including thyroid dysfunction, Cushing's disease, diabetes mellitus and polycystic ovarian disease.

There are also a number of cases of 'unexplained spontaneous abortions' that occur in healthy women without any evidence of chromosomal defects or structural defects in the mothers. Research is ongoing to identify the causes of spontaneous abortion in such circumstances.

5.2.2 Risk Factors for Spontaneous Abortion

Increasing maternal age is known to increase the risk of spontaneous abortion. Recently, increasing paternal age has also been cited to increase the risk of spontaneous abortion in women [2] due mainly to an increased likelihood of chromosomal damage, but there is much limited data on this. Previous experience of spontaneous abortion increases subsequent risk of abortions, with the risk rising to 28% after two abortions, and 43% after three abortions [3], in conceptions occurring with the same partners.

Behavioural risk factors for spontaneous abortion include smoking, alcoholism and the use of illicit drugs. Smoking more than ten sticks of cigarettes increases the likelihood of spontaneous abortion by at least twofold, while the consumption of more than three alcoholic drinks a day also increases the risk. However, the data on smoking and alcohol intake may be confounded by other behaviours as well as the under-reporting of the use of alcohol and cigarettes. Also, the use of illicit drugs may also be under-reported; however, reports indicate that the use of drugs such as cocaine increases the risk of spontaneous abortion in at-risk populations.

Non-steroidal anti-inflammatory drugs taken around the time of implantation may also increase the likelihood of spontaneous abortion mainly due to the possibility that such drugs may interfere with the production of prostaglandins that play crucial functions in the process of implantation. Also, accurate data is lacking, but the intake of caffeine at the time of pregnancy may also interfere with implantation and lead to a higher probability of pregnancy loss.

High fever as a cause of spontaneous abortion has been proposed, with some reporting higher rates of abortion with temperatures of over 37.80 Celsius [4], while others have not reported such increases [5]. However, in countries with a higher prevalence of acute episodes of fever such as malaria fever, more caution needs to be taken.

Other risk factors for spontaneous abortion include prolonged time to pregnancy [6], low levels of folate [7] and maternal obesity [8]. More research is required to specify and quantify the extent to which these risk factors contribute to abortion in various populations of women.

5.2.3 Clinical Presentation

The clinical features of spontaneous abortion include amenorrhea, vaginal bleeding and lower abdominal pain occurring in that order in a woman of reproductive age. The type of bleeding and the occurrence of abdominal pain will, however, depend on the type and stage of evolution of the abortion process. There are at least three clinical types of spontaneous abortion – threatened abortion, inevitable/incomplete abortion/complete abortion and missed abortion.

Threatened abortion is when the abortion process appears to have started, but there is still a chance that the pregnancy would continue. Thus, threatened abortion is characterised by amenorrhea, positive pregnancy test and vaginal bleeding. The bleeding often consists of fresh blood and is usually mild to moderate. Abdominal pain is frequently absent – which means that uterine contractions to expel the foetus have not started. A vaginal examination would show a closed cervical os and a uterine size that is compatible with the gestation age. An ultrasound scan would frequently show a viable foetus or a viable gestational sac with the live embryo or live foetal echoes.

Inevitable abortion, on the other hand, means that the abortion has progressed to a stage beyond which the pregnancy can be salvaged. The main features are amenorrhea, followed by heavy vaginal bleeding and abdominal pain. The presence of abdominal pain suggests that the process of emptying the uterus of the products of conception have started. This process may be incomplete (incomplete abortion), may have been completed (complete spontaneous abortion). Clinical examination often shows the presence of heavy blood or blood clots in the vagina and an open cervical canal that admits the tip of the index finger. More frequently, in incomplete abortion, products of conception could be found in the vagina or the cervical canal, and the uterine size would be much less than the gestational age as determined from the duration of amenorrhea.

Other varieties of inevitable abortion include early loss of the products of conception – when an ultrasound scan after 6 weeks of pregnancy does not show a foetal echo (called blighted ovum) or shows a foetal echo without demonstrable foetal heart (missed abortion). Such pregnancies have no chance of continuing beyond the dates the diagnoses are first made. Also, in cases when drainage of amniotic fluid occurs in women with second-trimester pregnancies, it is safe to assume that such pregnancies cannot continue and would inevitably be expelled.

5.2.4 Differential Diagnosis

The differential diagnosis of spontaneous abortion includes secondary amenorrhea from other causes, bleeding after prolonged anovulation, ectopic pregnancy, gestational trophoblastic disease and cervical/uterine pathology. The diagnosis of spontaneous abortion can often be made by a thorough history and clinical examination. However, a pregnancy test, sometimes made more sensitive by a beta-subunit pregnancy test provides further confirmatory evidence.

The results of recent research from the Glasgow Centre for Reproductive Medicine (first reported in the London Times of July 2, 2017) [9] suggest that the quantification of beta-subunit human chorionic gonadotropin (B-HCG) in early pregnancy can predict the risk of miscarriage. According to the report, when blood concentrations of B-HCG are less than 30 units per litre, there is only a 2% chance that the pregnancy would reach 8 weeks. A level of between 30 and 40 gives a 24% chance; levels of 50–70 give a probability of 52%; while levels above 70% imply a likelihood of 86% that the foetus would survive. Such an approach would be beneficial in women undergoing pregnancy by in vitro fertilisation (IVF) as well as those with history of previous spontaneous abortion.

Following a positive pregnancy test, transvaginal ultrasound should be carried out soon after to confirm the presence of a gestational sac with live embryonic echoes, and to ensure that it is appropriately cited within the uterus. Subsequent ultrasound scans, when compared to the early scan, will confirm the viability and sustenance of the pregnancy. A standard ultrasound scan would show a gestational sac around about 4–5 weeks, with foetal echoes detectable at around 5–6 weeks, while foetal heartbeat could be identified at 6 weeks.

Indications for subsequent ultrasound in the first or second trimester include the presence of mild to moderate bleeding of bright red blood (to exclude threatened abortion) and altered blood that presents as brownish discharge (which might indicate the presence of missed abortion). Additionally, ultrasound is indicated when there is watery discharge, especially at the beginning of the second trimester (which might indicate the presence of cervical incompetence). Severe vaginal bleeding with lower abdominal pain that suggests the presence of incomplete abortion is not an indication for an ultrasound scan. Gentle speculum and digital examination will usually confirm this diagnosis, while the immediate removal of any extruding products of conception will reduce the bleeding.

5.2.5 Management

Threatened abortion is best managed with ‘expectant management’ since it is difficult to predict its natural course. However, women should be counselled to be on bed rest and to avoid sexual intercourse for the time being. Pharmacological agents such as oestrogens and progestogens that have been tried in the past are often not useful, unless there is evidence that progesterone deficiency, for example, may be responsible for this or past episodes. However, there is something to be said for giving folic acid to the patients, although if congenital malformation has already occurred, this may be unhelpful.

A complete abortion needs no further management. However, patients with severe blood loss may require blood transfusion or other blood products. Incomplete abortion (before 13 weeks of pregnancy) requires immediate treatment to reduce or eliminate continuing blood loss. This is now better done with a suction curettage, such as a manual vacuum aspiration (MVA) after intravenous oxytocin rather than with the more traumatic dilatation and curettage (D&C) method. However, for patients that are not bleeding severely at the time of the diagnosis of incomplete abortion, randomised controlled trials have shown that misoprostol is an alternative effective medical treatment. In one study [10], patients were randomised between oral misoprostol (600 μg) or manual vacuum aspiration with success rates of 93.3% and 91.5%, respectively. The complication rate was only 0.9% for misoprostol.

However, in our experience, the treatment of missed abortion in the first trimester – blighted ovum (with or without a foetal pole), and no foetal heart when the foetal pole is present – is trickier. As the gestational membranes tend to be adherent to the uterine wall, they are not easily removed with MVA. A study investigated the use of misoprostol in such cases and also found less successful results [11]. The study used an initial dose of 800 μg of misoprostol inserted vaginally and re-evaluated on day three. When the expulsion had not occurred, another dose of 800 μg of misoprostol was re-inserted vaginally. The results showed complete removal of the conception in 71% of cases on day three after the first insertion, and 84% success rate after the second insertion. The remaining instances of non-success with medical treatment could then be effectively treated with MVA. Thus, we strongly recommend that in cases of missed abortion in the first trimester, medical treatment should be tried first, followed by an ultrasound scan to determine the continued presence or absence of retained products. Any retained products can then be removed with MVA. This systematic approach reduces the risks of bleeding, infection and possible uterine synechiae (Asherman syndrome) after the procedure.

Missed abortion occurring in the second trimester also needs to be handled with care. Such cases are often difficult to manage with MVA – and attempts to use surgical treatment have often been the cause of preventable morbidity and mortality, especially in the hands of inexperienced practitioners. We have shown a 100% success rate using repeated administration of low doses of misoprostol (400 μg initially, followed by 200 μg every 6 h) until the foetus is expelled [12]. The key word in the use of misoprostol for managing the second trimester missed abortion is patience, and for practitioners not to worry about the delay in the expulsion of the foetus. We had sometimes waited for 36 h before the foetus was expelled, whereas in some cases, the foetus was discharged within a few hours (<6 h) of insertion of misoprostol. As long as the foetal membranes are not ruptured, and there are not repeated vaginal examinations, the risk of infection is minimal.

5.2.6 Prevention of Spontaneous Abortion

Spontaneous abortion is difficult to prevent since a majority of cases are due to congenital malformations. However, women with past experiences of spontaneous abortions would need to be counselled to take peri-conceptional folic acid supplements to reduce the chances of a recurrence. Also, modifiable risk factors for spontaneous abortion that need to be attended to include smoking, alcohol, intake of illicit drugs and possibly caffeine intake. Additional risk factors such as existing illnesses such as thyroid disease and diabetes mellitus. would need to be treated before embarking on a planned pregnancy.

5.3 Induced Abortion

Induced abortion occurs in both developed and developing countries. But it is in developing countries, that induced abortion has profound implications for women's health and social development. Induced abortion may be 'safe' or 'unsafe'. The WHO has defined unsafe abortion as 'the termination of a pregnancy by persons lacking the necessary skills, or in an environment lacking minimal medical standards or both'. By contrast, safe abortion refers to abortion done by persons with the necessary skills in an environment where appropriate medical standards are met. Indeed, the WHO has developed standards and guidelines for safe abortion practices within national health systems [13]. Unsafe abortion carries a massive burden of immediate and long-term complications for women's reproductive health. The WHO and several international meetings and treaties recommend the adoption of safe abortion practices as a human right imperative needed to protect the life and social well-being of women.

5.3.1 Prevalence

The Guttmacher Institute estimates that about 73.3 million cases of induced abortion were recorded worldwide between 2015 and 2019 [14]. This was an increase from the 50 million cases recorded between 1990 and 1994. Although there appears to be an increase in the absolute number of abortions, due to increasing population growth, the actual abortion incidence rate declined from 40 per 1000 women in 1990–1994 to 35 per 1000 in 2010–2014 and increased to 39.0 per 1000 in 2015–2019. However, abortion numbers increased significantly in developing countries, especially in Africa and Latin America/the Caribbean during the period; the increase was not significant in Asia, while it decreased significantly overall in developed countries. Similarly, although high abortion rates occurred in Africa and Latin America/Caribbean, the increases were not statistically significant. By contrast, significant decreases in abortion rates occurred in developed countries overall, and in Europe and North America during the periods.

Of the total numbers of induced abortion worldwide, up to 49% are unsafe, occurring in countries with restrictive abortion laws and where physical and social hindrances to abortion exist. Up to 98% of all unsafe abortions occur in developing (low and middle income) countries, while only 2% occur in developed (high-income) countries. Put differently, up to 75% of all induced abortions performed in developing countries are categorised as unsafe. Thus, the burden of unsafe abortion with its consequences for harmful effects on women is located mostly in developing countries.

Comparing the world regions, up to 97% of induced abortions in Africa are unsafe, compared to 95% in Latin America, 40% in Asia and 13% in Eastern Europe. By contrast, only about 0.5% of all induced abortions in developed countries are classified as unsafe. Estimates of the trends, numbers and rates of abortion have also been calculated for different countries and regions. In Nigeria, with a restrictive abortion law, nearly all cases of induced abortion are unsafe. The estimated numbers of induced abortion increased from 610,000 abortions/year in 1998/1999 [15, 16] to 760,000 abortions/year in 2006 [17], to an estimated 1.2 million induced abortions in 2015 [18]. These increases may be due to the increasing population in the country but may also be due to an absolute increase in the numbers of abortion [19]. The abortion rate in Nigeria remains high at 40/1000 [18], one of the highest in the developing world. However, it is possible that the abortion estimates in the country are under-estimates of the true rates. When women attending antenatal clinics in Benin City, Nigeria were interviewed about their experiences of induced abortion as part of clinical care, up to 70% reported that they had induced abortion previously, with many reporting repeat episodes of abortion [20]. Thus, more research using innovative and value-free methods are needed to estimate the actual rates of abortion, especially in countries where abortion is not discussed openly because of social and legal restrictions.

5.3.2 Legal and Policy Context

It is clear that official policies and laws determine the extent to which abortion may be safe or unsafe and accounts for its impact on women. Marge Berer concluded from a recently detailed review [21] that 'abortion can only be safe for women if it is available on the woman's request and is universally affordable and accessible'. Sadly, this is not the case in many parts of the world. Available data indicate that up to 68 countries prohibit abortion entirely or permit it only to save a woman's life; 60 countries allow a woman to decide whether or not to terminate a pregnancy; while 57 countries permit abortion to protect a woman's life or health [22]. By contrast, 14 countries permit abortion for socio-economic motives.

Overall, nearly 39% of the world's population lives in countries with highly restrictive abortion laws [23]. Only 19% of developing countries allow abortion based on social or economic circumstances, many of which are in the more developed regions of the world. Sub-Saharan Africa has some of the most draconian abortion laws in the world. However, a ray of hope has recently arisen, indicating that many African countries are showing more dispassionate attitudes abortion laws and policy. South Africa made abortion liberal in the early 1990s, with positive results for women's health and social well-being. Some other African countries with increasingly liberal abortion laws include Tunisia, Ghana, Uganda, Mozambique and Ethiopia. However, despite the liberal laws, many women still do not have access to safe abortion practices as a result of existing cultural norms that stigmatise the use of abortion, and also because of poorly organised services. It is hoped that with increasing liberalisation, appropriate health systems will be put in place to improve women's access to safe abortion to reduce the negative impact of unsafe abortion on women's reproductive health.

One reason often put forward by those opposed to abortion reform is that it will increase the use of abortion in countries where abortion is liberal. However, this has not to be borne out to be available evidence, as the WHO has demonstrated a negative correlation between abortion liberalisation and the incidence of abortion [24].

With increasing liberalisation, available evidence suggests that abortion incidence and abortion rates would decline [25]. This is because the countries that liberalise are also more likely to put in place mechanisms to prevent unwanted pregnancies and to counsel women effectively to avoid repeat abortions. By contrast, countries with restrictive abortion laws also restrict access to family planning services, and indeed, some prevent the universal adoption of comprehensive sexuality education.

An example is the Netherlands, which has one of the most liberal abortion laws in the world. The abortion rate in the Netherlands is only 5 per 1000, with a contraceptive prevalence rate exceeding 80%. In contrast, Nigeria, with a restrictive abortion law, has an abortion rate of 40 per 1000 and a contraceptive prevalence rate of only 10%.

5.3.3 Risk Factors

Induced abortion frequently occurs because the resulting pregnancies are mistimed or unwanted. Estimates indicate that about 121 million unintended pregnancies occur annually in developing countries (64 unintended pregnancies per 1000 women), out of which 73.3 million end up in induced abortion. Thus, failure to use contraceptives when women are sexually active and at risk of a pregnancy at an inappropriate time in their lives is the essential reason for induced abortion. The appropriateness of the timing of pregnancy is best left in the hands of women because they are the end-incubators of such pregnancies and are better able to determine the effects of the pregnancies on their life, health and social well-being. This concept of the right to decision-making by women on pregnancy onset and progression is encompassed in the word 'choice', which is currently the most active focus of debates relating to abortion in many parts of the world. In choice, we see a determination based on human rights and social justice principles that women are allowed to decide as to whether to become pregnant, when to become pregnant, and whether or not to continue with an unwanted pregnancy. The opposite doctrine is referred to as 'anti-choice' when extraneous factors are considered in women's decision to continue or not continue a pregnancy.

Some of the reasons that women consider a pregnancy as 'unwanted' include health reasons – the woman may be harbouring a disease that could be worsened by a pregnancy, for example, pre-existing hypertension or diabetes mellitus, or the pregnancy may occur at a socially inconvenient time such as the woman not having a job, not being married or being in school. We know that in many parts of Africa, girls may be sent out of school should they become pregnant. The fear of not completing school, thereby jeopardising their future may, therefore, be a reason for girls to seek induced abortion for a mistimed pregnancy. Other reasons include pregnancy as a result of rape, incest, or as a result of the failure of contraception. A recent report from a study of Demographic and Health Surveys (DHS) in 20 countries [26] showed that one in four unwanted pregnancies occurred as a result of failed contraception. In four countries, more than 50% of the pregnancies took place while the women were taking contraceptives. Unwanted pregnancy and induced abortion may also be due to the need for a woman to end childbearing or due to cultural and religious reasons.

It is now recognised that abortion occurs in all women and all populations of women around the world. Both married and unmarried women, as well as young and older women, often resort to abortion as a means of resolving an unwanted pregnancy. However, young women, especially unmarried adolescents and those less than 25 years of age, are more likely to report that their pregnancies are unintended and therefore to report that they have used induced abortion. Women with higher levels of education and those living in urban and semi-urban areas are also at higher risk of induced abortion as compared to women with lower levels of education or those living in rural areas [10, 26, 27].

5.3.4 Consequences of Induced Abortion

Worldwide, the WHO estimates that between 4.7% and 13.2% of maternal deaths are attributable to complications of induced and unsafe abortion, accounting for about 40,000 annual deaths [28]. This was a decline compared to the 56,000 deaths that occurred in 2003 and 69,000 deaths in 1990. A further 5 million women suffer major disabilities, while about 220,000 children are motherless as a result of deaths from unsafe abortion. Several lines of research have shown that maternal mortality due to unsafe abortion is higher in countries with major restrictions to abortion, and lower in countries where abortion is available upon request or under broad conditions. Most deaths from unsafe abortion are due to acute complications including severe haemorrhage; injury to adjacent organisations such as the bladder, the small and large intestines, and even the rectum; and septic abortion.

In regions where abortion laws are restrictive, induced abortions are often self-induced by women or are done by unskilled professionals using dangerous instruments or methods. Methods used for induced abortion in such settings include the lifting of heavy weights, abdominal massage, attempted piercing of the foetus with a knitting needle, coat hanger or similar devices, ingesting harmful abortifacients [29]. However, with the advent of effective medical abortion methods such as misoprostol, women have been known to take such medications and then report themselves in hospital as experiencing miscarriages which are then handled within the formal health care system. This has significantly reduced complications and deaths from unsafe abortion in South America, but the effect has yet to be noticed in sub-Saharan Africa. Many cases of severe complications of induced abortion have been reported where women had perforated uterus with herniation of internal viscera through the uterus to the vagina, and severe infections leading to severe irreversible shock and death [30].

Induced and unsafe abortions also lead to long-term gynaecological and reproductive health complications in women. These include chronic pelvic pain from chronic pelvic inflammatory disease, secondary infertility, cervical incompetence and severe psycho-sexual problems [24, 30, 31]. It is now widely recognised that efforts to make induced abortion safe would reduce the rates of morbidity and mortality from use of harmful and dangerous abortion methods.

5.3.5 Prevention

Prevention of unsafe abortion is broadly divided into primary prevention, the prevention of unwanted pregnancies that lead to induced abortion; and secondary prevention, ensuring that women are counselled when they experience an unintended pregnancy within the limits of the circumstances under which they experience the pregnancies and their own choices and preferences. By contrast, tertiary prevention, also referred to as post-abortion care is the management of women after they have experienced complications of induced and unsafe abortion.

Primary prevention is anchored mainly on increasing women's access to contraceptives on a universal access basis. In countries where the lack of access to sexual and reproductive health information is a significant reason for women's poor use of contraceptives, providing information on sexual and reproductive health would be a necessary and critical intervention to prevent unwanted pregnancies and unsafe abortion.

Adolescents in developing countries often have poor access to reproductive health information and services, which puts them at higher risk of unwanted pregnancies and unsafe abortion. Such at-risk populations, including women in rural and hard to reach areas, would benefit from comprehensive sexuality education as an essential entry point, and also from special efforts devoted to increasing access to contraceptives. Ways to improve access to contraception, especially for adolescents, is currently a daunting task in many parts of Africa. Approaches include peer-to-peer counselling, youth-friendly services (especially in primary health care settings), clinic-based facilities, mobile clinics, community-based distribution and social marketing. Efforts must be made to determine the best approach to deliver contraceptive services to at-risk groups that are socially and culturally acceptable and context specific.

Secondary prevention of unsafe abortion includes efforts made to increase women's access to safe abortion when they have identified termination as the only option. The WHO has published general recommendations on policies and guidelines for safe abortion care [22]. Undergraduate and post-graduate health professionals seeking specific knowledge and skills in this aspect are encouraged to read the guidelines which itemise the most effective and reliable methods for terminating unwanted pregnancies in the first and second trimesters of pregnancy. Two broad methods are now available – medication abortion methods and manual vacuum aspiration.

In the first trimester, the WHO recommends mifepristone and misoprostol as the most effective option, followed by manual vacuum aspiration (MVA) and the misoprostol alone (in countries where mifepristone is not registered) [32]. By contrast, mifepristone and misoprostol, misoprostol alone and dilatation and evacuation are most effective for second-trimester abortion.

The details, as recommended by the WHO [33], include the use of medication abortion in the first and part of the second trimester. Especially in developing countries where abortion safety is less than optimal, medical abortion should routinely be used in the first trimester, with guided use of surgical abortion (MVA, and D&E) with misoprostol in the second trimester (Table 5.1).

Tertiary prevention of unsafe abortion, also called post-abortion care (PAC) is well accepted within the health systems of all countries, including those with restrictive abortion laws. The principle to compassionately manage women after they experience complications of unsafe abortion has been enshrined in several international conferences and documents since the 1990s. These include the treatment of incomplete abortion and severe abortion complications as well as the linkage of women to effective contraceptive methods after they experience unsafe abortion – also called post-abortion family planning.

Table 5.1 Methods for safe abortion in the first and second trimesters

Duration of pregnancy	Recommended method for safe abortion
Medication abortion	
<7 weeks (49 days)	Oral mifepristone – 200 mg followed by Oral misoprostol – 400 µg, 24–48 h after administration of mifepristone
7–9 weeks (63 days)	Oral mifepristone – 200 mg followed by Vaginal, buccal or sub-lingual misoprostol 800 µg, 24–48 h after Or Vaginal or sub-lingual misoprostol alone – 800 µg every 3–12 h for 3 doses
9–12 weeks (63–84 days)	Oral mifepristone – 200 mg followed by Vaginal or sub-lingual misoprostol 800 µg stat, followed by 400 µg every 3 h up to 5 doses
>12 weeks (84 days)	Oral mifepristone – 200 mg followed by Vaginal, then vaginal or sub-lingual misoprostol – 800 µg, then vaginal or sublingual misoprostol. Or Misoprostol alone – 400 µg every 4 h up to 5 doses
Surgical methods	
≤12–14 weeks	Manual vacuum aspiration (MVA) Electric vacuum aspiration (EVA) However, the priming of the cervix with oral misoprostol 400 µg 4–6 h before the procedure after 10 weeks would ease the procedure
≥12–14 weeks	Dilatation and evacuation (D&E). The priming of the cervix with oral misoprostol 400 µg 4–6 h before the procedure will greatly ease the procedure

World Health Organization. Clinical practice handbook for safe abortion, 2014. WHO. ISBN 978 92 4 154871 7

Table 5.2 Recommendations for post-abortion care and post-abortion contraception

Specific task to be performed	Recommended method	Recommended health worker
Management of incomplete abortion in the first trimester	Manual vacuum aspiration (MVA) Misoprostol	Nurses, midwives, non-specialist doctors, specialist doctors
Management of incomplete Abortion in the second trimester	Dilatation and evacuation (D&E) Mifepristone and misoprostol, or misoprostol alone	Non-specialist doctors, Specialist doctors
Recognising and managing non-life-threatening complications	Initial management of post-abortion haemorrhage Initial management of post-abortion sepsis	Auxiliary nurses, nurses, midwives, non-specialist doctors, specialist doctors
Counselling and information Provision	Provision of information on safe methods and providers and how to recognise and deal with Complications. Also, contraceptive counselling	Pharmacists, auxiliary nurses, nurses, midwives, non-specialist doctors, specialist doctors
Post-abortion contraception	Insertion and removal of IUDs Insertion and removal of implants Injectable contraceptives Tubal ligation Others	Pharmacists, auxiliary nurses, nurses, midwives, non-specialist doctors, specialist doctors

World Health Organization. Health worker roles in providing safe abortion care and post-abortion family planning. WHO, 2015. ISBN 978 92 4 154926 4

The WHO has provided guidelines to health care workers on the management of abortion complications as well as the provision of post-abortion contraception [34]. The guidelines are summarised in Table 5.2 and would need to be carefully followed within health systems to ensure the proper management of women experiencing abortion complications and to prevent the need for repeat abortions.

Most medical doctors can efficiently utilise these basic methods of post-abortion care and post-abortion family planning, but as recommended by the WHO, some of the tasks can be delegated to midlevel providers. However, severe complications such as septic abortion complicated by gram-negative septicaemia and septic shock would require treatment by specialists in referral hospitals. Such patients might require treatment with effective antibiotics which would be selected based on blood cultures and laboratory testing for antibiotic sensitivities, transfusion of fluids and blood, intensive emergency care and extensive surgeries including laparotomy to drain abdominal abscesses, and in some cases total abdominal hysterectomy. Most abortion-related deaths occur in women experiencing significant complications, which means that competent hands should manage such difficulties in well-equipped secondary and tertiary health care institutions.

5.3.6 Human Rights and Gender Implications

Induced abortion is a significant cause of death and disability in women. One in four women who undergo unsafe abortion experiences is likely to develop a temporary or permanent disability and infirmity that can compromise the attainment of her full lifelong potentials. Since it occurs only in women, it is considered one of the most profound gender-based issues in contemporary times. Induced abortion is also a major issue in human rights. Abortion is addressed indirectly in several treaties and through key international documents. Africa leads the world in recognising women's right to abortion in its Protocol on the Rights of Women in Africa (part of the African Charter on Human and Peoples' Rights), which was the only human rights treaty that mentions explicitly abortion as of 2013 [34]. After approval by the African Union in July 2003, it was only in November 2005 that the minimum required 15 countries ratified the Protocol so that it became legally binding. As of January 2014, 28 African States had ratified the Protocol [34].

Other necessary rights related to abortion that have been enshrined in several international documents include the following: (1) the right to life; (2) the right to health, reproductive health and family planning; (3) the right to freedom from discrimination; (4) the right to liberty and security of person; and (5) the right to the benefits of scientific progress [35, 36, 37].

Many of these treaties and documents were signed and agreed to by national governments in Africa. It is therefore imperative that health providers and human rights advocates should push for the implementation of these treaties in their various countries to ensure that women have the knowledge and the wherewithal to access modern family planning and safe abortion methods. Health providers, in particular, should be able to interpret national laws on abortion within the lenses provided by these treaties, so as not to deny access to safe abortion and post-abortion care to women experiencing unwanted pregnancies and unsafe abortion.

5.4 Conclusion

Abortion (spontaneous and induced), when it occurs, is a significant event in the reproductive life of a woman and is often associated with psychological, traumatic, physical and health consequences, which may remain with the woman for a long time. Health providers are advised to manage these events with care and thoughtfulness and following human and social justice principles. Improving the management of women experiencing unwanted pregnancies and the consequences of spontaneous and induced abortion is one of the most critical contributions that policymakers and health providers can make towards the promotion of the health and social well-being of women in all countries.

References

1. LFY H. Prenatal diagnosis of chromosomal anomalies through amniocentesis. In: Milunsky A, editor. Genetic disorders and the fetus. 4th ed. Baltimore: The Johns Hopkins University Press; 1998. p. 179.
2. Nybo Andersen AM, et al. Maternal age and fetal loss: population-based register linkage study. Br Med J. 2000;320:1708.
3. Regan L, Brande PR, Trembath PL. Influence of past reproductive performance on risk of spontaneous abortion. Br Med J. 1989;299:541.
4. Kline J, Stein Z, et al. Fever during pregnancy and spontaneous abortion. Am J Epidemiol. 1985;121:832.
5. Andersen AM, Vastrup P, et al. Fever in pregnancy and the risk of fetal death: a cohort study. Lancet. 2002;360:1552.
6. Axmon A, Hagner L. Time to pregnancy and pregnancy outcome. Fertil Steril. 2005;84:966.
7. George L, Mills L, et al. Plasma folate levels and the risk of spontaneous abortion. J Am Med Assoc. 2002;288:1867.
8. Landres N, Milki AA, Lathi RB. Karyotype of miscarriages in relation to maternal weight. Hum Reprod. 2010;25:1123.
9. Templeton Sarah-Kate. New test for risk of pregnancy failing. The Sunday Times of London, UK, 2017, 14.
10. Weeks A, Alia G, Blum J, et al. A randomised trial of misoprostol compared with manual vacuum aspiration for incomplete abortion. Obstet Gynecol. 2005;106(3):540–7.
11. Zhang J, Gilles JM, Barnhart K, et al. A comparison of medical management with misoprostol and surgical management for early pregnancy failure. N Engl J Med. 2005;353(8):761–9.
12. Okonofua FE, Menakaya U, Otoide V, Omo-Aghoja L, Odunsi K. Experience with misoprostol in the management of missed abortion in the second trimester. J Obstet Gynecol. 2005;25(6): 583–5.
13. World Health Organization. Safe abortion: technical and policy guidance for health systems. 2nd ed; 2008. ISBN 978 92 4 154843 4 (NLM Classification: WQ 440).
14. Bearak J, Popinchalk A, Ganatra B, et al. Unintended pregnancy and abortion by income, region, and the legal status of abortion: estimates from a comprehensive model for 1999–2019. Lancet Global Health. 2020; https://doi.org/10.1016/s2214-109x(20)30342-6.
15. Henshaw SK, et al. The incidence of induced abortion in Nigeria. Int Fam Plan Perspect. 1998;24(4):156–64.
16. Okonofua FE, Odimegwu C, Ajabor H, Daru H, Johnson A. Assessing the prevalence and determinants of unwanted pregnancy and induced abortion in South West Nigeria. Stud Fam Plan. 1999;30(1):67–77.
17. Sedgh C, et al. Unwanted and associated factors among Nigerian women. Int Fam Plan Perspect. 2006;32(4):175–84.
18. Bankole A, Adewole IF, Hussain R, Awolude V, Singh S, Akinyemi JO. The incidence of abortion in Nigeria. Int Perspect Sex Reprod Health. 2015;41(4):170–81.
19. Okonofua FE. Is abortion incidence rising in Nigeria? Afr J Reprod Health. 2015;19(4):9–13.
20. Okonofua FE, Omo-Aghoja L, Bello Z, Osughe M, Agholor K. Self-reporting of induced abortion by women attending antenatal clinics in urban Nigeria. Int J Obstetrics Gynaecol. 2010;111:122–5.
21. Marge B. Abortion law and policy around the world. Health Hum Rights. 2017;19(1):13–27.
22. Centre for Reproductive Rights. The abortion laws, 2012. https://www.worldabortionlaws.com. Accessed 8 Jul 2017.
23. Centre for Reproductive Rights. The world's abortion laws, 2011 (New York, 2011).
24. World Health Organization, 2011: whqlibdoc.who.int/publications/2011/9789241501118_eng.pdf
25. Grimes DA, Benson J, Singh S, Romero M, Ganatra B, Okonofua FE, Shah I. Unsafe abortion: the preventable pandemic. Lancet. 2006:65–76.
26. Bradley SEK, Croft TN, Rutstein SO. The impact of contraceptive failure on unwanted births and induced abortion estimates and strategies for reduction. Demographic and Health Research Division, ICF Macro, 11785, Beltsville Drive, Calverton, Maryland 20705, USA. https://iussp.org/sites/default/files/event_call_for_papers/contraceptives. Accessed 12 Jul 2017.
27. Mitsunaga TM, Larsen UM, Okonofua FE. Risk factors for complications of induced abortions in Nigeria. J Womens Health (Larchmt). 2005;14(6):515–28.
28. World Health Organization. Unsafe abortion – global and regional estimates of the incidence of unsafe abortion and associated mortality in 2008. 6th ed. WHO; 2008. ISBN 978 92 4 150111 8.
29. Okonofua FE, Ilumoka T. Prevention of morbidity and mortality from induced and unsafe abortion in Nigeria. New York: Report of a seminar presented to the Population Council; 1992.
30. Oye-Adeniran BA, Umoh AV, Nnatu SNN. Complications of unsafe abortion: a case study and the need for abortion law reform in Nigeria. Reprod Health Matters. 2002;10(19):18–21.
31. Okonofua FE. Induced abortion: a risk factor for infertility in Nigerian women. J Obstet Gynaecol. 1994;12:272–6.
32. World Health Organization. Safe abortion: technical and policy guidance for health systems. 2nd ed; 2012. ISBN 978 92 4154843 4.
33. World Health Organization. Clinical practice handbook for safe abortion. WHO; 2014. ISBN 978 92 4 154871 7.
34. World Health Organization. Health worker roles in providing safe abortion care and post-abortion family planning. WHO; 2015. ISBN 978 92 4 154926 4.
35. African Commission on Human and Peoples' Rights. Protocol to the African charter on human and peoples' rights on the rights of women in Africa, 2014. http://www.achpr.org/instruments/women-protocol/
36. Cook RJ, Dickens BM. Upholding pregnant women's right to life. Int J Gynecol Obstet. 2012;117:90–4.
37. Ipas. Maternal mortality, unwanted pregnancy and abortion as addressed by international human rights bodies – part one. Chapel Hill: Ipas; 2013. http://www.ipas.org/en/Resources/Ipas%20Publications/Maternal-mortality%2D%2Dunwanted-pregnancy-and-abortion-as-addressed-by-international-human-ri-2.aspx;

6 Female Circumcision/Mutilation/Cutting

Friday Okonofua

Learning Objectives

At the end of this chapter, the learner will be able to:

- Describe the different types of female genital cutting (FGC) and its epidemiology.
- Understand the plausible cultural reasons for its practice.
- Comprehend its obstetrics, psychological and social consequences for women.
- Recognise the human rights context of the practice, and the importance of its elimination for the promotion of women's rights and social justice.
- Identify that medical practitioners should never promote its practice.
- Fathom the various approaches applied to its prevention and elimination.
- Know the skills and methods for clinical counselling, management and rehabilitation of women affected by FGC.
- Understand how applied research can be tailored to eliminate the practice in communities where it is still common.

6.1 Introduction

Female circumcision is the deliberate removal of the clitoris or the female external genital organs for cultural and non-therapeutic reasons rather than for sensible therapeutic reasons. Initially referred to as 'female circumcision' by practitioners, it became known as 'female genital mutilation (FGM)', when its harmful effects on women became more widely evident. However, to enable broader engagement with stakeholders in efforts to eliminate the practice, the less combative term 'female genital cutting' has been suggested as a replacement and is now more generally used. Thus, throughout this chapter, the term 'female genital cutting (FGC)' will be used.

Female genital cutting is now recognised by several international organisations as a human rights violation, as violence against women, and as one of the most vivid testimonies of the abuse of women's rights and social well-being in communities where it is practiced. Several lines of research have shown that FGC is harmful to women and serves no useful purpose. As such, there is currently a world-wide call for its complete elimination, as a critical strategy to promote women's rights, social justice and equality with men.

This chapter will review the terminology and epidemiology of FGC, explain its harmful effects and consequences for obstetrics and gynaecological practice and specify ways to prevent and reduce its adverse impacts and manage its consequences.

6.2 Operational Definitions

In 2007, the World Health Organization (WHO) revised its earlier definition of FGC as follows: 'the partial or total removal or other injury to the female genital organs for cultural or other non-therapeutic reasons' [1]. This definition is now widely recognised throughout the world. Since the most dominant aspect of the practice is the removal of the female external genitalia, the WHO further identified the four most common types of FGC, in order of their severity as types I, II, III and IV (see Fig. 6.1). The typical female external genitalia consist of the introitus, the clitoris and clitoridal hood (prepuce), the labia minoria and labia majoria, whose removal has been termed FGC.

Type I FGC: This is the partial or total removal of the clitoris and the prepuce (clitoridectomy). This type is further

F. Okonofua (✉)
Centre of Excellence in Reproductive Health Innovation, Department of Obstetrics and Gynaecology, University of Benin, Benin City, Nigeria

Women's Health and Action Research Centre, Benin City, Nigeria

University of Medical Sciences, Ondo City, Ondo State, Nigeria

F. Okonofua et al. (eds.), *Contemporary Obstetrics and Gynecology for Developing Countries*,
https://doi.org/10.1007/978-3-030-75385-6_6

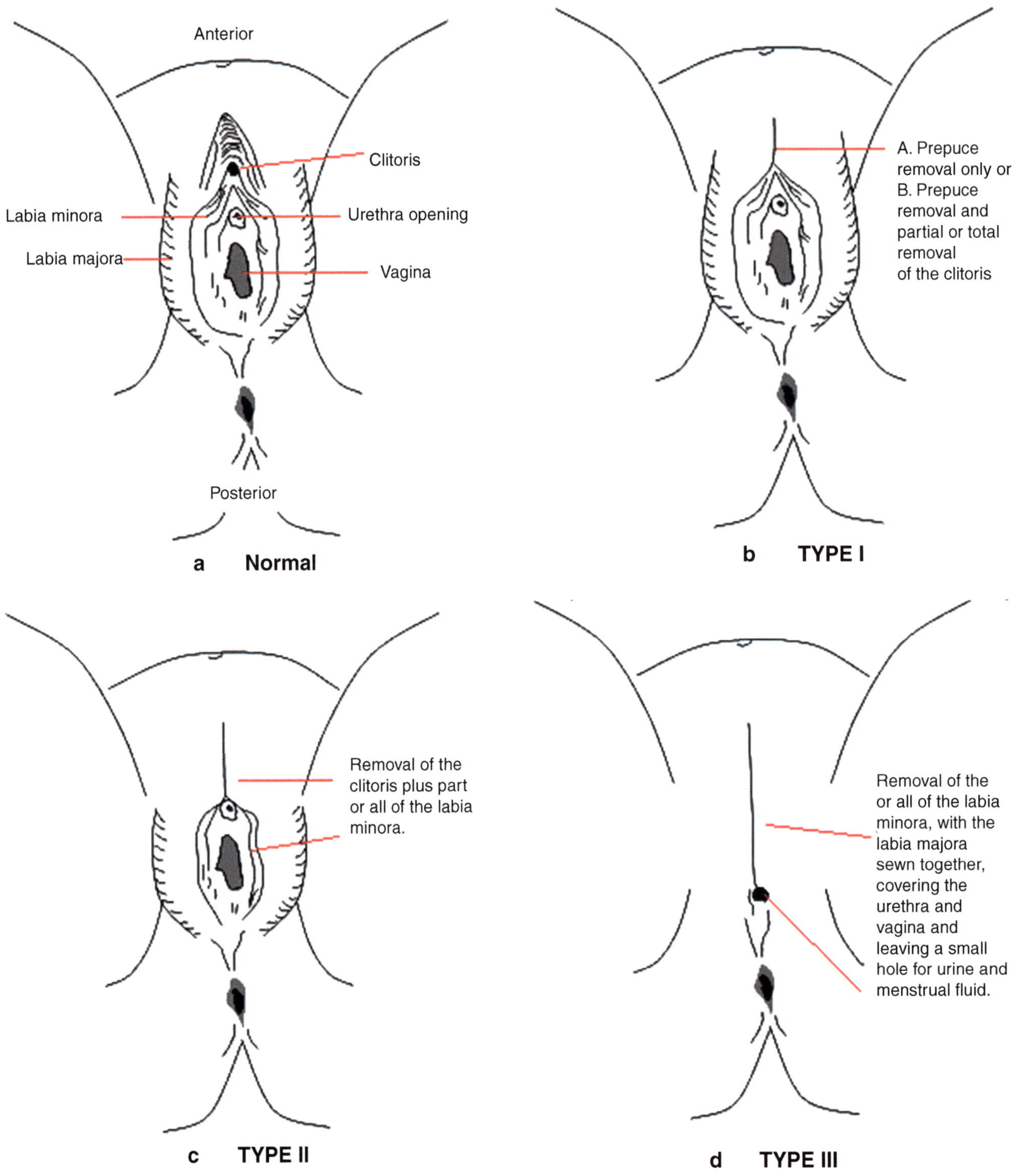

Fig. 6.1 Pictorial representation of female genital cutting types

divided into two sub-types: type Ia and type Ib. Type Ia is the removal of the hood or prepuce of the clitoris, supposedly the mildest form of FGC. However, this type still leaves in its wake, extreme damage to the blood vessels, which irreparably reduces the functionality of the clitoris. By contrast, type Ib is the removal of the prepuce (hood) as well as the clitoris.

Type II FGC: This type is the partial or total removal of the clitoris and the labia minora, with or without removal of the labia majora. This type is further sub-divided when necessary into three sub-types. Type IIa is the removal of the labia minora only, while type IIb consists of the partial or total removal of the clitoris and the labia minora. By contrast, type II c is the partial or complete removal of the clitoris, the labia minora and the labia majora.

Type III FGC: is the tightening of the vaginal orifice associated with the cutting and positioning the labia minora and the labia majora, with or without the excision of the clitoris. This procedure results in the extreme narrowing of the vaginal orifice (introitus) and is also known as infibulation. Type III FGC is further divided into two types. Type III a is the removal and apposition of the labia minora, while type IIIb is the removal and apposition of the labia majora.

Type IV FGC: is also referred to as the 'unclassified FGC' and consists of any other mishandling or manipulation of the external genitalia that is not done for medical reasons. These include cultural practices of pricking, piercing or incising of the clitoris or the labia, the burning of the clitoris or surrounding tissues, scraping of the tissues surrounding the introitus (also called Angurya cuts) or the cutting of the vaginal wall (also called Gishiri cut). It also includes massage for elongation of the clitoris or the labial minora, the introduction of corrosive substances or herbs into the vagina and the cultural tightening of the vagina.

6.3 Epidemiology of Female Genital Cutting

The Population Reference Bureau [2] and the WHO [3] estimated that between 150 and 200 girls and women worldwide have undergone FGC and that nearly three million girls are at risk of the procedure each year. The practice is concentrated mainly in countries in sub-Saharan Africa (SSA), especially north-east Africa, West and Central Africa and East Africa. However, due to migration, the practice has now spread to other parts of the world.

Regarding the incidence and prevalence of FGC, there are high prevalence countries in these regions with rates of FGC exceeding 80% in the countries. Prevalence data are often obtained from national surveys which are reviewed periodically. High prevalence countries include Egypt, Burkina Faso, Eritrea, Sudan and Mali. Countries such as Egypt and Mali have country prevalence levels higher than 95%.

Within the same region, countries with relatively lower prevalence levels of FGC (<40%) include the Central African Republic, Kenya, Nigeria and Yemen. Despite the overall national levels, the prevalence rates also vary by sub-groups within the countries. A country like Nigeria that has a national FGC prevalence rate of about 40% has rates as high as 80–90% in Oyo and Ebonyi states and low rates in the north-west and north-east regions.

Countries with the lowest prevalence rates of FGC in Africa include Democratic Republic of Congo (5%), Zaire (5%), Uganda (<5%) and South Africa (<2%). Data from the United Nations Children's Fund (UNICEF) suggest that the types of FGC performed also vary by region, countries and ethnicity [4]. It is of interest that countries with high prevalence rates also present the most severe forms of FGC. Infibulation (the most severe type) is practiced mainly in the north-east region of Africa – Djibouti, Eritrea, Ethiopia, Somalia and Sudan – where the overall prevalence of FGC is high. By contrast, the milder forms of FGC (types I and II) are practiced more in the low to medium prevalence countries.

6.3.1 Risk Factors for Female Genital Cutting

Several articles have been published that explain why FGC is practiced by communities where it is common [5–8]. Some of the documented reasons include as rites of passage into adulthood or entry into marriage, to reduce sexual promiscuity in women, as necessary to increase sexual pleasure for men and to improve the cleanliness of the external genital organs. Unfortunately, none of these reasons often proffered by practitioners have been proven in the real scientific sense.

However, what is true is that FGC is not a religious practice – many religions do not support it. Indeed, the incidence and prevalence of FGC have not to be shown to be different between the significant religions [9]. In Nigeria, the prevalence of FGC is lower in the Muslim North as compared to the Christian South, whereas FGC is ubiquitous in north-east African countries dominated predominantly by Muslims – Egypt, Sudan and northern Mali.

It is now generally agreed that FGC is mostly a cultural practice that has been handed down several generations, but its first origin remains a matter of conjecture till this day. It is therefore not surprising that the incidence and prevalence of FGC are higher in rural as compared to urban areas. Most traditional practitioners of FGC reside in rural communities. With modernisation and increasing rural-urban migration, the practice of FGC diminishes.

Indeed, the most modulating and auto-regulatory factor against the practice is education. Both increased education of parents and girls significantly reduces the incidence of FGC in moderate to high incidence countries. Indeed, ensuring that girls are in school reduces the likelihood of FGC among girls with the prevalence of FGC higher in out-of-school girls as compared to in-school girls in all communities.

Due to the combined effects of education, modernity and increasing international efforts to ban the practice, a secular trend towards declining incidence of FGC has been demonstrated [9]. Thus, emphasis needs to be placed on the universal education of girls and the specific health education of communities to sustain this trend over time.

6.3.2 Practice of Female Genital Cutting

Female genital cutting is often carried out by traditional circumcisers, mainly elderly women and relatives of the affected girls or women or by traditional birth attendants who may be men or women. It is usually carried out without anaesthetic and antisepsis and with a variety of instruments such as traditional knives, unsterilised blades, scissors, broken glass and other sharp tools. Cases have been described showing adults holding down the little infants who agonise in severe pain, while the circumciser carries out the procedure. It is often associated with moderate to heavy bleeding, while the use of herbs at the site of incision often exacerbates pain and bleeding and predisposes to infection.

There is an increasing trend for hospitals to perform the procedure in countries like Ethiopia and Egypt. In Egypt, up to 75% of FGCs are done by health professionals, with health providers arguing that medicalisation would be more neatly done and would reduce the rate of complications. However, both the WHO [10] and the International Federation of Obstetricians and Gynaecologists (FIGO) have strongly recommended that medical and health care providers should never perform FGC. The statement of FIGO was specific and is as follows: 'FIGO condemns all forms of female genital mutilation/cutting performed by traditional and medical personnel in all countries and all communities around the globe, as they are harmful, unethical, with no benefits whatsoever and are against the code of medical practice' [11].

The emphasis is on the ethical aspect. With the recommendation in all ethical codes of health professionals that 'they shall do no harm', FGC which has no benefit but has several health and social consequences, its performance by any health professional amounts to a severe breach of relevant ethical codes.

6.4 Health Consequences of Female Genital Cutting

Due to the unprofessional and crude methods for FGC, it is not surprising that it is associated with several short-term and longer-term health, social and psychological consequences. Klein et al. [12] recently reviewed the health and social consequences of FGC in 41 full-length articles published between 1994 and 2017. The reviewed articles included systematic reviews, cohort studies, case-control studies, case series analyses, cross-sectional studies, case reports and randomised controlled trials that focused on FGC and its complications.

Short-term consequences: The short-term implications of FGC widely reported in the review included significant bleeding, difficulties with micturition, considerable pain, shock and infections. Acute infections with *Staphylococcus aureus* and *Clostridium tetani* have been documented with variously reported severity of outcomes. Deaths have been reported from severe haemorrhage, shock and infections, with an estimate of one death per 500 procedures.

The question as to whether FGC results in greater likelihood of infection with sexually transmitted infections such as HIV/AIDS, Chlamydia trachomatis and herpes simplex virus has now been resolved with the review showing a higher prevalence of these infections in infibulated women as compared to controls. Presumably, such a higher incidence of infections is attributable to the use of unsterilised instruments or sexuality in the presence of trauma and wounds in infibulated women.

Longer-term consequences: These are manifold and can be divided into gynaecological, obstetrical and psychosexual consequences.

Gynaecological consequences include keloid formation and the development of clitoridal cysts. Urinary tract infection may also be a consequence due to retention of urine in the bladder due to difficulty in passage of urine through a scarred urethral outlet. Haematocolpos has also been reported in type III FGC (infibulation), when there is a complete closure of the vaginal introitus, preventing menstrual effluent from getting out of the uterus. This leads to secondary amenorrhea, which can only be corrected through surgical excision of the scarred vaginal outlet. Occasionally, coitus may become difficult or impossible due to severe narrowing of the vagina from scar tissues. This may lead to infertility or sub-fertility. A report from the Sudan showed that infertility is common in infibulated women and may also be due to sexual maladjustment in severely affected women [13].

Obstetric consequences: Several studies have reported the significant association of FGC with adverse pregnancy outcomes. Initial studies were small and uncontrolled and reported in single countries [14–17], but the large multicountry study conducted by the WHO in 2006 provided reliable evidence which showed that even mild types of FGC have adverse obstetric consequences [18]. The study consisted of the clinical examination of 28,393 pregnant women in 28 referral centres in Burkina Faso, Ghana, Kenya, Nigeria, Senegal and Sudan to determine whether they have had or not had FGC. Prospective information on demographic, pregnancy and health factors were obtained, while the participants and their infants were followed up until the women were discharged from the hospital. The results showed that compared with women without FGC, women with types II and III FGC were significantly more likely to be delivered by caesarean section, to experience primary postpartum haemorrhage and prolonged maternal hospital stay and to require the resuscitation of their infants, after controlling for confounding variables. It was noteworthy that types II and III FGC did not increase the likelihood of stillbirth, early neonatal deaths and low birth weight. In particular, there were no significant differences between type I FGC and women without FGC in all categories of adverse pregnancy outcomes. The authors concluded that 'women with FGC are significantly more likely than those without FGC to have adverse obstetric outcomes. The risks appear to be greater with more extensive FGC' [18]. From this study, it became evident that special care needs to be taken by health practitioners to determine the FGC status of women presenting in pregnancy and to take pro-active measures to prevent adverse maternal and perinatal outcomes.

Psycho-sexual consequences: The possible psychological consequences of FGC have been investigated. Researchers have linked FGC with various psychological effects including post-traumatic stress disorders, anxiety, depression, psychosis, memory problems and predilection to mental disorders in later life [19]. This may be due to the direct experiences of the procedure or to the associated life course changes. More empirical data is needed to document the nature of any possible association between FGC and psychological consequences.

The possible effects of FGC on psychological and sexual outcomes have been investigated. Initial results reported the increased likelihood of dysmenorrhea, vaginal dryness during sexual intercourse, lack of sexual desire, less frequency of sexual desire per week and less frequency of sexual orgasms in circumcised as compared to non-circumcised [20]. However, in a careful hospital-based study where we clinically examined women to confirm the presence or absence of FGC and then interviewed the women, we found no difference between circumcised compared to uncircumcised women in the self-reported rates of orgasmic sex [21]. The study concluded that although FGC was frequently carried out to reduce 'sexual promiscuity' in women, there was no scientific evidence to justify the procedure on this basis [21].

In particular, since the study found more self-reported episodes of sexual intercourse in circumscribed as compared to uncircumcised women, it concluded that circumcised women might be seeking more sexual episodes to achieve orgasm. This finding suggests that contrary to community opinions, FGC may increase the risk of 'promiscuity', rather than reduce it. Indeed, two published reviews concluded that FGC does not significantly reduce the enjoyment of sexual relationships [22, 23]. Further qualitative (phenomenological) studies are needed to illuminate this conclusion.

6.5 Medical Management of Female Genital Cutting

The WHO, the FIGO, the UNICEF, the UNFPA and all leading international bodies now recognise FGC as a human rights abuse and have called for the complete elimination of its practice throughout the world. The abolition of FGC has also been included in all major international consensus documents since the early 1990s including the 4th International Conference on Population and Development in Cairo, Egypt, the Beijing Conference on Women, the Millennium Development Goals and now the Sustainable Development Goals.

Since this textbook is targeted at health providers, clinicians and specialist obstetricians and gynaecologists (Ob-Gyns), we will approach the management of FGC from three perspectives. The approach includes **primary prevention** – the prevention of FGC from occurring in the first place; which consists of efforts aimed at eradicating FGC in communities, as we believe that health professionals have important roles to play in this regard. **Secondary prevention** encompasses the management of complications arising from FGC. We consider that health professionals, especially Ob-Gyns are best positioned to manage the complexities of FGC in pregnant and non-pregnant women, while they may refer affected women to related professionals – psychologists, psychiatrists, urologists, sexual medicine experts and social counsellors – to manage other associated complications. **Tertiary prevention**, by contrast, is the rehabilitation of women after they have been managed for FGC, so that they can return to regular sex and marital life.

6.5.1 Primary Prevention of Female Genital Cutting

Although medical practitioners first drew the attention of the world to the harmful effects of FGC, in recent times they have played less prominent roles in championing the abandonment of the practice. Notable Egyptian physicians like Nahid Toubia [24, 25], who was later followed by prominent Ob-Gyns in Egypt and Sudan [26] first worked tirelessly to document the harmful effects of FGC and suggested ways to manage its consequences medically. Unfortunately, in more recent times, women rights activists, civil society organisations and youth advocates have played more prominent roles in campaigning for its elimination and abolishment. Health professionals have crucial roles to play as they are respected opinion holders, and ought to function as champions and change-agents in bringing about the necessary reform to abolish FGC in their areas of influence.

Because of the limited scope of this article, it will not be possible to review all the strategies adopted in many parts of the world to prevent FGC. It will be sufficient to itemise them here, while the interested reader is encouraged to read various articles and publications that address the primary prevention of FGC [27–29]. Some of the most successful interventions that have been adopted for the primary prevention of FGC included the following:

- There is a need for assessment and documentation of FGC prevalence and practices in specific communities, including the identification of circumcisers, reasons for circumcision and the enabling factors. The findings from the study will promote the design of community-specific interventions for ending the practice.
- Leveraging government support and commitment. This proposal is crucial for policy development and implementation. It also provides an enabling opportunity for right activists to work on the issue.
- Promoting and enforcing legislation. Several legislations and laws have passed in many parts of Africa over the past two decades for the abolition of FGC. However, the extent to which the laws have been implemented, and have reduced the practice still needs to be investigated.
- Overcoming cultural norms and common barriers. This challenge appears to be the most challenging aspect, but when communities are adequately educated about its harmful effects, they can take steps to stop the practice.
- Promoting open discussion about the problem. Open dialogue such as 'community conversations' as first reported from Ethiopia, and other parts of Africa [30–33] can help to reduce the community tensions around the practice. We used the open discussion method in Edo State of Nigeria through debates on radio and television to build community consensus on the needlessness of the practice. Thus, when a bill to abolish the practice was eventually brought to the State House of Assembly, it received overwhelming support and was signed into law by the State Governor [33, 34].
- Seeking children's life skills, knowledge and participation – building the skills of children to resist the practice is critical to success. Also, ensuring that all school-age children are in school is one of the most effective deterrents to FGC.
- Building the capacity of families to address the problem – is crucial as, without family support, FGC will not take place. A major component of this is community education designed to enable community members to come to terms with the harmful effects of the practice.
- Monitoring, reporting and oversight functions. These should always be included in all FGC primary prevention programmes at community, national and regional levels. This recommendation will enable the collation of relevant empirical evidence and best practices that would guide the expansion and scale-up of such programmes.

6.6 Management of Female Genital Cutting Complications (Secondary Prevention)

Due to the high prevalence of short and long-term complications of FGC, it is essential that clinicians, especially Ob-Gyns are knowledgeable and skilled in ways to properly rectify the situation and restore the genitalia to normal or near-normal states of functionality. Both the Royal College of Obstetricians and Gynaecologists (RCOG) [35] and the WHO [36] have issued guidelines for the management of complications arising from FGC complications.

Due to its comprehensiveness and specificity for health professionals, we recommend the RCOG guidelines, especially Ob-Gyns. The RCOG stipulates that all professionals should be conversant 'with the female genital mutilation act 2003 in England, Wales and Northern Ireland, and the prohibition of the Female Genital Mutilation Act 2005 in Scotland' [35]. The specific recommendations include the non-medicalisation of the practice (i.e. recommendations to clinicians not to carry out genital cutting when not clinically required), the total prohibition of re-infibulation among practitioners (i.e. that re-infibulation should never be carried out under any circumstance), and the need for respectful treatment of women who have undergone FGC [35]. The RCOG guidelines [35] further require that clinicians and practitioners (especially those in gynaecological practice) understand the principles of the management of FGC, especially how recent FGC is managed, and the roles of de-infibulation and clitoral re-construction. Additionally, the guidelines provide for how FGC is managed in pregnancy, how pregnant women with FGC are identified, the place of proper antenatal documentation, the importance of screening for co-infections, and how intrapartum and postnatal care is managed in women with FGC. Some of these guidelines are summarised below.

6.6.1 Management of Short-Term Complications

For acute complications of FGC, the RCOG recommends the initial appraisal to assess the degree of blood loss and shock, the presence of infection and the severity of pain [35]. Specific treatments include replacement of intravascular volume with intravenous fluids and blood, tetanus toxoid immunisation, antibiotic prophylaxis, use of analgesics and urinary catheterisation to prevent retention of urine. Also, it is essential especially in countries where FGC is illegal for practitioners to properly document their findings at the time of presentation, if possible, with photographs and video-recording, as these may be needed for legal purposes in the future.

6.6.2 Management of Long-Term Complications

The treatment of long-term complications of FGC may involve different procedures and multiple disciplines. As such, clinicians are advised to be aware of the physical, sexual and psychological implications of the practice and to respond appropriately, promptly to the needs of patients, and if necessary, refer such patients to appropriate specialists. In particular, health care workers need to be aware that in patients with type III FGC, internal pelvic examination (including cervical cytology) and the conduct of simple pelvic procedures may be impossible without a general anaesthetic.

Some procedures that have been used for treating long-term complications of FGC include clitoridal cystectomy (the removal of clitoridal cysts), drainage and marsupialisation of clitoridal abscesses, vaginal and labial adhesiolysis (the removal of labial and vaginal adhesions), neo-vaginoplasty (reconstruction of a completely occluded vagina) and defibulation (reversal of a previously infibulated external genitalia). It also includes comprehensive counselling, referral for psychotherapy or sex therapy and the social rehabilitation of the women.

6.6.3 Management of Female Genital Cutting in Pregnancy

In high prevalence countries, clinical practitioners should be able to examine women at their first antenatal attendance to determine the presence or absence of FGC, regardless of whether or not this has been pointed out by the women during clinical interviews. With an early diagnosis made, clinicians will be able to counsel the women and also determine the best modes of care and plans for delivery. During antenatal care, screening for co-infections with chlamydia, HIV, hepatitis and syphilis should be managed according to existing protocols. Hopefully, if the women presented for antenatal care, the appropriate mode of delivery should have been identified and discussed. However, if the women present first in labour, a new assessment of the external genitalia and their potential to deliver vaginally should be made. Where or considerations for vaginal delivery fail, and especially in women with co-existing obstetric complications, caesarean section should be considered for the safety of the mother and the baby.

Clear guidelines have been provided in the RCOG guidelines [35] for a defibulation operation. Defibulation is best done during antenatal care (at about 28 weeks) or preferably during labour. Clinicians need to offer appropriate advice including recommendations about the place of birth. In particular, in cases where difficult surgery is anticipated or where fertility is delayed as a result of apareunia or dyspareunia, women should be advised to undergo defibulation before conception. Ancillary treatment of women needing defibulation includes referral to centres with experience in management, and preparations made for carrying out the procedure in a suitable outpatient room equipped with minor procedures or in an operating theatre.

The technique of defibulation involves the identification of the urethra and the passage of urethral catheter, the development of a preliminary incision along the vulvar excision scar with cutting diathermy (if available) to reduce bleeding. It also involves the use of excellent absorbable suture material (e.g. polyglactin, Vicryl or Ethicon) to ensure proper closure of the edges and prevent further bleeding. The administration of prophylactic antibiotics is essential to reduce the risks of infection, while adequate pain relief is essential to limit additional psychological effects.

In pregnant women known to have severe types of FGC, the recommendation is that they should be advised to deliver in maternity units with immediate access to facilities for emergency obstetric care, including caesarean section. However, women who have undergone successful defibulation and a previous uncomplicated vaginal delivery should be considered for delivery in midwives-led units. Epidural anaesthesia should be offered to women unable to tolerate vaginal examination as well as those requiring an anterior episiotomy.

Post-natal care in women with FGC should be conducted appropriately and should as much as possible involve professionals that managed the women during antenatal and delivery care. Efforts should be made to ensure proper counselling of the women, providing that they are pain-free and are as comfortable as possible. If defibulation has been done, the wound should be allowed to heal before the women are discharged, and the women should be counselled not to request re-fibulation as this would jeopardise their future health and obstetric career.

6.7 Tertiary Prevention (the Rehabilitation of Victims of Female Genital Cutting)

The purpose of secondary prevention of FGC which often involves reconstructive surgery is to restore women to proper sex life and functional reproductive health. Therefore, it is essential that women treated are supported to return to the life that enables them to forget the trauma of FGC. Women that have undergone clitoral or vaginal reconstruction and defibulation are particularly vulnerable and should be supported with guidance, clinical advice and counselling. As an example, women that underwent defibulation during pregnancy may be pressured to re-fibulate after delivery by their partners, family members or by cultural gatekeepers. This is a challenge, but practitioners must be brave and find ways to counsel such women to resist such pressures as it would be harmful to their future life and social well-being. If possible, a psychologist or counsellor should be engaged who may have to undertake specific home visits to explain the harmful effect of such a procedure.

Also, women that have undergone vaginal reconstruction or defibulation may experience gradual narrowing or spontaneous closure of the vaginal orifice if they are not sexually active. Thus, continued sexual activity should be discussed, if possible, with inactive lubricants initially, followed by normal regular intercourse at a later stage. However, if sexual intercourse is not immediately possible, the use of plastic vaginal dilators should be considered.

6.7.1 Health Workers Training

The training of health workers is critical to enable the appropriate prevention and management of FGC. Studies have documented the perceptions and practices of health practitioners towards FGC [37] and the WHO has made recommendations on ways to engage health professionals in the process of eradicating the practice [38]. The major issues include the need to build the knowledge and skills of health providers on FGC so that they can act in multiple ways as (1) advocates and community change agents, (2) providers of care to women who have experienced complications of FGC, and (3) counsellors to women and couples. Similarly, health providers can act as respected opinion leaders and influencers in communities on matters relating to FGC, and fathers, mothers and relatives with independent opinions on whether or not to undertake FGC. The health providers should be exemplary in ensuring that their immediate relatives are not exposed to FGC.

Female genital cutting training curricula for health workers should be comprehensive and broad-based and should include the following components:

- Types of FGC – prevalence in various regions, and its historical, cultural, social, economic and religious contexts
- Review of existing government laws, policies and legislation
- Prevention, identification and management of complications of FGC
- Health education strategies for FGC, including behaviour change communication and counselling techniques
- Appropriate documentation, monitoring and evaluation of FGC practices, experiences and complications

Health workers have tremendous influences in sub-Saharan Africa. They can leverage such controls to build political and social commitment for the abandonment of FGC. Going forward, the extent to which health workers are involved will be an essential indicator for measuring the success of FGC prevention programmes, especially in high prevalence countries. Guidelines should be developed and made available in such countries, and health professionals should be held accountable for the use of ethical principles in FGC prevention.

6.8 Gaps in Applied Research Relating to Female Genital Cutting

Most research relating to FGC in sub-Saharan Africa has been formative in describing the nature, epidemiology and extent of the problem. By contrast, there has been limited research that provides in-depth information about the rational and deep-seated reasons for the practice. As a result of the deficit of existing knowledge, it has been difficult to develop solutions based on empirical research for stemming the practice. Going forward, we recommend the following types of research especially in high prevalence countries with the objective to enable the effective prevention of FGC at scale.

- Qualitative research especially through community conversations and phenomenology that investigate communities' and individual experiences of FGC. Such analysis will determine how community and personal experiences of the consequences of FGC can be used to gain community ownership of efforts to abolish the practice.
- Intervention research based on quasi-experimental or randomised controlled studies that show the effectiveness of carefully selected complex or single interventions in preventing various components of the dependent variables relating to the practice and prevention of FGC.
- Translational research that involves the knowledge transfer of FGC research findings to community stakeholders, policymakers and affected individuals to enable behavioural change and active policy formation and implementation.
- Multi-centre clinical trials that involve the testing of similar methods of treatment of FGC.

These lines of treatment hold promise for finding a lasting solution to the high prevalence of FGC in sub-Saharan Africa.

6.9 Summary

Female genital cutting is an essential developmental challenge with serious negative consequences for the health and emotional well-being of sub-Saharan women. Violence against women is now globally recognised as a serious human rights abuse. Its complete eradication in all communities and countries around the world has been recommended by various international instruments, documents and agreements. This chapter strongly supports these recommendations and provides a framework for the understanding of the harmful effects of FGC by health professionals. It is a call to action for all health professionals to join in the fight for the elimination of FGC through research, evidence-based advocacy, service delivery, health education and dissemination of information to families and stakeholders.

References

1. World Health Organization (WHO). Eliminating female genital mutilation: an interagency statement. UNAIDS, UNDP, UNECA, UNESCO, UNHCHR, UNICEF, UNIFEM, WHO. Geneva: WHO; 2008.
2. Population Reference Bureau (PRB). Female genital cutting: prevalence, attitudes, and efforts to end the practice. PRB 2018. www.measurecommunication.org
3. WHO. Female genital mutilation, 2019. Accessed at: https://www.who.int/reproductivehealth/topics/fgm/prevalence/en
4. United Nations Children's Fund (UNICEF). Female genital Mutilation/Cutting. A global concern. UNICEF, New York 2016.
5. Shell-Duncan B, Hernlund Y, Herlind Y. Cutting without ritual and ritual without cutting: female "circumcision" and re-ritualization in the Gambia. In: Shell-Duncan B, Hernlund Y, editors. Circumcision in Africa. Culture, controversy and change. Boulder: Lynne Rienner; 2000. p. 235–52.
6. Shell-Duncan B, Herlund Y, Ahmadu F. Rights and Wrongs: an outsider/insider reflects on power and excision. In: Shell-Duncan B, Hernlund Y, editors. Circumcision in Africa. Culture, controversy and change. Boulder: Lynne Rienner; 2000. p. 283–12.
7. Odukogbe ATA, Afolabi BB, Bello OO, Adeyanju AS. Female genital mutilation in Africa. Transl Androl Urol. 2017;6(20):138–48.
8. Okeke TC, Anyaelue USB, Ezenyeaku CCK. An overview of FGM in Nigeria. Ann Med Health Sci Res. 2012;2(1):70–3. https://doi.org/10.4103/2141-9248.96942.
9. Snow RC, Slanger TE, Okonofua FE, Oronsaye F, Wacker J. Female genital cutting in southern urban and peri-urban Nigeria: self-reported validity, social determinants and secular decline. Trop Med Int Health. 2002;7(1):91–100.
10. World Health Organization. Global strategy to stop health providers from performing female genital mutilation. A Joint UNAIDS, UNDP, UNFPA, UNHCR, UNICEF, UNIFEM, WHO, FIGO, ICN, IOM, MMIA, WCPT, MWA Statement. WHO/RHR/10.9 2010. Accessed at: http://whqlibwho.int/hq/2010/who_RHR_10.9doc
11. FIGO. Statement by the FIGO President on medicalisation of female genital mutilation. June 2010. Accessed at http://www.figo.org/news/statement-figo-presidency
12. Klein E, Helzner E, Shayowitz M, Kohlhoff D, Smith-Norowitz TA. Female genital mutilation: health consequences and complications. Obstet Gynaecol Int. 2018:7365715. https://doi.org/10.1155/2018/7365715.
13. Lightfoot-Klein H. The sexual experience and marital adjustment of genital circumcised and infibulated females in the Sudan. J Sex Res. 1989;26:357–92.
14. Slanger TE, Snow RC, Okonofua FE. The impact of female genital cutting on first delivery in southwest Nigeria. Stud Fam Plan. 2002;23(2):173–84.
15. Larsen U, Okonofua FE. Female circumcision and obstetrics complications. Int J Gynaecol Obstet. 2002;77(3):255–65.
16. De Silva S. Obstetric sequelae of female circumcision. Eur J Obstet Gynecol Reprod Biol. 1989;32:233–40.
17. Oduro AR, Ansah P, Hodgson A, Afful TM, Daiden F, Adongo P, Adongo P. Trends in the prevalence of female genital mutilation and its effects on delivery outcomes in the Kassena-Nankana district of northern Ghana. Ghana Med J. 2008;40(3):87–92.
18. World Health Organization. Female genital mutilation and obstetric outcome: WHO collaborative prospective study in six African countries. Lancet. 2006;367:1835–41.
19. Behrendt A, Moritz S. Post-traumatic stress disorders and memory problems after female genital mutilation. Am J Psychiatry. 2005;162:100–2.
20. Almroth L, Bedri H, El Musharaf E, Satti A, Idris T, Hashom M, Suliman GI, Bergstrom S. Urogenital complications among girls with genital mutilation: a hospital-based study in Khartoum. Afr J Reprod Health. 2005;9(2):118–24.
21. Okonofua FE, Larsen U, Oronsaye F, Snow RC, Slanger TE. The association between female genital cutting and correlates of sexual and gynaecological morbidity in Edo State, Nigeria. Br J Obstet Gynaecol. 2002;109:1089–96.
22. Obermeyer CM. The consequences of female circumcision for health and sexuality: an update on the evidence. Cult Health Sex. 2005;7(5):443–61.
23. Alsibani SA, Rouzi AA. Sexual function in women with female genital mutilation. Fertil Steril. 2010;93(3):722–4.
24. Toubia N, Izett S. Female genital mutilation: an overview. Geneva: WHO; 1995.
25. Toubia N. Female genital mutilation: a call to action. New York: RAINBO; 1995. p. 4.
26. El-Defrawi MH, Lotfy G, Dandash KF, Refaat AH, Eyada M. Female genital mutilation and its psychosexual impact. J Sex Marital Ther. 2001;27(5):465–73.
27. Okonofua FE. Female genital cutting and reproductive health in Africa. In: Okonofua F, editor. Reproductive health challenges in Africa: textbook for students and development practitioners. Springer; 2014.
28. Program for Appropriate Technology for Health. Female genital mutilation in Africa: an analysis of current abandonment approaches. Nairobi: PATH; 2005.
29. World Health Organization. Global strategy to stop health providers from performing female genital mutilation. A Joint UNAIDS, UNDP, UNFPA, UNHCR, UNICEF, UNIFEM, WHO, FIGO, ICN, IOM, MMIA, WCPT, MWA Statement. WHO/RHR/10.9 2010.
30. UNDP. Upscaling Community Conversations in Ethiopia 2014: Unleashing capacities of communities for the HIV/AIDS response. Addis Ababa: UNDP; 2004.
31. Campbell C, Nhamo M, Scott K, Madnhire C, Nyamukapa C, Skovdel M, Gregson S. The role of Community Conversations in facilitating local HIV competence: case study from rural Zimbabwe. BMC Public Health. 2013;13:354. https://doi.org/10.1186/1471-2458-13-354.
32. Moulton PL, Miller ME, Offutt SM, Gibbens BP. Identifying rural health needs using Community Conversations. J Rural Health. 2007;23(1):90–6. https://doi.org/10.1111/j.1748-0361.2006.00074.
33. Women's Health and Action Research Centre. Advocacy for the abandonment of female genital mutilation in Edo State, Nigeria. Annual Report, 1999–2000, WHARC, Benin City, Nigeria website: www.wharc-online.org
34. Edo State Government. Bill to prohibit the genital mutilation of girls and other matters arising therefrom. Edo State, Nigeria 1999.
35. RCOG. Female genital mutilation and its management. Green-top guideline No. 53, July 2016. NICE accredited www.nice.org.uk/accreditation
36. World Health Organization. Guidelines on the management of the health complications from female genital mutilation, policy brief. Geneva: WHO; 2016.

37. Kaplan-Marcusan A, Del Rio NF, Moreno-Navarro J, Castany-Fàbregas MJ, Nogueras MR, Muñoz-Ortiz L, Monguí-Avila E, Torán-Monserrat P. Female genital mutilation: perceptions of healthcare professionals and the perspective of immigrant families. BMC Public Health. 2010;10:193.
38. World Health Organization (WHO). Female genital mutilation: Integration the prevention and the management of health complications in the curricular of nursing and midwifery: a teacher's guide. Geneva: World Health Organization; 2001.

Reproductive Epidemiology, Health Status and Burden of Disability

7

Joseph A. Balogun

Learning Objectives

After reading this chapter, the learner will be able to:

- Define reproductive health.
- Discuss reproductive epidemiology in Africa.
- Differentiate between Millennium and Sustainable Development Goals.
- Differentiate between the Alma-Ata and the Abuja Declaration Goals.
- Describe the health status of African women.
- Articulate the burden of disability among African women.
- Identify the level of funding needed by African countries to achieve the United Nations Sustainable Development Goals.

7.1 Introduction

Good health is central to human existence and the ability to handle stress and live a long and productive life. The World Health Organization (WHO) defined health as the 'state of complete physical, mental, and social well-being, and not merely the absence of disease or infirmity' [1]. There are seven major components to human health – physical, emotional, social, mental, spiritual, environmental and reproduction. But reproductive health, otherwise known as sexual health/hygiene, is often not discussed within the context of good health [2]. Reproductive health is the condition of complete physical, social and mental well-being and not just the absence of disease but include issues about the reproductive system, its functioning and processes.

Poor reproductive health services account for up to 18% of the global burden of disease among women of childbearing age. In Africa, the problem is even more insidious as it accounts for 32% of the total burden of illness. This unacceptable situation is due to the lack of access to family planning services needed to improve reproductive health [3]. The challenge is compounded further because the distribution and determinants of reproductive disorders and its sequelae are under-reported. There is presently limited information on pubertal development, gynaecologic disorders, female reproductive cancers, sexually transmitted infections, menstruation, menopause, female and male fertility, and assisted reproductive technologies in the region. Moreover, there are challenges in family planning, contraceptive safety and efficacy, maternal morbidity and mortality, perinatal and infant health, adolescent sexual behaviour, domestic violence, HIV/STDs and population-based reproductive health surveys [4]. More relevant information is therefore needed to understand better the prevalence, causes and prevention of reproductive health conditions in Africa.

People with disabilities are the most significant minority in the world. Approximately, 15% of the global population (over a billion people) have a disability, and the prevalence is higher for developing countries [5]. All over the world, women, children, older people and indigent adults are more prone to disability. In patriarchal societies, which are the norms in the developing nations, women and girls are more likely to have a disability due to gender-based violence, limited access to health care and poor working conditions. The impairment profoundly impacts the sexuality and quality of life of women and girls of all ages. Unfortunately, in Africa, because of limited information about disability, the plights of people with disabilities are often ignored by frontline clinicians and policymakers.

J. A. Balogun (✉)
Chicago State University, Chicago, IL, USA

University of Medical Sciences, Ondo City, Nigeria

Centre of Excellence in Reproductive Health Innovation,
University of Benin, Benin City, Nigeria
e-mail: jbalogun@csu.edu; jbalogun@unimed.edu.ng

F. Okonofua et al. (eds.), *Contemporary Obstetrics and Gynecology for Developing Countries*,
https://doi.org/10.1007/978-3-030-75385-6_7

To adequately address this unacceptable situation, this chapter discusses reproductive epidemiology, health status and burden of disability among African women. The information should be of interest to healthcare professional students, policymakers and clinicians working with women in Africa.

7.2 Operational Definitions

The terms Millennium and Sustainable Development Goals featured prominently in this chapter, and they warrant clarification here. Between 2000 and 2015, the United Nations championed eight Millennium Development Goals to fight global poverty in its many dimensions. In January 2016, after the successes of the Millennium Development Goals, the United Nations set in motion the 17 Sustainable Development Goals to provide universal healthcare and end poverty by the year 2030, and ensure that the global community protects the planet, enjoys peace and prosperity. The 17 global goals incorporated new interconnected ideas on economic inequality, innovation, climate change, peace and justice, and sustainable consumption.

7.3 Reproductive Epidemiology in Africa

Reproductive health implies having satisfying and safe sex life vis-à-vis the rights to make crucial choices about family welfare, procreative choices and be able to set future conceptive goals [1, 6] (Fig. 7.1).

Reproductive and sexual ill-health is responsible for 20% of the global burden of ill-health among women, and 14% for men [6]. Exposure to environmental pollutants is a major threat to reproductive health. For example, exposure to lead is associated with reduced fertility in both genders, and exposure to mercury is linked to congenital disorders and neurological diseases. Exposure to chemicals that impact hormonal activity may contribute to fertility, pregnancy and other aspects of reproduction [7]. Women need access to accurate preventative information on affordable and acceptable contraception method to maintain satisfying sexual and reproductive health. Making choices about sexual and reproductive health include family planning, the capability to reproduce and the fundamental right of every human being [8].

Around the world, caesarean section is the most frequently performed surgical operation, and the procedure has surged in the last two decades [9]. The WHO recommended 10–15% of deliveries to be a caesarean section; other experts advocated 19%. The average caesarean section rate is 27% in many high-income countries and between 3% and 29% in low- to middle-income countries. The surge in the caesarean section procedure is due to improved safety of the operation, suspected cephalopelvic disproportion, fewer vaginal births after the process, more high-risk pregnancies, preferred method of delivery in cases of breech presentation, an increase in the operation performed at the maternal request, the medicolegal environment and changes in practice patterns of obstetrics [1, 6].

Adhesion is a frequent complication of caesarean section and it clinically presents as abdominal discomfort, pain and associated lower quality of life. Long term, adhesion often complicates future caesarean section because of the increased difficulty of the operation resulting in complications such as bladder damage, prolonged duration of the procedure, maternal exhaustion, adverse perinatal and maternal outcomes such as birth asphyxia [9]. Pelvic floor injury is a significant determinant for a caesarean section as the preferred delivery mode [10].

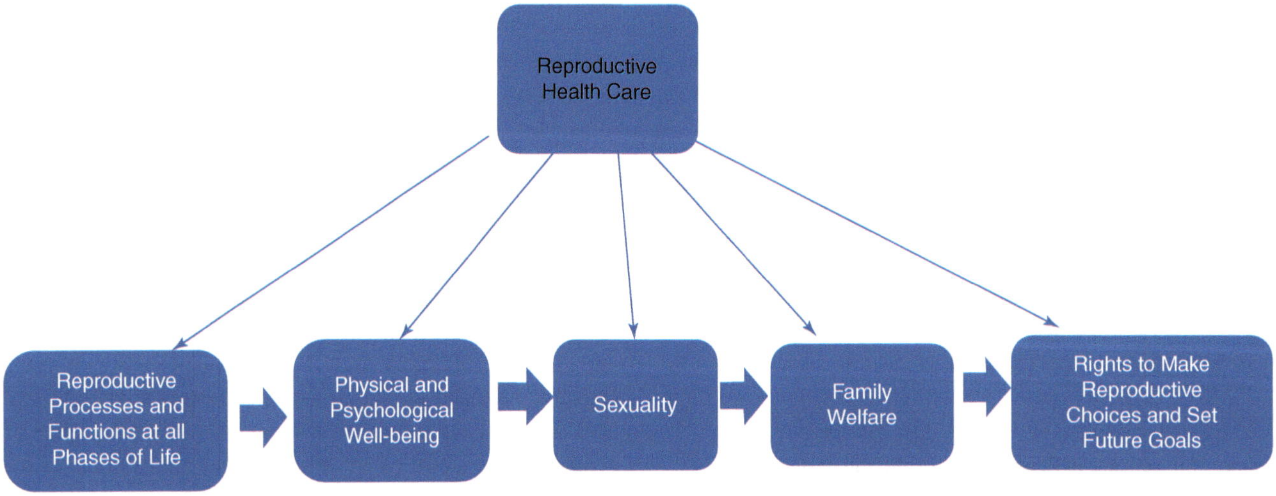

Fig. 7.1 Reproductive health care framework

The primary causes of death among women in sub-Saharan Africa are severe bleeding (haemorrhage), infection (sepsis), eclampsia, obstructed labour and unsafe abortion. And increasingly more women now die from HIV/AIDS, tuberculosis, malaria and anaemia. Because the HIV/AIDS pandemic in Africa is still on the increase, the prevention of mother-to-child transmission of the virus is critical to controlling the spread of the epidemic [3].

The prevention of reproductive tract infections is another crucial component of sexual and reproductive health that needs urgent action in Africa. Cervical cancer, with a 25% prevailing rate, is one of the leading causes of death among African women. Although 80% of these deaths are preventable if the diagnosis is made timely; unfortunately, 50% of the cases are detected too late [3].

Worldwide, cancer of the breast is the leading cause of carcinoma in women. Although recent advances in chemotherapy, surgical and radiation therapies have improved the survival rates, the three well-known cancer treatment options are associated with significant side effects [11]. Breast cancer survivors often experience treatment complication side effects that include musculoskeletal pain, post-mastectomy syndrome, shoulder dysfunction, axillary cording, chemotherapy-induced peripheral neuropathy and lymphedema.

Like women with breast cancer, African American men have one of the highest incidences of prostate cancer in the world (80.0–195.3, per 100,000 person-years, age-adjusted world standard), but the rates in indigenous African men are unclear because population-based data are quite limited in Africa. However, recent data from the International Agency for Research on Cancer showed regional differences; the rates were highest in East Africa (10.7–38.1) and lowest in West Africa (4.7–19.8). The disparities are due to variation in access to health care, screening services, registry quality, genetic diversity and westernisation [12]. The complications associated with prostatectomy include urinary incontinence and erectile dysfunction; both of which are amenable to physiotherapy intervention.

Both men and women have different types of cancer and they are managed with drugs, radiation and surgery. The treatment modalities have significant side effects which are managed in a cancer rehabilitation programme – a holistic treatment process that allows cancer survivors and their family to maintain the highest physical, social, psychological and vocational functioning levels within limits created by the disease and the various treatments. Despite the demonstrated effectiveness of cancer rehabilitation in the management of the treatment complication side effects, the service is underutilised. The reasons for this phenomenon are broad, but primarily due to lack of knowledge on the part of patients and referring physicians and limited access to health care services [13].

Compared to women in other parts of the world, women in sub-Saharan Africa face the greatest sexual and reproductive challenges in the world. They have the highest fertility, HIV infection rates, the risk of dying during childbearing and the top unmet need for contraception [14]. One-tenth of the world's population and 20% of global births are in Africa, where approximately 50% of the mothers who die during childbirth live. More than 50% of the global 536,000 maternal deaths are from sub-Saharan Africa, and 13 out of the 14 (93%) countries with maternal mortality rates of at least 1000 are in the region. The high child and maternal mortality rates are mostly due to inadequate access to quality medical care in the rural and remote areas and shortage of physicians and midwives. Despite the shocking child and maternal mortality rates, less than 10% of the health budget is allocated by most African countries to primary health care and over 80% to curative care delivered in the tertiary (teaching/specialist) institutions.

In Africa, adolescents continue to be victims of sexually transmitted diseases, HIV/AIDS, unwanted pregnancy, and demand for abortions from unprotected sex. The adolescents are exposed to risky health behaviours such as substance abuse and smoking, which continue into adult life [3]. Also, the increasing incidence of cardiovascular diseases and diabetes among adults is associated with the lack of proper diet and sedentary lifestyles during adolescence [12]. In addition, religion (measured by denominational affiliation) is a significant factor in maternal health service utilisation after controlling for socioeconomic factors. Women of Islamic faith and traditional women are less likely to use maternal health services compared with women who are Christians [15].

7.4 The Health Status of African Women

Health systems are part and parcel of the fabric of social and civic life. But most African countries are yet to fully achieve the Alma-Ata Declaration goal which entrenched the idea of health care as a fundamental human right issue adopted at the first international conference on primary health care held on September 6–12, 1978 at Almaty (formerly Alma-Ata) in Kazakhstan (formerly Kazakh Soviet Socialist Republic). The conference advocated the need for urgent action to protect and promote the health of all people by the world community. Since this landmark development, the concept of primary health care and the goal of achieving 'Health for All' has been accepted by the WHO's member countries. The idea was first recommended for developing countries and 5 years later applied to all other nations around the world [16].

Between 1970 and 1980, the health status of African children aged 1 month to 5 years improved, but the health status of newborns less than 4 weeks old remained unchanged, unfortunately. Around the world, neonates represent about 27% of children who die before their fifth birthday, and 29% of these deaths are in Africa [3]. Children born in sub-Saharan Africa confront the gravest survival challenge in the world. About 44% of the global under-five mortality is in Africa, where the leading causes of death are HIV/AIDS, neonatal complications, respiratory infections, malaria and diarrhoea. At least 50% of underage deaths in Africa are due to malnutrition. Of the 60 countries around the world responsible for 94% of child mortality rate, 37 of them are from Africa [17–20].

African women are more likely than women in other parts of the world to die from infectious diseases (such as HIV, tuberculosis and malaria), maternal and perinatal conditions, and nutritional deficiencies. About 468 million women between 15 and 49 years of age (30% of all women) around the world are anaemic due in most part due to iron deficiency, and 48–57% of the pale women are Africans. Among adult African women, 1 in 4 deaths is due to noncommunicable diseases such as heart disease, cancer and diabetes. Tobacco is a leading risk factor for noncommunicable diseases, and its use is increasing among the young and elite adult African women [5, 21].

About 62% of the 47,000 women who die annually from unsafe abortion are Africans because access to the procedure is severely restricted. The unmet need for contraception is highest in sub-Saharan Africa; only 32% of married African women compared to 68% Latin American and Caribbean women and 63% in industrialised countries use an effective modern contraceptive method. The overwhelming majority of the global HIV-infection is in sub-Saharan Africa, and over 58% of adults living with HIV in the region are women [23, 24]. Seventy-six percent (3.8 million) of young people with HIV or AIDS are in Africa. Young women compared to young boys are more vulnerable to HIV infection because they face higher risks of sexual violence, forced marriage, trafficking and less likely to have the information needed to protect themselves, and less empowered to use the information provided [5, 22, 23].

Currently, only 18% of married women in Africa use modern family planning devices, and 5% use traditional contraceptive approach. A significant number of women (25%) have unmet needs – they would prefer to stop having children or delay their next birth but are not using any family control method. Meeting this unmet need is an essential step toward improving reproductive health in sub-Saharan Africa. But other factors (extreme poverty and violence) affecting women's health, including the availability of modern health care services during childbirth, need to be addressed [25].

The significant impediments to the amelioration of African women's health challenges are due to gender inequity, poverty, weak economic capacity, sexual and gender-based violence, and female genital mutilation. Globally, women are twice unlikely to find employment, while 75% are excluded from the workforce. Women are more likely not to attend school, and they often drop out when they start menstruating as there is no assistance at school to deal with their periods [17]. To ensure equal access of both geneders to the opportunities needed to achieve full health potential and health equity, the health bureaucrats and policymakers around the world must, henceforth, recognise the social and biological differences - women and men experience different health risks, health-seeking behaviour, outcomes and responses from the healthcare systems [5].

Young people between the ages of 10 and 24 constitute the most substantial proportion (about one-third) of the population in sub-Saharan Africa. When compared to the other parts of the world, sub-Saharan Africa is the only region that young people continue to grow significantly. By 2025, the young people (aged 10–24) population living in sub-Saharan Africa is expected to increase to 436 million and by 2050 it will further increase to 605 million. Adolescents in the region particularly have reproductive health vulnerabilities such as gender inequality, high birth rate, early marriage, traditional draconic practices (such as female genital mutilation), unwanted and closely spaced pregnancies, unsafe abortions, abduction and sexually transmitted infections [22].

Over the years, African nations have failed to allocate enough funds to provide primary health care for their citizenry. For this reason, in April 2001, African Heads of State held a meeting at Abuja where they pledged to devote at least 15% of their annual budget to health care; a landmark event often referred to as the Abuja Declaration. Two decades after the pledge, most African countries are yet to achieve this goal. To date, only four African countries (Zambia, Malawi, Liberia and Rwanda) have met the 15% health budget allocation.

Sub-Saharan Africa is notably lagging behind other regions in the world in meeting the Sustainable Development Goals; particularly goals which focus on universal healthcare and how to reduce child mortality, improve maternal health and combat HIV/AIDS, and malaria and other diseases by the year 2030 [26]. To realise these goals that were not met by the 2015 target date, concerted scaled up double efforts are needed to educate women and improve newborn health, as well as promote universal access to reproductive health services which must include health care that spans the life cycle and enlivens linkages between the community and health facilities. A lot of work in reproductive health is needed, particularly in slowing the spread of HIV/AIDS, reducing maternal mortality and improving family planning. Around the world, many countries are making a concerted effort in reaching their targets, but in sub-Saharan Africa region, the pace of development is slow; there are still significant needs and opportunities to do more [24, 25].

7.5 The Burden of Disability Among African Women

Disability is defined in this chapter as any cognitive, physical, developmental, or mental disorder that impairs, or limits a person's ability to engage in specific tasks or the routine activities of daily living. There are many different types of disabilities faced by African women which fall into the following four broad categories [17].

1. Cognitive disabilities include difficulty communicating, learning and retaining information. They include Down syndrome, Fragile X syndrome, Prader-Willis syndrome and developmental delays.
2. Physical disability may affect temporarily or permanently, a person's physical capacity and/or mobility. They include multiple sclerosis, cerebral palsy, spina bifida, brain or spinal cord injury, epilepsy and muscular dystrophy.
3. Sensory disabilities affect one or more senses, sight, hearing, smell, touch, taste, or spatial awareness. They include autism, blindness and hearing loss.
4. Mental illness affects a person's thinking, emotional state and behaviours. They include bipolar, depression, schizophrenia and eating disorders [17].

Although African women with disabilities face double discrimination of stigma and marginalisation, yet only 26–55% of people who are disabled in developing countries receive the medical rehabilitation services that they need, and only 17–37% have the assistive devices (wheelchairs, prostheses and hearing aids) that they need for mobility [5]. In low- and middle-income countries, three-quarters of people with disabilities are women [18, 19].

African women and girls with disabilities experience various forms of abuses and physical violence that are often unreported. Gender-based violence is more pernicious among women and girls with disabilities, and they are less likely to seek help because they are usually not believed, and services are not accessible. Compared to adults, children with disabilities are four times more likely to experience violence, and girls are more at risk compared to boy [27]. For example, people with albinism in Africa face discrimination; but more horrific they are tortured and murdered. The stigma around mental health, learning difficulties and depression is pervasive, and these issues are often not discussed. These concerning issues need to be addressed globally to achieve Article 16 of the United Nations Convention on the Rights of Persons with Disabilities which is consistent with the Sustainable Development Goal 16 on peace and justice [28]. The Republic of Malawi, a landlocked country located in Southeast Africa, took the lead in Africa to pass legislation in 2012 to protect the rights of persons with disabilities in response to the increasing cases of exploitation, violence and abuse against women with disabilities [29].

The socioeconomically disadvantaged citizens have less access to education and health care, and they are more likely to become disabled by disease, illness and injury. Similarly, because they typically do not have extensive education, people living with disabilities are often unemployed, and in abject poverty. Notwithstanding, people living with disabilities everywhere in the world, want the same chance to participate fully and contribute to their communities, but they lack the skills needed for gainful employment and career mobility.

In developing countries, due to poverty, 90% of children with disabilities do not attend school [18]. In Africa, the problem is even direr as less than 5% of adults with disabilities have the requisite skill for reading or writing [19]. The issue of poverty is not going away anytime soon, and it is now occurring in unusual places. Extreme poverty is on the increase and gaining grounds in nations previously thought to be making progress in eradicating the problem. Recently, Nigeria, one of the two wealthiest countries in Africa, has overtaken India as the world's largest concentration of extreme poverty. Today, over 87 million Nigerians live in extreme poverty, compared to 73 million Indians. In the next 12 years, Africans would make up nine out of every ten poor people in the world [20].

Developmental and physical disabilities are common (8.4%) in young women, and reproductive health issues such as puberty, sexuality and menstruation are more complicated for teenagers with disabilities and their families due to concerns about menstrual hygiene, abuse risk, vulnerability, changes in seizure pattern and altered mood. Teenagers with disabilities have gynaecologic health care needs that are similar to their peers without limitation, but they have unique needs that are related to their physical and cognitive challenges [30]. Treatment of the impairments associated with physical disabilities is one of the core functions of the medical rehabilitation team that includes physicians, physiotherapists, occupational therapists, speech therapists, clinical psychologists and social workers.

African women and girls because of their gender and disability find it more difficult to form relationships and get married. The society perceives them as unable to fulfil the traditional family roles of having sex, bearing children and cooking food and caring for families. Although both women and men with disabilities face oppression, pervasive stereotypes and misconceptions that worsen their lives, women have very different experiences. The unfortunate stereotypic words used in Africa to describe women with disabilities include the following: 'asexual, hyper-sexual, unattractive, infertile, useless, unemployable, stupid, abnormal, defective, not good wife material, suffering innocent, a burden to carry and the will of God' [17].

7.6 Conclusion

This chapter discusses the reproductive health challenges, health status and the burden of disability among African women. Despite the horrific health indicators presented, most African countries presently allocate less than 10% of their national budgets to health. Compared to other public health programmes, funding for maternal, newborn and child survival programmes are limited. The WHO regional office must continue to provide technical support to strengthen planning capacities, evaluate and implement reproductive health services to improve reproductive services in Africa. Also, WHO must promote the utilisation of evidence-based practices for the application of reproductive health services and support the use of research outcomes designed to improve the sexual and reproductive health care programmes and services in Africa.

To effectively address the myriad of reproductive health challenges in Africa and to achieve the United Nations' Sustainable Development Goals to end poverty and provide universal healthcare by the year 2030. Furthermore, African countries must recommit to the 2011 Abuja Declaration treaty to annually allocate at least 15% of their national budget to health care.

References

1. World Health Organization. Sexual and reproductive health https://www.who.int/reproductivehealth/en/ 2018. Accessed 28 May 2019.
2. Nordqvist C. Health: what does good health really mean? https://www.medicalnewstoday.com/articles/150999.php. 2017. Accessed 28 May 2019.
3. United Nations. Reproductive health in the African region. What has been done to improve the situation? UN Chronicle. 2007;XLIV(4)
4. https://unchronicle.un.org/article/reproductive-health-african-region-what-has-been-done-improve-situation. Accessed 28 May 2019.
5. Reproductive Epidemiology (n.d.) https://www.omicsonline.org/scholarly/reproductive-epidemiology-journals-articles-ppts-list.php https://www.cdc.gov/reproductivehealth/global/rhepi.htm. Accessed 28 May 2019.
6. World Health Organization. Disabilities – Africa https://www.afro.who.int/health-topics/sexual-and-reproductive-health 2017. Accessed 28 May 2019.
7. WHO Reproductive Health (n.d). https://www.who.int/westernpacific/health-topics/reproductive-health. Accessed 28 May 2019.
8. National Institute of Environmental Health Sciences (NIEHS). Reproductive health. https://www.niehs.nih.gov/health/topics/conditions/repro-health/index.cfm 2018. Accessed 28 May 2019.
9. United Nations Foundation (n.d). https://unfoundation.org/blog/post/mdg-mondays-millennium-development-goals-4-5-6/. Accessed 28 May 2019.
10. Nuamah MA, Browne JL, Öry AV, Damale N, Klipstein-Grobusch K, Rijken MJ. Prevalence of adhesions and associated postoperative complications after cesarean section in Ghana: a prospective cohort study. Reprod Health. 2017;14:143. https://www.docphin.com/research/article-detail/19251217/PubMedID-29096649/Prevalence-of-adhesions-and-associated-postoperative-complications-after-cesarean-section-in-Ghana-a-prospective-cohort-study. https://reproductive-health-journal.biomedcentral.com/articles/10.1186/s12978-017-0388-0. Accessed 28 May 2019.
11. McLennan MT, Melick CF, Alten B, Young J, Hoehn MR. Patients' knowledge of potential pelvic floor changes associated with pregnancy and delivery. Int Urogynecol J Pelvic Floor Dysfunct. 17(1):22–6. https://www.ncbi.nlm.nih.gov/pubmed/16003482 2006. Accessed 28 May 2019.
12. Chu LW, Ritchey J, Devesa SS, Quraishi SM, Zhang H, Hsing AW. Prostate cancer incidence rates in Africa. Prostate Cancer, 947870. https://www.ncbi.nlm.nih.gov/pmc/articles/PMC3200287/ 2011. Accessed 28 May 2019.
13. Stubblefield MD. The underutilisation of rehabilitation to treat physical impairments in breast cancer survivors. PMR. 2017;9(9S2):S317–23.
14. Madise N. Reproductive health in Africa: major challenges and opportunities. https://www.gov.uk/dfid-research-outputs/reproductive-health-in-africa-major-challenges-and-opportunities 2007. Accessed 28 May 2019.
15. Obeng S, Baffour G, Takyib K, Addaic I. Challenges to the reproductive-health needs of African women: On religion and maternal health utilisation in Ghana. Soc Sci Med. 2006;62(12):2930–44. https://www.sciencedirect.com/science/article/abs/pii/S0277953605006295. Accessed 28 May 2019.
16. Therithal info, Chennai Health. Alma Ata Declaration and the goal of "Health for all." BrainKart.com. https://www.brainkart.com/subject/Sociology-of-Health_289/ 2018. Accessed 28 May 2019.
17. Lowrie MB (n.d.). Neurological disorders and their main causes. http://www.icsmsu.com/exec/wp-content/uploads/2011/12/ABS-Neuroscience.pdf. Accessed 28 May 2019.
18. Nagarajan C. The abilities of women with disabilities. https://thisisafrica.me/abilities-women-disabilities/ 2016. Accessed 28 May 2019.
19. Lime A. Disability in Africa: I'm no longer ashamed of my disabled daughter. https://www.bbc.co.uk/news/amp/world-africa-45220690. 2018. Accessed 28 May 2019.
20. Africa Educational Trust (n.d). Our work with people living with disabilities. https://africaeducationaltrust.org/disability. Accessed 28 May 2019.
21. Brookings Institution, USA. Oil-rich Nigeria outstrips India as a country with most people in poverty. https://www.theguardian.com/global-development/2018/jul/16/oil-rich-nigeria-outstrips-india-most-people-in-poverty. 2017. Accessed 28 May 2019.
22. Lukale N. Adolescent reproductive health concerns in Sub-Saharan Africa. https://www.girlsglobe.org/2015/12/15/adolescent-reproductive-health-concerns-in-sub-saharan-africa/ 2015. Aeccessed: May 28, 2019.
23. Erhabor O, Adias TC and Akani CI. Reproductive health challenges of living with HIV-infection in Sub Saharan Africa, In: Current Perspectives in HIV Infection, Shailendra K. Saxena. 2013.
24. Ibis (n.d). Reproductive health in sub-Saharan Africa. https://ibisreproductivehealth.org/where-we-work/sub-saharan-africa. Accessed 28 May 2019.
25. Gribble J, Haffey J. PRB – Reproductive health in sub-Saharan Africa. https://www.prb.org/reproductivehealthafrica/. 2018. Accessed 28 May 2019.
26. United Nations Population Fund (n.d.). Sexual and reproductive health. https://www.unfpa.org/sexual-reproductive-health. Accessed 28 May 2019.
27. Arroyo C, Thampoe E. Africa: children and women with disabilities, more likely to face discrimination. https://allafrica.com/stories/201808160405.html. 2017. Accessed 28 May 2019.

28. DIWA. Disabled women in Africa curbs violence against women and girls with disabilities. http://www.diwa.ws/?p=101. 2017. Accessed 28 May 2019.
29. Disability Rights Funds (n.d.). Disabled women in Africa http://disabilityrightsfund.org/grantees/disabled-women-in-africa/. Accessed 28 May 2019.
30. Quint EH. Menstrual and reproductive issues in adolescents with physical and developmental disabilities. Obstet Gynecol. 2004;124(2):367–75.

Part II

Obstetrics

Preconception Counselling and Prenatal Care

8

Kingsley N. Agholor and Nosakhare O. Enaruna

Learning Objectives

At the conclusion of this chapter, the reader will be able to:

- Define, in clear terms, the concept of preconception care.
- Explain the rationale for advocating for preconception care.
- Distinguish between informal and formal pre-pregnancy counselling.
- Identify the components of preconception care as well as the core components of prenatal care.
- Articulate the issues of interest for preconception counselling in well women.
- Identify the target population to improve preconception health and pregnancy outcome.
- Discuss preconception interventions that have been identified to be of proven benefits.
- Critically evaluate the constraints to establishing preconception care programme in Nigeria and the rest of West Africa.
- Discuss the pitfalls of prenatal care in the West African Sub-region.
- Provide evidence-based prenatal advice to pregnant women.

K. N. Agholor (✉)
Central Hospital, Warri, Nigeria

N. O. Enaruna
University of Benin, Benin City, Nigeria

University of Benin Teaching Hospital, Benin City, Nigeria

8.1 Preconception Care

8.1.1 Introduction

By the beginning of the 1980s, it became increasingly obvious that prenatal care was not able to guarantee favourable pregnancy outcomes in many cases. This conclusion was largely supported by the continued observation of increasing rates of adverse pregnancy outcomes, namely, major birth defects, low birth weight, preterm delivery, infant mortality and maternal mortality. In addition, it was often noted that a wide range of risk factors was prevalent among pregnant women and women likely to become pregnant [1]. Perhaps, it also became painfully obvious to many observers that the most critical periods of intrauterine development are not observed judging by the late presentation of many pregnant women for prenatal care [2]. Hence some interventions available during the prenatal period have been considered too late! In an attempt to deliver on the promise of prenatal care to improve pregnancy outcome, early proponents of preconception care had to devise a strategy believed to be remedial, though without much evidence, by leaning on the visibility of the folic acid research [3]. Researchers involved with the folic acid study had argued that 'there is necessarily uncertainty over when a woman will become pregnant, and she may seek medical attention only some weeks after her first missed menstrual period, which would be too late for folic acid supplementation to be effective. The general advice to women, therefore, must be to take folic acid supplementation from the time they decide to try to become pregnant' [4]. Although global acceptance remained slow, these arguments were helpful in pushing the boundaries of limitation to the practice. Over the course of time, preconception care as a routine practice has gained pre-eminence as a health goal in many countries especially as a healthy mother and a healthy baby remain valued hopes of many cultures around the world.

Today, however, there is good and consistent evidence [5] to show that 'the greatest opportunities for further improvement

F. Okonofua et al. (eds.), *Contemporary Obstetrics and Gynecology for Developing Countries*,
https://doi.org/10.1007/978-3-030-75385-6_8

Table 8.1 Risk factors found in pregnant and intending mothers [1]

Pregnant or gave birth	Smoke during pregnancy	11.0%
	Consumed alcohol in pregnancy (55% at risk of pregnancy)	10.1%
	Pre-existing medical conditions	4.1%
	Rubella seronegative	7.1%
	HIV/AIDS	0.2%
	Received inadequate prenatal care	15.9%
At risk of getting pregnant	Cardiac disease	3%
	Hypertension	3%
	Asthma	6%
	Dental caries or oral disease (women 20–39)	>80%
	Diabetic	9%
	On teratogenic drugs	2.6%
	Overweight or obese	50%
	Not taking folic acid	69%

in pregnancy outcomes – in improving the health of women and their children – lie in prevention strategies that must be implemented prior to conception to be effective'. As shown in Table 8.1, 11.0% of pregnant women smoke while pregnant; 10.1% consumed alcohol in pregnancy while a significant proportion of women at risk of getting pregnant were found to be diabetic or consuming alcohol. These maternal health conditions and behaviours are recognised as risk factors for adverse perinatal outcomes, for example, the association of alcohol with foetal alcohol syndrome, the association of smoking with low birth weight and the association of diabetes with congenital malformations. Obviously, the risk harvesting of these adverse outcomes of pregnancy remains high if these maternal health conditions and behaviours are not detected, managed, modified and controlled before the onset of pregnancy [3]. Clearly, this corroborates the argument that early prenatal care is too late. Therefore, in recognition of the importance of delivering these interventions before the onset of pregnancy, it was recommended that 'as the key physician/primary care provider, the obstetrician/gynaecologists must take advantage of every health encounter to provide preconception care and risk reduction before and between conceptions – the time when it really can make a difference' [6]. It is evident that the goal of preconception care is to promote the health of women at risk of pregnancy before they achieve conception so as to make pregnancy-related outcomes better. The relative simplicity and the promise of the concept led to its wide adoption and implementation by many industrialised countries especially following the publication of the 'Recommendations to Improve Preconception Health and Healthcare' [7, 8].

Despite the documented benefits of this practice, it is almost non-existent in developing countries like Nigeria. In fact, studies in developing countries have described the relative newness of preconception care, the poor knowledge of the practice and stressed the need for its urgent implementation [9, 10]. Findings of one study indicate that less than half of the antenatal attendees interviewed were aware of the concept of preconception care [9]. Regardless of this sub-optimal level of awareness as well as the reported low level of utilisation, the majority of the respondents in one of the studies were of the view that implementation of preconception care will lead to an improvement in maternal and child health [10]. This viewpoint is consistent with solid scientific evidence indicating that interventions targeted at improving pregnancy outcomes will best achieve their goals if delivered before the onset of pregnancy. Clearly, efforts in developing countries must be targeted at the development of clinics dedicated to the provision of preconception care. This can be easily achieved by incorporating preconception care into already existing programmes. Additionally, stakeholders in maternal and child health in these countries must 'be involved in vigorous, targeted and sustained women-centred education to improve knowledge and utilisation of preconception care by women in the reproductive age group' [10].

Taken together, it is crucial that preventive care of this nature be made available to all couples desiring pregnancy globally. This is important if the promise of preconception care is to be achieved. Unfortunately, inequities remain; whereas preconception care remains in its infancy in developing countries, it has now become firmly established as the first phase of comprehensive maternity care which also has antenatal (prenatal), intrapartum and postnatal phases in many industrialised countries. In such clime, the care emphasises screening, health education and effective interventions intertwined with prenatal care in a continuum.

In this section, the objectives of preconception care will be highlighted and the key components of a successful programme will be presented. The reasons for the slow take-off of preconception care in developing countries will be explored and the current constraints to having effective administration of preconception care will be also discussed.

8.1.2 Definition of Preconception Care

Preconception care has been defined as a set of interventions that aim to identify and to modify biomedical, behavioural and social risks to a woman's health or pregnancy outcome through prevention and management, emphasising those factors which must be acted on before conception or early in pregnancy to have a maximal impact [1].

8.1.3 The Rationale for Advocating for Preconception Care

The primary goal of preconception care is to promote the health of women of reproductive age before conception thereby improving pregnancy-related outcomes. This approach has called for a paradigm shift from 'healthy mothers to healthy babies' towards 'healthy women through healthy mothers to healthy babies'. This is important because evidence abounds that poor pregnancy outcomes continue to be at alarming levels and a good proportion of women enter pregnancy 'at-risk' for adverse pregnancy outcomes (see Table 8.1).

There is also evidence supporting the widespread consensus that intervening before pregnancy will help to improve outcome.

Adverse pregnancy outcomes remain common (see Table 8.2), especially in developing countries. Notably, pregnancy complications have increasingly become one of the leading causes of infant mortality worldwide. In specific terms, areas of interest for intervention in preconception counselling in our environment include women who have been exposed to alcohol and illicit drugs as well as 'herbal preparations', those with pre-existing medical conditions like chronic hypertension, diabetes mellitus, epilepsy and coagulation disorders, those who are socially disadvantaged or those with evidence of nutritional deficiencies.

Several studies investigating the knowledge of preconception care among antenatal attendees in Southern Nigeria revealed significantly poor knowledge of the concept [9, 10]. In one study, only a third of the women attending the antenatal clinic were aware of preconception care [9]. Hence, many pregnancies, in developing countries like Nigeria, continue to develop unplanned, resulting in little or no benefit from preconception care [11]. These reports indicate a positive association between preconception care, educational status and women's parity, suggesting that a woman's knowledge of the concept increased with educational status and an increasing number of deliveries. The association with parity may be due to the informal education received in the antenatal clinic. Indeed, Bastani et al. [12] in a randomised trial to evaluate the impact of a health education workshop noted that short-term health education can empower women to adapt to healthy lifestyles.

While it is common knowledge that preconception care as a structured practice is almost non-existent in developing countries, a review of the first 1000 cases in a structured practice at the University of Lagos, Nigeria illustrated the importance of accurate assessment of prior and existing health problems [13]. For example, routine investigations in that practice revealed significant serological and positive antibody carrier rates for toxoplasmosis, rubella, cytomegalovirus, herpes simplex I and herpes simplex II (TORCH). Clearly, preconception counselling is a useful strategy for determining foeto-maternal risks in subsequent pregnancies.

Table 8.2 Rates of some adverse pregnancy outcomes [1]

Major birth defects	3.3% of births
Foetal alcohol syndrome	0.2–1.5/1000 live births
Low birth weight	7.9% of births
Preterm delivery	12.3%
Complications of pregnancy	30.7%
C-section	27.6%
Unintended pregnancies	49%
Unintended births	31%

8.1.4 Informal Versus Formal Pre-pregnancy Counselling

A good number of the interventions which constitute part of structured preconception care, such as screening for HIV, assessment for family history for diabetes, counselling on folic acid consumption and vaccinations for tetanus toxoid are currently being offered to women and to couples when indicated in many developing countries. Nevertheless, the delivery of service remains non-formalised.

However, an informal form of preconception care has been shown not to be effective in the improvement of pregnancy outcomes. For example, diabetic women who had non-formalised preconception care had higher rates of hyperglycaemia during the first trimester, while structured pre-pregnancy care was demonstrated to improve metabolic control in diabetic women in the first and subsequent trimesters, thereby reducing the incidence of spontaneous abortions [14], major congenital abnormalities [15, 16], preterm births [14], small for gestational age [14], macrosomia [17], admission to neonatal intensive care [14] and early neonatal death [18]. Well-structured preconception care for diabetic women has been proven to be cost-effective by reducing the length of hospitalisation for the mothers and intensity of care for their babies [19, 20].

8.1.5 Components of Preconception Care

According to the ACOG and AAP, the components of preconception care are as follows [1]:

1. Maternal assessment
2. Vaccination
3. Screening
4. Counselling

8.1.6 Maternal Assessment

This aspect of the clinic should focus on the following areas:

- Family planning and pregnancy spacing
- Family history
- Genetic history (maternal and paternal)
- Medical, surgical, pulmonary and neurologic history
- Current medications (prescription, self-prescribed, or over-the-counter)

- Substance use, including alcohol, tobacco and illicit drugs
- Nutrition
- Domestic abuse and violence
- Environmental and occupational exposures
- Immunity and immunisation status
- Risk factors for STDs
- Obstetric history
- Gynaecologic history
- General physical exam
- Assessment of socio-economic, educational and cultural context

8.1.7 Vaccination

Vaccinations should be offered to women found to be at risk for or susceptible to certain infections, namely, rubella, varicella and hepatitis B.

8.1.7.1 Screening Tests

Screening should target specific conditions relevant to the individual (see Table 8.3) counselling.

Patients should be counselled regarding the benefits of the following activities:

- Exercising
- Reducing weight before pregnancy, if overweight
- Increasing weight before pregnancy, if underweight
- Avoiding food additives
- Preventing HIV infection
- Determining the time of conception by an accurate menstrual history
- Abstaining from tobacco, alcohol and illicit drug use before and during pregnancy
- Consuming folic acid

Table 8.3 Screening tests in preconception care [1]

Screening for HIV should be strongly recommended.
A number of tests can be performed for specific indications:
Screening for STDs
Testing to assess proven aetiologies of recurrent pregnancy loss
Testing for specific diseases based on medical or reproductive history
Mantoux skin test with purified protein derivative for tuberculosis.
Screening for other genetic disorders based on family history: cystic fibrosis (CF), fragile X, mental retardation and Duchenne muscular dystrophy.
Screening for genetic disorders based on racial/ethnic background:
Sickle haemoglobinopathies (Africans, African-Americans)
B-Thalassemia (Mediterranean, SE Asia)
α-Thalassemia (Asians)
Tay-Sachs disease (Ashkenazi Jews, French Canadians)
Gaucher's, Canavan and Niemann–Pick disease (Ashkenazi Jews)
Cystic fibrosis (Caucasians and Ashkenazi Jews)

- Maintaining good control of any pre-existing medical condition

8.1.8 Preconception Interventions of Proven Benefits [1]

Preconception care has been shown repeatedly to impact positively on the outcome of pregnancies in the following situations:

1. Folic acid supplements: Reduce the occurrence of neural tube defects by two-thirds.
2. Rubella seronegativity: Rubella immunisation provides protective seropositivity and prevents the occurrence of congenital rubella syndrome.
3. HIV/AIDS: Timely antiretroviral treatment can be administered; pregnancies can be better planned.
4. Hepatitis B: Vaccination is recommended for men and women who are at risk for acquiring hepatitis B virus (HBV) infection.
5. Diabetes: A threefold increase in birth defects among infants of women with Type 1 and Type 2 diabetes without management.
6. Hypothyroidism: Dosage of levothyroxine should be adjusted in early pregnancy to maintain levels needed for neurological development.
7. Maternal PKU: Low phenylalanine diet before conception and throughout pregnancy prevents mental retardation in infants born to mothers with PKU.
8. Obesity: Associated adverse outcomes include neural tube defects, preterm birth, caesarean section and hypertension and thromboembolic disease.
9. STDs: Have been strongly associated with ectopic pregnancy, infertility and chronic pelvic pain.
10. Alcohol use: Foetal alcohol syndrome (FAS) and other alcohol-related birth defects can be prevented.
11. Anti-epileptic drugs: Some anti-epileptic drugs are known as teratogens.
12. Accutane use: Use of Accutane in pregnancy results in miscarriage and birth defects.
13. Oral anticoagulants: Warfarin is a teratogen; medications can be switched before the onset of pregnancy.
14. Smoking: Associated adverse outcomes include preterm birth and low birth weight (Table 8.4).

Table 8.4 Common conditions amenable to preconception care [1]

Diabetes	STDs
Hypertension	Repetitive pregnancy losses
Seizure disorder	Eating disorders
Thyroid disorders	Alcohol, tobacco and other drug use
Thromboembolic disease	Domestic violence
Haemoglobin disorders	Poor nutrition

8.1.9 Organisation of Preconception Care Service

A preconception care clinic should provide a framework for health promotion and disease prevention that is designed to reach all women of child-bearing age in the community [21]. Obstetricians and gynaecologists should coordinate such clinics, involving other specialists as necessary such as specialist physicians, midwives, clinical geneticists and genetic counsellors to achieve the best level of care [22].

Patients for preconception care can be recruited from the family practice clinic, family planning clinic, well-women clinics (see Table 8.5) and postnatal clinic so as to achieve adequate coverage for the community. In addition, some categories of individuals should necessarily be offered preconception care (see Table 8.6).

Constraints to Establishing Preconception Care Programme in Nigeria and the Rest of West Africa

Considering the increasing evidence for the efficacy of preconception care in improving pregnancy outcomes, it is surprising that it is yet to be introduced into routine maternity care in the West African Sub-region. Quite a number of reasons have been adduced for the slow take-off. Firstly, it has been opined that preconception care is not being implemented today in our environment because many providers are not convinced enough to offer it, health insurance is very poorly organised and many consumers lack the appropriate information about it. So, scepticism about its value is prevalent. Pregnancies occur mostly unplanned, leaving no preconception period where the women can present for care. Yet another reason could be an extension of the overall disinterest and mistrust that patients express due to their perceived negative attitude of healthcare providers [23]. Moreover, the quality of the already established forms of care, namely, prenatal care and postnatal care leaves a lot to be desired. Even then, the utilisation of antenatal care services remains very remarkable. Perhaps strengthening the provision of antenatal care will serve as a necessary attraction for introducing preconception care to our population.

The need for community education cannot be overemphasised. This is important to create awareness about preconception care and to promote the involvement of primary care physicians including medical officers in the propagation of this knowledge as well as in the provision of care. Furthermore, the critics of preconception care on the grounds that it protects every woman as a 'potential mother' should be assuaged in that preconception care is intended to foster the health of the community which includes the males, though the concept was originally built around the 'mothers'. Even then, culturally sensitive guidelines and specific indicators for tracking progress must be established in different regions of the world. Wholesale adoption of the content and delivery of preconception care from other parts of the globe may be unrealistic at this time [24].

International commitment and collaboration have grown tremendously in the last decade with various consensus statements emerging (see Table 8.7). It is our hope that Nigeria and the rest of black Africa do not remain laggards in reaping the fruit of a few bold and faithful innovators who pushed ahead with the concept of preconception care at a time when evidence for its efficacy was totally non-existent!

Goals for improving preconception care have been outlined by the CDC [1] to include the following:

- Goal 1. Improve the knowledge and attitudes and behaviours of men and women related to preconception health.
- Goal 2. Assure that all women of childbearing age in the United States receive preconception care services (i.e. evidence-based risk screening, health promotion and interventions) that will enable them to enter pregnancy in optimal health.
- Goal 3. Reduce risks indicated by a previous adverse pregnancy outcome through interventions during the interconception period, which can prevent or minimise health problems for a mother and her future children.
- Goal 4. Reduce the disparities in adverse pregnancy outcomes.

Recommendations for improving preconception health by the CDC [1] include the following:

Table 8.5 Issues of interest for preconception counselling in well women [1]

Family planning
Genetic risks: familial, ethnic and racial
Nutrition and weight
Tobacco, alcohol, medications and illicit drugs
Occupational and environmental hazards
Domestic violence
Infections and immunisation
Screening for unapparent medical disease

Table 8.6 Target population to improve preconception health and pregnancy outcome [1, 21]

Ensure all women and men of childbearing age have high reproductive awareness
Ensure all women have a reproductive life plan
Ensure all pregnancies are intended and planned
Ensure all women of childbearing age have health coverage
Ensure all women of childbearing age are screened prior to pregnancy for risks related to outcomes
Ensure women with a prior pregnancy loss have access to intensive interconception care aimed at reducing their risks
Target women with chronic medical conditions, advanced age, and women with adverse family, social, obstetric and medication history

Table 8.7 International efforts to promote preconception care

American Diabetes Association (Diabetes – 2004)
American Association of Clinical Endocrinologists (Hypothyroidism – 1999)
American Academy of Neurology (Anti-epileptic drugs)
American Heart Association/American College of Cardiologists (Anti-epileptic drugs – 2003)
The key physician/primary care provider and the obstetrician/gynaecologist should take advantage of every health encounter to provide preconception care and risk reduction before and between conceptions, the time when health encounters can improve health status (The March of Dimes Foundation)
Increase to at least 60% the proportion of primary care providers who provide age-appropriate preconception care and counselling (Healthy People 2000).
Every woman (and, when possible, her partner) contemplating pregnancy within one year should consult a prenatal care provider. Because many pregnancies are not planned, providers should include preconception counselling, when appropriate, in contacts with women and men of reproductive age.... Such care should be integrated into primary care services (USPHS Expert Panel on the Content of Prenatal Care, 1989).
All health encounters during a woman's reproductive years, particularly those that are a part of preconception care should include counselling on appropriate medical care and behaviour to optimise pregnancy outcomes (ACOG/AAP Guidelines for Perinatal Care, 5th edition, 2002).

- Recommendation 1. Individual responsibility across the life span: Encourage each woman and every couple to have a reproductive life plan.
- Recommendation 2. Consumer awareness: Increase public awareness of the importance of preconception health behaviours and increase individuals' use of preconception care services using information and tools appropriate across varying age, literacy, health literacy and cultural/linguistic contexts.
- Recommendation 3. Preventive visits: As a part of primary care visits, provide risk assessment and counselling to all women of childbearing age to reduce risks related to the outcomes of pregnancy.
- Recommendation 4. Interventions for identified risks: Increase the proportion of women who receive interventions as follow up to preconception risk screening, focusing on high priority interventions.
- Recommendation 5. Interconception care: Use the interconception period to provide intensive interventions to women who have had a prior pregnancy ending in adverse outcomes (e.g. infant death, low birth weight or preterm birth).
- Recommendation 6. Pre-pregnancy checkups: Offer, as a component of maternity care, one pre-pregnancy visit for couples planning pregnancy.
- Recommendation 7. Health coverage for low-income women: Increase Medicaid coverage among low-income women to improve access to preventive women's health, preconception and interconception care.
- Recommendation 8. Public health programmes and strategies: Infuse and integrate components of preconception health into existing local public health and related programmes, including an emphasis on those with prior adverse outcomes.
- Recommendation 9. Research: Augment research knowledge related to preconception health.
- Recommendation 10. Monitoring improvements: Maximise public health surveillance and related research mechanisms to monitor preconception health.

8.2 Prenatal Care

Prenatal care as it exists today started almost 100 years ago. The main goal at the outset was to reduce maternal mortality and morbidity. It later evolved into a programme involved with screening to assess and obviate the risk of complications in the mother and foetus. The introduction of ultrasound technology to observe the growing foetus further revolutionised prenatal care. Attending a scan session has become for many women the sole reason for attending the hospital prenatal clinic [25].

The traditional form of prenatal care is still being practiced in many parts of West Africa today, even though most of the measures and interventions included have not been proven to be beneficial. However, proof of benefit has been difficult to obtain considering the multiplicity of measures of outcome involved in prenatal schedule. Consequently, many variations of care models have been proposed to streamline the activities to what have been substantiated by available evidence to be of benefit.

Focused antenatal care model probably fits into the description of an ideal prenatal care schedule but many criticisms have also emerged [26]. In this section, we will present the traditional approach or standard model of prenatal care, discuss variations of care promoted to improve the outcome of pregnancy and consider emerging issues that may modify current practice.

8.2.1 Definition of Prenatal Care

Prenatal care is a planned programme of risk assessment, clinical observation, health education and medical management aimed at ensuring a satisfactory experience and a healthy outcome in pregnancy, labour and puerperium for both the mother and her baby.

8.2.2 Aims of Prenatal Care [27]

The aims of prenatal care include the following:

- To prevent, detect and manage those factors that adversely affect the health of mother and baby

- To provide advice, reassurance, education and support for the woman and her family
- To deal with the 'minor ailments' of pregnancy
- To provide general health screening

8.2.3 The Core Components of Prenatal Care [28]

1. Risk assessment and screening
2. Health education and medical management
3. Complication readiness
4. Birth preparedness

These objectives are aimed at early diagnosis of abnormalities and detection of asymptomatic, potentially threatening conditions in either the mother or the foetus so that the ultimate goal of ANC is to reduce maternal and perinatal mortality. Hence, the value of antenatal care in developing countries can hardly be overemphasised. Such visits may be the only opportunities available to the woman to be seen by a qualified health worker. For the 'unbooked' patient (the parturient who had no antenatal care), the complications of pregnancy remain undiagnosed and unattended as they are unlikely to be seen at the appropriate health facility when they go into labour. The unbooked status is therefore regarded as a major risk factor as associated maternal mortality is consistently more than in patients who had antenatal care [28].

8.2.4 Classification of Prenatal Care [27]

Prenatal care is organised to allow the joint provision of care between hospital consultant, general practitioner (GP) and community midwives. When the pregnant woman 'books' with a hospital consultant, continue care with either the GP or community midwife, whether or not she returns for review later in the pregnancy by the consultant's team, this is referred to as shared care. However, if potential problems are detected, an appointment with the consultant is organised.

Community-based care is anchored by the community midwife. Routine scans and investigations are requested and interpreted by them, only occasionally involving the GPs. If potential problems arise, a referral to a hospital may become necessary. This form of care is ideal only for 'low-risk' women.

Hospital-based care is really an extension of shared care. It mostly involves a structured plan of a visit to a hospital prenatal clinic for specialised care such as diabetes clinic.

Considering that a problem-free low-risk pregnancy at initial assessment may soon progress to one of high risk, it is instructive to regard risk assessment as an ongoing exercise throughout the pregnancy so that the type of care offered to a woman can change if her level of risk changes.

8.2.5 Schedule of Prenatal Clinic Visits [28]

At least three visits are recommended by the WHO with the first ideally taking place early in the pregnancy.

8.2.5.1 Booking Visit

It should preferably not be later than 12 weeks gestation. However, research has shown that most women in our environment book for prenatal care between 16 and 26 weeks gestation [2, 27, 28].

Booking History

History should include age, parity and marital status. Women at the extremes of reproductive ages are at greater risk of certain pregnancy complications (like foetal chromosomal abnormalities in older women). Past medical, obstetric and gynaecological histories are explored in details, as these may have a major impact on the pregnancy risk assessment. Family and social history may be insightful and these too should be adequately evaluated.

Examination

- General examination should emphasise pallor, oedema, varicosities and dental hygiene.
- Blood pressure check is mandatory.
- Complete physical examination, which must include auscultation of heart sounds and breast palpation.
- Examination of the abdomen: This should include an inspection for fullness, surgical and scarification scars, obvious masses and herniae, striae gravidarum, linea nigra and foetal movements. In patients whose pregnancies are less than 20 weeks gestation, general superficial palpation for tenderness would be followed by an examination of the nine regions of the abdomen for masses or deep tenderness. In more advanced pregnancies, the latter step is not performed. Instead, the liver, spleen and kidneys are examined in the usual manner.

The abdominal examination is completed by the evaluation of the uterus and its contents.

Booking Investigations

All pregnant women are encouraged to undergo screening for a number of health problems which can adversely affect the pregnancy or the foetus. The blood and urine tests and other investigations frequently performed are shown in Table 8.8.

Table 8.8 Prenatal care investigations [28]

Haemoglobin concentration and packed cell volume
Blood group and genotype
Rhesus status and indirect Coomb's test for Rhesus negative women
Venereal disease research laboratory (VDRL) test
Hepatitis B surface antigen (HBsAg)
Human immunodeficiency virus test
Rubella antibody (optional)
Urine analysis for acetone, sugar and protein
Cervical smear (optional)
Ultrasound scan (optional)
Fasting blood sugar and post-prandial sugar test (optional)

Prophylactic Drugs in Pregnancy [28]

Supplemental folic acid, 5 mg and 200 mg of ferrous sulphate (60 mg elemental iron) should be given daily.

Prophylactic antimalarial drugs: Recommended drug is Fansidar (sulphadoxine and pyrimethamine combination), three tablets at once, giving at least three doses in the course of pregnancy, at least 4 weeks apart and commencing in the second trimester. Other drugs include proguanil, pyrimethamine and chloroquine especially in patients who do not tolerate Fansidar.

Some patients may also require vitamin A, calcium and iodine supplementation, antihelminthics for hookworm infestation, antibiotic prophylaxis for immunosuppression, and tetanus toxoid immunisation.

8.2.5.2 Subsequent Prenatal Visits

These are scheduled for:

- Every 4 weeks up to 28 weeks
- Every 2 weeks up to 36 weeks
- Thereafter, weekly visits until delivery

8.2.5.3 At Every Visit

- · Determine her general condition of health.
- · Encourage her to express any complaints and uncertainties.
- · Evaluate weight, blood pressure and urine analysis. Haemoglobin evaluation should be done every 4 weeks.

General Examination for Pallor, Pedal Oedema

· Abdominal examination: for the uterus and its contents. The symphysis-fundal height (estimated in centimetres) must be correlated with the presumed gestational age. The mother should start to feel the baby's movements (quickening) by 18–20 weeks.

After 26 weeks, using Leopold's manoeuvres, palpate for the lie, presentation and the position of the foetus. Appropriate action should be taken if there is any disparity by more than two estimated weeks. By this time, the foetal heart sounds should be audible with a Pinard's stethoscope; whilst with the Sonicaid Doppler monitor, it would be audible by 14 weeks gestation.

Continued education on hygiene, diet and antenatal exercises should be ensured; preparation for delivery and mothercraft should be discussed.

At 36 weeks gestation:

- An overview of the course of pregnancy should be carried out.
- A pelvic assessment may be indicated.
- A tentative decision of mode of delivery including special instructions with regards to the course of labour and puerperium should be clearly documented and the patient counselled.

Prenatal Advice

- Diet should be adequate, balanced and easily digestible to accommodate the extra requirement of a baby. Advice must, however, be realistic with due consideration of the socio-economic conditions and food habits of the community.
- The pregnant mother must complete her immunisation schedules (see antenatal immunisation below).
- The use of sensible clothing and shoes should be advised.
- Avoidance of smoking, alcohol, caffeine and self-medication should be emphasised.
- Coitus may take place according to her inclinations. Nevertheless, the process should be gentle. The male superior position should, however, be discouraged in the third trimester of pregnancy.
- Explain the physiological basis for the minor ailments of pregnancy and how to recognise and take appropriate action when significant signs occur.
- In the presence of the serious symptoms, namely, persistent headaches, labour pains, bleeding per vaginam and passage of fluid per vaginam, diminished or excessive foetal movements, they should report immediately to the hospital.
- Breasts and nipple hygiene should be taught including regularly lifting nipples up if they are retracted.
- Need for completion of her immunisation schedule should be stressed.
- Prenatal exercises for physical and mental relaxation.
- Dental hygiene should be emphasised, and counselling on the increased tendency of bleeding gums during pregnancy given.

Minor Ailments in Pregnancy [29]

Nausea and vomiting: Early sign of pregnancy. The symptom is usually worse before midday. This should usually disappear by 12 to 16 weeks of gestational age. Advise patient to take small, dry, frequent, non-oily meals. Anti-emetics may be prescribed.

Heartburn: Quite a common complaint during pregnancy. Due to reflux oesophagitis following upward displacement and compression of the stomach by the uterus in addition to the relaxation of the lower oesophageal sphincter caused by increased progesterone levels in pregnancy. Advise on the need for smaller meals and sitting up rather than lying flat or bending. Antacids may be indicated.

Backaches: Secondary to hormone-induced pelvic relaxation and the dragging weight of the uterus. Advise regular rest, mild analgesia, for example, paracetamol (1 g) three times a day for not more than a 3-day course at any one occasion.

Constipation: This is usually due to reduced gastric emptying and slow bowel transition. The patient should be asked to increase roughage (vegetables and fruits) in her diet. Prescribe stool softeners with reluctance.

Leg cramps: Periodic numbness and 'pricks and needles', usually worse at bedtime. Calcium or magnesium supplements may be helpful.

Vaginal discharge: Leucorrhoea of pregnancy. This may be copious but not foul-smelling and not associated with pruritus. The patient should be able to distinguish this from an abnormal discharge and leaking membranes.

Haemorrhoids: Worse during pregnancy; usually, would retract after pregnancy. Analgesic ointments may be indicated.

Pica: Irrational cravings for unusual and normally inedible products like clay, sand, ice lumps and soap. The cause is unknown; although there may be an association with iron deficiency. Patients need to be counselled on possible dangers.

Prenatal Immunisation [28]

In most developing countries, routine tetanus immunisation is indicated. This consists of five doses of intramuscular Tetanus toxoid (0.5 ml).

- First dose (T1) should be given at the first antenatal visit
- Second dose (T2) 4 weeks later
- Third dose (T3) 6 months after T2
- Fourth dose (T4) 1 year after T3 or next pregnancy
- Fifth dose (T5) one year after T4 or next pregnancy

Live vaccines (e.g. smallpox, varicella, HPV, measles, mumps, rubella, zoster and oral polio) are contraindicated in pregnancy. Killed vaccines (e.g. typhoid and cholera) when indicated are best given from the second trimester. Tetanus toxoid, diphtheria toxoid, Hepatitis B, influenza and meningococcal vaccines are safe in pregnancy. A pregnant woman who is non-immune to measles, hepatitis A or B, chicken pox or rabies and comes in contact with any of these, may be given 2 ml of human gamma globulin within 3 days of the exposure (for passive immunity) irrespective of the gestational age.

Focused Antenatal Care (FANC)

Focused antenatal care (FANC) is a woman-centred, goal-oriented care model which emphasises evidenced-based interventions in pregnancy, encouraging good quality service rather than quantity of visits. It recommends four visits for basic care clients with specific targets and interventions tied to each visit. Women who have indications for specialised care are appropriately linked based on their specific requirements. FANC could possibly reduce the cost of implementation of the standard schedule of care currently undertaken with an average of 10–14 visits per patient during pregnancy. However, criticisms of this model have highlighted the limited list of conditions used to classify the women into basic or specialised care; the observation that conditions specific to West African Sub-region such as malaria and sickle cell anaemia were not given prominence in the qualifying form, as well as the design, to have the postnatal visit schedule on the 7th day post-delivery, which often bears the socio-cultural significance of being the day for 'naming ceremony' in our environment.

Traditional Versus Modified Form of Prenatal Care

At the beginning of the modern-day prenatal care in England, there were reports of observation that women who were reviewed between 10 and 24 times in pregnancy had lower perinatal mortality rates. And so the drive to continue to reduce mortality (both maternal and perinatal) allowed the introduction of various procedures and interventions without necessarily establishing their need or safety [24]. With this came newer technologies like ultrasound scan, continuous foetal monitoring, and the ability to induce labour. However, the fact that these new interventions had not undergone proper proofs of benefit before introduction to practice meant that benefit to the whole population of women was never established [25, 30]. This realisation gradually paved the way for consumer groups and some professional groups to start to question the utility of the procedures, the need to attend hospital as well as the need for prenatal care.

Since the 1990s, these agitations regarding the pattern of maternity care provision entered the political arena culminating in the 'Changing Birth' document that among its other indicators outlined the need to reduce the number of prenatal visits for low-risk mothers, as well as improve choice, information and continuity of care for all women [25].

There is yet no evidence that fewer visits will compromise the pregnancy outcome. However, the initial risk evaluation of the pregnancy at booking is vital to determine women with a higher risk of complications and target them for a more intensive level of care. If pregnancy is deemed to be 'low-risk', the basic standard of care is warranted.

Pitfalls of Prenatal Care in West African Sub-region [28]

Although prenatal care is of immense benefit to the patient, there are pitfalls that nevertheless tend to reduce its overall value. These include:

High-risk pregnancies that would best benefit from prenatal care (especially associated with low socio-economic status) are the least likely to present for care. Its execution requires enormous medical and nursing time and patience. It involves endless waiting for patients who in fact have a physiological condition. Quite recently, it has been demonstrated (in low-risk pregnancies) that the number of prenatal visits may be safely reduced to a total of four throughout the duration of the pregnancy (see FANC above). Prenatal care may increase unnecessary interventions like induction of labour or caesarean section from misdiagnosis of intrauterine growth restriction or foetal distress. Painfully, an uneventful prenatal period does not necessarily guarantee an uncomplicated intrapartum or postnatal period.

8.3 Conclusion

Many pregnancies are at risk of complications. It is now obvious that reducing this risk of complications can best be achieved by establishing a continuum of care spanning from preconception, through prenatal to intrapartum and postnatal periods. Interconception health has also begun to gain prominence and may add value to the output of maternity care in the nearest future.

What is most striking in this spate of interesting revelations regarding emerging issues in maternity care is that Africa and the rest of the developing world have yet to imbibe the spirit of wholesome maternity care, especially in the area of preconception care. Joining the progressives in the debate is the best way to ensure that healthy women become healthy mothers and to increase the chance of producing healthy babies.

8.4 Summary

Preconception counselling is still in its infancy in developing countries. Many barriers to its establishment have been noted to include poor infrastructure and a low level of motivation on the part of the healthcare provider, as well as poor knowledge of the unique role of pre-pregnancy management in the overall outcome of maternity care. Preconception counselling mainly involves maternal assessment, screening, vaccination and specific counselling; prenatal care revolves around risk assessment and screening. It also involves health education, medical management, complication readiness and birth preparedness. Perhaps, the organisation of shared care programme by the midwives and obstetricians in the prenatal period will provide a template for introducing a preconception counselling programme as a part of a well-coordinated and properly conducted comprehensive maternity care that will guarantee the much-needed improvements in maternal and perinatal mortality in Africa and the rest of the developing world.

References

1. Centres for Disease Control and Prevention. Recommendations to improve preconception health and health care shared care p. MMWR Recommend Rep. 2006;55(RR-06):1–23.
2. Gharoro EP, Igbafe AA. Antenatal care: some characteristics of the booking visit in a major hospital in the developing world. Med Sci Monit. 2000;6(3):519–22.
3. Waggoner MR. Motherhood preconceived: the emergence of the preconception health and health care initiative. J Health Polit Policy Law. 2013;38(2):345–71.
4. Wald N. Folic acid and the prevention of neural tube defects. Ann N Y Acad Sci. 1993;678:112–29.
5. Atrash H, Adams M, Cordero J, Howse J. Time to act on missed opportunities to improve perinatal outcomes. Mat Child Health J. 2006;10:S3–S11.
6. March of Dimes Birth Defects Foundation. March of Dimes updates: is early prenatal care too late? Contemp Ob/Gyn. 2002;12:54t wi.
7. Atrash H, Jack BW, Johnson K. Preconception care: a 2008 update. Curr Opin Obstet Gynecol. 2008;6:581–9.
8. Wildschut HI, van Vliet-Lachotzki EH, Boon BM, Lie Fong S, Landkroon AP, Steegers EA. Preconception care: an essential part of the care for mother and child. Ned Tijdschr Geneeskd. 2006;150(24):1326–30.
9. Oranu EO, Ojule JD, Nnah EW. Preconception care in a southern Nigeria tertiary institution. Niger J Med. 2015;24(1):58–63.
10. Ezegwui HU, Dim C, Dim N, Ikeme AC. Preconception care in South Eastern Nigeria. J Obstet Gynaecol. 2008;28(8):765–8.
11. Vause T, Jones L, Evans M, Wilkie V. Preconception health awareness in infertility patients. J Obs Gynaecol Can. 2009;31(8):717–20.
12. Bastani F, Hashemi S, Bastani N, Haghani H. Impact of preconception health education on health locus of control and self-efficacy in women. East Mediterr Health J. 2016;16(4):396–401.
13. Ajayi GO, Popoola AT, Dina T, Okorie N. Pre-pregnancy counselling in Lagos: a report on the first 1,000 cases. Clin Exp Obstet Gynecol. 2013;40(3):359–60.
14. Jensen D, Korsholm L, Ovesen P. Peri-conceptional AIC and risk of serious adverse pregnancy outcome in 933 women with Type 1 diabetes. Diabetes Care. 2009;32:1046–8.
15. Schaefer-Graf M, Buchanan T, Xiang A. Patterns of congenital anomalies and relationship to initial maternal fasting glucose levels in pregnancies complicated by Type2 and gestational diabetes. Am J Obstet Gynaecol. 2000;182:313–20.
16. Correa A, Gilboa S, Besser L. Diabetes mellitus and birth defects. Am J Obstet Gynaecol. 2008;199:237 e1oll.
17. Rey E, Attie C, Bonin A. The effects of first trimester diabetes control on the incidence of macrosomia. Am J Obstet Gynaecol. 1999;181:202–6.
18. Tennant PW, Glinianaia SV, Bilous RW, Rankin J, Bell R. Preexisting diabetes, maternal glycated Haemoglobin, and

the risks of fetal and infant death: a population-based study. Diabetologia. 2014;57:285–94.
19. American Diabetes Association. Preconception care of women with diabetes. Clin Diab. 2000;18(3). Accessed from: http://journal.diabetes.org/clinicaldiabetes/V18N32000/pg124.htm 30 April, 2016.
20. Nafisehsadat N, Shahnaz K, Ashraf K. Preconception care in diabetic women. J Educ Health Promot. 2015;4:8.
21. Omigbodun A. Preconception and antenatal care. In: Kwawukume EY, Emuveyan EE, editors. Comprehensive obstetrics in the tropics. 1st ed. Dansoman: Asante and Hittscher Printing Press Ltd; 2002. p. 7t–14.
22. Preconception care: a guide for optimising pregnancy outcome. American College of Obstetrician and Gynaecologist, District II, Newyork and the New York State Department of Health. 2001. Accessed from: www.health.ny.gov//publications//2026.pdf. 30 April 2016.
23. Suleman H, Sambo M, Ibrahim M. Barriers to utilisation of maternal health services in a semi urban community in Northern Nigeria: the clientsst, rspective. Niger Med J. 2013;54(1):27–32.
24. Christiansen C, Chandra-mouli V, Ogbaselassie L, Willumsen J. Meeting to develop a global consensus on preconception care to reduce maternal and childhood mortality and morbidity. Geneva: WHO Headquarters; 2013.
25. Baker PN. Modern maternity care. In: Obstetrics by ten teachers. 18th ed. London: Hodder Arnold; 2006. p. 14r–19.
26. Ekele BA, Shehu CE, Ahmed Y, Fache M. What is the place of the new WHO antenatal care model in a teaching hospital setting? Trop Dr. 2008;38(1):21–4.
27. Baker PN. Antenatal care. In: Obstetrics by ten teachers. 18th ed. London: Hodder Arnold; 2006. p. 72r–81.
28. Okpere E. Protocol for antenatal care. In: Okpere E, editor. Clinical obstetrics. Revised ed. Benin City: UNIBEN Press; 2004. p. 1E–7.
29. Arulkumaran S. Minor symptoms in pregnancy. In: Arulkumaran S, Symonds IM, Fowlie A, editors. Oxford handbook of obstetrics and gynaecology, 2nd impression. New Delhi: Oxford University Press; 2004. p. 57d–66.
30. Stirrat GM. Obstetric care. In: Aids to obstetrics and gynaecology for MRCOG. 4th ed. Bristol: Churchill Livingstone; 1997. p. P3–10.

9 Ultrasound in Labour and Delivery

Morounfolu Olaleye Thompson

Learning Objectives

After reading this chapter, the learner will be able to:

- Describe the indications for an ultrasound scan during labour and delivery.
- Define the primary terminologies pertinent to the use of ultrasound.
- Describe the basic and advanced applications of ultrasound during labour and delivery.
- Discuss the evidence and limitations of intrapartum ultrasound.
- Evaluate the future utilisation of ultrasound during labour and delivery.

9.1 Introduction

Diagnostic ultrasound has a well-established safety record [1] and is appropriate for use in both developed and developing countries [2]. The utility of ultrasound in labour and delivery spans antenatal, intrapartum and immediate postpartum applications, and although assessments of the health impact of ultrasound use in obstetrics have mainly been carried out in the western world, where there is strong evidence for its selective use, there is also good evidence of benefit in developing countries [3].

Abnormal, difficult, and prolonged labour are associated with an increased maternal risk of complications such as intrapartum haemorrhage, uterine rupture, and sepsis [4], and this holds particularly for the areas in developing countries where healthcare infrastructure is minimal or lacking. The associated neonatal complications include low Apgar scores, neonatal hypoxia, acidosis, neonatal seizures, hypoxic ischaemic encephalopathy and stillbirth [5].

Prolonged and difficult labour and delivery are associated with the risks of neonatal encephalopathy, cerebral palsy, with possible long-term disability [5], as well as the risk of losing either mother or child or, worse still, both. There are published reports on other attendant intrapartum and immediate postpartum complications including maternal infection, urinary retention, haematoma and wound dehiscence, many of which relate to the high-income countries [6]. The reports from developing countries when access to skilled personnel is limited, or infrastructure inadequate, reflect the graver significance of such labour and delivery complications where severe complications such as obstetric fistula may result [7, 8].

Early recognition of dysfunctional labour and prompt implementation of corrective measures are important but depend on the accuracy and reliability of currently available means of obstetric diagnosis and assessment. The superiority of ultrasound in identifying problems once they have occurred is well documented [9–12]; however, its accuracy in prediction remains a challenge in antenatal and intrapartum care probably because it is highly operator dependent.

Assisted vaginal delivery and caesarean section are solutions to prolonged or difficult labour, but each bears associated risks and determining which is the safer route in different circumstances remains an inexact science. Short- and long-term complications of prolonged or difficult vaginal delivery include obstetric anal sphincter injuries, urinary and faecal incontinence [13]. There are, however, also severe long-term maternal morbidity and mortality risks associated with multiple caesarean deliveries which make prevention of the index caesarean section an important responsibility for modern obstetricians [14, 15].

M. O. Thompson (✉)
Fetal Medicine, Queens University Hospital, Romford, UK

Institute of Health Sciences, Barts and The London School of Medicine and Dentistry, Queen Mary University of London, London, UK
e-mail: moethompson@doctors.net.uk

F. Okonofua et al. (eds.), *Contemporary Obstetrics and Gynecology for Developing Countries*,
https://doi.org/10.1007/978-3-030-75385-6_9

9.2 Basic Considerations – Equipment and Safety

There is no requirement for overly expensive or sophisticated equipment; however, a machine with basic colour Doppler capability is preferable [16], and portability (mobility and versatility) are quite important considerations [17]. Acceptability of ultrasound examinations by women in developing countries is reportedly very high, often for non-clinical reasons [18, 19]. To promote a wider, more appropriate and effective application of ultrasound while maintaining safety and good standards in this environment, intensive training of qualified physicians in ultrasound is essential [3].

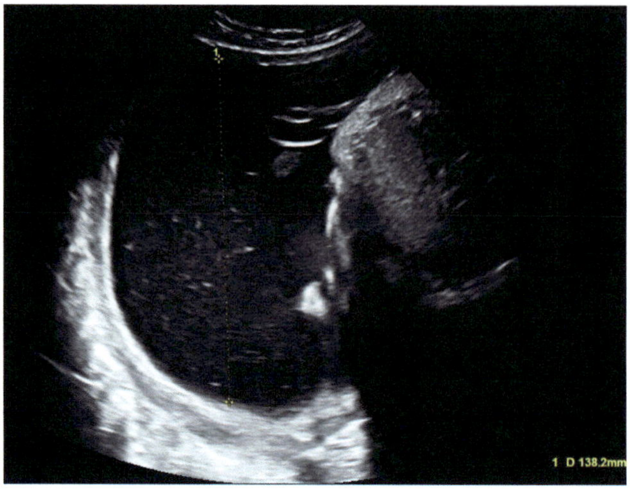

Fig. 9.1 Abnormally increased amniotic fluid volume (Polyhydramnios)

9.3 Indications for Ultrasound Use on Labour and Delivery

9.3.1 Antepartum

What Are We Trying to Achieve?

1. Assess maternal and fetal status before the onset of labour particularly where women present in late gestation for pregnancy care.
2. Prediction and diagnosis of preterm delivery with its highly significant public health burden.
3. Assessment of gestational age and fetal size, especially in unbooked patients in late pregnancy.
4. Determine fetal and uteroplacental abnormalities that may have an impact on labour outcome, cause deviation from the normal pattern of labour or indicate a different mode of delivery.
5. Diagnose conditions that indicate urgent delivery or immediate in utero transfer to units with more appropriate care facilities.

Indications for ultrasound examination on labour and delivery can be maternal or foeto-placental. In the most basic form, ultrasound in labour and delivery should include an assessment of fetal presentation, heart activity, number of fetuses, placental location, amniotic fluid and basic measurements.

9.3.1.1 Maternal Conditions

A maternal body mass index >30 makes abdominal palpation and foetal monitoring difficult and occasionally impossible and ultrasound assessment may be required prior to or during labour. Maternal diabetes predisposes to significantly above average fetal size or macrosomia and excessive amniotic fluid volume (see Fig. 9.1) which increase the risks of

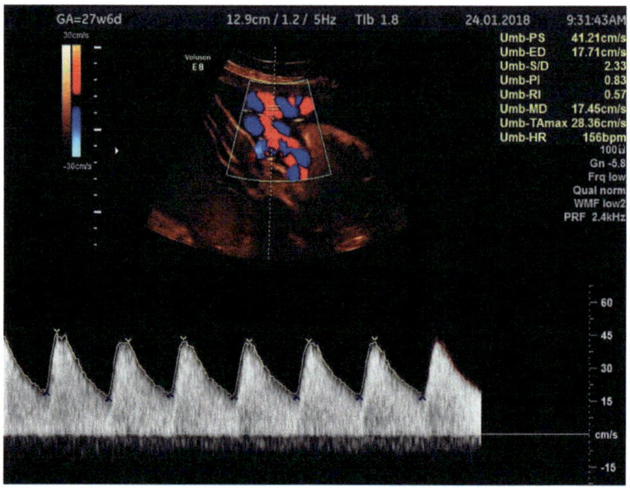

Fig. 9.2 Normal umbilical artery Doppler waveform

labour and delivery, and both can be assessed using ultrasound. However, even with ultrasound scan use, morbid maternal obesity could still prove technically difficult and such a limitation should not be overlooked but clearly reported.

The hypertensive disorders of pregnancy may be complicated by intra-uterine foetal growth restriction (IUGR) making an ultrasound assessment of fetal size, amniotic fluid volume and umbilical artery Dopplers (Fig. 9.2) important in the assessment of perinatal risk. Where available, Doppler ultrasound helps to predict and assess maternal and fetal complications, and the role of abnormal uterine artery Dopplers in predicting uteroplacental complications is well established [20].

Other maternal medical conditions such as viral infections and blood group incompatibility with fetal sensitisation

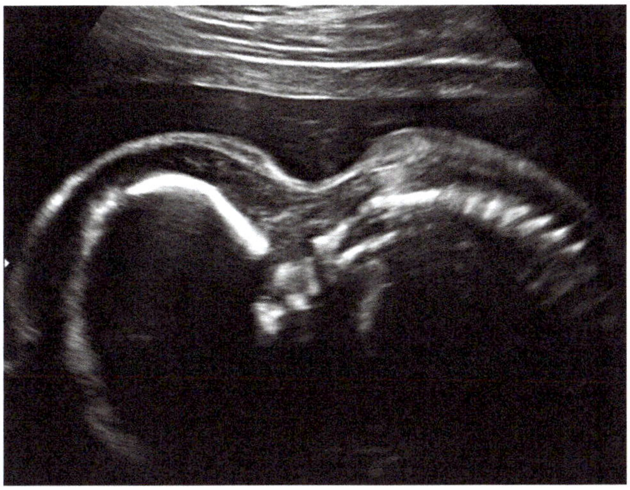

Fig. 9.3 Severe non-immune fetal hydrops

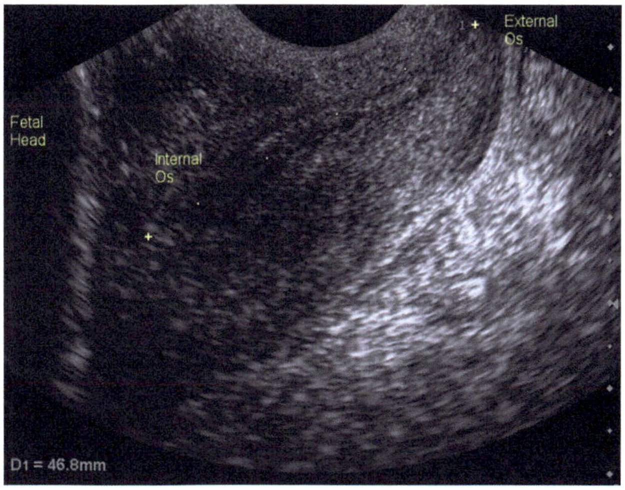

Fig. 9.4 A normal cervix length at 20 weeks

indicate preliminary assessments in labour and delivery to exclude the presence of fetal anaemia or hydrops as a matter of urgency (Fig. 9.3).

9.3.1.2 Prediction and Diagnosis of Preterm Labour

Preterm birth is the greatest contributor to neonatal deaths and disability [35], and accurate prediction will assist in finding effective prevention. Newham et al. [36] conducted serial digital assessments and compared the Bishop score with the cervical score (cervix length minus cervical diameter above the internal os) in 2916 singleton pregnancies. A correlation was found for preterm birth <35 weeks with a Bishop score > 4 or cervical score < 1.5 at 22–24 weeks gestation [36]. Recently, the most useful parameter identified is the measurement of the cervical length [37, 38], and in a study of 58,807 pregnancies, the best prediction of extreme spontaneous preterm birth at 24–28 weeks gestation was obtained by combining cervical length with a maternal history of previous preterm birth, high BMI, black ethnicity and cigarette smoking with an area under the receiver-operating characteristics curve (AUC) of 0.903 [35]. The close association demonstrated with ethnicity implies higher chances of successful screening for preterm labour in this environment, which is crucial considering the wide variation in availability and quality of neonatal care services. Active management is advised in women with a short cervix of 15 mm or less based on the very high likelihood of spontaneous preterm delivery ensuing (Figs. 9.4 and 9.5).

9.3.1.3 Assessing Gestational Age

Uncertain dates are a major issue in developing countries because of the widespread lack of early pregnancy dating; additionally some women calculate their periods based on lunar months, while others do not keep a clear record. Measurements of the fetal head, abdomen and long bones provide a reasonable estimate of fetal size and, when obtained serially, the growth. The performance and applications of basic fetal ultrasound biometry are well covered in standard ultrasound texts and will not be discussed further.

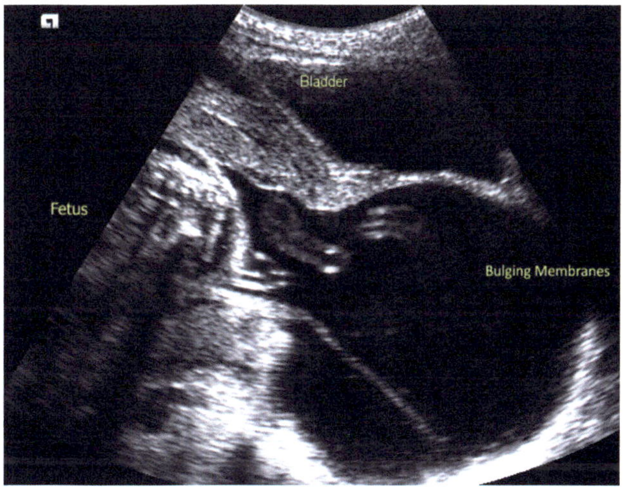

Fig. 9.5 A severely shortened dilated cervix with bulging membranes

9.3.1.4 Novel Late Pregnancy Dating Markers

Women in developing countries often present for the first time in the third trimester, a period when standard fetal biometric estimates of gestational age are least accurate. Women who attend late in pregnancy can create difficulty in establishing dates, particularly those presenting with suspected preterm labour where dating is essential to assess whether or not to use tocolysis to permit steroid prophylaxis or to expedite in utero transfer. The circumstances may therefore dictate a different approach to the use of ultrasound in labour and delivery in high-income countries.

9.3.1.5 Fetal Epiphyseal Ossification Centres

The use of fetal ossification centres can be helpful. The main fetal ossification centres are visualised on ultrasound as egg-shaped echoic areas [21] (Fig. 9.6). Chinn et al. assessed the reliability of ultrasound visualisation of fetal lower limb epiphyseal ossification during the last trimester of pregnancy and reported 95% accuracy for the distal femoral epiphyseal ossification centre (DFE) and the proximal tibial epiphyseal ossification centre (PTE) in estimating gestational age [22]. The presence of a DFE indicated a gestational age ≥33 weeks, and the presence of the PTE was highly predictive of a gestational age ≥35 weeks.

Similar findings are reported by Birang et al., following a study of 312 normal pregnancies between 20 and 40 weeks, who confirmed that the calcaneal ossification centre was detectable by 24 weeks of gestation, the talar ossification centre from 26 weeks and the distal femoral epiphyseal and proximal tibial epiphyseal ossification centres, from 32 to 36 weeks, respectively [23].

In a further study by Goldstein et al., the presence of a DFE measuring 1–2 mm was associated with a gestational age of >33 weeks in 87.0% of fetuses, and when ≥3 mm, it was associated with a gestational age >37 weeks in 85% of fetuses. The PTE, which is always absent before 34 weeks' gestation, was observed in 100% of fetuses at 39 weeks of gestation [24].

Areas of clinical concern where the use of ossification centres may help in the assessment of fetal maturity are in cases of threatened preterm labour, suspected IUGR, or where induction of labour (IOL) is contemplated for maternal reasons in pregnancies with uncertain dates or late presentation. Other specific clinical situations include oligohydramnios (Fig. 9.7), where fetal head and abdominal compression create difficulty in obtaining measurements.

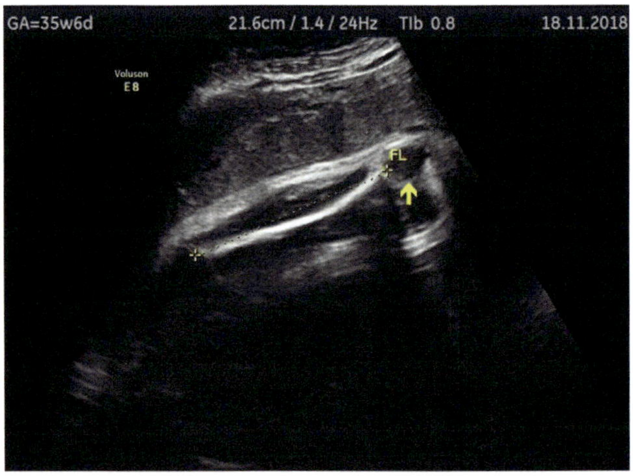

Fig. 9.6 A distal femoral epiphysis approaching 36 weeks gestation (yellow arrow)

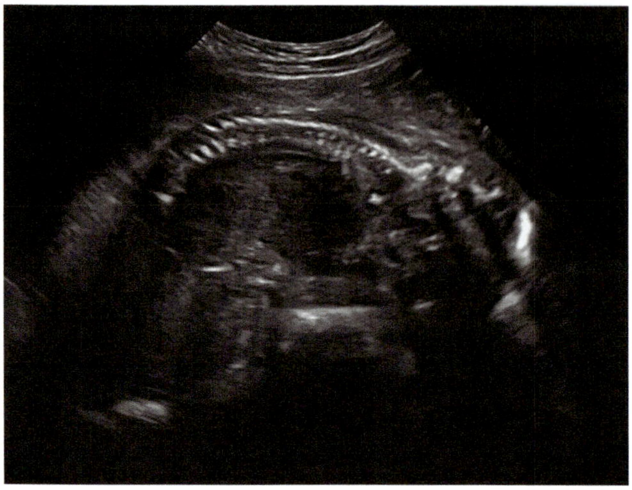

Fig. 9.7 Severely reduced amniotic fluid volume (oligohydramnios)

9.3.1.6 Trans Cerebellar Diameter (TCD)

The normal fetal cerebellum has a transverse diameter (TCD) that maintains constancy in its growth irrespective of the fetal growth pattern, is independent of fetal head shape and demonstrates less biological variation than other intracranial structures [25]. Cerebellar growth appears to be spared in asymmetrical intrauterine growth restriction (IUGR) and therefore remains a good marker for pregnancy dating even with this pregnancy complication [26]. It may also be useful in conditions where routine biometry is not useful, limb defects, skeletal abnormalities and abdominal wall defects.

The cerebellum appears like a horizontally rotated figure eight in the intracranial posterior fossa behind the thalami and in front of the cisterna magna. Measurements are traditionally obtained in an axial view, placing the calipers on the outer, lateral edges of the cerebellar hemispheres (see Fig. 9.8). As a rule of thumb, the TCD in millimetres correlates with the gestational age in weeks up to 22–24 weeks, and after this time, the direct correlation no longer exists [25]. When charted on a normogram, there is a 1–2 week difference between TCD and gestational age at 28–30 weeks and a 4–6 week difference at 32 weeks or greater [25]. The TCD is particularly valuable when the gestational age is unknown or asymmetrical IUGR is suspected provided aneuploidy is excluded [25] and has been shown to be of good predictive accuracy [26] and reproducibility in an African

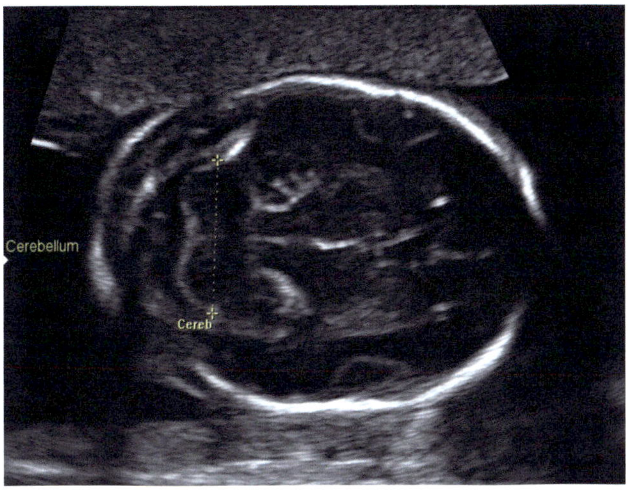

Fig. 9.8 Measurement of the Trans-Cerebellar Diameter

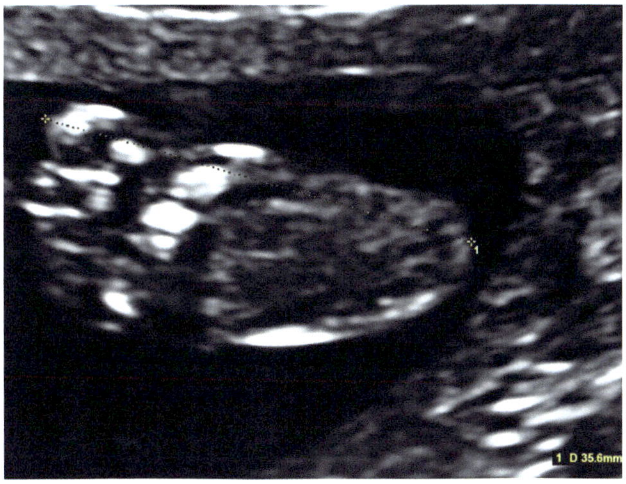

Fig. 9.9 Fetal foot length

population [27]. Caution is advocated in assessing suspected assymetric IUGR [28].

9.3.1.7 Foot Length

Foetal foot length can be measured from 12 weeks by placing the calipers from the outer margin of the posterior heel to the outer margin of the great toe in either the plantar or longitudinal plane (Fig. 9.9). Although fetal foot length is reported to correlate linearly with the gestational age with an accuracy similar to the fetal biparietal diameter and femur length, it may be less useful in IUGR [25].

Other approaches such as the use of biometric ratios, orbital diameters, fetal kidney length and fetal long bones other than the femur are reported but with limited application [25, 29–31].

9.3.1.8 Placental Localisation

A crucial step in modern obstetric care, now undertaken routinely at the mid-trimester scan, is placental localisation to exclude placenta praevia which is defined as partial or complete placental implantation in the lower segment of the uterus. It is classified by ultrasound imaging according to clinical relevance: if the placenta lies over the internal cervical os, it is considered a major praevia; if the leading edge of the placenta is in the lower uterine segment but not covering the cervical os, minor or partial praevia exists (see Figs. 9.10 and 9.11).

Despite the awareness that the distance between the placental edge and cervical os is inversely proportional to the risks of antepartum and intrapartum bleeding, and chances of avoiding a Caesarean delivery, accurate localisation is not always accomplished and clinical judgment remains paramount [32]. The cut-off of 2.0 cm held in RCOG guidelines

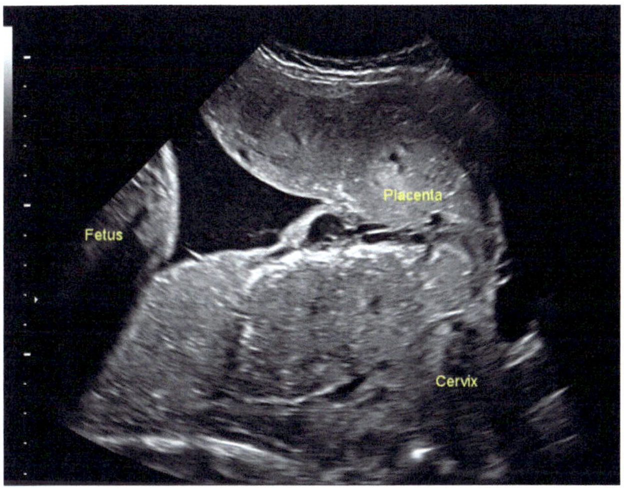

Fig. 9.10 A placenta in the lower uterine segment completely covering the internal cervical os

is still subject to intra- and inter-observer variation and even with the recommended trans-vaginal third-trimester ultrasound scan in uncertain cases, selection of the appropriate cut-off for a trial of vaginal delivery remains difficult with a false negative rate of 2.3% [32]. There are a number of reasons for this variation, including bladder filling, the dynamic nature of the cervix and posterior or lateral placentation to mention a few. In addition, the vaginal bleeding risk remains significant even with low lying placentas within 2–4 cm of the cervix [33] and in one series hysterectomy was required in 3.4% of these [34]. Despite these issues, it is important to ensure that placental site is determined prior to or on arrival in the labour and delivery room before undertaking any procedures to avoid provoking genital tract bleeding.

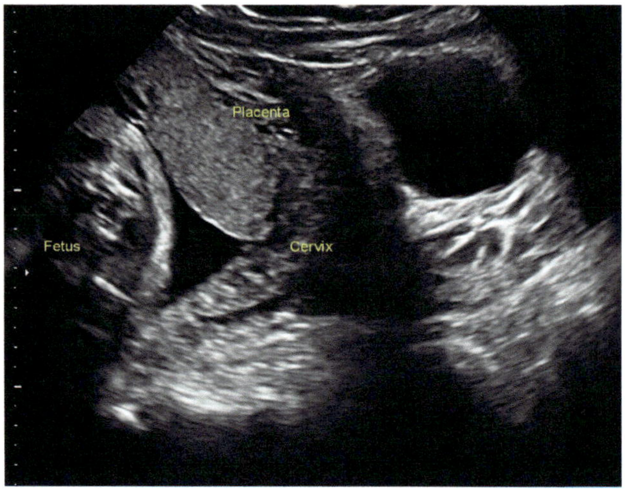

Fig. 9.11 An anterior low lying placenta encroaching on the edge of the internal cervical os

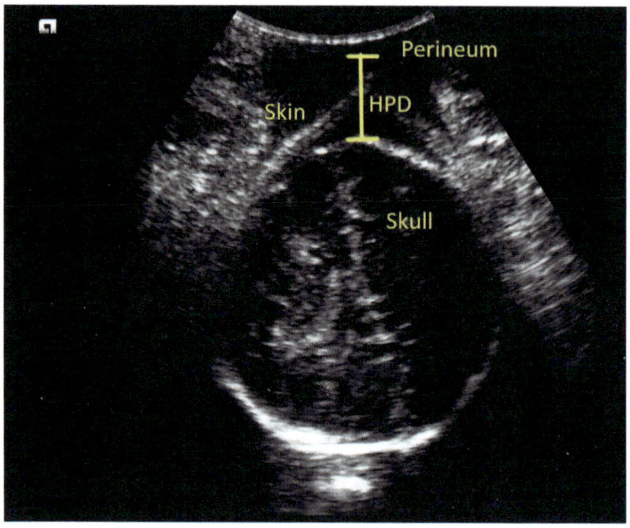

Fig. 9.12 Fetal head engagement - head perineal distance measurement

9.3.2 Intrapartum

What are we trying to achieve?

1. Prediction of successful induction of labour
2. Prediction of dystocia, difficult or prolonged labour and assisted delivery
3. Assessment of progress in labour, diagnosis of prolonged or arrested labour
4. Prediction of mode of delivery
5. Prediction of fetal size/birth weight/risk of uterine rupture

9.3.2.1 Prediction of Successful Induction of Labour

The artificial initiation of labour is a common obstetric intervention, which in a WHO Global Survey on Maternal and Perinatal Health of 373 healthcare facilities in 24 countries and nearly 300,000 births, and it was undertaken in 9.6% of the deliveries [39]. In low- to-medium-income countries, this relatively lower rate compared with the average figure of 25% for high-income countries may partly reflect the confidence of clinicians assessing gestational age and monitoring pregnancy reliably in an environment with presentation often late in gestation [39–41].

The traditional method of predicting a successful induction of labour is based on favourability of the cervix as assessed by the Bishop score [42]. This method is subjective and systematic review has shown a poor predictive value for the outcome of induction [43]. Pandis et al. demonstrated in a multicentre study where trans-vaginal ultrasound (TVUS) measurements were compared with the different components of the Bishop score and that only the cervical length measurement provided any significant contribution to predicting the likelihood of vaginal delivery within 24 hours [44]. This was corroborated by later studies even after including factors such as fetal head position and maternal body mass index (BMI) [45, 46]. Trans-perineal ultrasound (TPU) measurements of the fetal head-perineum distance (Fig. 9.12) have also shown promise in predicting successful labour induction ending in vaginal delivery within 24 hours [47]. Crane et al. having conducted a review of these methods reported that both TVUs and Bishop score reasonably predicted successful labour induction [likelihood ratio (LR) = 1.82, 95% confidence interval (CI) = 1.51–2.20 and LR = 2.10, 95% CI = 1.67–2.64, respectively] [48]. The vagino-cervical fetal fibronectin (fFN) and Bishop score also predicted successful induction (LR = 1.49, 95% CI = 1.20–1.85 and LR = 2.62, 95% CI = 1.88–3.64, respectively). However, neither TVUS nor fFN was shown to be significantly superior to the Bishop score, therefore whether ultrasound techniques can replace the digital assessment of the cervix for this purpose remains debatable [48, 49].

9.3.2.2 Prediction of Dystocia, Difficult or Prolonged Labour and Delivery

Labour progression and arrest disorders are common, occurring in 20.8% of labours ending in a vaginal birth [50]. The key components of advancing labour are progressive cervical dilatation along with progressive rotation and descent of the presenting part. These are in turn dependent on the strength and effectiveness of uterine contractions. Anthropological comparisons with non-human primates suggest that the necessity for human babies to negotiate the curvatures in the human birth canal is a major contributory factor.

Although progress in labour is mainly influenced by uterine contractions, maternal pelvic capacity and fetal size, added factors that play a role in determining labour outcome include the fetal lie, presentation, position and attitude. The fetal lie is the relation of the fetal longitudinal axis/fetal spine to the axis of the maternal spine; the fetal presentation is defined as the fetal part which occupies the lower uterine pole and is in closest proximity to the internal cervical os, and the fetal position is the relationship between the fetal presenting part and the anterior, posterior and lateral axes of the pelvis [51].

The current means of assessing labour progression is through serial digital examination by trained midwives and doctors with partographic charting along the traditional "Friedman curves" modified following research conducted in Zimbabwe in the 1970s [52, 53]. The argument has arisen that considerable subjectivity and individual variation exist with these traditional assessments, and the current standards are being challenged as underestimates of active labour duration with a resultant overestimate in labour progress [54, 55]. Others advocate individualised, serial assessment for estimating the likelihood of a safe vaginal delivery [56].

9.3.2.3 Assessment of Progress in Labour, Diagnosis of Protracted or Arrested Labour

The diagnosis of established labour remains difficult to date and with the variation in facilities available for managing dysfunctional labour in developing countries, objective methods for assessing progress in labour will be invaluable. A study from Nigeria revealed that dystocia-related complications are among the top five causes of maternal morbidity and mortality in the country and are associated with delayed senior intervention associated with inadequacies in triaging [57]. A practical remedial measure that has been proposed is to utilise the average presentation-to-delivery interval in benchmarking for prolonged labour [58]. This could help avoid prolonged and obstructed labour in developing countries by enabling appropriate, earlier intervention by senior clinicians [57].

Prolonged labour is usually due to poor uterine activity, while the arrest is more often secondary to fetopelvic disproportion. Prediction of either is difficult and a diagnosis can only be made after a period of trial of labour and this is usually late. It would be valuable to make an earlier diagnosis but this requires reliable objective assessments. Operative vaginal delivery after prolonged labour is associated with significantly higher neonatal intracranial haemorrhage rates [59, 60] and important determinants of successful and safe use of vacuum and forceps include correct diagnosis of the fetal head position and appropriate application of the instrument. With more accurate prediction and avoiding attempts at difficult assisted delivery, this complication should be reduced.

Cervical Dilatation

Assessment of cervical dilatation is essential to determine labour progression, but current digital assessments are observer dependent and more intrusive, with a higher risk of maternal distress and infection than ultrasound examination [61]. Although ultrasound assessment of cervical dilatation in labour has previously been unsuccessful in its application to clinical practice, a trans-perineal technique reported for measuring cervical dilatation antero-posteriorly with intact membranes shows good accuracy and correlation with digital assessment and appears promising [62]. Although high-resolution equipment is required which may be beyond the means of many maternity units in low-to-medium-income countries, measuring cervical dilatation remains feasible (Fig. 9.13).

Head Engagement or Head Progression Distance

In a seminal pilot study from Australia, Dietz demonstrated that fetal head engagement assessed using trans-labial ultrasound in late pregnancy correlated with the mode of delivery at a predictive value that exceeded any previously investigated parameters [63]. Defined by the minimal distance from a line through the infero-posterior symphyseal margin (parallel to the main transducer axis) and the leading edge of the fetal skull (Fig. 9.14), this team established the significance of the symphysis pubis as a good landmark for antepartum pre-labour trans-labial ultrasound and showed excellent reproducibility [64]. In a subsequent multivariate study of 202 nulliparous women, the best predictive model for vaginal delivery ($c = 0.87$) incorporated the maternal age, history of caesarean section, Bishop score and bladder position on Valsalva combined with the BMI [65]. This established the feasibility of the identification of women at increased risk of operative delivery using ultrasound.

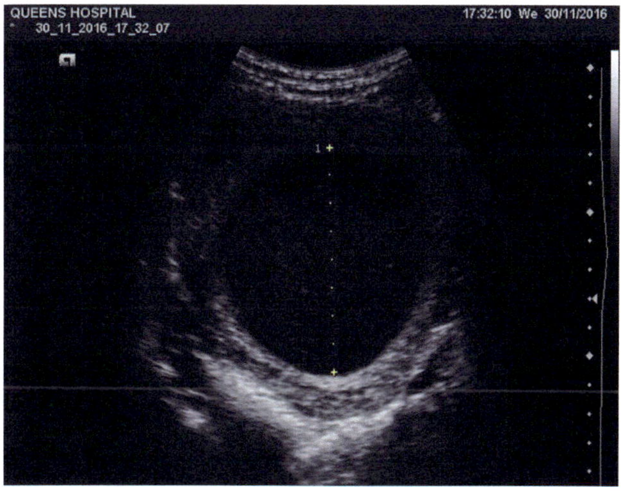

Fig. 9.13 A dilating cervix - trans perineal ultrasound

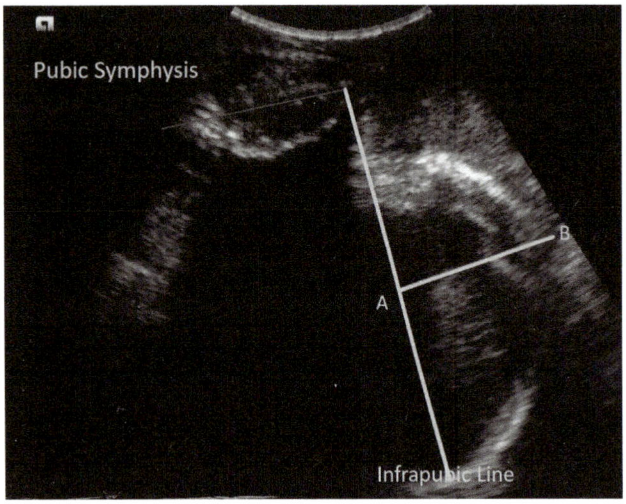

Fig. 9.14 Translabial ultrasound measurement of fetal head engagement - fetal head perineal distance

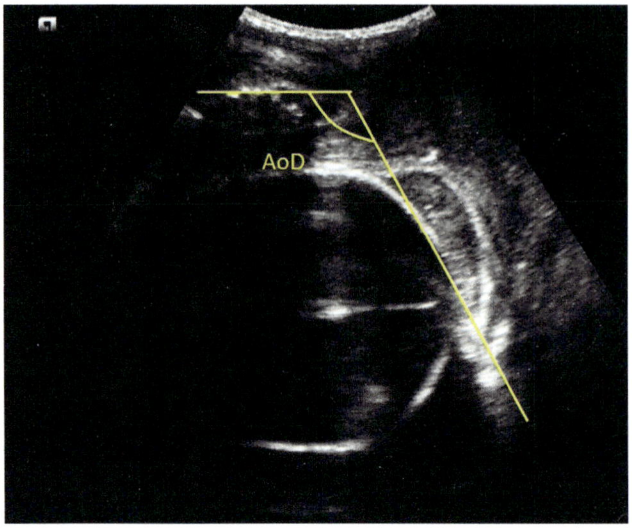

Fig. 9.15 Fetal head progression transperineal ultrasound measurement of angle of descent

It is noteworthy that the Australian studies were initially conducted using 2D ultrasound machines with 4–7 MHz curved array transducers, with the transducer placed on the perineum in a mid-sagittal direction after being covered with an unpowdered glove and ultrasound gel [63–65]. The near-vertical hypoechogenic line of the urethra was used to identify this plane. All imaging was undertaken immediately after bladder emptying and in the supine position. The quantification of head engagement was performed using two methods. For method A, a line was drawn through the posterior-inferior symphyseal margin, parallel to the main transducer axis, as reference, identical to the vertical line used to measure bladder neck descent on Valsalva manoeuvre. The shortest distance between this line and the presenting part was measured in millimetres. For method B, the line of reference was a line perpendicular to the central axis of the symphysis pubis, placed through the caudal end of the symphysis; this line was later called the 'infrapubic line'. Head engagement was defined as the minimal distance between the presenting part and this line. The presenting part has been clarified in definition as the most distal part of the hyper-echogenic curvature signifying fetal skull and scalp [61].

Various other linear measurements such as the head-perineum distance and head progression distance, and angles, such as the head direction, head progression angle also described as the angle of progression or angle of descent (see Fig. 9.15), and midline angle have all been studied using either 2D or 3D ultrasound which latter has the advantage of storage of acquired datasets for off-line analysis later [47, 66–71]. However, 3D machines are expensive and not readily available for use on most labour wards even in high-income countries, special training is required for their use and they have not demonstrated any extra benefit over two-dimensional ultrasound for this purpose [70–72]. At the moment, there is a lack of consensus as to the method of choice for assessing labour progression, and the current profusion of different published methods is an indicator of the uncertainty regarding what is accurate or clinically useful. The global objective by whatever means is to prevent poor labour and delivery outcomes by enabling good clinical assessments and decision making, and with improved case selection, allowing better operative skills to be developed. Ultrasound potentially holds the advantage for this purpose.

Head Station

Head station can be clinically assessed abdominally, and digitally or sonographically from below. A suggested approach is to assess station in the transverse plane trans-abdominally at high stations, and to use a ongitudinal trans-abdominal approach after head engagement to show the foetal occiput and cervical vertebrae, and finally, scan trans-perineally or trans-labially with fetal heads low in the pelvis [11].

Henrich and co-workers made further efforts to improve assessment and prediction of labour progression using intrapartum trans-labial ultrasound (ITU) assessments in 2006 [73]. Head station was defined on ITU as the measurement between the intersections of the infrapubic line and the deepest bony part of the fetal head along the longest visible axis of the fetal head, after subtracting 3 cm for the level of the ischial spines [66]. The plane indicated by the infrapubic line being reportedly 3 cm cranial to a parallel plane passing through the ischial spines [73, 74]. This measurement has been queried because of the difficulty in delineating the 'imaginary plane' drawn between the ischial spines by its definition [75]. A closer reference to the original studies by Dietz clarifies where the disputed measurements should be made, i.e. by a line drawn through the inferio-posterior margin of the symphysis pubis [64] and predictive value with successful operative vaginal delivery has been demonstrated [73]. In addition, MRI studies appear to correlate well with these measurements [76–78]. Another cogent experimental finding is that that the head station and angle of progression appear so closely related as to be possibly interchangeable [66].

Head Direction

This is defined as the angle between the infrapubic line of the pelvis (a line perpendicular to the longer diameter of the pubis starting from the inferior border) and another line drawn perpendicular to the widest diameter of the fetal head [73] (Fig. 9.16). There are three types of head direction: head down, horizontal and head up (Figs. 9.17, 9.18 and 9.19). 'Head up' is when the line drawn perpendicular to the widest diameter of the fetal head points ventrally at an angle of $\geq 30°$; head down is when this angle is $<0°$; all other angles are considered 'horizontal'. Also definable as the direction of the longest visible axis of the fetal head measured with regard to the long axis of the symphysis pubis; positive angles signify upward directions, and negative angles signify downward directions [73].

As the fetal head descends along the curved birth canal, changes in head station and head direction during a contraction have been shown to depend on the absolute head station, underlining the importance of the Valsalva manoeuvre when conducting assessments [66]. This measurement has shown good reproducibility, with angles >22° reported in 97% of women with successful vaginal deliveries [66].

Angle of Progression, Angle of Descent

This is defined as the angle between a line drawn through the pubic symphysis in the midline and the tangent of the fetal skull [76] (Fig. 9.15). The plane of the ischial spines is a clinically important reference point representing the zero station at which ultrasound-derived measurements have been correlated with computed tomography (CT) scans for the angle of progression [79] and magnetic resonance imaging (MRI) for the angle of progression and head station [77] concluding that an angle of 99° correlates with zero station [76]. There, however, appears to be no consensus cut-off for the angle of progression with angles wider than 92° [71], 100° [77], 110° [79] and 135° [66] that are quoted for good correlation with successful vaginal birth.

Head Perineum (Head Progression) Distance

Defined as the shortest distance from the perineal skin to the outermost limit of the fetal bony skull measured on a transverse plane [47], this is measured by applying a transducer

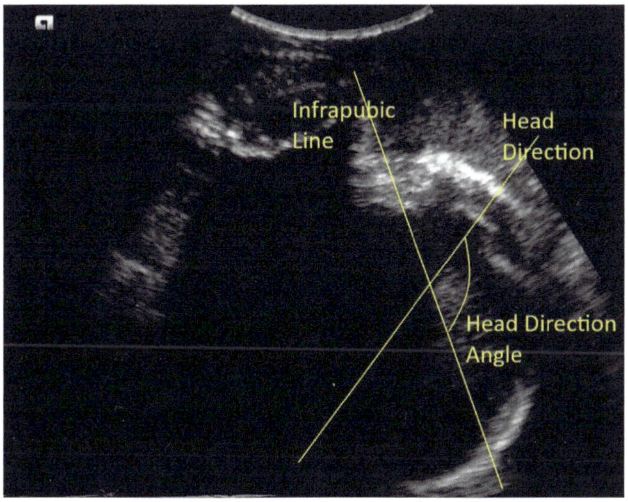

Fig. 9.16 Fetal head direction - transperineal measurement of the fetal head direction angle

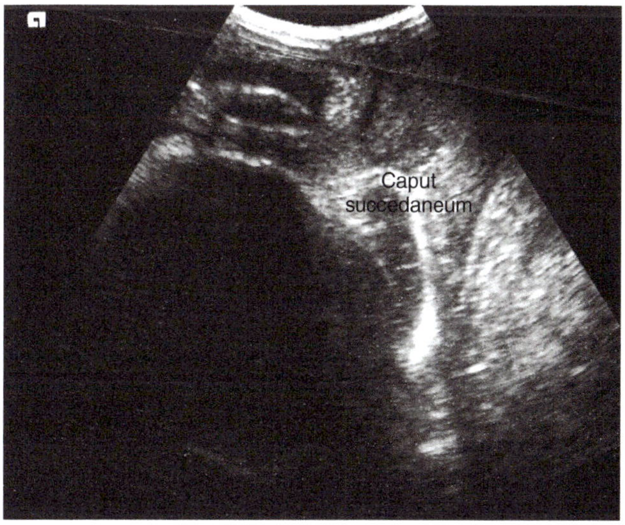

Fig. 9.17 Fetal head direction; downwards direction with prominent caput succedaneum

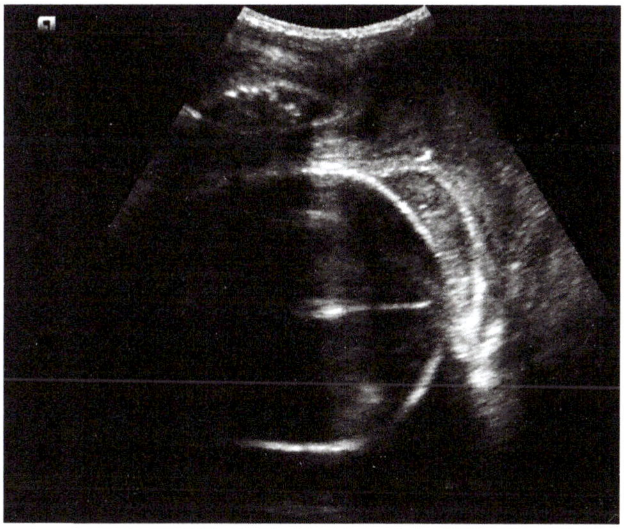

Fig. 9.18 Fetal head direction; horizontal direction with prominent caput succedaneum

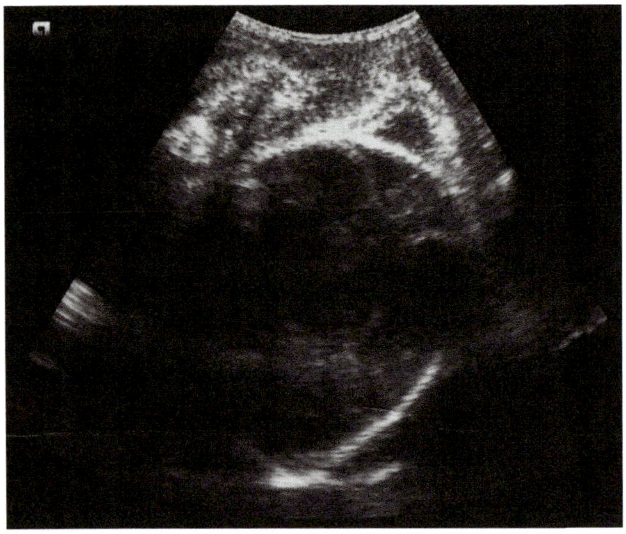

Fig. 9.19 Fetal head direction; upward direction with moderate caput succedaneum

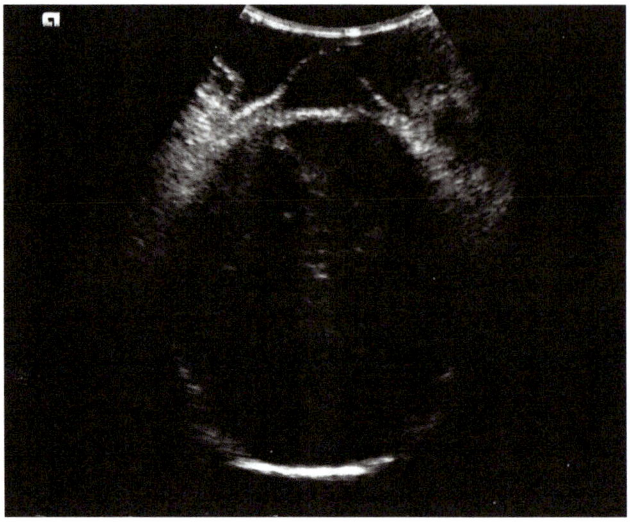

Fig. 9.20 Assessing the sub-pubic arch or angle

firmly against the posterior fourchette and clearly visualising the anterior pelvic and fetal bony structures (Fig. 9.12). This distance between the infrapubic line and the lowest part of the fetal skull was initially tested for associations with time from membrane rupture to delivery or need for operative delivery in a group of women with spontaneous pre-labour membrane rupture [80] and subsequently for the prediction of successful induction of labour [47]. At a cut-off of 45 mm, more women with a shorter distance had gone into labour by 36 hours in the former; while in the latter study, head-perineal distance was shown to have a similar predictive ability to the cervical length and the Bishop score [47, 80].

9.3.2.4 Clinical and Ultrasound Pelvimetry, Sub-Pubic Arch Angle, Midline Angle

In 1932, Caldwell and Molloy contended that an accurate knowledge of the pelvic size and shape would help predict the course of labour and assist in deciding where to offer operative delivery [81]. Using postpartum pelvic radiography, they studied pelvises in women who had required operative delivery, then followed up with intrapartum studies. The objectives were to (a) deduce the appropriate station in transverse or occipito-posterior arrest of the head to attempt rotational delivery based on pelvic shape and diameters, (b) ascertain the normal position in which a fetal head should descend through the lower pelvis and (c) develop accuracy in the prediction of the probable mechanism of labour with each particular pelvic shape [81].

These authors reported four basic pelvic shapes with wide anatomical variations in between, and their studies gave rise to the concept of a clinically important conjugate obstetric diameter through which a fetal presenting part passed to become engaged in the pelvis. A key point is that this diameter between the sacral promontory and upper symphyseal border could not be measured clinically and a digitally measured surrogate, the diagonal conjugate, was used in clinical pelvimetry. While some studies showed benefit [82, 83] systematic reviews revealed the lack of large randomised controlled trials and concluded that there is insufficient evidence to support clinical pelvimetry with cephalic presentations [84, 85]. EOS BiPlanar X-Ray imaging *(Electronic imaging of low-dose ionising radiation with gases), CT, MRI and ultrasound have also been tried [86–90]. EOS BiPlanar X-Ray imaging was of particular interest because it apparently acquires simultaneous lateral and anteroposterior images with a radiation dose that is one-third to one-tenth that of conventional X-ray imaging, a major concern with traditional X-ray pelvimetry being the high radiation exposures required for the pelvic bone. There have been varying reports of usefulness with these techniques.

The pelvimetry concept was recently re-explored by Gilboa et al. [91] who evaluated the subpubic (pubic arch) angle using transperineal ultrasound in 62 term pregnancies following a diagnosis of failure to progress in the second stage (Fig. 9.20). They found that women with occipito-transverse positions had significantly smaller angles than occipito-anterior positions (94.3° vs. 103.2°), and those who required operative delivery had significantly smaller angles than those that ended in normal delivery (97.1° vs. 110.1°). Their reported correlations with fetal malposition and the need for operative delivery suggest a role in the prediction of delivery mode and potential value in avoiding unnecessary interventional delivery [91].

Ghi et al. defined the midline angle (MLA) as the angle between the anteroposterior axis of the maternal pelvis and the head midline [92]. They combined the MLA with the angle of progression (AoP) which is currently the most reproducible parameter for fetal head station in the sagittal plane and demonstrated that poor fetal head descent as assessed by the AoP seems to be an early finding in cases with a higher risk of operative delivery, whereas slow head rotation, as assessed by the MLA, seems to be a late finding [93]. Unfortunately because all the study participants had successful vacuum-assisted deliveries, a direct clinical application of their findings to predicting delivery outcome was not possible [93]. This group has also demonstrated the effectiveness of ultrasound in the diagnosis of face presentation and asynclitism in labour [94–96]. However, their studies all utilised 3D ultrasound which holds limitations as previously noted, particularly, for low- to-medium-income countries.

Although ultrasound determined fetal head position has proven to be more accurate than digital assessment and prediction of dystocia is well reported using the head perineal distance, these significant findings have so far not shown direct clinical benefit in studies on perinatal outcome [97]. The data available are, however, limited and larger; more widespread studies in different populations are required. The recent International Society of Ultrasound in Obstetrics and Gynaecology guidelines on intrapartum ultrasound summarise by affirming the global uncertainty regarding how current knowledge impacts on the management of labour and maternal and neonatal outcomes [97].

9.4 Summary

We have reviewed the recent literature on ultrasound in labour and delivery, with particular regard to its clinical significance and utility in developing countries. In conclusion, the ideal ultrasound labour assessment method in this circumstance should be suited to purpose, simple to perform, easy to learn, accurate, reliable, easily repeatable clinically irrespective of fetal position or station, universally applicable and widely acceptable to women. Ideally, it should not be operator dependent. Clearly, there is a great deal of work to be done in this field as none of these criteria has been fully satisfied to date. There is also currently no consensus as to what constitutes the best means of ultrasound labour assessment.

9.5 Recommendations

Judging by the literature, routine use of labour and delivery ultrasound should initially be directed at objective ultrasound definition of fetal gestational age, estimated size and placental location and function to help identify fetuses at risk of compromise in labour. In the future, those ultrasound parameters identified to accurately predict the mode of delivery will enhance the safety of childbirth. It is emphasised that high-quality training and monitoring of qualified physicians will be essential to ensure patient safety by avoiding complications associated with missed diagnoses and misdiagnosis of potentially dangerous conditions.

References

1. Torloni MR, Vedmedovska N, Merialdi M, et al. Safety of ultrasonography in pregnancy: WHO systematic review of the literature and meta-analysis. Ultrasound Obstet Gynecol. 2009;33(5):599–608.
2. Groen RS, Loew JJ, Sadasivam V, Kushner AL. Review: indications for ultrasound use in low- and middle-income countries. Tropical Med Int Health. 2011;16(12):1525–35.
3. Wanyonyi SZ, Mariara CM, Vinayak S, et al. Opportunities and challenges in realising universal access to obstetric ultrasound in sub-Saharan Africa. Ultrasound Int Open. 2017;3(02):E52–9.
4. Harrison K. The struggle to reduce high maternal mortality in Nigeria. Afr J Reprod Health. 2009;13(3):9–20.
5. Badawi N, Kurinczuk JJ, Keogh JM, Alessandri LM, O'Sullivan F, Burton PR, Pemberton PJ, Stanley FJ. Intrapartum risk factors for newborn encephalopathy: the Western Australian case-control study. BMJ. 1998;317:1554–8.
6. Stephansson O, Sandström A, Petersson G, Wikström AK, Cnattingius S. Prolonged second stage of labour, maternal infectious disease, urinary retention and other complications in the early postpartum period. BJOG. 2016;123(4):608–16.
7. Coombes R. Supporting surgery for obstetric fistula. BMJ. 2004;329(7475):1125.
8. Wall LL. Obstetric vesicovaginal fistula as an international public-health problem. Lancet. 2006;368(9542):1201–9.
9. Dupuis O, Silveira R, Zentner A, Dittmar A, Gaucherand P, Cucherat M, Redarce T, Rudigoz RC. Birth simulator: reliability of transvaginal assessment of fetal head station as defined by the American College of Obstetricians and Gynecologists classification. Am J Obstet Gynecol. 2005;192(3):868–74.
10. Dupuis O, Ruimark S, Corinne D, Simone T, André D, René-Charles R. Fetal head position during the second stage of labor: comparison of digital vaginal examination and transabdominal ultrasonographic examination. Eur J Obstet Gynecol Reprod Biol. 2005;123(2):193–7.
11. Akmal S, Tsoi E, Kametas N, Howard R, Nicolaides KH. Intrapartum sonography to determine fetal head position. J Matern Fetal Neonatal Med. 2002;12(3):172–7.
12. Akmal S, Kametas N, Tsoi E, Hargreaves C, Nicolaides KH. Comparison of transvaginal digital examination with intrapartum sonography to determine fetal head position before instrumental delivery. Ultrasound Obstet Gynecol. 2003;21(5):437–40.
13. Sultan AH, Kamm MA, Hudson CN, Thomas JM, Bartram CI. Anal-sphincter disruption during vaginal delivery. N Engl J Med. 1993;329(26):1905–11.
14. Eichelberger KY. A prolonged second stage should prompt increased vigilance for postpartum maternal complications. BJOG. 2016;123(4):617.
15. Thompson MO, Otigbah C, Kelkar A, Coker A, Pankhania A, Kapoor S. The management of placenta accreta at Queen's Hospital, Romford, UK. In: A comprehensive textbook of postpartum haemorrhage. 2nd ed. London: Sapiens Publishing Limited; 2012. p. 247–58.
16. Kiserud T. Global reproductive health: is diagnostic ultrasound appropriate technology? Ultrasound Obstet Gynecol. 2012;40:123–5.
17. Sayasneh A, Preisler J, Smith A, Saso S, Naji O, Abdallah Y, Stalder C, Daemen A, Timmerman D, Bourne T. Do pocket-sized

ultrasound machines have the potential to be used as a tool to triage patients in obstetrics and gynaecology? Ultrasound Obstet Gynecol. 2012;40:145–50.
18. Ramphul M, Kennelly M, Murphy DJ. Establishing the accuracy and acceptability of abdominal ultrasound to define the fetal head position in the second stage of labour: a validation study. Eur J Obstet Gynecol Reprod Biol. 2012;164(1):35–9.
19. Oboro V, Oboro O, Awopetu O. P16.09: psychological acceptability of transvaginal scan among Nigerians attending for early pregnancy ultrasound. Ultrasound Obstet Gynecol. 2015;46(S1):174.
20. Papageorghiou AT, Christina KH, Nicolaides KH. The role of uterine artery Doppler in predicting adverse pregnancy outcome. Best Pract Res Clin Obstet Gynaecol. 2004;18(3):383–96.
21. Gentili P, Trasimeni A, Giorlandino C. Fetal ossification centres as predictors of gestational age in normal and abnormal pregnancies. J Ultrasound Med. 1984;3(5):193–7.
22. Chinn DH, Bolding DB, Callen PW, Gross BH, Filly RA. Ultrasonographic identification of fetal lower extremity epiphyseal ossification centres. Radiology. 1983;147(3):815–8.
23. Goldstein I, Lockwood C, Belanger K, Hobbins J. Ultrasonographic assessment of gestational age with the distal femoral and proximal tibial ossification centres in the third trimester. Am J Obstet Gynecol. 1988;158(1):127–30.
24. Birang S, Ameri AA, Najmi Z. Distal femoral epiphyses ossification centre diameter and third trimester gestational age in Iranian population. Ginekol Pol. 2013;84(12):1025–9.
25. Gottlieb AG, Galan HL. Nontraditional sonographic pearls in estimating gestational age. Semin Perinatol. 2008;32(3):154–60.
26. Adeyekun AA, Orji MO. Predictive accuracy of trans-cerebellar diameter in comparison with other fetal biometric parameters for gestational age estimation among pregnant Nigerian women. East Afr Med J. 2014;91(4):138–44.
27. Eze CU, Onwuzu QE, Nwadike IU. Sonographic reference values for fetal transverse cerebellar diameter in the second and third trimesters in a Nigerian population. J Diagn Med Sonography. 2017;33(3):174–81.
28. Lee W, Barton S, Comstock CH, et al. Transverse cerebellar diameter: a useful predictor of gestational age for foetuses with asymmetric growth retardation. Am J Obstet Gynecol. 1991;165:1044–50.
29. Mayden KL, Tortora M, Berkowitz RL, et al. Orbital diameters: a new parameter for prenatal diagnosis and dating. Am J Obstet Gynecol. 1982;144:289–97.
30. Konje JC, Abrams KR, Bell SC, et al. Determination of gestational age after the 24th week of gestation from fetal kidney length measurements. Ultrasound Obstet Gynecol. 2002;19:592–7.
31. Jeanty P, Rodesch F, Delbeke D, et al. Estimation of gestational age from measurements of fetal long bones. J Ultrasound Med. 1984;3:75–9.
32. Green Top Guideline No 27. Placenta praevia, placenta praevia accreta and vasa praevia: diagnosis and management. London: RCOG; 2011.
33. Wortman AC, Twickler DM, McIntire DD, Dashe JS. Bleeding complications in pregnancies with low-lying placenta. J Matern Fetal Neonatal Med. 2015;4:1–5.
34. Kollmann M, Gaulhofer J, Lang U, Klaritsch P. Placenta praevia: incidence, risk factors and outcome. J Matern Fetal Neonatal Med. 2015;4:1–4.
35. Celik E, To M, Gajewska K, Smith GC, Nicolaides KH. Cervical length and obstetric history predict spontaneous preterm birth: development and validation of a model to provide individualised risk assessment. Ultrasound Obstet Gynecol. 2008;31(5):549–54.
36. Newman RB, Goldenberg RL, Iams JD, Meis PJ, Mercer BM, Moawad AH, Thom E, Miodovnik M, Caritis SN, Dombrowski M, Thurnau GR. Preterm prediction study: comparison of the cervical score and Bishop score for prediction of spontaneous preterm delivery. Obstet Gynaecol. 2008;112(3):508.
37. Iams JD, Goldenberg RL, Meis PJ, Mercer BM, Moawad A, Das A, Thom E, McNellis D, Copper RL, Johnson F, Roberts JM. The length of the cervix and the risk of spontaneous premature delivery. N Engl J Med. 1996;334(9):567–73.
38. Heath VC, Southall TR, Souka AP, Elisseou A, Nicolaides KH. Cervical length at 23 weeks of gestation: prediction of spontaneous preterm delivery. Ultrasound Obstet Gynecol. 1998;12(5):312–7.
39. World Health Organization. WHO recommendations for induction of labour. Geneva: World Health Organization; 2011. http://apps.who.int/iris/bitstream/10665/70730/1/WHO_RHR_11.10_eng.pdf
40. Orhue AAE. Induction of labour. Trop J Obstet Gynaecol. 1997;14(1):1–4.
41. Ade-Ojo IP, Akintayo AA. Induction of labour in the developing countries – an overview. J Med Med Sci. 2013;4(7):258–62.
42. Bishop EH. Pelvic scoring for elective induction. Obstet Gynecol. 1964;24(2):266–8. Bishop Score.
43. Kolkman DG, Verhoeven CJ, Brinkhorst SJ, Van der Post JA, Pajkrt E, Opmeer BC, Mol BW. The Bishop score as a predictor of labor induction success: a systematic review. Am J Perinatol. 2013;30(8):625–30.
44. Pandis GK, Papageorghiou AT, Ramanathan VG, Thompson MO, Nicolaides KH. Preinduction sonographic measurement of cervical length in the prediction of successful induction of labor. Ultrasound Obstet Gynecol. 2001;18(6):623–8.
45. Peregrine E, O'Brien P, Omar R, Jauniaux E. Clinical and ultrasound parameters to predict the risk of cesarean delivery after induction of labor. Obstet Gynecol. 2006;107(2, Part 1):227–33.
46. Rane SM, Guirgis RR, Higgins B, Nicolaides KH. The value of ultrasound in the prediction of successful induction of labor. Ultrasound Obstet Gynecol. 2004;24(5):538–49.
47. Eggebø TM, Heien C, Økland I, Gjessing LK, Romundstad P, Salvesen KA. Ultrasound assessment of fetal head-perineum distance before induction of labor. Ultrasound Obstet Gynecol. 2008;32:199–204.
48. Crane JM. Factors predicting labor induction success: a critical analysis. Clin Obstet Gynaecol. 2006;49(3):573–84.
49. Eggebø TM, Økland I, Heien C, Gjessing LK, Romundstad P, Salvesen KÅ. Can ultrasound measurements replace digitally assessed elements of the Bishop score? Acta Obstet Gynecol Scand. 2009;88(3):325–31.
50. Zhu BP, Grigorescu V, Le T, et al. Labor dystocia and its association with interpregnancy interval. Am J Obstet Gynecol. 2006;195:121.
51. Simm A, Woods A. Fetal malpresentation. Curr Obstet Gynaecol. 2004;14:231–8.
52. Friedman EA. Cervimetry: an objective method for the study of cervical dilatation in labor. Am J Obstet Gynecol. 1956;71(6):1189–93.
53. Philpott RH, Castle WM. Cervicographs in the management of labor in primigravidae. J Obstet Gynaecol Br Commonw. 1972;79:599–602.
54. Zhang J, Troendle JF, Yancey MK. Reassessing the labor curve in nulliparous women. Am J Obstet Gynecol. 2002;187:824–8.
55. Neal JL, Lowe NK, Ahijevych KL, Patrick TE, Cabbage LA, Corwin EJ. "Active labor" duration and dilation rates among low-risk, nulliparous women with spontaneous labor onset: a systematic review. J Midwifery Womens Health. 2010;55(4):308–18.
56. Cohen WR, Friedman EA. Perils of the new labor management guidelines. Am J Obstet Gynecol. 2015;212(4):420–7.
57. Oladapo OT, Adetoro OO, Ekele BA, Chama C, Etuk SJ, Aboyeji AP, Onah HE, Abasiattai AM, Adamu AN, Adegbola O, Adeniran AS. When getting there is not enough: a nationwide cross-sectional study of 998 maternal deaths and 1451 near-misses in public tertiary hospitals in a low-income country. BJOG. 2016;123(6):928–38.
58. Silas O. Basic indices for labour and delivery management in Nigeria. Trop J Obstet Gynaecol. 2013;30:1.

59. Towner D, Castro MA, Eby-Wilkens E, Gilbert WM. Effect of mode of delivery in nulliparous women on neonatal intracranial injury. N Engl J Med. 1999;341(23):1709–14.
60. Benedetti TJ. Birth injury and method of delivery. N Engl J Med. 1999;341(23):1758–9.
61. Hassan WA, Tutschek B. Intrapartum sonography: an opportunity for objective assessment of labour. Fetal Matern Med Rev. 2013;24(01):2–17.
62. Hassan WA, Eggebø TM, Ferguson M, Lees C. Simple two-dimensional ultrasound technique to assess intrapartum cervical dilatation: a pilot study. Ultrasound Obstet Gynecol. 2013;41(4):413–8.
63. Dietz HP, Bennett MJ. Can we predict the course of labour? Aust N Z J Obstet Gynaecol. 2002;42:S16.
64. Dietz HP, Lanzarone V. Measuring engagement of the fetal head: validity and reproducibility of a new ultrasound technique. Ultrasound Obstet Gynecol. 2005;25:165–8.
65. Dietz HP, Lanzarone V, Simpson JM. Predicting operative delivery. Ultrasound Obstet Gynecol. 2006;27(4):409–15.
66. Tutschek B, Braun T, Chantraine F, Henrich W. A study of progress of labour using intrapartum translabial ultrasound, assessing head station, direction, and angle of descent. BJOG. 2011;118:62–9.
67. Kalache KD, Duckelmann AM, Michaelis SA, Lange J, Cichon G, Dudenhausen JW. Transperineal ultrasound imaging in prolonged second stage of labor with occipitoanterior presenting foetuses: how well does the "angle of progression" predict the mode of delivery? Ultrasound Obstet Gynecol. 2009;33:326–30.
68. Dückelmann AM, Bamberg C, Michaelis SA, Lange J, Nonnenmacher A, Dudenhausen JW, Kalache KD. Measurement of fetal head descent using the "angle of progression" on transperineal ultrasound imaging is reliable regardless of fetal head station or ultrasound expertise. Ultrasound Obstet Gynecol. 2010;35(2):216–22.
69. Pereira S, Frick AP, Poon LC, Zamprakou A, Nicolaides KH. Successful induction of labor: prediction by preinduction cervical length, angle of progression and cervical elastography. Ultrasound Obstet Gynecol. 2014;44(4):468–75.
70. Cho GJ, Hong HR, Seol HJ, Koo BH, Hong SC, Oh MJ, Kim HJ. Use of the angle of progression on ultrasonography to predict spontaneous onset of labor within 7 days. J Perinat Med. 2015;43(2):185–9.
71. Gillor M, Vaisbuch E, Zaks S, Barak O, Hagay Z, Levy R. Transperineal sonographic assessment of the angle of progression as a predictor of a successful vaginal delivery following induction of labor. Ultrasound Obstet Gynecol. 2017;49(2):240–5.
72. Iliescu D, Antsaklis P, Paulescu D, Comanescu A, Tudorache S, Antsaklis A, Ceausu I, Novac L, Cernea N, Kurjak A. Applications of ultrasound in prelabor and labor. Donald School J Ultrasound Obstet Gynecol. 2012;6(3):257–69.
73. Henrich W, Dudenhausen J, Fuchs I, Kamena A, Tutschek B. Intrapartum translabial ultrasound (ITU): sonographic landmarks and correlation with successful vacuum extraction. Ultrasound Obstet Gynecol. 2006;28(6):753–60.
74. Salomon N, Siedentopf J, Grieser C, Henrich W. 3D reconstruction of the female pelvis to estimate the distance between the infrapubic line and the plane of ischial spines. J Perinat Med. 2009;37(s1):296.
75. Simon EG, Arthuis CJ, Perrotin F. Ultrasound in labor monitoring: how to define the plane of ischial spines? Ultrasound Obstet Gynecol. 2013;42(6):722–3.
76. Barbera AF, Pombar X, Perugino G, Lezotte DC, Hobbins JC. A new method to assess fetal head descent in labor with transperineal ultrasound. Ultrasound Obstet Gynecol. 2009;33:313–9.
77. Bamberg C, Scheuermann S, Fotopoulou C, Slowinski T, Dückelmann AM, Teichgräber U, Streitparth F, Henrich W, Dudenhausen JW, Kalache KD. Angle of progression measurements of fetal head at term: a systematic comparison between open magnetic resonance imaging and transperineal ultrasound. Am J Obstet Gynecol. 2012;206(2):161–e1.
78. Armbrust R, Henrich W, Hinkson L, Grieser C, Siedentopf JP. Correlation of intrapartum translabial ultrasound parameters with computed tomographic 3D reconstruction of the female pelvis. J Perinat Med. 2016;44(5):567–71.
79. Arthuis CJ, Perrotin F, Patat F, Brunereau L, Simon EG. Computed tomographic study of anatomical relationship between pubic symphysis and ischial spines to improve interpretation of intrapartum translabial ultrasound. Ultrasound in Obstetrics & Gynecology. 2016;48(6):779–85.
80. Eggebø TM, Gjessing LK, Heien C, Smedvig E, Økland I, Romundstad P, Salvesen KÅ. Prediction of labor and delivery by transperineal ultrasound in pregnancies with prelabor rupture of membranes at term. Ultrasound Obstet Gynecol. 2006;27(4):387–91.
81. Caldwell WE, Moloy HC. Sexual variations in the pelvis. Science. 1932;76:37–40.
82. Adadevoh SW, Hobbs C, Elkins TE. The relation of the true conjugate to maternal height and obstetric performance in Ghanaians. Int J Gynaecol Obstet. 1989;28(3):243–51.
83. Liselele HB, Boulvain M, Tshibangu KC, Meuris S. Maternal height and external pelvimetry to predict cephalopelvic disproportion in nulliparous African women: a cohort study. BJOG. 2000;107(8):947–52.
84. Pattinson RC, Cuthbert A, Vannevel V. Pelvimetry for fetal cephalic presentations at or near term for deciding on mode of delivery. Cochrane Database of Systematic Reviews. 2017;(3):1–30.
85. Rozenberg P. Is there a role for X-ray pelvimetry in the twenty-first century? Gynecol Obstet Fertil. 2007;35(1):6–12.
86. Sigmann MH, Delabrousse E, Riethmuller D, Runge M, Peyron C, Aubry S. An evaluation of the EOS X-ray imaging system in pelvimetry. Diagn Interv Imaging. 2014;95(9):833–8.
87. Lenhard MS, Johnson TR, Weckbach S, Nikolaou K, Friese K, Hasbargen U. Pelvimetry revisited: analyzing cephalopelvic disproportion. Eur J Radiol. 2010;74(3):e107–11.
88. Spörri S, Hänggi W, Braghetti A, Vock P, Scheider H. Pelvimetry by magnetic resonance imaging as a diagnostic tool to evaluate dystocia. Obstet Gynaecol. 1997;89(6):902–8.
89. Spörri S, Thoeny HC, Raio L, Lachat R, Vock P, Schneider H. MR imaging pelvimetry: a useful adjunct in the treatment of women at risk for dystocia? Am J Roentgenol. 2002;179(1):137–44.
90. Daghighi MH, Poureisa M, Ranjkesh M. Association between obstetric conjugate diameter measured by transabdominal ultrasonography during pregnancy and the type of delivery. Iran J Radiol. 2013;10(3):185.
91. Gilboa Y, Kivilevitch Z, Spira M, Kedem A, Katorza E, Moran O, Achiron R. Pubic arch angle in prolonged second stage of labor: clinical significance. Ultrasound Obstet Gynecol. 2013;41(4):442–6.
92. Ghi T, Youssef A, Maroni E, Arcangeli T, De Musso F, Bellussi F, Nanni M, Giorgetta F, Morselli-Labate AM, Iammarino MT, Paccapelo A. Intrapartum transperineal ultrasound assessment of fetal head progression in active second stage of labor and mode of delivery. Ultrasound Obstet Gynecol. 2013;41(4):430–5.
93. Ghi T, Maroni E, Youssef A, Morselli-Labate AM, Paccapelo A, Montaguti E, Rizzo N, Pilu G. Sonographic pattern of fetal head descent: relationship with duration of active second stage of labor and occiput position at delivery. Ultrasound Obstet Gynecol. 2014;44(1):82–9.
94. Ghi T, Bellussi F, Azzarone C, Krsmanovic J, Franchi L, Youssef A, Lenzi J, Fantini MP, Frusca T, Pilu G. The "occiput–spine angle": a new sonographic index of fetal head deflexion during the first stage of labor. Am J Obstet Gynecol. 2016;215(1):84–e1.
95. Ghi T, Maroni E, Youssef A, Cariello L, Salsi G, Arcangeli T, Frasca C, Rizzo N, Pilu G. Intrapartum three-dimensional ultrasonographic imaging of face presentations: report of two cases. Ultrasound Obstet Gynecol. 2012;40(1):117–8.
96. Ghi T, Youssef A, Pilu G, Malvasi A, Ragusa A. Intrapartum sonographic imaging of fetal head asynclitism. Ultrasound Obstet Gynecol. 2012;39(2):238–40.
97. Ghi T, Eggebø T, Lees C, Kalache K, Rozenberg P, Youssef A, Salomon LJ, Tutschek B. ISUOG practice guidelines: intrapartum ultrasound. Ultrasound Obstet Gynecol. 2018;52(1):128–39.

Evidence-Based Antenatal Care

10

Olufemi A. Olatunbosun and Lindsay Edouard

Learning Objectives

At the conclusion of this chapter, the reader will be able to discuss the following:

- Approach to a focused and evidence-based antenatal care that is cost-effective and efficient for developing countries
- Current protocols for regular assessment, diagnostic testing, interventions and preventive care in each trimester of pregnancy
- The relevance of incorporating research evidence from developed countries and of due consideration for prevailing local conditions and circumstances in the provision of antenatal care
- The value of an expanded, multidisciplinary, community-based maternal health programme that includes birth centres, well-woman clinics, teen pregnancy care and family planning services

10.1 Introduction

Antenatal care (ANC) is a major component of integrated maternal health within sexual and reproductive health which is a vital element of primary healthcare. It is preventive healthcare the goal of which is to identify and treat potential pregnancy-related health problems throughout the course of the pregnancy while promoting healthy lifestyles that benefit both mother and child [1]. The improved access to family planning and contraceptive services and availability of routine antenatal care have played a large part in reducing maternal and perinatal morbidity and mortality, low birth weight infants and other preventable health problems in both developed and developing countries [2, 3]. Comprehensive maternity care includes the following:

1. Appropriate diagnosis of pregnancy followed by an initial thorough assessment in early pregnancy.
2. Periodic examination including screening tests as appropriate through the course of gestation.
3. Patient education addressing pregnancy care, labour and delivery, nutrition and exercise, and early infant care.
4. Provision of emergency obstetric care and management of the patient during labour, delivery and the postpartum period. Ideally, obstetric care should commence before pregnancy as preconception visits where family and medical history for both parents and a physical examination of the prospective mother are done. Pre-existing conditions that may influence conception and/or pregnancy are identified, and appropriate management plans are formulated with the goal of achieving a 'normal' low-risk pregnancy.

The concept of pre-pregnancy evaluation is particularly relevant to developing countries with a substantial proportion of unplanned pregnancies and where individuals initially seek care after pregnancy has begun. Besides poor care during pregnancy, delivery and the puerperium, the high maternal and perinatal mortality and morbidity in most developing countries are partly due to many women becoming pregnant with underlying undiagnosed and untreated medical and surgical conditions [2, 3].

While global strategies seek to reduce maternal mortality through universal access to antenatal care [4, 5], progress has been slow in developing countries where antenatal care coverage is often less than 50% [6]. Some investigators have suggested that there may be a lack of congruency between service provision and the social and cultural context of some women in low- and middle-income countries [7]. Therefore, it is imperative to design the process and structure of antenatal care in developing countries to (1) promote access to care;

O. A. Olatunbosun (✉) · L. Edouard
Department of Obstetrics and Gynaecology, College of Medicine, University of Saskatchewan, Saskatoon, SK, Canada
e-mail: femi.olatunbosun@usask.ca

F. Okonofua et al. (eds.), *Contemporary Obstetrics and Gynecology for Developing Countries*,
https://doi.org/10.1007/978-3-030-75385-6_10

(2) enhance patient education and involvement in their care; (3) provide a team approach to ongoing maternal and foetal surveillance and (4) establish uniform protocols for screening for high-risk conditions, along with organised plans to address complications that may arise in pregnancy.

Several aspects of antenatal care are becoming evidence-based rather than relying on traditional models of care that are not supported by rigorous scientific evidence [8, 9]. The purpose of this chapter is to discuss the provision of antenatal care that is practically and contextually consistent with local beliefs, experiences and resources, and would be well utilised at both secondary and tertiary care centres in countries. The challenge for healthcare professionals working in rural and district hospitals and health centres is to tailor their practices to limited resources while maintaining an appropriate standard of care. As much as possible, an evidence-based approach that is grounded in achieving the best outcomes for both mother and infant must form the basis for antenatal care rather than long-standing traditional practices. Recognising the relative dearth of well-conducted randomised clinical trials to guide the provision of antenatal care, the Cochrane Pregnancy and Childbirth Database has been aggressively seeking ways to rectify the gap in evidence through a partnership with researchers in developing countries [10, 11]. Although the research output of developing country authors has increased to 40%, many health problems relevant to the developing world and the best ways to address them remain largely neglected [12]. While it could be argued that developing countries should obtain evidence for prevailing health problems locally, existing databases from developed countries provide a framework for such efforts. Healthcare professionals in low-resource countries must appreciate the limitations of local circumstances in using such evidence and evidence-based clinical guidelines for decision making.

Antenatal care is an excellent example of preventive healthcare, as it deals mainly with healthy individuals with an emphasis on the practice of health promotion. Besides, it includes the application of the principles of screening and early treatment of clinical complications. Rather than being limited to clinical interventions within a health facility, preventive actions can occur at various levels – from the home for family decisions to the community, and for public-wide actions such as the availability of transportation to health facilities. While some progress has been made toward meeting the United Nations Millennium Development Goal 5 targets of reducing maternal deaths by three quarters and universal access to reproductive health, the World Health Organization (WHO) reported that while maternal mortality has declined worldwide by 45%, in 2015 around 830 women die every day from problems in pregnancy and childbirth [13]. Only 5% of the women who died lived in high-income countries, the rest of the women lived in low-income countries [13]. Action for safe maternal care remains an urgent health priority in most developing countries.

Recently, a series of evidence-based algorithms and practice guidelines were developed for effective pregnancy and childbirth care [14]. The guidelines have the potential to improve outcomes of antenatal care for mothers and their newborns, particularly, in low resource countries. Caution should be exercised when using such guidelines and databases in the provision of care because of the limited contribution of the small number of patients from developing countries to their development. Present and planned contribution of studies from developing countries would improve the applicability of such clinical practice guidelines to local circumstances. This is most likely to occur when physicians take an active role in understanding and responding to the process of evidence-based practice based on the application of research-derived evidence to achieve the most effective clinical outcomes [10].

10.2 Preconception Care

Preconception care aims at identifying and reducing modifiable factors that can adversely affect pregnancy outcomes. Major professional organisations worldwide have endorsed pre-conception counselling as an integral component of care for all women contemplating pregnancy. A preconception care programme has the potential to assist women who want to become pregnant by advising them about risk factors, healthy lifestyles and assessing readiness for pregnancy. It includes a comprehensive history and physical examination with the initiation of health promotion interventions prior to conception. Preconception care operates within a variety of settings and modalities to achieve the following:

- Evaluation of medical conditions such as hypertension and diabetes that may adversely affect pregnancy outcomes.
- Risk assessment of high-risk health behaviours and counselling on health promotion activities such as smoking and alcohol cessation, cessation of non-prescription drugs and review of prescription medications with adverse effects on pregnancy.
- Dietary counselling including treatment of anaemia, pre-pregnancy weight problems and use of folic acid (400 μg) daily by women of childbearing age, preconception and during the first trimester. This is associated with a reduced incidence of first and subsequent neural tube defects.

- Screening for infectious diseases is important for patients at risk including tuberculosis that remains prevalent in many developing countries. Vaccination for the prevention of congenital infections such as congenital rubella syndrome, varicella and similar perinatal infections. Screening, prevention and treatment of infections such as hepatitis and acquired human immunodeficiency virus (HIV) can be achieved at this time to improve birth outcomes and prevent mother-to-child transmission of infection.
- Genetic counselling for conditions such as sickle cell disease and thalassaemia that are prevalent in some populations in developing countries should be an integral component of preconception care.

Counselling is tailored to the educational level of the patient, and risk factor reduction is emphasised as an important component of counselling. Healthcare providers must address the social as well as medical ramifications of pregnancy for both the mother and the foetus. A large proportion of pregnancies are unintended and unplanned in both developed and developing countries. Comparison of women whose pregnancies were intended to those with unintended pregnancies shows that the latter are more likely to report cigarette smoking and less likely to report daily vitamin intake. Women with unintended pregnancies are less likely to decrease consumption of caffeinated beverages [14]. Preconception care can further enhance pregnancy outcomes by optimising health during the most critical period of organogenesis, that is, between 17 and 56 days after conception.

A multidisciplinary approach to preconception and antenatal care can be achieved and effective in developing countries. Preconception care is most cost-effectively provided as an integral part of primary care services during routine health promotion. It may be introduced during routine screening, through patient education literature, family planning clinics, pre-employment assessment and in group health promotion classes. Nurses, midwives, social workers, nutritionists and health educators complement physicians in providing preconception care. This cost-effective approach appears to be acceptable to most women of childbearing age in developing countries.

Research data supporting the efficacy of preconception care are limited, but it has been shown to reduce perinatal mortality and morbidity in certain populations [15]. Much of the research on maternal outcomes focus on the events of pregnancy and delivery. Good maternal healthcare requires attention to physical, psychological and social factors. The rapport that often develops between patients and healthcare providers in the preconception period assists during difficult decision-making in pregnancy. Preconception programmes play an important role in reducing maternal and infant mortality and require appropriate priority in the allocation of resources for maternal health.

10.3 Organisation and Standardisation of Antenatal Care

Antenatal visits are embraced by pregnant women for the reassurance they receive besides providing opportunities for improving confidence and building rapport between healthcare providers and pregnant women. Continuity of care is promoted as being vital to good care. Medical surveillance throughout pregnancy is the foundation of antenatal care and is enhanced by emotional and psychosocial support. Organising integrated antenatal care is a challenge for most developing countries in view of the need to adapt to prevailing local circumstances. The philosophy of antenatal care developed mainly after the proposals of Ballantyne in 1902 and was originally for surveillance of medical complications during pregnancy and for preventing preterm labour [1]. Current models of antenatal care have evolved and expanded to include educational evaluation, psychological, social and financial support and health promotion, with little research to support their effectiveness. For more than three decades, there has been increasing scepticism of many tasks that are routinely included in antenatal care [16, 17]. Unfortunately, much of the controversy regarding antenatal care has focused on the timing and frequency of antenatal visits, whereas the content of antenatal care and the effectiveness of its actual delivery are more important. It is evident that much of the improvement in maternal health during the last century can be attributed to increased standards of living, and improved hygiene and nutrition. Nevertheless, the role of medical care should not be underestimated as exemplified by the higher levels of preventable maternal mortality among a North American religious group that opposed the provision of such care [18]. With continuing emphasis on evidence-based care, it is most appropriate to critically assess antenatal care with the aim of proposing an objective framework of care after considering local circumstances and implementation challenges.

Healthcare professionals including specialists must have a community perspective in their work, and in the case of antenatal care, constantly seek out unbooked patients, that is, patients lacking antenatal care, who are at increased risk of experiencing complications during pregnancy and delivery [14]. Further, the involvement of healthcare professionals in health centres and dispensaries increases access to antenatal services besides improving supervision and on-the-job training for staff based in peripheral and rural clinics. The value of home-based maternal record cards should not be underestimated. Quality of care should be a central feature of tasks, and clinical audit should be performed regularly to promote optimum utilisation of limited resources. Clinical management of difficult cases is facilitated by the availability of protocols for dealing with those situations.

Standardised antenatal care has been shown to minimise variability of care and ensure the quality and cost-effectiveness of care. Other potential applications include the education of individuals or groups developing quality indicators, improving the allocation of resources such as insurance payment decisions and reducing the risk of liability for care that is perceived to be substandard. For example, some pregnant women are eager to have supplementary care and certain tests, as substantiated by their willingness to pay for ultrasound examinations [19]. In the context of publicly provided services, the value of any intervention should be seen from the perspective of clinical needs relative to available resources. Throughout this chapter, we emphasise the philosophy of cost-effective, evidence-based antenatal care for developing countries.

A standardisation of antenatal medical records for primary care physicians is urgently needed in most developing countries. Antenatal records document the medical risks, behaviour and psychosocial situations of the patient and serve as a reminder for testing, counselling, and educational and medical services that are needed. Most antenatal records have a flow sheet that allows the clinician to follow important parameters during pregnancy. It is essential that women be given their antenatal records to have control over their health besides serving as an important tool of communication for healthcare teams [20]. Measurement processes are evolving to focus on how healthcare systems function in an integrated fashion instead of strictly on the approach or belief of individual physician or healthcare provider. Medical records are essential to evidence-based care, standardisation of care, and communication among healthcare professionals, especially using current information communication technologies. Whereas patient-held records are valuable to increase the involvement of pregnant women in their care, it is crucial to exploit linkages between databases of health facilities, especially with laboratories and imaging units, for efficient effective delivery of clinical services through improvement of quality of care.

10.4 Education, Counselling and Support

In general, pregnant women have certain expectations from the healthcare providers including respect for their sociocultural values, being treated with respect, and psychosocial and emotional support, besides education, counselling and medical treatment. Information from providers is more likely to be positively received in the aforementioned context by women as part of a consultation process. Therefore, antenatal care should offer great potential for behavioural changes for health promotion. Reducing or ceasing unhealthy personal habits such as smoking, alcohol consumption and the use of untested local herbal remedies should be encouraged. Foetal alcohol syndrome characterised by microcephaly, mental retardation, facial deformities and growth restriction is well-established preventable sequelae of alcohol consumption during pregnancy. Furthermore, smoking cessation efforts have been shown to be beneficial through individual or group counselling, supplemented by information booklets and community-wide approach for smoking control.

Similarly, appropriate advice is provided to pregnant women for improved nutrition. This nutritional support includes education on breastfeeding of the baby and the promotion of healthy nutrition throughout the course of pregnancy. This approach is of paramount importance in developing countries with high infant mortality attributable to infant nutritional deficiencies, besides infection from the unsafe water supply. Given the rising prevalence of single mothers in developing countries, access to social services and financial and psychological support are needed to assist individual mothers.

10.5 Antenatal Care Plans

Antenatal care must be tailored to each woman's needs and local circumstances. It is important to develop a care plan appropriate to the woman's situation and integrate antenatal care into the existing healthcare system to achieve its effectiveness. Current efforts focus on designing antenatal care involving fewer routine visits for low-risk women. This approach may lead to patient convenience and reduce costs besides enhancing compliance with ongoing care. The WHO recommends that pregnant women should all receive four antenatal visits to identify and treat clinical problems and give immunisations and appropriate medical interventions [21].

Several studies [21–23] have suggested that in women who book early for antenatal care, it might be possible to reduce the total number of antenatal visits without having any negative effect on infant health. As part of its work to help define and strengthen antenatal care, the WHO convened a working group to formulate recommendations for prenatal care at health centre levels. In a published report [22], the group agreed on the timing and content of focused prenatal care for all women as well as risk factors for medical conditions that would require special care. There is a need for a reduced schedule of visits (Table 10.1) for low-risk women in developing countries and a focus on greater maternal and professional satisfaction with this care plan.

Table 10.1 Frequency of antenatal visits in low-risk pregnancy

Visit	Gestational age (weeks)
First visit	16
Second visit	24–28
Third visit	32
Fourth visit	36

Emphasis must be placed on the role and appropriateness of midwives and allied health workers as providers of antenatal care services in developing countries. Also, it is imperative to educate and empower the entire community to address factors that contribute to maternal morbidity and mortality. Uncertainty remains as to the clinical effectiveness of reduced visit schedules for rare pregnancy problems. Operational research and evaluation of prenatal care practices are underway to identify the most effective and efficient way to provide antenatal care services [23, 24].

10.6 The Initial (Booking) Visit (Up to 16-Weeks Gestation)

Following the diagnosis of pregnancy, the first prenatal visit should occur during the first trimester. The focus of this visit, as for most of the antenatal care, is to identify all risk factors involving the mother and foetus. Once identified, high-risk pregnancies require individual specialised care beyond what could be provided by the community nurse, midwife or general physician. A thorough comprehensive medical history is necessary with particular attention to chronic illness, surgical procedures with attention to abdominal and pelvic operations and blood transfusions. It is important to obtain a detailed menstrual and gynaecological history including a history of sexually transmitted infections. Details of previous pregnancies and deliveries are important to ascertain risk. Genetic risk factors include maternal and paternal age, and past and family history of birth defects. Finally, social history must include substance use, nutrition, and lifestyle factors and stresses.

10.7 World Health Organization [22]

A comprehensive physical examination is performed at the first visit. Most pregnant women in developing countries might not have had a thorough physical examination since early childhood. Abnormal general physical findings such as anaemia, high blood pressure or heart murmur require further evaluation. A pelvic examination is carried out at the booking visit. Besides estimating the gestational age using uterine size, pelvic examination provides a unique opportunity for women in developing countries to have a Papanicolaou smear for cervical cancer screening. The common myth that a vaginal examination in pregnancy may be associated with spontaneous abortion has no scientific basis.

Appropriate laboratory investigations are ordered at the booking visit; again, the focus is on risk identification (Table 10.2). Abnormalities noted by history or on physical examination may require direct laboratory testing and follow-up. For example, women with uncertain dates may require ultrasonography for pregnancy dating. Routine counselling and education and the offering of HIV testing for pregnant women in developing countries have a great potential for reducing mother-to-infant transmission. With the proven effectiveness of antiretroviral agents in reducing the risk of vertical transmission of HIV from mother to foetus, there is a good reason to screen all pregnant women for HIV so that appropriate therapy can be administered. Initial management during the first antenatal visit includes advice on diet, exercise, work and lifestyle. Appropriate tests are requested and an outline of a formal plan for the rest of the pregnancy and how to access support services are discussed.

Table 10.2 Laboratory tests during antenatal care

Test	Rationale
(First trimester)	
Blood group and type	Determines ABO and RH incompatibility
Blood antibody screen	Detects isoimmunisation
Haematocrit	Detects maternal anaemia
Haemoglobin	
Electrophoresis	Screens for haemoglobinopathy
Hepatitis B, C surface	
Antigen	Screens for infection
Wasserman test	Screens for maternal infection
HIV test	Screens for maternal infection
Rubella titre	Detects maternal immunity
Chlamydia test	Screens for maternal infection
Gonorrhoea test	Screens for maternal infection
Urine culture	Detects asymptomatic bacteriuria
Papanicolaou smear	Screens for cervical cancer
(Second trimester)	
Maternal serum screen	
Or cell-free DNA	Screens for chromosomal anomalies and neural tube defect
Ultrasonography	Pregnancy dating, placental localisation, screens for major structural anomalies
(Third trimester)	
Glucose screen (50–	Screens for gestational diabetes
Blood antibody screen	Screens for isoimmunisation
Group B streptococcus	Detects carriers

10.8 Risk Scoring

Serious attempts to develop a scoring system for identifying risk factors in pregnancy began in the 1970s [23]. While risk scoring systems enable risk groups to be identified, they were too crude to be of value regarding caring for the individual woman. Current obstetric risk scoring systems do not make a precise prediction of an abnormal outcome, and therefore, cannot be used in formal decision analysis. An accurate assessment of foetal risk using a risk scoring system is limited by geographic and individual factors and the interdependency of most obstetric variables. However, where obstetrical care resources are limited and large numbers of high-risk pregnant women are scattered throughout remote areas, it would appear that risk scoring assists positively with decisions regarding the best use of resources.

Although clear evidence is lacking, there is a strong indication that favours the application of a modification of the WHO criteria for classifying women for the basic component of the new antenatal care model (Table 10.3) in developing countries, with limited availability of experienced caregivers to provide antenatal care [22, 23]. Risk scoring has also been proposed as a means of best utilisation of sparse human and material resources. It may be used to identify women who do not require an intensive programme of antenatal care that may be triaged to various healthcare providers based on the risk score.

10.9 Second Visit (24–28 weeks)

For patients with normal findings at the initial visit, our proposed care schedule of subsequent visits is shown in Table 10.1. Evidence from developing countries suggests that early onset of antenatal care and having subsequent three to four visits provide significant consistent and effective care for preventing perinatal problems [24–26]. Patients with high-risk pregnancies and those with ongoing complications are seen more frequently. During the visits, the results of routine tests are reviewed, health behaviour is reinforced and appropriate therapy provided as needed. Physical examination is limited to checking the blood pressure, maternal weight, assessing foetal growth by measuring the symphysis-fundal height in centimetres, verifying foetal cardiac activity and assessing peripheral oedema. The only routine laboratory test performed at every antenatal visit is the determination of proteinuria and glycosuria. Education continues to be important and patients must be made aware of warning signs such as vaginal bleeding, abnormal vaginal discharge, swelling and headaches. When appropriate, genetic testing is offered and performed at this time. Recent studies suggest that early amniocentesis and chorionic villus sampling are associated with a significant increase of foetal loss as compared to later amniocentesis. Second trimester (15–18 weeks) screening of a pregnant woman's serum for markers of congenital anomalies such as trisomy 21 (Down's syndrome) and neural tube defects is increasingly being utilised in developing countries as an important component of antenatal care. While assessing maternal blood for foetal cell-free DNA testing is new and limited to specialised centres, the most commonly utilised protocol is the triple marker screen, which measures serum levels of alpha-foetoprotein (AFP), unconjugated estriol (uE3) and beta human chorionic gonadotropin (beta-HCG). The results of these tests are used to derive a value known as a multiple of the median (MoM). An algorithm that combines maternal age with the test value can be used to calculate the risk for chromosomal disorders such as trisomy 21 and 18. Alpha-foetoprotein alone corrected for maternal weight, race, insulin-dependent diabetes, and multiple pregnancies can be used to predict the risk of neural tube defect.

Prenatal screening is best performed within an integrated programme providing biochemical testing in conjunction with knowledgeable, experienced counsellors, expert ultrasonographers and physicians with special expertise in maternal-foetal medicine and neonatal care. Prenatal screening provides patients with the information they need to make informed pregnancy decisions and, when necessary, organise support and resources essential to the care of an infant with special needs.

Routine ultrasound examination for congenital anomalies consists of a screening procedure performed on the total obstetrical population usually at 18–20 weeks of gestation, as opposed to the selective use of ultrasound that might provide more information for a problem that is suspected on clinical grounds. As the risk for foetal malformation is present in all pregnant women, many experts hold the opinion that antenatal ultrasound screening should be universal. However, screening may either lead to unnecessary anxiety if there is a false positive result or a false sense of security if there is a false negative result. There is extensive published work showing neither improvement in perinatal morbidity nor an overall reduction in unnecessary intervention with routine ultrasound. The role of ultrasonography and its validity as a screening test for foetal malformation in a low-risk population remains the subject of debate [27].

Notwithstanding the beneficial impact of prenatal screening, developing countries with limited financial and human resources must be cautious in introducing widespread screening services for pregnant women. In view of doubtful value in the investment of scarce resources, because the outcome might not justify the input, consideration must be given to health economics and health resource utilisation.

Table 10.3 Classifying form. Criteria for classifying women in the basic component of the new antenatal care model [22, 23]

Name of patient: ____________________ **Clinic record number:** ☐☐☐☐☐☐

Address: ____________________ **Telephone:** ____________________

INSTRUCTIONS: Answer all of the following questions by placing a cross mark in the corresponding box.

OBSTETRIC HISTORY		**No**	**Yes**
1.	Previous stillbirth or neonatal loss?	☐	☐
2.	History of 3 or more consecutive spontaneous abortions?	☐	☐
3.	Birthweight of last baby < 2500 g?	☐	☐
4.	Birthweight of last baby < 4500 g?	☐	☐
5.	Last pregnancy: hospital admission for hypertension or pre-e clampisa/e clampisa?	☐	☐
6.	Previous surgery on reproductive tract? (Myomectomy, removal of septum, cone biopsy, classical CS, cervical cerclage)	☐	☐

CURRENT PREGNANCY		**No**	**Yes**
7.	Diagnosed or suspected multiple pregnancy?	☐	☐
8.	Age less than 16 years?	☐	☐
9.	Age more than 40 years?	☐	☐
10.	Isoimmunization Rh (-) in current or in previous pregnancy?	☐	☐
11.	Vaginal bleeding?	☐	☐
12.	Pelvic mass?	☐	☐
13.	Diastolic blood pressure 90mm Hg or more at booking?	☐	☐

GENERAL MEDICAL		**No**	**Yes**
14.	Insulin-dependent diabetes mellitus?	☐	☐
15.	Renal disease?	☐	☐
16.	Cardiac disease?	☐	☐
17.	Known 'substance' abuse (including heavy alcohol drinking)?	☐	☐
18.	Any other severe medical disease or condition?	☐	☐

Please specify ____________________

____

A "Yes" answer to any ONE of the above questions (i.e. ONE shadd box marked with a cross) means that the Woman is not eligible for the basic component of the new antenatal care model.

Is the woman eligible? (circle) **NO** **YES**

If NO, she is referred to ____________________

Date ____________ Name ____________ Signature ____________

(staff responsible for ANC)

10.10 Third Visit (32 weeks)

During this period, advice and counselling provided during earlier visits are reinforced. Physical examination during the visit includes measurement of blood pressure, foetal growth by fundal height, documentation of foetal heart activity, and assessment of the presentation of the foetus. Foetal movement awareness and charting are initiated. The status of screening procedures for gestational diabetes remains highly controversial in view of the lack of evidence regarding the various strategies such as glycosuria testing, blood glucose levels and oral glucose challenge or tolerance tests. The situation is made more complex by conflicting recommendations from various respected organisations [28]. Therefore, the approach should be based on clinical acumen and the appropriate use of resources, a good example of the practical limitations of an evidence-based approach. It seems reasonable to screen for diabetes based on risk factors such as older age, obesity, family history and previous history of conditions such as prematurity, foetal macrosomia, congenital anomalies or intrauterine foetal death. Because diabetes has a devastating effect on pregnancy, screening for diabetes at 26–28 weeks' gestation with a 50-g 1-hour glucose challenge test seems prudent.

In Rhesus negative women, a repeat indirect Coomb's test is performed and, if negative, rhesus (D) immune globulin is given to prevent sensitisation to the Rhesus antigen. Repeat haematocrit and HIV screening are done in high-risk women during the period. Common causes of pregnancy-related anaemia consist of deficiencies of iron and folic acid besides infections such as malaria and helminths such as hookworms. Given the widespread prevalence of iron deficiency in developing countries, it is reasonable to recommend oral iron supplementation on a routine basis. As oral iron therapy is associated with minor side effects such as constipation especially in early pregnancy, it is best to await the beginning of the second trimester before initiating daily supplementation with 30 mg of elemental iron in the ferrous form. Patients with anaemia require appropriate therapy and those with folate deficiency which occurs mostly in multiple gestations require daily supplementation with 5 mg of folic acid orally for prevention. This approach regarding supplementation does not replace the value of an appropriate diet even prior to pregnancy. It is even more important for the primary prevention of neural tube defects through an adequate intake of folic acid.

10.11 Fourth Visit (36 weeks)

In developing countries, the major causes of morbidity and mortality for the mother, foetus and newborn are haemorrhage, hypertensive disorders, infections, obstructed labour, prematurity and anaemia. Therefore, it is appropriate that antenatal care addresses the preventive issues associated with these conditions. Third-trimester antenatal care focuses on maternal blood pressure and weight as well as surveillance of foetal wellbeing. Hypertensive disorders account for much of the maternal and perinatal morbidity and mortality in developing countries. Transient hypertension is a clinically benign condition characterised by isolated high blood pressure in late pregnancy; its significance lies in the difficulty in distinguishing it from early pre-eclampsia. Chronic hypertension is a risk factor for intrauterine foetal growth restriction and intrauterine foetal demise, as well as for pre-eclampsia. Management of gestational hypertension at earlier stages of gestation requires balancing the risks of immediate delivery of an immature infant against the risks to both mother and infant of a complication of pre-eclampsia. The management strategy consists of control of maternal blood pressure, ongoing antepartum assessment of foetal wellbeing, and surveillance for superimposed pre-eclampsia. Prompt recognition can prevent adverse outcomes in most cases. Early detection enables treatment to avoid complications such as eclampsia and stroke [26].

The third trimester is the time to discuss the birth plan. A detailed review of labour and delivery prepares the patient for the labour experience. Pain control methods are discussed (or taught in special education classes) as they reduce the need for pain medication by as much as 30%.

10.12 Foetal Surveillance

As part of meticulous antenatal care, multiple methods of foetal health surveillance provide enormous means to improve foetal outcomes. Antepartum foetal assessment is used in pregnancies at risk for perinatal morbidity and mortality. Current testing options include the foetal movement count, non-stress test, contraction stress test and biophysical profiles. Vibroacoustic stimulation and umbilical as well as mid-cerebral artery Doppler velocimetry studies are useful adjunctive procedures in women with pregnancy complications. All these modalities have limitations. A strict protocol for antepartum foetal surveillance that is applicable to all patients is not feasible. However, testing based on general principles and guidelines can be followed. Although few practitioners working in specialised centres in developing countries have experience and expertise with these complex tests, knowledge is growing with the increased availability of modern facilities. Current evidence suggests that antepartum assessment by foetal biophysical profile scoring is associated with a significant reduction in the incidence of cerebral palsy in tested high-risk patients compared to untested patients [29]. Nevertheless, the extent of testing needs to be tailored to local resources and available expertise.

Pregnant women and their families usually become more apprehensive as delivery approaches and have several concerns that require sensitive explanation and reassurance. A common concern relates to the health of the foetus as labour approaches, particularly regarding delivery and perinatal infectious complications. Group B streptococcal infection is the most common cause of neonatal sepsis and is responsible for significant neonatal morbidity and mortality. Approximately 25% of women have asymptomatic Group B streptococcal infection at some time during pregnancy, but the neonatal infection rate is only about 2 per 1000 deliveries [30]. Nevertheless, it is important for all pregnant women to be tested for group B streptococcus between 35 and 37 weeks of every pregnancy. To help protect their newborns from infection, pregnant women who test positive for Group B strep in the current pregnancy should receive prophylactic antibiotics intravenously during labour.

Detailed counselling of women during the last weeks of pregnancy includes childbirth preparations (labour, monitoring plans, support, pain relief and questions about episiotomy). It is critically important that skilled birth attendants are available during labour regardless of the type of birthing centre, maternity unit or hospital undertaking the delivery. It is particularly important to plan for the place of birth especially for the 10–20% of women who will need to have an emergency transfer in late pregnancy or during labour to facilities where blood transfusion and procedures such as caesarean section are available. In patients with gestation exceeding 40 weeks, an explanation is provided about the significance of a postdate pregnancy. Of concern to women is uteroplacental insufficiency and increased size of the baby, which can make delivery more difficult. Assessment of the cervix is conducted, and education is provided on foetal surveillance and the methods of induction of labour when needed. While routine induction of labour is not recommended, available evidence shows that it is beneficial after 41 completed weeks in reducing the risk of perinatal death.

10.13 Unbooked Patients (With no Antenatal Care)

A pregnant woman is classified as 'booked' or having had appropriate care if she has attended at least four antenatal visits. Unbooked patients presenting for the first time late in the third trimester or in labour are a common occurrence in developing countries. When a patient who has had no antenatal care presents late in pregnancy or in labour, it is essential to rapidly assess the pregnancy risk factors. A focused history, physical examination and laboratory assessment are conducted. The profile that emerges from various studies is that the unbooked mother is young, unmarried, unemployed, has a low income, and has no permanent relationship with the father of the infant. However, she knows about antenatal care and knows that is important to seek such care [31]. The reasons for not seeking care are usually varied and non-specific. It has been suggested that an important difference between booked and unbooked patients is the personality and attitude toward pregnancy and parenthood. Obstetric complications in unbooked patients include anaemia, hypertensive disorders, preterm labour, preterm rupture of the membranes, antepartum haemorrhage and intrauterine foetal death. In reviewing published work, one can detect a higher obstetric risk profile in booked mothers with poor obstetric history, which probably influenced their decision to seek antenatal care. Unbooked mothers tend to be at lower risk, often presenting 'unbooked' because of antenatal complications [31]. Several studies found a statistically significant association between the absence of antenatal care and adverse maternal and foetal outcomes [32]. This emphasises the need for regular antenatal visits and underscores the utilisation of antenatal care services to avoid the complications of pregnancy. The provision of antenatal and emergency obstetric care has played a vital role in reducing maternal, perinatal and infant mortality in developing countries during the past 60 years and must continue to be promoted as an important component of safe maternal health.

10.14 Effectiveness of Different Antenatal Care Models

There is not a lot of evidence to justify a specific antenatal care model among the different ones that are currently used. There is a dearth of objective evidence to enable comparative assessment of the various existing models for antenatal care: focused visits versus the traditional number of visits; midwife-led continuity care versus shared care with the general practitioner or consultant-led care. Midwife-led care for low-risk women is where a midwife team leads the care a woman receives (with general physician back-up when needed) or with specialist back-up [33]. Group ANC is a model that brings together a healthcare provider, usually a midwife, and a group of women in the same stage of pregnancy to receive care. This model is highly utilised in low- and medium-resource countries. Group antenatal care has a couple of obvious benefits: it costs less than one-to-one visits and the women have more hours of care as a group than on their own. Only small studies have been conducted looking at group care, but they have found that mothers knew more about pregnancy, birth and parenting in the group setting. The mothers reported liking the group care and the review found no difference between how the pregnancies developed between the group and individual setting [34, 35].

A meta-analysis of models of antenatal care by Fernandez and colleagues found no significant differences in different models of antenatal care regarding maternal and foetal outcomes in low risk women [36].

10.15 Barriers and Enablers to Utilisation of Antenatal Care

Although antenatal care is important for improving the health of the mother and baby, many women do not receive the recommended four visits. Barriers that exist to effective antenatal care include: (1) inadequate infra-structural resources, (2) lack of knowledge of services, (3) ignorance of the importance and value of antenatal services, (4) cultural, religious and traditional practices (including beliefs in traditional healers, (5) lower women's autonomy, in making their own healthcare decisions, (6) poverty and lack of transportation resources and (7) household responsibilities. Aniebue and colleagues [24] found that while most women who utilised fewer focused antenatal visits did so because of its convenience and low cost. On the contrary, 45% feared the new model might be inadequate for their learning, familiarisation with care providers and for early detection of disease. The authors suggested 'an extensive health education campaign, social mobilisation and involvement of relevant stakeholders in the design, execution and monitoring of focused antenatal care from the inception of the programme' [24]. There are additional strategies to assist women to access antenatal care such as new health policies, educating health workers and promote health service reorganisation. Community interventions to help people change pregnant women's behaviour can also play a part. Examples of these interventions are media campaigns reaching many people, enabling communities to take control of their own health, informative-education-communication interventions or financial incentives [37, 38]. These interventions used together are more effective and have the potential to improve the number of women receiving antenatal care and reduce maternal mortality in early infant deaths in developing countries.

10.16 Summary

Antenatal care has various facets, ranging from the prevention of morbidity and mortality to the promotion of maternal and foetal wellbeing and their medical and psychosocial implications. Developing and industrialised countries have much in common and can learn from each other in terms of programme development to enhance maternal health. It would not be appropriate for programmes of developed countries to be adopted by developing countries without evaluation of their relevance. Instead, they should be adapted for utilisation after considering local circumstances. As detailed in this chapter, it is easy to agree on certain procedures for antenatal care such as routine assessment of blood pressure for early detection of hypertensive disease of pregnancy but difficult to obtain consensus on others, such as an appropriate number of antenatal visits, the extent of prenatal genetic screening, and the need for routine use of ultrasound for the monitoring of foetal growth. Nevertheless, the promotion and availability of an appropriate framework should enhance the improvement of antenatal care delivery.

With the rationalisation of healthcare resources and a paradigm shift towards evidence-based care, communities in developing countries must work together to improve access to reproductive healthcare. We have reviewed an approach to a focused and evidence-based antenatal care that is cost-effective and efficient. However, caution must be exercised in adopting a narrow focus toward evidence-based care that incorporates research evidence from developed countries without due consideration for prevailing local conditions and circumstances. We suggest an expanded, community-based maternal health initiative that includes birth centres, well-woman clinics, teen pregnancy programmes and family planning services. The staff of such programmes must include nurses, certified midwives, social workers, general medical practitioners, and specialist obstetricians and gynaecologists. Pregnant women need the support of caring family members, friends and health professionals. As noted by East and colleagues [39] 'while programmes that offer additional social support during pregnancy are unlikely to have a large impact on the proportion of low birthweight babies or birth before 37 weeks' gestation and little impact on stillbirth or neonatal death, they may be helpful in reducing the likelihood of caesarean birth and antenatal hospital admission'. Through innovative and well-coordinated healthcare delivery by health professionals, it is anticipated that the incidence of pregnancy complications would continue to decrease, and thereby improve maternal health, newborn and infant outcomes in developing countries.

References

1. Cunningham EG, MacDonald PC, Leveno KJ, et al. Prenatal care. In: Williams obstetrics. 24th ed. Stamford: Appleton and Lange; 2014. p. 227.
2. Hogan MC, Freeman K, Naghavi M, et al. Maternal mortality for 181 countries, 1980-2008: a systematic analysis of progress towards Millennium Development Goal 5. Lancet. 2010;375:1609–23.
3. Bingham D, Suplee PD, Morris HM, McBride M. Healthcare strategies for reducing pregnancy-related morbidity and mortality in the postpartum period. J Perinat Neonatal Nurs. 2018;32(3):241–9.
4. Bollini P, Quack-Lotscher K. Guidelines-based indicators to measure quality of antenatal care. J Eval Clin Pract. 2013;19(6):1060–6.
5. Chavane L, Merialdi M, Betran AP, et al. Implementation of evidence-based antenatal care in Mozambique: a cluster randomised controlled trial: study protocol. BMC Health Serv Res. 2014;14:228.
6. Finlayson K. Global access to antenatal care: a qualitative perspective. Pract Midwife. 2015;18(2):10–2.

7. Finlayson K, Downe S. Why do women not use antenatal services in low- and middle-income countries. A meta-synthesis of qualitative studies. PLoS Med. 2013;10:1373.
8. Dowswell T, Carrolli G, Gates S, et al. Alternative versus standard packages of antenatal care for low-risk pregnancy. Cochrane Database Syst Rev. 2015;(7):CD000934. https://doi.org/10.1002/14651858.CD000934.pub3.
9. Vogel JP, Oladapo OT, Manu A, et al. New WHO recommendations to improve the outcome of preterm birth. Lancet Glob Health. 2015;3(10):e589–90.
10. Olatunbosun OA, Edouard L. The teaching of evidence-based reproductive health in developing countries. Int J Obstet Gynaecol. 1997;56:171–6.
11. Mbuagbaw L, Medley N, Darzi AJ, et al. Health system and community level interventions for improving antenatal care coverage and health outcomes. Cochrane Database Syst Rev. 2015;(12):CD010994. https://doi.org/10.1002/14651858.CD010994.pub2.
12. Abalos E, Chamilard M, Diaz V, et al. Antenatal care for healthy pregnant women: a mapping of interventions from existing guidelines to inform the development of new WHO guidance on antenatal care. BJOG. 2016;123(4):519–28.
13. Say L, Chou D, Gemmill A, et al. Global causes of maternal death: a WHO systematic analysis. Lancet Glob Health. 2014;2(6):e323–33.
14. World Health Organization. Preconception care to reduce maternal and childhood mortality and morbidity. Meeting report and packages of interventions. Geneva: World Health Organization; 2013.
15. Dean SV, Lassi ZS, Imam AM, et al. Preconception care: closing the gap in the continuum of care to accelerate improvements in maternal, newborn and child health. Reprod Health. 2014;11(suppl 1):S1.
16. Ali AAA, Osman MM, Abbaker AO, et al. Use of antenatal care services in Kassala, eastern Sudan. BMC Pregnancy Childbirth. 2010;10:67. https://doi.org/10.1186/1471-2393-10-67.
17. Tayebi T, Zahrani ST, Mohammadpour R. Relationship between adequacy of prenatal care utilisation index and pregnancy outcomes. Iran J Nurs Midwifery Res. 2013;18(5):360–6.
18. Kanunitz AM, Spence C, Danielson TS, et al. Perinatal and maternal mortality in a religious group avoiding obstetric care. Am J Obstet Gynecol. 1984;150(7):826–31.
19. Whitworth M, Bricker L, Mullan C, et al. Ultrasound for fetal assessment in early pregnancy. Cochrane Database Syst Rev. 2015;(7):CD007058. PMID 26171896.
20. Hawley G, Janamian T, Jackson C, Wlkinson SA. In a maternity shared-care environment, what do we know about paper hand-held and electronic health record: a systematic literature review. BMC Pregnancy Childbirth. 2014;14:52.
21. World Health Organization. WHO statement on antenatal care. WHO/RHR/11.12. 2011.
22. World Health Organization. WHO antenatal care randomised trial manual for the implementation of the new WHO programme to map best reproductive health practices. WHO/RHR/01.30. 2002.
23. Yeoh PL, Hometz K, Dahlui M. Antenatal care utilisation between low-risk and high-risk pregnant women. PLoS One. 2016;11(3):e0152167. https://doi.org/10.1371/journal.pone.0152167.
24. Aniebue UU, Aniebue PN. Women's perception as a barrier to focused antenatal care in Nigeria: the issue of fewer antenatal visits. Health Policy Plan. 2011;26:423–8.
25. Ekele BA. What is the place of the new WHO antenatal care model in a teaching hospital setting? Trop Dr. 2008;36:21–4.
26. Ezeonu PO, Lawani LO, Iyoke CA, et al. The preference and practice of Nigerian obstetricians regarding focused versus standard models of antenatal care. Int J Gynaecol Obstet. 2015;128:232–5.
27. Honore KD, Garne E. Trends in prenatal diagnosis of congenital anomalies among live births over a 30-year period. J Reprod Biol Health. 2014;2(1):1. http://www.hoajonline.com
28. Simmons D, Moses RG. Gestational diabetes mellitus: to screen or not to screen? Is this really a question? Diabetes Care. 2013;36:2877–8.
29. Okusanya BO. Antenatal cardiotocography for fetal assessment. RHL The WHO Reproductive Health Library. Geneva: World Health Organization; 2010.
30. John AK, Lata H, Yaday P, et al. Epidemiology of group B streptococcus in developing countries. Vaccine. 2013;31(Suppl):D43–5.
31. Chigbu B, Onwere S, Kamanu CI, et al. Pregnancy outcome in booked and unbooked mothers in south eastern Nigeria. East Afr Med J. 2009;86(6):267–71.
32. Guerrier G, Oluyide B, Keramarou M, Grais R. High maternal and neonatal mortality rates in northern Nigeria: an 8-month observational study. Int J Women's Health. 2013;13(5):495–9.
33. Sandall J, Soltani H, Gates S, et al. Midwife-led continuity model versus other models of care for child-bearing women. Cochrane Database Syst Rev. 2015;(9):CD004667. PMID 26370160.
34. Catling CJ, Medley N, Foureur M, et al. Group versus conventional antenatal care for women. Cochrane Database Syst Rev. 2015;(2):CD007622. https://doi.org/10.1002/14651858. PMID 25922865.
35. Gareau S, Lopez-De Fede A, Loudermilk BL, et al. Group prenatal care results in Medicaid savings with better outcomes: a propensity score analysis of centreing/pregnancy participation in South Carolina. Matern Child Health J. 2016;20(7):1384–93.
36. Fernandez TC, Sandal J, Peacock JL. Models of antenatal care to reduce and prevent preterm birth: a systematic review and meta-analysis. BMJ Open. 2016;6(1):e009044. https://doi.org/10.1136/bmjopen-2015-009044.
37. Basani DG, Surkan PJ, Olinto MTA. Inadequate use of prenatal services among Brazilian women: the role of maternal characteristics. Int Perspect Sex Reprod Health. 2009;35:15–20.
38. Tuncalp O, Were WM, McLennan C, et al. Quality of care for pregnant women and newborns: the WHO vision. BJOG. 2015;122(8):1045–9.
39. East CE, Biro MA, Fredericks S, Lau R. Support during pregnancy for women at risk of low birthweight babies. Cochrane Database Syst Rev. 2019;(4):CD000198. https://doi.org/10.1002/14651858.

11 Fetal Growth Abnormalities: Intrauterine Growth Restriction and Macrosomia

Jedidiah Dase Kingsley Sodje

Learning Objectives

At the end of this chapter, the reader should be able to:

- Define the terms IUGR, SGA, LGA, AGA and SGA.
- List the causes of the various foetal growth abnormalities especially IUGR and LGA foetuses.
- Identify the specific features and clinical and sonologic diagnostic tools for evaluating the IUGR and LGA foetuses and pregnancies.
- Differentiate between constitutionally small or large foetuses and IUGR and LGA foetuses, respectively.
- Contrast between AGA, IUGR and LGA foetuses.
- Discuss the pathology of IUGR and macrosomia and their management.
- Review and manage foetal macrosomia and IUGR pregnancies.

11.1 Introduction

Birth weight is an important determinant of pregnancy outcome. Normal standards of weight matched for gestational age (GA) in utero and weight at birth have been developed for the different races of the world [1]. Normal standards for other parameters of foetal growth measurement such as biparietal diameter, head circumference, foetal length, abdominal circumference and femur length have also been developed. Abnormalities in foetal growth are measured in percentiles of these values for each sex, race and population [1]. Foetuses or newborns whose weights are more than the 90th percentile are said to be large for gestational age (LGA) while those whose weights are less than the tenth percentile for that population are described as small for gestational age (SGA). These foetuses may be suffering from intrauterine growth restriction (IUGR) and may be constitutionally small or small due to chromosomal or environmental causes. Intrauterine growth restriction refers to a situation where the progressive growth of a foetus has reduced or is failing to reach its optimal potential and is usually due to a pathological condition [2].

Small for gestational age and LGA foetuses and newborns are associated with increased likelihood of complications that result in perinatal morbidity and mortality especially in developing countries having inadequate facilities for diagnoses and treatment. Intrauterine growth restriction, in particular, contributes significantly to foetal death, preterm deliveries, need for intervention (including surgical), perinatal and early neonatal deaths [2, 3]. They may also result in immediate, medium and long-term consequences and complications for the babies who survive.

Normal birth weights for most races and populations are generally determined to be ≥2500 g to <4500 g (some in the developing world use <4000 g). Outside these accepted normal values are the babies with disproportionate foetal growths of foetal macrosomia or LGA and low birth weight babies. These babies even when appropriate for gestational age (AGA) or not growth restricted may also develop pathologies that will require close attention. The specialist obstetrician, family physician and health professionals who care for pregnant women need to be abreast with the various pathologies and differentials that could lead to IUGR and LGA babies. They need to know how to prevent, investigate, diagnose and treat these pathologies that result in disproportionate foetal growth in settings with standard diagnostic and therapeutic tools as well as in under-resourced settings.

J. D. K. Sodje (✉)
Department of Obstetrics & Gynaecology, University of Benin and University of Benin Teaching Hospital, Benin City, Nigeria
e-mail: jedidiah.sodje@uniben.edu

F. Okonofua et al. (eds.), *Contemporary Obstetrics and Gynecology for Developing Countries*,
https://doi.org/10.1007/978-3-030-75385-6_11

11.2 Intrauterine Growth Restriction

A foetus is said to be intrauterine growth restricted when the weight or other biophysical parameters are less than the tenth percentile for that gestational age, sex and race or population due to a pathological condition or causes [1, 2, 4]. This assumes that there is the correct determination of GA which may require a reliable calendar record of last menstrual period or better still a first or second trimester ultrasound scan dating of the pregnancy. The incidence of IUGR depends on the population being studied. It is thought to be 4–8% in developed and 6–30% in developing countries [5, 6]. IUGR is a condition that does not allow the developing foetus to achieve its highest growth potential and is second only to prematurity as a leading cause of perinatal morbidity and mortality [7, 8].

IUGR foetuses may be symmetrically or asymmetrically growth restricted [7]. Symmetrical growth restriction results from early assaults on growth (usually before 28 weeks) affecting all biophysical parameters while asymmetrical growth restriction results from late assaults which mostly spare the brain and head. The Ponderal index (PI), an indicator of asymmetrical foetal growth, is the ratio of the birth weight of a newborn to the cube root of the length. It may be normal in symmetrical IUGR. Genetic and chromosomal abnormalities, congenital, teratogenic and infectious causes usually cause growth restriction early and result in symmetrical growth restriction. Conditions resulting in placental abnormalities and insufficiency usually occur later (usually after 28 weeks), and these cause asymmetrical growth restriction with large head to body ratios. The PI in asymmetric IUGR is low [8]. Approximately 50–70% of foetuses with estimated foetal weight below the tenth percentile are correctly constitutionally small [10, 11]; the terminology IUGR is, therefore, inappropriate for them.

SGA and IUGR are terms occasionally used to discuss foetuses with disproportionate growth. SGA often used to describe the newborn and IUGR to describe the foetus.

11.2.1 Pathology of IUGR

IUGR foetuses when compared with appropriate for gestational age foetuses have altered body constitution. They have decreased total body fat, protein, glycogen, free fatty acids, DNA, RNA and altered distribution of weight amongst the organs of the body [12]. Twenty per cent of IUGR infants are symmetrically small while another 80% are asymmetrically small, the brain-head to body ratio being proportionately larger. This is due to late assault causing the IUGR. Brain weight is only slightly reduced in asymmetrical IUGR babies compared to the symmetrical IUGR [7–9, 12]. Asymmetric IUGR newborns have slightly decreased brain weight compared to appropriate for gestational weight newborns due to decreased brain cell size not due to decreased number of brain cells. Brain abnormalities include reduced myelination, reduced ability to utilise metabolic substances like fat and amino acids but are able to utilise glucose. They have reduced ability for protein synthesis by the brain cells. These abnormalities most likely affect cerebellar and brainstem functions. The brain sparing is most pronounced when the assault causing IUGR occurred late in pregnancy [12, 13]. IUGR newborns with symmetric disproportionate growth have much smaller brains than the asymmetric. This is caused by the reduced number of brain cells.

Pulmonary and renal blood flow is reduced in IUGR foetuses, reducing the contribution of the lungs and kidneys to amniotic fluid and resulting in oligohydramnios. The lungs of IUGR foetuses mature earlier and produce surfactant at an earlier gestational age than would appropriate for gestational age babies.

It is estimated that maternal factors influence about 50%, foetal factors influence about 20% and unknown factors influence another 30% of foetal growth.

11.3 Risk Factors and Causes of IUGR [7, 11, 12]

Foetal Causes

(a) Genetic/Chromosomal Disorders
   (i). Autosomal genetic disorders – trisomy 13, 18, 21, deletions
   (ii). Sex chromosomes – Turner syndrome
(b) Structural Congenital Abnormalities
   (i). Cardiovascular anomalies
   (ii). Abdominal wall defects – gastroschisis, omphalocele
   (iii). Gastrointestinal anomalies
   (iv). Genitourinary system anomalies
   (v). Skeletal/dysmorphic syndromes, e.g. osteogenesis imperfecta
   (vi). CNS anomalies – Neural tube defects – spinal bifida
(c) Placental/Umbilical Cord Abnormalities
   (i). Placenta previa
   (ii). Placental malformations
   (iii). Twin-twin transfusion syndrome
   (iv). Placental infarction
(d) Multiple Gestation
(e) Congenital Infections
   (i). Rubella
   (ii). Cytomegalovirus

(iii). Varicella zoster
(iv). Herpes
(v). Listeriosis
(vi). Syphilis
(vii). Malaria
(viii). Toxoplasmosis

I. Maternal Causes
(a) Pre-eclampsia/eclampsia
(b) Chronic hypertension
(c) Anaemia
(d) HBSS
(e) Malnutrition
(f) Cardiac disease.
(g) Chronic obstructive airway disease
(h) Renal disease
(i) Substance abuse – alcohol, cigarette and hard drugs
(j) Anticonvulsants
(k) Anticoagulants

II. Maternal Constitutional Make Up. Constitutionally small newborns

III. Maternal Infections
(a) Malaria
(b) Tuberculosis
(c) HIV/AIDS

11.3.1 Foetal causes of IUGR

11.3.1.1 Genetic/Chromosomal Anomalies

Genetic and chromosomal disorders are found in over 38% of IUGR newborns with 8–19% of them having an associated major congenital anomaly [12–14]. They usually cause symmetrical growth restrictions. Down syndrome (trisomy 21) is the most frequent trisomy in the newborn with the incidence of 1.6 per 1000 live births with higher incidence with increasing maternal age. Down syndrome newborns have four times the frequency of IUGR found in normal babies. Edward's syndrome (trisomy 18) and Patau's syndrome (trisomy 13) are less common. Almost all Edward's syndrome and 50% of Patau's syndrome foetuses suffer from IUGR. Sex chromosome anomalies such as Turners cause the foetus to be growth restricted [12–14].

11.3.1.2 Foetal Structural Abnormalities

Newborns with structural abnormalities have IUGR in 22% [15]. Foetuses with neural tube defects (such as spina bifida) and anencephaly are usually growth restricted with the anencephalic being up to 1000 g less than normal newborns at birth [14, 15].

Foetuses with dysmorphic syndromes such as osteogenesis imperfecta and achondroplasia may be IUGR foetuses. Abdominal wall defects such as gastroschisis cause IUGR newborns. Foetuses with renal agenesis (Potters syndrome), urinary outflow obstruction, duodenal atresia and pancreatic agenesis frequently have IUGR [12].

11.3.1.3 Congenital Infections

Congenital infections are reported by authors to be the cause of 5–10% of IUGR pregnancies. The most microbial cause is cytomegalovirus, said to be present in 0.5–2% of all neonates in the United States and Europe [16]. Foeto-placental infections result in cell destruction, inflammation, calcification and reduced placental function and exchange. They thus cause growth restriction. Congenital pneumonia, hepatosplenomegaly, thrombocytopenia, microcephaly and intracranial calcifications may suggest congenital infection.

Congenital rubella infection increases the risk of IUGR and congenital abnormalities significantly, especially with first trimester infections. Anomalies include central nervous system anomalies like microcephaly, blindness, deafness, mental retardation and structural problems of the cardiovascular system.

Listeriosis caused by Listeria monocytogenes is a notable bacterial cause of IUGR with associated congenital pneumonia, hepatosplenomegaly, jaundice, petechial haemorrhage and encephalitis. Other bacterial infections majorly cause preterm labour and delivery.

Malaria is a frequent cause of IUGR in Sub-Saharan Africa, the Latin Americas and Asia. The incidence of maternal, umbilical cord blood and placental parasitaemia in malarial endemic regions are 33.2%, 22% and 21.7%, respectively [17]. Cord blood and placenta parasitaemia both correlate with a twofold higher risk of IUGR. These outcomes are more pronounced in the primigravida. Toxoplasmosis gondii transmitted through improperly cooked meat also predisposes to IUGR.

11.3.1.4 Placental/Umbilical Cord Disorders

Placental causes of IUGR include placenta previa, placental infarction, mild chronic abruptio placenta, calcifications in placenta, malformations of the umbilical cord or placenta and single umbilical artery.

11.3.1.5 Multiple Gestation

Multiple pregnancies are high risk pregnancies associated with increased risk of IUGR (20–30%) [9], congenital anomalies and preterm delivery; all of which may result in delivery of LBW babies, some of which will be growth restricted. IUGR in multiple pregnancies may result from placental insufficiency, twin-twin transfusion syndrome and inadequate nutrient intake by the mother for more than one foetus [9, 18, 19].

11.3.1.6 Foetal Sex

Male foetuses averagely weigh 5% more and measure 2% more than female foetuses at term.

11.3.2 Cautionary Tale

A 2-year-old child attending daycare was noticed by her 30-year-old mother to have rash assumed to be measles. The mother later had a similar rash and was at that time 6 weeks pregnant. The mother sought medical advice and was treated for 'measles' which was assumed would pose no serious threat to the pregnancy. In the third trimester, the foetus was noted to be growth restricted and ultrasound did not detect gross abnormalities. The baby was born at 38 weeks weighing 2000 g and was shortly noted to have poorly developed eyes, hearing and mental defects. Further investigation and enquiries confirmed that the IUGR and birth defects were in keeping with rubella infection which if suspected in early pregnancy could have been confirmed and termination of pregnancy recommended to the woman.

11.3.2.1 Maternal Causes of IUGR

Maternal factors predisposing to IUGR cause impaired blood flow to the placenta and placental insufficiency. A woman who has had an IUGR foetus before has about two- or four-fold risk for another IUGR foetus after 1 or 2 IUGR births, respectively [12]. Maternal hypertensive disorders in pregnancy including pre-eclampsia are the most common intrinsic maternal factors resulting in IUGR [3]. Hypertension frequently causes placental infarction.

In the developing world, the most important aetiologic factors for IUGR are poor maternal nutrition, malaria, pre-eclampsia, poor pregnancy weight gain, low pre-pregnancy weight and intestinal parasites. In the developed world, maternal cigarette smoking is the single most important aetiologic factor for IUGR.

11.3.2.2 Maternal Lifestyle/Habits

Significant alcohol consumption in pregnancy could cause foetal alcohol syndrome with IUGR. Cigarette smoking causes one-third of the IUGR cases in USA and is the most easily identifiable and preventable cause of IUGR [20, 21]. There is 3–4 times increased incidence of IUGR in foetuses of mothers who smoke. Mothers who use recreational drugs such as Indian hemp, cocaine and heroin also have their foetuses prone to IUGR.

Women in developing countries engage in strenuous work activities such as subsistence farming and its related heavy lifting. This along with the associated malnutrition of poverty predispose to IUGR.

11.3.2.3 Maternal Prescription Drugs

Warfarin (anticoagulant) and immunosuppressive agents like azathioprine, corticosteroids, cyclosporine and anticonvulsants are possible causes of IUGR.

11.3.2.4 Maternal Malnutrition and Malabsorption

Malnutrition with decreased provision of protein (amino acids), glucose, lipids (fatty acids and triglycerides), vitamins (including folate) and minerals (including iron) are common causes of IUGR particularly in the developing world [22]. Poverty is an associated aetiologic factor for IUGR. Poor maternal weight gain in pregnancy, hyperemesis gravidarum, intestinal parasites, inflammatory bowel diseases and tropical sprue are causes of IUGR. Adolescent pregnancies are also noted to have nutrition-related IUGR [14, 23].

11.3.2.5 Maternal Anaemia

Chronic maternal anaemia is still very prevalent in the developing countries of the world, particularly, in sub-Saharan Africa. Incidence of sickle cell disease is still high with associated chronic anaemia and vascular occlusion. These states predispose to IUGR [22].

11.3.2.6 Vascular Disorders

Diseases that affect the blood supply to the placenta bed particularly affecting the microvasculature frequently cause IUGR. These include complicated insulin-dependent diabetes mellitus, pre-eclampsia and antiphospholipid syndrome (collagen vascular disease).

11.3.2.7 Maternal Infections

Maternal infection with malaria, HIV/AIDS and tuberculosis are noted to be associated with increased incidence of IUGR. These diseases are still prevalent in parts of the developing world [22].

11.3.2.8 Uterine Abnormalities

Uterine abnormalities like uterine fibroids and uterine synechiae may result in impaired blood flow to the foetus causing IUGR.

11.3.2.9 Constitutionally Small Mother

The mother may be constitutionally small, belong to a race or population with a small body physique and thus deliver essentially normal newborns who are small. These babies will have a normal Pondera index.

$$\text{Pondera Index is Birthweight}(\text{g}) \times 100 / \left[\text{crown heel length}(\text{cm})\right]^3.$$

The Pondera index for a normal foetus at 28 weeks is 1.8 and value increases by 0.2, 4 weekly. The Pondera index can be used to distinguish a constitutionally small baby (whose PI will, therefore, be normal) from an IUGR baby. The normal PI range for the neonate is 2.32–2.85 g/cm^3.

11.3.2.10 Maternal Parity

Birth weights of newborns of a particular woman progressively increase up to a parity of 4. This will of course be influenced by the sex of the babies as male babies tend to weigh more at birth.

11.3.2.11 Maternal Hypoxic Conditions

Conditions such as chronic obstructive airway disease like asthma, chronic bronchitis and cyanotic heart disease as well as high altitudes such as mountain ranges could also predispose to IUGR [4, 9].

11.3.2.12 Clinical presentation and Antenatal Diagnosis of the Intrauterine Growth Restricted Foetus

Certainty of GA is key to the diagnosis of IUGR. Twenty to 40% of pregnant women are, however, unsure of their last menstrual periods. Clinicians can reduce the enormity of this problem by probing into the menstrual history: Have the menses been regular in recent times; was the last menstrual period normal in terms of flow volume and number of days? Can the date of quickening be related to the GA for more reliable calculation of GA? When was the first palpation of fundal height in relation to land marks? Was an ultrasound scan done before 24 weeks? The answers to these highlighted issues will go a long way to help in certifying GA in poor resource settings. IUGR may be suspected antenatally when the symphysio-fundal height (SFH) measurement in the clinic is less than the known gestational age in weeks by more than 3 cm especially after the 20th week of gestation [24, 25]. This simple tool of regular SFH measurement is invaluable in the suspicion and diagnoses of IUGR in resource poor settings and is associated with 70–85% diagnostic sensitivity and 96% specificity [26]. Suspected cases in primary healthcare centres can be sent for biophysical assessments with an ultrasound scan (USS) in referral centres.

Pregnancies at risk of IUGR should have a baseline and serial studies. GA must be ascertained with good certainty particularly with first trimester USS. Serial clinic examination findings, biochemical pregnancy confirmation and quickening should also be taken note of. USS examination in the first trimester is accurate to within 1 week in establishing GA and may also point out congenital and genetic causes of IUGR. Serial USS is invaluable in diagnosis and monitoring growth in the IUGR foetus as well as assessing congenital abnormalities. Birth weight calculations by USS formulas are known to have a 10–20% error margin [12, 27].

Deciding on the biophysical measure to use depends on the GA of the foetus. The crown rump length (CRL) dates pregnancy best in the first trimester. The head circumference (HC) and biparietal diameter (BPD) are used in the second trimester (reliable to within 7–11 days). HC is more helpful in assessing gestational age in the third trimester. Abdominal circumference measurement (AC) is the most useful tool for investigating IUGR but is less accurate than the previous methods for dating. It reflects the volume of fat stored subcutaneously and the liver size which reveals the extent of foetal nutritional wellbeing. Femur length is useful in detecting skeletal abnormalities. The trans-cerebellar diameter, though not commonly used, could also be used to date pregnancies [9, 12, 28, 29].

Reduced amniotic fluid volume is clinically noted as a common feature of IUGR and must be assessed by ultrasound while evaluating IUGR. It is usually the earliest sign of IUGR detectable by ultrasound.

Doppler velocimetry of the umbilical artery (UA) can predict the likelihood of adverse perinatal outcomes where available and is useful in monitoring the IUGR foetus [3]. In the IUGR foetus, diastolic flow in the umbilical artery is reduced or absent. Reverse UA end diastolic flow is an ominous sign of severe hypoxemia and acidemia and is a good pointer of the urgent need to deliver [3, 8, 9, 28].

Doppler studies are more predictive of worsening IUGR and can help prevent unnecessary interventions such as caesarean delivery and improve the outcome of IUGR pregnancies [3]. Middle cerebral artery (MCA) and UA systolic/diastolic ratios are strong pointers to delivery at an early GA and closely correlate with foetal distress, LBW and UA acidemia [30, 31]. Abnormality in Doppler cerebro-placental ratio (MCA pulsatility index/UA pulsatility index) shows high association with a significant rise in perinatal morbidity and mortality. Intracranial haemorrhage and respiratory distress syndromes are, however, not predictable by Doppler studies [8, 12, 29–31].

Redistribution of blood supply in the IUGR foetus in favour of the brain at the expense of the abdominal organs causes increased vascular resistance in the perfusion regions of the descending aorta and decreased vascular resistance in the cerebrum. Thus, an elevated pulsatility index in the descending aorta is associated with a higher chance of foetal distress, acidemia, caesarean delivery and perinatal mortality [29, 30].

Maternal serum alpha foetal protein (MSAFP) at increased levels are predictive of worsening outcomes for the IUGR foetus and predict elevated risks for abruptio placenta, pre-eclampsia, preterm delivery and intrauterine foetal death.

Clinical evidence suggestive of infection should be investigated using maternal immunoglobulin M antibodies produced by the mother against CMV, rubella and toxoplasmosis. If levels suggest recent infection, detailed anomaly ultrasounds should be done to assess congenital abnormalities particularly involving the central nervous system.

11.3.2.13 Complications of IUGR

Complications of IUGR may affect the mother or foetus. They may be due to the underlying disease causing the IUGR or the management of the disease. The mothers with IUGR and the newborn that had IUGR will need intensive prenatal, neonatal care and sometimes intensive maternal postnatal care. IUGR foetuses are already undergoing insults and are sometimes unlikely to be able to withstand the stress of labour; hence, a significant number are delivered by caesarean section. The lower the birth weight of IUGR foetuses, the more the attendant perinatal morbidity and mortality. With improved antenatal foetal surveillance in recent decades, perinatal mortality rate for IUGR babies has reduced to 2–3 times than that of appropriate for gestational age babies [8, 9, 29].

11.3.2.14 Maternal Complications

These include complications of underlying diseases such as pre-eclampsia, hypertensive disorders renal disease and diabetes. Other complications include preterm labour and caesarean delivery.

Foetal Complications

- Hypoxia (foetal distress)
- Acidosis
- Foetal heart rate abnormalities
- Significant foetal malformations
- Oligohydramnios
- Iatrogenic prematurity
- Intrauterine foetal death (IUFD).

Immediate/Short-Term Neonatal Complications

- Hypoxia (manifesting with poor Apgar scores)
- Acute respiratory distress syndrome
- Need for intubation
- Need for exogenous surfactant
- Meconium aspiration
- Hypoglycaemia
- Acidosis
- Hypothermia
- Hypocalcaemia
- Polycythaemia
- Prone to infections
- Apnoeic attacks
- Congenital abnormalities
- Early neonatal death
- Neonatal jaundice

Long-Term Complications

These include mental retardation, delayed developmental milestones, cerebral palsy, seizure disorders, significant neurologic handicaps, learning and behaviour abnormalities, low intelligent quotient, hypertension and heart disease in adult life (Barker hypothesis) [8, 13, 29, 32, 33].

The Management of the pregnancy with IUGR

The cause of a significant number of IUGR may not be known. Diagnosis is often difficult particularly in the resource poor setting of the developing world. Even in the face of good history, serial physical and serial ultrasound scan examinations, diagnosis may be uncertain and many IUGR pregnancies may be missed. The management of an IUGR pregnancy to a large extent depends on the following:

- The GA at diagnosis
- The aetiologic factor
- The level of expertise and facilities available
- The chances of foetal survival

Underlying maternal conditions such as chronic hypertension, pre-eclampsia and diabetes should be identified and controlled [34]. All pregnant women should be advised to discontinue cigarette smoking and the use of recreational drugs like Indian hemp, cocaine, heroin and alcohol. Ideally, the advice to stop these preventable causes of IUGR should be at a preconception clinic especially with the history of a previous IUGR baby. Research evidence does not prove that bed rest improves foetal weight for IUGR foetuses, although this is a common recommendation.

IUGR foetuses have a significant risk for antepartum and intrapartum complications and death. They should thus be monitored closely. Depending on the cause of IUGR, the mothers are seen more frequently [1, 2]; weekly or admitted. Tools for assessing foetal wellbeing and monitoring include the following:

- Foetal kick charts
- Non-stress test
- Biophysical profile
- Modified biophysical profile
- Umbilical artery Doppler
- USS evaluation of foetal growth 2–3 weekly

The foetal kicks chart is an invaluable, low-cost tool for foetal monitoring especially in resource poor settings. This tool gives the mother a sense of partnership with her obstetrician or family physician in the management of her condition.

Non-stress test and amniotic fluid volume assessment in a modified biophysical profile once to twice weekly give some assurance that sudden foetal death is unlikely. When UA Doppler and other studies are added as previously discussed, it increases the sensitivity in detecting worsening foetal condition and the need for intervention such as immediate delivery [8, 29].

The detailed biophysical profile as originally enunciated includes the following:

- A non-stress test
- Amniotic fluid volume/index assessment
- Gross foetal body movement
- Foetal tone
- Foetal breathing movements

Scores of 0 or 2 are allotted in an all or none manner. Poor biophysical scores may indicate immediate delivery, while good biophysical test scores of 8–10 including a reactive non-stress test and normal amniotic fluid volume are reassuring.

Serial ultrasound of BPD, HC, AC and femur length to assess foetal growth should be done 2–4 weekly. Femur length/abdominal circumference ratios of >0.24 are suggestive of an asymmetric IUGR foetus. If foetal structural anomalies not compatible with extra-uterine life are found, the situation is explained to the woman who may then wish to terminate the pregnancy. Whatever her choice is after detailed counselling, it *must* be respected (with regard to the prevailing laws in the country or territory where care is being provided).

IUGR cases that have nutritional deficiency should be managed with nutritional supplementation.

Amniocentesis may be necessary for assessing foetal karyotype and foetal infection testing. This is particularly useful in suspected HBSS foetus in sub-Saharan Africa.

Foetuses below 34 weeks will benefit from maternal glucocorticoids (betamethasone or dexamethasone) administration. This will aid the production of pulmonary surfactant and lung maturity. Exogenous surfactant administered at birth to babies born before 34 weeks is becoming increasingly available in developing countries and is improving survival of IUGR and SGA babies.

It is imperative that each confirmed IUGR pregnancy be evaluated for when best to deliver the foetus [35, 36]. This decision is normally taken when it is adjudged that the newborn will do better or as well outside as in utero. This is either when monitoring suggests foetus is at 38 weeks, maturity demonstrated or imminent foetal compromise. There may be a need for intrauterine transfer of the foetus to a centre with better neonatal facilities before delivery. It may be necessary to deliver some foetuses with IUGR at 34 weeks' gestation [3].

Intrapartum complications are a common feature of IUGR pregnancies. Good obstetric care, operative, anaesthetic and neonatal care should be readily available in a centre managing IUGR pregnancies [35, 36]. Caesarean delivery may be the best recommendation and the attending neonatologist must anticipate meconium aspiration and be prepared to use a laryngoscope and suction meconium from the throat and larynx before the baby inspires it into the lungs.

If labour is the agreed route of delivery with the mother, continuous electronic foetal monitoring where available *must* be performed with the cardiotocograph [9, 35, 36].

Prognosis/Expected Outcome of IUGR Pregnancies

IUGR is a continued threat to foetal wellbeing and survival but on its own is not a threat to the mother's life. Some underlying causes of IUGR, however, may pose threat to the mother. These include severe pre-eclampsia/eclampsia [3], diabetes and renal disease. IUGR infants with LBW have comparatively high morbidity and mortality. Birth weights below the third percentile are associated with high rates of neonatal death, UA pH <7.0, Apgar scores at 5 minutes of ≤3, seizures in the first day, and increased need for intubation.

Long-term prognosis studies of IUGR infants show that they tend to catch up in weight within 6 months. They are however generally smaller, shorter, less weighty and have smaller head circumference than appropriate for gestational age infants. IUGR babies generally have more neurologic and intellectual defects, lower IQs, learning and behavioural difficulties than their counterparts appropriate for gestational age babies [8, 9, 13].

Mental retardation, cerebral palsy, seizures and sudden infant death are common in IUGR infants [8, 12, 13]. The Barker hypothesis notes that IUGR babies in adulthood have higher risk of having ischaemic heart disease, hypertension, cardiovascular accidents and hypercholesterolaemia [8, 13, 29, 33].

11.3.2.15 Prevention of IUGR

Most causes of IUGR as have been enumerated are not preventable, so there are few proven interventions to prevent IUGR occurrence. Notable interventions with proven benefit include haematinics (iron and folate), correction of maternal anaemia, anti-helminths in settings prone, antimalarial chemoprophylaxis and treatment, good protein-rich diets and cessation of smoking [20, 22, 37]. Smoking, a common problem in the developed world, is increasingly becoming a problem in the developing world as more and more women are taking to smoking as a habit [21]. Smoking is said to be the single most preventable cause of IUGR in the United States of America. Nutritional supplementation will benefit women in severe poverty and adolescent pregnancies [23]. Programs on food supplementation in pregnancy will benefit women most in countries of sub-Saharan Africa with extreme poverty and some countries in Latin America and Asia.

Pre-pubertal girls should be immunised against rubella (German measles) and pregnant women should avoid close contact with persons known or suspected to have rubella or cytomegalovirus. Populations exposed to Toxoplasma gondii should be encouraged to eat properly cooked meat only and when a pregnant woman or woman of childbearing age is suspected of Toxoplasmosis or rubella infection, she should be properly screened and diagnosis confirmed.

Low dose aspirin has been shown to be of some benefit in preventing, delaying and modulating the complications of pre-eclampsia and IUGR. Women with a history of previous pre-eclampsia and primigravida may thus benefit from low dose aspirin at an early gestation of about 10 weeks till term. This was demonstrated in the CLASP as well as other studies [38, 39].

Though therapeutic medications are not a frequent cause of IUGR, all drugs being used especially long-term by a woman should be reviewed in a pre-pregnancy clinic, so teratogenic drugs and other drugs that may be harmful to a developing foetus are stopped or replaced by safer ones. Women of childbearing age should be evaluated for possible pregnancy before being given drugs that may be teratogenic or being exposed to ionising radiation.

Timely treatments of the maternal diseases that cause IUGR are bound to reduce the incidence and severity of IUGR.

11.4 Large For Gestational Age (LGA) Foetuses/Foetal Macrosomia

A foetus is said to be large for gestational age when the weight or other biophysical parameters are more than the 90th percentile for that gestational age, sex and race or population. Foetal macrosomia is said to occur when a newborn has a weight equal to or in excess of 4500 g. Some consider foetal macrosomia to be birth weight equal to or in excess of 4000 g especially in developing countries like Nigeria. Morbidity and mortality for large for gestational age foetuses is increased in LGA newborns when compared to appropriate for gestational age foetuses and newborns. This risk becomes even more pronounced when foetus is both macrosomic and LGA.

11.4.1 Pathology of LGA/Macrosomia

Pregnancy is associated with endocrinological changes that promote adequate nutrient supply to the growing foetus. This is more so in regards to glucose. Pregnancy causes a somewhat diabetogenic state through the increase in levels of human placental lactogen, prolactin and cortisol which cause a degree of maternal insulin resistance which instigates postprandial insulinaemia [12]. Gestational diabetes may develop in mothers who are unable to respond to this hyperglycaemia with hyperinsulinaemia. In these mothers, foetal hyperglycaemia develops as glucose will easily cross the placenta. The foetus responds to this hyperglycaemia with hyperinsulinaemia leading to more glucose transfer into foetal cells resulting in large for gestational age babies and or foetal macrosomia. Maternal diabetes is the most significant factor for foetal macrosomia [6, 40, 41].

11.5 Risk Factors and Causes of LGA/Macrosomia

Risk factors for LGA/macrosomia can be foetal or maternal. The most preventable causes are maternal. However, the cause of some macrosomia may not be known as in over 40%; no obvious risk factors are identified.

11.5.1 Foetal Factors of LGA/Macrosomia

- Postdate pregnancy
- Genetic and congenital disorders
- Constitutionally large foetus
- Male gender
- Racial
- Foetus-to-foetus transfusion

11.5.2 Maternal Factors for LGA/Macrosomia

- Gestational diabetes
- Pre-gestational diabetes
- Obesity
- Large maternal stature.
- Previous LGA/Macrosomic newborn

- 'Postdatism'
- Advanced maternal age
- Multiparity

11.5.3 Foetal Factors of LGA/Macrosomia

11.5.3.1 Postdate Pregnancy

A foetus that is ascertained to be postdated has an increased chance of being macrosomic.

11.5.3.2 Genetic and Congenital Disorders

Many congenital and genetic disorders are known to be causal for foetal macrosomia, such as pancreatic cell hyperplasia in the foetus (the Beckwith–Wiedemann syndrome). Newborns may suffer concomitant hypoglycaemia, omphalocele, visceromegaly and macroglossia. Fragile X syndrome and Carpenter's syndrome may also be associated with LGA babies (Fragile X syndrome is a genetic condition caused by a mutation in the FMR1 gene, inherited in an X-linked dominant pattern thus affecting males more than females and causing problems with development, learning abilities, cognitive impairment and macrosomia. Carpenter's syndrome manifests with the fusion of some skull bones, abnormalities of fingers and toes, developmental problems and macrosomia and is caused by mutations in RAB23 or MEGF8 gene and is inherited in an autosomal recessive pattern).

11.5.3.3 Constitutional Large Foetus

Some constitutionally large foetuses are born to mothers with large maternal stature as foetal weight correlates more evidentially with maternal height than maternal weight.

11.5.3.4 Male Gender

Male foetuses are averagely 150 g weightier than female foetuses at same gestational age. There is a 60–65% more frequency of male foetal macrosomia than female [12].

11.5.3.5 Racial

Some races manifest with macrosomia than others. Caucasians have more macrosomia than the Negroid race.

11.5.3.6 Maternal Factors for LGA/Macrosomia

One of the most noted maternal causes of macrosomia is diabetes whether gestational or pre-gestational. Good control of diabetes before and during pregnancy may reduce the incidence of foetal macrosomia. The Pedersen hypothesis suggests that poor maternal diabetic control is the cause of foetal macrosomia. Recent studies suggest that better correlate with macrosomia are cord blood concentrations of acquired maternal anti-insulin IgG antibodies, increased serum levels of free fatty acids, triglycerides, plasma leptin, cord epidermal growth factor concentrations and the amino acids – serine, alanine and isoleucine.

11.5.3.7 Maternal Obesity and Large Stature

A three- to fourfold increase in macrosomia is associated with maternal obesity. Large maternal stature is also associated with foetal macrosomia [40, 41]. Pre-pregnancy body mass index >30 kg/m^2 has been shown to have a clear association with foetal macrosomia.

11.5.3.8 Previous LGA/Macrosomic Newborn

A mother who has had a previous LGA or macrosomic baby has a higher chance of having more LGA/macrosomic babies.

11.5.3.9 'Postdatism'

This should actually be a foetal cause but a mother whose pregnancy is postdated has a higher chance of her foetus being macrosomic.

11.5.3.10 Advanced Maternal Age and Multiparity

More incidence of macrosomia occurs amongst mothers in advanced ages and at higher parities.

Cautionary Tale

A booked 30-year-old woman with a previous history of LGA foetus and a family history of diabetes was attended by a junior cadre resident doctor at 31 weeks in the antenatal clinic of a hospital in a developing country with poor resources. The symphysiofundal height measurement was 4 cm larger than the calculated GA. The junior doctor requested an oral glucose tolerance test (OGTT) and gave the woman a 2-week appointment. She was seen at 33 weeks by a senior resident doctor who noted the previous request for OGTT. The woman was yet to perform the investigation because she did not have money for the test. She promised to carry out the investigation and was given a 1-week appointment. She only returned to the clinic 3 weeks after, at 36 weeks and the senior resident drew the attention of the managing consultant to the fact that the woman had defaulted from the clinic and had still not carried out the requested OGTT. The consultant counselled the woman and arranged hospital admission but the woman declined the admission and promised to carry out the test and come with the result the next week. At 37 weeks, she presented to the labour ward in active phase of labour before the appointment date. The senior resident in the labour ward noted all previous documentations and the fact that the woman was yet to carry out the requested OGTT. There was no functional glucometer available in the labour ward at the time of her admission, so blood was collected and sent to the chemistry laboratory without stating that the test was an emergency. The woman was observed to be physically normal. The labour progressed fast and she was delivered of a live 4.55 kg female newborn. By this time fresh doctors had resumed duties in the labour ward and no one remembered the yet-to-be retrieved random blood sugar result. Two hours after delivery, with all seemingly well with the woman, she was transferred to the maternity ward while her baby was placed under the paediatricians watch list because of the macrosomia. The blood glucose test for the baby revealed hypoglycaemia which was corrected with glucose infusion. Two hours after the woman was transferred to the maternity ward; she was noticed to be delirious, sweating and confused. The attending doctor saw all previous documentation and the fact that a blood glucose result was yet to be retrieved. The doctor assumed a sense of urgency and danger, collected fresh samples, put up glucose solution (assuming that the woman may be suffering from hypoglycaemia) and quickly dispatched a junior doctor to hurriedly take the fresh sample to the chemistry laboratory and retrieve the previously sent sample result. Meanwhile, the laboratory scientist who had since run the first sample random blood sugar test recorded 565 mg of per 100 ml of blood. He did not register the implication of the result and did not immediately inform the managing physicians. By the time the result got to the patient's bed side, the patient had lapsed into a coma. The glucose infusion was immediately stopped and insulin regimen was instituted. The woman died 30 minutes later. This is a true story of a classical example of a woman failing herself or rather a health system failing a pregnant woman whose manifestation of clear signs of foetal macrosomia if it had been properly investigated and managed would have prevented the maternal death and the incidence of hypoglycaemia in the macrosomic newborn. Unfortunately, this is all too common in under-resourced settings with poor facilities and hectic work schedules.

11.5.3.11 Complications of LGA/Macrosomia

Complications exist for both the LGA/macrosomic foetus and the mother. These complications may be related to the cause of the macrosomia, the treatment of the cause or the delivery process of the macrosomic foetus.

11.5.3.12 Maternal complications of Foetal Macrosomia

Need for caesarean section, shoulder dystocia (5–24% in macrosomia), severe perennial tears (five times more in macrosomia), operative vaginal delivery, postpartum haemorrhage and maternal death are all possible complications of foetal macrosomia, especially in developing countries with poor resources. Primigravida delivering a macrosomic baby is at more risk for complications than a multiparous woman [12].

11.5.3.13 Foetal Complications

Associated congenital foetal anomalies, foetal distress, delayed lung maturity (from diabetes), shoulder dystocia, brachial plexus injury, clavicular fracture and perinatal mortality are common with foetal macrosomia and LGA babies. Babies with truncal obesity (abdominal circumference/biparietal diameter ratio) measured by USS have increased incidence of shoulder dystocia and birth trauma. This is more so in babies born to mothers with diabetes in pregnancy (prepregnancy or gestational). Apart from macrosomia and maternal diabetes (3–4 times more frequency of shoulder dystocia than in non-diabetic mothers), another risk factor for shoulder dystocia is a previous history of shoulder dystocia in mother [42].

LGA newborns born to diabetic mothers have a disproportionately higher incidence of cardiac septal hypertrophy.

11.5.3.14 Neonatal Complications

Poor Apgar scores, need for intubation, birth injuries, polycythaemia, jaundice, hypoglycaemia, hypocalcaemia and difficulty with feeding are known complications in the first few days of life.

11.5.3.15 Long-Term Complications

LGA and macrosomic babies may suffer long-term consequences of birth injury such as cerebral palsy. Obesity, Type 2 diabetes mellitus, neurologic and behavioural abnormalities are more common in LGA/macrosomia than in appropriate for gestational age babies.

11.5.3.16 Treatment

The causes of foetal macrosomia and LGA should be thoroughly evaluated, investigated and managed.

Recommendations of early delivery by the induction of labour to prevent macrosomia and LGA are not backed by evidence. Most studies recommend a routine caesarean section for delivery in confirmed foetal macrosomia of 5 kg and above. In diabetics, 4.5 kg and above is the recommended cut-off for caesarean section.

Timing of delivery for diabetic mothers should be at 38th weeks. The American Diabetes Association in their 2004 clinical practice recommendations noted that in GDM, 'prolongation of gestation past 38 weeks increases the risk of fetal macrosomia without reducing cesarean rates, so that delivery during the 38th week is recommended. [42] Whatever the decision on timing and route of delivery, all effort should be made to achieve euglycaemia before delivery. Co-management of the patient with an endocrinologist if available may be necessary to achieve euglycaemia. Decisions regarding the route of delivery are best based on clinical grounds. Maternal age, parity and her choices should always be strong considerations when taking decisions on the route of delivery. Instrumental deliveries should note the increase in the risk of shoulder dystocia. Therefore, when the second stage is unduly delayed in mothers with foetuses weighing ≥4 kg, caesarean delivery may be considered in such scenarios [12].

Women at risk of LGA and foetal macrosomia are advised to be delivered in facilities with the full range of obstetric, anaesthetic, blood banking and neonatal services. This will reduce the need of emergency referrals, incidence of obstructed labour and birth trauma.

In the most unfortunate event of the development of shoulder dystocia, the accoucheur should apply a dynamic controlled and non-panic approach. There should be no haste. The most experienced accoucheur physically present should take charge. The bladder should be emptied, adequate episiotomy given and McRoberts manoeuvre instituted (hyperflexion of the legs and abduction of the thighs) [12, 43]. This should be accompanied by suprapubic pressure to help reduce the bis-accromial diameter and bring the foetal anterior shoulder under the pubic symphysis. This manoeuvre many a time resolves the situation but when it fails, more complex manoeuvres outside the scope of this chapter may be tried.

11.5.3.17 Prognosis of Macrosomia/LGA Pregnancies

Women who have delivered LGA/macrosomic babies should be made aware of the high chance of recurrence (2.5–4 times). They should be screened for diabetes at delivery and 6 weeks post-delivery. Subsequent pregnancies should receive specialist care and follow up.

Obese women should ideally attend pre-pregnancy clinics and be encouraged to shed weight before pregnancy.

Babies born with macrosomia, particularly those born to diabetic mothers are at higher risk of obesity and Type 2 diabetes in later life [40–43].

11.5.3.18 Prevention of LGA/Macromia

Women with conditions known as risk factors for foetal macrosomia should attend pre-pregnancy clinics so that conditions such as diabetes and obesity can be controlled and good weight loss achieved before pregnancy. Blood glucose level controls in pre-conception and antenatal period are best with monitoring of postprandial glucose levels. Euglycaemia is essential in the first trimester [6, 12, 42, 43].

Other risk factors to be identified early in pregnancy are advanced maternal age, previous delivery of a macrosomic newborn and multiparity. Birth weights are known to increase for successive pregnancies up to a parity of 4. Advanced maternal age and multiparity are associated with diabetes and obesity. Family history of diabetes in the woman should also be taken note of as these women have a higher risk of developing pre-pregnancy diabetes and gestational diabetes.

The gestational ages of pregnancies with maternal risk factors for macrosomia should be ascertained early in the first trimester by USS and serial 4 weekly USS used to monitor estimated foetal weight compared to normative values for the GA, gender and race. Sensitivity and specificity of USS weight estimations are noted to be 24–88% and 60–98%, respectively. The best measurement in assessing macrosomia and LGA foetuses in mothers with diabetes is abdominal circumference. Initial abdominal circumference above the 70th percentile is noted to be associated with the delivery of an LGA newborn.

Good control of maternal glucose levels prevents the development of macrosomia [42–45]. Pregnancy weight and weight gain in pregnancy are associated with macrosomia. In diabetics, essential principles of management are proper nutrition and aerobic exercises starting in the preconception period. Infants of women who participate in regular aerobic exercises have lower average weights.

11.6 Summary

Pregnancies associated with IUGR, LGA and foetal macrosomia are high risk pregnancies that need detailed considerations in their care and management. Knowledge of the causative pathologies, their control, investigating the pathology and pregnancy course and appropriate decision on when and how to deliver the at-risk foetuses contribute significantly to reducing perinatal morbidity and mortality in the foetuses, mothers and their newborn. The management of pregnancies with foetal growth anomalies and their causative pathologies frequently requires collaboration amongst specialists of different disciplines of medical care along with the cooperation of the pregnant woman.

References

1. Groom KM, Poppe KK, North RA, McCowan LM. Small-for-gestational-age infants classified by customized or population birth weight centiles: impact of gestational age at delivery. Am J Obstet Gynecol. 2007;197(3):239.e1–5.
2. Bernstein IM, Horbar JD, Badger GJ, et al. Morbidity and mortality among very-low-birth-weight neonates with intrauterine growth restriction. The Vermont Oxford Network. Am J Obstet Gynecol. 2000;182(1 Pt 1):198–206.
3. Enaruna NO, Sodje JDK. Early-onset severe preeclampsia in Nigerian women: determining a balance between maternal wellbeing and fetal survival in a resource-limited setting. Br J Med Med Res. 2015;10(3):1–9.

4. Morrison JL. Sheep models of intrauterine growth restriction: fetal adaptations and consequences. Clin Exp Pharmacol Physiol. 2008;35:730–43. https://doi.org/10.1111/j.1440-1681.2008.04975.
5. Krammer MS. Determinations of low birth weight: methodological assessment and met analysis. Bull WHO. 1987;65:663.
6. Gossett D, Gurewtsch E. Gestational complications; In: Bankowski BJ, Hearne AE, Lambrou NC, Fox HE, Wallach EE (Eds) The Johns Hopkins manual of gynaecology and obstetrics , 2nd ed. 2002. Pg 40–44. Lippincott Williams and Wilkins Publishers; Philadelphia, PA.
7. Peleg D, Kennedy CM, Hunter SK. Intruterine growth restriction: identification and management. Am Fam Physician. 1998;58920:453–60.
8. Cosmi E, Fanelli T, Visentin S, Trevisanuto D, Zanardo V. Consequences in infants that were intrauterine growth restricted. J Pregnancy. 2011;2011:6. Article ID 364381, 6 pages. https://doi.org/10.1155/2011/364381.
9. Figueras F, Gardosi J. Intrauterine growth restriction: new concepts in antenatal surveillance, diagnosis, and management. Am J Obstet Gynecol. 2011;204:288–300.
10. Small-for-Gestational-Age Foetus, Investigation and Management; Royal College of Obstetricians and Gynaecologists Green top guideline (Mar 2013).
11. Baschat AA, Galan HL, Gabbe SG. Intrauterine growth restriction. Chapter 16. In: Gabbe SG, Niebyl JR, Simpson JL, Landon MB, Galan HL, Jauniaux ERM, Driscoll DA (Eds.). Obstetrics: normal and problem pregnancies. 6th ed Churchill Livinstone, Elsevier Inc. Philadelphia, PA: 2012, ; pg 706–741.
12. Rahimian J, Varner MW. Disproportionate fetal growth. Chapter 16. In: DeCherny AH, Nathan L, Goodwin TM, Laufer Neri (Eds.). Current obstetrics and gynaecologic diagnosis and treatment 10th ed. McGraw Hill's Access Medicine, The McGraw Hill Company. New York, USA: 2006, Pg 301–314.
13. Tideman E, Marsal K, Ley D. Cognitive function in young adults following intrauterine growth restriction with abnormal fetal aortic blood flow. Ultrasound Obstet Gynecol. 2007;29(6):614–8.
14. Mekonen HK, Nigatu B, Lamers WH. Birth weight by gestational age and congenital malformations in Northern Ethiopia. BMC Pregnancy Childbirth. 2015;15:76. Pulished online 2015 Mar 29. https://doi.org/10.1186/s12884-015-0507-2.
15. Resnick R. Intrauterine growth restriction. Obstet Gynecol. 2002;99:490–6.
16. Schleiss MR, Cytomegalovirus in the neonate: immune correlates of infection and protection. Clin Dev Immunol. 2013;2013:14, Article ID 501801. https://doi.org/10.1155/2013/501801.
17. Adebami OJ, Owa JA, Oyedeji GAO, Oyelami OA, Omoniyi-Esan GO. Associations between placental and cord blood malaria infection and fetal malnutrition in an area of malaria holoendemicity. Am J Trop Med Hyg. 2007;77(2):209–13.
18. Kilby MD, Oepkes D. Multiple pregnancy. In: Edmonds DK, editor. Dewhurst textbook of obstetrics and gynaecology. 8th Edition, Wiley-Blackwell, Oxford, UK; 2012. p. 230–46.
19. Onyiriuka AN. Incidence of delivery of low birth weight infants in twin gestation. Niger J Clin Practice. 2010;13(4):365–70.
20. Milnerowicz-Nabzdyk E, Bizon A. How does tobacco smoke influence the morphometry of the foetus and the umbilical cord?-research on pregnant women with intrauterine growth restriction exposed to tobacco smoke. Reprod Toxicol. 2015;58:79–84.
21. Fourn L, Ducic S, Seguin L. Smoking and intrauterine growth retardation in Republic of Benin. J Epidemiol Community Health. 1999;53:432–3.
22. Lawoyin TO, Oyediran AB. A prospective study on some factors which influence the delivery of low birth weight babies in a developing country. Afr J Med Sci. 1992;21(1):33–9.
23. Wallace JM, Aitken RP, Milne JS, Hay WW Jr. Nutritionally mediated placental growth restriction in the growing adolescent: consequences for the foetus. Biol Reprod. 2004;71:1055–62.
24. Gardosi J, Francis A. Controlled trial of fundal height measurement plotted on customised antenatal growth charts. Br J Obstet Gynaecol. 1999;106(4):309–17.
25. Jelks A, Cifuentes R, Ross MG. Clinician bias in fundal height measurement. Obstet Gynecol. 2007;110(4):892–9.
26. Singh A. Intrauterine growth restriction. In: Puri M, Trivedi SS, editors. Management of high risk pregnancy – a practical approach. Jaypee Brothers; New Delhi, India: 2011. p. 176–98.
27. Turan OM, Turan S, Buhimschi IA, Funai EF, Campbell KH, Ozan MB, Harman CR, Copel JA, Baschat AA, Buhimschi CS. Camparative analysis of 2-D versus 3-D ultrasound estimation of the fetal adrenal gland volume and prediction of preterm birth. Am J Perinatol. 201229(9). https://doi.org/10.1055/s-0032-1314887.
28. Yoshida S, Unno N, Kagawa H, et al. Prenatal detection of a high-risk group for intrauterine growth restriction based on sonographic fetal biometry. Int J Gynaecol Obstet. 2000;68(3):225–32.
29. Harman CR, Baschat AA. Arterial and venous Dopplers in IUGR. Clin Obstet Gynecol. 2003;46(4):931–46.
30. Mandruzzato GP, Bogatti P, Fischer L, Gigli C. The clinical significance of absent or reverse end-diastolic flow in the fetal aorta and umbilical artery. Ultrasound Obstet Gynecol. 1991;1(3):192–6.
31. Mari G, Hanif F, Kruger M, Cosmi E, Santolaya-Forgas J, Treadwell MC. Middle cerebral artery peak systolic velocity: a new Doppler parameter in the assessment of growth-restricted foetuses. Ultrasound Obstet Gynecol. 2007;29(3):310–6.
32. Zubrick SR, Kurinczuk JJ, McDermott BM, et al. Fetal growth and subsequent mental health problems in children aged 4 to 13 years. Dev Med Child Neurol. 2000;42(1):14–20.
33. Barker DJP, Adult consequences of Fetal growth restriction, Clin Obstet Gynaecol, 2006;49(2):270–283. View at Publisher · View at Google Scholar · View at Scopus.
34. Kanaka-Gantenbein C, Mastorakos G, Chrousos GP. Endocrine-related causes and consequences of intrauterine growth retardation. Ann N Y Acad Sci. 2003;997:150–7.
35. Boers KE, Vijgen SM, Bijlenga D, et al. Induction versus expectant monitoring for intrauterine growth restriction at term: randomised equivalence trial (DIGITAT). BMJ. 2010;341:c7087.
36. Siristatidis C, Salamalekis E, Vitoratos N, et al. Intrapartum surveillance of IUGR foetuses with cardiotocography and fetal pulse oximetry. Biol Neonate. 2003;83(3):162–5.
37. Say L, Gulmezoglu AM, Hofmeyr GJ. Maternal nutrient supplementation for suspected impaired fetal growth. Cochrane Database Syst Rev. 2003;1:CD000148.
38. Collaborative Low-dose Aspirin Study in Pregnancy Collaborative Group. CLASP: a randomised trial of low-dose aspirin for the prevention and treatment of pre-eclampsia among 9364 pregnant women. CLASP (Collaborative Low-Dose Aspirin Study in Pregnancy) Collaborative Group. Lancet. 1994;343(8898):619–29.
39. Sibai BM, Caritis SN, Thom E, et al. Prevention of preeclampsia with low-dose aspirin in healthy, nulliparous pregnant women. The National Institute of Child Health and Human Development Network of Maternal-Fetal Medicine Units. N Engl J Med. 1993;329(17):1213–8.
40. Catalano PM. Management of obesity in pregnancy. Obstet Gynecol. 2007;109(2 Pt 1):419–33.

41. Gaudet L, Ferraro ZM, Wen SW, et al. Maternal obesity and occurrence of fetal macrosomia: a systematic review and meta-analysis. Biomed Res Int. 2014;2014:640291.
42. American Diabetes Association. Gestational diabetes mellitus. Diabetes Care. 2004 ; 27(Suppl 1):S88–90.
43. Nippita T, Forster K, Morris J. Obstetric emergencies. In: Abbott J, Bowler L, Martha F, editors. Obstetrics and gynaecology and evidence based guide. Churchill Livingstone; Philadelphia, PA: 2013. p. 201–18.
44. Catalano PM, Sacks DA. Timing of indicated late preterm and early term birth in chronic medical complications: diabetes. Semin Perinatol. 2011;35(5):297–301. https://doi.org/10.1053/i.semperi.2011.05.003.
45. Spong CY, Mercer BM, D'alton M, Kilpatrick S, Blackwell S, Saade G. Timing of indicated late-preterm and early-term birth. Obstet Gynecol. 2011;118(2 Pt 1):323–33. https://doi.org/10.1097/AOG.0b013e3182255999.

Management of Normal and Abnormal Labour

12

Olusegun Badejoko and Uchenna Onwudiegwu

Learning Objectives

At the end of reading this chapter, individuals should be able to:

- Acquaint themselves with developmental highlights in the concept of active management of labour.
- Describe and elaborate on the importance of the partograph in labour management.
- Review abnormal labour and its management.

12.1 Introduction

Labour is the entire physiological process leading up to the expulsion of the products of conception (i.e. the foetus, placenta and membranes) par vaginam, after the age of viability. It is characterised by the onset of rhythmic painful uterine contractions of increasing frequency, intensity and duration, associated with cervical effacement and dilatation, along with progressive descent of the foetus, all culminating in the vaginal delivery of the products of conception.

This process is somewhat unique in humans compared to other species. Labour in humans appears to be the most painful, prolonged, and prone to cephalopelvic disproportion [1, 2]. The reason for this is postulated in the anthropological concept of the obstetric dilemma [3–5]. This hypothesises that the human bony pelvis has had to undergo structural changes to make the erect posture required for bipedal locomotion possible. These evolutionary changes are thought to have resulted in a bony pelvis with smaller dimensions. Similarly, to cater for the species' higher intelligence, human babies had to be born with a larger brain size, and consequently, larger skull diameters. The combination of the foregoing set the stage for cephalopelvic disproportion, which has given rise to an increased need for assistance during labour in humans. Indeed, while other primates are known to seek seclusion during childbirth, humans usually require assistance, a trend which is thought to underlie the evolution of midwifery [6, 7].

The provision of assistance during labour and the ultimate medicalisation of the labour process were advanced even further with the advent of active management of labour, which can be defined as a constellation of procedures and interventions aimed at preventing prolonged labour and its complications in nullipara, by ensuring cervical dilatation at a rate of at least 1 cm per hour in the active phase of labour, as a means of achieving the delivery of a healthy baby to a healthy mother. This concept was enunciated and popularised by Kieran O'Driscoll and colleagues at the National Maternity Hospital, Dublin, Ireland, in 1969 [8]. In their pioneering work involving 1000 consecutive nulliparous pregnant women, O'Driscoll and colleagues sought to debunk three widely held obstetrical myths at the time:

1. That cephalopelvic disproportion was the usual cause of prolonged labour.
2. That the primigravid uterus may rupture with the use of oxytocin.
3. That a real difference existed in the correct mode of treatment between so-called hypotonic and hypertonic uterine action.

In 1968, the team put together a package of interventions assuring nulliparous mothers of delivery within 24 hours of hospital admission. They further revised this in 1973 to in fact guarantee delivery within 12 hours of admission, while keeping operative delivery to a minimum [9]. Eligibility for this protocol was limited to nulliparous women in spontaneous labour with singleton pregnancies in cephalic

O. Badejoko (✉) · U. Onwudiegwu
Department of Obstetrics, Gynaecology and Perinatology, Obafemi Awolowo University, Ile-Ife, Nigeria

F. Okonofua et al. (eds.), *Contemporary Obstetrics and Gynecology for Developing Countries*,
https://doi.org/10.1007/978-3-030-75385-6_12

presentation. The components of their package included the following:

1. Antenatal education: This involved counselling eligible women about the protocol and allowing them to make an informed choice between the active management protocol and routine intrapartum care.
2. Strict definition of labour: The diagnosis of labour was only made by the healthcare provider, and that, only when the cervix was >3 cm dilated, thus disregarding the latent phase of labour. Women presenting before labour was well established were sent back home. About 50% of these women re-presented in established labour within 24 hours.
3. One-to-one nursing care: Every parturient undergoing the active management protocol was assigned a midwife for proper monitoring and companionship in labour.
4. Partographic monitoring: The progress of cervical dilatation was plotted on a partograph with an expected minimum cervical dilatation rate of at least 1 cm/hr. Cervical dilatation was assessed by hourly vaginal examinations for the first 3 hours and two-hourly thereafter.
5. Early amniotomy: This was routinely performed 1 hour after admission to enhance the uterine contractions and monitor the colour of the amniotic fluid.
6. Oxytocin augmentation of labour: Oxytocin infusion was frequently employed after amniotomy to enhance uterine contractions and prevent prolonged labour in the active management protocol. Its use was only limited by the occurrence of foetal distress. The infusion was commenced 1 hour after amniotomy if the cervical dilatation had not increased by at least 1 cm. Women who had ruptured membranes spontaneously at home were also augmented if cervical dilatation had not gained at least 1 cm 1 hour after admission. Oxytocin infusion was routinely continued until after the placenta had been delivered. O'Driscoll believed that oxytocin had been falsely implicated in uterine rupture and that with proper monitoring, it was safe and in fact beneficial.

With this protocol, O'Driscoll and co-workers were able to achieve a low caesarean section rate of 4% and forceps delivery rate of about 19%. Virtually all the women delivered within 24 hours, except for one subject in whom the decision to augment labour had been delayed. They also observed no increase in need for analgesia in actively managed labour, as most of the women were more interested in the prospect of an expeditious delivery than in an analgesic which was also often associated with drowsiness and nausea – pethidine being the only analgesic option used. The foetal outcomes of the study were also very commendable. The only intrapartum foetal death following oxytocin infusion was in a delayed second twin. There was also no increase in the rate of neonatal neurological deficits with the use of oxytocin [8].

O'Driscoll's active management of labour has interestingly been met with a lot of criticism [10, 11]. To start with, the low caesarean section rates he reported in Dublin had made the active management protocol highly attractive worldwide, most especially in the United States where an astronomical caesarean section rate had become a major problem [10]. Unfortunately, several attempts that have been made to replicate this study in different centres around the world have by and large failed to reproduce similar results to O'Driscoll's [10–14]. It must however be borne in mind that the Dublin protocol was never originally designed for avoidance of caesarean section but rather for prevention of prolonged labour, in which case it has been proven indisputably to be effective. In a recent randomised-controlled trial, active management of labour was shown to reduce the duration of labour by an average of 2.7 hours and also reduce the rate of maternal infectious morbidity by about 50% [10].

Another important criticism of active management of labour is its implementation of strict medicalisation of the delivery process, which is easily deemed by many to constitute meddlesome obstetrics. For instance, the practice of artificial rupture of membranes which is an integral component of the active management protocol is strongly opposed by many critics because of its attendant risks albeit small, of complications such as cord prolapse, abruptio placentae and foetal distress. Indeed, current best available evidence has demonstrated no clear benefit or justification for the routine use of amniotomy [15–18]. Similarly, the routine use of oxytocin is not supported by current evidence [12, 18]. However, companionship in labour as encapsulated in the O'Driscoll protocol and more recently provided by Doulas, has been shown to cause remarkable reduction in the duration of labour, need for analgesia and operative intervention. In fact, it is currently thought to have been the single biggest contributor to the positive foeto-maternal outcomes of the O'Driscoll active management package [10].

Globally, the practice of active management of labour has been dwindling, especially in the developed world [19]. This is probably due to the continuing emergence of convincing evidence regarding the attainability of low caesarean section and instrumental delivery rates, good foeto-maternal outcomes, and high maternal satisfaction with the entire delivery experience; with the use of simple midwife-centred natural childbirth models [20–24]. Typically, these models involve minimal medical interventions which are usually evidence-based. This narrative is however substantially reversed in sub-Saharan Africa and perhaps many other under-developed regions of the world, where the doctor–patient relationship still remains highly paternalistic, and facility-based delivery is still considered the ultimate goal if maternal and perinatal mortality and morbidity are to be prevented [25, 26].

Many contemporary labour management guidelines do not recommend the use of O'Driscoll's active management of labour [27, 28]. Rather, some of the components of the protocol have been adapted with significant modifications, based on current best available evidence. For example, the threshold for artificial rupture of foetal membranes and use of oxytocin infusion for labour augmentation is significantly higher in current guidelines, compared to the Dublin protocol [27–31]. Also, the frequency of vaginal examinations is reduced, while the options of analgesia in labour are much expanded to include epidural analgesia [27, 28, 32]. With respect to the positions for delivery in the second stage of labour, women are encouraged to adopt any position they find comfortable, while as much as possible avoiding the traditional dorsal and lithotomy positions [33, 34]. Indeed, in addition to all the foregoing, many new elements of intrapartum care, such as ultrasonography, electronic foetal monitoring, and foetal blood sampling for pH and lactate, have made it all the more challenging to resolve the uncertainty regarding the place for O'Driscoll's active management of labour protocol in modern day obstetric practice.

12.2 Partograph

The partograph or partogram is a single page graphical representation of the salient events occurring in labour, plotted against time. At a glance, the partograph shows various important parameters of intrapartum monitoring such as the foetal heart rate, cervical dilatation, foetal descent, as well as the frequency and duration of uterine contractions, among other things. Several types of partographs have been developed over the years, some of which are still in use today. Some examples include the old and new WHO partographs, Studd's labour stencil, the round partograph, the electronic partograph and even a second stage partograph [35–40].

Historically, the origin of the partograph can be traced back to the pioneering work of Dr. Emmanuel Friedman of Boston, United States, who incorporated this science into the art of labour management [41, 42]. Friedman in 1954 analysed the progress of cervical dilatation against time in 500 women and with this generated the sigmoid-shaped normogram which is popularly referred to as the Friedman's curve (Fig. 12.1). He observed that labours that progressed along this normogram typically resulted in normal delivery, while those that deviated from it often ended in caesarean section. The Friedman's curve was made up of four phases, namely the latent, acceleration, maximum slope and deceleration phases of the first stage of labour.

Friedman explained the phases of the cervical dilatation curve based on the mechanics of the interaction between the foetal head and the cervix. The latent phase was attributed to the slow process of cervical effacement up until cervical dilatation of 3 cm. Dilatation from 3 to 4 cm was marked by acceleration in the rate of dilatation as the foetal head became better applied to the cervix. Progress from 4 to 9 cm cervical dilatation occurred at the peak rate, hence its appellation the phase of maximum slope. This was attributed to the optimisation of the mechanical dilating effect of the well applied foetal head on the cervix. Lastly, he described a deceleration

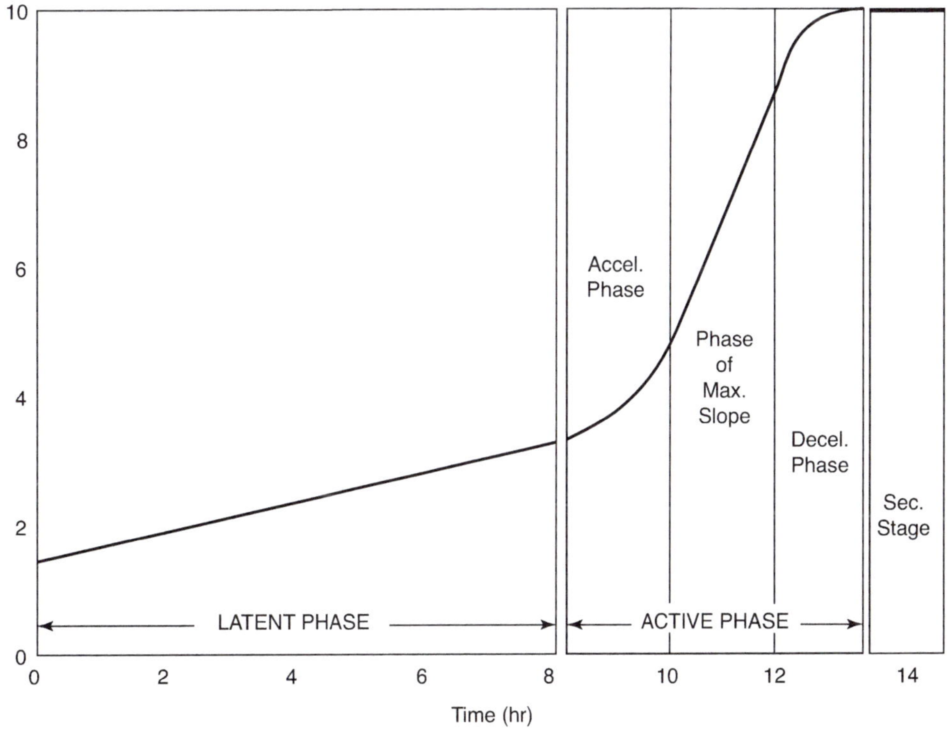

Fig. 12.1 Friedman's curve. (*Source*: http://resources.ama.uk.com/glowm_www/graphics/figures/v2/0680/001f.gif. Accessed on 20/8/2016)

phase between 9 cm and full cervical dilatation, which was attributed to the loss of mechanical advantage as the cervix turned the bend along the fringes of the foetal head.

Friedman's work formed the foundation upon which several other investigators have built. Although their findings authenticated most of Friedman's observations, they consistently failed to demonstrate the deceleration phase of the Friedman's curve. In particular, Hendricks et al. in 1969 established that there was in fact no deceleration phase in the first stage of labour, and that the cervical dilatation rate was similar for both primigravidae and multiparae [43].

In 1972, R.H. Philpott and W.M. Castle working in the East African nation Rhodesia (now Zimbabwe) developed a cervicograph which was also partly based on the work of Friedman [44–46]. Their cervicograph featured a pre-printed cervical dilatation slope called the alert line, which corresponded to a cervical dilatation rate of 1 cm per hour. This represented the mean rate of cervical dilatation among the slowest 10% of primigravidae who subsequently achieved normal delivery. The cervicograph also had a second predrawn arbitrary line called the action line, which was 4 hours to the right of the alert line and parallel to it.

Philpott and Castle observed that most of the Rhodesian parturients they studied progressed along or to the left of the alert line; and all who did so were able to achieve a normal delivery. However, about 22% of their study subjects crossed to the right of the alert line. Although half of these women delivered within the succeeding 4 hours, while the remaining 11% invariably crossed the action line, and subsequently needed special interventions. In practice, the 4 hours between the alert and action lines were found to be sufficient time for the transfer of these women from peripheral centres to central facilities where the needed special interventions were available. The alert line therefore proved effective in the early identification of poor progress of labour, most especially in the peripheral centres, where it prompted timely referral to the central facilities.

At the central facilities, the referred women were assessed for possible underlying causes of poor labour progress. Those women whose cervicographs did cross the action line were mostly found to have identifiable problems such as inadequate uterine contractions requiring oxytocin augmentation, or cephalopelvic disproportion requiring caesarean section. Thus, the action line marked an important decision point regarding the need for appropriate intervention for women with poor progress in labour.

In 1988, soon after the 1987 launch of the Safe Motherhood Initiative, the World Health Organization adapted Philpott and Castle's cervicograph to develop the WHO partograph, for use in the prevention of prolonged and obstructed labour globally [47–49]. The composite WHO partograph had a cervicograph with latent phase of 8 hours, alongside Philpott and Castle's alert and action lines (Fig. 12.2). In a large multicentre study involving over 35,000 women in Indonesia, Malaysia and Thailand, the WHO evaluated the impact of this partograph on labour and delivery outcomes. The study revealed that partograph use was associated with significant reduction in the occurrence of prolonged labour, need for oxytocin augmentation, rate of caesarean delivery and incidence of infections [47]. Based on these findings, a global campaign was launched to promote partograph use for monitoring of all labours. Many high- and mid-level personnel were trained in its use. Indeed, in combination with institutional labour management protocols, the partograph has been found over the years to be an indispensable tool for the prevention of prolonged/obstructed labour and its complications, especially in resource-challenged environments, with high maternal mortality and morbidity from prolonged and obstructed labour [47–49].

Despite its benefits however, many centres around the world did not adopt the use of the partograph [50–52]. Some of the reasons given for this include difficulty in keeping up with the stipulated frequency of observations, due to manpower shortages. Some middle and low-level personnel also found parts of it to be rather confusing. For example, the required transfer of the cervicograph plot from the latent phase on to the alert line when the parturient progressed from latent to active phase of labour proved in practice to be quite confusing for many users. In addition, the eight-hour duration allotted to the latent phase of labour in the composite WHO partograph was rather inadequate, considering the wide variation in the normal length of the latent phase of labour [53]. This invariably would have led to many unnecessary labour augmentations and avoidable caesarean sections.

In addressing some of these perceived shortcomings, the WHO in 2002 released the modified WHO partograph (Fig. 12.3). In this modern partograph, the latent phase of labour had been completely expunged. This modified partograph is only to be commenced when a woman is already in the active phase of labour, thus eliminating the need for the confusing transfer of plots from latent phase to alert line. In addition, the active phase of labour was redefined as commencing from 4 cm cervical dilatation and not 3 cm as in the old partograph. This effectively eliminated the worrisome regimentation of the latent phase of labour associated with the use of the composite WHO partograph [54].

In a recent Cochrane review examining the effect of utilisation of the partograph on the outcome of spontaneous labour at term, Lavender et al. pooled six studies involving a total of 7706 women [55]. Two of the studies (n = 1590) compared use versus non-use of the partograph, while the

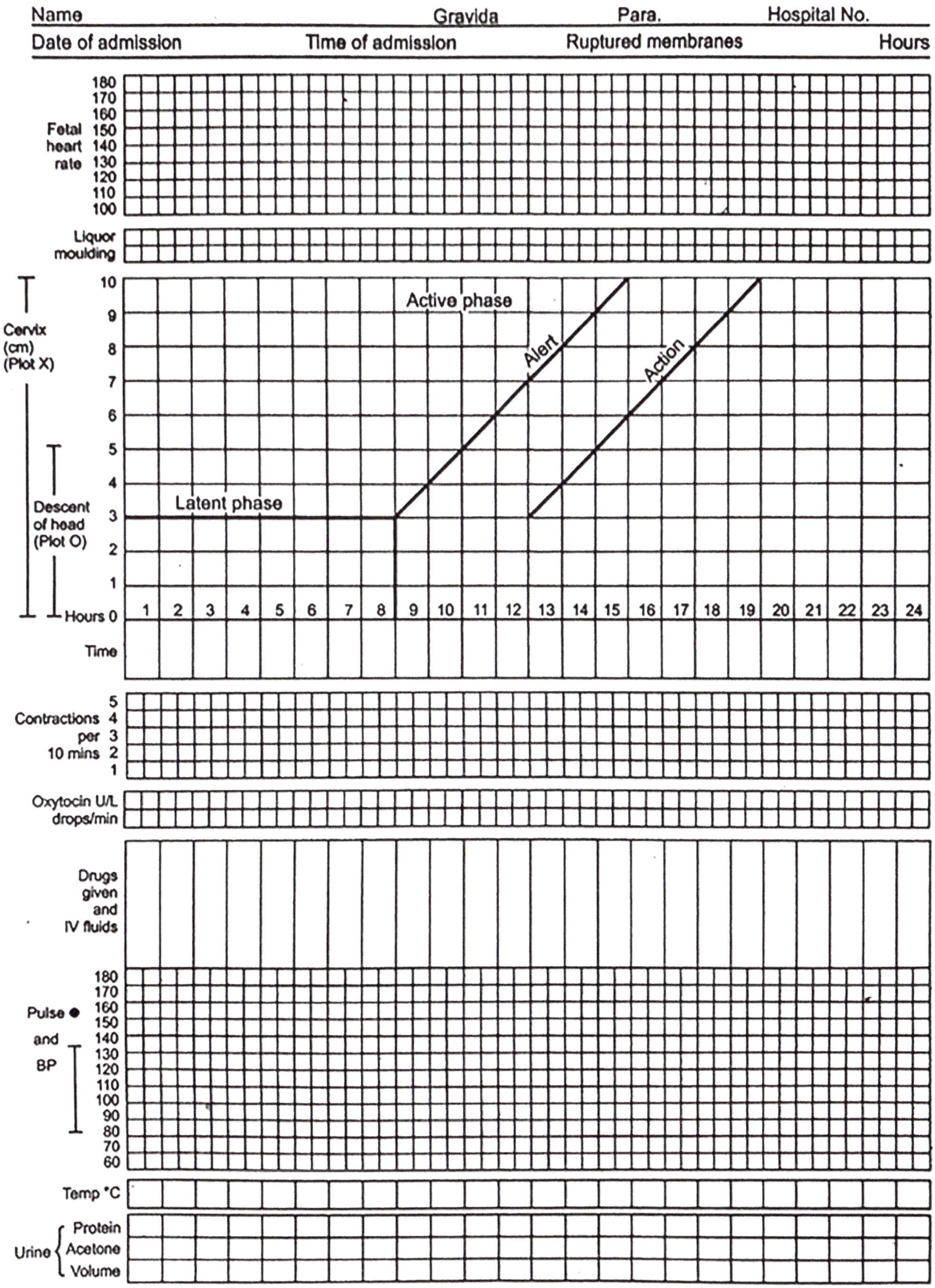

Fig. 12.2 The composite WHO partograph

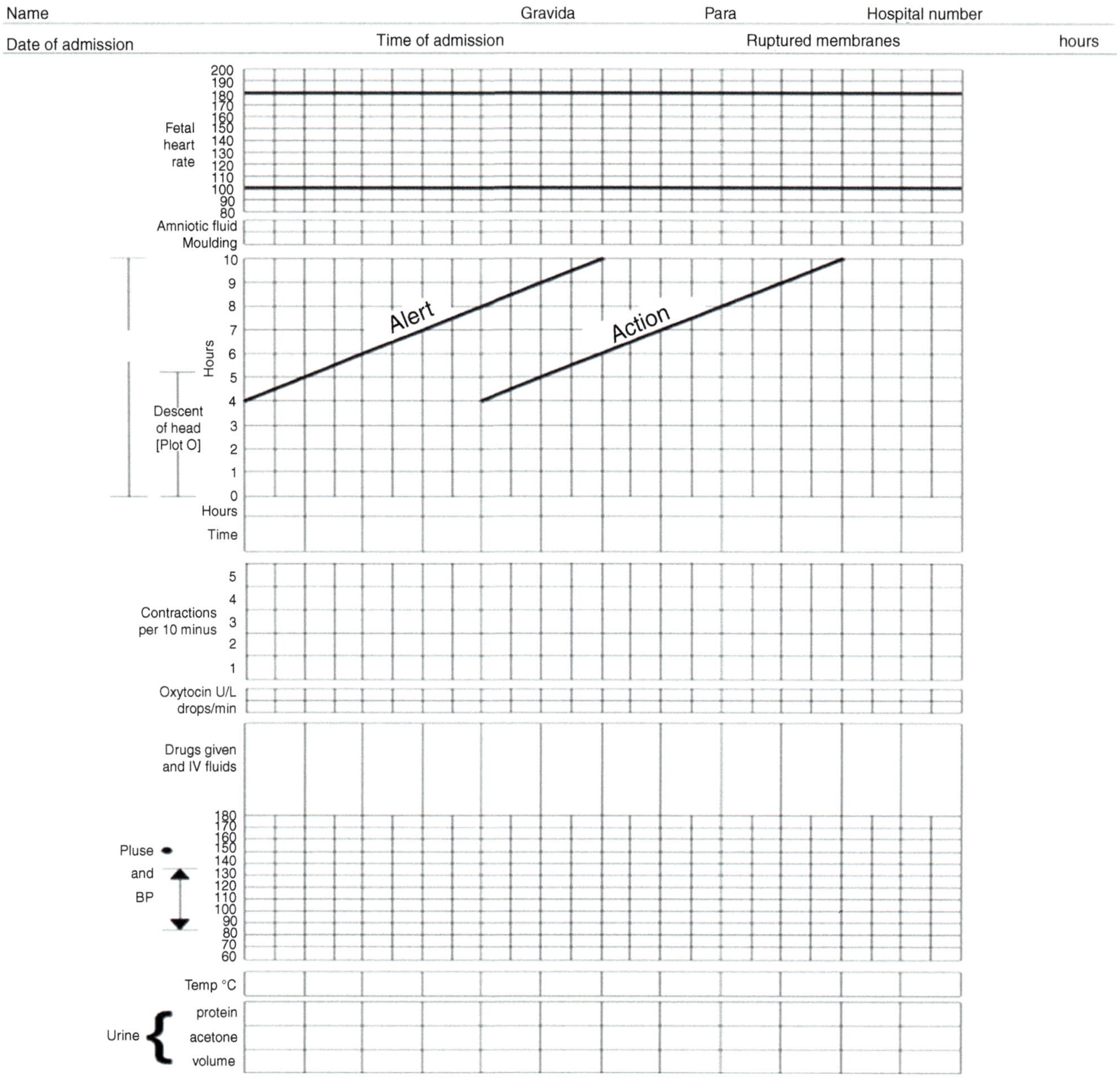

Fig. 12.3 The modified WHO partograph

rest compared different partograph designs. The results showed that partograph use was not associated with any significant difference in the rate of caesarean section, instrumental delivery or five-minute Apgar score <7, when compared to non-use of the partograph. Furthermore, compared to the four-hour action line, partographs with the two-hour action line were associated with a higher rate of oxytocin augmentation of labour in two trials involving 3601 women (risk ratio (RR) = 1.14; 95% CI = 1.05–1.22). A comparison of the 3- and 4-hour action line partographs in one trial (n = 613) revealed that the former was associated with a statistically significant increase in caesarean section rate (RR = 1.70; 95% CI = 1.07–2.70). When a composite partograph containing the latent phase was compared to a modern partograph with no latent phase in one trial (n = 694), the caesarean section rate was observed to be significantly lower in the latter (RR = 2.45; 95% CI = 1.73–2.50). Based on these findings, the authors concluded that routine partographic monitoring cannot be recommended as part of standard labour management and care. While calling for more trials, they suggested that partograph use should be locally determined, pending the arrival of stronger evidence.

This review is not without criticism. First, quite a few of the observations were based entirely on the findings of single trials. Also, resource-poor environments were under-represented, as only two out of the six studies were conducted in developing countries (Mexico and South Africa). Ultimately, changing from an existing practice requires strong evidence demonstrating the superiority of a suggested alternative. This systematic review, however, did not demonstrate this, hence discontinuation of partograph use cannot be justifiably recommended based on this review. As recommended by the authors, there is indeed a great need for well-designed randomised-controlled trials, especially in under-resourced settings, to provide conclusive evidence regarding the role of the partograph in present-day labour management. In the meantime, however, the partograph should continue to be used, most especially in the developing world, where the burden of prolonged and obstructed labour and the attendant morbidity and mortality is still significant.

12.3 Plotting the Modified WHO Partograph

The modified WHO partograph should only be commenced when a woman is in the active phase of labour, i.e. cervical dilatation ≥4 cm [56, 57]. Contraindications to its use include cervical dilatation >8 cm at admission, preterm labour <34 weeks and the presence of indications for emergency caesarean section. After entering the patient's relevant information in the bio data section, the next entry to be made in the partograph is the cervical dilatation. This must be plotted as an X at the appropriate point ON THE ALERT LINE! Entry of all the other parameters (both foetal and maternal) should then be commenced along the same vertical line as this first cervical dilatation plot. Vaginal examinations are to be performed four-hourly, or at a shorter interval if so indicated, and the cervical dilatation so obtained appropriately plotted against time.

The foetal heart rate should be auscultated half-hourly and represented with a dot on the appropriate line, and successive dots should be connected to create a foetal heart rate tracing. The state of the amniotic fluid should be indicated using C for clear, M for meconium stained, B for bloody, A for absent liquor and I for intact membranes. Moulding should be indicated as – for absent, and 1+, 2+ and 3+ for grades 1, 2 and 3 moulding, respectively. Descent should be indicated with a O in the cervicogram section, and consecutive plots joined using straight lines. The number of uterine contractions in 10 minutes is represented as the number of boxes shaded in a stack of five, starting from the bottom. To depict the duration of the contractions, the boxes are filled with dots if contractions last <20 seconds, diagonal bars are used if contractions last 20–40 seconds, while solid shading is employed for contractions >40 seconds.

In the section for oxytocin, the concentration of the base solution in units/litre should be entered in the upper row and the drop rate per minute in the bottom row. Any fluids or medications given to the woman should be recorded in the fluid and drugs section. Maternal pulse should be recorded half-hourly as dots and the blood pressure four-hourly as vertical arrows, while the temperature should also be documented 2-hourly in the maternal vital signs section. Finally, the volume of any urine passed and the urinalysis result (protein and acetone) should be recorded in the section provided in the partograph.

12.4 Abnormal Labour

Normal labour is a retrospective diagnosis which is only made when a physiological process occurring spontaneously at term results in the timely and safe vaginal delivery of a healthy baby to a healthy and satisfied mother.

For convenience, labour is divided into three stages:

1. First stage of labour: from onset of painful uterine contractions up till full (10 cm) cervical dilatation. This is further subdivided into the following:
   (a) Latent phase (0–3 cm cervical dilatation)
   (b) Active phase (4–10 cm cervical dilatation)
2. Second stage of labour: from full cervical dilatation to the delivery of the foetus. This is also subdivided into the following:
   (a) Propulsive phase
   (b) Expulsive phase
3. Third stage of labour: this is from the delivery of the foetus to the delivery of the placenta and foetal membranes. It is subdivided into the following:
   (a) Latent phase
   (b) Contraction phase
   (c) Detachment phase
   (d) Expulsion phase

Clearly, deviation from normal can easily occur in this complex process, and when this happens, it is termed abnormal labour. In general, abnormal labour may result from problems with the powers (i.e. uterine contractions), the passenger (i.e. the foetus) or the passage (i.e. the birth canal). However, the commonest cause of abnormal labour is dystocia (i.e. difficult labour) which manifests as poor progress in the rate of cervical dilatation or descent of the presenting part, despite uterine contractions [57, 58]. Multiple gestation, malpresentation, malposition, induction of labour and presence of uterine scar(s) are some other factors, the presence of which renders labour abnormal [57].

There are various classifications of abnormal labour. Some of them are shown in Table 12.1 [59, 60]. In addition, the ACOG classifies abnormal labour into protraction disor-

Table 12.1 Classification of the disorders of the first stage of labour

Fields	Philpott	Freidman	Schifrin & Cohen
Hypotonic dysfunction	Prolonged latent phase	Prolonged latent phase	Disorders of dilatation
Prolonged latent phase	Primary dysfunctional labour	Protraction disorders	Prolonged latent phase
Prolonged active phase	Secondary arrest	Protracted active phase	Protracted active phase
Prolonged deceleration phase		Protracted descent	Secondary arrest
Prolonged 2nd stage		Arrest disorders	Disorders of descent
Hypertonic dysfunction		Secondary arrest of cervical dilatation	Failure of descent
		Prolonged deceleration phase	Protracted descent
		Arrest of descent	Arrest of descent
		Failure of descent	

ders and arrest disorders – the protraction disorders being those associated with abnormally slow progress, while the arrest disorders are associated with abrupt cessation after initial progress of labour [61]. The various abnormalities of labour can be more conveniently considered under each of the three stages of labour during which they occur [62].

12.4.1 Abnormalities of the First Stage of Labour

Aetiology of abnormal first stage of labour comprises of problems of the latent phase and problems of the active phase of labour.

12.4.2 Problems of the Latent Phase of Labour

Latent phase disorders have been a source of controversy and confusion with respect to their definition and management for almost as long as the disorders have been recognised. Significant among these disorders are prolonged latent phase and spurious labour.

Prolonged Latent Phase This was defined by Friedman as duration of latent phase exceeding the 95th centile which was 20 hours in the nulliparous and 14 hours in the parous women [62]. Philpott, however, defined prolonged latent phase as >6 hours after admission in labour in nullipara and 4 hours in parous women [46]. In the composite partograph, the WHO also defined prolonged latent phase as exceeding 8 hours regardless of parity [47]. The latter two definitions are thought to have led to a high rate of interventions for prolonged latent phase, such as oxytocin augmentation and caesarean sections, many of which in retrospect could have been avoided, leaving well alone. Indeed, the latent phase of labour is now known to be quite innocuous, especially if the foetal membranes are still intact [62]. This explains the present tendency to allow a much longer duration of latent phase of labour without unnecessary interventions.

The management of persistent prolonged latent phase of labour must take into account any identifiable cause present. In particular, a thorough assessment should be performed to exclude inlet or gross cephalopelvic disproportion, which if present is an indication for prompt caesarean section. Other causes of prolonged latent phase, however, include excessive sedation, prelabour rupture of membranes and wrong diagnosis of labour. Also, the condition is quite often idiopathic. Generally, in the absence of cephalopelvic disproportion, prolonged latent phase of labour should be managed with bed rest and analgesics. If the condition, however, still persists after this, then oxytocin augmentation is indicated [62, 63].

Spurious (False) Labour When women admitted in prolonged latent phase of labour are given sedative analgesics, the uterine contractions cease altogether in about 10% of them. This matches the diagnosis of spurious labour, in which case, there is no need for any further intervention, and the woman may be discharged home. It is, however, interesting to note that 85% of the women given sedatives because of prolonged latent phase of labour actually progress to active phase, while in the remaining 5% the prolonged latent phase persists [62, 63].

12.4.3 Problems of the Active Phase of Labour

Active phase abnormalities are the most common abnormalities in labour, affecting about 25% of nulliparous and 15% of parous women in labour. These disorders are made up of the protraction disorders (e.g. primary dysfunctional labour) and the arrest disorders (e.g. secondary arrest of labour) [60–63].

Primary Dysfunctional Labour This is defined as a cervical dilatation rate that is less than 1 cm per hour in the active phase of labour. The usual causes of primary dysfunctional labour include poor (incoordinate) uterine contractions, unrecognised cephalopelvic disproportion and foetal malpresentation such as breech or malposition such as persistent occipitoposterior position. The condition is characterised by slow progress of labour, such that the patient's cervical dilatation plot on the partograph crosses to the right of the alert line and possibly also, the action line. If not properly managed, primary dysfunctional labour could lead to prolonged labour, foetal distress and possible foetal demise, maternal anxiety, dehydration and acidosis, obstructed labour, genital sepsis, as well as uterine rupture and postpartum haemorrhage.

The management of primary dysfunctional labour entails thorough clinical evaluation to rule out cephalopelvic disproportion. If there is evidence of cephalopelvic disproportion or foetal distress, then emergency caesarean section is indicated. If, however, these are absent, then oxytocin augmentation should be commenced, especially if the uterine contractions are not adequate, i.e. contractions fewer than three in 10 minutes and/or lasting less than 40 seconds each. If an intrauterine pressure catheter is in place, intrauterine pressure of less than 200 Montevideo units per 10-minute period is considered inadequate.

Secondary Arrest of Labour Secondary arrest of labour is defined as the absence of any progress in cervical dilatation over two consecutive hours, following an initially normal progress of labour in the active phase. It is usually a manifestation of cephalopelvic disproportion or foetal malposition, and mostly occurs at cervical dilatation of about 5–7 cm. It complicates some 2% of parous and 6% of nulliparous labours. Secondary arrest is usually associated with features of exaggerated foetal squeeze such as moulding and caput succedaneum, and progresses if not promptly relieved, to obstructed labour, foetal distress and possible foetal demise. If neglected, it could also lead to uterine rupture in the parous patients, and postpartum haemorrhage.

In the management of secondary arrest of labour, every effort should be made to detect cephalopelvic disproportion if present; the finding of which should prompt an emergency caesarean section. However, in the absence of cephalopelvic disproportion, artificial rupture of membranes and oxytocin augmentation of labour should be considered. Other means of correcting malposition such as manual rotation or instrumental delivery may later be required. If, however, there is no progress after 4 hours, an emergency caesarean section should be performed.

12.4.4 Problems of the Second Stage of Labour

Prolonged Second Stage of Labour In the absence of epidural anaesthesia, the second stage of labour is considered to be prolonged when it lasts longer than 1 hour in the parous and 2 hours in the nulliparous woman. However, this definition is extended by 1 hour, to become 2 hours in the parous and 3 hours in the nulliparous woman, if epidural anaesthesia had been administered [62]. Causes of prolonged second stage include maternal or uterine exhaustion, as well as foetal malposition and unrecognised cephalopelvic disproportion. In addition to frequent monitoring of the foetal heart rate (every 5 minutes) for early detection of foetal distress in the second stage of labour, foetal descent should be assessed frequently (every 30 minutes) to confirm that the foetus is descending at a rate of at least 1 cm per hour [63].

The management of prolonged second stage of labour might entail correction of dehydration if present, change of the maternal position, e.g. changing from the supine to the upright childbirth positions, and oxytocin augmentation if not contraindicated by foetal distress or cephalopelvic disproportion. If the foetal head is engaged, then instrumental vaginal delivery using the vacuum device or the obstetric forceps may be performed, with full observance of the necessary precautions and strict adherence to the criteria for their use. The increased risk of shoulder dystocia associated with such deliveries must also be borne in mind and anticipatory measures instituted accordingly. If the foregoing measures are contraindicated or fail, then an emergency caesarean should be performed.

12.4.5 Abnormalities of the Third Stage of Labour

The commonest problem of the third stage of labour is retained placenta. This has been defined as failure to deliver the placenta within 30 minutes after the delivery of the foetus. However, the placenta is also regarded as retained if the cord should snap or detach from its attachment to the in situ placenta, or if reasonable attempts using the Brandt-Andrew's manoeuvre fail to deliver the placenta. Retained placenta is a leading cause of postpartum haemorrhage due to uterine atony. It is occasionally due to morbid adherence disorders such as placenta accreta, increta or percreta. Management of retained placenta entails appropriate resuscitation followed by manual removal of the placenta. However, in the absence of bleeding, the less invasive Papinga's technique could be used to deliver the placenta [64, 65].

References

1. Fathalla MF. How evolution of the human brain shaped women's sexual and reproductive health. Reprod Biol Insights. 2013; 6:11–8.
2. Dunsworth H, Eccleston L. The evolution of difficult childbirth and helpless hominin infants. Annu Rev Anthropol. 2015;44:55–69.
3. Rosenberg K, Trevathan W. Bipedalism and human birth: the obstetrical dilemma revisited. Evol Anthropol. 1995;4:161–8.
4. Wells JC, DeSilva JM, Stock JT. The obstetric dilemma: an ancient game of Russian roulette, or a variable dilemma sensitive to ecology? Am J Phys Anthropol. 2012;149:40–71.
5. Wittman AB, Wall LL. The evolutionary origins of obstructed labor: bipedalism, encephalization, and the human obstetric dilemma. Obstet Gynecol Surv. 2007;62(11):739–48.
6. Rabinerson D, Horowitz E. [The evolution of midwifery]. Harefuah 2007;146(5):380–4, 405. [Article in Hebrew].
7. Weiner S, Monge J, Mann A. Bipedalism and parturition: an evolutionary imperative for cesarean delivery? Clin Perinatol. 2008;35:466–78.
8. O'Driscoll K, Jackson RJ, Gallagher JT. Prevention of prolonged labour. Br Med J. 1969;2(5655):477–80.
9. O'Driscoll K, Stronge JM, Minogue M. Active management of labour. Br Med J. 1973;3(5872):135–7.
10. Frigoletto FD, Lieberman E, Lang JM, Cohen A, Barss V, Ringer S, Datta S. A clinical trial of active management of labour. NEJM. 1995;333(12):745–50.
11. Rogers R, Gilson GJ, Miller AC, Izquierdo LE, Curet LB, Qualls CR. Active management of labor: does it make a difference? Am J Obstet Gynecol. 1997;177(3):599–605.
12. Fraser W, Venditelli F, Krauss I, Breart G. Effects of early augmentation of labour with amniotomy and oxytocin in nulliparous women: a meta-analysis. Br J Obstet Gynaecol. 1998;105: 189–94.
13. Dencker A, Berg M, Bergqvist L, Ladfors L, Thorsén LS, Liljaa H. Early versus delayed oxytocin augmentation in nulliparous women with prolonged labour—a randomised controlled trial. Br J Obstet Gynaecol. 2009;116:530–6.
14. Sadler LC, Davison T, McCowan LM. A randomised controlled trial and meta-analysis of active management of labor. Br J Obstet Gynecol. 2000;107:909–15.
15. Smyth RM, Markham C, Dowswell T. Amniotomy for shortening spontaneous labor. Cochrane Database Syst Rev. 2013;6: CD006167.
16. Fraser WD, Turcot L, Krauss I, Brisson-Carrol G. Amniotomy for shortening spontaneous labor. Cochrane Database Syst Rev. 2006;3:CD000015.
17. Wei S, Wo BL, Xu H, Luo ZC, Roy C, Fraser WD. Early amniotomy and early oxytocin for prevention of, or therapy for, delay in first stage spontaneous labor compared with routine care. Cochrane Database Syst Rev 2009; 2:CD006794.
18. Cammu H, Van Eeckout E. A randomised controlled trial of early versus delayed use of amniotomy and oxytocin infusion in nulliparous labor. Br J Obstet Gynecol. 1996;103:313–8.
19. Impey L, Boylan P. Active Management of Labour Revisited. Br J Obstet Gynaecol. 1999;106:183–7.
20. Nijagal M, Kuppermann M, Nakagawa S, Cheng Y. Two practice models in one labor and delivery unit: Association with caesarean delivery rates. Am J Obstet Gynecol. 2015;212(4): 491.e1–491.e8.
21. Wax JR, Lucas FL, Lamont M, et al. Maternal and newborn outcomes in planned home birth vs planned hospital births: a meta-analysis. Am J Obstet Gynecol, 2010;203:243.e1–8.
22. Zeldes K, Norsigian J. Encouraging women to consider a less medicalised approach to childbirth without turning them off: challenges to producing our bodies, ourselves: pregnancy and birth. Birth. 2008;35(3):245–9.
23. Wagner M. Fish can't see water: the need to humanize birth. Int J Gynecol Obstet. 2001;75(1):S25–37.
24. Hutton EK, Reitsma AH, Kaufman K. Outcomes associated with planned home and planned hospital births in low-risk women attended by midwives in Ontario, Canada, 2003–2006: a retrospective cohort study. Birth. 2009;36(3):180–9.
25. De Brouwere V, Tonglet R, Van Lerberghe W. Strategies for reducing maternal mortality in developing countries: what can we learn from the history of the industrialised West? Tropical Med Int Health. 1998;3(10):771–82.
26. Ronsmans C, Etard JF, Walraven G, Høj L, Dumont A, de Bernis L, et al. Maternal mortality and access to obstetric services in West Africa. Tropical Med Int Health. 2003;8(10):940–8.
27. National Collaborating Centre for Women's and Children's Health. Intrapartum Care. Care of healthy women and their babies during childbirth. Clinical Guideline 190 Methods, evidence and recommendations. NICE 2014.
28. World Health Organization. WHO recommendations for augmentation of labour. Geneva 2014.
29. Smyth RMD, Markham C, Dowswell T. Amniotomy for shortening spontaneous labour. Cochrane Database Syst Rev 2013;6:Art. No.: CD006167. https://doi.org/10.1002/14651858.CD006167.pub4.
30. Downe S, Gyte GM, Dahlen HG, Singata M. Routine vaginal examinations for assessing progress of labour to improve outcomes for women and babies at term. Cochrane Database Syst Rev. 2013;7:CD010088. https://doi.org/10.1002/14651858.CD010088.pub2.
31. Nunes VD, Gholitabar M, Sims JM, Bewley S. Intrapartum care of healthy women and their babies: summary of updated NICE guidance. BMJ. 2014;349:g6886.
32. Chua S, Arulkumaran S. Intrapartum care. ANZJOG. 1997;37(1):25–35.
33. Gupta JK, Hofmeyr GJ, Shehmar M. Position in the second stage of labour for women without epidural anaesthesia. Cochrane Database Syst Rev. 2012;5:Art. No.: CD002006. https://doi.org/10.1002/14651858.CD002006.pub3.
34. Badejoko OO, Ibrahim HM, Awowole IO, Bola-Oyebamiji SB, Ijarotimi AO, Loto OM. Upright or dorsal? Childbirth positions among antenatal clinic attendees in southwestern and northwestern Nigeria. Trop J Obstet Gynaecol. 2016;33:172–8.
35. Kwast BE, Lennox CE, Farley TMM, Olayinka I, et al. World Health Organization partograph in management of labour. Lancet. 1994;343(8910):1399.
36. Studd J. Partograms and nomograms of cervical dilatation in management of Primigravid labour. Br Med J. 1973;4:451–5.
37. Wacker J, Utz B, Kyelem D, Lankoande J, Bastert G. Introduction of a simplified round Partogram in rural maternity units: Seno Province, Burkina Faso. West-Africa Trop Doct. 1998;28(3):146–52.
38. Reproductive care program of Nova Scotia. A Companion Guise for Completion of the Nova Scotia Labour Partogram. Halifax, 2010.
39. Bhatt BMR. Designing interfaces for healthcare workers: a case study of the electronic partogram. APCHI '13 Proceedings of the 11th Asia Pacific Conference on Computer Human Interaction. ACM New York, 2013. p. 187–191. https://doi.org/10.1145/2525194.2525268.
40. Sizer AR, Evans J, Bailey SM, Wienera J. Second-stage Partogram. Obstet Gynecol. 2000;96:678–83.
41. Friedman EA. Primigravid labor: a graphicostatistical analysis. Obstet Gynaecol. 1955;6(6):567–89.

42. Friedman EA. The graphic analysis of labour. Am J Obstet Gynecol. 1954;68(6):1568–75.
43. Hendricks CH, Brenner WE, Kraus G. Normal cervical dilatation pattern in late pregnancy and labor. Am J Obstet Gynecol. 1970;106(7):1065–82.
44. Phillpott RH, Castle WM. Cervicographs in the management of labour in primigravidae 1: the alert line for detecting abnormal labour. J Obstet Gynaecol Br Commonwealth. 1972;79:592–8.
45. Phillpott RH, Castle WM. Cervicograms in the management labour in primigravidae II: the action and treatment of abnormal labour. J Obstet Gynaecol Br Commonwealth. 1972;79:599–602.
46. Phillpott RH. Graphic records in labour. Br Med J. 1972;4:163–5.
47. WHO. World Health Organization partograph in management of labour. Lancet. 1994;343:1399–404.
48. Walraven GE. WHO Partograph. Lancet. 1994;344:617.
49. WHO. World Health Organization partograph cuts complications of labour and childbirth. Safe Mother. 1994;15:10.
50. Orhue AAE, Ande ABA, Aziken ME. Barriers to the universal application of the partograph for labour management: a review of the issues and proposed solutions. Trop J Obstet Gynaecol. 2011;28(1):32–42.
51. Orhue AAE, Aziken ME, Osemwenkha AP. Partograph as a tool for team work management of spontaneous labour. Niger J Clin Pract. 2012;15(1):1–8.
52. Orhue AAE, Aziken ME, Osemwenkha AP. Spontaneous latent phase labour: a review of issues, definition, classification and management options. Trop J Obstet Gynaecol. 2010;27(2): 13–22.
53. Ollerhead E, Osrin D. Barriers to and incentives for achieving partograph use in obstetric practice in low- and middle-income countries: a systematic review. BMC Pregnancy Childbirth. 2014;14:281. https://doi.org/10.1186/1471-2393-14-281.
54. Mathews JE, Rajaratnam A, George A, Mathai M. Comparison of the two WHO partographs. Int J Gyaecol Obstet. 2007;96: 147–50.
55. Lavender T, Hart A, Smyth RM. Effect of partogram use on outcomes for women in spontaneous labour at term. Cochrane Database Syst Rev. 2012;8:CD005461. https://doi.org/10.1002/14651858.CD005461.pub3.
56. Fatusi AO, Makinde ON, Adeyemi AB, Orji EO, Onwudiegwu U. Evaluation of health workers' training in use of the partogram. Int J Gynaecol Obstet. 2008;100(1):41–4.
57. WHO. Preventing prolonged labour: a practical guide. The partograph – Part 1: Principles and strategy. Maternal Health and Safe Motherhood Programme Division of Family Health, World Health Organization, Geneva, 1994.
58. Duncan T, McEwan A. An evidence-based approach to the management of abnormal labour. Curr Obstetr Gynaecol. 2004;14(4):277–84.
59. Drennan K, Blackwell S, et al. Glob Libr Women's Med, (ISSN: 1756–2228) 2008; https://doi.org/10.3843/GLOWM.10132.
60. Ness A, Goldberg J, Berghella V. Abnormalities of the first and second stages of labor. Obstet Gynecol Clin N Am. 2005;32: 201–20.
61. Practice Bulletin Number ACOG 49, December 2003. Dystocia and augmentation of labor. Obstet Gynecol 2003;102:1445–1453.
62. Friedman E. Labor: clinical evaluation and management. 2nd ed. New York: Appleton-Century-Crofts; 1978.
63. Bowes WA, Thorp JM. Clinical aspects of normal and abnormal labor. In: Creasy CK, Resnick R, Iams JD, editors. Maternal-fetal medicine: principles and practice. 5th ed. Philadelphia: WB Saunders; 2004. p. 671–705.
64. Pipingas A, Hofmeyr JG, Sesel KR. Umbilical vessel oxytocin administration for retained placenta: In vitro study of various infusion techniques. Am J Obstet Gynecol. 1993;168(3 Part 1) :793–5.
65. Rogers MS, Yuen PM, Wong S. Avoiding manual removal of placenta: evaluation of intra-umbilical injection of uterotonics using the Pipingas technique for management of adherent placenta. Acta Obstet Gynecol Scand. 2007;86(1):48–54.

Premature Rupture of Membranes (PROM)

13

Osric Banfegha Navti

Learning Objectives

At the end of this chapter, the learner will be able to:

- Explain the concept of premature rupture of membranes (PROM)
- Distinguish between:
  - Premature rupture of membranes (PROM)
  - Term prelabour rupture of membranes (term PROM)
  - Preterm prelabour rupture of membranes (PPROM)
- Evaluate the risk factors of preterm birth and the contribution of PROM to this
- Describe the diagnostic strategy for premature rupture of membranes (PROM)
- Discuss the management of premature rupture of membranes (PROM)
- Critically examine offering conservative or active management to patients with premature rupture of membranes (PROM)
- Understand the principles behind antenatal corticosteroids, tocolysis and the place of magnesium sulphate in women with premature rupture of membranes (PROM)

13.1 Introduction

Premature rupture of membranes (PROM) – more commonly referred to now as prelabour rupture of membranes is defined as membrane rupture before the onset of uterine contractions. Spontaneous preterm rupture of membranes (SROM) is defined as rupture of membranes occurring after or with the starting of labour before 37 weeks gestation. Prolonged rupture of membranes describes ruptured membranes persisting for more than 24 hours and occurring before the onset of labour.

Term prelabour rupture of membranes (term PROM) is defined as rupture of the membranes before the onset of labour at or beyond 37 weeks of completed gestation. Preterm prelabour rupture of membranes (PPROM) refers to PROM before 37 + 0 weeks of gestation. PPROM occurs in 2–4% of pregnancies: approximately 0.5% of pregnancies <27 weeks, 1% of pregnancies 27–34 weeks, and 1% of pregnancies 34–37 week [1, 2]. It is the single most common identifiable factor associated with preterm delivery with up to 40% of these cases resulting in preterm delivery [3]. 85% of neonatal morbidity and mortality is due to prematurity. The incidence of term PROM is 8%. Spontaneous labour follows term PROM at 12, 24, 48 and 96 hours in 50%, 70%, 85% and 95% of women, respectively [4–7]. In women with preterm PROM remote from term, 50% will go into labour within 24–48 hours and 70–90% within 7 days [4, 5, 8, 9]. For women with preterm PROM at 24–28 weeks of gestation, the latency period tends to be longer than those with preterm PROM closer to term.

13.2 Pathogenesis

The pathogenesis of spontaneous membrane rupture is not entirely understood. PPROM arises from complex, multifaceted pathways. Epidemiological and clinical factors considered precursors to PPROM are summarised in the Table 13.1.

Biochemical signals arising from the foetus, including endocrine signals that promote foetal membrane apoptosis, have also been implicated in the initiation of PPROM [10–13]. More recently PPROM has been described as a disease of the foetal membranes where the inflammation-oxidative stress axis plays a significant role in producing pathways that can result in membrane weakening through a variety of processes [14]. Recent data provides molecular evidence for the ageing of foetal membranes in response to oxidative stress (physiologically at term and pathologically at pre-

O. B. Navti (✉)
Al Wakra Hospital, Hamad Medical Corporation, Doha, Qatar
e-mail: onavti@doctors.org.uk

F. Okonofua et al. (eds.), *Contemporary Obstetrics and Gynecology for Developing Countries*,
https://doi.org/10.1007/978-3-030-75385-6_13

Table 13.1 Epidemiological and clinical factors considered precursors to PPROM

Factors	Examples
Maternal reproductive tract infections	Bacterial vaginosis [BV], trichomoniasis, gonorrhoea, chlamydia and occult chorioamnionitis
Behavioural factors	Substance abuse, smoking, poor nutritional status and coitus during pregnancy
Obstetric complications	History of previous PPROM Multiple gestation, polyhydramnios, cervical weakness, antepartum haemorrhage, prior cervical surgery and antenatal trauma
Environmental factors	Stress, toxin exposure
Genetic predisposition	Several genetic polymorphisms of genes related to infection, inflammation and collagen degradation

term). Our current understanding of the pathogenesis of spontaneous membrane rupture is incomplete. Rupture of the foetal membranes may occur for several reasons. When membranes rupture at term, it results from a physiologic weakening of the foetal membranes combined with shearing forces from uterine contractions. Preterm PROM can result from a wide range of pathologic mechanisms that act individually or in concert. Recent data provide molecular evidence for the ageing of foetal membranes in response to oxidative stress (physiologically at term and pathologically at preterm) causing a telomere dependent, p38MAPK signaller-driven senescence activation of the foetal membranes [15]. Senescence, a mechanism contributing to ageing of foetal membranes, produces sterile inflammation that can cause further damage to foetal membranes leading to weakening and or rupture [16]. The major function of foetal membranes is to protect the foetus during its growth and development in utero. Specifically, the foetal membrane functions to provide mechanical [17, 18] and immune protection and acts as a barrier for microbial access [19, 20]. This protective role is supported by the biomarkers that are produced by foetal membranes during gestation and parturition [21]. Compromise in the immune and mechanical properties of the foetal membranes allows for microbial invasion from genital tract [22], activation of host inflammatory response leading to collagenolysis-mediated mechanical disruption [17, 23–25], and membrane weakening predisposing the membranes to PPROM.

13.3 Risk Factors

Maternal physiologic, genetic, and environmental factors predispose to the development of PPROM in a good number of cases. These risk factors mirror those for preterm labour (Table 13.1), but most patients have no identifiable risk factors. Factors with a strong association with PPROM include a personal history of previous PPROM, genital tract infection, antepartum bleeding and cigarette smoking.

Previous PPROM has consistently been shown to be associated with a risk of recurrence. A large prospective study, the Preterm Prediction Study, observed that women with a history of PPROM leading to preterm birth had a threefold higher frequency of PPROM in a subsequent pregnancy compared with women with no such history (13.5% versus 4.1%; relative risk [RR] 3.3, 95% CI 2.1–5.2) [26]. Moreover, in the subsequent pregnancy, women with a history of PPROM leading to preterm birth were at high risk of PPROM and preterm birth before 28 weeks (1.8% versus 0.13% in women with no history of preterm birth due to PPROM; RR 13.5, 95% CI 23.0–80.3). Others studies have reported recurrence rates as high as 32 [27].

Genital tract infection This is the single most identifiable risk factor for PPROM. Epidemiological evidence strongly supports this association in three ways:

- Women diagnosed with PPROM are significantly more likely to have pathogenic microorganisms in the amniotic fluid than women with intact membranes
- Rate of histologic chorioamnionitis is significantly higher with PPROM than in those who deliver preterm without PPROM
- The rate of PPROM is significantly higher in ladies with certain lower genital tract infections (particularly bacterial vaginosis) than in those who are not infected [28].

A number of the microorganisms that colonise the lower genital tract can produce phospholipases, which can stimulate the production of prostaglandins, thereby leading to the onset of uterine contractions. Besides, the immune response of the host to bacterial invasion of the endocervix and/or foetal membranes can lead to the production of multiple inflammatory mediators that can cause localised weakening of the foetal membranes and result in PPROM [28]. The genetic regulation of the host's immune and inflammatory responses appears to play a significant role in the susceptibility and response to infections associated with PPROM.

Antepartum haemorrhage (APH) Bleeding in the first trimester is associated with a small but statistically significant increased risk of PPROM [29]. When APH occurs in more than one trimester the risk is increased three to seven-fold [30–32]. Abruption-associated thrombin, matrix metalloproteinase activation and collagenolytic processes have been reported in foetal membrane weakening and PPROM [33].

Cigarette smoking The mechanism of the association is unclear, but cigarette smoking is associated with a two to four-fold increased risk of PPROM compared to non-smokers. This risk persists after adjustment for known confounders [34].

Clinical presentation The classic clinical presentation of PPROM is a sudden gush of fluid from the vagina, which may soak through clothing. The fluid is typically clear or pale yellow. In some women, the presentation may be atypical with leaking small amounts intermittently or of the dampness of the vagina and perineum and under clothing. This can happen if the hole in the membranes is small or not directly in front of the baby's head (also called a hind-water leak).

The diagnosis of PPROM is typically based on the characteristic history and findings on clinical examination. A sterile vaginal speculum exam will confirm pooling of amniotic fluid in the posterior vaginal vault. This is the gold standard for diagnosis. When pooling is not observed, asking the patient to cough, bear down or perform a Valsalva's manoeuvre may enhance the flow of amniotic fluid through the cervix and confirm the diagnosis. For women who are not in active labour, an examination of the cervix and vagina should be performed using a sterile speculum. A digital examination *should be avoided* because it may decrease the latency period (i.e. time from PROM to delivery) and increase the risk of intrauterine infection [35–37].

The role of ultrasound in the diagnosis of PPROM is controversial. Ultrasound examination of the foetus demonstrating oligohydramnios may be useful to support the clinical impression of PPROM. Case-control studies have shown that women with a clinically diagnosed PPROM who also have reduced amniotic fluid volumes on scan are more likely to give birth within 7 days from the rupture of the membranes [38]. In the presence of a good history, the presence of oligohydramnios on ultrasound may be suggestive of ruptured membranes. Oligohydramnios may be defined as a maximum vertical pocket (MVP) of amniotic fluid <2 cm in depth or an amniotic fluid index (AFI) ≤5 cm (some use ≤2 cm and <5 cm, respectively). In a prospective study of 290 singleton pregnancies with PPROM at 24–34 weeks of gestation, 67% had AFI <5 cm and 47% had an MVP <2 cm [39]. Other causes of oligohydramnios should, of course, be excluded.

Laboratory Haematology and blood chemistry are typically normal in the absence of infection or other complications of pregnancy. A number of tests that are designed to assist with confirming a diagnosis of PROM are commercially available. These include insulin-like growth factor binding protein-1 (IGFBP-1 – Actim® PROM) and placental alpha microglobulin-1 (PAMG-1 – AmniSure®). Analysis shows that the accuracy of Actim® PROM and AmniSure® for the detection of PROM are comparable if used in the same clinical population [40–42]. In a 2013 meta-analysis of prospective observational or cohort studies investigating insulin-like growth factor binding protein 1 (IGFBP-1 [Actim PROM]) and placental alpha microglobulin-1 protein assay (PAMG-1 [AmniSure]) for diagnosis of rupture of membranes, data was retrieved from 17 studies; 10 for Actim® PROM (n = 1066), four for AmniSure® (n = 1081) and another three studies in which both biomarker tests were directly compared. When pooled, the analysis showed that the specificity and positive predictive value were statistically significantly higher for AmniSure® when compared with Actim® PROM. When, however, 762 and 1385 mothers with known or suspected ROM, respectively, were evaluated, AmniSure® remained significantly superior in the latter group only. Furthermore, when these two tests were directly compared in the same study, there were no statistically significant differences observed. It was of note that women with a history or evidence of vaginal bleeding were excluded in all the four studies for AmniSure®, in two Actim® PROM studies and in two of the three studies reporting on both tests. The authors, therefore, concluded that both tests appeared equally useful for clinical use to aid in the diagnosis of PROM, as no significant differences were observed between them when compared side by side in the same study. The exclusion of women with vaginal bleeding from all but one of the AmniSure® studies may have limited the direct comparison of studies evaluating the two biomarkers. There is no doubt that some degree of bleeding may be present in a good number of women presenting with suspected PROM in real clinical settings. Further studies are essential to consider the performance of AmniSure® in such conditions [43].

Another test, ROM plus (combination of Placental protein 12 and alpha-foetoprotein) in a prospective observational study in comparison with conventional clinical assessment (speculum examination plus both fern and nitrazine tests) for diagnosis of rupture of membranes in 285 patients at 15–42 weeks of gestation found that the immunoassay had higher sensitivity (99% versus 85%) and lower specificity (91% versus 98%) [44]. A limitation of this study was that confirmation of PROM was based on a review of the medical records following delivery.

Several tests have been used to confirm PPROM by measuring the pH; the most widely used is the nitrazine test, which detects pH change [45, 46] and has a sensitivity of 90% and specificity of 83% [47]. Nitrazine paper is used only to test the pH of vaginal fluid. Amniotic fluid generally has a pH range of 7.0–7.3, which is different from the normal vaginal pH of 3.8–4.2 and often different from the pH of urine, which is typically <6.0 but may be higher [48]. False-negative and false-positive nitrazine test is observed in up to 5% of cases [46, 49]. False-negative test results can occur when leaking is intermittent, or the amniotic fluid is diluted by other vaginal fluids. False-positive results can be due to the presence of alkaline fluids in the vagina, such as blood, seminal fluid or soap.

Other tests that have been widely used include microscopic examination of vaginal fluid for characteristic ferning of a crystalline pattern of dried amniotic fluid owing to its sodium chloride and protein content [50] with a reported sensitivity of 98% and specificity of 88.2% [51]. A fingerprint on the microscope slide or oestrogenised cervical mucus may cause a false positive fern test. False negatives can result from inadequate amniotic fluid on the swab or heavy contamination with vaginal discharge and/or blood. In the United Kingdom, a home test, an absorbent pad (AmnioSense) that changes colour at pH >5.2 is used in the form of a panty liner is marketed to pregnant women as a test for ruptured membranes. Antibiotic therapy or vaginal infections with BV or TV can lead to an elevated vaginal pH level, which may result in a false-positive test. Tap water can also interfere with the test and may give a false-positive result [52]. Other reasons for vaginal/perineal wetness include urinary incontinence, excessive vaginal discharge (normal or related to infection), cervical mucus and perspiration and should be excluded.

Pregnancy complication	Potential consequences for offspring	Potential maternal consequences
Intrauterine infection	Neonatal sepsis Long-term neurodevelopmental abnormalities, particularly cerebral palsy	Chorioamnionitis Postpartum endometritis Septicaemia
Umbilical cord compression	Foetal asphyxia and demise	Caesarean delivery
Oligohydramnios	Limb restriction deformities and pulmonary hypoplasia (mainly with severe oligohydramnios in the early to mid-second trimester). Rare when membrane rupture occurs after 23 weeks	
Foetal malpresentation		Caesarean delivery
Umbilical cord prolapse	Foetal asphyxia and demise	Caesarean delivery
Abruptio placentae	Foetal asphyxia and demise	Caesarean delivery Coagulopathy
Preterm birth	Morbidity of prematurity, including respiratory abnormalities, intraventricular haemorrhage, necrotising enterocolitis, retinopathy of prematurity, patent ductus arteriosus	

Management of PROM is influenced by gestational age, and the presence of complicating factors, such as clinical infection, abruptio placentae, labour or non-reassuring foetal status. An accurate assessment of gestational age of patients and knowledge of the maternal, foetal and neonatal risks are essential for appropriate evaluation, counselling and care of patients with PROM.

Controversial aspects of the management include the following:

- Accurate diagnosis in problematic cases
- Expectant management versus intervention
- Use of tocolytics
- Duration of administration of antibiotic prophylaxis
- Timing of administration of antenatal corticosteroids
- Methods of testing for maternal/foetal infection
- Timing of delivery

PROM may occur at term (≥37 weeks of gestation) or preterm (<37 weeks of gestation); the latter is designated preterm PROM (PPROM). Mid-trimester PROM typically refers to PPROM at 16–26 weeks of gestation; this is an arbitrary definition, which varies slightly among investigators. The frequencies of term, preterm and mid-trimester PROM are approximately 8%, 3%, and <1% of pregnancies, respectively.

PROM at term A clinician should evaluate women with suspected PROM. There is no clear data supporting the safety of delaying evaluation, the most prudent approach is a prompt assessment to confirm membrane rupture, determine foetal position, evaluate maternal and foetal status and discuss options for further management. A digital vaginal examination should be avoided; foetal presentation should be determined by abdominal palpation +/− ultrasound and foetal wellbeing assessed by CTG. Maternal assessment should rule out any signs of infection and include a review of the patient's obstetric history.

Following ruptured membranes at term, the primary concerns are increased risks of maternal and newborn infection. This is particularly so with expectant management. Prompt intervention may also reduce the risk for other serious but less common complications during expectant management, such as cord prolapse or abruption, and was the most cost-effective approach in one model [7]. However, labour tends to be longer with induction than when labour begins spontaneously.

A 2017 systematic review of 23 randomised trials of women with PROM at ≥37 weeks of gestation compared pregnancy outcome of planned early intervention versus expectant management (*n* = 8615 women) [53].

Planned early intervention resulted in the following:

- A reduction in time from membrane rupture to birth (mean difference −10 hours, 95% CI −12 to −8 hours)
- A reduction in maternal chorioamnionitis and/or endometritis (54/1000 versus 110/1000, relative risk [RR] 0.49, 95% CI 0.33–0.72)
- A reduction in admission to special neonatal care or intensive care unit (RR 0.75, 95% CI 0.66–0.85)
- No increase in caesarean delivery (126/1000 versus 150/1000, RR 0.84, 95% CI 0.69–1.04)
- Trends in reductions in definite early-onset neonatal sepsis (12/1000 versus 22/1000, RR 0.57, 95% CI 0.24–1.33) and perinatal mortality (1/1000 versus 2/1000, RR 0.47, 95% CI 0.13–1.66)

The authors concluded that there is poor quality evidence to suggest that a planned early delivery (with labour-induction methods such as oxytocin or prostaglandins) reduces the risk of maternal infectious morbidity when compared with expectant management of PROM at 37 weeks' of pregnancy or later, without an apparent increased risk of Caesarean section. Evidence was mainly downgraded because the majority of studies contributing the data had some serious design limitations, and most outcomes' estimates were imprecise. There is an urgent need to assess the benefits or harms of planned early birth compared with expectant management. Consideration must be given to maternal, neonatal, foetal and long-term childhood outcomes, and the use of health services, in these two lines of management. Any future trials should be adequately designed and powered to evaluate the effects on short- and long-term outcomes. The standardisation of outcomes and their definitions, including for the assessment of maternal and neonatal infection, would be very beneficial. For patients who choose expectant management, it is critical to provide a time limit for expectant management through shared decision-making. There are no robust data on which to base a recommendation for the maximum duration of expectant management in women with no pregnancy complications warranting delivery. In the term PROM study, which limited expectant management to 96 hours post rupture, the risk of chorioamnionitis appeared to increase significantly after 24 hours [54], suggesting that 24 hours is a reasonable limit. However, waiting longer would increase the number of women who would begin to labour spontaneously. In the term PROM trial, 50% of women with PROM managed expectantly were in active labour by approximately 17 hours, and 95% were in active labour by approximately 75 hours after membrane rupture [54]. Active management should be initiated if there are signs of infection or other pregnancy complications, and delivery completed by the most appropriate method for the clinical situation.

Active management Current evidence suggests that active management of term PROM with induction of labour is associated with a reduction in maternal infective morbidity and increased maternal satisfaction without increasing the rate of Caesarean sections or operative vaginal birth rates. There were fewer infants being admitted to NICU and fewer infants were requiring postnatal antibiotics. Nevertheless, following preliminary assessment, some women and/or clinicians may reasonably elect for a short trial of expectant management (e.g. for up to 24 hours) in highly selected and well-supervised cases. The available evidence on prostaglandins versus oxytocin for induction following term PROM is limited and has failed to show a clear benefit. The previous Cochrane meta-analysis suggested an increased risk of chorioamnionitis and neonatal infection with the administration of prostaglandins [55]. Concerns regarding the risk of hyperstimulation and tachysystole may be part of the reason that drug information on commonly used prostaglandin preparations lists ruptured membranes as a contraindication to use. In a Cochrane review to determine the effects of vaginal misoprostol in third-trimester cervical ripening or induction of labour, it was concluded that vaginal misoprostol administered in doses above 25 μg 4-hourly was much more effective than conventional methods of labour induction. However, it resulted in more uterine hyperstimulation. Lower doses of misoprostol were similar to conventional methods in effectiveness and risks. The authors request that the vaginal route should not be researched further as another Cochrane review has shown clearly that the oral route of administration of misoprostol is preferable to the vaginal route. Professional and governmental bodies should agree on guidelines for the use of misoprostol, based on the best available evidence and local circumstances [56]. For these reasons, therefore, oxytocin remains the method of choice as it is also easier to titrate and may be less expensive. For a subset of women with an unfavourable cervix, prostaglandins may, however, have a significant role. This has been further evaluated in one small trial where dinoprostone was followed by infusion of oxytocin 6 hours later in women with a Bishop score of less than five. This resulted in a significantly increased rate of vaginal delivery within 24 hours when compared to those induced with oxytocin alone [57]. Further trials in this area are clearly indicated, but where the cervix is not favourable, the risks and benefits need to be considered very carefully. Prostaglandins (including misoprostol) may have a valuable role in the clinical management of induction for term PROM [58].

In mothers known to have vaginal Group B streptococcus (GBS) colonisation, prophylactic antibiotics and early induction of labour are recommended. For women known to be GBS negative, a recent meta-analysis [59] reported that the use of routine antibiotic administration in women with PROM after 36 weeks had a reduction in the rate of chorioamnionitis which was not statistically significant (2.7% versus 3.7%; RR 0.73, 95% CI 0.48–1.12), neonatal sepsis (1.0% versus 1.4%; RR 0.69, 95% CI 0.34–1.39), maternal infection (3.1% versus 4.6%; RR 0.48, 95% CI 0.19–1.21) and neonatal death (0.4% versus 0.9%; RR 0.44, 95% CI 0.18–1.10). The use of routine antibiotics in women with term PROM, therefore, needs to be weighed against the increased risk of antibiotic resistance. In a subset analysis of the same meta-analysis, women with latency of 12 hours or more, who received antibiotics had a lower rates of chorioamnionitis (2.9% versus 6.1%; RR 0.49, 95% CI 0.27–0.91) and endometritis (0% versus 2.2%; RR 0.12, 95% CI 0.02–0.62) when compared with the control group that did not receive antibiotics. Overall, this suggests that in women with latency longer than 12 hours, prophylactic antibiotics seem to be associated with statistically significant lower rates of chorioamnionitis by 51% and endometritis by 88%.

A sub-analysis of term PROM concluded that expectant management of women at home was associated with a further rise in the risk of maternal need for antibiotics (OR 1.52) and neonatal infections (OR 1.97) [60]. In preterm PROM, women who are managed as an outpatient face additional risks associated with rapid delivery [61]. Women being considered for expectant management at home must, therefore, be carefully selected with no evidence of maternal or foetal compromise but also live close to the hospital, have adequate support at home and dependable transport.

Management of preterm pre-labour rupture of membranes PPROM refers to PROM before 37 + 0 weeks of gestation and is among the most controversial issues in perinatal medicine.

Points of contention include the following:

- Accurate diagnosis in problematic case
- Expectant management versus intervention
- Use of tocolytics
- Duration of administration of antibiotic prophylaxis
- Timing of administration of antenatal corticosteroids/rescue courses
- Methods of testing for maternal/foetal infection
- Timing of delivery

The management is based upon consideration of several factors, which are assessed upon presentation:

- Gestational age
- Presence or absence of maternal/foetal infection
- Presence or absence of labour
- Foetal presentation
- Foetal wellbeing
- Cervical status (by visual inspection)
- Availability of appropriate level of neonatal care

The duration of the latency period (i.e. time from PROM to delivery) inversely correlates with gestational age at membrane rupture. The majority of pregnancies with PPROM nevertheless deliver within 1 week of membrane rupture. The median latency after PPROM is similar when membrane rupture occurs from 24 to 28 + 6 weeks of gestation (approximately 9 days), but shortens with membrane rupture from 29 weeks of gestation [62]. Prolonged latency after PPROM at 23–34 weeks does not worsen neonatal prognosis [63–65]. The early preterm foetus (<34 weeks), who is otherwise stable, will benefit by prolonging the time it remains in the uterus if the duration is sufficient for a significant reduction in gestational age-related morbidity. However, this benefit needs to be balanced with the risks of PPROM-associated complications and their sequelae in expectantly managed pregnancies: intrauterine infection, placental abruption and cord prolapse/compression. One of the most concerning risks associated with PPROM is ascending infection leading to chorioamnionitis.

The National Institute of Clinical Excellence (NICE) in the United Kingdom recommends that a combination of clinical assessment (pulse, blood pressure, temperature and symptoms), maternal blood tests (C-reactive protein and white cell count) and foetal heart rate using cardiotocography, should be employed to diagnose and monitor clinical infection. If the results of the clinical assessment or any of the tests are not consistent with each other, it is recommended that the woman should continue to be observed and consideration should be given to repeating the tests [66]. An investigation of several maternal serum markers for predicting histological chorioamnionitis after PPROM concluded that C-reactive protein was the most informative [67]. When managed as an inpatient, women with PPROM should have their vital signs, including pulse, blood pressure and temperature, recorded on an obstetric early warning chart. The women should also be observed for clinical symptoms and signs of infection. When managed as an outpatient, women should be advised of the symptoms of chorioamnionitis and be reviewed regularly (including blood tests, clinical recordings and cardiotocography), for example, in a day care unit, maternity triage or antenatal ward, three times each week; if the woman has any concerns, she should attend the hospital immediately. In the absence of complications, patients are monitored closely and managed expectantly before 34 weeks of gestation. Most patients who are initially managed expectantly should be delivered at about 34 weeks of gestation. The American College of Obstetricians and Gynaecologists (ACOG) suggests delivery for all PPROM patients at ≥34 + 0 weeks of gestation. If expectant management is continued beyond 34 weeks of gestation, the balance between benefit and risk should be carefully considered and discussed [68]. The Royal College of Obstetricians and Gynaecologists or the Royal Australian and New Zealand College of Obstetricians and Gynaecologists, guideline states: 'Delivery should be considered at 34 weeks of gestation. Where expectant management is considered beyond this gestation, women should be informed of increased risk of chorioamnionitis and the reduced risk of respiratory problems in the neonate' [69].

A 2017 meta-analysis of randomised trials of management of women with PPROM prior to 37 weeks concluded that, in the absence of either foetal or maternal compromise, expectant management until 37 weeks of gestation was preferable to timed early delivery (*n* = 12 trials, 3617 women, 3628 neonates) [70].

Compared with expectant management until 37 weeks, planned early birth increased the risk of several adverse newborn outcomes:

- Respiratory distress syndrome (relative risk [RR] 1.26, 95% CI 1.05–1.53)
- Need for mechanical ventilation (RR 1.27, 95% CI 1.02–1.58)
- Admission of babies to neonatal intensive care unit (RR 1.16, 95% CI 1.08–1.24)
- Perinatal death (RR 2.55, 95% CI 1.17–5.56)

It did not reduce the risk of some outcomes of concern, such as neonatal sepsis (RR 0.93, 95% CI 0.66–1.30), positive neonatal blood cultures (RR 1.24, 95% CI 0.70–2.21), overall perinatal mortality (RR 1.76, 95% CI 0.89–3.50) or foetal death (RR 0.45, 95% CI 0.13–1.57).

For the mother, planned early birth resulted in the following:

- Lower rate of chorioamnionitis (RR 0.50, 95% CI 0.26–0.95)
- Shorter total length of hospitalisation (mean difference −1.75 days, 95% CI −2.45 to −1.05)
- Higher caesarean delivery rate (RR 1.26, 95% CI 1.11–1.44)
- Higher frequency of endometritis (RR 1.61, 95% CI 1.00–2.59)

A 2018 individual participant data meta-analysis of trials of late PPROM (34 + 0 to 36 + 6 weeks) with randomisation to immediate delivery or expectant management included three of the trials in the above meta-analysis (*n* = 2563 women) [71].

Major findings were as follows:

The two clinical approaches resulted in similar rates of the composite adverse neonatal outcome (probable or definitive neonatal sepsis, necrotising enterocolitis, neonatal respiratory distress syndrome, stillbirth or neonatal death; 9.6% with immediate delivery versus 8.3% with expectant management; RR 1.20, 95% CI 0.94–1.55).

For the mother, immediate delivery reduced the risk of antepartum haemorrhage (1.7% versus 3.0%; RR 0.57, 95% CI 0.34–0.95) and chorioamnionitis (1.3% versus 6.4%; RR 0.21, 95% CI 0.13–0.35) but modestly increased the risk of caesarean delivery (22% versus 18%; RR 1.26, 95% CI 1.08–1.47).

The rate of endometritis (0.2% versus 0.6%) and the length of hospitalisation (3.45 versus 3.39 days) were not statistically different between groups. Current evidence remains inconclusive, and individualisation of care is important, taking into account the patient's specific circumstances after detailed counselling.

13.4 Expectant Management

A course of corticosteroids should be administered to pregnancies that present with PPROM between 23 and 34 weeks of gestation. Data from systematic reviews of randomised trials show that neonatal death, respiratory distress syndrome, intraventricular haemorrhage, necrotising enterocolitis and duration of neonatal respiratory support were significantly reduced by antenatal corticosteroid treatment without an increase in either maternal or neonatal infection [72, 73]. Mean risk reduction for these adverse events ranged from 30% to 60%.

Administration of antenatal steroids for PPROM from 22nd week of gestation is also reasonable if delivery is anticipated over the next 7 days, and the family desires aggressive neonatal intervention after thorough consultation with maternal-foetal medicine and neonatology specialists. There is some evidence of benefit of short-term benefit in neonatal morbidity from repeated courses of steroids in women who remain at risk of very preterm birth 7 or more days after an initial course with no long-term adverse effects in children followed up to 6–8 years of age [74, 75]. There is a lack of consensus on this with the American College of Obstetricians and Gynaecologists (ACOG) declining to make a recommendation for or against a rescue dose of corticosteroids at any gestational age in patients with PPROM [68].

Patients with PPROM should be screened for infection, including GBS, on admission since these pregnancies are at high risk of preterm delivery. Women with positive results are managed, as appropriate. In some cases, the prophylactic antibiotic therapy administered to prolong latency will provide adequate treatment. Chemoprophylaxis specifically for GBS is indicated if GBS test results are positive or unknown and delivery is imminent.

Infection can be a cause or a consequence of PPROM. The goal of antibiotic therapy is to reduce the rate of maternal and foetal infection and thereby delay the onset of preterm labour (i.e. prolong latency) and the need for indicated preterm delivery. The importance of reducing neonatal infection is underscored by studies suggesting a sort of relationship between chorioamnionitis, duration of rupture of membranes and the development of cerebral palsy or neurodevelopmental impairment in the baby.

A 2013 systematic review of 22 placebo-controlled randomised trials involving over 6800 women evaluated the use of antibiotics following PPROM before 37 weeks of gestation [76]. Compared with placebo/no treatment, antibiotic use was associated with significant reductions in the following:

- Chorioamnionitis (relative risk [RR] 0.66, 95% CI 0.46–0.96)
- Infants born within 48 hours (RR 0.71, 95% CI 0.58–0.87) and 7 days (RR 0.79, 95% CI 0.71–0.89) of randomisation
- Neonatal infection (RR 0.67, 95% CI 0.52–0.85)
- Use of surfactant (RR 0.83, 95% CI 0.72–0.96)
- Neonatal oxygen therapy (RR 0.88, 95% CI 0.81–0.96)
- Abnormal cerebral ultrasound scan prior to hospital discharge (RR 0.81, 95% CI 0.68–0.98)

The authors concluded that Routine prescription of antibiotics for women with preterm rupture of the membranes is clearly associated with prolongation of pregnancy and improvements in a number of short-term neonatal morbidities, but no significant reduction has been proven in perinatal mortality. Despite the lack of evidence of longer-term benefit in childhood, the advantages of short-term morbidities are such that antibiotics are routinely prescribed. The WHO recommends Erythromycin as the antibiotic of choice for prophylaxis in women with preterm prelabour rupture of membranes [77]. The choice of erythromycin was based on the findings of the ORACLE I trial (with over 2000 women), which showed that erythromycin reduces the risk of necrotising enterocolitis (NEC) in the newborn compared to co-amoxiclav [78]. The recommendation was made conditional simply because antibiotic choice may be dependent on local availability of the drug and sensitivities of prevalent local organisms. The recommended regimen is oral erythromycin 250 mg four times a day for 10 days (or until delivery). Penicillins (excluding amoxicillin) have been used in other pooled trials that showed benefits of antibiotics in this context. Therefore, where erythromycin is not available, penicillin (e.g. amoxicillin) can be used. Ongoing studies to determine the optimal prophylactic antibiotic regimen are needed, given changes in bacterial sensitivities over time [79].

The principal indication for tocolysis in the setting of PPROM is to delay delivery for 48 hours to allow administration of a course of corticosteroids. As a general rule, tocolytics should not be administered for more than 48 hours.

In a 2014 systematic review of randomised trials evaluating pregnancy outcomes of women with PPROM who received or did not receive tocolytic therapy (prophylactic or therapeutic), tocolysis for pregnancies <34 weeks resulted in the following:

- Fewer births within 48 hours (RR 0.59, 95% CI 0.34–1.00; four trials, $n = 243$ women)
- An increase in chorioamnionitis (RR 1.79, 95% CI 1.02–3.14; three trials, $n = 168$ women)
- No significant improvement in perinatal morbidity or mortality [80]

Limitations to these data included the small number and size of the trials and the fact that patients did not consistently receive antenatal corticosteroids to reduce neonatal morbidity or antibiotics to prolong latency, which diverges with current standards of care and may explain the lack of improvement in clinically important outcomes.

There is currently no conclusive evidence determining the best location for managing women with PPROM. A meta-analysis of currently available trials found no significant differences in maternal or neonatal outcomes between the hospital and home care groups, although the home group had lower maternal costs [81]. However, these small trials did not have sufficient statistical power to detect meaningful differences between groups. The decision to offer outpatient management to women with PPROM should be made on an individual basis. Factors including the woman's preferences, past obstetric history, support at home and distance from the hospital should be taken into account and markers of delivery latency should be assessed (cervical length on transvaginal ultrasound scan, amniotic fluid volume, gestational age at which PPROM occurs and clinical and laboratory markers of infection) [82, 83].

Maternal and foetal wellbeing are essential for expectant management with PPROM. Some form of foetal monitoring is employed to assure wellbeing. Options include foetal movement monitoring, CTGs. A Cochrane review on the best methods to monitor the foetus following PPROM found insufficient evidence (three randomised controlled trials) to allow recommendations to be made for any method [84]. Women with PPROM should clearly be monitored for signs of infection. However, there is no consensus on the best approach. At a minimum, routine clinical parameters (e.g. maternal temperature, presence of uterine tenderness, and frequency of contractions, maternal and foetal heart rate) should be monitored. Periodically monitoring white blood cell counts or other markers for inflammation/infection has not been proven to be useful [85].

13.5 Prelabour Rupture of Foetal Membranes at Limits of Viability

Prelabour rupture of the foetal membranes (PROM) before or at the limit of viability is associated with substantial serious paediatric morbidity and mortality. The aetiology, diagnosis and complications of PROM in this period, which can loosely be defined as <23 weeks of gestation.

PROM before or at the limit of viability complicates 0.1–0.7% of pregnancies [86–88].

Causes and risk factors Pathogenesis of PPROM at limits of foetal viability is poorly understood. The major risk factors appear to be a prior history of preterm labour, PROM before or at the limit of viability, cervical insufficiency or a current pregnancy complicated by multiple gestation or antepartum bleeding. It is likely that both PROM before or at the limit of viability and preterm labour are expressions of a more general process of intrauterine inflammation and thus share many antecedents [89]. Since the foetal membranes are avascular, they may be particularly vulnerable to the local effects of inflammatory reactions. Evidence is accumulating to suggest that aberrant trophoblastic development in the late first trimester, a pathology more traditionally associated with preeclampsia, may be associated with up to half of the cases of membrane rupture in this gestational interval [90].

It can occur spontaneously or be iatrogenic (during/after an invasive procedure that breaches the foetal membranes, e.g. amniocentesis, foetoscopy, foetal surgery, percutaneous umbilical vein blood sampling and cervical cerclage). Patients with iatrogenic PROM before or at the limit of viability after amniocentesis usually reseal membranes within a week and have good pregnancy outcomes. The relatively discrete and focal nature of the iatrogenic membrane disruption, when compared with the more ragged and more substantial defect that occurs with spontaneous membrane rupture likely, contributes to these differences in resealing rates.

Up to 14% of women with spontaneous PROM periviability eventually stop leaking amniotic fluid, presumably due to resealing of the foetal membranes [91–93]. Cessation of leakage is unlikely due to actual repair and regeneration of the membranes, but rather to changes in the decidua and myometrium that block further leakage [94]. This subgroup of pregnancies has outcomes comparable to pregnancies uncomplicated by PPROM [91]. Approximately 25% of patients with PROM before or at the limit of viability reaccumulate fluid on ultrasound examination during expectant management [95, 96].

Some authors have suggested an inverse relationship between latency and gestational age at rupture with ruptures occurring earlier in pregnancy appearing to have longer latencies [9, 95, 97–101]. This inverse relationship is likely to be due to the fact that patients who deliver shortly after arriving on the labour floor are often excluded from latency studies. These patients are also more likely to be at an advanced gestational age.

13.6 Pregnancy Complications and Outcome

Chorioamnionitis	30–40%	Maternal sepsis complicates approximately 5% PROM between 20 and 24 weeks [102] and 1.2% PROM between 14 and 23 weeks [103]
Placental abruption	2–44% versus 0.4–1.3% [96] in general obstetric population	Correlates inversely with gestational age at rupture
Cord prolapse	1.9% incidence	
Foetal death	Up to 33% Termination of pregnancy up to 27%	The risk appears to be inversely related to gestational age at PROM [104]
Caesarean delivery	Increased incidence often classical	Due to an increased prevalence of foetal heart rate abnormalities and foetal malpresentation
Retained placenta	Increased manual removal rates from 9% to 18%	Especially true in PPROM before 20 weeks
Postpartum endometritis	Occurs in up to 40%	
Postpartum maternal sepsis	0–3%	Related to latency period

13.7 Paediatric Outcomes

Neonatal morbidity Short- and long-term morbidity is common and primarily related to gestational age at birth [86, 87]. The National Institute of Child Health and Human Development (NICHD) Neonatal Research Network provides an online calculator to estimate the risk of neurodevelopmental impairment of extremely preterm birth based on gestational age at birth, birth weight, sex, singleton birth and exposure to antenatal glucocorticoids within 7 days [105]. It does not account for the specific effects of pregnancy complications such as PROM before or at the limit of viability, which increases the risks of pulmonary hypoplasia and infection. Infection-related morbidities include sepsis, meningitis and pneumonia.

The prognosis for intact survival after PROM before or at the limit of viability is only fair. In one study, early PROM was associated with greater composite severe childhood morbidity at age 2 years than later PROM, even after controlling for delivery gestational age and other confounders [87]. In two studies of pregnancies complicated by PROM before or at the limit of viability, approximately 50% of offspring had no severe morbidity at 2 years of corrected age [102, 106]. However, in another study, 90% and 64% of 22- and 23-week PROM survivors were diagnosed with some form of cerebral palsy [104]. Multiple gestations do not appear to affect outcome [107].

Neonatal death post-PPROM is related primarily to gestation and latency period post-diagnosis. In a review of three studies of PROM at 14 or 16 to 24 weeks, neonatal survival after conservatively managed PROM at <22 weeks was significantly lower than PROM at 22–24 weeks 14.4% versus 57.7% [86]. A study of pregnancies with PROM at 20–23 weeks and latency of at least 7 days reported neonatal survival in 90% [108]. However, these data likely overstate survival because of exclusion of patients who delivered soon after PROM or elected pregnancy termination for persistent fluid leakage, oligohydramnios, abnormal ultrasound findings or other issues associated with a poor prognosis. A study of PROM between 20 and 24 weeks that did not exclude patients with latency less than 7 days reported neonatal survival in 49% [102]. The risk of neonatal mortality is also correlated with residual amniotic fluid volume [96, 109–111]. In one study, for neonates delivering at the same gestational age, neonatal survival was 98% when the largest amniotic fluid pocket was ≥2 cm but only 31% when <2 cm [96]. The survival rate for pregnancies associated with iatrogenic PROM before or at the limit of viability is several-fold higher than that for spontaneous PROM before or at the limit of viability [112]. This may be related to a lower rate of infection, higher residual amniotic fluid volume, higher rate of resealing or other factors.

The prevalence of pulmonary hypoplasia in neonates of pregnancies complicated by PROM before or at the limit of viability is approximately 30% [113]. The mortality rate for these neonates is 70–90% [99, 109, 114–116]. The gestational age at the time of membrane rupture is the critical factor in the risk of subsequent neonatal pulmonary hypoplasia [101, 109, 114, 117–119]. Several series had reported a low incidence (less than 1.4%) of pulmonary hypoplasia when PROM occurred after 26 weeks of gestation [99, 101, 114, 116, 118]. The degree of oligohydramnios is an additional risk factor for pulmonary hypoplasia; lower volumes of residual fluid confer the highest risk [109, 110, 115].

Asymmetric intrauterine pressure and associated with PROM before or at the limit of viability can lead to deformities of variable severity in previously normally formed extremities [48]. An increased likelihood of skeletal deformities has been observed among infants diagnosed with pulmonary hypoplasia [101, 114, 116], suggesting that the two disorders have a common aetiology. Limb deformations related to PROM before or at the limit of viability generally do not require surgical correction as they gradually resolve with postnatal growth and development [114].

The challenges presented in the management of PROM peri-viability are quite different from later gestation. The limit of viability is defined as the stage of foetal maturity that ensures a reasonable chance of survival. Determining the limit of viability is vital so that costly and futile painful interventions can be avoided. However, deciding upon a threshold of viability is challenging because it remains uncertain which extremely preterm newborn has a reasonable chance of survival. Institutional variability in survival at the limit of viability is due, at least in part, to varying levels of aggressive management. The pros and cons of expectant management versus pregnancy termination should be discussed openly with senior obstetricians and neonatologists. Most women at this gestational age who are stable and choose to continue their pregnancies are not admitted to the hospital and not given antenatal corticosteroids or tocolytics, swabs to rule out infection are obtained. Antibiotics can be considered as early as 20 weeks of gestation [120]. Treatment for a positive GBS culture is initiated when the patient has reached a viable gestational age and is in labour with a high likelihood of delivery. Neonatology input is critical to set clear expectations with the parents. A common practice among neonatologists is not to offer or provide neonatal resuscitation to neonates <22 weeks of gestation due to the low chance of intact survival. Beyond 22 weeks, it is common practice among neonatologists to offer neonatal resuscitation to parents if there is at least a small chance of survival. These decisions on resuscitation are based on available information including estimated fetal weight from ultrasound, gestational age and are taken in consultation with the parents. Administration of antenatal corticosteroids in the 22nd week is reasonable if delivery at 23 weeks is anticipated and the family desires aggressive neonatal intervention after thorough consultation with maternal-foetal medicine and neonatology specialists [121]. Antibiotic prophylaxis to prolong latency should be considered from 23 weeks according to the same protocol used in patients who present with preterm PROM at later gestational ages. Mothers should be monitored for signs of infection and foetal wellbeing assessed by foetal auscultation and ultrasound. Magnesium sulphate for neuroprotection is administered when delivery appears to be imminent.

Management of pregnancy complications Clinical infection, abruptio placenta and foetal compromise are indications for delivery, as expectant management in these situations can increase maternal or neonatal morbidity. When there is an expectation of neonatal survival, the route of delivery is determined by the obstetric indication [121].

Coexistent cerclage It is unclear whether foreign material in the cervix after cerclage placement increases the risk of maternal or neonatal sepsis in the setting of PROM before or at the limit of viability; the most appropriate management in this clinical setting remains controversial. If there are any signs of infection, the cerclage should be removed.

Delayed interval delivery of multiple gestations Management of multiple gestations with PROM periviability presents unique challenges. It may be reasonable to consider delayed interval delivery with close foeto-maternal monitoring after detailed counselling of parents with regard to the potential risks.

Women with PROM before or at the limit of viability are at high risk of recurrence in subsequent pregnancies. An early prior spontaneous preterm delivery appears to be more predictive of recurrence than late preterm delivery and highly associated with a subsequent early spontaneous preterm delivery [80]. Given this increased risk of recurrence, modifiable risk factors such as cigarette smoking and short interpregnancy interval should be addressed, and progesterone prophylaxis against recurrent spontaneous preterm birth in a subsequent pregnancy should be considered.

References

1. Mercer BM. Preterm premature rupture of the membranes: current approaches to evaluation and management. Obstet Gynecol Clin N Am. 2005; https://doi.org/10.1016/j.ogc.2005.03.003.
2. Smith GN, Rafuse C, Anand N, et al. Prevalence, management, and outcomes of preterm prelabour rupture of the membranes of women in Canada. J Obstet Gynaecol Can. 2005; https://doi.org/10.1016/S1701-2163(16)30711-3.
3. Mercer BM. High-risk pregnancy series: an expert's view. Preterm premature rupture of the membranes. Obstet Gynecol. 2003;101:178–93.
4. American College of Obstetricians and Gynaecologists. ACOG practice bulletin. Premature rupture of membranes. Clinical management guidelines for obstetrician-gynaecologists. Number 1, June 1998. American College of Obstetricians and Gynaecologists. Int J Gynaecol Obstet. 1998;63(1):75–84.
5. ACOG Committee on Practice Bulletins-Obstetrics. ACOG Practice Bulletin No. 80: premature rupture of membranes. Obstet Gynecol. 2007; https://doi.org/10.1097/01.AOG.0000263888.69178.1f.
6. Duff P. Premature rupture of the membranes in term patients. Semin Perinatol. 1996; https://doi.org/10.1016/S0146-0005(96)80007-3.
7. Ohlsson A, Gafni A, Willan AR, et al. Induction of labour versus expectant management for prelabour rupture of the membranes at term: an economic evaluation [TERMPROM (Term Prelabor Rupture of the Membranes) Study Group report]. Can Med Assoc J. 1997;157(11):1519–25.
8. Dale PO, Tanbo T, Bendvold E, Moe N. Duration of the latency period in preterm premature rupture of the membranes. Maternal and neonatal consequences of expectant management. Eur J Obstet Gynecol Reprod Biol. 1989; https://doi.org/10.1016/0028-2243(89)90010-5.
9. Bengtson JM, VanMarter LJ, Barss VA, Greene MF, Tuomala RE, Epstein MF. Pregnancy outcome after premature rupture of the membranes at or before 26 weeks' gestation. Am J Obstet Gynecol. 1989; https://doi.org/10.1097/00006250-198906000-00002.
10. R. Menon. Spontaneous preterm birth, a clinical dilemma: etiologic, pathophysiologic and genetic heterogeneities and racial disparity. Acta Obstet Gynecol Scand. 2008; 87(6):590-600.
11. Macones GA, Parry S, Elkousy M, Clothier B, Ural SH, Strauss JF. A polymorphism in the promoter region of TNF and bacterial vaginosis: preliminary evidence of gene-environment interaction in the etiology of spontaneous preterm birth. Am J Obstet Gynecol. 2004; https://doi.org/10.1016/j.ajog.2004.01.001.
12. Burns DN, Landesman S, Muenz LR, Nugent RP, Goedert JJ, Minkoff H, Walsh JH, Mendez H, Rubinstein WA. Cigarette smoking, premature rupture of membranes, and vertical transmission of HIV-1 among women with low CD4+ levels. J Acquir Immune Defic Syndr. 1994;7(7):718–26.
13. Silverman RK, Wojtowycz M. Risk factors in premature rupture of membranes. Prim Care Update Ob Gyns. 1998;5(4):–181.
14. Menon R, Richardson LS. Preterm prelabor rupture of the membranes: a disease of the fetal membranes. Semin Perinatol. 2017; https://doi.org/10.1053/j.semperi.2017.07.012.
15. Dutta EH, Behnia F, Boldogh I, et al. Oxidative stress damage-associated molecular signaling pathways differentiate spontaneous preterm birth and preterm premature rupture of the membranes. Mol Hum Reprod. 2015; https://doi.org/10.1093/molehr/gav074.
16. Coppé JP, Patil CK, Rodier F, et al. Senescence-associated secretory phenotypes reveal cell-nonautonomous functions of oncogenic RAS and the p53 tumour suppressor. PLoS Biol. 2008; https://doi.org/10.1371/journal.pbio.0060301.
17. Kumar D, Moore RM, Mercer BM, Mansour JM, Redline RW, Moore JJ. The physiology of fetal membrane weakening and rupture: insights gained from the determination of physical properties revisited. Placenta. 2016; https://doi.org/10.1016/j.placenta.2016.03.015.
18. Moore RM, Mansour JM, Redline RW, Mercer BM, Moore JJ. The physiology of fetal membrane rupture: insight gained from the determination of physical properties. Placenta. 2006;27(11–12):1037–5.
19. Keelan JA, Wang K, Chaiworapongsa T, et al. Macrophage inhibitory cytokine 1 in fetal membranes and amniotic fluid from pregnancies with and without preterm labour and premature rupture

of membranes. Mol Hum Reprod. 2003; https://doi.org/10.1093/molehr/gag068.
20. King AE, Kelly RW, Sallenave JM, Bocking AD, Challis JRG. Innate immune defences in the human uterus during pregnancy. Placenta. 2007; https://doi.org/10.1016/j.placenta.2007.06.002.
21. Menon R, Nicolau NN, Bredson S, Polettini J. Fetal membranes: potential source of preterm birth biomarkers. In: General methods in biomarker research and their applications; 2015. https://doi.org/10.1007/978-94-007-7696-8_28.
22. DiGiulio DB, Romero R, Kusanovic JP, et al. Prevalence and diversity of microbes in the amniotic fluid, the fetal inflammatory response, and pregnancy outcome in women with preterm pre-labor rupture of membranes. Am J Reprod Immunol. 2010;64(1):38–57.
23. Grobman WA, Bailit J, Lai Y, et al. Defining failed induction of labor. Am J Obstet Gynecol. 2018;218(1):122.e1–8. https://doi.org/10.1016/j.ajog.2017.11.556.
24. Arechavaleta-Velasco F, Ogando D, Parry S, Vadillo-Ortega F. Production of matrix metalloproteinase-9 in lipopolysaccharide-stimulated human amnion occurs through an autocrine and paracrine proinflammatory cytokine-dependent system. Biol Reprod. 2004; https://doi.org/10.1095/biolreprod.102.004721.
25. Fortunato SJ, Menon R. IL-1β is a better inducer of apoptosis in human fetal membranes than IL-6. Placenta. 2003; https://doi.org/10.1016/S0143-4004(03)00160-7.
26. Mercer BM, Goldenberg RL, Moawad AH, et al. The preterm prediction study: effect of gestational age and cause of preterm birth on subsequent obstetric outcome. Am J Obstet Gynecol. 1999; https://doi.org/10.1016/S0002-9378(99)70111-0.
27. Asrat T, Lewis DF, Garite TJ, et al. Rate of recurrence of preterm premature rupture of membranes in consecutive pregnancies. Am J Obstet Gynecol. 1991; https://doi.org/10.1016/0002-9378(91)90481-6.
28. Parry S, Strauss JF. Premature rupture of the fetal membranes. N Engl J Med. 2002; https://doi.org/10.1056/nejm199803053381006.
29. Lykke JA, Dideriksen KL, Lidegaard Ø, Langhoff-Roos J. First-trimester vaginal bleeding and complications later in pregnancy. Obstet Gynecol. 2010; https://doi.org/10.1097/AOG.0b013e3181da8d38.
30. Harger JH, Hsing AW, Tuomala RE, et al. Risk factors for preterm premature rupture of fetal membranes: a multicentre case-control study. Am J Obstet Gynecol. 1990; https://doi.org/10.1016/S0002-9378(11)90686-3.
31. Ekwo EE, Gosselink CA, Woolson R, Moawad A. Risks for premature rupture of amniotic membranes. Int J Epidemiol. 1993; https://doi.org/10.1093/ije/22.3.495.
32. Berkowitz GS, Blackmore-Prince C, Lapinski RH, Savitz DA. Risk factors for preterm birth subtypes. Epidemiology. 1998; https://doi.org/10.1097/00001648-199805000-00011.
33. Puthiyachirakkal M, Lemerand K, Kumar D, et al. Thrombin weakens the amnion extracellular matrix (ECM) directly rather than through protease activated receptors. Placenta. 2013;34(10):924–31.
34. Williams MA, Mittendorf R, Stubblefield PG, Lieberman E, Schoenbaum SC, Monson RR. Cigarettes, coffee, and preterm premature rupture of the membranes. Am J Epidemiol. 1992; https://doi.org/10.1093/oxfordjournals.aje.a116385.
35. Alexander JM, Mercer BM, Miodovnik M, et al. The impact of digital cervical examination on expectantly managed preterm rupture of membranes. Am J Obstet Gynecol. 2000; https://doi.org/10.1067/mob.2000.106765.
36. Schutte MF, Treffers PE, Kloosterman GJ, Soepatmi S. Management of premature rupture of membranes: the risk of vaginal examination to the infant. Am J Obstet Gynecol. 1983; https://doi.org/10.1016/0002-9378(83)90819-0.
37. Imseis HM, Trout WC, Gabbe SG. The microbiologic effect of digital cervical examination. Am J Obstet Gynecol. 1999; https://doi.org/10.1016/S0002-9378(99)70257-7.
38. Mehra S, Amon E, Hopkins S, Gavard JA, Shyken J. Transvaginal cervical length and amniotic fluid index: can it predict delivery latency following preterm premature rupture of membranes? Am J Obstet Gynecol. 2015; https://doi.org/10.1016/j.ajog.2015.01.022.
39. Mercer BM, Rabello YA, Thurnau GR, et al. The NICHD-MFMU antibiotic treatment of preterm PROM study: impact of initial amniotic fluid volume on pregnancy outcome. Am J Obstet Gynecol. 2006;194(2):438–45.
40. Tagore S, Kwek K. Comparative analysis of insulin-like growth factor binding protein-1 (IGFBP-1), placental alpha-microglobulin-1 (PAMG-1) and nitrazine test to diagnose premature rupture of membranes in pregnancy. J Perinat Med. 2010; https://doi.org/10.1515/JPM.2010.099.
41. Marcellin L, Anselem O, Guibourdenche J, et al. Comparison of two bedside tests performed on cervicovaginal fluid to diagnose premature rupture of membranes. J Gynecol Obstet Biol Reprod (Paris). 2011; https://doi.org/10.1016/j.jgyn.2011.06.007.
42. Albayrak M, Ozdemir I, Koc O, Ankarali H, Ozen O. Comparison of the diagnostic efficacy of the two rapid bedside immunoassays and combined clinical conventional diagnosis in prelabour rupture of membranes. Eur J Obstet Gynecol Reprod Biol. 2011; https://doi.org/10.1016/j.ejogrb.2011.04.041.
43. Palacio M, Kühnert M, Berger R, Larios CL, Marcellin L. Meta-analysis of studies on biochemical marker tests for the diagnosis of premature rupture of membranes: comparison of performance indexes. BMC Pregnancy Childbirth. 2014; https://doi.org/10.1186/1471-2393-14-183.
44. Thomasino T, Levi C, Draper M, Neubert A. Diagnosing rupture of membranes using combination monoclonal/polyclonal immunologic protein detection. J Reprod Med. 2013;58:187–94.
45. Baptisti A. Chemical test for the determination of ruptured membranes. Am J Obstet Gynecol. 2015; https://doi.org/10.1016/s0002-9378(38)90265-0.
46. Abe T. The detection of the rupture of fetal membranes with the nitrazine indicator. Am J Obstet Gynecol. 1940; https://doi.org/10.1016/S0002-9378(40)90571-3.
47. Friedman ML, McElin TW. Diagnosis of ruptured fetal membranes. Clinical study and review of the literature. Am J Obstet Gynecol. 1969; https://doi.org/10.1016/S0002-9378(16)34244-2.
48. Seeds AE, Hellegers AE. Acid-base determinations in human amniotic fluid throughout pregnancy. Am J Obstet Gynecol. 1968; https://doi.org/10.1016/0002-9378(68)90196-8.
49. Davidson KM. Detection of premature rupture of the membranes. Clin Obstet Gynecol. 1991; https://doi.org/10.1097/00003081-199112000-00007.
50. Volet B, Morier-Genoud J. Le test de cristallisation dans le liquide amniotique. Gynecol Obstet Investig. 1960; https://doi.org/10.1159/000305941.
51. de Haan HH, Offermans JPM, Smits F, Schouten HJA, Peeters LL. Value of the fern test to confirm or reject the diagnosis of ruptured membranes is modest in nonlaboring women presenting with nonspecific vaginal fluid loss. Am J Perinatol. 1994; https://doi.org/10.1055/s-2007-994535.
52. Mulhair L, Carter J, Poston L, Seed P, Briley A. Prospective cohort study investigating the reliability of the AmnioSense™ method for detection of spontaneous rupture of membranes. BJOG. 2009; https://doi.org/10.1111/j.1471-0528.2008.01828.x.
53. Middleton P, Shepherd E, Flenady V, McBain RD, Crowther CA. Planned early birth versus expectant management (waiting) for prelabour rupture of membranes at term (37 weeks

or more). Cochrane Database Syst Rev. 2017; https://doi.org/10.1002/14651858.CD005302.pub3.
54. Hannah ME, Ohlsson A, Farine D, et al. Induction of labor compared with expectant management for prelabor rupture of the membranes at term. TERMPROM Study Group [see comments]. N Engl J Med. 1996;334(16):1005–10.
55. Tan BP, Hannah ME. Prostaglandins versus oxytocin for prelabour rupture of membranes at or near term. Cochrane Database Syst Rev. 2000; https://doi.org/10.1002/14651858.CD000158.
56. Hofmeyr GJ, Gülmezoglu AM, Pileggi C. Vaginal misoprostol for cervical ripening and induction of labour. Cochrane Database Syst Rev. 2010; https://doi.org/10.1002/14651858.cd000941.pub2.
57. Güngördük K, Asicioglu O, Besimoglu B, et al. Labor induction in term premature rupture of membranes: comparison between oxytocin and dinoprostone followed 6 hours later by oxytocin. Am J Obstet Gynecol. 2012;206(1):60.e1–8.
58. Weekes CR, Mahomed K. Management of pre-labour rupture of membranes at term – a survey of current practice in Australia. Aust New Zeal J Obstet Gynaecol. 2010;50(5):428–31.
59. Saccone G, Berghella V. Antibiotic prophylaxis for term or near-term premature rupture of membranes: metaanalysis of randomised trials. Am J Obstet Gynecol. 2015; https://doi.org/10.1016/j.ajog.2014.12.034.
60. Hannah ME, Hodnett ED, Willan A, Foster GA, Di Cecco R, Helewa M. Prelabor rupture of the membranes at term: expectant management at home or in hospital? The TermPROM Study Group. Obstet Gynecol. 2000;96(4):533–8.
61. Ellestad SC, Swamy GK, Sinclair T, James AH, Heine RP, Murtha AP. Preterm premature rupture of membrane management-inpatient versus outpatient: a retrospective review. Am J Perinatol. 2008; https://doi.org/10.1055/s-2007-1004830.
62. Peaceman AM, Lai Y, Rouse DJ, et al. Length of latency with preterm premature rupture of membranes before 32 weeks' gestation. Am J Perinatol. 2015; https://doi.org/10.1055/s-0034-1373846.
63. Lorthe E, Ancel PY, Torchin H, et al. Impact of latency duration on the prognosis of preterm infants after preterm premature rupture of membranes at 24 to 32 weeks' gestation: a National Population-Based Cohort Study. J Pediatr. 2017; https://doi.org/10.1016/j.jpeds.2016.11.074.
64. Manuck TA, Maclean CC, Silver RM, Varner MW. Preterm premature rupture of membranes: does the duration of latency influence perinatal outcomes? Am J Obstet Gynecol. 2009; https://doi.org/10.1016/j.ajog.2009.07.045.
65. Frenette P, Dodds L, Armson BA, Jangaard K. Preterm prelabour rupture of membranes: effect of latency on neonatal and maternal outcomes. J Obstet Gynaecol Can. 2013; https://doi.org/10.1016/S1701-2163(15)30861-6.
66. National Institute for Health and Care Excellence (NICE). NICE guideline on preterm labour and birth. London: National Institute for Health and Care Excellence; 2015.
67. Caloone J, Rabilloud M, Boutitie F, et al. Accuracy of several maternal seric markers for predicting histological chorioamnionitis after preterm premature rupture of membranes: a prospective and multicentric study. Eur J Obstet Gynecol Reprod Biol. 2016; https://doi.org/10.1016/j.ejogrb.2016.08.022.
68. Kuba K, Bernstein PS. ACOG practice bulletin no. 188: prelabor rupture of membranes. Obstet Gynecol. 2018; https://doi.org/10.1097/AOG.0000000000002663.
69. Royal College of Obstetricians and Gynaecologists. Preterm prelabour rupture of membranes. Green–top guideline no. 44. London: Royal College of Obstetricians and Gynaecologists. https://doi.org/10.1136/adc.66.7_Spec_No.812.
70. Bond DM, Middleton P, Levett KM, et al. Planned early birth versus expectant management for women with preterm prelabour rupture of membranes prior to 37 weeks' gestation for improving pregnancy outcome. Cochrane Database Syst Rev. 2017; https://doi.org/10.1002/14651858.CD004735.pub4.
71. Quist-Nelson J, de Ruigh AA, Seidler AL, et al. Immediate delivery compared with expectant management in late preterm prelabor rupture of membranes: an individual participant data meta-analysis. Obstet Gynecol. 2018; https://doi.org/10.1097/AOG.0000000000002447.
72. Park CK, Isayama T, Mcdonald SD. Antenatal corticosteroid therapy before 24 weeks of gestation a systematic review and meta-analysis. Obstet Gynecol. 2016; https://doi.org/10.1097/AOG.0000000000001355.
73. Roberts D, Brown J, Medley N, Dalziel SR. Antenatal corticosteroids for accelerating fetal lung maturation for women at risk of preterm birth. Cochrane Database Syst Rev. 2017; https://doi.org/10.1002/14651858.CD004454.pub3.
74. Crowther CA, Anderson PJ, McKinlay CJD, et al. Mid-childhood outcomes of repeat antenatal corticosteroids: a randomised controlled trial. Paediatrics. 2016; https://doi.org/10.1542/peds.2016-0947.
75. Crowther CA, Haslam RR, Hiller JE, Doyle LW, Robinson JS. Neonatal respiratory distress syndrome after repeat exposure to antenatal corticosteroids: a randomised controlled trial. Lancet. 2006;367(9526):1913–9.
76. Kenyon S, Boulvain M, Neilson JP. Antibiotics for preterm rupture of membranes. Cochrane Database Syst Rev. 2013; https://doi.org/10.1002/14651858.CD001058.pub3.
77. WHO Reproductive Health Library. WHO recommendation on the prophylactic antibiotic of choice in women with preterm prelabour rupture of membranes, The WHO Reproductive Health Library. Geneva: World Health Organization; 2015.
78. Kenyon SL, Taylor DJ, Tarnow-Mordi W. Broad-spectrum antibiotics for preterm, prelabour rupture of fetal membranes: the ORACLE I randomised trial. Lancet. 2001; https://doi.org/10.1016/S0140-6736(00)04233-1.
79. Wolf MF, Miron D, Peleg D, et al. Reconsidering the current preterm premature rupture of membranes antibiotic prophylactic protocol. Am J Perinatol. 2015; https://doi.org/10.1055/s-0035-1552935.
80. Mackeen AD, Seibel-Seamon J, Muhammad J, Baxter JK, Berghella V. Tocolytics for preterm premature rupture of membranes. Cochrane Database Syst Rev. 2014; https://doi.org/10.1002/14651858.CD007062.pub3.
81. Abou El Senoun G, Dowswell T, Mousa HA. Planned home versus hospital care for preterm prelabour rupture of the membranes (PPROM) prior to 37 weeks' gestation. Cochrane Database Syst Rev. 2014; https://doi.org/10.1002/14651858.CD008053.pub3.
82. Dussaux C, Senat MV, Bouchghoul H, Benachi A, Mandelbrot L, Kayem G. Preterm premature rupture of membranes: is home care acceptable? J Matern Fetal Neonatal Med. 2018; https://doi.org/10.1080/14767058.2017.1341482.
83. Phupong V, Kulmala L. Factors associated with latency period in preterm prelabor rupture of membranes. J Matern Fetal Neonatal Med. 2016; https://doi.org/10.3109/14767058.2015.1095884.
84. Sharp GC, Stock SJ, Norman JE. Fetal assessment methods for improving neonatal and maternal outcomes in preterm prelabour rupture of membranes. Cochrane Database Syst Rev. 2014; https://doi.org/10.1002/14651858.CD010209.pub2.
85. Tita ATN, Andrews WW. Diagnosis and management of clinical chorioamnionitis. Clin Perinatol. 2010; https://doi.org/10.1016/j.clp.2010.02.003.
86. Waters TP, Mercer BM. The management of preterm premature rupture of the membranes near the limit of fetal viability. Am J Obstet Gynecol. 2009; https://doi.org/10.1016/j.ajog.2009.06.049.
87. Manuck TA, Varner MW. Neonatal and childhood outcomes following early vs later preterm premature rupture of membranes (PPROM). Am J Obstet Gynecol. 2014;211(3):308.e1–6.

88. Linehan LA, Walsh J, Morris A, et al. Neonatal and maternal outcomes following midtrimester preterm premature rupture of the membranes: a retrospective cohort study. BMC Pregnancy Childbirth. 2016; https://doi.org/10.1186/s12884-016-0813-3.
89. McElrath TF, Hecht JL, Dammann O, et al. Pregnancy disorders that lead to delivery before the 28th week of gestation: an epidemiologic approach to classification. Am J Epidemiol. 2008; https://doi.org/10.1093/aje/kwn202.
90. Nijman TAJ, van Vliet EOG, Benders MJN, et al. Placental histology in spontaneous and indicated preterm birth: a case control study. Placenta. 2016; https://doi.org/10.1016/j.placenta.2016.10.006.
91. Beydoun SN, Yasin SY. Premature rupture of the membranes before 28 weeks: conservative management. Am J Obstet Gynecol. 1986;155(3):471–9.
92. Fortunato SJ, Welt SI, Eggleston MK, Bryant EC. Active expectant management in very early gestations complicated by premature rupture of the fetal membranes. J Reprod Med. 1994;39(1):13–6.
93. Shenker L, Reed KL, Anderson CF, Borjon NA. Significance of oligohydramnios complicating pregnancy. Am J Obstet Gynecol. 1991; https://doi.org/10.1016/0002-9378(91)91442-Y.
94. Devlieger R, Millar LK, Bryant-Greenwood G, Lewi L, Deprest JA. Fetal membrane healing after spontaneous and iatrogenic membrane rupture: a review of current evidence. Am J Obstet Gynecol. 2006; https://doi.org/10.1016/j.ajog.2006.01.074.
95. Hibbard JU, Hibbard MC, Ismail M, et al. Pregnancy outcome after expectant management of premature rupture of the membranes in the second trimester. J Reprod Med Obstet Gynecol. 1993;38(12):945–51.
96. Hadi HA, Hodson CA, Strickland D. Premature rupture of the membranes between 20 and 25 weeks' gestation: role of amniotic fluid volume in perinatal outcome. Am J Obstet Gynecol. 1994;170(4):1139–44.
97. Taylor J, Garite TJ. Premature rupture of membranes before fetal viability. Obstet Gynecol. 1984;64(5):615–20.
98. Rib DM, Sherer DM, Woods JR Jr. Maternal and neonatal outcome associated with prolonged premature rupture of membranes below 26 weeks' gestation. Am J Perinatol. 1993;10(5):369–73.
99. Farooqi A, Holmgren PA, Engberg S, Serenius F. Survival and 2-year outcome with expectant management of second- trimester rupture of membranes. Obstet Gynecol. 1998; https://doi.org/10.1016/S0029-7844(98)00287-7.
100. Kurkinen-Räty M, Koivisto M, Jouppila P. Perinatal and neonatal outcome and late pulmonary sequelae in infants born after preterm premature rupture of membranes. Obstet Gynecol. 1998; https://doi.org/10.1016/S0029-7844(98)00213-0.
101. Nimrod C, Varela-Gittings F, Machin G, Campbell D, Wesenberg R. The effect of very prolonged membrane rupture on fetal development. Am J Obstet Gynecol. 1984; https://doi.org/10.1016/0002-9378(84)90743-9.
102. Kibel M, Asztalos E, Barrett J, et al. Outcomes of pregnancies complicated by preterm premature rupture of membranes between 20 and 24 weeks of gestation. Obstet Gynecol. 2016; https://doi.org/10.1097/AOG.0000000000001530.
103. Dotters-Katz SK, Panzer A, Grace MR, et al. Maternal morbidity after previable prelabor rupture of membranes. Obstet Gynecol. 2017; https://doi.org/10.1097/AOG.0000000000001803.
104. Lorthe E, Torchin H, Delorme P, et al. Preterm premature rupture of membranes at 22–25 weeks' gestation: perinatal and 2-year outcomes within a national population-based study (EPIPAGE-2). Am J Obstet Gynecol. 2018; https://doi.org/10.1016/j.ajog.2018.05.029.
105. https://www1.nichd.nih.gov/epbo-calculator/Pages/epbo_case.aspx.
106. Pristauz G, Bauer M, Maurer-Fellbaum U, et al. Neonatal outcome and two-year follow-up after expectant management of second trimester rupture of membranes. Int J Gynecol Obstet. 2008; https://doi.org/10.1016/j.ijgo.2007.12.007.
107. Wong LF, Holmgren CM, Silver RM, Varner MW, Manuck TA. Outcomes of expectantly managed pregnancies with multiple gestations and preterm premature rupture of membranes prior to 26 weeks. Am J Obstet Gynecol. 2015; https://doi.org/10.1016/j.ajog.2014.09.005.
108. Brumbaugh JE, Colaizy TT, Nuangchamnong N, et al. Neonatal survival after prolonged preterm premature rupture of membranes before 24 weeks of gestation. Obstet Gynecol. 2014; https://doi.org/10.1097/AOG.0000000000000511.
109. Shumway JB, Al-malt A, Amon E, et al. Impact of oligohydramnios on maternal and perinatal outcomes of spontaneous premature rupture of the membranes at 18-28 weeks. J Matern Fetal Neonatal Med. 2009; https://doi.org/10.3109/14767050909063148.
110. Kilbride HW, Thibeault DW. Defining limits of survival: lethal pulmonary hypoplasia after midtrimester premature rupture of membranes. Am J Obstet Gynecol. 1996;175(3 Pt 1):675–81.
111. Grisaru-Granovsky S, Eitan R, Kaplan M, Samueloff A. Expectant management of midtrimester premature rupture of membranes: a plea for limits. J Perinatol. 2003; https://doi.org/10.1038/sj.jp.7210880.
112. Chauleur C, Rochigneux S, Seffert P, Chene G, Billiemaz K, Collet F. Neonatal outcomes and four-year follow-up after spontaneous or iatrogenic preterm prelabor rupture of membranes before 24 weeks. Acta Obstet Gynecol Scand. 2009; https://doi.org/10.1080/00016340902971433.
113. Kiver V, Boos V, Thomas A, Henrich W, Weichert A. Perinatal outcomes after previable preterm premature rupture of membranes before 24 weeks of gestation. J Perinat Med. 2018; https://doi.org/10.1515/jpm-2016-0341.
114. Blott M, Greenough A. Neonatal outcome after prolonged rupture of the membranes starting in the second trimester. Arch Dis Child. 1988; https://doi.org/10.1136/adc.63.10_Spec_No.1146.
115. Vergani P, Ghidini A, Locatelli A, et al. Risk factors for pulmonary hypoplasia in second-trimester premature rupture of membranes. Am J Obstet Gynecol. 1994; https://doi.org/10.1016/S0002-9378(94)70156-3.
116. Rotschild A, Ling EW, Puterman ML, Farquharson D. Neonatal outcome after prolonged preterm rupture of the membranes. Am J Obstet Gynecol. 1990;162(1):46–52.
117. Moretti M, Sibai BM. Maternal and perinatal outcome of expectant management of premature rupture of membranes in the midtrimester. Am J Obstet Gynecol. 1988; https://doi.org/10.1016/S0002-9378(88)80092-9.
118. Falk SJ, Campbell LJ, Lee-Parritz A, et al. Expectant management in spontaneous preterm premature rupture of membranes between 14 and 24 weeks' gestation. J Perinatol. 2004; https://doi.org/10.1038/sj.jp.7211163.
119. Lauria MR, Gonik B, Romero R. Pulmonary hypoplasia: pathogenesis, diagnosis, and antenatal prediction. Obstet Gynecol. 1995;86(3):466–75.
120. Practice bulletin no. 160 Summary: premature rupture of membranes. Obstet Gynecol. 2016; https://doi.org/10.1097/AOG.0000000000001261.
121. Raju TNK, Mercer BM, Burchfield DJ, Joseph GF. Periviable birth: executive summary of a joint workshop by the Eunice Kennedy Shriver National Institute of Child Health and Human Development, Society for Maternal-Fetal Medicine, American Academy of Paediatrics, and American College of Obstetricians and Gynecologists. Obstet Gynecol. 2014; https://doi.org/10.1097/AOG.0000000000000243.

Induction of Labour

14

Osric Banfegha Navti and Victor N. Chilaka

Learning Objectives

At the end of the chapter, the reader will be able to:

- Define induction of labour.
- Identify the methods of induction of labour.
- Critically evaluate the different options available.
- Discuss specifically induction of labour in patients with previous Caesarean section or intrauterine foetal death.

14.1 Introduction

Induction of labour (IOL) refers to methods used to initiate uterine contractions to accomplish delivery before the onset of spontaneous labour. Induction of labour is a relatively common practice. The proportion of births where labour was induced increased from 20.4% in 2007–2008 to 32.6% in 2017–2018 in the United Kingdom [1]. Between 1990 and 2012, the frequency of induction of labour in the United States more than doubled from 9.5% in 1990 to 23.3% in 2012 [2].

Induction of labour is indicated when the maternal/foetal risks of the pregnancy continuing outweigh the risks associated with delivery. The determination of maternal/foetal risks is often imprecise and is influenced mainly by the gestational age and the severity of the maternal/foetal indication for the induction of labour. The treatment and care of the woman should take into account women's individual needs and preferences [3]. When women are having or are being offered induction of labour, they should have the opportunity to make informed decisions on their care and treatment, in partnership with their healthcare professionals. The only two interventions that can affect delivery before spontaneous onset of labour are the induction of labour and caesarean delivery. Induction is preferred unless there are contraindications to a vaginal birth due to the relatively increased maternal risks from Caesarean section and the implications for future birth and fertility.

O. B. Navti (✉)
Al Wakra Hospital, Hamad Medical Corporation, Doha, Qatar
e-mail: onavti@doctors.org.uk

V. N. Chilaka
Women's Wellness and Research Centre, Hamad Medical Corporation, Doha, Qatar

14.2 Indications for Induction of Labour

14.2.1 High Priority

- Preeclampsia ≥37 weeks
- Significant maternal disease not responding to treatment
- Significant but stable antepartum haemorrhage
- Chorioamnionitis
- Suspected foetal compromise
- Term pre-labour rupture of membranes with maternal GBS colonisation

14.2.2 Other Indications

- Postdates (>41 + 0 weeks) or post-term (>42 + 0 weeks) pregnancy
- Uncomplicated twin pregnancy ≥38 weeks
- Diabetes mellitus (glucose control may dictate urgency)
- Alloimmune disease at or near term
- Intrauterine growth restriction
- Oligohydramnios
- Gestational hypertension ≥38 weeks
- Intrauterine foetal death
- PROM at or near term, GBS status

F. Okonofua et al. (eds.), *Contemporary Obstetrics and Gynecology for Developing Countries*,
https://doi.org/10.1007/978-3-030-75385-6_14

- Other logistical problems (history of rapid labour, distance to a hospital)
- Intrauterine death in a previous pregnancy (Induction may be performed at times to alleviate parental and social anxiety, but there has been no proven medical or outcome advantage for mother or baby.)

14.2.3 Unacceptable Indications

- Care provider or patient convenience.
- Suspected foetal macrosomia (estimated foetal weight >4000 gm) in a non-diabetic woman – there is no evidence of reduction in the incidence of shoulder dystocia but twice the risk of CS [4–6].

14.2.4 Contraindications

Induction should be avoided if there are contraindications to labour and or normal vaginal delivery.

These include, but not limited to, the following:

- Placenta praevia, vasa praevia, cord presentation
- Abnormal lie or foetal presentation (e.g. transverse lie or footling breech)
- Category III foetal heart tracing
- Previous classical or inverted T-shaped uterine incision
- Significant prior uterine surgery (e.g. full-thickness myomectomy)
- Active genital herpes at the time of labour
- Pelvic structural deformities
- Invasive cervical carcinoma
- Previous uterine rupture with an incision into the uterine cavity

Whenever possible, patients with previous uterine incisions or surgery should have their operative report reviewed and/or the opinion of the previous surgeon obtained.

The National Institute of Clinical Excellence (NICE) in the United Kingdom recommends that women with uncomplicated pregnancies should be offered an induction of labour between 41 and 42 weeks to avoid the risks of prolonged pregnancy [3]. The exact timing of induction of labour should take into account the woman's preferences and the local circumstances. A recent Cochrane review looking at the induction of labour in women with normal pregnancies at or beyond term concluded that a policy of induction of labour for pregnancies at or near term when compared with expectant management is associated with fewer perinatal deaths as well as fewer caesarean sections, but more operative vaginal deliveries. Neonatal Intensive Care Unit (NICU) admissions seemed lower and fewer babies had low Apgar scores with term induction of labour. There were no significant differences observed for most of the other maternal and infant outcomes – the optimal timing of offering induction at or beyond term warrants further investigation [7]. Although not recommended by currently available guidelines, induction of labour is being used increasingly at the request of pregnant mothers to shorten the duration of pregnancy and/or to time delivery to the convenience of the mothers and/or the healthcare workers [8–10].

Induction is considered elective when no medical indications are suggesting that the benefits of delivery at that point outweigh the risks.

14.2.5 Induction at 39 Weeks or More

Potential advantages of elective induction at term include reductions in stillbirths, reduction in macrosomia and its potential consequences. Elective induction may also be of benefit in women with a history of previous precipitate deliveries or who dwell far away from the hospital and are concerned about the risks of birth before arrival in hospital [11–13]. Despite these potential advantages, elective induction before 41 weeks is controversial primarily because of concerns about increased caesarean section rates and other adverse maternal outcomes as well as increased costs [14]. Recent studies comparing electively induced nulliparous or multiparous women with those managed expectantly showed no convincing evidence that elective induction is associated with an increase in caesarean section delivery whether the cervix is favourable or not. The multicentre ARRIVE trial evaluated the perinatal and maternal consequences of planned induction of labour at 39 + 0 to 39 + 4 weeks of pregnancy versus expectant management in over 6100 low-risk nulliparous women across the United States [15]. Induction reduced the chances of caesarean delivery (18.6% versus 22.2%; relative risk [RR] 0.84; 95% CI 0.76–0.93), hypertensive disorders of pregnancy (9.1% versus 14.1%; RR 0.64, 95% CI 0.56–0.74) and neonatal respiratory support (3.0% versus 4.2%; RR 0.71, 95% CI 0.55–0.93), and resulted in a statistically similar frequency of the composite outcome of perinatal death or severe neonatal complications (4.3% versus 5.4%; RR 0.80, 95% CI 0.64–1.00) [15]. However, induction also increased the median duration of stay on the labour unit (20 versus 14 hours). Following the results of this trial, the American College of Obstetricians and Gynecologists (ACOG) concluded that offering elective induction of labour to low-risk nulliparous women at 39 weeks of pregnancy is a reasonable option that may be considered and as a shared decision of a woman and her obstetric provider, with consideration of available resources [15].

Although the overall incidence of stillbirth at term in women is low, it seems to be higher in women with advanced maternal age. The stillbirth rate at 39–40 weeks of gestation is about to 2 in 1000 for women ≥40 years of age when compared to 1 in 1000 for women <35 years old [16]. Women who are 40 years of age have a similar stillbirth risk at 39 weeks of gestation to women who are in their mid-20s at 41 weeks of pregnancy [17]. The consensus, therefore, is that induction of labour should be offered to them to prevent late stillbirth [17, 18]. There is, therefore, a good argument for offering induction of labour at 39–40 weeks of gestation to women who are ≥40 years of age. Available evidence suggests this practice will reduce late antenatal stillbirths as well as maternal risks such as pre-eclampsia in ongoing pregnancies. The argument is even stronger when concurrent medical comorbidities such as nulliparity or Afro Caribbean ethnicity exist, which are known to be associated with higher stillbirth rates [16]. However, at present, there are insufficient data available on the effect such a policy would have on surgical deliveries and perinatal mortality, specifically in older mothers. There is growing evidence that such a policy would not increase the number of operative vaginal deliveries or emergency caesarean sections. Such issues should be discussed with women who are older and pregnant [19]. Women who are older and potentially nulliparous may request elective caesarean section as a form of elective delivery rather than induction of labour. A discussion of risks and benefits of induction of labour versus elective caesarean section is appropriate in these circumstances.

Elective induction of labour before 39 weeks should be avoided [20]. The morbidity of preterm birth (<37 weeks) is well established as early preterm birth (37 + 0 to 38 + 6) is associated with higher neonatal morbidity. There is also more increased healthcare utilisation during the first year of life than delivery at 39–40 weeks. In order to emphasise the importance of avoiding elective induction prior to 39 weeks ('the 39 week rule'), the National Quality Forum, the Joint Commission and the Leapfrog Group in the United States made elective delivery prior to 39 + 0 weeks a maternal performance measure and collect data from hospitals on elective deliveries performed at >37 and < 39 weeks of gestation [21]. The American College of Obstetricians and Gynaecologists (ACOG) has also stated that maternal anxiety or discomfort related to normal pregnancy, the distance lived from the hospital, and a previous pregnancy with shoulder dystocia are not appropriate indications for early-term induction [20], although they may be appropriate reasons for induction at ≥39 weeks.

Prior to the onset of induction of labour, a thorough evaluation needs to be made to ensure that the induction is appropriately indicated and to rule out any contraindications to induction of labour. ACOG has published a patient safety checklist to facilitate the process of pre-induction assessment [22].

This evaluation includes the following:

- Reviewing the expected date of delivery and gestational age
- Determining foetal presentation
- Estimating foetal weight
- Performing a cervical examination to decide if a cervical ripening agent is required
- Assessing the foetal heart rate pattern
- Reviewing the patient's history and pregnancy course to ensure there are no contraindications to induction and identify any relevant risk factors for labour and delivery

In addition

- Perform baseline maternal observations (e.g. temperature pulse, respiratory rate and blood pressure)
- Vaginal examination (VE) to assess the cervix and check if membranes are intact
- Assess foetal wellbeing: FHR and CTG
- If CTG is abnormal, escalate as per local protocol
- Consider urgency for IOL

Factors associated with a higher chance of successful induction of labour

- Cervical status (Bishop's score)
- Multiparity (best predictor) [22]
- Term gestation (GA <34 weeks less likely to deliver vaginally than those ≥34 weeks)
- Ruptured membranes
- Foetal weight < 4000 g
- Lower body mass index (BMI)
- Maternal height (taller)
- Absence of comorbidities associated with placental insufficiency, e.g. preeclampsia

The status of the cervix is used to assess the chances of successful induction of labour with the Bishop's score being the most commonly used clinical tool for cervical assessment worldwide. This offers the best prognostic index of successful induction of labour. If the Bishop score is high, reflecting a high degree of cervical ripeness, induction of labour usually can be achieved with very simple types of intervention. If, on the other hand, the Bishop score is very low (regardless of the gestational age of the pregnancy), induction is much more likely to fail [23, 24]. There is no universal definition of a favourable or unfavourable cervix. Most obstetricians associate a score of ≥ six as favourable and a score ≤3 as unfavourable. When the cervix is considered unfavourable, cervical ripening is employed. When the cervix is favourable, an artificial rupture of membranes with or without oxytocin is preferred.

Score	0	1	2	3
Dilation, cm	Closed	1 to 2	3 to 4	≥5 to 6
Effacement, %	0 to 30	40 to 50	60 to 70	≥80
Station[a]	−3	−2	−1, 0	+1, +2
Cervical consistency	Firm	Medium	Soft	
Position of the cervix	Posterior	Mid position	Anterior	

[a]Based on a −3 to +3 scale

There are two main methods for cervical ripening. These are non-pharmacological or pharmacological. Non-pharmacological methods include mechanical methods like the insertion of a balloon catheter or less commonly hygroscopic dilators, amniotomy (artificial rupture of membranes – ARM), membrane sweeps or stripping.

Mechanical methods are thought to act by applying direct pressure on the internal os, causing the release of prostaglandins from the adjacent membranes, decidua and cervix. These combined effects then lead to cervical ripening and increased myometrial contractility. Advantages of mechanical methods include a lower risk of foetal heart rate abnormalities, low risk of uterine hyperstimulation and other systemic side effects and convenient storage [25, 26]. Disadvantages include discomfort during insertion and possible antepartum haemorrhage. In the absence of prelabour rupture of membranes, mechanical methods for IOL do not result in an increased risk of ascending infection or chorioamnionitis [27, 28]. GBS colonisation is not a contraindication, and standard chemoprophylaxis is recommended.

Balloon catheter There are two options. The double-balloon catheter specifically designed for cervical ripening or the single balloon catheter, e.g. Foleys urinary bladder catheter. Current evidence [29, 30] from meta-analysis of comparative trials does not show any clinically significant difference in outcomes [29, 30]. The single balloon catheters are less expensive and readily available.

Procedure Balloon catheter insertion should follow aseptic techniques.

Single balloon catheter

- Pass deflated catheter through the internal os and into the extra-amniotic space using a ring forceps.
- Inflate the balloon with 30–80 mL of saline. Meta-analysis of trials comparing larger (60–80 mL) versus smaller (30 mL) volumes found that larger volumes resulted in shorter induction to delivery intervals (mean difference 1.97 hours, 95% CI −3.88 to −0.06) but had a similar caesarean delivery, time to catheter expulsion and maternal and foetal complication rates [31]. Current data suggest that either volume is reasonable. A randomised trial noted a decrease in time to balloon expulsion when traction was used, but no effect on the time to delivery [32]. Some clinicians attach a weight (e.g. a catheter bag with 1 litre of fluid) to the end of the catheter and suspend it from the end of the bed. Weighted traction may shorten the time to spontaneous expulsion but has not been shown to reduce the time to delivery in two randomised trials [33, 34].

Leave the catheter in place till extruded or remove 12 hours after insertion. A randomised trial found that removing non-extruded catheters after 12 hours and beginning oxytocin resulted in significantly more vaginal births within 24 hours than waiting 24 hours before removal and oxytocin induction (60 versus 21%) and did not result to an increased risk of caesarean delivery [32]. There is, however, no absolute contraindication to leaving the catheter in place for more than 12 hours.

Double balloon catheter
Procedure for insertion is similar to that for a single balloon.

- The catheter is inserted until the proximal balloon is in the cervical canal, at which point the distal balloon should be intrauterine and in the extra-amniotic space.
- The intrauterine balloon is inflated with 40 mL saline and gently retracted so that it rests against the internal os.
- The proximal balloon should now be placed outside the external cervical os and is inflated with 20 mL saline.
- If the balloons are correctly situated on either end of the cervix, the balloons can now be inflated with up to 80 mL saline per balloon.

Once the balloon is extruded, amniotomy should be performed, followed by oxytocin. If following removal of the catheter, an amniotomy is not technically possible, oxytocin can be commenced. Oxytocin can also be started concomitantly with the balloon in situ. This was shown to increase the delivery rate within 24 hours in one trial [33], but this has not been a consistent finding [34].

Evidence Use of balloon catheters has been associated with a mean change in Bishop score of 3.3 to 5.3 [34]. A

Cochrane systematic review in 2012 of mechanical methods for induction of labour reported an unfavourable cervix was still present after 12 hours in only 6% of women treated with a balloon catheter compared with 86% of women in the no-treatment group (relative risk [RR] 0.07, 95% CI 0.03–0.19) [27]. This meta-analysis also compared outcomes with the use of a balloon catheter versus a prostaglandin (prostaglandin E2 [PGE2], misoprostol PGE1]). Delivery outcomes (e.g. the proportion of women who did not achieve vaginal delivery within 24 hours, caesarean delivery) were similar for both approaches, but women who received a balloon catheter were more likely to receive oxytocin augmentation (RR 1.51, 95% CI 1.15–1.97; 6 trials, 613 women) and less likely to experience tachysystole with FHR changes (RR 0.19, 95% CI 0.08–0.43; 9 trials, 1931 women). Tachysystole without FHR changes was less frequent as well, although the difference did not reach statistical significance (RR 0.78, 95% CI 0.26–2.33; 11 trials, 1578 women). The proportion of multiparous mothers who did not achieve spontaneous vaginal delivery within 24 hours was higher when compared with vaginal PGE2. Compared with oxytocin, mechanical methods of IOL reduced the risk of caesarean section.

The WHO recommends the use of balloon catheters for induction of labour. The combination with oxytocin is an alternative when prostaglandins are not available or are contraindicated [35]. NICE guidelines, however, recommended that mechanical procedures, e.g. balloon catheters and laminaria tents, should not be used routinely for IOL, citing limited evidence for their efficacy and possibly increased risk of neonatal infection [3].

Hygroscopic dilators There are two types of hygroscopic dilators: One, made from natural seaweed (laminaria tents), and the other, a synthetic product (e.g. Dilapan-S). They are designed to absorb moisture and thus gradually expand within the cervical canal and may function by disrupting the chorion amnion decidual interface, causing lysosomal destruction and prostaglandin release. These events lead to changes in cervical tissue beyond the passive mechanical stretching provided by the tent itself. Hygroscopic dilators are considered as safe and effective as other cervical ripening agents [36, 37], although they are more commonly used during pregnancy termination rather than for pre-induction cervical ripening of term pregnancies. There is no evidence to recommend hygroscopic dilators rather than balloon catheters in patients with a prior caesarean delivery who are scheduled for induction of labour.

14.3 Procedure

- Prep the cervix and vagina with an antiseptic.
- The cervix is held with a non-traumatic clamp, if necessary, and as many dilators as possible are inserted into the endocervical canal without using excessive force; some cramping is common. Dipping the laminaria in a sterile lubricant before insertion may facilitate placement. The dilators can be packed in place with two 4-by-4-inch gauze sponges tucked into the fornices; the number of dilators and gauze sponges that were inserted should be recorded in the patient's chart at insertion and removal.
- Laminaria typically is removed 12 to 24 hours after placement, whereas synthetic dilators can be removed sooner, after 6 to 8 hours.

Efficacy In a meta-analysis of randomised trials, the risk of tachysystole with FHR changes was lower in women who received laminaria compared with those who received prostaglandins (RR 0.13; 95% CI 0.04 to 0.48; five studies, 538 women). The caesarean delivery rate was similar for women receiving laminaria and those receiving any prostaglandin (vaginal PGE2, intracervical PGE2 or misoprostol) or balloon catheters [27]. Addition of either prostaglandins or oxytocin to laminaria during cervical ripening did not appear to improve outcomes.

Balloon catheter combined with prostaglandins Combining mechanical and pharmacologic ripening methods may confer modest added benefits over use of a single method alone. A combination of two cervical ripening techniques appears to achieve more vaginal deliveries within 24 hours compared with the use of one technique but does not appear to affect the overall caesarean delivery rate or offer a benefit compared with the concurrent use of a balloon catheter and oxytocin.

A meta-analysis of randomised trials has revealed that the combination of a balloon catheter and prostaglandins lowered the chance of not achieving a vaginal delivery within 24 hours compared with prostaglandins alone (RR 0.45, 95% CI 0.28–0.71; 3 trials, 698 women) but did not significantly impact the chance of caesarean delivery (RR 0.92, 95% CI 0.79–1.08; 8 trials, 1295 women) [27, 28]. Somewhat surprisingly, combination therapy decreased the risk of uterine tachysystole with FHR changes (RR 0.53, 95% CI 0.35–0.78).

A subsequent randomised trial demonstrated that women who received combination therapy (misoprostol and a balloon catheter) delivered more quickly than those who received either misoprostol alone (hazard ratio [HR] 1.92,

95% CI 1.42–2.59) or a balloon catheter alone (HR 1.87, 95% CI 1.39–2.52) [28]. There were, however, no significant differences in the rate of caesarean delivery or adverse maternal or neonatal health outcomes [38]. The time to delivery with combination therapy was similar to that in women who had a balloon catheter placed and received oxytocin concurrently rather than after extrusion [38].

Amniotomy (ARM – Artificial Rupture of Membranes) This is the deliberate rupture of the membranes using amnihooks. This procedure may avoid the need for further pharmacological treatment. Amniotomy works best when the cervix is at least 3 cm dilated and is favourable. Amniotomy has been used to prime the cervix and induce labour with up to 60–80% of women going into labour within 24 hours. NICE in the United Kingdom currently states that amniotomy, alone or with oxytocin should not be used as a primary method for IOL unless there are specific clinical reasons for not using PGE2, in particular, the risk of uterine hyperstimulation [3].

Sweeping membranes This involves the examining finger passing through the cervix to rotate against the uterine wall separating the chorionic membrane from the decidua. If the cervix does not admit a finger, massaging around the cervix in the vaginal fornices may achieve a similar effect.

NICE recommends that:

1. Before IOL, women should be offered a vaginal exam for membrane sweeping.
2. At the 40 and 41 week antenatal visits, nulliparous women should be offered a VE for cervical sweeping.
3. At the 41 week visit, parous women should be offered a membrane sweep.
4. When a VE is carried out to assess the cervix, the opportunity should be taken to offer the woman a membrane sweep.
5. Additional membrane sweeps may be offered if labour does not start spontaneously.

A recent systematic review and meta-analysis of membrane sweeping at term to promote spontaneous labour and reduce the likelihood of a proper IOL for postmaturity included a total of seven studies consisting of 2252 participants. The results revealed that membrane sweeping is advantageous in promoting spontaneous labour (RR = 1.205, 95% CI: 1.133–1.282, p = <0.001), and reduction of formal induction of labour for postmaturity (RR = 0.523, 95% CI: 0.409–0.669, p = <0.001) [39]. The results suggest that this positive effect is significant from 38 weeks of gestation and is neither dependent on the number of times nor the timing of membrane sweeps performed. There is no evidence to support any increase in maternal or foetal morbidity, suggesting that membrane sweeping is a safe and simple procedure to offer to all low-risk pregnant women who will accept the examination. The author suggests therefore that there could be a reduction in the gestation at which membrane sweeping is offered from 40 weeks to primiparous women and 41 weeks to multiparous women down to 38 weeks onwards for all low-risk women without any increased risk of maternal or foetal morbidity. This may result in a reduced number of women requiring a formal induction of labour for postmaturity [39].

Currently, available evidence lends no support the use of the following non-pharmacological methods for induction of labour: herbal supplements, castor oil, hot baths, enemas, breast stimulation, sexual intercourse, acupuncture, acupressure or transcutaneous nerve stimulation.

14.4 Pharmacological Methods of IOL

Dinoprostone (PGE2) This is the most commonly used vaginal prostaglandin for IOL in women with an unfavourable cervix when there are no contraindications to IOL or risk of hyperstimulation. PGE2 can be administered as a gel, tablet or slow-release pessary. Prostaglandins promote several biochemical and biophysical changes that lead to cervical ripening and an increase in myometrial contractility [40]. NICE recommends one cycle of vaginal PGE2 tablet or gel followed by a second dose after 6 hours if labour has not established (up to a maximum of 2 doses) or 1 cycle of vaginal PGE2 controlled-release pessary over 24 hours [3]. In practice, a third dose may be administered of gel or tablet 6 hours later following cervical assessment. If oxytocin is required after PGE2, 6 hours must elapse after the last PGE2 dose to reduce the risk of hyperstimulation. Adverse reactions are uncommon with PGE2 and include vomiting, nausea and diarrhoea. Rarer adverse effects include uterine hyperstimulation, bronchospasm, backache, rash and extremely rarely amniotic fluid embolism.

Evidence A Cochrane database systematic review in 2014 to determine the effects of vaginal prostaglandins E2 and F2α for third-trimester cervical ripening or induction of labour in comparison with placebo/no treatment or other vaginal prostaglandins (except misoprostol) concluded that prostaglandins PGE2 probably increase the chance of vaginal delivery in 24 hours [41]. There was an increased risk of uterine hyperstimulation with foetal heart changes, but there was about a 10% reduction in caesarean section rates. They increase the likelihood of cervical changes that favour the onset of labour, with no increase in operative delivery rates. PGE2 tablets, gels and pessaries appear to be as effective as each other; any differences between formulations are marginal but may be necessary.

WHO guidelines recommend using low dose PGE2. Low-dose prostaglandin E2 has been compared with higher-dose counterparts in seven trials. The use of lower doses seems to present comparative advantages over the higher doses:

(i) Lower risk of uterine tachysystole with foetal heart rate changes (two trials, 140 participants, RR 0.18, 95%, CI 0.03–0.99)
(ii) Similar risk of caesarean sections (seven trials, 1466 participants, RR 1.07, 95% CI 0.8–1.42) and Apgar score of less than seven at 5 minutes of life (three trials, 1064, RR 0.51, 95% CI 0.2–1.31)
(iii) Trend to reduced neonatal intensive care unit admissions (one trial, 955 participants, RR 0.51, 95%, CI 0.24–1.09) [42]

14.5 Gel Versus Tablets or Pessary

A UK RCT involving 165 pregnant women with cephalic presentation undergoing induction of labour after 37 weeks of gestation compared with prostaglandin E2 vaginal tablets (3 mg) or vaginal gel (1 mg/2 mg) administered at 6-hourly intervals until the cervix was suitable for amniotomy. There were significant dissimilarities between the two treatment groups in the primary outcomes [43]. The mean induction-to-delivery interval was significantly shorter in women who received the gel. The rate of failed induction of labour (IOL) was significantly higher in women who received tablets (10.84 versus 1.22%; $p = 0.01$). When subjected to a subanalysis, it was revealed that these observed differences were only representative of variations in the groups of primigravid women. There were no significant differences observed for any of the secondary outcomes, including the number of women who required oxytocin augmentation, the rate of uterine hyperstimulation, the need for epidural analgesia, meconium staining of liquor, the need for intrapartum foetal blood sampling or delivery by caesarean section. There were no differences observed for adverse maternal and neonatal outcomes. The authors concluded that prostaglandin E2 vaginal gel is superior to vaginal tablets for the induction of labour [43].

Some studies have compared vaginal prostaglandin E2 gel with vaginal prostaglandin E2 suppository/pessary. In this comparison, the E2 gel was associated with a reduction in uterine hyperstimulation (2 trials, 159 participants, RR 0.16, 95% CI 0.03–0.87). There was no statistically difference observed between E2 gel and suppository/pessary in terms of influencing the risk of caesarean section (2 trials, 159 participants, RR 0.65, 95% CI 0.38–1.11) and an Apgar score of less than seven at 5 minutes of life (one trial, 69 participants, RR 0.21, 95% CI 0.01–4.13) [44]. There was limited, low-quality evidence revealing no statistically significant differences between controlled-release prostaglandin E2 and other prostaglandin E2 formulations (8 trials, 929 participants, five priority outcomes evaluated) [44].

Misoprostol (PGE1) It is a prostaglandin E1 analogue first marketed in the 1980s to prevent gastric ulcers. Because of its effect on uterine contractility and cervical ripening, several randomised trials and systematic reviews have evaluated its use in obstetrics and gynaecology. It is stable at room temperature, cheap and available in more than 80 countries, making it particularly useful in resource-poor settings [45]. It is available for use as tablets, 100 or 200 μg and can be broken to provide 25 or 50 μg doses. It can be administered orally, vaginally or rectally with rapid absorption. A Cochrane review on oral misoprostol for induction of labour concluded that oral misoprostol is an induction agent that is effective at achieving vaginal delivery. It is more effective than placebo, as effective as vaginal misoprostol and vaginal dinoprostone and results in fewer caesarean sections than oxytocin alone [46]. The WHO recommends a dose of 25 μg orally 2 or 6 hourly PV for induction of labour at term in women who have not had a caesarean delivery [45]. It is vital that women using misoprostol for induction of labour are never left unattended because the procedure carries the risk of uterine tachysystole, uterine rupture and foetal distress. Induction with misoprostol should therefore only be carried out in facilities where the wellbeing of mother and baby can be closely monitored and where caesarean deliveries can be performed urgently. It is also suggested that rather than cutting pills which makes dosing problematic, a 200 μg pill should be dissolved in 200 mL of water and 25 mL of that solution administered as a single dose [36]. Uniform concentration and accurate drug delivery are, however, not guaranteed.

For women with dead or anomalous foetuses in the third trimester, oral or vaginal misoprostol is recommended for IOL by the WHO at the same doses or regimens recommended for the use of misoprostol for IOL for live babies at term.

Evidence Compared with placebo, oral misoprostol is an effective induction agent. For all women irrespective of parity, membranes and cervical status, caesarean birth was less likely to occur with oral misoprostol (50–100 μg) when compared with vaginal PGE2 (RR 0.88, 95% CI 0.76–1.01; 6 RCTs) although this was not statistically significant [47]. Maternal and foetal outcomes were comparable between oral misoprostol (50–200 μg) and intracervical PGE2. Meconium stained liquor was more likely with oral misoprostol than with oxytocin (RR 0.72, 95% CI 1.08–2.74; 6 RCTs).

Compared with vaginal misoprostol (25 μg every 4 hours, maximum dose 150 μg), primiparous women with an unfavourable cervix given oral misoprostol (50 μg every 4 hours, max dose 300 μg) were significantly less likely to achieve vaginal delivery within 24 hours (RR 1.25, 94% CI 1.01–1.55, 1 RCT). Maternal and foetal outcomes were comparable between oral and vaginal misoprostol in women with an unfavourable cervix [47].

Titrated low dose oral misoprostol (25 μg) was more effective than standard regimen (vaginal PGE2 plus intravenous oxytocin) in terms of achieving vaginal birth within 24 hours and reduced the caesarean birth rate, in women with pre-labour rupture of membranes. There were significantly more maternal side effects with the use of misoprostol (19% versus 13%, RR 1.42, 95% CI 1.02–1.98). These side effects include nausea, vomiting, diarrhoea, shivering and pyrexia in labour [48].

Mysodelle is a 200-μg misoprostol, vaginal delivery system. It is a PGE1 analogue and authorised for induction of labour in women with an unfavourable cervix from 36 weeks pregnancy in whom induction is clinically indicated. A routine EU review of the use of mysodelle investigated reports from a study in which 13% of women (90 of 678 patients) were randomly assigned to the 200-μg misoprostol vaginal pessary developed uterine tachysystole requiring intervention. In 5 cases (0.7% of women), hyperstimulation did not subside with the use of tocolysis [49].

Uterine tachysystole has been associated with poor uteroplacental perfusion leading to a decrease in foetal oxygenation and eventually foetal compromise. In the study, irrespective of the higher incidence of tachysystole requiring intervention recorded in women given the misoprostol vaginal insert than those given a dinoprostone vaginal insert (13% versus 4%, respectively), neonatal outcomes did not appear to differ.

NICE currently recommends that misoprostol should only be offered as a method of induction of labour to women who have intrauterine foetal death or in the context of a clinical trial [3].

Oxytocin is a hormone released naturally from the pituitary gland that stimulates the contraction of the uterus during labour and facilitates the ejection of milk from the breasts during nursing. Synthetic oxytocin is the most common and proven method of IOL [50, 51]. In a recent meta-analysis of ways to induce labour, use of IV oxytocin plus amniotomy and the use of vaginal misoprostol were the most likely methods to achieve vaginal delivery within 24 hours (55). NICE does not recommend IV oxytocin alone for IOL. In clinical practice, in the presence of ruptured membranes, IV oxytocin is an alternative initiating agent to prostaglandins [3].

Exogenous oxytocin administration produces periodic uterine contractions first demonstrable at approximately 20 weeks of gestation. Myometrial responsiveness increases with advancing gestational age, and at about 34 weeks, it levels off until spontaneous labour begins when it increases rapidly [52]. Increases in myometrial sensitivity are due primarily to increases in myometrial oxytocin receptor binding sites [53]. Receptor activation triggers signalling events that stimulate contractions, primarily by elevating intracellular calcium [54]. Progress during spontaneous labour is not related to increasing oxytocin concentration, uterine contractions are not associated with changes in plasma oxytocin concentration, and hypo-contractile labour does not appear to be the result of a deficit of oxytocin [55]. However, variations in genes related to the oxytocin receptor appear to be associated with the amount of oxytocin required during induction and the duration of labour [56].

Oxytocin cannot be administered orally because the polypeptide is degraded into small, inactive forms by gastrointestinal enzymes. It is administered intravenously; its plasma half-life estimated at three to 6 minutes [57]. Oxytocin is given as an intravenous infusion of a dilute solution (10 mU/mL) and has a time to uterine response of 3–4 minutes with steady levels being achieved by 40 minutes [58]. Generally, the dose is titrated increasing every 30 minutes until regular contractions occur lasting 45 seconds to 1 minute. Ideally, there should be 3 or 4 contractions every 10 minutes. Oxytocin should be administered intravenously by an infusion pump to allow continuous, precise control of the dose administered. Hospitals should implement a standardised protocol to minimise errors in oxytocin administration [59–61].

See tables below for commonly used regimens of oxytocin infusion.

14.6 Regimen for Oxytocin (Syntocinon®) Infusion via a Volumetric Pump

14.6.1 Standardised Dilutions and Dose Regimes

Time after starting (mins)	**Oxytocin Dose (mU/min)**	**Volume infused (mU/hour)**	
		Dilution 10 units oxytocin in 500mls normal saline 0.9% or Hartmann's	Dilution 30 units oxytocin in 500mls normal saline 0.9% or Hartmann's **(Refer to point 13.0)**
0	1	3	1
30	2	6	2
60	4	12	4
90	8	24	8
120	12	36	12
150	16	48	16
180	20	60	20
210	24	72	24
240	28	84	28
270	32	96	32

Shaded doses only to be administered following review by a senior obstetrician

14.6.2 Regimen for Oxytocin (Syntocinon®) Infusion via a Syringe Driver

Time after starting (min)	Oxytocin dose (mU/min)	Volume infused (mL/hour) Dilution 10 units in 49 mL normal saline or Hartmann's
0	2	0.6
30	4	1.2
60	8	2.4
90	12	3.6
120	16	4.8
150	20	6.0
180	24	7.2
210	28	8.4
240	32	9.6

Side effects of oxytocin include tachysystole, defined by ACOG as more than five contractions in 10 minutes averaged over a 30 minute period [62]. It is essential to note the presence or absence of foetal heart changes. Tachysystole is commoner when higher doses of oxytocin or prostaglandins are used. If tachysystole occurs when oxytocin is being infused, the dose should be reduced or discontinued until the tachysystole resolves even if FHR suggests foetal wellbeing. If oxytocin is discontinued, there is no clear evidence on when to resume the drug if contractions remain suboptimal. A pragmatic approach would be to resume at least 30 minutes later and at the next lower dose. Other side effects of oxytocin include hyponatraemia and hypotension.

14.6.3 Evidence

A Cochrane review in 2009 including 61 trials (12,819 women) [50] found that when oxytocin inductions were compared with expectant management (wait and see), fewer women failed to deliver vaginally within 24 hours (8.4% versus 53.8%, Risk Ratio (RR) 0.16, 95% confidence interval (CI) 0.10–0.25). There was a significant increase in the number of mothers requiring epidural analgesia (RR 1.10, 95% CI 1.04–1.17). Fewer women were dissatisfied with the use of oxytocin induction of labour in the one trial reporting this outcome (5.9% versus 13.7%, RR 0.43, 95% CI 0.33–0.56). Compared with vaginal prostaglandins, the use of oxytocin increased unsuccessful vaginal delivery within 24 hours in the two trials reporting this outcome (70% versus 21%, RR 3.33, 95% CI 1.61–6.89). There was a small increase in the use of epidurals when oxytocin alone was used (RR 1.09, 95% CI 1.01–1.17) [50].

Most of the studies with ruptured membranes, and there was some evidence that vaginal prostaglandin increased infection in women (chorioamnionitis RR 0.66, 95% CI 0.47–0.92) and in their babies (use of antibiotics RR 0.68, 95% CI 0.53–0.87). These data should be interpreted with a lot of caution as the infection was not pre-specified in the original review protocol [50].

The authors concluded that comparison of oxytocin with either intravaginal or intracervical PGE2 reveals that the prostaglandin agents probably increased the chances of achieving a vaginal birth within 24 hours. Oxytocin induction may increase intervention rates during labour. For women with pre-labour rupture of membranes, that induction of labour with vaginal prostaglandins may increase the risk of infection in both mother and babies needs further studies [63].

14.7 Special Situations

14.7.1 Previous CS

A quarter of women with previous caesarean section require early delivery for various medical indications [63]. This presents a challenge as the best method to ripen cervix/ induce labour is not established with available evidence being inconclusive [64]. No RCTs have compared the outcomes of induction of labour in women with prior caesareans to those of women who undergo either planned repeat caesarean delivery or expectant management. Data are limited to findings from observational studies, which have several limitations including inconsistent definitions of uterine rupture and dehiscence, wide variation in induction protocols (e.g. timing and dosage of prostaglandins and/or oxytocin administration), heterogeneity in patient populations, and inconsistency in primary outcome measures [65]. In women considering induction following a previous caesarean section, the odds of success appear to be similar in those with one or 2 previous caesarean sections. Factors associated with a higher chance of vaginal birth (e.g. prior vaginal delivery, favourable cervix) when labour is induced are similar for women undergoing a trial of labour after previous caesarean delivery (TOLAC) and women who have not had a prior caesarean [66].

The overriding concern with VBAC is the risk of uterine rupture. The 2010 Nation Institutes of Health Consensus Development Conference Statement on Vaginal Birth After Caesarean reported that the frequency of uterine rupture in women at term who had their labour induced was significantly higher than the frequency in women whose labour started spontaneously (1.5 versus 0.8%) [67]. When women undergoing expectant management were compared with those induced at 39 weeks, the risk of uterine rupture also was statistically higher among women undergoing induction (1.4 versus 0.5%, respectively) [68].

Two factors associated with an increased risk of rupture during induction in women with prior caesarean deliveries are an unfavourable cervix and use of prostaglandins.

- Unfavourable cervix – In a nested case-control study, an unfavourable cervix (defined initial cervical dilation <2 cm) was significantly associated with higher risk of uterine rupture during induction (hazard ratio [HR] 4.09, 95% CI 1.82–9.17), whereas women with a favourable cervix (defined as initial cervical dilation >4 cm) had a statistically similar risk of rupture as women who entered labour spontaneously (HR 1.5, 95% CI 0.97–2.36) [69]. It should be noted, however, that this association has not been reported consistently: In one study of over 11,000 women, an unfavourable cervix at the time of labour induction was not associated with an increased risk of uterine rupture [66].
- Use of prostaglandins – Induction with prostaglandins appears to be associated with a higher risk for uterine rupture than induction with oxytocin. A prior vaginal delivery is a favourable prognostic factor [65, 69]

Evidence A large prospective study evaluated the risk of rupture by labour status in women with one or more caesarean deliveries (n = 17,898 TOLACs and 15,801 planned repeat caesarean deliveries [PRCDs]). Women who underwent induction with oxytocin alone had a threefold higher risk of uterine rupture than those in spontaneous labour (odds ratio [OR] 3.01, 95% CI 1.66–5.46) [70], although the absolute differences in frequency of rupture were relatively small:

- PRCD without labour – 0.
- Spontaneous labour – 4 ruptures per 1000.
- Augmented labour – 9 ruptures per 1000.
- Induced labour (oxytocin alone) – 11 ruptures per 1000.
- Induced labour (mechanical dilation with or without oxytocin) – 9 ruptures per 1000 women.
- Induced labour (prostaglandin with or without oxytocin) – 14 ruptures per 1000.

Concern regarding the use of prostaglandins arose after the publication of a population-based cohort study that analysed data from 20,095 primiparous women who gave birth after a single prior caesarean [71]. In this study, the rate of uterine rupture was similar for women in spontaneous labour and those who were induced without the use of prostaglandin but was significantly higher among women induced with prostaglandins. Specifically, the rate of uterine rupture by category was:

- PRCD without labour – 1.6 ruptures per 1000.
- Spontaneous labour – 5.2 ruptures per 1000.
- Induced labour (no prostaglandins) – 7.7 ruptures per 1000.
- Induced labour (with prostaglandins) – 24.5 ruptures per 1000.

Compared with PRCD, the relative risk (RR) of rupture with the use of prostaglandins was 15.6 (95% CI 8.1–30.0). However, all of the information in this study was derived from a database using hospital discharge coding and birth certificates; individual chart reviews were not performed to verify the uterine ruptures or medications administered. Thus, there is significant potential for missing and inaccurate data [72].

A randomised trial on the use of misoprostol for cervical ripening or labour induction in women with previous caesarean births was stopped early because of safety concerns [73]. This trial and several case reports have led many investigators to conclude that misoprostol may be associated with a higher risk of rupture of the uterus than other prostaglandins and therefore should not be used in women attempting TOLAC [64, 74–76].

14.8 Intra-Uterine Foetal Death (IUFD)

Vaginal birth is the preferred option following intrauterine foetal deaths. More than 85% of women with intrauterine foetal death tend to labour spontaneously within 3 weeks of diagnosis [3, 76] If the woman is physically well, her membranes are intact, and there is no evidence of pre-eclampsia, infection or bleeding, the risk of expectant management for 48 hours is low [3, 76–78] There is a 10% chance of maternal DIC within 4 weeks from the date of foetal death and an increasing chance thereafter [79]. Vaginal birth can be achieved within 24 hours of induction in about 90% of women [80]. Recommendations about labour and delivery should take into account the mother's preferences as well as her medical condition and previous intrapartum history. Women should be strongly advised therefore to take immediate steps towards delivery if there is sepsis, pre-eclampsia, placental abruption or rupture of the membranes, but a more flexible approach can be discussed if these factors are not present. Well women with intact foetal membranes and no laboratory evidence of DIC should be advised that they are unlikely to come to significant physical harm if they delay labour for a short period, but prolonged intervals may be associated with the development of severe medical complications, and they may also suffer more considerable anxiety. Women who postpone labour for periods longer than 48 hours should be advised to have testing for DIC twice a week. Women contemplating extended expectant management should be advised that the value of post-mortem may be reduced. Women considering prolonged expectant management should be advised that the appearance of the baby may deteriorate. Vaginal birth is recommended as the preferred mode of delivery for most women, but caesarean birth will need to be considered with some.

The RCOG recommends a combination of mifepristone and a prostaglandin preparation as the first-line intervention for induction of labour. Misoprostol can be used instead of prostaglandin E2 because of equivalent safety and efficacy with lower cost but at doses lower than those currently marketed in the United Kingdom. Women should be advised that the use of vaginal misoprostol is as effective as oral therapy but associated with fewer adverse effects. The addition of Mifepristone appears to reduce the time interval to delivery [80]. NICE has endorsed the use of misoprostol for induction of labour in women with IUFD. NICE recommended that the choice and dose of vaginal prostaglandins should take into account the clinical circumstances, availability of preparations and local protocols. A review of misoprostol use for late IUFD recommended that the dose should be adjusted according to gestational age (100 μg 6-hourly before 26^{+6} weeks, 25–50 μg 4-hourly at 27^{+0} weeks or more, up to 24 hours) [73].

If delivery does not occur after the first course of misoprostol, the following may be considered as the next options:

- Repeat a course of misoprostol 24 hours or more after starting treatment.
- Oxytocin infusion with intact membranes (oxytocin should only be started at least 4 hours after the last dose of prostaglandin).
- Amniotomy and oxytocin.
- Surgical uterine evacuation if under 24 weeks, hysterectomy or CS.

In a 2009 systematic review of 14 randomised trials on the use of misoprostol for termination of pregnancy in antepartum foetal death, misoprostol was 100% effective in achieving uterine evacuation within 48 hours [81].

In women with a previous caesarean section, mifepristone can be used alone to increase the chances of labour significantly within 72 hours (avoiding prostaglandins). Mechanical methods for induction of labour in women with an IUFD should be used only in the context of a clinical trial. Women with a single lower segment scar should be advised that, in general, induction of labour with prostaglandin is safe but carries some risks. Misoprostol can safely be used for induction of labour in a single previous LSCS and an IUFD but with lower doses than those marketed in the United Kingdom [82]. No safety studies have been done on women with previous caesarean births and an IUFD. In women with two previous LSCS and a live foetus, the absolute risk of induction of labour with prostaglandin is only slightly higher than for women with a single previous LSCS [83]. Induction of labour was the significant risk factor. The safety of induction in women with 3 or more LSCS deliveries or atypical scars is unknown.

Failed IOL The definition remains controversial with no agreed consensus. A recently proposed definition is: failure to generate regular (e.g. every 3 minutes) contractions and cervical change after at least 24 hours of starting oxytocin infusion with artificial membrane rupture as soon as feasible and safe [84]. The time devoted to cervical ripening is not included when calculating the length of induction or diagnosing failed induction [85]. Because rupture of membranes is an important factor in the duration of induced labour, oxytocin generally should be administered for at least 12 hours after membrane rupture before considering the induction to have failed, given the results of two analyses [85–90]

- For nulliparous women with an unfavourable cervix, 40% who remained in the latent phase after 12 hours of oxytocin administration and membrane rupture delivered vaginally [88]. Of note, approximately 70% exited the latent phase after 6 hours of oxytocin and membrane rupture, 20% between 6 and 12 hours, and 5% remained in the latent phase more than 12 hours.
- For parous women, the 12-hour criteria virtually eliminated failed labour induction as an indication for a caesarean birth [87].

A retrospective review of the Consortium of Safe Labor study, including over 18,000 patients, focused on neonatal morbidity and concluded that in an otherwise uncomplicated induction with membranes ruptured, after initiation of oxytocin, a latent phase of at least 12 hours for nulliparous women and 15 hours for multiparous women is a reasonable criterion for diagnosing a failed induction [86]. In an analysis of a multicentre cohort involving over 10,000 nulliparous women undergoing induction of labour, 96% reached the active phase of labour within 15 hours [90]. The authors, members of the National Institute of Child Health and Human Development Maternal-foetal Medical Units Network, concluded that caesarean should not be performed for a failed induction in the latent phase before at least 15 hours after starting oxytocin and rupturing the membranes.

14.9 Setting and Timing of Induction

NICE in the United Kingdom recommends the following: In the outpatient setting, induction of labour should only be carried out if safety and support procedures are in place. Current data are limited to evaluate the efficacy or potential hazards of outpatient induction. It is therefore not yet possible to confirm outpatient induction as safe [91]. The practice of induction of labour in an outpatient setting should be audited continuously. In the inpatient setting, induction of labour using vaginal PGE_2 should be carried out in the morning because of higher maternal satisfaction [92].

References

1. NHS Digital. NHS Maternity Statistics, England 2016–17. November 09, 2017.
2. Osterman MJK, Martin JA. Recent declines in induction of labor by gestational age. NCHS Data Brief. 2014;155:1–8.
3. Inducing Labour Inducing Labour Clinical Guideline. 2008.
4. Boulvain M, Irion O, Dowswell T, Thornton JG. Induction of labour at or near term for suspected fetal macrosomia. Cochrane Database Syst Rev. 2016;2016(5) https://doi.org/10.1002/14651858.CD000938.pub2.
5. Sanchez-Ramos L, Bernstein S, Kaunitz AM. Expectant management versus labor induction for suspected fetal macrosomia. Obstet Gynecol. 2016;100(5, Part 1):997–1002. https://doi.org/10.1097/00006250-200211000-00030.
6. American College of Obstetricians and Gynaecologists. fetal Macrosomia.Practice Bulletin No. 173. Obstet Gynecol. 2016. https://doi.org/10.1097/AOG.0000000000001767.
7. Gülmezoglu AM, Crowther CA, Middleton P. Induction of labour for improving birth outcomes for women at or beyond term. Cochrane Database of Systematic Reviews 2006, Issue 4. Art. No.: CD004945. https://doi.org/10.1002/14651858.CD004945.pub2.
8. Cartwright A. The dignity of labour?: A study of childbearing and induction. London: Tavistock Publications, 1979.
9. Benoit C, Oakley A. The captured womb: a history of the medical care of pregnant women. Can J Sociol/Cah Can Sociol. 2006; https://doi.org/10.2307/3340861.
10. Out JJ, Vierhout ME, Verhage F, Duivenvoorden HJ, Wallenburg HCS. Characteristics and motives of women choosing elective induction of labour. J Psychosom Res. 1986; https://doi.org/10.1016/0022-3999(86)90016-4.
11. Ehrenthal DB, Hoffman MK, Jiang X, Ostrum G. Neonatal outcomes after implementation of guidelines limiting elective delivery before 39 weeks of gestation. Obstet Gynecol Surv. 2012;67(3):135–6. https://doi.org/10.1097/OGX.0b013e318249febc.
12. Mishanina E, Rogozinska E, Thatthi T, Uddin-Khan R, Khan KS, Meads C. Use of labour induction and risk of cesarean delivery: a systematic review and meta-analysis. CMAJ. 2014;186(9):665–73. https://doi.org/10.1503/cmaj.130925.
13. Rosenstein MG, Cheng YW, Snowden JM, Nicholson JM, Caughey AB. Risk of stillbirth and infant death stratified by gestational age. Obstet Gynecol. 2012; https://doi.org/10.1097/AOG.0b013e31825bd286.
14. Grobman WA. Costs of elective induction of labor. Clin Obstet Gynecol. 2014; https://doi.org/10.1097/GRF.0000000000000022.
15. Eisenberg Centre at Oregon Health & Science University. Elective Induction of Labor: Safety and Harms. 2007.
16. Reddy UM, Ko CW, Willinger M. Maternal age and the risk of stillbirth throughout pregnancy in the United States. Am J Obstet Gynecol. 2006; https://doi.org/10.1016/j.ajog.2006.06.019.
17. Dhanjal M, Kenyon A. Scientific Impact Paper No. 34 – Induction of Labour at Term in Older Mothers.; 2013.
18. Page JM, Snowden JM, Cheng YW, Doss AE, Rosenstein MG, Caughey AB. The risk of stillbirth and infant death by each additional week of expectant management stratified by maternal age. Am J Obstetr Gynaecol. 2013. https://doi.org/10.1016/j.ajog.2013.05.045.
19. Walker KF, Bugg GJ, Macpherson M, et al. Randomised trial of labor induction in women 35 years of age or older. Obstet Gynecol Surv. 2016; https://doi.org/10.1097/01.ogx.0000488681.91547.73.
20. American Congress of Obstetricians and Gynaecologists. ACOG committee opinion no. 561: Nonmedically indicated early-term deliveries. Obstet Gynecol. 2013. https://doi.org/10.1097/01.AOG.0000428649.57622.a7.
21. Main EK. New perinatal quality measures from the National Quality Forum, the joint commission and the leapfrog group. Curr Opin Obstet Gynecol. 2009; https://doi.org/10.1097/gco.0b013e328332d1b0.
22. American College of Obstetricians and Gynaecologists. Patient Safety Checklist no. 5: scheduling induction of labor. Obstet Gynecol 2011;118(6):1473–1474. https://doi.org/10.1097/AOG.0b013e318240d429.
23. Bishop EH. Pelvic scoring for elective induction. Obstet Gynecol. 1964;24:266–8.
24. Kolkman DGE, Verhoeven CJM, Brinkhorst SJ, et al. The Bishop score as a predictor of labor induction success: a systematic review. Am J Perinatol. 2013;30(8):625–30. https://doi.org/10.1055/s-0032-1331024.
25. Vaknin Z, Kurzweil Y, Sherman D. Foley catheter balloon vs locally applied prostaglandins for cervical ripening and labor induction: a systematic review and metaanalysis. Am J Obstet Gynecol. 2010;203(5):418–29. https://doi.org/10.1016/j.ajog.2010.04.038.
26. Fox N, Saltzman D, Roman A, Klauser C, Moshier E, Rebarber A. Intravaginal misoprostol versus Foley catheter for labour induction: a meta-analysis. BJOG An Int J Obstet Gynaecol. 2011;118(6):647–54. https://doi.org/10.1111/j.1471-0528.2011.02905.x.
27. Jozwiak M, Bloemenkamp KW, Kelly AJ, Mol BWJ, Irion O, Boulvain M. Mechanical methods for induction of labour. Cochrane Database Syst Rev. 2012; https://doi.org/10.1002/14651858.CD001233.pub2.
28. McMaster K, Sanchez-Ramos L, Kaunitz AM. Evaluation of a Transcervical Foley catheter as a source of infection: a systematic review and meta-analysis. Obstet Gynecol. 2015;126(3):539–51. https://doi.org/10.1097/AOG.0000000000001002.
29. Yang F, Huang S, Long Y, Huang L. Double-balloon versus single-balloon catheter for cervical ripening and labor induction: a systematic review and meta-analysis. J Obstet Gynaecol Res. 2018;44(1):27–34. https://doi.org/10.1111/jog.13551.
30. Salim R, Schwartz N, Zafran N, Zuarez-Easton S, Garmi G, Romano S. Comparison of single- and double-balloon catheters for labor induction: a systematic review and meta-analysis of randomised controlled trials. J Perinatol. 2018;38(3):217–25. https://doi.org/10.1038/s41372-017-0005-7.
31. Schoen CN, Saccone G, Backley S, et al. Increased single-balloon Foley catheter volume for induction of labor and time to delivery: a systematic review and meta-analysis. Acta Obstet Gynecol Scand. 2018;97(9):1051–60. https://doi.org/10.1111/aogs.13353.
32. Schoen CN, Grant G, Berghella V, Hoffman MK, Sciscione A. Intracervical Foley catheter with and without oxytocin for labor induction. Obstet Gynecol. 2017;129(6):1046–53. https://doi.org/10.1097/AOG.0000000000002032.
33. Pettker CM, Pocock SB, Smok DP, Lee SM, Devine PC. Transcervical Foley catheter with and without oxytocin for cervical ripening. Obstet Gynecol. 2008;111(6):1320–6. https://doi.org/10.1097/AOG.0b013e31817615a0.
34. Gelber S, Sciscione A. Mechanical methods of cervical ripening and labor induction. Clin Obstet Gynecol. 2006;49(3):642–57.
35. WHO Recommendations for Induction of Labour.
36. Gilson GJ, Russell DJ, Izquierdo LA, Qualls CR, Curet LB. A prospective randomised evaluation of a hygroscopic cervical dilator, Dilapan, in the preinduction ripening of patients undergoing induction of labor. Am J Obstet Gynecol. 1996;175(1):145–9. https://doi.org/10.1016/S0002-9378(96)70264-8.
37. Saad A, Villareal J, Eid J, et al. 21: a randomised controlled trial of pre-induction cervical ripening comparing dilapan-s versus Foley balloon (DILAFOL trial). Am J Obstet Gynecol. 2018; https://doi.org/10.1016/j.ajog.2018.11.024.
38. Levine LD, Downes KL, Elovitz MA, Parry S, Sammel MD, Srinivas SK. Mechanical and pharmacologic methods of labor induction: a randomised controlled trial. Obstetr Gynaecol. 2016. https://doi.org/10.1097/AOG.0000000000001778.

39. Avdiyovski H, Haith-Cooper M, Scally A. Membrane sweeping at term to promote spontaneous labour and reduce the likelihood of a formal induction of labour for postmaturity: a systematic review and meta-analysis. J Obstet Gynaecol (Lahore). 2019; https://doi.org/10.1080/01443615.2018.1467388.
40. Yount SM, Lassiter N. The pharmacology of prostaglandins for induction of labor. J Midwifery Women's Heal. 2013; https://doi.org/10.1111/jmwh.12022.
41. Boulvain M, Kelly AJ, Irion O. Intracervical prostaglandins for induction of labour. Cochrane Database Syst Rev. 2008; https://doi.org/10.1002/14651858.CD006971.
42. Kelly AJ, Malik S, Smith L, Kavanagh J, Thomas J. Vaginal prostaglandin (PGE2 and PGF2a) for induction of labour at term. In: Kelly AJ, editor. Cochrane database of systematic reviews. Chichester, UK: John Wiley & Sons, Ltd; 2009. https://doi.org/10.1002/14651858.CD003101.pub2.
43. Taher SE, Inder JW, Soltan SA, Eliahoo J, Edmonds DK, Bennett PR. Prostaglandin E2 vaginal gel or tablets for the induction of labour at term: a randomised controlled trial. BJOG An Int J Obstet Gynaecol. 2011; https://doi.org/10.1111/j.1471-0528.2011.02901.x.
44. WHO Reproductive Health Library. World Health Organisation recommendation on use of vaginal misoprostol for induction of labour. Geneva; 2011.
45. Tang J, Kapp N, Dragoman M, de Souza JP. WHO recommendations for misoprostol use for obstetric and gynaecologic indications. Int J Gynecol Obstet. 2013;121(2):186–9. https://doi.org/10.1016/j.ijgo.2012.12.009.
46. Alfirevic Z, Aflaifel N, Weeks A. Oral misoprostol for induction of labour. Cochrane Database of Systematic Reviews. Cochrane Libr. 2014. https://doi.org/10.1002/14651858.CD001338.pub4.
47. Langenegger EJ, Odendaal HJ, Grové D. Oral misoprostol versus intracervical dinoprostone for induction of labor. Int J Gynecol Obstet. 2005; https://doi.org/10.1016/j.ijgo.2004.12.005.
48. Bricker L, Peden H, Tomlinson A, et al. Titrated low-dose vaginal and/or oral misoprostol to induce labour for prelabour membrane rupture: a randomised trial. BJOG An Int J Obstet Gynaecol. 2008;115(12):1503–11. https://doi.org/10.1111/j.1471-0528.2008.01890.x.
49. Wing DA, Brown R, Plante LA, Miller H, Rugarn O, Powers BL. Misoprostol vaginal insert and time to vaginal delivery: a randomised controlled trial. Obstet Gynecol. 2013. https://doi.org/10.1097/AOG.0b013e31829a2dd6
50. Alfirevic Z, Kelly AJ, Dowswell T. Intravenous oxytocin alone for cervical ripening and induction of labour. Cochrane Database Syst Rev. 2009;4:CD003246. https://doi.org/10.1002/14651858.CD003246.pub2.
51. Alfirevic Z, Keeney E, Dowswell T, et al. Which method is best for the induction of labour? A systematic review, network meta-analysis and cost-effectiveness analysis. Health Technol Assess (Rockv). 2016;20(65):1–584. https://doi.org/10.3310/hta20650.
52. Calderyro-Barcia RSJ. The response of human uterus to oxytocin throughout pregnancy. In: Calderyro-Barcia R, Heller H, editor. Oxytocin. London: Pergamon Press; 1959.
53. Fuchs AR, Fuchs F, Husslein P, Soloff MS. Oxytocin receptors in the human uterus during pregnancy and parturition. Am J Obstet Gynecol. 1984;150(6):734–41.
54. Arrowsmith S, Wray S. Oxytocin: its mechanism of action and receptor Signalling in the myometrium. J Neuroendocrinol. 2014;26(6):356–69. https://doi.org/10.1111/jne.12154.
55. Thornton S, Davison JM, Baylis PH. Plasma oxytocin during the first and second stages of spontaneous human labour. Acta Endocrinol. 1992;126(5):425–9.
56. Grotegut CA, Ngan E, Garrett ME, Miranda ML, Ashley-Koch AE, Swamy GK. The association of single-nucleotide polymorphisms in the oxytocin receptor and G protein-coupled receptor kinase 6 (GRK6) genes with oxytocin dosing requirements and labor outcomes. Am J Obstet Gynecol. 2017;217(3):367.e1–e9. https://doi.org/10.1016/j.ajog.2017.05.023.
57. Rydén G, Sjöholm I. The metabolism of oxytocin in pregnant and non-pregnant women. Acta Obstet Gynecol Scand Suppl. 1971;9(Suppl 9):37.
58. Seitchik J, Amico J, Robinson AG, Castillo M. Oxytocin augmentation of dysfunctional labor. IV. Oxytocin pharmacokinetics. Am J Obstet Gynecol. 1984;150(3):225–8.
59. Hayes EJ, Weinstein L. Improving patient safety and uniformity of care by a standardised regimen for the use of oxytocin. Am J Obstet Gynecol. 2008;198(6):622.e1–e7. https://doi.org/10.1016/j.ajog.2008.01.039.
60. Clark S, Belfort M, Saade G, et al. Implementation of a conservative checklist-based protocol for oxytocin administration: maternal and newborn outcomes. Am J Obstet Gynecol. 2007;197(5):480.e1–e5. https://doi.org/10.1016/j.ajog.2007.08.026.
61. Freeman RK, Nageotte M. A protocol for use of oxytocin. Am J Obstet Gynecol. 2007;197(5):445–6. https://doi.org/10.1016/j.ajog.2007.08.025.
62. ACOG Practice Bulletin No. 106: intrapartum fetal heart rate monitoring: nomenclature, interpretation, and general management principles. Obstet Gynecol. 2009;114(1):192–202. https://doi.org/10.1097/AOG.0b013e3181aef106.
63. Kehl S, Weiss C, Rath W. Balloon catheters for induction of labor at term after previous cesarean section: a systematic review. Eur J Obstet Gynecol Reprod Biol. 2016;204:44–50. https://doi.org/10.1016/j.ejogrb.2016.07.505.
64. Jozwiak M, Dodd JM. Methods of term labour induction for women with a previous caesarean section. In: Jozwiak M, editor. Cochrane database of systematic reviews. Chichester, UK: John Wiley & Sons, Ltd; 2013:CD009792. https://doi.org/10.1002/14651858.CD009792.pub2
65. Grobman WA, Gilbert S, Landon MB, et al. Outcomes of induction of labor after one prior cesarean. Obstet Gynecol. 2007;109(2, Part 1):262–9. https://doi.org/10.1097/01.AOG.0000254169.49346.e9.
66. Miller ES, Grobman WA. Obstetric outcomes associated with induction of labor after 2 prior cesarean deliveries. Am J Obstet Gynecol. 2015;213(1):89.e1–e5. https://doi.org/10.1016/j.ajog.2015.02.003.
67. Cunningham FG, Bangdiwala SI, Brown SS, et al. NIH consensus development conference draft statement on vaginal birth after cesarean: new insights. NIH Consens State Sci Statements. 2010;27(3):1–42.
68. Palatnik A, Grobman WA. Induction of labor versus expectant management for women with a prior cesarean delivery. Am J Obstet Gynecol. 2015;212(3):358.e1–e6. https://doi.org/10.1016/j.ajog.2015.01.026.
69. Harper LM, Cahill AG, Boslaugh S, et al. Association of induction of labor and uterine rupture in women attempting vaginal birth after cesarean: a survival analysis. Am J Obstet Gynecol. 2012;206(1):51.e1–5. https://doi.org/10.1016/j.ajog.2011.09.022.
70. Landon MB, Hauth JC, Leveno KJ, et al. Maternal and perinatal outcomes associated with a trial of labor after prior cesarean delivery. N Engl J Med. 2004;351(25):2581–9. https://doi.org/10.1056/NEJMoa040405.
71. From the Centres for Disease Control and Prevention. Use of hospital discharge data to monitor uterine rupture–Massachusetts, 1990–1997. JAMA. 2000;283(16):2098–100.
72. Wing DA, Lovett K, Paul RH. Disruption of prior uterine incision following misoprostol for labor induction in women with previous cesarean delivery. Obstet Gynecol. 1998;91(5 Pt 2):828–30.
73. Gómez Ponce de León R, Wing D, Fiala C. Misoprostol for intrauterine fetal death. Int J Gynaecol Obstet. 2007;99(Suppl 2):S190–3. https://doi.org/10.1016/j.ijgo.2007.09.010.
74. Sanchez-Ramos L, Gaudier FL, Kaunitz AM. Cervical ripening and labor induction after previous cesarean delivery. Clin Obstet Gynecol. 2000;43(3):513–23.

75. Plaut MM, Schwartz ML, Lubarsky SL. Uterine rupture associated with the use of misoprostol in the gravid patient with a previous cesarean section. Am J Obstet Gynecol. 1999;180(6 Pt 1):1535–42.
76. Goldstein DP, Reid DE. Circulating fibrinolytic activity--a precursor of hypofibrinogenemia following fetal death in utero. Obstet Gynecol. 1963;22:174–80.
77. Silver RM. Fetal death. Obstet Gynecol. 2007;109(1):153–67. https://doi.org/10.1097/01.AOG.0000248537.89739.96.
78. Goldstein D, Johnson J, Gynaecology DR-O&, 1963 undefined. Management of intrauterine fetal death. journals.lww.com.
79. Parasnis H, Raje B, Hinduja IN. Relevance of plasma fibrinogen estimation in obstetric complications. J Postgrad Med. 38(4):183–5.
80. Wagaarachchi PT, Ashok PW, Narvekar NN, Smith NC, Templeton A. Medical management of late intrauterine death using a combination of mifepristone and misoprostol. BJOG. 2002;109(4):443–7.
81. Dodd JM, Crowther CA. Misoprostol for induction of labour to terminate pregnancy in the second or third trimester for women with a fetal anomaly or after intrauterine fetal death. Cochrane Database Syst Rev. 2010;4:CD004901. https://doi.org/10.1002/14651858.CD004901.pub2.
82. Late Intrauterine Fetal Death and Stillbirth Green-Top Guideline No. 55.; 2010.
83. Macones GA, Cahill A, Pare E, et al. Obstetric outcomes in women with two prior cesarean deliveries: is vaginal birth after cesarean delivery a viable option? Am J Obstet Gynecol. 2005;192(4):1223–8. https://doi.org/10.1016/j.ajog.2004.12.082.
84. Spong CY, Berghella V, Wenstrom KD, Mercer BM, Saade GR. Preventing the first cesarean delivery: summary of a joint Eunice Kennedy Shriver National Institute of Child Health and Human Development, Society for Maternal-Fetal Medicine, and American College of Obstetricians and Gynaecologists Workshop. Obstet Gynecol. 2012;120(5):1181–93. https://doi.org/10.1097/AOG.0b013e3182704880.
85. American College of Obstetricians and Gynaecologists and the Society for Maternal-Fetal Medicine. Safe Prevention of the Primary Cesarean Delivery: Obstetric care consensus no. 1: Safe prevention of the primary Cesarean delivery. Obstet Gynecol. 2014;123(3):693–711. https://doi.org/10.1097/01.AOG.0000444441.04111.1d. PMID: 24553167.
86. Kawakita T, Reddy UM, Iqbal SN, et al. Duration of oxytocin and rupture of the membranes before diagnosing a failed induction of labor. Obstet Gynecol. 2016;128(2):373–80. https://doi.org/10.1097/AOG.0000000000001527.
87. Rouse DJ, Owen J, Hauth JC. Criteria for failed labor induction: prospective evaluation of a standardised protocol. Obstet Gynecol. 2000;96(5 Pt 1):671–7.
88. Rouse DJ, Weiner SJ, Bloom SL, Varner MW, Spong CY, et al. Failed labor induction: toward an objective diagnosis. Obstet Gynecol. 2011; https://doi.org/10.1097/AOG.0b013e318207887a.
89. Simon CE, Grobman WA. When has an induction failed? Obstet Gynecol. 2005; https://doi.org/10.1097/01.AOG.0000157437.10998.e7.
90. Grobman WA, Bailit J, Lai Y, et al. Defining failed induction of labor. Am J Obstet Gynecol. 2018;218(1):122.e1–e8. https://doi.org/10.1016/j.ajog.2017.11.556.
91. Kelly AJ, Alfirevic Z, Ghosh A. Outpatient versus inpatient induction of labour for improving birth outcomes. Cochrane Database Syst Rev. 2013;11:CD007372. https://doi.org/10.1002/14651858.CD007372.pub3.
92. Guid Oei S, Jongmans L, Mol BWJ. Randomised trial of administration of prostaglandin E2 gel for induction of labor in the morning or the evening. J Perinat Med. 2000;28(1):20–5. https://doi.org/10.1515/JPM.2000.003.

15 Electronic Fetal Monitoring

Ehigha Enabudoso

Learning Objectives

At the conclusion of this chapter, the learner will be able to:

- Define electronic fetal monitoring (EFM)
- Describe the process of fetal oxygenation and intrauterine adaptation
- Describe the pathophysiology of fetal distress
- Understand the different fetal heart rate patterns and the underlying control mechanisms
- Identify the indications for EFM
- Describe and interpret a CardioTocoGraphy (CTG) trace
- Determine basic resuscitative measures and interventions following a pathologic CTG trace
- Differentiate between an antenatal and an intrapartum CTG
- Enumerate potential challenges and some mitigating factors in EFM in LMIC
- Describe some basic steps in setting up a CTG unit in a low-resource setting

15.1 Introduction

Electronic fetal monitoring (EFM) refers to the use of medical equipment that has the ability to detect, record, analyse and present the records of the fetal heart rate changes with time. These recordings can then be used as assessment of the fetal health in utero for the purpose of reassurance/intervention/management in order to prevent fetal injury/death chiefly from hypoxia. EFM is often also called cardiotocographic (CTG) monitoring.

15.2 History

Electronic fetal monitoring dates back to the 1960s and 1970s. Prior to this time, the standard of care for intrapartum monitoring of the foetus was intermittent auscultation (IA). In one of the earliest published studies, it was observed that abnormal fetal heart patterns, especially prolonged fetal bradycardia, was associated with fetal hypoxia and fetal death [1]. It was already known that the autonomic nervous system controlled the fetal heart rate pattern. It was hypothesised that fetal hypoxia led to changes in the autonomic nervous system outflow, hence leading to abnormalities in the fetal heart rate pattern. This fetal heart rate pattern could be easily documented by the emerging technology of EFM. It was therefore believed that this new technology would be the panacea for avoidable fetal morbidity and mortality, especially the long-term handicap from hypoxia – cerebral palsy.

Numerous studies over the years however, have been unable to detect real statistical benefit of EFM over IA in improving fetal outcome and at best have reported slightly conflicting results [2–5]. However, it has been recommended that for low-risk pregnancies, EFM increased Caesarean section rate with no improvement in neonatal outcome. Caesarean section rates have been found to increase by about a third following introduction of EFM in many obstetric centres [6]. Therefore, more recent studies have concentrated on high-risk pregnancies and on improving the technology. In addition, there have been reviews of guidelines to further standardise cardiotocographic (CTG) criteria suggestive of fetal compromise [7, 8].

Subjectivity in criteria interpretation was also considered as a limiting factor to achieving the ideal aim of EFM. Attempts to eliminate human bias in CTG trace interpretation led to introduction of computerised interpretation of EFM tracings. Another innovation that was introduced was the computerised interpretation of specific components of the electrocar-

E. Enabudoso (✉)
Department of Obstetrics & Gynaecology, University of Benin Teaching Hospital, Benin City, Nigeria
e-mail: ehigha.enabudoso@uniben.edu

F. Okonofua et al. (eds.), *Contemporary Obstetrics and Gynecology for Developing Countries*,
https://doi.org/10.1007/978-3-030-75385-6_15

diographic (ECG) trace such as the 'ST-segment' analysis. This ECG trace required the use of fetal scalp electrodes. While these have added more available information and knowledge on fetal monitoring and physiology, they are yet to solve the unequivocal superiority dilemma of the new technologies of EFM over IA in the detection of fetal hypoxia [9].

15.3 Basic Fetal Physiology Relating to Oxygen Consumption

Oxygen is essential for the production of energy. Energy is necessary for the survival of the foetus. Energy is derived as shown in the following schema:

$$\text{Glucose} + \text{Oxygen} \rightarrow \text{Energy} + \text{Carbon Dioxide} + \text{water}$$

15.3.1 Delivery of Oxygen to Reach the Foetus

The oxygen supply to the foetus is derived entirely from the mother through the placenta. Essentially, the mother inhales oxygen which is carried in her blood mainly as oxyhaemoglobin eventually getting to the placenta through the uterine arteries and its branches to reach the placenta sinuses. This oxygen in maternal blood diffuses through the placenta sinuses to reach the foetus through the umbilical vein. At the tissue level, the oxygen is utilised for energy production and carbon dioxide is released into the blood. The oxygen-depleted/carbon dioxide-rich blood is transported through the umbilical arteries to reach the placenta where carbon dioxide diffuses freely through the membrane and is carried out of the uterus through the uterine veins.

15.3.2 Oxygen Saturation Across the Placenta

The placenta acts as a transport organ for exchange of materials between the mother and the baby. Blood on the maternal side of the placenta is usually almost 100% saturated with oxygen. However, the placenta being a living organ requires energy for its activities, hence it also requires oxygen. So the placenta consumes part of the oxygen that is presented to it for transfer to the foetus. The placenta consumes as much as 40% of the oxygen presented to it, hence the oxygen saturation of the blood after it has passed through the placenta and getting to the umbilical vein is drastically reduced. In addition, the placenta membrane is a very thin one allowing easy transport of gases. However, in certain abnormal conditions, chiefly exemplified by preeclampsia, thickening of the membrane could occur resulting in impedance to transfer of substances including oxygen across the placenta membrane, further worsening the level of oxygen saturation getting to the foetus – a prelude to fetal hypoxaemia.

15.4 Clinical Implications of Hypoxia

- *Fetal distress* – Antenatal or intrapartum fetal compromise resulting from fetal hypoxia.
- *Hypoxaemia* – This refers to reduced oxygen tension in the fetal blood.
- *Hypoxia* – This is more severe and refers to reduced oxygen tension in the fetal blood and tissues. This in turn can lead to acidaemia and acidosis.
- *Acidaemia* – The increase in fetal H^+ concentration in fetal blood or the reduction in the pH of fetal blood.
- *Acidosis* – This is a serious condition and refers to the increased H^+ concentration in fetal blood and tissues or the reduction of the pH in fetal blood and tissues.
- *Asphyxia* – This refers to the clinical manifestations due to inability of the foetus to respire and take in adequate oxygen at birth. This usually results in brain damage and damage to other tissues.

Hypoxaemia can lead to fetal hypoxia which in turn can lead to birth asphyxia, hypoxic ischaemic encephalopathy and then to cerebral palsy. Fetal hypoxia can also lead to damage of other organs and tissues including:

- Gastrointestinal tract – Necrotising enterocolitis
- Renal – Acute renal failure
- Heart – Myocardial ischaemia, etc.

It is in a bid to reduce or mitigate these effects that it is essential to reduce the incidence of fetal hypoxia through adequate use of electronic fetal monitoring.

15.5 Determinants of Severity of Fetal Damage From Fetal Hypoxia

1. Severity of the hypoxia
2. Duration of the hypoxia
3. Repetitive nature of the hypoxia
4. Availability and adequacy of fetal reserve
5. Individual capacity of the foetus to cope

15.6 Fetal Coping Mechanisms to Avoid Fetal Hypoxia

A reduction in oxygen supply to the foetus, whether acute or chronic, does not lead immediately to deleterious effect. This is because the baby has developed various coping mechanisms that enable it deal with the inevitable occasional drop in oxygen tension reaching it. This is even more necessary in labour when the blood flow to the placenta is momentarily shut down during uterine contractions. It is these coping mechanisms that allow most foetuses to remain calm during these upheavals in oxygen supply.

On a basic level, the foetus is 'oversupplied' with oxygen in utero despite the reduction in oxygen tension reaching it across the placenta. This may be likened to the mechanisms developed in persons living in high altitude regions of the world. These regions have been known to produce world record holders in the long distance races as exemplified by athletes from Kenya and Ethiopia. Like these, the babies have:

- A higher hematocrit (compare fetal hematocrit of over 60% to adult hematocrit of less than 50%).
- The foetuses also have a comparatively faster heart rate, hence a cardiac output for body weight that is far higher than the adult (compare a fetal heart rate of 140/minute to the adult of about 80/minute).
- Foetuses also have fetal haemoglobin (HBF) that has a higher affinity for oxygen, especially at low oxygen tension than the adult haemoglobin (HBA). This enables the fetal haemoglobin to extract more oxygen from an already oxygen-depleted blood that reaches it.
- The fetal haemoglobin has a higher level of 1,3-DPG unlike the adult haemoglobin that has a higher level of 2,3-DPG. 1,3-DPG results in a shift of the oxygen dissociation curve to the left, hence a higher affinity for oxygen by fetal haemoglobin.

Once this basic coping mechanism of being oversupplied is overstretched, the baby starts to manifest with certain signs all in a bid to reduce its oxygen usage. These will include features like:

- Reduction in growth referred to as intrauterine growth restriction (IUGR)
- Reduction in fetal movement (the mothers often giving the complaints of not feeling the baby's kicks as previously)

Often too, the foetuses start to use up their glycogen reserves. These reserves are majorly in the liver and the heart. So, there may be:

- Reduction in fetal abdominal circumference (this can be accurately detected by ultrasonography).

As the hypoxaemia persists/worsens, there is prioritisation of blood flow to the more essential areas of the brain, heart and adrenal glands. Conversely, blood is shunted away from the kidneys (hence oligohydramnios), skin and gastrointestinal tract [hence increased risk of Necrotising-Entero-Colitis (NEC)]. In these instances, there may be:

- A reduction in the amniotic fluid index (AFI).
- A reduction of the pulsatility index (PI) in the middle cerebral artery (MCA). This implies increased flow of blood to the brain. This is referred to as placenta-cerebral redistribution.
- Reversal of the ratio of the umbilical artery PI to MCA PI. This implies shunting of blood away from the peripheral circulation to supply the brain. This is referred to as centralisation of fetal blood flow. These latter two features can be demonstrated on fetal Doppler studies.

If the hypoxia worsens, then the foetus, in its attempt to survive, starts to use anaerobic respiration to produce energy. This is wasteful as it produces one-nineteenth of the equivalent amount of energy that aerobic respiration will produce for the same amount of glucose. Worse still, this process results in the production of lactic acid which is injurious to the tissues, giving acidaemia and subsequent acidosis.

In anaerobic respiration:

$$\text{Glycogen} \rightarrow \text{Glucose} \rightarrow \text{Energy} + \text{lactic acid} \rightarrow \text{Lactate} + \text{H}+$$

These mechanisms listed above are called upon in the long term when chronic hypoxaemia/hypoxia occurs. The worse the condition is, the more the manifestations seen. This manifestation of fetal hypoxia is referred to as fetal distress.

In acute or acute-on-chronic fetal distress, the predominant fetal reaction is somewhat different. In dire circumstances of severe oxygen lack, as already stated above, anaerobic respiration is resulted to. Anaerobic respiration, while helping the foetus stay alive, unfortunately leads to the production of the harmful lactic acid and subsequent acidosis. The predominant reaction of the foetus in these acute cases is in abnormality of the fetal heart rate pattern. The type and extent of the fetal heart rate reaction depends on the factors listed above including the prior state of health of the foetus and the severity and the duration of onset of the insult.

15.7 Regulation of Fetal Heart Rate and Rhythm in Pregnancy

The Sino-Atrial (S.A) node is the pacemaker of the heart. Electrical impulses are generated from the S.A node and are transmitted to the musculature of the heart leading to myocardial contraction. The S.A node is primarily responsible for the determination of the fetal heart rate. However, the S.A node is responsive to influences, both nervous and humoral. The nervous influences are mainly autonomic. The vagus nerve, which is parasympathetic, is the main autonomic nervous supply to the heart. Its influence on the

S.A node is the reduction of the fetal heart rate. The myocardium also has a lot of sympathetic fibres supplying it. Sympathetic impulses through its adrenergic influence lead to increase in the fetal heart rate. Humoral influences are mainly adrenergic from the adrenal gland which leads to increase in the fetal heart rate. Fetal movement gives rise to stimulation of the sympathetic nervous system and also release of adrenaline both having positive chronotropic effect on the heart.

Optimal regulation of these influences requires an intact fetal central nervous system (CNS) which is in turn dependent on the gestational age of the foetus. Generally, the CNS is fully developed for this function by 28 to 30 weeks of gestation. In the resting stable fetal state, all the nervous and humoral influences continuously come to play. They result in moment-by-moment change in the duration between consecutive heart beats. The Doppler transducer of the CTG machine (see below) is able to detect these changes which are reflected in the continuous subtle changes in the fetal heart rate referred to variability. The CTG Doppler feature of autocorrelation is majorly responsible for the accuracy of this. Adrenergic response is excited by fetal movement and this results in momentary increase in the fetal heart rate referred to as acceleration (see below).

Acute transient reduction in oxygen tension in the foetus is detected by the chemoreceptors located at the carotid sinus of the carotid arteries and the aortic arch. This leads to stimulation of the brain stem to activate the sympathetic nervous system and the release of adrenergic substances resulting in a positive chronotropic and inotropic effect on the heart. The ensuing increased heart rate attempts to restore fetal perfusion especially to the vital organs of the brain, heart, adrenals and the placenta and the reduction of blood flow to the peripheral organs. This later action is usually due to vasoconstriction of the vessels supplying these peripheral tissues and organs.

If the hypoxia persists, the increased peripheral resistance and consequent increased blood pressure results in the stimulation of the baroreceptors also in the carotid arteries and the aortic arch. This, in turn, leads to stimulation of the vagus nerve leading to the reduction of the fetal heart rate. There is also concurrent hormonal influence from release of adrenergic hormones from the adrenal gland. These complex events give rise to varying changes in the fetal heart rate pattern of the affected foetus. This pattern can be detected by the CTG used in EFM.

15.8 Factors That Could Affect Fetal Heart Rate Pattern Include

Gestational age: The fetal heart rate reduces with advancing gestational age from an average of 140 to 160 beats per minute at less than 26 weeks gestation to an average of about 120 to 140 beats per minute at term.

Cord compression: This leads to interruption of blood supply to the foetus and can result in varying fetal heart rate pattern changes chief of which is the presence of decelerations.

Drugs: The effect of the drugs will depend on their effect on the autonomic nervous system. Atropine will reduce vagal stimulation, hence leading to increased fetal heart rate. Salbutamol, a sympathomimetic drug, will increase the fetal heart rate.

Hypoxia: This can have profound changes in the fetal heart rate pattern as discussed.

Cerebral activity: Increased activity leads to increased fetal heart rate and presence of accelerations. Fetal sleep can give rise to absence of accelerations and reduction in variability. (Sleep cycles can last up to 50 minutes).

Maternal blood pressure: Maternal hypotension can give rise to fetal heart rate changes as seen in fetal hypoxia. Similar changes can also occur in severe maternal hypertension.

Maternal pyrexia: This can lead to increased baseline fetal heart rate called fetal tachycardia.

Maternal pH: Maternal acidosis could result in fetal acidosis leading to profound fetal heart rate pattern as seen in fetal distress including prolonged and persistent late decelerations and fetal bradycardia.

15.9 Indications for Electronic Fetal Monitoring

Maternal

- Previous Caesarean section
- Preeclampsia
- Post-term pregnancy
- Prolonged rupture of membranes
- Induced labour
- Diabetes mellitus
- Antepartum haemorrhage

Other maternal medical conditions:

- Fetal
  - Intrauterine growth restriction
  - Breech presentation
  - Oligohydramnios
  - Abnormal Dopplers
  - Meconium stained liquor
  - Multiple pregnancy
- Intrapartum
  - Augmentation of labour
  - Fresh meconium stained liquor
  - Abnormality in intermittent auscultation
  - Antepartum haemorrhage
  - Maternal pyrexia
  - Epidural analgesia

15.10 Cardiotocography (CTG)

This is electronic fetal monitoring using the CTG machine. The CTG is the continuous measurement of the fetal heart rate and uterine contractions with the aim of preventing death and/or serious morbidity from hypoxia. The CTG machine, otherwise called the *cardiotocograph*, is a device that monitors and plots on a graph the various changes in the fetal heart rate and also the uterine contractions with time. The graphical plot of the fetal heart rate pattern and uterine contractions is called the *cardiotocogram*. There are two types of transducers attached to the machine:

- The Doppler transducer that acquires the fetal heart rate
- The tocodynamometer that acquires the uterine contractions

A careful look at the trace will easily reveal the fetal heart rate changes which are then analysed to detect the presence and the severity of fetal distress.

15.10.1 The CTG Procedure

This requires a comfortable room with the CTG machine and a couch. The rested patient lies in the semi-recumbent or right lateral position to avoid the supine hypotension syndrome which could affect the CTG trace. It is more convenient for the patient to have an empty bladder before the procedure but this is not essential. The position of the fetal back is identified and the fetal heart confirmed either with a Pinard stethoscope or a sonicaid. Thereafter, ultrasonic gel is gently applied to the surface of the Doppler probe which is then applied over the region where the fetal heart tone was loudest and confirmed to be picking up the fetal heart tone. This is then strapped in place with the elastic belt tied loosely around the paturient's abdomen. Thereafter, the tocodynamometer is applied towards the fundus of the uterus without application of the ultrasonic gel. This is also strapped loosely in place with the elastic belt. In the event of twin gestation and having a machine that has double Doppler probe, the procedure is similar. However, it is expedient to use a scan to identify the position where the different fetal heart tones can be assessed. In the absence of an ultrasound scan, clinical means can be used to identify these and then place the probes simultaneously over the areas. The trace can then be obtained continuously as previously described. Occasionally, contact is temporarily lost. The probe position can then be adjusted to re-establish contact and continue the acquisition of the trace.

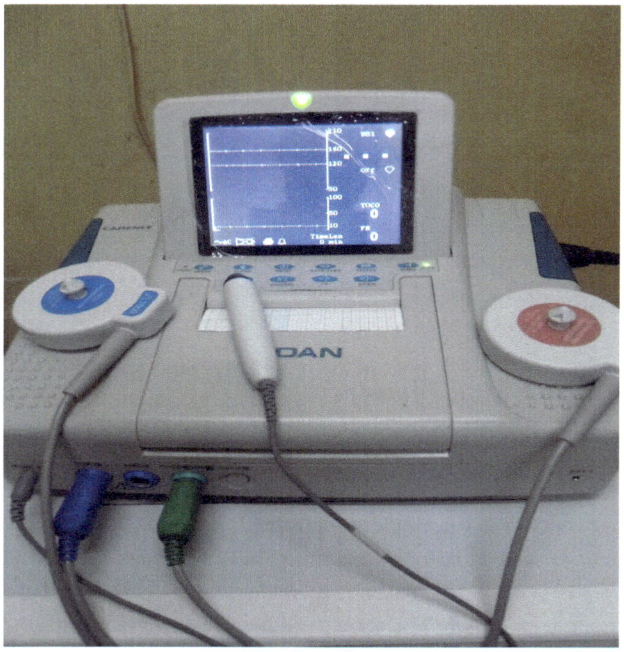

Picture of CTG machine (the cardiotocograph) with the Doppler probe, the event marker and the tocodynamometer (from left to right of picture)

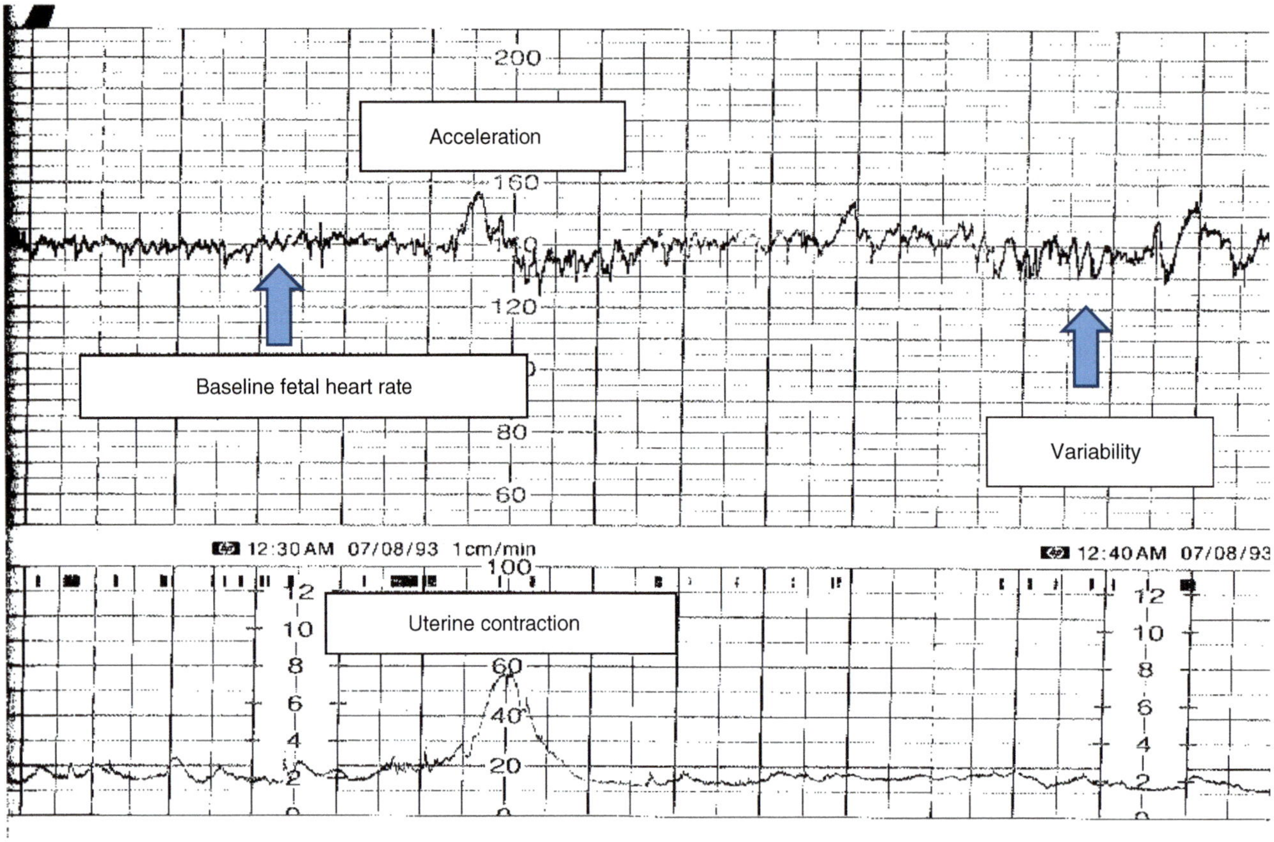

- Baseline fetal heart rate
- Variability
- Uterine contraction
- A typical normal CTG trace

15.10.2 Basic Features of the CTG

Baseline fetal heart rate (bFHR) This refers to the mean level of the most horizontal and less oscillatory FHR segments over a 10-minute period. It is recorded as beats/minute. It is the basic feature from which the other features derive. The normal baseline fetal heart rate is 110–160 beats/minute [10]. A bFHR above 160 beats/minute is referred to as fetal tachycardia while that below 110 beats/minute is referred to as fetal bradycardia. Common causes of fetal tachycardia include:

- Maternal pyrexia
- Intrauterine infection like chorioamnionitis
- Maternal drug ingestion like Beta 1 receptor agonist, e.g. Salbutamol
- Excessive fetal movement
- Fetal hypoxia

While causes of fetal bradycardia include:

- Fetal hypoxia
- Fetal heart block
- Administration of B-blockers like propranolol

Baseline variability This refers to the oscillations of the fetal heart rate above and below the baseline. It is evaluated as the average bandwidth of this oscillation in a one-minute period (that is the width between the peak and the trough of the oscillation). It is recorded as beats/minute. The normal value is between 5 and 25 beats/minute. The presence of variability is a strong factor favouring fetal health and absence of fetal hypoxia. Reduced baseline variability is variability less than 5 beats/minute. Causes of reduced baseline variability include:

- Fetal sleep
- Maternal drugs use including anxiolytics
- Fetal hypoxia

Increased baseline variability above 25 beats/minutes is uncommon and could be due to excessive fetal movement.

Acceleration This refers to an increase in the fetal heart rate of at least 15 beats/minute above the baseline lasting at least

15 seconds. In foetuses less than 32 weeks gestation, acceleration occurs at an increase of 10 beats/minute lasting at least 10 seconds. A CTG trace that shows the presence of at least 2 accelerations over a 20-minute period is referred to as being reactive. Reactivity is a sign of an intact central nervous system control of fetal heart rate, hence a sign of fetal health and absence of fetal hypoxia.

It is a reassuring sign in electronic fetal monitoring. Accelerations may be absent in conditions such as:

- Fetal sleep
- Maternal use of central nervous system depressants
- Fetal hypoxia

Deceleration This refers to a decrease in the fetal heart rate of at least 15 beats/minute below the baseline lasting at least 15 seconds. In routine antenatal CTGs, decelerations are absent. Deceleration most times denotes fetal response to stress and not necessarily to fetal distress. This is commonly encountered in intrapartum CTG. There are different types of deceleration. The type and duration of the deceleration may signify the clinical significance.

Early deceleration – This is one of the common types of decelerations encountered in labour. It is usually short lasting, shallow, a mirror image of the contraction and there is presence of variability throughout the deceleration. It is caused by fetal head compression with consequent fetal vagal nerve stimulation and is considered innocuous. It is a common accompaniment of contractions in labour.

Variable deceleration – This is believed by many to be the commonest type of deceleration. It is characterised by not being in phase with contractions, is 'V' shaped and has good variability during the period of deceleration. It is believed to be caused by fetal cord compression during labour and does not signify fetal hypoxia, especially if it is non-repetitive.

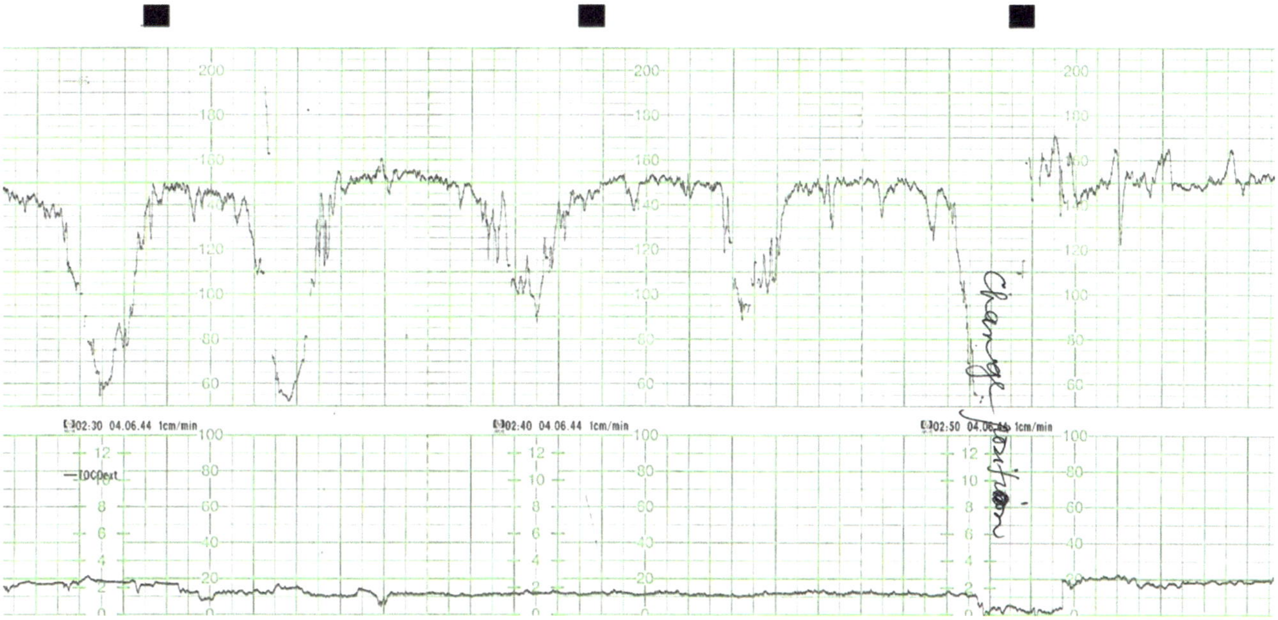

Variable deceleration (which also shows very deep troughs which could be disturbing)

Late deceleration – This type of deceleration is commonly 'U' shaped, has absence of variability during the deceleration and is not in phase with the uterine contraction. It commences at least 20 seconds after the onset of the contraction and the nadir occurs after the peak of the contraction with the return to the baseline at least 20 seconds after the end of the contraction. It is a strong indicator of fetal hypoxia. Features that heighten its indication of fetal hypoxia are absence of variability and the duration of more than 3 minutes. This latter feature is referred to as prolonged deceleration.

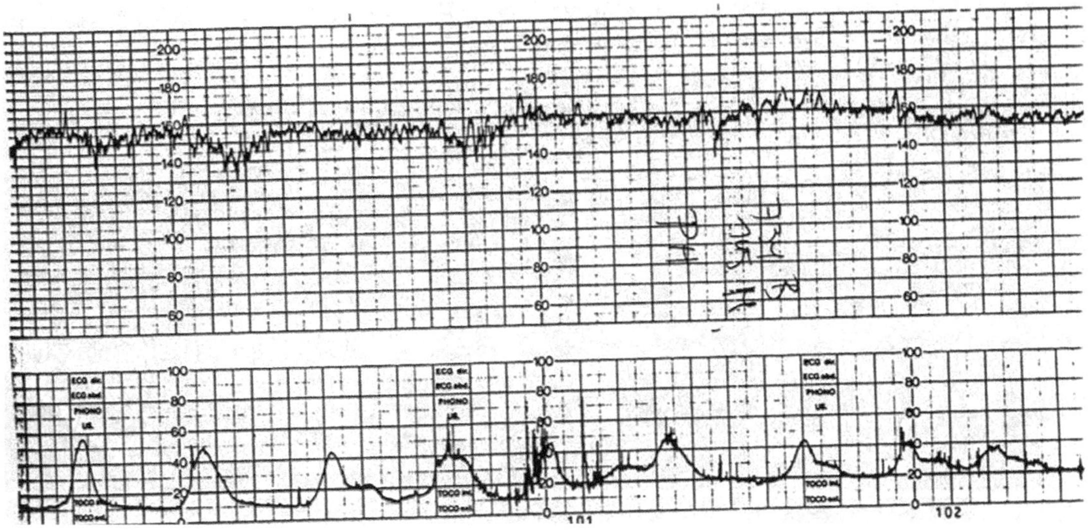

Late deceleration (however with good variability)

Sinusoidal CTG pattern – This is an uncommon but peculiar type of CTG trace. It is characterised by the presence of a regular undulating pattern resembling a sine wave. It has amplitude of 5–15 beats/minute, a frequency of 3–5 cycles/minute and has neither variability nor acceleration. The duration is usually more than 30 minutes. It is believed to be indicative of fetal anaemia.

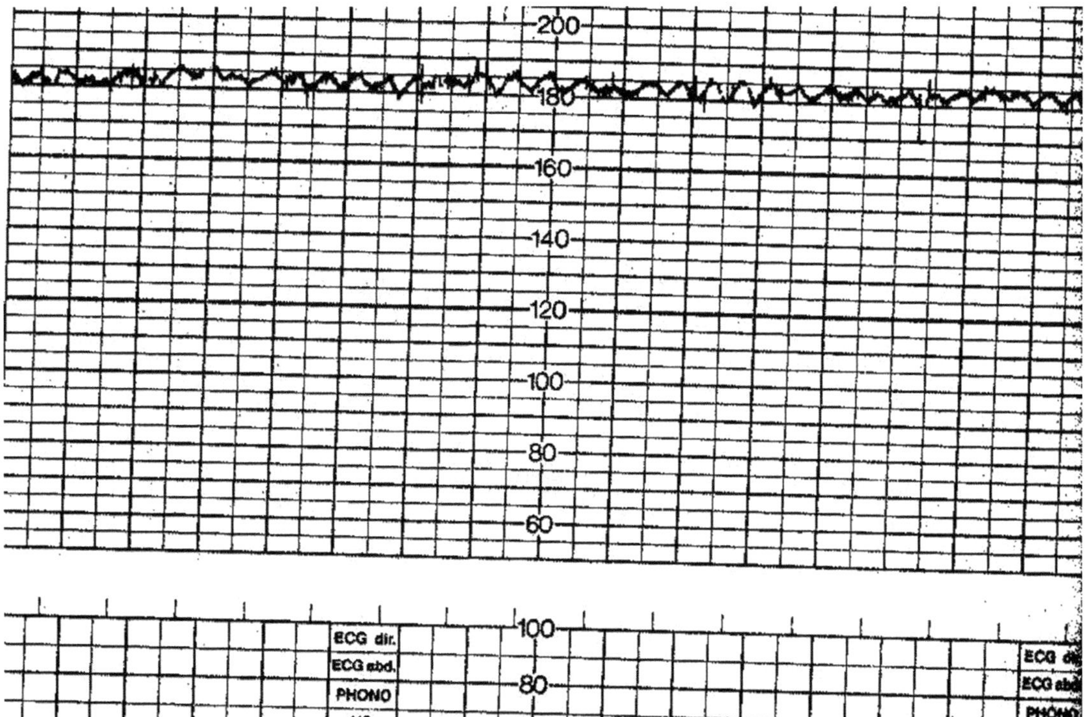

Sinusoidal CTG pattern

Contractions – This is the trace acquired by the tocodynamometer. These are indicated by bell-shaped tracings at the bottom of the CTG trace. They are, at best, indicators of the presence of contractions and the frequency of these contractions. They cannot reliably indicate strength or duration of a contraction. A contraction frequency of greater than 5 in 10 minutes averaged over 30 minutes is referred to as tachysystole and may be associated with fetal hypoxia. Uterine hypertonus refers to a contraction lasting more than 90 seconds. It is also abnormal and can cause fetal heart rate abnormality. However, this condition cannot be reliably diagnosed using the CTG.

15.11 Types of CTG Evaluation

Cardiotocography can be either antenatal or intrapartum.

15.11.1 Antenatal CTG

There are two basic types of antenatal CTG – the non-stress test (NST) which is the conventional CTG and the contraction stress test (CST).

Notable high-risk cases indicating antenatal CTG will include:

- Previous bad obstetric history
- Hypertensive disorders of pregnancy
- Disparity in fetal growth (disparity in symphysiofundal measurement)
- Poor growth detected by ultrasound scan
- Oligohydramnios
- History of reduced fetal movement
- Abdominal trauma
- Multiple gestation
- Antepartum haemorrhage
- Chronic medical disorders including diabetes mellitus

The NST is carried out during the pregnancy in the absence of contractions. It is recommended that antepartum fetal monitoring with the non-stress test (NST) commences at least after the attainment of gestational age not less than the salvage gestational age for the centre. However, due to the confounding factor of prematurity on the CTG findings, commencing monitoring at least at 28 weeks gestation is advised. Interventions based on the CTG findings will depend on various factors including the severity of the CTG abnormality, the gestational age, the salvage gestational age at the centre, the maternal clinical features and the obstetric history of the parturient.

The fetal gestational age is a strong factor affecting the interpretation and guiding the intervention following a CTG trace. Due to immaturity of the fetal brain including immature development of the vagus nerve and its connections, the fetal heart rate is higher, acceleration is less frequent with less amplitude and duration and the fetal heart variability is also less before 28 weeks gestation. These must be considered in deciding on the intervention to be instituted. However, the presence of repetitive decelerations is a strong factor that can be relied upon for intervention even in the preterm foetus. In deciding on delivery in these cases, apart from the severity of the CTG pattern, worsening maternal clinical state is a useful factor. Deciding on conservative management to improve gestational age is a useful consideration if the gestational age is well below the expected fetal salvage age in the centre.

A bad obstetric history may indicate earlier intervention with a non-reassuring CTG. Historically, fetal monitoring is expected to commence at least 4 weeks before the gestational age at which the last fetal demise occurred with the aim of achieving delivery of the foetus before it gets to the same gestational age, especially if the same complication is seen in the mother that may have led to the previous fetal demise. However, the condition may not be recurrent and a normal CTG is reassuring in such circumstances. The CTG should be repeated at regular intervals to ensure it remains normal in such pregnancies with bad obstetric history in which the event may not have recurred.

Worsening maternal illness or clinical state is an indication for delivery irrespective of the features seen in the CTG. However, if the maternal condition warrants it, then fetal monitoring can continue at reasonable intervals. While there is no specific recommendation to the timing interval for repeating the CTG in high-risk cases, the interval could be from 6 hourly to weekly. The timing interval should be dictated not only by the prevailing circumstances as above but also by the availability of resources for the repeat tests and system infrastructural concerns.

A non-reassuring CTG finding at term or at least after 34 weeks requires a definite action. In the absence of contractions, an NST finding of persistent bradycardia or repetitive decelerations of any kind is worrisome. Delivery by Caesarean section is a recommendation. Other abnormalities of the CTG in similar circumstances may be less worrisome. The finding of absence of accelerations or variability should indicate use of other ancillary testing if available including ultrasound scans to assess growth (if not already done), liquor and fetal Dopplers if available. These could assist in decision making. Reactivity of the NST at this gestational age is reassuring. Repeat of the test will be indicated by the clinical features and may range from a few days to weekly.

The contraction stress test (CST) is a test of utero-placental function and relies on eliciting uterine contractions and assessing the fetal heart rate pattern. The uterus is stimulated to achieve 3 uterine contractions in 10 minutes. This stimulation more commonly is achieved using dilute oxytocin solution or less commonly by nipple stimulation. In the latter, the parturient gently massages one or both nipples until 3 uterine contractions in 10 minutes are elicited. The fetal heart rate pattern is then assessed. The result could either be positive or negative. A positive CST refers to the presence of repetitive late or variable decelerations while a negative result is the absence of this. The test is said to be unsatisfactory when there are fewer than 3 contractions in 10 minutes or in the presence of poor tracing. The test could also be additionally described as reactive or non-reactive (see previous notes). A negative CST precludes fetal hypoxia in over 99% of cases and requires no further action other than repeat tests at regular intervals depending on the risk factor elicited. However, a positive CST indicates fetal hypoxia in about 50% of cases and could indicate further testing or delivery.

The CST is rapidly falling out of favour. This is because it is time consuming, quite cumbersome, more expensive and more invasive. It could also get complicated by preterm labour and delivery. It is contraindicated in conditions that preclude vaginal delivery like placenta praevia, more than one previous Caesarean section and abnormal fetal lie. Furthermore, not many studies have been able to demonstrate any superiority over the simpler and commoner NST.

15.11.2 Intrapartum CTG

In this instance, the trace is obtained from a parturient in labour, based on indication. The procedure, interpretation and decision-making following intrapartum CTG are more challenging. There is a higher incidence of signal loss, especially in the second stage due to the inherent nature of maternal change of position, fetal descent and pain during labour. EFM is recommended to be reserved for the high-risk intrapartum parturient (see indications above). Intermittent CTG monitoring for the high-risk patient may suffice. However, in the event of a suspicious or abnormal CTG finding, then continuous CTG is recommended. In addition, the finding of abnormal fetal heart rate and/or rhythm on intermittent auscultation indicates confirmation with the CTG. If the abnormal finding is not confirmed after at least 20 to 40 minutes of the CTG, then reversion to the previous monitoring regime is recommended provided it is normal. If it is still abnormal, then CTG monitoring is continued. Persistence of abnormal findings, especially if it is remote from delivery, is an indication for Caesarean section.

15.11.3 Interpretation of a CTG Trace

In the interpretation of a CTG trace, it is important to appreciate that though the cardiotocogram is similar, the interpretation and implication of findings differ between the antenatal CTG and the intrapartum CTG. Understanding these differences is essential to avoid pitfalls in management decisions based on the CTG trace. Some of the important differentiating features in terms of clinical relevance are as below.

The antenatal CTG In this, the presence of accelerations is very important in the classification of the CTG and the determination of the health of the foetus, hence the CTG is classed as either reactive or not reactive. The presence of all the other reassuring features further contributes to this diagnosis. These other reassuring features are baseline fetal heart rate of 110–160 beats/minute and variability of 5–25 beats/minute. Decelerations are generally absent in antenatal CTGs and even if present, they are infrequent. The presence of repetitive decelerations could be an ominous sign here as there is generally no uterine contraction.

The intrapartum CTG In this, the absence of accelerations is of uncertain significance. While the baseline heart rate and the variability give confidence of the fetal health as in the antenatal CTG, there is major focus on the decelerations. Unlike in the antenatal CTG, decelerations are not infrequently seen here and the presence of type 1 decelerations show normal fetal reaction to intermittent labour contractions and are considered innocuous. Emphasis is placed then on the type of deceleration and the frequency. Presence, duration and repetitiveness of variable and type 2 decelerations are associated with presence of fetal hypoxia. The absence of the other non-reassuring features, especially the variability, strengthens this association.

CTG classification

2015 revised FIGO guidelines on intrapartum fetal monitoring

	Normal	Suspicious	Pathological
Baseline	110-160 bpm	Lacking at least one characteristic of normality, but with no pathological features	< 100 bpm
Variability	5-25 bpm		Reduced variability. Increased variability. Sinusoidal pattern.
Decelerations	No repetitive* decelerations		Repetitive* late or prolonged decelerations for > 30 min (or > 20 min if reduced variability). Deceleration > 5 min
Interpretation	No hypoxia/acidosis	Low probability of hypoxia/acidosis	High probability of hypoxia/acidosis
Clinical management	No intervention necessary to improve fetal oxygenation state	Action to correct reversible causes if identified, close monitoring or adjunctive methods	Immediate action to correct reversible causes, adjunctive methods, or if this is not possible expedite delivery. In acute situations immediate delivery should be accomplished

*Decelerations are repetitive when associated with > 50% contractions.
Absence of accelerations in labour is of uncertain significance.

The above table is a recent (2015) FIGO classification of CTG. Following the interpretation of the CTG features as itemised earlier, the next step is the classification into normal, suspicious and pathologic. It is noteworthy that in many centres, especially in the United States, the terminology used is Category 1, 2 and 3, respectively.

It is important to note that the CTG is a screening tool for fetal hypoxia and NOT a diagnostic tool. There are features seen on CTG that may strongly suggest fetal hypoxia but the diagnosis of fetal hypoxia is by fetal blood pH estimation. It is worth emphasising that a CTG trace that shows acceleration and/or variability denotes a foetus that does not have hypoxia. Put more scientifically, the CTG has a high sensitivity of about 99%. This therefore means that the risk of a foetus having hypoxia following a normal reactive CTG is very slim. However, the contrary is not the case. A foetus that does not have acceleration and/or variability is not equivalent to a foetus with fetal hypoxia. More scientifically, the CTG has a low specificity of about 40 to 60%. This therefore means that for a non-reactive CTG, only about 40% of the foetuses may be hypoxic with the remaining being false positive.

In the interpretation of the CTG, it is important to consider:

- The clinical condition
- The features of the trace
- Other associated features like recent positional change, drug administration, insertion of epidural analgesia.

15.11.4 Clinical Implication

The CTG is a very useful tool for giving reassurance in the case of a foetus with normal features. In other words, it is very sensitive. However, the specificity is much lower in that it being abnormal does not necessarily imply a foetus with fetal hypoxia. This therefore underscores the need for training and retraining in CTG interpretation to avoid unnecessary maternal morbidities through unwarranted interventions.

In deciding the best approach to management, it is worth considering the following:

- Maternal background history.
- The features of the CTG trace preceding the abnormal trace.
- Any inciting event. If the trace had been previously normal and suddenly showed features of abnormality, there is likely to be an inciting event that should be explored.
- Progress of labour.
- Presence of Fetal Scalp Blood Sampling (FBS) facilities or other ancillary tests including ultrasound Dopplers.
- *Stage of labour.*
- Station of the fetal presentation.

Normal CTG trace – This gives reassurance of fetal health. There is no extra intervention. It is important to note that in cases where there is reduced baseline variability and absence of accelerations, this may be due to fetal sleep. Fetal deep sleep could last up to 50 minutes [11], hence there may be need to continue the CTG monitoring for beyond 50 minutes if other parameters are normal.

Suspicious or pathologic CTG trace – This is an indication for action. The actions may include:

- Reversing any identified cause. This could be abnormal positioning, especially maternal dorsal position causing aorto-caval compression. In this situation, the mother should adjust her position to a lateral position. It could also be as a result of the use of the bed pan or administration of epidural anaesthesia with consequent maternal hypotension. If it follows epidural analgesia, rapid intravenous infusion may reverse the hypotension and its effects. The action taken could also involve putting off any oxytocic agent being used, especially if hyperstimulation is observed.
- Institution of palliative/resuscitative measures. One of these is the administration of tocolysis if there is uterine tachysystole. The use of bolus dose of intravenous infusion has only been shown to benefit those cases with fluid deficit [12] while the routine administration of oxygen to the mother has not been shown to be beneficial [13].
- Reassessment to see the impact of the above resuscitative measures.
- Closer monitoring of foeto-maternal status. This involves maintenance on continuous EFM, especially after the institution of the above measures.
- Institution of other methods to evaluate fetal oxygenation if available. This includes fetal scalp stimulation which results in FHR acceleration indicating good health. Another measure could be fetal scalp blood sampling (FBS) to assess fetal blood pH if the cervix is dilated.
- If following these adjunctive tests, the foetus is adjudged not to be hypoxic, labour is allowed to continue with more astute monitoring.
- If following the above resuscitative measures, there is no improvement in the fetal state or there is deterioration, then plans for delivery should be made.
- The mode of delivery will depend on the aetiology of the fetal distress, the severity and the stage of labour. If delivery is imminent, then instrumental vaginal delivery is an option if all favourable conditions are met.
- If the aetiology of the abnormal CTG trace is identified as an acute severe event like abruptio placentae, uterine rupture or cord prolapse, immediate delivery preferably by Caesarean section should immediately be undertaken as the features obviate the need for any other confirmatory test.

15.12 Controversies Surrounding the Use of EFM

While EFM finds use in most centres in the high-income countries and many low-income countries, there still is no concrete scientific proof of benefit over intermittent auscultation. Presently, there is also no scientific proof of benefit of continuous EFM against intermittent use of EFM, especially in the low-risk patients. In one of the largest studies that involved almost 35,000 patients, there was no reported benefit of continuous over-intermittent EFM in terms of stillbirth rate, Apgar scores, assisted ventilation at birth, NICU admission or seizures [14]. EFM was also not found to confer any significant benefit in parturients with preterm labour in terms of Caesarean section rate, fetal acidosis, neonatal seizures, respiratory distress syndrome and intracranial haemorrhage [15, 16].

There have been criticisms of these reported studies. They were carried out in the earlier days of EFM when a lot of the available information now was still sketchy. Studies have also shown a high degree of inter- and intra-observer variability in CTG interpretation [17]. It is also believed that most of the studies lacked the statistical power to detect differences in the rates sought. These studies were carried out in high income countries where the perinatal mortality rates are quite low, hence it will require very large study population. However, conducting large-scale studies in contemporary obstetric practice is an ethical challenge. In present day practice, it is considered unethical to randomise patients to not having what may be considered as adequate intrapartum monitoring. Based on expert opinion and many medico-legal antecedents, it is imperative to offer EFM to women who qualify for its use.

In a recent review on possible reasons for the finding of absence of statistical benefit of EFM, it was opined that there is a need to always critically review the CTG trace preceding the abnormal trace. This will help in deciding if the foetus is responding to an insult from which it may recover or it is in a downward spiral to acidosis which requires major interventions like Caesarean section. In addition, it was suggested that the strict adherence to the written protocols without the full understanding of fetal behavioural pattern may be responsible for the increased Caesarean section rate following use of EFM [18]. It therefore behoves on individuals using EFM to constantly update their knowledge of fetal physiology and the changing guidelines and interpretations of EFM traces.

15.13 Relevance of EFM in Low- and Medium-Income Countries (LMIC)

As earlier stated, EFM has become the standard of care in most of the high-income countries exemplified by those in Europe and the United States of America. However, the same cannot be said of the resource-constrained countries mainly in Asia and sub-Saharan Africa. In most instances, fetal monitoring, especially in the intrapartum period, is by the use of intermittent auscultation with the Pinard stethoscope. In some centres, there has been the introduction of IA using the hand-held sonicaids. There have been attempts by some centres to introduce cardiotocography as a form of EFM.

It is estimated that up to 98% of stillbirths occur in low- and medium-income countries [19, 20]. Similar figures are believed to exist for early neonatal deaths in the region. Though there is dearth of reliable data, it is believed that a high percentage of this occurs due to actions and inactions in the intrapartum period. Impaired placental function and growth restriction are believed to account significantly to this. Improved care at birth has been proposed to be essential to prevent 1.3 million intrapartum stillbirths, end preventable maternal and neonatal deaths, and improve child development [20]. This underscores the need for improvement in intrapartum management of the parturient. While unequivocal benefits of EFM are presently unavailable, intuitively, it is believed that improved fetal monitoring is necessary to produce significant decline in perinatal mortality rates.

Antenatal electronic fetal monitoring is believed to be necessary in the management of high-risk pregnancies and in confirming the impact of complications occurring in pregnancy. It is also invaluable in the triaging of pregnancies to various levels of care and in confirmation of some complaints in pregnancy as exemplified by complains of reduced fetal movement by the parturient. It will be a useful tool in the monitoring of foetuses of mothers with bad obstetric history like those with previous intrauterine fetal death and those with previous still birth and also as useful tool in medical audit.

EFM will assist in early detection of fetal heart rate abnormalities, hence indicating adjustment of care in the clients before irreversible damage occurs. In addition, the recognition of the fact that there is an electronic record of the fetal heart rate will encourage greater attention to the care of the foetus in a parturient in labour. The records from EFM can also act as training and teaching tools, even in cases of fetal demise, to help prevent recurrence. While presently not so common in LMIC, records from EFM can assist in the resolution of medico-legal issues. In areas with severe labour ward staff lack, EFM can come to the rescue enabling a limited number of midwives monitor fetal health in such staff-constrained labour wards.

15.14 Challenges with EFM in Low- and Medium-Income Countries

While EFM is believed to be an important tool in the reduction of perinatal morbidity and mortality in low resource countries, there are major system and implementation challenges that potentially militate against its introduction. One of these is the cost of procurement of the machines. In many of the countries, health budgets are limited and various equipment compete for this lean budget. Based on some other pressing and established demands, such technologies may not be affordable on a large scale. Another important challenge is the supporting infrastructure – mainly electricity. With the lack of adequate electricity in many LMIC, the challenge becomes real that EFM may be a far-fetched technology. There also is lack of experience and training in EFM. Training has been shown to be essential to maximise the beneficial effect of introduction of new technology. EFM is not left out of this assertion. Many healthcare workers will have to be trained in the effective deployment of EFM. The maintenance of these equipment is also a challenge as they are not manufactured locally and service and maintenance services may be unavailable. Many centres in LMIC still lack expedient intervention to salvage cases requiring emergency intervention and also poor salvage rates for prematurity. In the absence of effective intervention when EFM detects a condition requiring such, one doubts the usefulness of its introduction.

15.15 Recommended Practical Approach for the Deployment and Use of EFM in LMIC

It is recommended that there should be antenatal and intrapartum CTG services in obstetric units in LMIC. These should be for specific indications and for high-risk obstetric patients. Realising that there is an essential learning curve for EFM and its introduction usually results in an increase in Caesarean section rates due to its high false positivity, limiting this technology to high-risk patients will result in reduction of this setback.

15.16 Setting Up a CTG Unit

This should be in two different sections if the availability of machines permits – the antenatal section should be domiciled in the antenatal clinic while the intrapartum service should be domiciled in the labour ward.

Setting up a new CTG monitoring unit comes with its challenges. Despite the lack of specific guidelines on this subject, it is pertinent to share experiences that have been beneficial in some centres. The first consideration is to have staff that will be dedicated to the care and maintenance of the machine and who will take responsibility for carrying out the test. Experience has shown that the doctors, based on pressure of work, are ill suited to maintain the service. Based on this, the nurses are recommended to supervise the acquisition of the CTG trace and the care of the machine. This is however not exclusive.

15.17 The Antenatal Unit: Recommendations Here Include

- A practical training workshop/seminar conducted by a professional experienced in the practice of the CTG. This should precede the commencement of the service in the centre.
- Provision of a dedicated room for the service. The room should be in the antenatal clinic with a comfortable couch and lighting. Having an air conditioner is desirable.
- Service should run a minimum of the full working hours. 24-hour service is ideal.
- There should be a dedicated nurse to run the service. She should have at least basic knowledge of trace acquisition and basic interpretation. Depending on manpower need, the nurse may be a member of the antenatal nursing team who is called upon to carry out the CTG when necessary. However, if the demand is high and manpower is not a challenge, the nurse can be stationed in the CTG monitoring unit.
- A CTG machine fit with a power surge protector and a UPS system to maintain power to the device in the event of power loss while the machine is already in use.
- Having a computer in place for record purpose is encouraged.
- Once a CTG evaluation is requested, the requisite request is made by the managing team and the test carried out by the nurse. It is recommended that there be a continuous 20-minute trace acquired per client. However, if the demand is high, a normal trace with at least two accelerations acquired in at least 10 minutes is sufficient. If however there is absence of accelerations in 20 minutes, the trace could be continued for up to 40 to 50 minutes during which time, at least two accelerations are expected in a normal healthy foetus. The trace is then sent back to the managing team for interpretation and action. However, if the nurse notices the trace to be pathologic or persistently lacks accelerations, it is advised that she takes direct action to alert the managing team for review and immediate action.
- Practice like this helps to build the system and maintain the equipment over time. Experience gathering also occurs in the process.

15.18 The Intrapartum Unit: Recommendations Here Include

- Ideally, every delivery suite should have a CTG machine. In practice, this is impracticable in many centres in LMIC. Each centre should provide the optimum number of machines it can reasonably afford depending on resources and need.
- Each machine should be equipped with a power surge protector and a UPS system. The unit should be on a movable trolley to prevent damage.
- If there is more than one machine, there should be some stationed in particular rooms while one could be mobile, again to prevent undue damage.
- As indicated, high-risk patients could be on intermittent CTG monitoring. If normal, this is continued at regular intervals without disrupting the regular intermittent auscultation using the Pinard stethoscope or the sonicaid. However, in the event of any abnormality in the tracing on intermittent CTG, the patient may then be commenced on continuous CTG monitoring.
- Depending on the local circumstances, the nurse/midwife carries out the CTG and the trace is reviewed by the attending doctor. This does not preclude the doctor from carrying out the CTG when necessary.
- Any abnormal trace requires prompt attention for either resuscitation or delivery as indicated.

15.19 Summary

Electronic fetal monitoring often also referred to as cardiotocography (CTG) is the use of a special Doppler device to monitor the fetal heart rate patterns. Abnormal patterns are associated with fetal hypoxia. The aim is early detection of these patterns and institution of corrective measures and/or delivery in order to prevent fetal damage or death. There is the antenatal and the intrapartum CTG. The non-stress test is a form of antenatal CTG that is recommended after the age of viability in pregnancies complicated by features suggestive of bad fetal outcome from hypoxia. The contraction stress test is a less common form of antenatal CTG that assesses the placenta reserve and relies on the eliciting of 3 contractions in 10 minutes and assessment of the ensuing heart rate changes. The features of a CTG are the baseline fetal heart rate, variability, acceleration and deceleration. A CTG trace (cardiotocogram) with at least 2 accelerations is said to be reactive and is very reassuring of the fetal health. The CTG has a high sensitivity and a less impressive specificity. Therefore, a pathologic CTG is not diagnostic but may be indicative of further evaluation. Though there are obvious challenges to the deployment of the CTG in LMIC, it is a recommended form of care in the management of high-risk pregnancies.

References

1. Kubli FW, Hon EH, Khazin AF, Takemura H. Observations on heart rate and pH in the human foetus during labor. Am J Obstet Gynecol. 1969;104(8):1190–206.
2. Haverkamp AD, Thompson HE, McFee JG, Cetrulo C. The evaluation of continuous fetal heart rate monitoring in high-risk pregnancy. Am J Obstet Gynecol. 1976;125(3):310–20.
3. Kelso IM, Parsons RJ, Lawrence GF, Arora SS. An assessment of continuous fetal heart rate monitoring in labor.A randomised trial. Am J Obstet Gynecol. 1978;131(5):526–32.
4. Haverkamp AD, Orleans M, Langendoerfer S, McFee J, Murphy J, Thompson HE. A controlled trial of the differential effects of intrapartum fetal monitoring. Am J Obstet Gynecol. 1979;134(4):399–412.
5. MacDonald D, Grant A, Sheridan-Pereira M, Boylan P, Chalmers L. The Dublin randomised controlled trial of intrapartum fetal heart rate monitoring. Am J Obstet Gynecol. 1985;152(5):524–39.
6. Thacker SB, Stroup D, Chang MH. Continuous electronic heart rate monitoring for fetal assessment during labor. Cochrane Database Syst Rev. 2006;(3):Art. No.: CD000063. https://doi.org/10.1002/14651858.CD000063.pub2.
7. Electronic fetal heart rate monitoring: research guidelines for interpretation. National Institute of Child Health and Human Development research planning workshop. Am J Obstet Gynecol. 1997;177(6):1385–90.
8. American College of Obstetricians and Gynaecologists. ACOG practice bulletin No. 106: intrapartum fetal heart rate monitoring: nomenclature, interpretation, and general management principles. Obstet Gynecol. 2009;114(1):192–202.
9. Stout MJ, Cahill AG. Electronic fetal monitoring: past, present and future. Clin Perinatol. 2011;38(1):127–42.
10. Ayres-de-Campos D, Spong CY, Chandraharan E, Byaruhanga R, Enabudoso E, Anthony J, et al. FIGO consensus guidelines on intrapartum fetal monitoring: Cardiotocography. IJGO. 2015;131(1):13–24.
11. Suwanrath C, Suntharasaj T. Sleep–wake cycles in normal fetuses. Arch Gynecol Obstet. 2010; 281:449-54.
12. Simpson KR, James DC. Efficacy of intrauterine resuscitation techniques in improving fetal oxygen status during labor. Obstet Gynecol. 2005;105:1362–8.
13. Fawole G, Hofmeyr GJ. Maternal oxygen administration for fetal distress. Cochrane Database Syst Rev. 2012;12:CD000136.
14. Leveno KJ, Cunningham FG, Nelson S, Roark M, Williams ML, et al. A prospective comparison of selective and universal electronic fetal monitoring in 34,995 pregnancies. N Engl J Med. 1986;315(10):615–9.
15. Luthy DA, Shy KK, van Belle G, Larson EB, Hughes JP, et al. A randomised trial of electronic fetal monitoring in preterm labor. Obstet Gynecol. 1987;69(5):687–95.
16. Shy KK, Luthy DA, Bennett FC, Whitfield M, Larson EB, et al. Effects of electronic fetal-heart-rate monitoring as compared with periodic auscultation, on the neurologic development of premature infants. N Engl J Med. 1990;322(9):588–93.
17. Blackwell SC, Grobman WA, Antoniewicz L, Gyamfi BC. Interobserver and intraobserver reliability of the NICHD 3-tier fetal heart rate interpretation system. Am J Obstet Gynecol. 2011;205:378.e1bs.
18. Ugwumadu A. Are we (mis)guided by current guidelines on intrapartum fetal heart rate monitoring? Case for a more physiological approach to interpretation. BJOG. 2014;121:1063–70.
19. Blencowe H, Cousens S, Jassir FB, Say L, Chou D, Mathers C, et al. National, regional, and worldwide estimates of stillbirth rates in 2015, with trends from 2000: a systematic analysis. Lancet Glob Health. 2016;4:e98–108.
20. Lawn JE, Blencowe H, Waiswa E, Amouzou A, Mathers C, Hogan D, et al. Stillbirths: rates, risk factors, and acceleration towards 2030. Lancet. 2016;387(10018):587–603.

Further Reading

Ayres-de-Campos D, Spong CY, Chandraharan E, Byaruhanga R, EhighaEnabudoso JA, Mirza F, et al. FIGO consensus guidelines on intrapartum fetal monitoring: Cardiotocography. IJGO. 2015;131(1):13–24.

National Institute for Care and Health Excellence (NICE). Intrapartum Care for Healthy women and babies. 2014. Nice.org.uk/guidance/cg190.

The Royal Australian and New Zealand College of Obstetricians and Gynaecologists. Intrapartum Fetal Surveillance.Clinical Guidelines. 2014.*.

Operative Vaginal Delivery

16

Christopher O. Aimakhu and Abiodun O. Ilesanmi

Learning Objectives

At the end of this chapter, readers will learn the following:

- The incidence and types of operative deliveries (forceps, ventouse, destructive operations, symphysiotomy and episiotomy), especially within the context of developing countries
- The clinical indications and contraindications for use of the identified operative delivery methods
- The methods of use and complications arising from inappropriate use of operative deliveries
- Special considerations for use of operative delivery in developing countries
- The research gaps with respect to use of operative deliveries in developing countries

16.1 Introduction

Majority of deliveries occur spontaneously per vaginam and the aim of obstetric practice is to achieve a good outcome for both the pregnant woman and her baby. In some cases to achieve a safe vaginal delivery, an operative instrumental vaginal delivery has to be performed.

An operative vaginal delivery is an obstetric procedure in which active measures with specialised instruments are required to accomplish the delivery of the foetus through the vaginal route and without such measures, progress and delivery will be delayed to such an extent as to be deleterious for the parturient mother or her baby or both [1]. The instruments used commonly are the forceps and the vacuum extractor (ventouse). These instruments are designed to assist the delivery process by applying traction to the fetal head. Obstetricians should be confident and competent in the use of both instruments.

Other forms of operative vaginal delivery still practiced in some developing countries are destructive operations for dead foetuses and symphysiotomy.

An episiotomy is also an operative vaginal procedure to ensure delivery.

An understanding of the anatomy of the birth canal and the fetal head is a prerequisite to becoming skilled in the safe use of the forceps or vacuum extractor. It is strongly recommended that obstetricians achieve experience in spontaneous vaginal delivery prior to commencing training in operative vaginal delivery. The goal of operative vaginal delivery is to mimic spontaneous vaginal birth, thereby expediting delivery with minimal maternal or neonatal morbidity [2].

16.1.1 Incidence of Operative Vaginal Deliveries

There are large differences between countries in the frequency of operative vaginal deliveries [3]. In most countries, however operative delivery rates using the forceps and ventouse have fallen steadily since the mid-1970s [4]. This has been as a result of most obstetricians opting for a caesarean section, which they consider to be safer for the mother and foetus. The fear of litigation has also contributed to this.

While forceps delivery is widely used in Western Europe including the United Kingdom, the United States of America, and is still used in many developing countries, vacuum extractor has largely replaced forceps delivery in most developing countries and in many countries in Northern Europe [5]. Since the late 1980s the use of the vacuum extractor has increased whereas the use of the forceps has decreased [5].

C. O. Aimakhu (✉)
College of Medicine, University of Ibadan and University College Hospital, Ibadan, Nigeria

Society of Gynaecology and Obstetrics of Nigeria (SOGON), Kaura District Abuja, Nigeria

A. O. Ilesanmi
College of Medicine, University of Ibadan and University College Hospital, Ibadan, Nigeria

F. Okonofua et al. (eds.), *Contemporary Obstetrics and Gynecology for Developing Countries*,
https://doi.org/10.1007/978-3-030-75385-6_16

16.2 Forceps Delivery

Operative vaginal delivery using the obstetric forceps has been an important part of obstetric practice for nearly 400 years [6] and its history constitutes one of the richest aspects of our specialty's heritage [7, 8]. A pair of forceps is an instrument designed primarily for the delivery of the baby's head either to expedite delivery or to correct certain abnormalities in the cephalopelvic relationship that will impede further progress in labour such as asynclitism [8].

Many different forceps have been described and developed throughout time since the original instruments fashioned by the Chamberlain family came to public knowledge. There are over 700 different makes of forceps [6], but only a few are in clinical use today.

Forceps delivery has reduced in Nigeria [8] and the world in general since the introduction of the vacuum extractor and obstetricians opting for caesarean section. Applied by those skilled in their use, it can safely and quickly deliver the foetus. Unfortunately, it can be an instrument of harm for the woman or her baby.

At the University College Hospital in Ibadan the incidence of forceps delivery was 1.57% or 16 per 1000 deliveries and they were all low cavity deliveries [8].

16.2.1 History of the Procedure

The history of the obstetric forceps is long and often colourful [9]. The credit for the invention of the precursor of the modern forceps to be used on live infants goes to Peter Chamberlain of England. Modifications have led to more than 700 different types and shapes of forceps. In 1745, William Smellie described the accurate application to the occiput, rather than the previously performed pelvic application, regardless of the position of the head. In 1845, Sir James Simpson developed a forceps that was designed to appropriately fit both cephalic curvatures and pelvic curvatures. In 1920, Joseph DeLee further modified that instrument and advocated the prophylactic delivery. In an era in which many women laboured and delivered under heavy sedation, forceps deliveries became common.

In current obstetric practice, the use of forceps has become much less common. The availability of blood products and greater choices in antibiotics helped make caesarean delivery a safe alternative to operative vaginal deliveries. In the 1980s, information became available suggesting that some forceps deliveries (mid forceps deliveries) may be associated with an increased risk of fetal morbidity, though this issue remains controversial. These factors combined to greatly reduce the appeal of forceps delivery. Currently, many obstetric training programs in West Africa struggle to teach forceps delivery. Problems include the lack of adequate personal comfortable with teaching forceps-assisted vaginal deliveries, changes in consumer attitudes and the demand for natural delivery. In addition, many practitioners fear litigation if a forceps-assisted delivery results in a poor outcome.

16.2.2 The Instrument [5]

The forceps are a paired instrument made up of left and right parts or halves which mirror image each other and articulates by crossing of their shanks. There are several designs and types.

The parts of the forceps are Fig. 16.1:

(a) *The blades*

These are the parts of the instrument that are used to hold the fetal head. They are either oral or elliptical, and are mostly fenestrated but a few are solid. The blades of virtually all the obstetric forceps (with notable exception of the Kielland's) have two curves: the cephalic curve that fits the lateral aspects of the fetal head, and the pelvic curve that corresponds to the curvature of the maternal pelvis. Because the Kielland's forceps is used for rotation of the fetal head it has virtually no pelvic curve.

(b) *The Shanks*

The shanks connect the blades to the handles and provide length to the instrument. This is the position where the two halves cross each other and are articulated by the locks. The shanks may be generally parallel on overlapping/crossing. They may be short (e.g. Wrigley's and Simpson's forceps) or long (e.g. Kielland's forceps).

(c) *The Lock*

This is the point of articulation of the 2 halves of the forceps. The lock may be sliding or non-sliding. The Kielland's forceps has a sliding lock that allows it to be used to correct asynclitism of the fetal head.

(d) *The Handles*

These are where the operator or doctor holds the instrument. They often have finger grips (or finger guides), which enhance traction.

The two most common used obstetric forceps are the Wrigley's and the Kielland's forceps (Fig. 16.2a, b).

There are some special features of the Kielland's forceps that are worth noting. This forceps, which was first described by Kielland in 1956, was designed purposely for delivery of the incompletely rotated fetal hand. The shape is such that the axis of the blades lies parallel to the axis of the handle, hence traction follows direction of the handles, so-called axis traction. The blades hardly have any pelvic curve; hence it is very satisfactory for the rotation of the fetal head. It also has a sliding lock. These features make it possible to apply

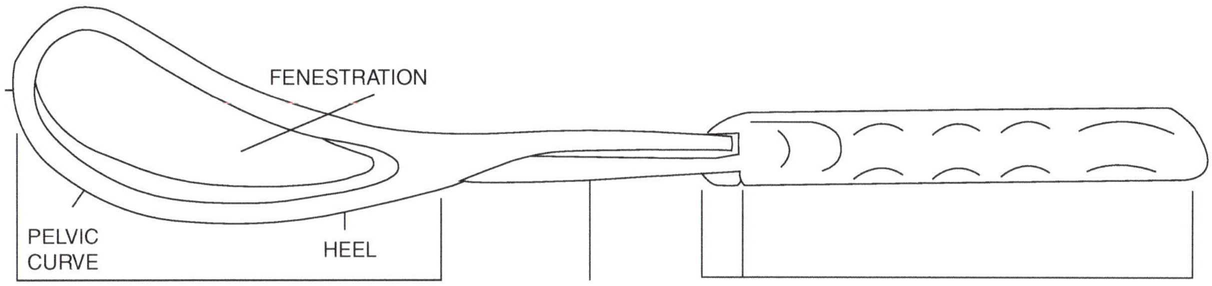

Fig. 16.1 Parts of the obstetric forceps

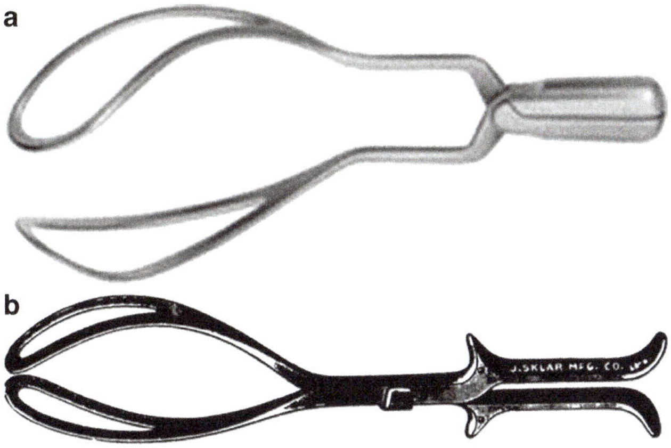

Fig. 16.2 (**a**) Wrigley's forceps. (**b**) Kiellands's forceps

the blades in cases of asynclitism. Finally, there is a knob on each finger grip (finger guide) that must point to the occiput when the forceps are applied.

16.2.3 Operative Classification

Forceps delivery is classified according to the station of the presenting part when the instrument is being applied. These are:

(i) Mid forceps delivery
(ii) Low forceps delivery
(iii) Outlet forceps delivery

High forceps delivery (when the fetal head is not engaged) is no more practiced due to significant complications to both the mother and the baby.

(i) *Mid Forceps*. This is when the forceps is applied on an engaged fetal head above station plus 2 (+2). The Kielland's forceps is usually used here.
(ii) *Low Forceps*. The fetal head is at station plus 2 (+2) or below but the fetal scalp is usually not visible at the vulva. Sub classified into Type A: rotation of the fetal head of equal or less than 45° and Type B: more than 45° rotation.
(iii) *Outlet Forceps*. The fetal head is on the perineum (station plus three) (+3) with the fetal scalp visible without separating the labia. The sagittal suture is in the antero-posterior diameter of the pelvis or the fetal head is in the right or left occipito-anterior, or occipito-posterior position with head rotation less than 45°. Outlet forceps is the simplest and this is what is recommend for non-specialist doctors.

Caution: It is easy to confuse low and outlet forceps and use these inter-changeably. The key is the position of the sagittal suture and the visibility of the fetal scalp without significant caput succedaneum [5].

16.2.4 Indications for Forceps Delivery

The use of forceps should be concise and timely. Unnecessary delays may defeat the intended intervention either for maternal or fetal interests.

A. *Maternal Indications for Forceps Delivery*
1. Prolonged or delayed second stage of labour.
   This includes nulliparous women with failure to deliver after 2 hours without and 3 hours with conduction anaesthesia. It also includes multiparous women with failure to deliver after 1 hour without and 2 hours with conduction anaesthesia.
2. Shortening of the second stage of labour.
   This is to minimise stress on the mother's cardiopulmonary system, e.g. patients with cardiac disease, severe hypertension, pre-eclampsia, eclampsia, severe anaemia, sickle cell disease in imminent crisis, pulmonary disease including tuberculosis and thyroid disease.
3. Maternal distress or exhaustion.
4. Intrapartum haemorrhage in the second stage of labour, e.g. abruptio placenta.

5. Perineal rigidity. With a rigid perineum, an episiotomy may not be enough to deliver the foetus and an operative delivery may be required.

B. *Fetal Indications for Forceps Delivery*

The fetal reasons are to avoid fetal morbidity and/or mortality.

1. Fetal distress in the second stage of labour.
2. Premature delivery.
3. Cord prolapse in second stage of labour.
4. The after-coming head in breech presentation.

16.2.5 Prerequisites for Forceps Delivery

To avoid or minimise complications to both the mother and the foetus, certain conditions must be met before an attempt at forceps delivery.

1. The cervix must be fully dilated.
2. The fetal membranes must be ruptured.
3. The fetal presenting part; mostly the vertex, infrequently the after coming head in breech deliveries; and occasionally with face mento-anterior presentation.
4. The position of the vertex must be known with certainty.
5. The fetal head must be well engaged.
6. There should be no cephalopelvic disproportion.
7. The estimated fetal weight must be less than 4 kilogrammes.
8. The bladder must be empty.
9. Adequate analgesia (general anaesthesia, regional, pudendal block or local infiltration of the perineum). Pudendal or local infiltration may suffice for outlet forceps, while regional or general anaesthesia is performed for low and mid cavity forceps, especially if rotation is required.
10. An episiotomy may be performed in most cases.
11. There must be adequate facilities for neonatal resuscitation and caesarean section.
12. Above all the experience and skill of the operator is crucial.

16.2.6 Contraindication to Forceps Delivery

The following are contraindications to forceps-assisted vaginal delivery.

1. Any contraindication to vaginal delivery.
2. Refusal of the patient to verbally consent to the procedure.
3. The cervix is not fully dilated.
4. Inability to determine the presentation of the fetal head position.
5. Inadequate pelvic size.
6. Confirmed cephalopelvic disproportion.
7. Unsuccessful trial of vacuum extractor (relative contraindication).
8. Absent of adequate anaesthesia or analgesia.
9. Inadequate facilities and support staff.

16.2.7 Patient Preparation for Forceps Delivery

The preparation for a patient for forceps delivery includes:

1. Obtaining a written informed consent from the patient.
2. Facilities for anaesthesia and caesarean section must be available.
3. The patient should be placed in the lithotomy position.
4. Prior to the application of the forceps:
   - Review indications and conditions for forceps delivery
   - Assemble the forceps (ensure parts fit and lock)
5. Anaesthesia should be administered.
   - Pudendal, spinal or epidural anaesthesia may be used.

16.2.8 Technique of Forceps Delivery (Fig. 16.3) [10]

- Once the second stage of labour has started, the patient should be given a regional anaesthetic by pudendal block or a general anaesthetic.
- Place her in the lithotomy position, clean and drape the area, and catheterise the bladder.
- Then check for the following before proceeding: full dilatation of the cervix, the absence of membranes, complete rotation of the fetal head, and the station of the head below the ischial spines.
- Check the forceps blades to ensure that they will lock correctly.
- Apply the left blade first, guiding it into the uterine cavity along your right palm (Fig. 16.3a–d). Similarly apply the right blade along the inserted left hand (Fig. 16.3e, f). Lock the forceps and apply traction during uterine contractions, first downwards and backwards (Fig. 16.3g, h), gradually levelling out, and finally upwards and forwards in the case of the occipito-anterior position (Fig. 16.3i–l).
- Perform an episiotomy with the crowning of the head. Once the head reaches the pelvic outlet, lift it out using the forceps.

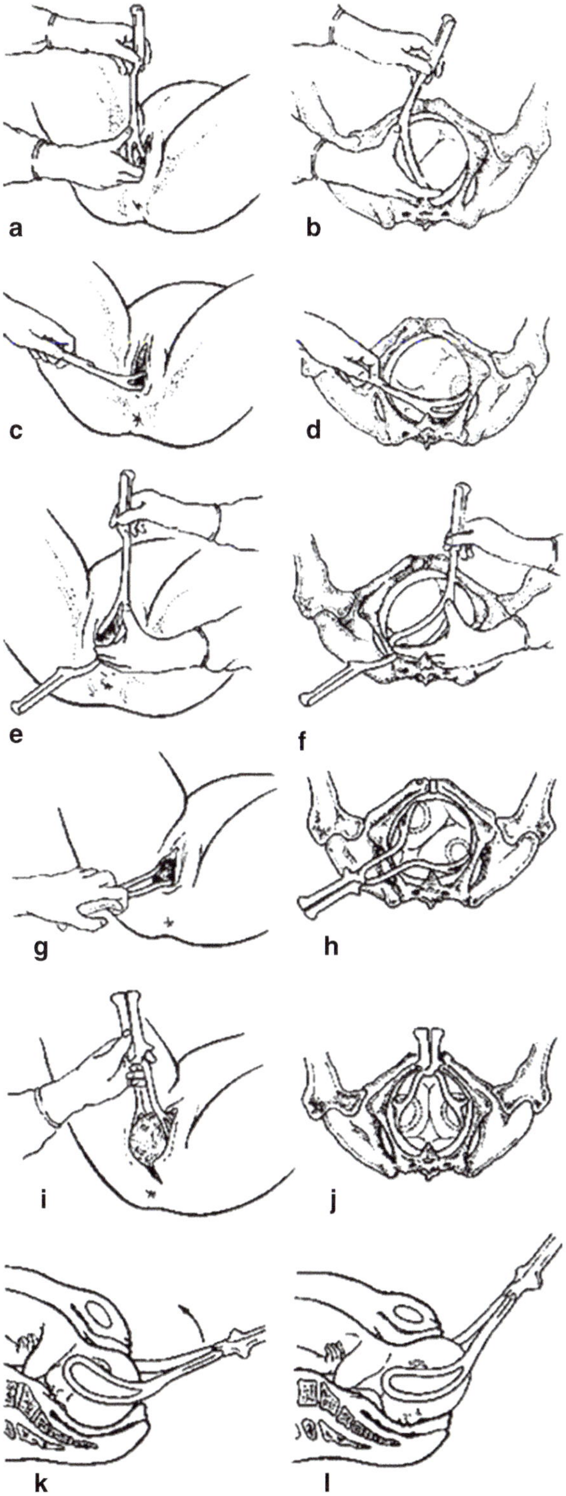

Fig. 16.3 Low forceps delivery. Applying the left blade of delivery forceps (**a**–**d**); applying the right blade (**e**, **f**). Right-hand illustrations show position of forceps in relation to fetal head and mother's pelvic bones. Locking the forceps and applying traction downwards and backwards (**g**, **h**); applying traction gradually upwards (**i**–**l**). Illustrations (**h**) and (**j**) show position of forceps in relation to fetal head and mother's pelvic bones

16.2.9 Failed Forceps Delivery

Unsuccessful attempt at forceps delivery and abandonment of efforts in favour of caesarean section is done if:

- The fetal head does not advance with each pull.
- The foetus is undelivered after 3 pulls with no descent.
- The foetus is undelivered after 30 minutes.

16.2.10 Trial of Forceps Delivery

Tentative cautions traction with forceps with the aim of abandoning attempts at delivery if undue resistance is encountered:

- Every application should be considered as trial of forceps.
- Do not persist if the head does not descend with every pull.
- If forceps delivery fails, perform a caesarean section.

16.2.11 Complications of Forceps Delivery [5, 9, 10]

A. *Maternal Complications of Forceps Delivery*

Maternal complications include:

- Complications of anaesthesia (especially if general anaesthesia is used).
- Episiotomy extension and perineal tears leading later to dyspareunia.
- Vaginal lacerations occurring during the application of the blades and during traction.
- Cervical laceration with upward extension leading to profuse haemorrhage or bladder damage which may result in vesico-vaginal fistula (VVF).

  These lacerations require prompt examination in theatre under anaesthesia and proper repair.
- Uterine rupture.
- Postpartum urine retention and bladder dysfunction.
- Urine incontinence, anal sphincter dysfunction.
- Sepsis predisposed by prolonged labour and genital tract trauma during the delivery.
- Spinal sprain and nerve root damage due to excessive traction force.
- Separation of the public symphysis.

B. *Fetal Complications of Forceps Delivery*

Common complications to the foetus include:

- Asphyxia
- Birth seizures
- Scalp lacerations
- Supratentorial haemorrhage

- Subdural and subarachnoid haemorrhage following skull fractures and compression
- Cephalohematoma
- Facial abrasion from undue compression or slipping of the forceps
- Facial nerve damage leading to facial palsy
- Fractures of the face and skull
- Rarely, clavicle fractures
- Intracranial haemorrhage, sometimes leading to death

Forceps delivery is associated with more complications than vacuum extraction [11].

16.2.12 Post-operative Care

- The patient's vital signs should be monitored closely.
- Observe for vaginal bleeding and vulval hematoma.
- Perineal toileting with cetrimide or chlorhexidine lotion twice daily.
- Antibiotics and analgesia are given as indicated.

16.3 Vacuum Extractor (Ventouse)

The vacuum extractor or ventouse is an instrument designed to assist vaginal delivery by applying traction on the fetal scalp.

The vacuum extractor uses suction as a means of assistance. A cup (which can either be hard or soft, metal or plastic) is attached to the top of the baby's head. This cup is connected to a suction device which once switched on will gently pull the baby from the vagina.

16.3.1 History of the Vacuum Extractor

The vacuum extractor was first described in 1705 by Dr. James Yonge who was an English Surgeon several decades before the invention of the obstetric forceps [9]. However, it did not gain widespread use until the 1950s, when it was popularised in a series of studies by the Swedish obstetrician Dr. Tage Maelstrom.

By the 1970s, the vacuum extractor had almost completely replaced the forceps for assisted vaginal deliveries in most Northern European countries, but its popularity in many English speaking countries, including the United States and the United Kingdom was limited. By 1992, however, the number of vacuum-assisted deliveries surpassed the number of forceps deliveries in West Africa, and by the year 2000 and more than 66% of all operative vaginal deliveries were by vacuum [9].

The choice to use the vacuum extraction depends on the Operator's experience and skill, fetal condition and the available resources (instruments).

16.3.2 Types of Vacuum Extractors

A. *Metal Cup*

The metal-cup vacuum extractor is a mushroom-shaped metal cup varying from 40 to 60 mm in diameter. A centrally attached chain connects the cup to a detachable handle that is used to apply traction. A mechanical or electrical suction device is attached to the metal cup via a peripherally located vacuum port [12].

The advantages of metal-cup vacuum extraction over soft-cup extraction include a higher success rate and easier cup placement in the occipito-posterior (OP) position, especially when an OP cup is used [13]. Unfortunately, the rigidity of metal cups can make application difficult and uncomfortable, and their use is associated with an increased risk of fetal scalp injuries [14]. Metal-cup vacuum extractors are rarely used in the United States.

B. *Soft Cups*

Compared with metal-cup devices, soft-cup vacuum extractors cause fewer neonatal scalp injuries. However, these instruments have a higher failure rate [13].

Soft-cup instruments can be used with a manual vacuum pump or an electrical suction device. Some have a built-in-vacuum-release value that allows pressure to be rapidly attained and accurately controlled. This results in easy manoeuvrability and simplicity of operation. Soft-cup vacuum extractions may be disposable or reusable.

Traditionally, the soft cups are bell or funnel shaped (Fig. 16.4). A newer variety, the mushroom-shaped vacuum cup, or M-cup, combines the advantages of soft and metal cups [15]. The soft sidewall of the M-cup minimises infant scalp trauma compared with the Maelstrom metal cup [16] (Figs. 16.5 and 16.6).

16.3.3 Indications for Vacuum Assisted Delivery

The indications for vacuum extraction are mostly the same as for forceps delivery. In addition the vacuum extractor can be used in situations where the forceps should not be used, such as in cases of cord prolapse or severe fetal distress when the cervix is not fully dilated but is about 8 cm dilated. It can

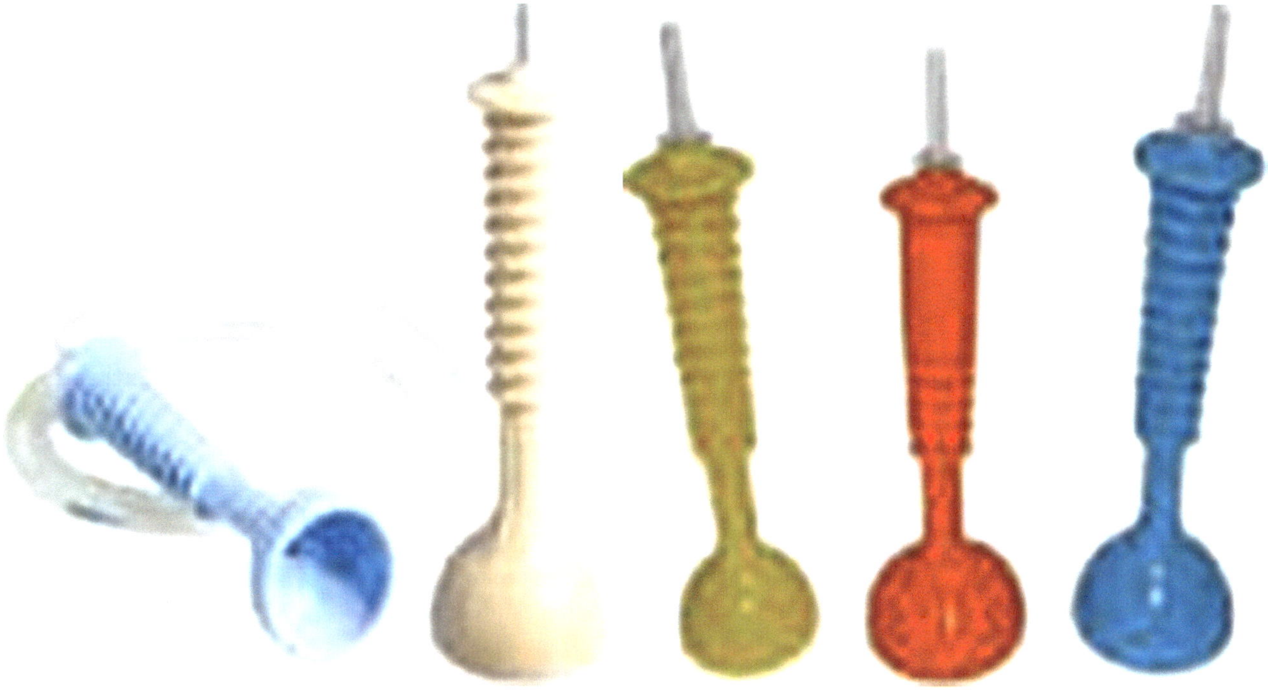

Fig. 16.4 Auto-clavable silicon cups

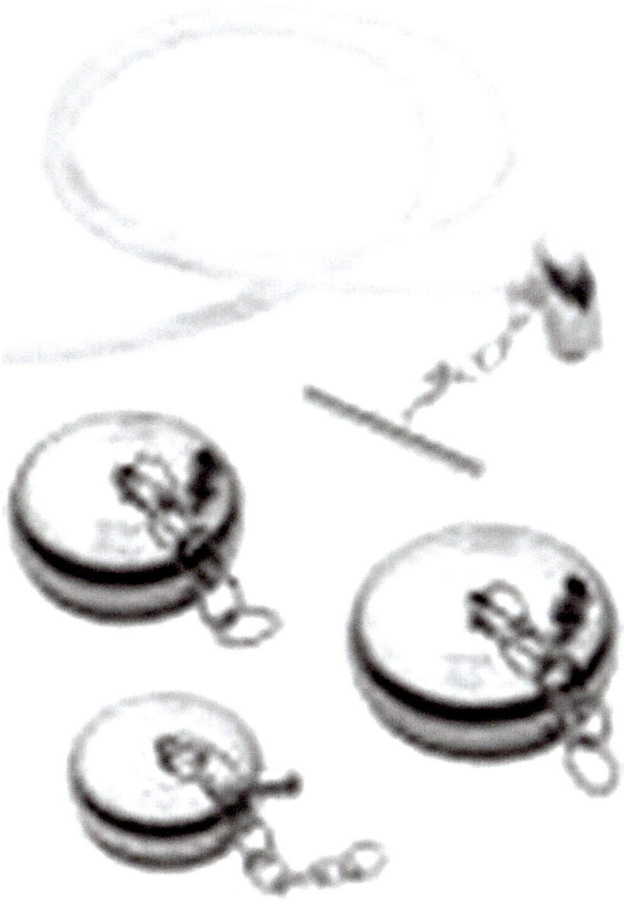

Fig. 16.5 Maelstrom suction cups

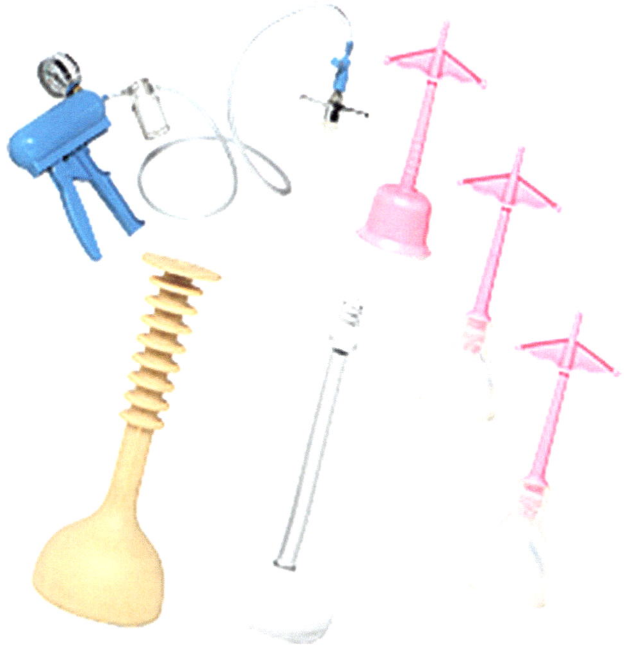

Fig. 16.6 Disposable polyethylene bell-shaped cups (disposable mushroom-shaped cups, reusable siliconebell-shaped cups, manual vacuum pumps, adaptors)

also be used to deliver the second twin in vertex presentation when the head is not engaged [5].

A. *Maternal Indications for Vacuum Extraction*
   1. *Elective Indications*
      In situations where excessive maternal expulsive effort could be detrimental to her cardio-pulmonary system and shortening of the second stage of labour is required.
- Cardiac disease
- Severe hypertension or pre-eclampsia
- Severe anaemia, including sickle cell anaemia in imminent crises
- Pulmonary disease including tuberculosis
- Thyroid disease
   2. *Emergency Indications*
- Maternal disease on exhaustion
- Intrapartum haemorrhage in the second stage of labour, for example abruptio placenta
- Delayed second stage of labour due to lack of, or delayed progress due to poor maternal expulsive effort, conduction anaesthesia
- Eclampsia
- Sickle cell disease patient in imminent crisis

B. *Fetal Indications for Vacuum Extraction*
Fetal indications which are almost always an emergency include:
Fetal distress in the second stage of labour
Cord prolapse when the cervix is 8 cm or more dilated
Abruptio placenta in second stage of labour
Second twin with vertex presentation
Fetal distress in the second stage of labour

16.3.4 Conditions That Must Be Fulfilled Before Embarking on Vacuum Extraction

The prerequisites for vacuum extraction are similar to forceps delivery.

1. The cervix must be at least 8 cm dilated.
2. The membranes must be ruptured.
3. The vertex must be presenting.
4. The position of the vertex must be known with certainty.
5. The fetal head must be engaged (except in cases of the second twin with vertex presentation).
6. There should be no significant cephalopelvic disproportion.
7. The bladder must be empty.
8. The operator must have the requisite experience or if he/she is now acquiring the skill, an experienced operator must be present.
9. The operator must have the willingness to abandon the procedure when it fails.
10. Anaesthesia and/or episiotomy are not always required for vacuum extraction.
11. Caesarean section and neonatal facilities must be available.

16.3.5 Contraindication for Vacuum Extraction

Vacuum delivery is contraindicated:

- If any of the above listed prerequisites is not met.
- Fetal malposition or malpresentation.
- Face or brow presentation.
- Breech presentation.
- Transverse lie.
- Prematurity. If the Gestational age <34 weeks. This is due to the increased risk of cephalohematoma.
- Cephalopelvic disproportion.
- It is also avoided in cases of fetal coagulopathy, and if fetal scalp blood sampling has been done due to increased likelihood of bleeding from the site.
- Patients with HIV.
- Suspected fetal macrosomia.

16.3.6 Technique of Vacuum Extraction

A successful vacuum-assisted vaginal delivery is dependent on several factors, including patient selection and a number of technical considerations. The goal is for correct placement of the vacuum cup on the fetal scalp. Application of a vacuum of up to 0.8 kg/cm^3 to suck part of the fetal scalp into the cup and create an artificial caput succedaneum (known as a chignon), and then application of a traction forceps to the foetus in concert with uterine contractions to expedite delivery.

A. *Preparation for Vacuum Delivery*
   Before attempting the procedure of vacuum delivery the following preparation should be done.
   1. The patient is counselled on the procedure, including the possibility of a caesarean section should it fail.
   2. Both the rigid and soft cup must ideally be available.
   3. If the fetal head is flexed and synclitic, the soft cup must be used. If the head is deflexed or asynclitic, or malpositioned the rigid or any metal cup is preferable.

4. Prior to applying the cup to the fetal head, the operator must assemble the vacuum and test it for sustained negative pressure on the palm of the gloved hand.
5. Anaesthetic requirements.

   These may include any of the following:

- None.
- Local infiltration.
- The line of the episiotomy is infiltrated with 10 mL of 1% lignocaine (Xylocaine).
- Pudendal block.

6. The patient must:

- Be positional in the lithotomy position and the thighs and vulva prepared and draped.
- The bladder should be empty.

B. *The Procedure*

This involves in:

1. Application of the vacuum cap
2. Creation of the negative pressure
3. Traction (Fig. 16.7)

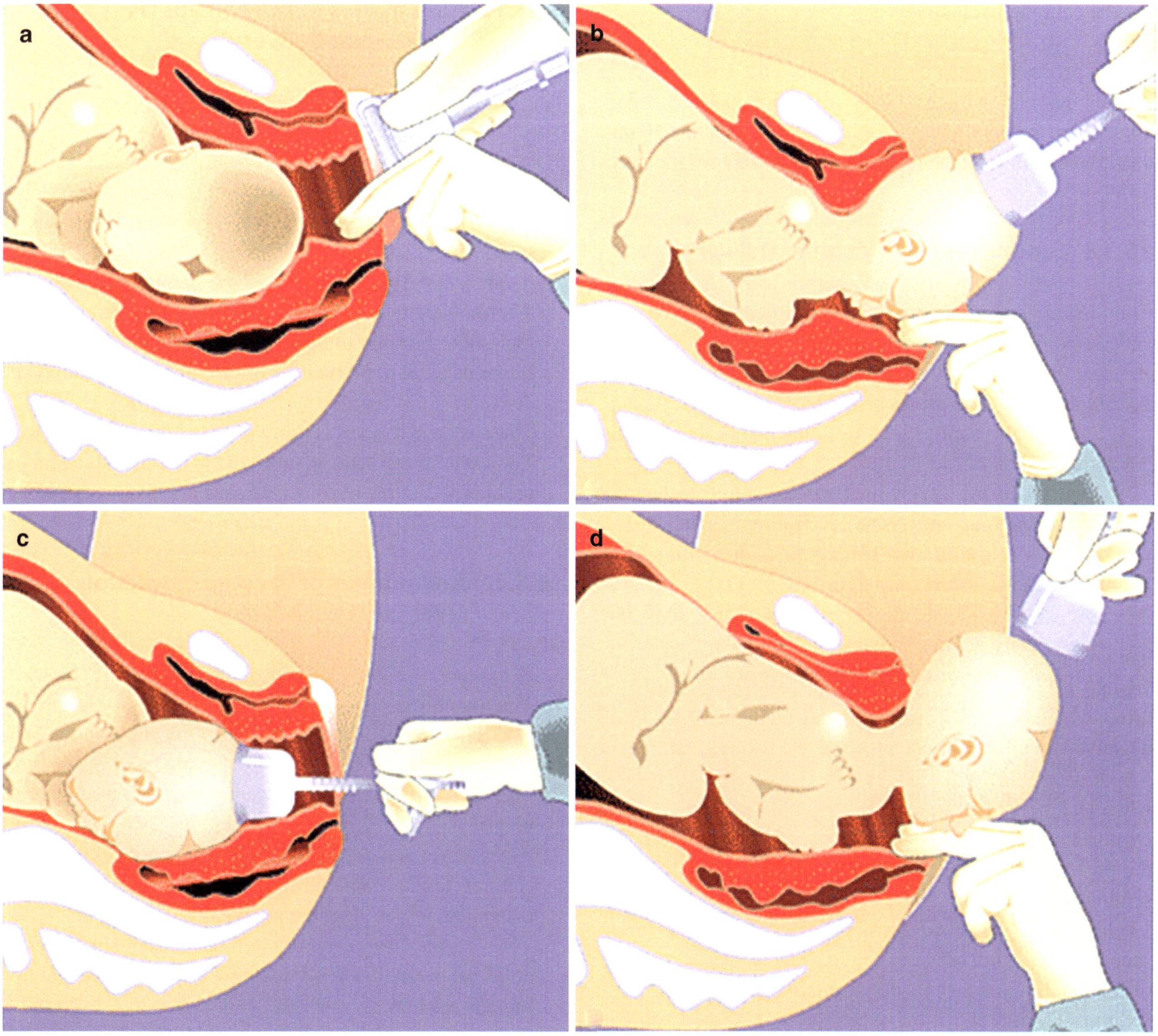

Fig. 16.7 Technique of vacuum delivery [17]. Using the vacuum device for delivery. After determining position of the head, (**a**) insert the cup into the vaginal vault, ensuring that no maternal tissues are trapped by the cup. (**b**) Apply the cup to the flexion point 3 cm in front of the posterior fontanel, centring the sagittal suture. (**c**) Pull during a contraction with a steady motion, keeping the device at right angles to the plane of the cup. In occipitoposterior deliveries, maintain the right angle if the fetal head rotates. (**d**) Remove the cup when the fetal jaw is reachable

16.3.7 Failed Vacuum Delivery

Failed vacuum delivery occurs when a vaginal delivery is not achieved after attempting a vacuum extraction. The causes of this are:

- Lack of experience
- Wrong patient selection as with cephalopelvic disproportion or an unanticipated greater degree of fetal head deflexion, e.g. brow presentation
- Traction not in the axis of the birth canal
- Not pulling hard enough or pulling too hard
- The equipment is faulty

The procedure must be abandoned in the absence of significant descent of the fetal head after three pulls. Similarly application delivery interval should not be more than 30 minutes. Beyond this the incidence of fetal morbidities increases.

16.3.8 Complications of Vacuum Delivery

Complications tend to be minimal if precautions are taken and prerequisites and contradictions are met.

A. *Maternal Complications of Vacuum Delivery*

   Maternal complications from the use of the ventouse include:
   - Injuries to the vagina and cervix leading to haemorrhage and may later cause cervical incompetence
   - Injuries to the urethra bladder and /or rectum which may lead to fistula formation
   - Weakening of the uterine support which may later cause utero vaginal prolapse

B. *Fetal Complications of Vacuum Delivery*

   Fetal complications from the use of the ventouse include:
   - Scalp abrasions are relatively common and are usually of no clinical significance
   - Cephalohematoma. This is more common in difficult vacuum deliveries
   - Sub-galeal haemorrhage
   - Fetal asphyxia with or without anoxic encephalopathy
   - Intracranial haemorrhage
   - Tentorial tears
   - Neonatal jaundice
   - Alopecia

16.3.9 Medico Legal Concerns in Operative Vaginal Delivery

Before an instrumental delivery is initiated, the patient and her husband should be given a clear explanation of the risks and benefits of the procedure for the mother and foetus. Advising the patient that an attempt at instrumental delivery may not result in vaginal delivery may avoid unrealistic expectations. Avoiding the use of these instruments when the foetus is high in the pelvis or the mother is not pushing can reduce the risk of complications.

Following an attempted assisted delivery, documentation should include the indication for the procedure, a record of the discussion with the patient and a detailed description of the procedure itself [12, 18].

16.3.10 Advantages of the Forceps Over the Vacuum Delivery

The forceps has some advantages over the vacuum extraction. These include:

1. In experienced and skilled hands it results in faster delivery of the foetus and hence is very useful in cases of severe fetal distress or cord prolapse.
2. It can be safety used to deliver the premature infant with a birth weight less than 1.5 kg where the ventouse is thought to be contraindicated.
3. It can be used to deliver the after-coming head in breech delivery.
4. The obstetric forceps is more portable than the ventouse.
5. The vacuum extractor is more likely to develop technical problems than the obstetric forceps.

16.3.11 Advantages of Vacuum Extraction Over Forceps Delivery

1. The technique of vacuum extraction is easily learnt and the skill more easily acquired compared to the forceps.
2. The vacuum cap does not occupy space in the maternal pelvis.
3. Anaesthesia is not a prerequisite for vacuum extraction.
4. Natural forces come into play. The mother pushes to assist delivery as it occurs in spontaneous delivery.
5. The vacuum has an inbuilt safety mechanism. The cap pulls off from the fetal scalp when excessive traction force is applied.
6. Failed vacuum delivery is associated with fewer complications to the mother and the baby.
7. Vacuum extraction can be used in the late first stage of labour.
8. Compared to forceps delivery, with vacuum extraction there are fewer maternal and fetal complications.
9. With a vacuum extractor, traction causes auto-rotation of the fetal head unlike with forceps delivery and hence is

useful in occipito-posterior and occipito-transverse positions.

16.3.12 Controversies in Operative Vaginal Deliveries [5]

There are some controversies associated with the use of both instruments. Some of these are:

1. *Should there be Trial of Operative Vaginal Delivery?*
   Careful and thorough patient evaluation is paramount. The skill of the operator cannot be over emphasised for a successful outcome.
2. *Should non-specialist doctors be taught and encouraged to practice forceps delivery?*
   The developing world is being encouraged to use operative vaginal deliveries.
3. *Creation of negative pressure in vacuum extraction.*
   Randomised controlled studies have shown that rapid creation of the vacuum significantly reduces the duration of a vacuum extraction procedure without compromising to efficiency and safety [5].
4. *Do we have to reduce the vacuum in-between contractions and does maintenance of vacuum and traction force in-between contractions (to prevent loss of fetal head station) lead to faster and better delivery outcome?*
   This will allow both the operator and the mother some rest and also enable the operator to recheck for any soft tissue entrapment, and descent of the fetal head with the previous traction.
5. *Does the use of the vacuum extraction in preterm babies increase the risk of intracranial haemorrhage?*
   Until better evidence becomes available, preterm babies of less than 34 weeks should continue to be a contraindication.

16.4 Destructive Operations

Obstructed labour is one of the common causes of maternal morbidity and mortality worldwide [19] and remains a common occurrence in developing countries such as Nigeria [20]. This is mainly as a result of some patients depriving themselves of antenatal care because of its cost despite increased awareness, and others choosing to deliver at home and in other places with no proper monitoring and supervision in labour and delivery.

In cases where the foetus is alive, an emergency caesarean section suffices to deliver the baby, but in others, fetal death may have occurred. The attendant sepsis of such neglect limits the use of caesarean section even when facilities are available [21].

In order to reduce maternal morbidity and mortality associated with caesarean section in these patients, destructive operations can be performed to deliver these dead foetuses per vaginam.

Destructive operations are procedures done to reduce the bulk of the foetus or divide it into parts to facilitate delivery per vaginam [19]. The procedures are unpleasant to perform and watch. In skilled hands and with the criteria for these procedures present, it is a safer and cheaper mode of delivery [22].

16.4.1 Prerequisites for Destructive Operations [23]

The following are prerequisites for destructive operations:

1. The foetus must be dead or malformed (not conducive to extra uterine life).
2. The operator must be skilled in the procedure.
3. The uterus must not be ruptured or at imminent rupture.
4. The cervix must be fully dilated.
5. The membrane must be ruptured.
6. The bladder must be empty.
7. Any metabolic disturbance must have to be corrected.

16.4.2 Contraindications to Destructive Operations [23]

There are basically three contraindications to destructive operations:

- Lack of necessary skills for the procedure.
- Rupture or an imminent rupture of the uterus.
- The baby is alive.

*None adherence to these and the prerequisites for destructive operations should be avoided.

16.4.3 Types of Destructive Operations

Destructive operations are fairly technical procedures requiring special training and some experience to ensure safety. The following are the main destructive operations.

1. *Craniotomy*
   Craniotomy is usually done for the delivery of a dead foetus following prolonged obstructed labour in a cephalic presenting foetus. In obstructed labour the head is usually driven down firmly into the pelvic brim where it becomes impacted. Craniotomy is advisable in such circumstances

but if the head is high above the brim especially in extreme degrees of pelvic contractions then craniotomy is difficult [24]. Dangerous and subsequent extraction of the foetus may be impossible and caesarean section is safer in such situations.

The Procedure [23]

In craniotomy the cervix must be at least 6 cm dilated and at least 2/5 of the head must have gone into the maternal pelvis. The objective is to reduce the size of the fetal head and achieve a vaginal delivery.

It is the commonest type of destructive operation done in Nigeria [22, 23].

The fetal head is perforated using the Simpson's perforator (or any other suitable instrument) and the foetus is extracted by traction using the Volselum. Kocher's forceps or any other strong forceps is attached to the edges of the perforation. Occasionally traction force on the Volselum provided through a pulley attached to a weighted object hanging down the perineum is utilised to achieve steady descent of the presenting part.

After delivery, the bladder should be on continuous drainage for 10 to 14 days to prevent development of a vesico-vaginal fistula.

2. *Cleidotomy*

   This procedure is indicated to complete the extraction of a large dead foetus by reducing the size of the shoulder girdle following the delivery of the head [24]. This is achieved by dividing the clavicle with a stout embryotomy scissors. The more accessible clavicle is usually divided first, thereby reducing the size of the shoulder girdle to facilitate the delivery of the baby.

3. *Embyotomy or Evisceration*

   The procedure is done for an abdominal tumour or a very large foetus following craniotomy or cleidotomy. The incision is made in the abdomen or thorax of the foetus if accessible using the embryotomy scissors. The contents are them removed manually. This leads to a reduction in the size of the foetus. It is most easily performed in breech presentation where the abdomen is easily approached. A caesarean section is advisable in cephalic presentations where the abdomen on thorax is not easily accessible.

4. *After-Coming Head of the Breech*

   Obstruction due to entrapped after-coming head of the breech can be delivered by craniotomy. This is done by perforating the head through the occiput and letting out some brain tissue. The head can then be delivered by using forceps as traction or by the Mauriceau–Smellie–Veit method.

5. *Decompression of a Hydrocephalic Head*

   The foetus with a hydrocephalic head can be decompressed by perforating the head at its most accessible point on vaginal examination. This can be done before full dilatation of the cervix. Any sharp instrument like the Simpson's perforator, Drew Smythe catheter, spinal bifida needle, a pair of scissors on surgical blade mounted on a scalpel can be used to perforate the head. A trans-abdominal route can also be employed with the aid of a spinal needle in a breech presenting foetus with spina bifida. Cerebrospinal fluid (CSF) can be withdrawn by exposing the spinal canal and passing a catheter into the canal and up into the cranium. The collapsed head is subsequently delivered vaginally.

6. *Decapitation*

   This procedure is usually done when obstructed labour is due to an impacted shoulder presentation and the foetus is dead. The neglected prolapsed arm soon becomes edematous giving an impression of a large foetus. (The foetus is lying transverse).

   The prolapsed hand is held (but if not prolapsed, is pulled out of the vagina) before the decapitation of the fetal head is done. Decapitation can be achieved using a stout scissors, Blond-Heidler Thimble and Saw or Jardine Decapitation Hook. After decapitation, the foetus (minus the head) is delivered by traction on the hand already held. The decapitated hand can be delivered.

16.4.4 Post-operative Management After a Destructive Operation

After a destructive operation, the following must be done [5]:

- The vagina, cervix and lower uterus must be explored for injuries.
- The bladder must be catheterised and the catheter should be kept in situ for 5–14 days. This is to rest the bladder and thus prevent fistula formation.
- Potent broad spectrum antibiotics must be given.
- Enough intravenous fluids must be given to correct dehydration, ensure adequate urinary output and bladder drainage. There should be no hurry in commencing oral intake since the patients are prone to paralytic ileus.
- The patient who has had a destructive operation should be managed post-operatively like a patient with obstructed labour.

16.4.5 Complications of Destructive Operations

The complications of destructive operations can due to the primary indications for the destructive operation, i.e. obstructive or difficult deliveries [24] or due to the procedure itself [23].

The complications of the destructive operations and obstructive labour may also overlap and indeed become undistinguishable [24].

These complications include maternal morbidities such as uterine rupture, puerperal sepsis, postpartum haemorrhage, vesico-vaginal and/or recto-vaginal fistulae, lacerations (vaginal or cervical laceration, perianal tear, bladder laceration) and dyspareunia [23, 24]. Others are endotoxic shock and puerperal psychosis [24].

Destructive Operations can also result in maternal death.

16.5 Symphysiotomy

Symphysiotomy is a surgical procedure in which the cartilage of the pubic symphysis is divided to widen the pelvis allowing childbirth when there is a mechanical problem. It is also known as pelviotomy [25], synchondrotomy [25], pubiotomy [26] and Gigli's operation after Leonardo Gigli, who invented a saw commonly used in Europe to accomplish the operation.

Symphysiotomy is intended to widen the maternal pelvis by dividing the fibro-cartilage of the symphysis pubis thereby facilitating vaginal delivery of the foetus in the presence of mild to moderate cephalic pelvic disproportion [27].

Historically, the first symphysiotomy was performed by Percival Willoughby in 1665 as an alternative to post mortem caesarean section. Its use was however first popularised in the Irish Roman Catholic community to forestall the possible limitation of family size by the use of caesarean section. Even in non-Catholic countries like Great Britain, symphysiotomy was performed in the first half of the twentieth century [28]. It has also been reported that the procedure was practiced by traditional healers in several parts of Africa [29, 30]. A review of literature showed that most communications on symphysiotomy since 1960 emanated from Africa [31] although one has been documented from Papua, New Guinea [32].

16.5.1 Technique

At present, the procedure is practiced using Seedat Crichton's method [33], which is based on Zarate's work [34]. It differs from Zarate's in the sense that complete division of the symphysis is done instead of the partial advocated by Zarate. This is to prevent forceful abduction that could occur in partial divisions. The forceful abduction damages the sacro-iliac joints, possibly resulting in permanent pelvic instability and pain. The authors also avoid hyaline cartilage by strict adherence to the midline during the divisions, as deviation from this will also result in osteitis pubis and subsequent difficulty in walking.

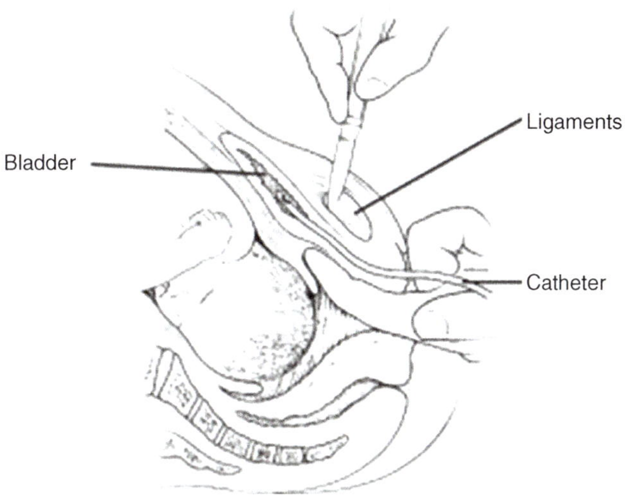

Fig. 16.8 Dividing the cartilage in symphysiotomy

Symphysiotomy increases the pelvic diameters, particularly the transverse diameters. The bottom ends of the symphyseal joints separate more than the upper ends, thus making the outlet diameters increase more than the inlet ones. This does not imply that symphysiotomy is only indicated in outlet disproportion as previously thought by some authors [28].

It is important to avoid undue strain on the sacro-iliac joints by avoiding forceful abduction of the thighs; complete separation should be brought about by the use of scalpel only (Fig. 16.8).

16.5.2 Indications for Symphysiotomy

- Cephalopelvic disproportion with vertex presentation and a live foetus.
- Failed trial of vacuum extraction or forceps delivery in second stage of labour.
- Breech presentation to prevent entrapment of the after coming head.
- Appropriate descent of fetal head. At least two-thirds should have entered the pelvic brim.
- Degree of overlap as a result of fetal head moulding, and dilatation of the cervix, which should be more than 6–7 cm in a primigravida according to Gebbie's rules [35].

16.5.3 Management Protocol [24, 35, 36, 37]

The following conditions are usually fulfilled when symphysiotomy is to be performed:

1. Decide to carry out symphysiotomy after the third failed vacuum extraction pull on the fetal head.
2. Empty the bladder and catheterise the patient.
3. Anaesthetise the perineum with the patient in the lithotomy position, ensure that the angles between the legs are not more than 80 degrees, and avoid excessive abduction with a resultant strain on the sacro-iliac joints.
4. Guard the urethra with the index and middle fingers of the left hand.
5. Perform symphysiotomy by closed method and complete the procedure by inserting thumb into the divided joint. This promotes further descent and further dilatation of the cervix, thereafter the expulsion of the foetus can start.
6. Perform a large episiotomy to relieve tension on the anterior vaginal wall, abduct the legs at the crowning of the head and apply the vacuum extractor to complete the delivery. Do not apply forceps.
7. After delivery of the foetus and placenta, compress the symphysis by the thumb above and index and middle fingers beneath for some minutes to express blood clots and achieve haemostasis.
8. Explore the uterus and genital tracts for evidence of uterine rupture or genital lacerations.
9. Close the skin incision of the symphyseal site before repairing the episiotomy.
10. Post-operatively, nurse the patient on her sides and strap the knees together. Catheterise for three days or for ten days if haematuria is present. In case of suspected fistulae, catheterise for six weeks.
11. Administer broad-spectrum antibiotics.
12. Encourage early mobilisation and physiotherapy.
13. On discharge, advice the patient to refrain from lifting heavy objects and hard physical work for three months.
14. Hospital deliveries are advocated for future pregnancies.

16.5.4 Maternal Mortality and Morbidity

Maternal mortality after symphysiotomy has been described as almost negligible. There were three maternal deaths from a total of 1752 Symphysiotomies (1.7/1000 births). The deaths were not related to the procedure of symphysiotomy: two were caused by eclampsia while one was due to complications following caesarean sections [34].

The maternal morbidities encountered are vesico-vaginal fistula (1.7%); urethral/ vestibular lesions (1.9%); osteitis pubis/retropubic abscess (0.6%); walking disability/pains (1.8%) and stress incontinence (2.0%). The quoted perinatal mortality following symphysiotomy varies. A range of 19–296 per 1000 has been reported with an overall rate of 112 [34].

Comparison of symphysiotomy with caesarean section has been done by some authors [32, 38, 39]. Caesarean section demonstrated higher rates of maternal mortality, morbidity and perinatal mortality. The outcome of labour in women with a history of previous symphysiotomy is also reviewed. Uncomplicated vaginal delivery occurred in 73% while operative vaginal delivery took place in 14%, with caesarean births in 11% and repeat symphysiotomy in 2% of the cases.

The vaginal delivery rate after previous symphysiotomy is higher than after previous caesarean section for disproportion: 85% versus 44% [40].

16.6 Episiotomy

An episiotomy, also known as perineotomy, is the surgical enlargement of the vaginal orifice by an incision of the perineum during the last part of the second stage of labour to facilitate the birth of the baby.

Carl Braun (1857) coined the term episiotomy [41] and a report as far back as 1741 suggested the first surgical opening of the perineum to prevent severe perineal tears [42].

Too frequent recourse to episiotomy suggests bad management of the second stage of labour [43]. An episiotomy must be performed at the right time and place and repaired properly within a short time after delivery. The primary reason to perform an episiotomy is to prevent a spontaneous large, irregular laceration of the perineum. A controlled surgical incision is usually easier to repair than a spontaneous laceration. The repair of a surgical incision is also more likely to be anatomically correct, and thus, less likely to result in long-term complications [43, 44].

16.6.1 Types of Episiotomy

There are four types of episiotomy. The first three are in common practice. Whichever type of episiotomy that is performed, the incision must start from the midline.

1. *Mediolateral episiotomy*. This is the commonest type of episiotomy. It is a cut given at an angle of 45 degrees from the midline towards the ischial tuberosity avoiding the anal sphincter. It can be made on the right or the left side of the perineum.

   The anatomical structures incised include the vaginal epithelium, transverse perineal and bulbocavernosus muscles and perineal skin. If the incision is large, adipose tissue within the ischiorectal fossa may be exposed.

Advantage

- Extension into the anal sphincter is not common

Disadvantages

- It is more difficult to repair (apposition of the tissues is not good)
- More painful in the puerperium (postapartum discomfort is more)
- Faulty healing is more common
- Dyspareunia occasionally follows
- Blood loss is greater
- Anatomical results are not satisfactory in a few cases.

2. . *Midline (central or median) episiotomy*. It is a vertical incision starting from the fourchette and extends caudally in the midline.

   The anatomical structures involved in the incision include the vaginal epithelium, perineal body and the junction of the perineal body with the bulbocavernosus muscle in the perineum.

Advantages

- Easy to repair
- Blood loss is less
- Wound healing is faster
- Faulty healing is rare
- Less pain in the postpartum period
- Dyspareunia rarely follows
- Anatomic result is almost always excellent

Disadvantages

- Extension through the anal sphincter and rectum is common
- Not suitable for manipulative deliveries (Table 16.1).

3. *The J-Shaped Incision*. The incision starts at the fourchette and is initially extended caudally in the midline and then curved laterally at an angle similar to the letter 'J'. It is not commonly used.

   The anatomical structures incised include the vaginal epithelium, perineal body and the junction of the perineal body with the bulbocavernosus muscle and perineal skin.

   The purpose of the 'J' incision is to combine the advantages of the median and mediolateral techniques, while avoiding their disadvantages.
4. *The Lateral Incision*. The incision starts from about 1 cm away from the centre of the fourchette and extends laterally. The drawbacks include the chance of injury to the Bartholin's duct, therefore some people have discouraged the lateral incision.

Table 16.1 Midline versus mediolateral episiotomy

	Type of episiotomy	
Characteristic	Midline episiotomy	Mediolateral episiotomy
Surgical repair	Easy	More difficult
Faulty healing	Rare	More common
Post-operative pain	Minimal	Common
Anatomical results	Excellent	Occasional faulty
Blood loss	Less	More
Dyspareunia	Rare	Occasional
Extensions	Common	Uncommon

16.6.2 Benefits of an Episiotomy

(a) *Maternal Benefits*
   - A clean cut surgical incision is easier to repair than a ragged perineal tear.
   - It prevents undue stretching of the vaginal walls which predispose to future cystocele, rectocele, uterine prolapse, deficient perineum, loose vaginal outlet, stress urinary incontinence, anal canal and rectal injuries, and periclitoral injuries.
   - Shortens the duration of the second stage of labour.
   - Spares the mothers bearing down efforts.

(b) *Fetal Benefits*
   - It spares the fetal head from the compressive forces prior to its exit.
   - It is of great benefit to prevent injuries to preterm babies and high risk babies.

16.6.3 Indications for Episiotomy

These include:

1. Arrest of the progress of labour because of a rigid or inelastic perineum.
2. Prophylactic when the perineum threatens to tear as in:
   - Persistent occipito-posterior position
   - Extensive scarring of the perineum from previous repair of tears or female genital mutilation or a very tight perineum
3. To facilitate instrumental assisted vaginal delivery.

   All cases of forceps require episiotomy but not all ventouse cases require it.
4. To prevent prolonged compression of the fetal head.
5. To shorten the second stage of labour in high risk pregnancies.
6. To reduce the strain of bearing down efforts in women with medical disorders.

7. Breech delivery.
8. To facilitate quick delivery in fetal distress and/or cord prolapse.
9. In preterm labour to minimise the stress on the fetal head.
10. With macrosomic babies to increase manoeuvrability in the event of shoulder dystocia.
11. Previous pelvic floor surgery.

16.6.4 Technique of Episiotomy

- Prior to performing the episiotomy, adequate analgesia is obtained by local infiltration with 10 mL of 1% plain xylocaine (lidocaine). When regional or general anaesthesia has been instituted already, there is no need for the local anaesthetic.
- The incision is made when the presenting part is distending the perineum with uterine contractions (crowning) but before sufficient bruising and devitalisation occurs and tearing of the perineum is imminent. If it is performed too early, blood loss from insidious oozing will be unnecessarily excessive. The site of the incision may be influenced by the presence of a previous scar or imminent rupture. If the perineum is already tearing it is better to continue the line of the tear than to create another competing wound.
- The operation varies from an incision 2 cm long to one extending the length of the perineum. A mediolateral episiotomy is performed with an 8 inch straight scissors with blunt points or an episiotomy scissors. The fingers of one hand are inserted behind the fourchette and a straight cut is made between them. It is important to make sure that the incision starts from the midpoint of the fourchette. Any oozing between contractions can be controlled by applying pressure with a perineal pad or artery forceps (Fig. 16.9).

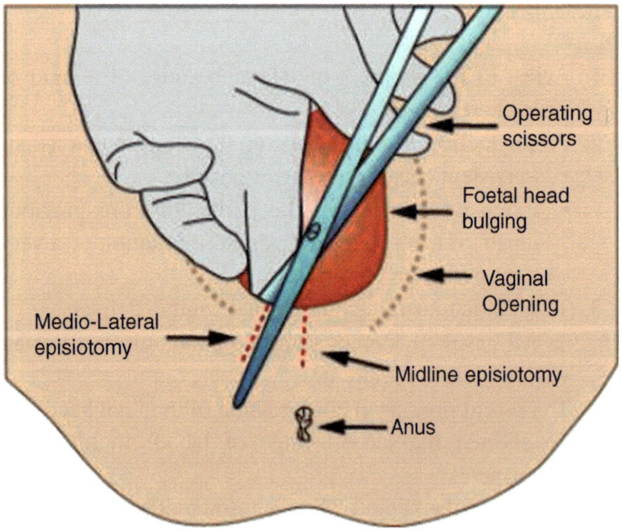

Fig. 16.9 Performing an episiotomy

16.6.5 Repair of an Episiotomy (Fig. 16.10)

- The repair should be taken with the same precautions as for any surgical procedure with very good light. The procedure should be explained to the mother and consent obtained.
- Prepare the instrument tray with all that is needed.
- The wound is cleaned with an antiseptic and all clots in the vagina are removed.
- A careful examination of the lower genital tract including the cervix, vaginal walls, and vulva and paraurethral areas is done looking out for any lacerations.
- The vagina is packed with gauze to prevent trickling of blood into the operation field from the genital tract above the wound.
- Local anaesthesia is then administered using infiltration of the operation area with 1% xylocaine.
- Identify the edges of the vaginal incision from the apex in the vaginal to the perineum; the incision is sutured in three layers beginning with the vaginal mucosa-suturing from the apex downwards using continuous sutures with 2/0 vicryl or chromic catgut. The second layer is the muscle, the cut edges of the perineal muscle are approximated with interrupted sutures of 1/0 vicryl or chromic catgut. Lastly the skin is sutured with interrupted 1/0 on subcuticular 2/0 vicryl or chromic catgut. Ensure haemostasis at the repair site.
- After the repair the vaginal gauge pack should be removed.
- A rectal examination is then done to feel for the stitch or defeat in the wall.
- Adequate pain relief with analgesics is important. Advice on perineal hygiene and vaginal toileting twice daily with chlorhexidine swabs or sitz-baths should be done and the perineum kept clean and dry with sanitary pads.
- Routine antibiotic prophylaxes are not indicated.
- Prior to discharge home all repairs should be evaluated.

16.6.6 After Care of an Episiotomy

Adequate pain relief with analgesia like paracetamol or ibuprofen is helpful. Perineal toileting is required after micturition and defecation. Patients are advised not to sit in warm or hot water, as is the practice. They could use tap water with a little salt or antiseptic solution. Antibiotics are not routinely given to patients with episiotomy. If pain is persistent or severe, it is essential to examine the perineum as this may signify a large vulval, paravaginal, or ischiorectalhaematoma or abscess.

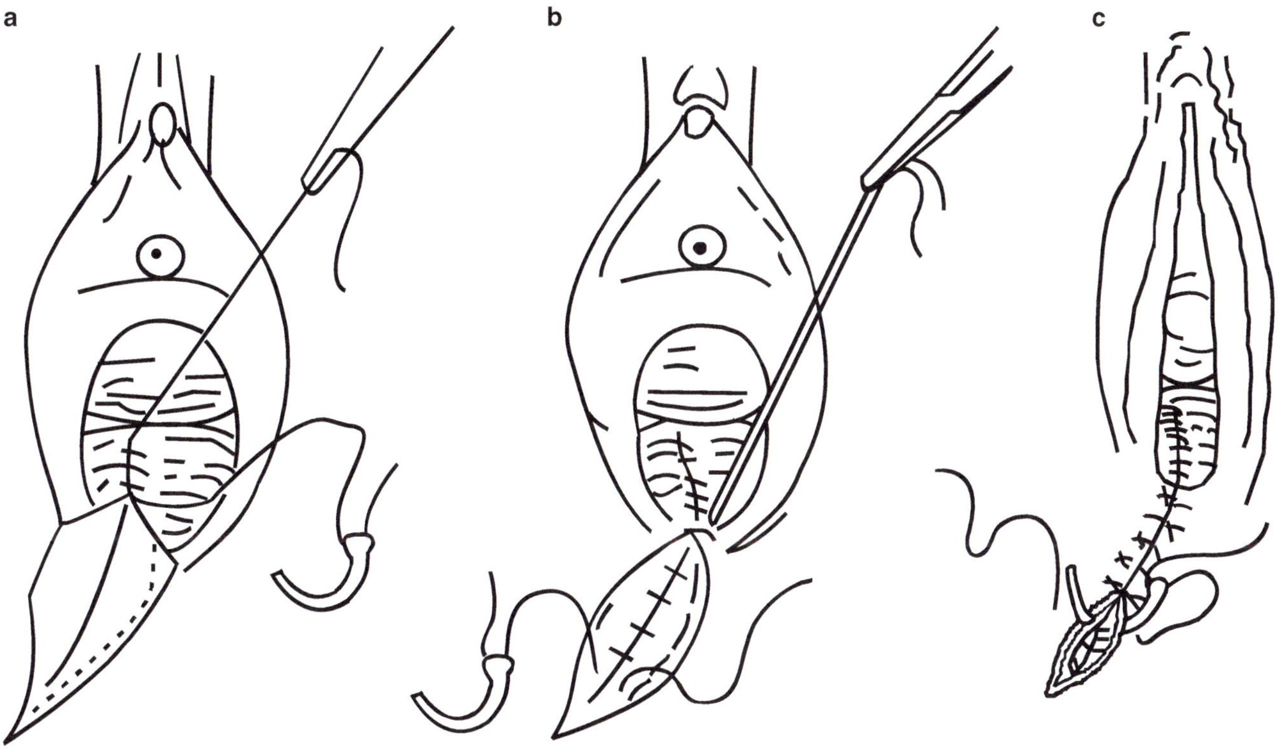

Fig. 16.10 Repair of episiotomy. (**a**) Vaginal mucosa. (**b**) Muscle layer. (**c**) Skin

16.6.7 Complications of Episiotomy

(a) *Maternal Complications*

Early complications

1. Haemorrhage. Bleeding may be very heavy.
2. Haematoma formation. Missing the apex of the episiotomy during repair can lead to haematoma formation.
3. Dehiscence or episiotomy breakdown. When an episiotomy breaks down, remove all stitches and open the entire wound. Debride wound and remove all necrotic tissues, evacuate haematoma and clean with hydrogen peroxide and hibitane daily. Re-suturing should be performed under adequate anaesthesia when the edges and floor of the wound is covered with pink granulation tissue.
4. Infection and wound breakdown. This is more likely when the episiotomy is contaminated or due to poor hygiene.
5. Extension to the anal sphincter or rectum causing a third degree tear.

Late complications

1. Pain and Dyspareunia. Very tight suturing, closing of skin over the fourchette can make the episiotomy very painful and on the long term patients may have superficial dyspareunia.
2. Psychosexual problems and a morbid fear of subsequent delivery.
3. Scar endometriosis can occur but is rare.
4. Possibility of perineal injuries in subsequent labour.

(b) *Fetal Complications*

1. Laceration of the fetal eye lid.
2. Castration (in breech delivery).
3. Increased risk of vertical transmission of HIV infection.
4. Risk of hypersensitivity to the local anaesthetic (xylocaine).

16.7 Conclusion

Operative vaginal deliveries still have a place in poor low resource and developing countries and are done to accomplish the delivery of the foetus through the vaginal route and thereby avoiding a caesarean section and its complications, morbidity and sometimes maternal mortality. In skilled hands they are fairly safe and easy procedures but the art is gradually dying as there is a decline in training of medical doctors and obstetricians on the use of these procedures.

Given the apparent association between difficult operative deliveries and increased morbidity, it is important that the operator attempts delivery only when vaginal delivery seems to be a safe option.

Operative vaginal deliveries can cause significant fetal morbidity and Paediatricians should be notified whenever any of these procedures is going to be performed.

References

1. Aimakhu CO, Olayemi O, Oladokun O, Iwe CAB, Umoh AV. Current practice of forceps and vacuum deliveries by Nigerian obstetricians. Trop J Obstet Gynaecol. 2014;21(1):40–3.
2. RCOG Green-top Guideline No. 26. Operative vaginal delivery, 2011.
3. Parazzini F, Cortinovis I, Restelli S, Bortolus R, Tozzi L. Vaginal deliveries in Italy. Acta Obstet Gynecol Scand. 1994;73:698–700.
4. Notzon FC, Bergsjo P, Coles S, Irgens LM, Daltveit AJ. International collaborative effort (ICE) on birth weight, plurality, perinatal, and infant mortality. IV. Differences in obstetrical delivery practice: Norway, Scotland and the United States. Acta Obstet Gynecol Scand. 1991;70:451–60.
5. Odoi AT, Opare HO. Operative vaginal delivery. In: Kwawukume EY, Ekele BA, Danso KA, Emuveyen EE, editors. Comprehensive obstetrics in the tropics. 2nd ed. Accra-North: Assemblies of God literature centre Ltd; 2015. Chapter 46. p. 422–34.
6. Gei AF, Belfort MA. Forceps assisted vaginal delivery. Obstet Gynecol Clin North Am. 1999;26(2):345–70.
7. Hankins GDV, Rowe TF. Operative vaginal delivery – year 2000. Am J Obstet Gynecol. 1996;175:272–82.
8. Aimakhu CO, Olayemi O, Enabor OO, Oluyemi FA, Aimakhu VE. Forceps delivery at the University College HospitalU.C.H., Ibadan, Nigeria. West Afr J Med. 2003;22(3):222–4.
9. Iklaki C. Operative Vaginal Delivery (OVD). In: Udoma ET, Ekanem EI, editors. Textbook of clinical obstetrics in the tropics for undergraduate and post-graduate students. Calabar alabar Pr: University of Calabar Press; 2014Chapter 45. p. 283–97.
10. Figure3: http://helid.digicollection.org/fr/d/Jwho43e/5.2.3.html# Jwho43e.5.2.3. From:Surgery at the District Hospital: Obstetrics, Gynaecology, Orthopaedics and Traumatology (WHO; 1991; 207 pages).
11. Demissie K, Rhoads GG, Smulian JC, et al. Operative vaginal delivery and neonatal and infant adverse outcomes: population based retrospective analysis. Br Med J. 2004;329:24–9.
12. Nargolkar S, Sexena M. Operative delivery. In: Puri R, Malhotra N, editors. Operative obstetrics and gynaecology. New Delhi: Jaypee Brothers Medical Publishers (P) Ltd; 2008. Chapter 21. p. 176–86.
13. Johanson R, Memom V. Soft versus rigid vacuum extraction cups for assisted vaginal delivery. Cochrane Database Syst Rev. 2000;2:CD 000446.
14. Kuit JA, Eppinga HC, Wallenburg HC, Huikeshoven FJ. A randomised comparison of vacuum extraction delivery with a rigid and a pliable cup. Obstet Gynecol. 1993;82:280–4.
15. Bofill JA, Rust OA, Schorr SJ, Brown RC, Martin RW, Martin JN, et al. A randomised prospective trial of the obstetric forceps versus the M-cup vacuum extractor. Am J Obstet Gynecol. 1996;175:1325–30.
16. Ross MG. Vacuum delivery by soft cup extraction. Contemp Obs Gyn. 1994;39:48–53.
17. Damos JR, Bassett R. Chapter H: assisted vaginal delivery. In: Advanced Life Support in Obstetrics (ALSO) provider syllabus. 4th ed. Leawood, Kan: American Academy of Family Physicians; 2003. p. 3–8.
18. Cutting your legal risk with vacuum – assisted vaginal delivery. OBG management 1999, March Page 22. Retrieved March 2016 from the World Wide Web.
19. World Health Organization. Reduction of maternal mortality. A Joint WHO/UNFPA /UNICEF /World Bank Statement, 1999.
20. Ozumba BC, Uchegbu H. Incidence and management of obstructed labour in Eastern Nigeria. Austr NZJ Obstet Gynaecol. 1991;31:231–6.
21. Aimakhu VE. The place of craniotomy in obstetric practice. Nig Med J. 1975;5(1):38–41.
22. Aimakhu CO, Olayemi O, Enabor OO, Ayinde OA. Destructive operations: still a relevant mode of delivery in developing countries. Nigerian Clin Rev. 2004;8(4):12–6.
23. Ande ABA. Instrument deliveries: destructive operations. In: Okepere EE, editor. Clinical obstetrics. Revised ed. Benin City: University of Benin Press; 2007. Section F4. p. 329–31.
24. Ilesanmi AO. Operative vaginal delivery. In: Okonofua F, Odunsi K, editors. Contemporary obstetrics and gynaecology for developing countries. Lagos: Inter Printers Limited; 2003. Chapter 26. p. 477–501.
25. Symphysiotomy (http://dictionary.reference.com/browse/symphysiotomy), The American Heritage Stedman's Medical Dictionary. Retrieved 15 April 2015, from Dictionary.com.
26. Hunter N. Asymphysiotomy victim's story. (http://www.irishhealth.com/article.html?id=16909), February 19, 2010. Irish Health.
27. Adeoye IS. Symphysiotomy. In: Okpere EE, editor. Clinical Obstetrics. Revised ed. Benin City, Nigeria: University of Benin Press; 2007.Section F5. p. 332–6.
28. Munro Kerr JM. The investigation and treatment of borderline cases of contracted pelvis. J Obstet Gynecol Br Emp. 1948;55:401–17.
29. Pereira JS. A sinfisiotomianaobstetricamoderna. Anals Inst Med Topical. 1964;21:153–9.
30. van der Linden AJ. Symphysiotomy and pubiotomy.Thesis, Utrect, 1961.
31. van Roosmalen J. Symphysiotomy – a reappraisal for the developing world. In: Studd J, editor. Progress in obstetrics and gynaecology, vol. 9. Edinburgh: Churchill Livingstone; 1991. p. 149–62.
32. Mola G, Lamang M, McGoldrick IA. A retrospective study of matched symphysiotomies and caesarean section at Port Moresby General Hospital, Papau. New Guinea Med J. 1981;24:103–12.
33. Seedat EK, Crichton D. Symphysiotomy: technique, indications and limitations. Lancet. 1962;1:554–9.
34. Zarate E. Subcutaneous partial symphysiotomy. Buenos Aires: TICA; 1992.
35. Gebbie DAM. Symphysiotomy. Trop Doct. 1974;4:69–75.
36. Gebbie DAM. Symphysiotomy. Clin Obstet Gynaecol. 1982;9:663–8.
37. Crichton D, Seedat EK. The technique of symphysiotomy. S Afr Med J. 1963;37:227–31.
38. van Roosmalen J. Symphysiotomy as an alternative to caesarean section. Int Gynaecol Obstet. 1987;25:451–8.
39. Hartfield VJ. A comparison of the early and late effects of subcutaneous symphysiotomy and of lower segment caesarean section. J Obstet Gynaecol Br Commonwealth. 1973;80:508–14.
40. van Roosmalen J. Maternal health care in the south western highland of Tanzania. PhD Thesis, Leiden, 1988.
41. Nungent FB. The primiparous perineum after forceps delivery. Am J Obstet Gynaecol. 1935;30:249–56.
42. Ould F. Atreatise of midwifery. London J Buckland. 1741:145–6.
43. Kwawukume EY, Samba A. Episiotomy and perineal tears. In: Kwawukume EY, Ekele BA, Danso KA, Emuveyen EE, editors. Comprehensive obstetrics in the tropics. 2nd ed. Accra-North, Ghana: Assemblies of God literature centre Ltd; 2015. Chapter 47. p. 435–9.
44. Robinson JN. Approach to episiotomy. Up to date version 17.3, Sept 2009.

Breech Presentation and Delivery

17

Uche A. Menakaya

Learning Objectives

At the conclusion of this chapter, the learner will be able to:

- Understand the different types of breech presentations at term
- Recognise the antenatal risk factors for a breech presentation at term
- Evaluate the intrapartum and postpartum risks associated with breech deliveries at term
- Understand the role of ultrasound in the management of term breech presentations
- Critically evaluate the evidence for and against the different options for managing term breech presentations
- Articulate the significant challenges facing the term breech foetus in resource restricted countries

17.1 Introduction

Breech presentation refers to the presence of the fetal buttocks, knees or feet at the lower pole of the gravid uterus during pregnancy. In most pregnancies, breech presentation at term appears to be a chance occurrence. However, it may be due to fetal, maternal or placental abnormalities in up to 15% of cases [1]. Vaginal delivery of a breech presentation at term could result in significant maternal and/or perinatal morbidity and mortality when compared to vertex presentation. These poorer outcomes associated with vaginal breech delivery are often the result of the underlying conditions causing the breech presentation and/or related to factors associated with the breech delivery.

17.2 Prevalence

Breech presentation is a common occurrence in early pregnancy. During this time the foetus is small and mobile relative to the large volume of amniotic fluid. With increasing gestational age and near term, a foetus with normal anatomy, activity, amniotic fluid volume and placental location adopts the cephalic presentation as this position is the best fit for the intrauterine space.

The prevalence of breech-presenting foetuses decreases from 20 to 25% under 28 weeks to about 7–16% at 32 weeks. At term, only 3–4% of fetal presentations are breech [2, 3].

17.3 Types of Breech Presentation

There are three main types of breech presentations:

17.3.1 Frank Breech (50–70%)

In this presentation both fetal hips are flexed and both knees are extended with the fetal feet lying adjacent to the fetal head.

17.3.2 Complete Breech (5–10%)

In this presentation, both the fetal hips and the knees are flexed.

17.3.3 Incomplete (Footling) Breech (10–40%)

In this presentation, one or both hips are not completely flexed. This presentation is also known as the footling breech presentation or partial breech presentation.

U. A. Menakaya (✉)
JUNIC Specialist Imaging and Women's Centre, Coombs, ACT, Australia

Calvary Public Hospital, Bruce, ACT, Australia

Calvary Private Hospital, Bruce, ACT, Australia
e-mail: info@junicimaging.com.au

F. Okonofua et al. (eds.), *Contemporary Obstetrics and Gynecology for Developing Countries*,
https://doi.org/10.1007/978-3-030-75385-6_17

Other rarer forms of breech presentation include compound breech presentation when a fetal extremity /part (i.e. arm/hand/umbilical cord) presents together with the breech at the lower uterine segment.

17.4 Antenatal Risk Categorisation

An assessment of the maternal risk for a breech presentation at term should be undertaken as part of routine antenatal care. For those identified to be at increased risk, surveillance for fetal presentation, especially in the third trimester, should be increased.

The frequency of recurrence of breech presentation following a first breech pregnancy is about 10% [4]. This risk increases to 25% after two consecutive breech pregnancies and up to 40% after three consecutive breech deliveries [4, 5]. In addition, parents who were breech at term were twice likely to have a first born in breech presentation compared to parents who were delivered in cephalic presentation suggesting a possible heritable component transmitted from either parent [6]. Other risk factors for breech presentation are presented in Table 17.1.

17.5 Clinical Assessment

The clinical assessment of fetal presentation is an essential component of antenatal examination in late pregnancy. This is because breech presentation influences the management of delivery and counselling of the patient. Women with a breech-presenting foetus may perceive fetal movements predominantly in the lower abdomen and may report upper abdominal/rib cage discomfort from the fetal head at the fundus [7].

Abdominal examination of the breech-presenting foetus may be characterised by the absence of the hard fetal skull in the lower uterine segment and the presence of a soft mass (i.e. buttocks). The fetal head in the upper segment of the uterus could be readily balloted.

Table 17.1 Risk factors for breech presentation

Fetal factors	Placental factors	Maternal factors
Preterm Gestation	Placental Previa	Previous Breech Presentation
Fetal Anomaly	Cornual Placental	Primiparity or Grand Multiparity
Multiple Gestation		Maternal Anticonvulsant Therapy
Short Umbilical Cord		Contracted Maternal Pelvis
Female Sex		Polyhydramnios/ Oligohydramnios
Extended Fetal Legs		Older maternal age
Growth Restricted Foetus		Uterine anomaly/fibroids

The ability to accurately diagnose a breech presentation at term may be limited by maternal obesity, full bladder, leiomyoma, polyhydramnios, anterior placenta and/or multiple gestation. In one study that examined 138 women at 30 to 41 weeks of gestation immediately before an ultrasound examination, the experienced examiner identified only three of eight breech presentations and falsely diagnosed six breech presentations [8].

17.6 Ultrasound Diagnosis of Breech Presentation

Transabdominal ultrasound plays an important role in the confirmation of the breech-presenting foetus at term. It is also useful for defining the type of breech, attitude of the fetal head, quantification of amniotic fluid volume and location of the placenta.

The information provided by trans-abdominal ultrasound in the third trimester is useful in planning the delivery of the persistent breech presentation at term and in counselling the woman as to her suitability for external cephalic version or vaginal breech birth.

17.7 Significance of Type of Breech in Planning Delivery

With the frank and complete breech presentations, the fetal position with the flexed hips and extended/flexed knees could enable the fetal thighs and trunk to pass through the birth canal simultaneously. Successful passage of this large presenting part through the birth canal improves the likelihood of easy passage of the after-coming shoulders and head, although a difficult breech delivery could still be possible.

On the other hand, with an incomplete or footling breech, one or both feet or knees may easily slip through an incompletely dilated cervix or an inadequate pelvis leading to entrapment of the shoulders or head because of their much larger diameters. This type of breech presentation is also associated with an increased risk of umbilical cord prolapse.

17.8 Antenatal Management of Breech Presentation

17.8.1 External Cephalic Version

External cephalic version (ECV) is an antenatal obstetric procedure in which a breech-presenting foetus at or near term is rotated from a breech position to a cephalic presentation by externally manipulating the gravid abdomen. In a systematic review of 84 studies involving nearly 13,000 attempts at ECV at term, the pooled success rate of ECV was 58% [9].

The clinical effectiveness of ECV is related to its ability to increase the proportion of foetuses in cephalic presentation during labour and reduce the rate of caesarean delivery for breech presentation at term. In one systematic review of eight randomised trials of ECV at term, 1308 women who attempted ECV approximately halved their risks of both non-cephalic deliveries (relative risk [RR] 0.42, 95% CI 0.29–0.61) and caesarean delivery (RR 0.57, 95% CI 0.40–0.82) when compared with women with breech foetuses who had no attempt at ECV [10].

However, the rate of caesarean deliveries after successful ECV was twice as high as the rate in women with cephalic-presenting foetuses with no ECV (21% vs 11%; RR 2.19, 95% CI 1.73–2.76) [11]. This increased risk of caesarean delivery was related to both dystocia and non-reassuring fetal heart rate patterns. It has been hypothesised that factors common to both breech presentation and successful ECV, such as an unengaged presenting part or small maternal pelvis, are also risk factors for dystocia [11].

The cost-effectiveness of ECV has been demonstrated in the United Kingdom and United States [12]. When compared with a scheduled caesarean delivery for breech presentation, ECV was more cost-effective when the probability of successful ECV was greater than 32% [12, 13].

The factors that reduce the success rate of ECV [14–20] include the following:

- Anterior placenta
- Nulliparity
- Tense uterus
- Fetal head not palpable
- Thinner myometrial thickness
- Ruptured membranes
- Posteriorly located fetal spine
- Obesity
- Descent of the breech into the pelvis
- Low birth weight
- Decreased amniotic fluid volume
- Lateral or cornual placenta
- Frank breech presentation

By contrast, the factors that increase the success rate for ECV are as follows [15, 21]

- Black race
- Posterior placental location
- Complete breech position
- Amniotic fluid index >10
- Multiparity
- Non-longitudinal lie

17.8.2 Risks Associated with ECV

In a systematic review of 84 ECV studies including 13,000 women with attempted ECV, the pooled complication rate was 6.1% (95% CI 4.7–7.8) [9]. These complications included emergency caesarean section, cord prolapse, transient abnormal fetal heart rate changes, vaginal bleeding, rupture of the fetal membranes, foeto-maternal haemorrhage.

The pooled risk of more serious complications like stillbirth and abruptio placenta was 0.24% (95% CI 0.17–0.34). Despite the limitation of this meta-analysis (differences in study design, patient populations, ECV techniques and definitions of outcomes), the results were comparable to those in the largest single study on the complications of ECV [22].

17.8.3 Contraindications to ECV

ECV is not recommended in the following clinical scenarios: indications for caesarean delivery irrespective of fetal presentation (e.g. placenta previa), severe oligohydramnios or ruptured membranes, non-reassuring fetal monitoring test results, hyperextended fetal head, significant fetal or uterine anomaly (e.g. hydrocephaly, septate uterus), placental abruption and multiple gestation. In women with multiple gestation, ECV may be considered for the second twin after delivery of the first twin.

Relative contraindications include maternal hypertension, maternal obesity, fetal growth restriction, decreased amniotic fluid volume and previous caesarean delivery. Despite the theoretical risk of fetal HIV transmission in HIV-infected women who undergo ECV, the risk appears to be small, comparing favourably with the risk of transmission in vaginal breech delivery (if caesarean delivery is unavailable) [23].

17.8.4 Timing of ECV

Most obstetrical societies recommend scheduling ECV for uncomplicated breech pregnancies at $\geq 37^{0/7}$ weeks of gestation [24, 25]. Advantages of ECV at term include: (1) it is often successful, (2) the foetus is likely to remain cephalic after successful ECV (i.e. the procedure is effective), (3) the foetus is mature or nearly mature in the event of complications necessitating urgent caesarean delivery [26].

A randomised multicentre trial involving 1543 women with a singleton breech foetus assessed whether attempting ECV before term (and repeating the procedure until delivery, if necessary) has any benefit over ECV at term [27]. In this large study, early ECV resulted in significantly fewer foetuses in non-cephalic presentation at delivery compared to late ECV (41.1% vs 49.1%; relative risk [RR] 0.84, 95% CI

0.75–0.94) and similar rates of complications with late ECV (overall complication rate of 3–4%) [27].

The Early ECV did not significantly increase the risk of preterm birth before 37 weeks (6.5% vs 4.4%; RR 1.48, 95% CI 0.97–2.26) with the median gestational age at delivery for both groups: 39.1 weeks. There were no significant reductions in the rates of caesarean delivery with early ECV (52% vs 56%; RR 0.93, 95% CI 0.85–1.02) [27–29].

17.9 Performing ECV

An ultrasound should be performed to confirm a non-cephalic presentation and define the type of breech presentation and location of placenta. It is also useful to exclude oligohydramnios, fetal or uterine anomalies. A biophysical profile with fetal heart rate monitoring should be undertaken to assess fetal well-being prior to performing an ECV.

17.9.1 Adequate Counselling and Obtaining Informed Consent

The use of a structured decision-making tool to aid counselling for ECV has been shown to be more effective in increasing the uptake of ECV with patients reporting a higher rate of satisfaction with the decision-making process [30]. Obtaining informed consent should include a description of the procedure and its related discomfort, the likelihood of spontaneous reversion to breech, the success rates of ECV (preferably using data from the local hospital) and the risks, benefits and alternatives to ECV. The risks associated with use of ancillary measures (e.g. tocolysis) to improve success rates should also be discussed.

In a systematic review of six randomised trials of ECV with versus without parenteral beta adrenergic agents, tocolysis was associated with an increased prevalence of cephalic presentation in labour (RR1.68, 95% CI 1.14–2.48) and a reduction in caesarean delivery rates (RR 0.77, 95% CI 0.67–0.88) in both nulliparous and multiparous women [31].

Women who are likely to undergo ECV are those who are well-informed, encouraged to undergo the procedure, believe in its safety and desire a vaginal delivery [32]. Conversely, incomplete information, fear of the procedure and a preference for scheduled caesarean delivery could limit a woman choice of ECV [32].

17.9.2 Technique of ECV

Ensure the woman is comfortable, lying supine with a left lateral tilt. First, disengage the breech from the pelvis by scooping the breech from the pelvis to a position above the sacral promontory. For a backward somersault, the breech is held with the edge of the left palm and pushed towards the woman's right flank and upward. If version is not completed by this manoeuvre, the head is gently manipulated towards the woman's left flank and downward with the edge of the right hand, taking care to apply most pressure to the breech so that a flexed posture is maintained. Slight back-and-forth movement between the two hands may help promote fetal movement, but generally, pressure on the foetus should be slow and steady rather than repeated pushing.

For a forward somersault, the operator is positioned on the side of the woman opposite to the fetal back. The procedure is similar to that described above, except that once the breech has been disengaged from the pelvis, more pressure is applied to the head than the breech, to maintain flexion of the baby.

The fetal heart rate is auscultated every two minutes, with interruption of the procedure if bradycardia occurs. In one large series, an abnormal fetal heart rate leading to discontinuation of the ECV occurred in approximately 5% of cases [29] (Fig. 17.1).

17.10 Antenatal Management After ECV

17.10.1 Fetal Heart Rate Monitoring

After an ECV, fetal well-being should be evaluated by monitoring the fetal heart rate until it is stable and reactive. Fetal heart rate may be monitored with a cardiotocogram. It is not uncommon for fetal heart rate tracings with the cardiotocogram to be non-reactive for up to 40 minutes after ECV. These changes probably reflect the fetal response to a transient period of stress caused by decreased utero-placental blood flow during the procedure [33].

17.10.2 Anti D Immune Globulin

Anti D immunoglobulin is recommended following ECV in Rhesus D Negative women.

17.11 Management After Unsuccessful ECV

When ECV is unsuccessful or the foetus reverts to breech following successful ECV, the woman may be offered a re-trial of ECV, a caesarean, or a vaginal breech birth. Up to two re-trials of ECV can be attempted, one or more days following an initial ECV [1].

Women who have unsuccessful ECV are often disappointed and worried about losing control over a desire to achieve vaginal birth [34]. In centres that do not offer vaginal breech deliveries, a post-procedure debriefing session with the involvement of a social worker is recommended [34].

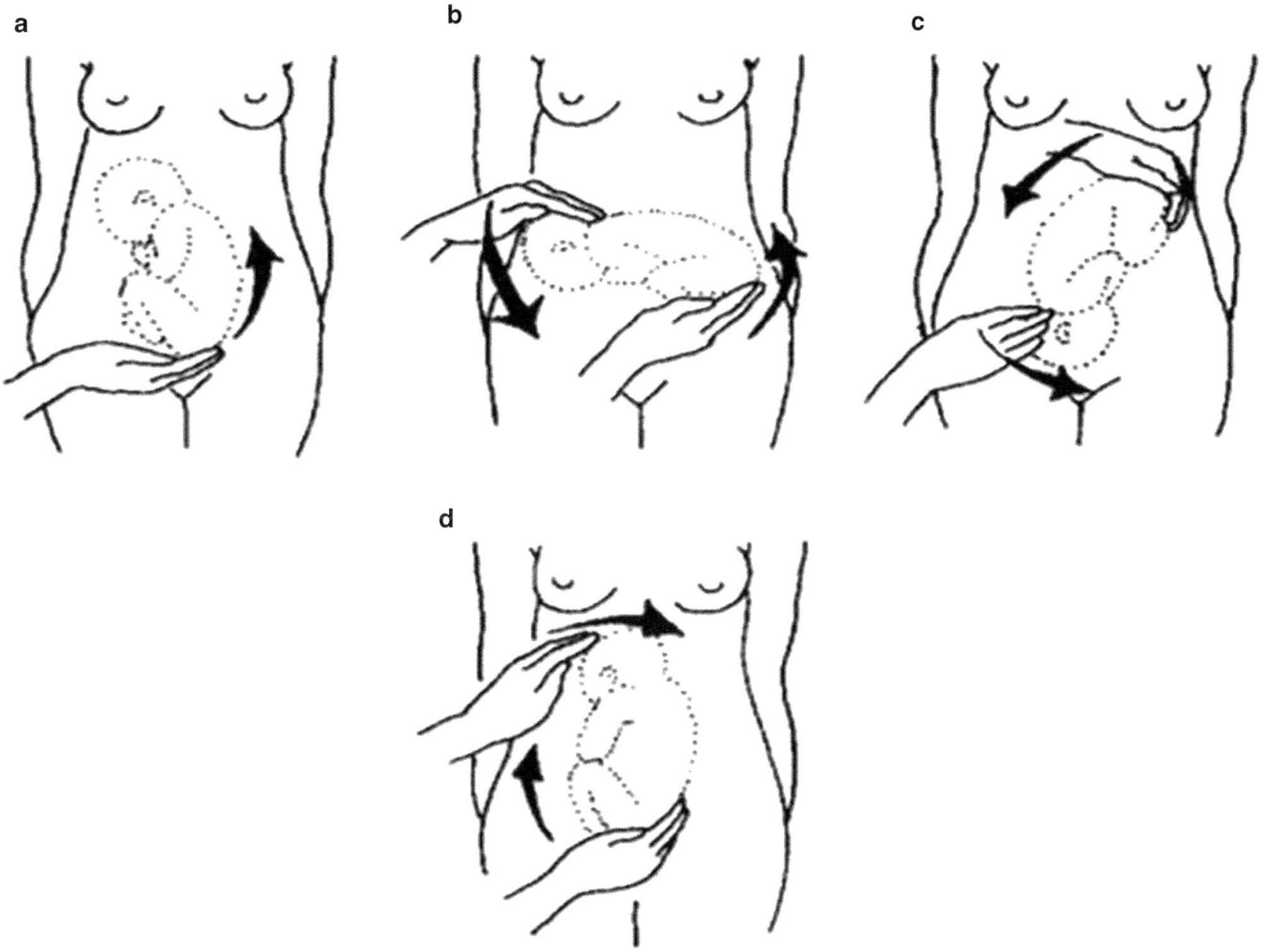

Fig. 17.1 Steps in performing an ECV. (**a**) Mobilization of the breech. (**b**) Manual forward rotation using both hands, one to push the breech and the other to guide the vertex. (**c**) Completion of forward roll. (**d**) Backward roll. (Reproduced from Managing complications in pregnancy and childbirth: a guide for midwives and doctors – 2nd ed. Geneva: World Health Organization; 2017. Licence: CC BY-NC-SA 3.0 IGO)

17.12 Management After Successful ECV

Routine antenatal care should be continued following a successful ECV. Elective induction of labour is not recommended as the risk of reversion to breech is small [35, 36]. However, subsequent antenatal visits should include a documented assessment of fetal presentation. Thereafter, delivery planning should be based on local protocols.

17.13 Alternatives to ECV

17.13.1 Expectant Management

Spontaneous cephalic version may occur at any time before delivery including at term [37]. There is a 25% likelihood of spontaneous version to cephalic presentation after 36 weeks [37]. Despite this likelihood of spontaneous version, it has been reported that the ratio of spontaneous version to successful ECV is 1: 3 [20].

17.13.2 Other Alternatives

There is no evidence that Moxibustion, acupuncture, positional changes and manoeuvres could facilitate spontaneous version from breech to cephalic at term [38, 39].

17.14 Delivery of Persistent Breech Presentation at Term

17.14.1 Choosing the Route of Delivery

A persistent breech presentation at term may be delivered via a planned caesarean section or vaginal breech delivery. The choice of route of delivery should be made with due consideration to the specific healthcare environment [40, 41]. It should also consider the patient's values and preferences, the obstetrician's experience, values and preferences while taking into account the risks and benefits of the various approaches.

17.14.2 Scheduled Caesarean Section for Breech Presentation at Term

Evidence for scheduling a planned caesarean delivery at 39 weeks' gestation for a persistent breech presentation has been provided by the term breech trial [42]. The trial was a large multicentre, international trial comparing planned caesarean delivery with planned vaginal delivery performed by an experienced clinician following agreed upon clinical guidelines [42]. A total of 121 centres in 26 countries involving 2088 women with a singleton foetus in a frank or complete breech presentation were randomly assigned planned caesarean section or planned vaginal birth [42].

The key findings from the term breech trial were a lower perinatal and neonatal mortality, and significantly lower serious neonatal morbidity in the planned caesarean section group compared with the planned vaginal birth group (1.6% vs 5.0%; RR 0.33 [95% CI 0.19–0.56]; $p < 0.0001$) [42]. There were no differences between groups in terms of maternal mortality or serious maternal morbidity (3.9% vs 3.2%; 1.24 [0.79–1.95]; $p = 0.35$). Other studies have estimated that 338 caesarean breech deliveries would be needed to prevent a single perinatal death [43]. However, a policy of planned caesarean breech delivery was not associated with a reduction in risk of death or neurodevelopmental delay in children at 2 years of age compared with vaginal breech delivery [44].

The findings from the term breech trial impacted clinical practice worldwide with the rate of planned vaginal breech birth falling since the publication of this trial [45–47]. There has also been an accompanied fall in morbidity and mortality associated with breech delivery with a policy of planned caesarean delivery especially if performed prior to onset of labour [43, 46, 48].

Criticisms of the term breech trial have included the heterogeneous skill levels of units involved in the study, presence of only 87% of licensed obstetricians for women undergoing trial of vaginal delivery compared with 98% of those delivered by caesarean section, suboptimal antenatal and intrapartum care with limited use of pre/early labour ultrasound and continuous fetal monitoring and the lack of intervention for relatively slow progress. Other criticisms relate to the inclusion of up to 16 stillbirths not associated with the delivery method in the final study analysis and the use of neonatal morbidity as a proxy for long-term neurodevelopmental outcome [40, 41, 49–53].

There are significant challenges with instituting a policy of planned caesarean delivery especially in low income, resource-poor settings where it may not be affordable or feasible. There may also be clinical circumstances where the maternal risks of caesarean and/or the mother's desire to avoid caesarean delivery outweigh the newborn's short-term risks of vaginal birth. Thirdly, there are risks associated with repeat caesarean sections (e.g. placenta accreta and uterine rupture) for women planning future pregnancies [54].

17.14.3 Planned Vaginal Breech Delivery for Persistent Breech Presentation at Term

Historically, vaginal delivery of the persistent breech presentation at term had been the tradition since the first century A.D. Although it was performed primarily for the safety of the mother, obstetricians of the time were aware of the hazards associated with the breech birth particularly those associated with the delivery of the after coming head [55, 56].

The manual skills required for breech extraction were well recognised and acknowledged.

Acquiring the skill necessary for breech delivery was also a measure of an obstetrician at the time. In 1939, Joseph B. Delee commented *"Let me watch a man conduct a breech case and I will give you his obstetrical rating. There are few operations in any discipline of medicine that are inherently so artistic. Every movement imparted by the hands to the fetal body has been worked out by the great accouchers of time and the complete delivery done by an expert can be likened to the technique of a violin virtuoso" (De Lee 1939)* [57].

There is now a general consensus that women who choose to undergo a trial of labour for vaginal breech birth should be at low risk of complications from vaginal breech delivery and their labour and delivery should be supervised by a clinician with experience in vaginal breech birth [50]. Current evidence to support vaginal breech birth in selected women is provided by the PREsentation et MODe d'Accouchement (PREMODA) study [49]. The study illustrated the magnitude of neonatal morbidity/mortality associated with planned vaginal birth and recommended that planned vaginal delivery of singleton foetuses in breech presentation at term remains a safe option that can be offered to women when strict criteria are met before and during labour [49, 58].

The selection criteria used for planned vaginal breech birth in the PREMODA study include normal X Ray/CT pelvimetry, non-hyperextended fetal head on ultrasound, frank breech presentation, continuous intrapartum use of cardiotocography and written informed consent for vaginal breech birth [49]. Additional factors associated with increased adverse perinatal outcomes in planned vaginal breech births include geographic origin, gestational age <39 weeks at birth, birthweight <10th percentile and annual number of maternity unit births <1500 [58].

17.14.3.1 Intrapartum Management of the Breech Birth

Spontaneous labour is preferable with induction of labour best avoided for breech presentations at term planning vaginal birth [35, 36]. Augmentation with oxytocin may be considered to optimise uterine contractility in the latent phase of labour or after epidural anaesthesia. Poor progress in the active phase may be an indicator of fetopelvic disproportion, therefore oxytocin augmentation is not recommended once active labour has begun [50, 59, 60].

Labour progress is monitored and recorded, as with a cephalic presentation. Caesarean section should be performed if progress is inadequate in the active phase of labour. The rationale for the guidelines for intrapartum management of breech deliveries is based on observational studies of vaginal breech birth using strict selection criteria, adherence to an intrapartum protocol with a low threshold for intervention, and with an experienced obstetrician in attendance [50, 60].

Adequate analgesia including epidural analgesia should be considered because it relieves pain, prevents the mother from pushing involuntarily before full cervical dilatation and provides anaesthesia if obstetrical manoeuvres are needed to facilitate delivery. However, the ability of the woman to push effectively when the breech descends to the pelvic floor should be maintained as effective maternal pushing is essential to safe vaginal breech delivery [50].

Descent of the breech is regarded as adequate if the breech reaches the level of the ischial spines when the cervix is 6 cm dilated and reaches the pelvic floor at full dilation [60]. A passive second stage (i.e. delayed pushing) for up to 90 minutes is acceptable [50]. However, once the woman starts bearing down, failure of the breech to descend and deliver within 30 to 60 minutes is managed by caesarean delivery rather than breech extraction [60].

The techniques for successful vaginal breech deliveries include allowing spontaneous descent and fetal expulsion to the level of the umbilicus. Subsequent manoeuvres should include rotation of the baby to the sacrum anterior position when appropriate with no attempts at fetal traction. Providing ongoing support for the expelled parts of the baby by holding the baby around the bony hips is necessary as the woman continues her expulsive efforts. A Pinard manoeuvre may be considered if the legs do not deliver spontaneously. The Pinard manoeuvres involve the flexion of the extended fetal knee to encourage delivery of the fetal lower limbs.

The delivery of the fetal arms could be facilitated with the Lovset manoeuvre. This involves the rotation of the fetal truck to enable delivery of the arms. It starts once the inferior angle of the scapula is visible below the pubic arch. Holding the foetus around its bony pelvis and keeping the fetal back anterior, the attendant should maintain a gentle downward traction while rotating the foetus through 90°to deliver the anterior arm. The truck is then rotated through 180° in the opposite direction to deliver the posterior arm under the symphysis pubis. Attempts should be made by an assistant to keep the fetal head in the flexed position by applying suprapubic pressure.

Finally, the delivery of the fetal head could be assisted with the Mauriceasu–Smellie–Veit (MSV) manoeuvre or with the Piper's forceps applied to facilitate the delivery of the after coming head. With the MSV manoeuvre, the fetal head is maintained in flexion by placing the attendant's fingers over the chin and malar eminences as downward traction is applied by the accoucheur. An assistant may help to maintain the fetal head in flexion by providing suprapubic pressure.

The Pipers forceps are designed for delivery of the after coming head in a breech delivery. The forceps help maintain the fetal head in flexion during extraction of the fetal head. It requires an assistant to hold the foetus while the operator kneels on one knee to apply the forceps from below.

17.15 Postpartum Care

17.15.1 Neonatal Examination and Care

Following a breech delivery, all newborns born will require a thorough paediatric examination. A paediatrician should be present at delivery because of the possibility of birth related injury. In addition, the risk of developmental dysplasia of the hip is increased with breech presentation [61]. Early detection and subsequent treatment of developmental dysplasia of the hip improves its prognosis [61].

17.16 Documentation

Clear and concise clinical documentation is necessary following a vaginal breech delivery. Documentation should include whether the breech delivery was planned or incidental emergency vaginal birth. These notes should be included in both the mother and child's clinical records. The documentation should include the manoeuvres performed to deliver the baby, time in second stage, APGAR scores and results of cord blood analysis. It should also include neonatal resuscitation activities and clear descriptions of maternal or neonatal traumas.

17.17 Conclusion

In resource limited countries, the term breech faces significant challenges. For example, ECV is not routinely performed in clinical practice because many health personnel lack its mastery or unduly perceive it to be associated with adverse perinatal outcomes [62]. Data on vaginal breech delivery for singleton term pregnancies are limited as such there is a lack of consensus on the management of this fetal presentation in the sub Saharan continent [63]. And a general health policy recommending caesarean delivery for all breech presentations would require significant investments of scarce resources in the health care system [63].

Fortunately, the PREMODA study provides evidence that planned vaginal delivery of singleton foetuses in breech presentation at term remains a safe option and can be offered to women [49, 58]. However, it requires that local hospitals develop protocols and policies for vaginal breech delivery consistent with the criteria as defined by the study. Such protocols must necessarily include clear pathways for refresher courses and practical workshops for health personnel involved in the management of the term breech foetus.

References

1. Hofmeyr GJ, Lockwood CJ, Barss VA. Overview of issues related to breech presentation: Uptodate Topic 6776 Version 24.0.
2. Scheer K, Nubar J. Variation of fetal presentation with gestational age. Am J Obstet Gynecol. 1976;125(2):269–70.
3. Hickok DE, Gordon DC, Milberg JA, Williams MA, Daling JR. The frequency of breech presentation by gestational age at birth: a large population-based study. Am J Obstet Gynecol. 1992;166(3):851–2.
4. Albrechtsen S, Rasmussen S, Dalaker K, Irgens LM. Reproductive career after breech presentation: subsequent pregnancy rates, inter pregnancy interval, and recurrence. Obstet Gynecol. 1998;92(3):345.
5. Ford JB, Roberts CL, Nassar N, Giles W, Morris JM. Recurrence of breech presentation in consecutive pregnancies. BJOG. 2010;117(7):830.
6. Nordtveit TI, Melve KK, Albrechtsen S, Skjaerven R. Maternal and paternal contribution to intergenerational recurrence of breech delivery: population based cohort study. BMJ. 2008;336(7649):872.
7. Hofmeyr GJ. Abnormal fetal presentation and position. In: Chapter 34, Turnbull's obstetrics; 2000.
8. Thorp JM Jr, Jenkins T, Watson W. Utility of Leopold maneuvers in screening for malpresentation. Obstet Gynecol. 1991;78(3 Pt 1):394.
9. Grootscholten K, Kok M, Oei SG, Mol BW, van der Post JA. External cephalic version-related risks: a meta-analysis. Obstet Gynecol. 2008;112(5):1143.
10. Hofmeyr GJ, Kulier R, West HM. External cephalic version for breech presentation at term. Cochrane Database Syst Rev. 2015 Apr;4:CD000083.
11. De Hundt M, Velzel J, de Groot CJ, Mol BW, Kok M. Mode of delivery after successful external cephalic version: a systematic review and meta-analysis. Obstet Gynecol. 2014;123(6):1327.
12. Tan JM, Macario A, Carvalho B, Druzin ML, El-Sayed YY. Cost-effectiveness of external cephalic version for term breech presentation. BMC Pregnancy Childbirth. 2010;10:3.
13. Gifford DS, Keeler E, Kahn KL. Reductions in cost and caesarean rate by routine use of external cephalic version: a decision analysis. Obstet Gynecol. 1995;85(6):930–6.
14. Ben-Meir A, Erez Y, Sela HY, Shveiky D, Tsafrir A, Ezra Y. Prognostic parameters for successful external cephalic version. J Matern Fetal Neonatal Med. 2008;21(9):660.
15. Kok M, Cnossen J, Gravendeel L, van der Post J, Opmeer B, Mol BW. Clinical factors to predict the outcome of external cephalic version: a meta-analysis. Am J Obstet Gynecol. 2008;199(6):630.e1.
16. Ebner F, Friedl TW, Leinert E, Schramm A, Reister F, Lato K, Janni W, De Gregorio N. Predictors for a successful external cephalic version: a single centre experience. Arch Gynecol Obstet. 2016;293(4):749.
17. Buhimschi CS, Buhimschi IA, Wehrum MJ, Molaskey-Jones S, Sfakianaki AK, Pettker CM, Thung S, Campbell KH, Dulay AT, Funai EF, Bahtiyar MO. Ultrasonographic evaluation of myometrial thickness and prediction of a successful external cephalic version. Obstet Gynecol. 2011;118(4):913–20.
18. Fortunato SJ, Mercer LJ, Guzick DS. External cephalic version with tocolysis: factors associated with success. Obstet Gynecol. 1988;72(1):59.
19. Boucher M, Bujold E, Marquette GP, Vezina Y. The relationship between amniotic fluid index and successful external cephalic version: a 14-year experience. Am J Obstet Gynecol. 2003;189(3):751.
20. Hofmeyr GJ, Sadan O, Myer IG, Galal KC, Simko G. External cephalic version and spontaneous version rates: ethnic and other determinants. Br J Obstet Gynaecol. 1986;93(1):13.
21. Hofmeyr GJ. Effect of external cephalic version in late pregnancy on breech presentation and caesarean section rate: a controlled trial. Br J Obstet Gynaecol. 1983;90(5):392.
22. Collins S, Ellaway P, Harrington D, Pandit M, Impey LW. The complications of external cephalic version: results from 805 consecutive attempts. BJOG. 2007;114(5):636.
23. Holmes WR, Hofmeyr GJ. Management of breech presentation in areas with high prevalence of HIV infection. Int J Gynaecol Obstet. 2004;87(3):272.
24. American College of Obstetricians and Gynaecologists. External cephalic version. Practice Bulletin No. 161. Obstet Gynecol. 2016;127:e54.
25. Royal College of Obstetrics and Gynaecology. External Cephalic Version (ECV) and Reducing the Incidence of Breech Presentation (Green-top Guideline No. 20a). https://www.rcog.org.uk/en/guidelines-researchservices/guidelines/gtg20a/. Accessed on 12 May 2016.
26. Ben-Meir A, Elram T, Tsafrir A, Elchalal U, Ezra Y. The incidence of spontaneous version after failed external cephalic version. Am J Obstet Gynecol. 2007;196(2):157.e1.
27. Hutton EK, Hannah ME, Ross SJ, Delisle MF, Carson GD, Windrim R, Ohlsson A, Willan AR, Gafni A, Sylvestre G, Natale R, Barrett Y, Pollard JK, Dunn MS, Turtle P. Early ECV2 Trial Collaborative Group. The Early External Cephalic Version (ECV) 2 Trial: an international multicentre randomised controlled trial of timing of ECV for breech pregnancies. BJOG. 2011;118(5):564.
28. Hutton EK, Hofmeyr GJ, Dowswell T. External cephalic version for breech presentation before term. Cochrane Database Syst Rev. 2015;7:CD000084.
29. Hutton EK, Kaufman K, Hodnett E, Amankwah K, Hewson SA, McKay D, Szalai JP, Hannah ME. External cephalic version beginning at 34 weeks' gestation versus 37 weeks' gestation: a randomized multicenter trial. Am J Obstet Gynecol. 2003;189(1):245.
30. Nassar N, Roberts CL, Raynes-Greenow CH, Barratt A, Peat B. Decision aid for breech presentation trial collaborators evaluation of a decision aid for women with breech presentation at term: a randomised controlled trial [ISRCTN14570598]. BJOG. 2007;114(3):325.
31. Cluver C, Gyte GM, Sinclair M, Dowswell T, Hofmeyr GJ. Interventions for helping to turn term breech babies to head first presentation when using external cephalic version. Cochrane Database Syst Rev. 2015 Feb;2:CD000184.
32. Rosman AN, Vlemmix F, Fleuren MA, Rijnders ME, Beuckens A, Opmeer BC, Mol BW, van Zwieten MC, Kok M. Patients' and professionals' barriers and facilitators to external cephalic version for breech presentation at term, a qualitative analysis in the Netherlands. Midwifery. 2014;30(3):324.

33. Hofmeyr GJ. Sonnendecker EW Cardiotocographic changes after external cephalic version. Br J Obstet Gynaecol. 1983;90(10):914.
34. Menakaya UA, Trivedi A. Qualitative assessment of women experiences with ECV. Women Birth. 2013;26(1):41–4.
35. ACOG Committee on Obstetric Practice ACOG Committee Opinion No. 340. Mode of term singleton breech delivery. Obstet Gynecol. 2006;108 (1):235.
36. Royal College of Obstetricians and Gynaecologist (RCOG). The management of breech presentation. London: RCOG; 2006.
37. Westgren M, Edvall H, Nordström L, Svalenius E, Ranstam J. Spontaneous cephalic version of breech presentation in the last trimester. Br J Obstet Gynaecol. 1985;92(1):19.
38. Coyle ME, Smith CA, Peat B. Cephalic version by moxibustion for breech presentation. Cochrane Database Syst Rev. 2012;5:CD003928.
39. Hofmeyr GJ, Kulier R. Cephalic version by postural management for breech presentation. Cochrane Database Syst Rev. 2012;10:CD000051.
40. Glezerman M. Five years to the term breech trial: the rise and fall of a randomized controlled trial. Am J Obstet Gynecol. 2006;194(1):20.
41. Menticoglou SM. Why vaginal breech delivery should still be offered. J Obstet Gynaecol Can. 2006;28(5):380.
42. Hannah ME, Hannah WJ, Hewson SA, Hodnett ED, Saigal S, Willan AR. Planned caesarean section versus planned vaginal birth for breech presentation at term: a randomised multicentre trial. Term Breech Trial Collaborative Group. Lancet. 2000;356(9239):1375.
43. Vlemmix F, Bergenhenegouwen L, Schaaf JM, Ensing S, Rosman AN, Ravelli AC, Van Der Post JA, Verhoeven A, Visser GH, Mol BW, Kok M. Term breech deliveries in the Netherlands: did the increased caesarean rate affect neonatal outcome? A population-based cohort study. Acta Obstet Gynecol Scand. 2014;93(9):888.
44. Whyte H, Hannah ME, Saigal S, Hannah WJ, Hewson S, Amankwah K, Cheng M, Gafni A, Guselle P, Helewa M, Hodnett ED, Hutton E, Kung R, McKay D, Ross S, Willan A, Term Breech Trial Collaborative Group. Outcomes of children at 2 years after planned cesarean birth versus planned vaginal birth for breech presentation at term: The International Randomized Term Breech Trial. Am J Obstet Gynecol. 2004;191(3):864–71.
45. Adegbola O, Akindele OM. Outcome of term singleton breech deliveries at a University Teaching Hospital in Lagos. Nigeria Niger Postgrad Med J. 2009;16(2):154–7.
46. Hartnack Tharin JE, Rasmussen S, Krebs L. Consequences of the term breech trial in Denmark. Acta Obstet Gynecol Scand. 2011;90(7):767.
47. Vistad I, Klungsøyr K, Albrechtsen S, Skjeldestad FE. Neonatal outcome of singleton term breech deliveries in Norway from 1991 to 2011. Acta Obstet Gynecol Scand. 2015;94(9):997.
48. Lyons J, Pressey T, Bartholomew S, Liu S, Liston RM, Joseph KS. Canadian Perinatal Surveillance System (Public Health Agency of Canada) Delivery of breech presentation at term gestation in Canada, 2003-2011. Obstet Gynecol. 2015;125(5):1153.
49. Goffinet F, Carayol M, Foidart JM, Alexander S, Uzan S, Subtil D, Bréart G, PREMODA Study Group. Is planned vaginal delivery for breech presentation at term still an option? Results of an observational prospective survey in France and Belgium. Am J Obstet Gynecol. 2006;194(4):1002.
50. Kotaska A, Menticoglou S, Gagnon R, Farine D, Basso M, Bos H, Delisle MF, Grabowska K, Hudon L, Mundle W, Murphy-Kaulbeck L, Ouellet A, Pressey T, Roggensack A. Maternal Fetal Medicine Committee, Society of Obstetricians and Gynaecologists of Canada. Vaginal delivery of breech presentation. J Obstet Gynaecol Can. 2009;31 (6):557.
51. Goffinet F, Blondel B, Breart G. Breech presentation: questions raised by the controlled trial by Hannah et al. on systematic use of caesarean section for breech presentations. J Gynecol Obstet Biol Reprod. 2001;30:187–90.
52. Glezerman M. Five years to the term breech trial: the risk and fall of a randomised controlled trial. Am J Obstet Gynecol. 2006;194:20–5.
53. Hauth JC, Cunningham FG. Vaginal breech delivery is still justified. Obstet Gynecol. 2002;99:1115–6.
54. Hull AD, Moore TR. Multiple repeat caesareans and the threat of placenta accreta: incidence, diagnosis, management. Clin Perinatol. 2011;38(2):285.
55. Moore WT, Steptoe PP. The experience of the John Hopkins hospital with breech presentation: an analysis of 1444 cases. South Med J. 1943;36:295.
56. Piper EB, Bachman C. The prevention of fetal injuries in breech delivery. J Am Med Assoc. 1929;92:217–21.
57. DeLee JB. Year book of obstetrics and gynaecology. Chicago: Year Book Medical Publishers; 1939.
58. Azria E, Le Meaux JP, Khoshnood B, Alexander S, Subtil D, Goffinet F. PREMODA Study Group Factors associated with adverse perinatal outcomes for term breech fetuses with planned vaginal delivery. Am J Obstet Gynecol. 2012;207(4):285.e1–9. Epub 2012 Aug 17
59. Alarab M, Regan C, O'Connell MP, Keane DP, O'Herlihy C, Foley ME. Singleton vaginal breech delivery at term: still a safe option. Obstet Gynecol. 2004;103(3):407.
60. Hofmeyr GJ, Lockwood CJ, Barss VA. Delivery of the fetus in breech presentation. Uptodate.com 2016 Topic 5384 version 18.
61. De Hundt M, Vlemmix F, Bais JM, Hutton EK, de Groot CJ, Mol BW, Kok M. Risk factors for developmental dysplasia of the hip: a meta-analysis. Eur J Obstet Gynecol Reprod Biol. 2012;165(1):8.
62. Kenfack B, Ateudjieu J, Ymele FF, et al. Does the advice to Assumethe knee-chest position at the 36th to 37th weeks of gestation reduce the incidence of breech presentation at delivery? Clin Mother Child Health. 2012;9:1–5.
63. Dobbit JS, Foumane P, Tochie JN, Mamoudou F, Mazou N, Temgoua MN, Tankeu R, Aletum V, Mboudou E. Maternal and neonatal outcomes of vaginal breech delivery for singleton term pregnancies in a carefully selected Cameroonian population: a cohort study. BMJ Open. 2017;7(11):e017198.

Caesarean Delivery and Peripartum Hysterectomy

18

Rotimi A. K. Jaiyesimi, Oluropo Ebenezer Ojo, and Aderonke F. Awe

Learning Objectives

After studying this chapter, you should be able to:

- Discuss the different indications for caesarean section.
- Describe the management of caesarean section in labour.
- Explain the surgical techniques of caesarean section.
- Understand the management of common complications of caesarean section.
- Define peripartum (caesarean/postpartum) hysterectomy and discuss its indication.
- List the risk management issues in caesarean section.

18.1 History of Caesarean Section

Caesarean section is the most commonly performed surgical operation in the world [1]. It is an operative technique by which a foetus is delivered through an incision in the uterus. It is performed for foetal or maternal benefit and is as old as modern obstetrics. Legend has it that Julius Caesar (100 BC) was born in this manner, and this may explain the origin of the name. However, there is no supporting evidence for this claim. Trolle's monograph provides a more comprehensive historical background. Caesarean section was popularised in the pre–World War II Britain following a paper published in 1931 by St George Wilson. Its use was associated with a high maternal mortality, with a rate of 3.5 per 1000 births in the UK in 1962. This was ten times that of the overall maternal mortality [2]. Caesarean section is now deemed a safe operation worldwide and this has led to substantial increase in its use. Improved operative techniques, thromboprophylaxis, availability of antibiotics and blood have resulted in a fall in maternal deaths associated with caesarean sections and maternal death is now quite rare. From 1988 to 1990, women undergoing elective caesarean sections were more than eight times likely to die than women having a vaginal delivery; from 1994 to 1996, they were approximately three times as likely to die; and by 1997 to 1999, the relative risk of death had decreased to slightly more than two. In Brazil, 'a middle income country with high caesarean section rate', caesarean section compared to vaginal delivery was associated with a significantly increased risk of postpartum maternal mortality, adjusted OR 2.9 [3].

18.2 The Incidence of Caesarean Section

There has been unprecedented increase in the use of caesarean section. Using the latest data from 150 countries, Betrán et al. calculated the incidence of caesarean to be 18.6%, ranging from 6% to 27.2% in the least and most developed regions, respectively. Latin America and the Caribbean region have the highest caesarean section (CS) rates (40.5%), followed by Northern America (32.3%), Oceania (31.1%), Europe (25%), Asia (19.2%) and Africa (7.3%). Based on the data from 121 countries, the trend analysis showed that between 1990 and 2014, the global average CS rate increased by 12.4% (from 6.7% to 19.1%) with an average annual rate of increase of 4.4%. The largest

R. A. K. Jaiyesimi (✉)
Mid and South Essex University Hospitals NHS Foundation Trust, Basildon, UK

Faculty of Law, University of Ibadan, Ibadan, Nigeria
e-mail: jaiyesimi@obs-gyn.org

O. E. Ojo
Cedarpark Healthcare Lincoln, Lincolnshire East CCG, Lincoln, UK

Elizade University Healthcare Centre, Ilara Mokin, Nigeria

A. F. Awe
Shrewsbury and Telford Hospitals NHS Trust, Shropshire, Shrewsbury, UK

Plymouth University, Plymouth, UK
e-mail: aderonke.awe@nhs.net

F. Okonofua et al. (eds.), *Contemporary Obstetrics and Gynecology for Developing Countries*,
https://doi.org/10.1007/978-3-030-75385-6_18

absolute increases occurred in Latin America and the Caribbean (19.4%, from 22.8% to 42.2%), followed by Asia (15.1%, from 4.4% to 19.5%), Oceania (14.1%, from 18.5% to 32.6%), Europe (13.8%, from 11.2% to 25%), Northern America (10%, from 22.3% to 32.3%) and Africa (4.5%, from 2.9% to 7.4%) [4]. Asia and Northern America were the regions with the highest and lowest average annual rate of increase (6.4% and 1.6% respectively). The gap between higher- and lower-resource settings remains despite an increase worldwide [4].

The increase in caesarean section rates is largely driven by a variety of factors. These include societal demands for improved foetal outcome and protection of the maternal pelvic floor, the aspirations of obstetricians to meet these demands and protect themselves himself from a highly litigating society. Potential difficult forceps delivery is a thing of the past, and similarly, the diagnosis of dystocia is more often managed by caesarean section. The advent of electronic foetal monitoring leads to the over-diagnosis of foetal distress and delivery of the foetus by caesarean section. Improved anaesthetic techniques, thromboprophylaxis and a wider choice of antibiotics for treatment of infection have made maternal deaths from caesarean section rare.

Unlike the developed nations, the caesarean section rate is low in low resource nations, as low as 1.4% in Niger; howbeit, the overall average has increased slightly to an average rate of 5.2% [5]. This is as a result of the poor access to the available facilities, lack of facilities and personnel. The high maternal and perinatal morbidity and mortality rate in this region is a reflection of the low caesarean section rate. This is a result of poor access to caesarean sections. There is suggestive evidence that a caesarean section rate of 3.6–6.5% is needed to address obstetric complications in West Africa, and that a rate of 2% is the required minimum [6]. J Ye et al. showed that the least developed countries in his study had the greatest relative changes of caesarean section rate (caesarean section rates increased 160% compared with the baseline), and this led to a phenomenal decline in maternal and neonatal mortality rate [5].

Conversely, the rising trend of caesarean section rates is gradually becoming the practice in some low resource nations and this has been shown to be driven by the private sector. A caesarean section rate of 55.6% was reported in Brazil [3]. There can be no medical justification for this and one hopes that medical needs and not financial gains will be the driving force for caesarean sections.

Studies suggesting that caesarean birth improved the outcomes of various complications of pregnancy led to use of caesarean delivery for certain conditions. As the primary caesarean rate rose due to more frequent increase in surgical intervention for these complications, the long-held tenets stating 'once a Caesarean, always a Caesarean' led to a rapid increase in the number of repeat caesarean births, as these women delivered subsequent pregnancies. The decision to perform a caesarean should involve calculating the trade-offs between risk and benefit to both the mother and foetus simultaneously. While caesarean delivery may be more morbid for the mother, it is often perceived as being the safest route of delivery for the infant [7]. Ideally, information about risks and benefits to both mother and infant, at least in the most common clinical situations, would be available to assist decision-making. However, in many cases such information does not exist [8].

Recent studies have shown that high caesarean section rates were associated with lower maternal and infant mortality until it gets to a specific point, at which caesarean section above these rates were not significantly associated with improved foetal outcomes. Hence this inflection point was considered as a necessary caesarean section rate from a medical viewpoint to minimise mortality. The significant and negative relationship between caesarean section rates and mortality was only found when the caesarean section rate was below 5–10%; hence, the study suggested that the aforementioned advantage of caesarean section reducing both maternal and neonatal mortality was lost once the caesarean section rate was greater than 10% [5].

The big question then is this, 'Is there really an optimal caesarean section rate'? Recently, a global online survey of medical doctors who had performed at least one caesarean in the last 5 years was conducted and respondents were asked to report their opinion of the optimal caesarean rate (defined as the caesarean rate that would minimise poor maternal and perinatal outcomes); there was sizeable disparity in their responses, and this further highlights a lack of consensus around which women are in need of a caesarean among obstetric care providers worldwide [9].

The WHO in 1985 suggested that a rate between 10% and 15% was ideal, however, in their most recent statement WHO concluded that:

1. Caesarean sections are effective in saving maternal and infant lives, but only when they are required for medically indicated reasons.
2. At population level, caesarean section rates higher than 10% are not associated with reductions in maternal and new-born mortality rates.
3. Caesarean sections can cause significant and sometimes permanent complications, disability or death particularly in settings that lack the facilities and/or capacity to properly conduct safe surgery and treat surgical complications. Caesarean sections should ideally only be undertaken when medically necessary.
4. Every effort should be made to provide caesarean sections to women in need, rather than to achieve a specific rate.
5. The effects of caesarean section rates on other outcomes, such as maternal and perinatal morbidity, paediatric outcomes and psychological or social well-being are still unclear. More research is needed to understand the health effects of caesarean section on immediate and future outcomes.

The WHO has also proposed that the Robson classification system be used as a global standard for assessing, monitoring and comparing caesarean section rates within and between healthcare facilities over time. The WHO plans to develop guidelines for the use, implementation and interpretation, including standardisation of terms and definitions of the Robson classification in order to assist healthcare facilities [10]. Further, JP Souza et al. using the WHO Multi-Country Survey on Maternal and Newborn Health created a mathematical model, the 'C-Model', a tool designed to guide obstetric teams, health managers and other stakeholders in the complex task of optimising the use of CS. They built their model including comparison of caesarean rates across different populations and institutions, they applied dynamic econometric models to assess aggregate level determinants of caesarean section rates in developed countries, and made adjustments for Robson's Ten-Group Classification System, as well as clinical and socio-demographic variables of the mother and the foetus for inter-hospital comparisons of CS rates. Through a customised estimate of CS rates, the C-Model may provide a locally relevant reference of what would be an optimal CS rate. Nevertheless, this should not be used to prevent a woman that needs a caesarean from having one or vice versa [1].

18.3 The Indications of Caesarean Section

The most common indications for caesarean section in the United States are previous caesarean section, failure to progress in labour and foetal distress, accounting for 35%, 30% and 8% of caesarean sections respectively [11]. The rising rates of caesarean section have led to questions being raised about the appropriate use of caesarean sections for many indications. These questions are motivated by several observations. First, the United States has higher rates of infant mortality than many developed countries in which caesarean rates are less than half of those in the United States [12]. Second, there is considerable variation in the use of caesareans between regions of the United States, and from hospital to hospital [13]. This variation does not appear to be explained by differences in clinical risk factors, since non-clinical factors such as hospital ownership, hospital teaching status, payment source and volume of deliveries have also been shown to influence the rate of caesarean births [14, 15]. All of these observations suggest that factors other than the health benefits to mother or infant may influence the decision to perform caesarean delivery [16].

We continue to witness a rise in caesarean section rate due to factors as maternal request for social reasons and perceived medical reasons such as the protection of the pelvic floor muscles. Some observers have suggested that the caesarean rate has been affected by other factors, such as defensive medicine and financial rewards in the private sector. Further research is required into these emerging indications.

18.4 Cephalopelvic Disproportion (CPD)

Failure to progress in labour or dystocia is a leading indication for primary caesarean section and has a major impact on escalating caesarean section rate (CSR) especially in the United States [17]. Studies have shown that the diagnosis of CPD has no prognostic value from one pregnancy to the next and generally should not exclude a patient from a trial of labour. In women with a cephalic presentation who had an arrest of descent in the second stage of labour during their first delivery, the chances of vaginal delivery in their next pregnancy are high, even after a failed instrumental vagina delivery, and a trial of labour can usually be pursued with success [18]. In the study of 132 women in their second pregnancy and who had a caesarean section in the first pregnancy, 29 (22%) underwent planned repeat caesarean section. Of the 103 women who were allowed a trial of labour, 82 (80%) were successful in having vaginal delivery, and 21 (20%) had a second caesarean section. Of the 74 women with failed trial of instrumental delivery during the previous labour, 19 had a planned repeat caesarean section while 41 of the remaining 55 (75%) had successful trial of labour.

18.5 Foetal Distress in Labour

This is an acceptable indication for caesarean section. Peter et al. [19] found that foetal distress was the indication for 25% of caesarean sections in their study. The diagnosis of 'fetal distress' is open to different interpretations. Initially, Apgar scores were used to determine the presence or absence of 'true' distress, but they have been shown to correlate poorly with other morbidity measures and with long term outcomes [20]. The development of procedures such as electronic foetal monitoring (EFM) for the diagnosis of foetal distress has been made difficult by the fact that they were introduced into clinical practice without being subjected to clinical trials and the lack of a 'gold standard' against which they can be assessed. Inter and intra-observer reliability of cardiotocography (CTG) interpretation is poor. In one study, four obstetricians were asked to read 50 different CTG tracings. Only 11 of the 50 tracings were assessed in the same way 'need for immediate delivery' by all four physicians. 21% of the tracings were interpreted differently by individual obstetricians when re-assessed 2 months later [21]. The diagnosis of hypoxia based on cardiotocography (CTG) alone has led to an increase in caesarean section rate (CSR). The use of foetal scalp pH to confirm the diagnosis of foetal distress in labour is recommended. Ayromlooi and Garfinkel

[23] found that foetal blood sampling has helped reduce the CSR. MacDonald et al. [24], however, have shown that electronic foetal monitoring did not influence the number of caesarean sections in low-risk pregnancies at the National Maternity Hospital, Dublin. Electronic foetal heart monitoring is indicated in high-risk women.

18.6 Breech Presentation

Breech babies are often prone to birth injuries and intrauterine hypoxia during vaginal deliveries. Kubli et al. [24], found that foetal acidosis was much more common in breech than cephalic presentations and concluded that all breeches should be delivered by caesarean section. The management dilemma of best mode of delivery persisted for years until when the term breech trial, a randomised control trial, recommended caesarean section as the safer option of delivery. The trial involved 2088 women from 121 centres in 26 countries, all of whom were at least 37 weeks pregnant with a single live foetus in a breech position between January 1997 and April 2000. The women were randomly assigned to have either a planned caesarean delivery or a planned vaginal birth. The trial showed that in pregnant women with breech presentation, planned caesarean section had a lower risk for perinatal mortality and serious morbidity than did planned vaginal birth [25]. This has changed the management of breech foetuses and has contributed to the rising rate of caesarean section. The trend in the UK in line with the RCOG guideline is to offer women who have an uncomplicated singleton breech pregnancy at 36 weeks' gestation external cephalic version with the exceptions of women in advanced labour and women with a uterine scar or major uterine abnormality, foetal compromise, ruptured membranes, recent vaginal bleeding, multiple pregnancy or medical conditions (Royal College of Obstetricians and Gynaecologists. The Management of Breech Presentation. Guideline No. 20. London: RCOG Press; 2001). This is aimed at reducing the need for caesarean section. If external cephalic version is contraindicated or unsuccessful, the women are offered caesarean section because it reduces perinatal mortality and neonatal morbidity [26].

Paul et al. [27], examined 72 patients with breech presentation and found that vaginal delivery was achieved in 46%, and 18% allowed a trial of labour. Access to a delivery suite with facilities for performing a caesarean section is not always possible in developing nations and the inevitability of carrying out vaginal breech deliveries exists. Schutte et al. [29] and O'Driscoll and Foley [28] showed that breeches could be safely delivered vaginally. However, certain criteria have to be met to improve the likelihood of a safe delivery. These criteria include the following:

(i) Anticipated foetal weight is 3.5 kg or less by ultrasound examination (or clinical estimation where ultrasound is not available)
(ii) Frank breech presentation with flexed head
(iii) The presence of an experienced obstetrician to conduct the delivery

Planned caesarean section compared with planned vaginal birth has been shown to reduce perinatal or neonatal death as well as the composite outcome death or serious neonatal morbidity, but this is at the expense of slightly increased maternal morbidity. Remarkably, a 2-year follow up, has identified that there were increased infant medical problems following planned caesarean section and there were no differences in long-term neurodevelopmental delay or the outcome of 'death although the numbers were too small to exclude the possibility of an important difference in either direction' [30]. Thus, the benefits need to be weighed against factors like the mother's access to a safe hospital for her future trial of labour (especially in a resource poor country with limited hospitals and obstetricians), her preference for vaginal birth, and the risks to her future pregnancy complications in the woman's specific healthcare setting.

18.7 Multiple Pregnancy

There is little evidence regarding the best mode or type of delivery for women with multiple pregnancy [31]. There is ongoing debate as to the optimum mode of delivery for multiple pregnancy. This has been due to the increasing recourse to caesarean section for the delivery of the second twin. One limited trial found no advantage of caesarean section for a second twin presenting other than as a vertex [32]. There is a place for advocating an elective caesarean section in high order multiple pregnancy in order to prevent birth trauma in the small foetuses.

It would be logical to think that the abdominal distension associated with multiple pregnancy may predispose to dehiscence or rupture of a previous caesarean section scar. Gilbert et al. [32], in a retrospective study showed that a transverse low uterine segment scar does not present a risk because of uterine distension secondary to a twin pregnancy. Strong et al. [33], studied the pregnancy outcome of 56 women with twin gestation and a previous section birth. In these patients, 31 (55%) underwent an elective repeat caesarean delivery and 25(45%) attempted a vaginal delivery. In the latter, 18 (72%) were vaginally delivered of both infants. The dehiscence rate among women with twin pregnancies who attempted a trial of labour was 4%, compared with 2% in women with a singleton pregnancy.

'The Twin Birth Study', a Randomised Trial of Planned Caesarean or Vaginal Delivery for Twin Pregnancy, as well as a Cochrane review have concluded that in twin pregnancy between 32 weeks 0 days and 38 weeks 6 days of gestation, with the first twin in the cephalic presentation, planned caesarean delivery did not significantly decrease or increase the risk of foetal or neonatal death or serious neonatal morbidity, as compared with planned vaginal delivery. Hence, there is insufficient evidence to support the routine use of planned caesarean section for term twin pregnancy with leading cephalic presentation [34, 35].

18.8 Very Low Birth Weight Babies (500–1499 g)

Increasing numbers of very low birth weight (VLBW) infants are being delivered by caesarean section in order to reduce the incidence of birth trauma. However, population-based data do not support the view that caesarean section enhances the neonatal survival of VLBW babies when obstetric complications are absent [36]. Caesarean section has been shown to be beneficial to LBWB with breech presentation [37]

18.9 Prevention of Mother-to-Child Transmission of Maternal Infections

Women with viral blood borne infections need to be given information as early as possible about the risks and benefits for them and their child as well as of the treatment options and mode of birth so that they can make an informed decision. They should not be routinely offered a caesarean section on the grounds of their infection. To prevent mother-to-child transmission of HIV offer vaginal birth to women on highly active anti-retroviral therapy (HAART) that have a viral load of less than 400 copies per mL or if on any anti-retroviral therapy with a viral load of less than 50 copies per mL as the risk of HIV transmission is the same for a CS and a vaginal birth [26].

They can either have a vaginal birth or a CS for women on anti-retroviral therapy (ART) if their viral load is between 50 and 400 copies per mL because there is insufficient evidence that a caesarean section prevents mother-to-child transmission of HIV. However, women with HIV who are not receiving any anti-retroviral therapy or are receiving any anti-retroviral therapy and have a viral load of 400 copies per mL or more should be advised to have a caesarean section [26].

Mother-to-child transmission of hepatitis B can be reduced if the baby receives immunoglobulin and vaccination. Hence, pregnant women with hepatitis B should not be offered an elective caesarean birth as there is insufficient evidence that this reduces mother-to-child transmission of hepatitis B virus [26]. Additionally, women who are infected with hepatitis C should not be offered a planned CS because this does not reduce mother-to-child transmission of the virus. Though, pregnant women who are co-infected with hepatitis C virus and HIV should be offered planned CS because it reduces mother-to-child transmission of both hepatitis C virus and HIV [26].

Women with primary genital herpes simplex virus (HSV) infection occurring in the third trimester of pregnancy should be offered planned CS because it decreases the risk of neonatal HSV infection. Conversely, if it is a recurrence of HSV the risk of transmission is less. Therefore, CS should not routinely be offered [26].

18.10 Maternal Request

A new trend is arising with women requesting caesarean section, where some women have a genuine fear of labour 'Tocophobia', others cannot be bothered to push for various reasons, 'the too posh to push group'. These women who request a caesarean section (when there is no clinical indication) need to have a documented discussion with members of the maternity team about the overall risks and benefits of a caesarean section compared with vaginal birth [38]. Those who request a caesarean section because of anxiety about childbirth should be referred to a healthcare professional with expertise in perinatal mental health support [38]. Two small randomised trials suggested that a nurse-led relaxation training programme for women with a fear or anxiety of childbirth as well as birth preparation sessions were effective in reducing caesarean section rates [39].

Sydsjö G et al. investigated the prevalence of psychiatric illness amongst women who requested for caesarean section and found psychiatric illnesses was significantly higher in women giving birth by caesarean section on maternal request. The most common diagnoses were 'Neurotic disorders, stress-related disorders and somatoform disorders' and 'Mood disorders'. Further, in his study, women giving birth by caesarean section on maternal request were older, smoked more, had a lower educational level, higher body mass index, were more often married, unemployed and their parents were more often born outside of Scandinavia [40]. It is imperative that patient-centred care is offered and patients provided with full information to aid them in decision-making about their care.

18.11 Classification of Caesarean Section

The National Institute of Health and Care Excellence (NICE) guidelines in the UK advised that the urgency of caesarean section should be documented using a standardised scheme in order to aid clear communication between healthcare professionals about the urgency of a CS. They classify caesarean section from category 1–4 [26].

1. Immediate threat to the life of the woman or foetus
2. Maternal or foetal compromise which is not immediately life-threatening
3. No maternal or foetal compromise but needs early delivery
4. Delivery timed to suit woman or staff

Obstetricians are advised to perform category 1 caesarean section as quickly as possible after making the decision, that is, the decision-to-delivery intervals should be within 30 min. Category 2 caesarean section in most situations should be performed within 75 min of making the decision. Nonetheless, care should be taken to consider the condition of the woman and the unborn baby when making decisions about rapid delivery, because rapid delivery may be harmful in certain circumstances. This is not a tool to measure the overall performance of an obstetric unit, or to judge multidisciplinary team performance for any individual caesarean section. It is to communicate urgency to the multidisciplinary, and it could also be used as a tool for audit standards [26].

In the developing countries, the recommendation of decision delivery interval of 30 min is not currently feasible; several studies have shown that in only between 0% and 6% of cases were the caesarean done within 30 min. Anaesthetic delay was the major cause of delay in carrying out emergency caesarean sections. The average interval in the studies were between 100 and 400 min, although the decision delivery interval was not deemed to correlate with perinatal outcome. The perinatal outcomes used were Apgar scores, admission to neonatal unit as well as perinatal death, but there is a great spectrum between a healthy baby and a dead one [41–43]. Nonetheless, effort should be made to expedite caesarean section when it is life threatening to either the mother or the foetus.

18.12 Elective Caesarean Section

The indications for an elective operation are often relative rather than absolute. Factors such as maternal age, relative infertility, past obstetric history, as well as foetal age and estimated weight are taken into consideration. Maternal request is increasingly becoming an acceptable indication for elective and emergency caesarean sections. In the developing world, cephalopelvic disproportion is fairly common due to the small underdeveloped pelvis in teenage brides. In Europe and other developed parts of the world, cephalopelvic disproportion is not common and not a usual indication for primary elective caesarean section. Elective caesarean section is usually performed following a previous caesarean section due to suspected cephalopelvic disproportion. However, a repeat caesarean section may not be necessary if the babies in subsequent pregnancies are much smaller than the baby born previously by caesarean section.

An elective caesarean section is justified whenever it is deemed that the uterus or foetus could be damaged during labour. Previous uterine surgery or injury normally constitute a real hazard though the degree of potential danger will often depend on the site of the scar, the clinical conditions influencing previous healing, for example, infection, and the site of the placenta in the current pregnancy.

If there is a uterine anomaly or anomaly of the lower genital tract, which precludes vaginal delivery or endangers nearby structures, for example, a successful vesico-vaginal fistula repair, or surgically treated stress incontinence, elective caesarean section may be preferable. Both minor and major degrees of placenta praevia or fulminating pre-eclampsia are special indications for elective caesarean section.

The usual time for an elective caesarean section for such reasons like cephalopelvic disproportion, breech presentation, placenta praevia, or previous caesarean section is after 37 completed weeks and not beyond 40 weeks gestation, preferably after the 39 weeks to reduce the risk of admission to neonatal unit. It is good clinical practice to ascertain foetal maturity by referring to the gestational age as calculated from a dating ultrasound scan to avoid the delivery of a premature baby.

In situations such as foetal growth restriction, the timing of the operation will require a careful judgment. One needs to balance the risks of prematurity and continued intrauterine existence. Antenatal cardiotocography with the addition of foetal umbilical artery Doppler studies, where available, will help to determine the optimum time for delivery. The administration of antenatal corticosteroids to the mother will help promote foetal lung maturation and is recommended.

18.13 Caesarean Section in Labour

It is sometimes necessary to abandon a proposed vaginal delivery in favour of an abdominal delivery. The indications for this change are usually fairly clear – obstructed labour occurring during labour or the appearance of foetal or maternal distress prior to full cervical dilatation. Before deciding to operate, it is important for the obstetrician to confirm that foetal distress is not being caused simply by the injudicious use of oxytocics over-stimulating uterine activity. Also, if maternal distress is being aggravated by pain, it may be sensible to consider introducing epidural analgesia before finally deciding upon the need for caesarean section.

Delay in the progress of labour, especially during the first stage, is probably the commonest reason for considering the need to deliver a baby abdominally. In this clinical situation, it is helpful to have partographic evidence of delay, as the visual evidence of a partograph often helps the obstetrician to distinguish between any sudden onset of delay after normal progress and the slow latent or first stage of labour.

In addition to partography, it is helpful to have some reliable quantitative measure of uterine activity. Simple clinical assessments of uterine activity are rather unreliable. Many potential caesarean sections for uterine inertia can probably be avoided by recognising quantitatively that uterine activity is sub-optimal. The restoration of optimal uterine activity by oxytocic stimulation may then be attempted. If optimal activity according to quantitative criteria cannot be restored, or if delay continues despite optimal uterine activity, the indications for caesarean section become much clearer. A common example of the value of using quantitative assessments of uterine activity is the slow rotation of a foetal head from the occipito-posterior position. This will often result from uterine inertia rather than from any disadvantageous cephalopelvic relationships. If optimal uterine activity can be secured, abdominal delivery may well be averted. Conversely, if delayed progress continues despite the stimulation of uterine activity that is quantitatively satisfactory, there is a clear indication to proceed to caesarean section. Delay in labour in a multiparous woman is to be viewed with extreme suspicion. This clinical situation always necessitates prompt and careful evaluation. Uterine inertia is a most uncommon cause.

In the developing countries with inherent lack of maternity services and facilities, obstructed labour complicated by significant delay and impaction of presenting part, maternal and foetal distress or even intrauterine foetal death, are not uncommon especially among unbooked patients. This is a situation almost unknown in the developed world. When the situation does occur, the patient presents a serious operative risk. Despite the need for haste in proceeding with the operation, adequate time must be spent to properly resuscitate the patient. Dehydration must be corrected as well as any electrolyte deficit or acidosis. Central venous pressure monitoring will be required if the patient is in shock, and in the presence of septicaemia, broad-spectrum antibiotics are necessary and probably steroid therapy as well. De Lee incision (a low vertical instead of a low transverse) in the uterus is recommended when, because of thinning and distension of the lower segment, there is a danger that any transverse incision may extend laterally and compromise major vessels or the uterus. A particularly dangerous circumstance is a neglected shoulder presentation with a prolapsed arm. In obstructed labour, the bladder is usually bruised and friable and may extend much higher into the abdomen than is usual. To avoid damage to the bladder, the parietal peritoneum must be entered higher than usual and the bladder must be reflected downwards with extreme caution.

18.14 Surgical Technique of Caesarean Section

Pre-operative preparations include haemoglobin estimation, blood group determination and saving for cross-match. The use of a lateral 15° wedge at caesarean section is now mandatory in order to reduce the effects of caval occlusion during surgery. Immediate pre-operative preparation also includes administration of sodium citrate by mouth or H_2 antagonist.

The commonest incision is a transverse incision on the lower segment of the uterus. The lower segment is approached through a Pfannenstiel incision, a transverse incision through the skin and external sheath of the recti muscles, about an inch above the pubes. It follows natural folds of the skin and curves over mons pubis in such a way that the pubic hairs cover the cicatrix.

More recently, the transverse incision of choice is the Joel Cohen incision (a straight skin incision, 3 cm above the symphysis pubis; subsequent tissue layers are opened bluntly and, if necessary, extended with scissors and not a knife), this is because it is associated with shorter operating times and reduced postoperative febrile morbidity [26]. A lower segment uterine incision is widely used, as it has a much lower risk of scar rupture than a classical incision (0.5% compared with 2.2%). Care must be taken to reflect the bladder downwards before incising the uterus; it is at this time that most bladder injuries occur. The classical incision that employs a midline uterine incision is rarely used today. It may be indicated in a few situations such as in the presence of cervical carcinoma, and with a transverse lie with a prolapsed arm [17]. It may also be indicated if the lower half of the patient's uterus is very vascular as may occur in placenta praevia, or inaccessible as the result of adhesions from a previous operation joining her lower segment to her abdominal wall. A classical incision may also be used in the delivery of pre-term infants at less than 28 weeks gestation when the lower segment is not sufficiently formed.

The De Lee incision is a modified classical incision. It is a vertical incision, two thirds of which are in the lower segment, and one-third in the upper one. It is thus a cross between the classical upper segment operation, and the ordinary lower segment one. It is advisable to make a De Lee incision if a lateral tear is likely, as can happen if the lower segment is very thin, or the baby is in an abnormal position, as in a transverse lie. It has the advantages of allowing easier access than the lower segment incision and causes less bleeding than a classical incision. Most studies of scar rupture do not differentiate between a classical and a De Lee incision but the risk of rupture of the latter incision is usually quoted as lying between that of the classical and lower segment incisions. Patients who have had a previous classical, low vertical incision or an inverted T-incision should be delivered by an elective caesarean section in subsequent pregnancies in order to minimise the risk of uterine rupture.

The number of layers to repair the uterus has been contentious; however, a recent meta-analysis found that 'the risk of uterine rupture during trial of labour after a single-layer closure was not significantly different from that after a double-layer closure'. However, a sensitivity analysis indicated that the risk of uterine rupture was increased after a locked single-layer closure but not after an unlocked single-layer closure, compared with a double-layer closure [44].

18.15 Peritoneal Closure

The sutures used to close the peritoneum may cause more adhesions than if the peritoneal edges were left unsutured. The traditional practice until recently was to close the peritoneum at caesarean section. It has been shown that for gynaecological procedures, omitting peritoneal closure does not increase the length of hospital stay or the subsequent development of adhesions [45]. It would therefore seem logical to apply this to caesarean section.

The Royal College of Obstetricians and Gynaecologists as well as the NICE guidelines in the UK recommend non-closure of the peritoneum at caesarean section. Studies have shown that non-closure of the parietal peritoneum results in significantly shorter operating time and post-operative hospital stay. It is also associated with lower post-operative febrile morbidity and postoperative use of analgesics [26]. A recent Cochrane review concluded that there is insufficient evidence of benefit to justify the additional time and use of suture material necessary for peritoneal closure [46].

18.16 Anaesthesia for Caesarean Section

Factors to be taken into consideration when choosing an anaesthetic for caesarean section include the safety of the mother, the safety of the foetus, the experience of the anaesthetist and the ability to perform the surgery under that anaesthetic technique. Caesarean section can be performed under general or regional anaesthesia. Regional anaesthesia includes both spinal and epidural anaesthesia. Increasing numbers of caesarean sections are performed under regional anaesthesia for safety reasons, and it is the preferred method when time is not as much of a factor [26].

Regional anaesthesia includes both spinal and epidural techniques. Contraindications to the use of regional anaesthesia include patients with bleeding and clotting abnormalities, patients with neurological problems and patients with infections that might be spread to the spinal area if regional anaesthesia is done.

Spinal anaesthesia is faster and simpler to place, works slightly faster and is less technically complicated than an epidural anaesthesia. A combined spinal epidural has a single injection like a spinal anaesthesia, as well as, an epidural catheter placed in the back; this allows the anaesthetic, Marcain, to be given repeatedly or continuously. If an epidural catheter is already in place for labour analgesia, then it makes sense to utilise this, should a caesarean become necessary. An epidural may also be used for postoperative pain control. Music is increasingly being used in theatre, current studies indicate that music during planned caesarean section under regional anaesthesia may improve pulse rate and birth satisfaction score [47].

The main disadvantages of general anaesthesia include the fact that the mother is unconscious and, therefore, unable to participate in the process of birth or interact with the baby once it is delivered. General anaesthesia is performed when there is an urgent need to deliver the baby. The advantages of general anaesthesia are that it can be given very quickly and the blood pressure is more easily controlled. The disadvantages of general anaesthesia include the fact that it wears off quickly, resulting in greater post-operative pain and increasing the need for postoperative analgesia. The other disadvantage is that there are some significant risks associated with general anaesthesia. Anaesthetic complications at present account for 5% of all direct deaths associated with caesarean section. Almost all of these are associated with general anaesthesia. The primary causes are failure of endotracheal intubation and inhalation of acidic stomach contents resulting in Mendelson's syndrome. Failure of intubation may be due to anatomical variations in the patient's neck or jaw or an abnormally small larynx or trachea.

It is recommended that an anaesthetist of at least registrar grade should cover a labour ward and a fully trained assistant (operating department personnel) should be present. The complications of a failed intubation can be minimised by regularly carrying out a failed intubation drill. Mendelson's syndrome accounted for 32 maternal deaths in the first report on confidential enquiries into maternal deaths in 1952. Better understanding of the disease process has led to the use of important therapeutic strategies to minimise the risks of aspiration and has led to a progressive reduction in the maternal death rate from aspiration syndromes to the extent that no maternal deaths were reported in the confidential enquiries into maternal deaths (1988–1990). The therapeutic strategies that have been adopted include the use of cricoid pressure at induction in association with pre-oxygenation and the use of a cuffed endotracheal tube to protect the airway. The administration of ranitidine, an H2 antagonist is used to raise the gastric pH and is more effective than sodium citrate at raising gastric pH. If used prior to elective caesarean section, two oral doses of ranitidine (150 mg) should be given, one the night before surgery and one on the morning of the operation. For emergency caesarean section, ranitidine 50 mg can be given intravenously. Sodium citrate should also be used. H2 antagonists may have the additional advantage of reducing gastric volume. The combined use of ranitidine and sodium citrate will raise gastric pH above 2.5 in the great majority of women in labour [48]. Women are also given anti-emetics to reduce nausea and vomiting during CS. General anaesthesia for emergency caesarean delivery should include pre-oxygenation, cricoid pressure and rapid sequence induction to reduce the risk of aspiration [26].

18.17 Complications of Caesarean Section

As with other surgical operations, caesarean section is not without its risk. The risks of caesarean section include maternal death, haemorrhage, venous thrombosis, infection, and anaesthetic complications. The latter has been dealt with in the preceding paragraph. Intraoperative surgical complications include damage to adjacent organs, for example: bladder, ureter or bowel, as well as inadvertent damage to the uterus or cervix. The occurrence of one or more of these complications is reported to be approximately 12% [49]. Caesarean sections performed during labour have overall complication rates greater than during a planned procedure (24% compared with 16%). Further, complication rates are higher at 9–10 cm dilatation when compared with 0–1 cm (33% compared with 17%) [50].

18.18 Maternal Death

The estimated risk of a woman dying after a caesarean section is less than one in 2500 (the risk of death after a vaginal birth is less than one in 10,000). The absolute risk of death in childbirth is small. In 1997–1999, there were two million births in the UK, of which 400,000 were by caesarean section. Sixty-nine women died at or shortly after giving birth; 40 of these deaths were after caesarean section, giving a fatality rate for caesarean section around five times greater than vaginal birth [38]. It cannot necessarily be concluded that caesarean section is more dangerous than vaginal birth because pre-existing conditions may have influenced the decision to carry out the CS and the outcome. Complications from caesarean section including maternal mortality and sepsis are, however, much higher in the developing countries. Ojo et al. [51] in a retrospective analysis of 27 maternal deaths after caesarean section over 5 years in Nigeria, found that caesarean section was 4.1%. Maternal mortality rate (MMR) following caesarean section was 18.1 per 1000 (81.5% from sepsis) while 1.89 per 1000 MMR from Egypt was equally high at 5% of all maternal mortality [52]. Factors contributing to this high maternal mortality include sepsis, obstructed labour, poor access to facilities, lack of equipment and poorly trained personnel. The risk of postpartum maternal death was almost threefold higher with caesarean than vaginal delivery, mainly due to deaths from postpartum haemorrhage and complications of anaesthesia [3].

Due to very low maternal mortality in developed countries, significant maternal morbidity is often used as an indirect means for maternal mortality which is described as 'near misses'. The overall incidence of near miss is about 7.1 per 1000 births and, irrespective of the mode of birth, advanced maternal age, high BMI and nulliparity were identified as significant risk factors. Any type of caesarean birth was associated with a five-times increased risk of near miss [53].

18.19 Haemorrhage

Blood loss at caesarean section is about twice as much as with vaginal delivery. However, the overall incidence of intra-operative blood transfusion for acute blood loss at caesarean section is between 0.6% and 1.0%. Haemorrhage accounts for 6% of deaths associated with caesarean section and an unknown proportion of postoperative morbidity. Risk factors include placenta praevia, placental abruption and uterine atony in multiple pregnancy or multiparous patients. Patients requiring a cross-match of blood prior to caesarean section include those with placenta praevia Grade IV and severe pre-eclampsia with evidence of coagulopathy. Disseminated intravascular coagulation is a rare cause but must be considered in cases of continuing haemorrhage.

Haemorrhage may be primary, delayed primary or secondary. Bleeding may come from the placental bed or may be due to a tear or extended uterine incision into major vessels. A rapid first line of uterine sutures must be placed to close the uterine incision taking care to include the angles in the suture. Delivering the uterus onto the abdomen may facilitate this. Bleeding tears should be repaired in two layers. Caution should be exercised to avoid injuring the ureter when repairing extended tears.

Uterine atony may be corrected by a bolus dose of 10 units of syntocinon given intravenously followed by a continuous infusion of 40 units of syntocinon in 500 mL of normal saline over 2 h. The use of Hemabate (carboprost tromethamine) should be considered if uterine atony and bleeding persists. Hemabate may be injected directly into the uterine muscle or given intra-muscularly. If haemorrhage continues, more radical surgical intervention is required. The B-Lynch suturing technique (brace suture) may be particularly useful because of its simplicity of application, life-saving potential, relative safety, and its capacity for preserving the uterus and, thus, fertility. Satisfactory haemostasis can be assessed immediately after application. The special advantage of this innovative technique is an alternative to major surgical procedures to control pelvic arterial pulse pressure or hysterectomy. This suturing technique has been successfully applied with no problems to date and no apparent complications documented [54].

If the B-Lynch suture fails, more radical surgical methods should be considered. These include tying off the uterine arteries and, if unsuccessful, ligating the internal iliac arteries. The long-term blood supply to the uterus is not compromised as an adequate collateral circulation is already present and takes effect immediately [55]. There is no compromise of the pelvic tissues following internal artery ligation, and subsequent normal pregnancies have been reported. If there is access to interventional radiologist, internal iliac catheters or embolisation could be used, this helps to reduce the bleeding and may completely stop the haemorrhage and prevent hysterectomy. The reader is referred to the treatment of the collapsed obstetric patients in other text.

18.20 Deep Venous Thrombosis and Pulmonary Thrombosis

Thrombosis and thromboembolism remains once again the leading cause of direct maternal death [56]. Pulmonary embolism is the major cause of maternal mortality following caesarean section accounting for 15% of direct deaths. Pregnant women and in particular those with a history of thromboembolic disease are at appreciable risk during pregnancy. The reported incidence of deep vein thrombosis (DVT) and non-fatal pulmonary embolism varies considerably because of the peculiar diagnostic difficulties in pregnancy. Real time ultrasound scanning combined with Doppler studies, being noninvasive, are the first line diagnostic techniques for DVT in pregnancy [57]. The majority of deaths from pulmonary embolism following caesarean section occur after the first week of the puerperium after discharge from hospital. All those involved with the care of women in the puerperium must be alert to this possibility. A clinically recognisable deep venous thrombosis precedes only 50% of cases of pulmonary embolus and, therefore, clinical suspicion must be high. The patient may present with a pyrexia, cough, shortness of breath, or acutely collapsed. It is essential that an accurate diagnosis be made, as inappropriate full anticoagulation carries risk to mother and foetus.

The Royal College of Obstetricians and Gynaecologists [57] recommend the following guidelines:

18.21 Prophylaxis Against Thromboembolic Disease in Patients Undergoing a Caesarean Section

- A risk assessment should be performed.
- Early mobilisation and adequate hydration are required.
- Patients at moderate risk should receive subcutaneous heparin or mechanical methods (Flowtrons).
- Patients at high risk should receive heparin prophylaxis and, in addition, leg stockings would be beneficial.
- Prophylaxis should be continued for 10 days or more depending on risk assessment.
- Subcutaneous heparin can be used after 4–6 h post operation in patients with an epidural or spinal block.

18.22 Caesarean Section and Chorioamnionitis

Chorioamnionitis is an overt intrauterine infection involving the amniotic fluid, placental membranes and the baby. The incidence of histologic chorioamnionitis (44%) is far larger than the incidence of culture positive amniotic fluid that is about 26% of clinical chorioamnionitis (9.6%) [58]. These are European figures and it would be expected to be much higher in the African setting in view of the general state of poor hygiene and sterility.

Premature rupture of the membranes is the commonest antecedent of significant intra-amniotic infection. Foetal and maternal tachycardia associated with low-grade pyrexia, and possibly offensive liquor, may be the earliest signs of developing infection. Broad-spectrum parental antibiotics should be commenced immediately. The mode of delivery will depend on the gestational age, state of the cervix and the foetal condition. Caesarean section should be considered if foetal maturity exceeds 26 weeks and the foetus is normal.

Extraperitoneal caesarean section is indicated if there is established chorioamnionitis. The presence of antibiotics, particularly metronidazole, has made the need for extraperitoneal approach unnecessary. Its use is recommended in the absence of antibiotics as it greatly reduces the incidence of life-threatening peritonitis. Excluding the incision in the uterus from the peritoneal cavity reduces the risk of peritonitis. To do this, the parietal peritoneum is reflected from the inside of the abdominal wall, the visceral peritoneum from the front of the lower uterine segment, and both tied together. This seals off the peritoneal cavity from the incision that is then made into the infected uterus. Suction evacuation of liquor following an incision into the uterus also minimises the risk of spreading infection by spillage. Irrigation of the extraperitoneal space should be performed post-operatively.

18.23 Peripartum (Caesarean/Postpartum) Hysterectomy

Postpartum hysterectomy (PH) refers to hysterectomy done either after vaginal delivery or skin closure after caesarean section, while caesarean hysterectomy is done in the same surgical case as caesarean delivery. Peripartum hysterectomies are largely unplanned and usually performed to control life-threatening haemorrhage and often done as an emergency. The most common indication for peripartum hysterectomy is uncontrollable maternal haemorrhage especially associated with a morbidly adherent placenta. It may also be performed for co-existing cervical or uterine carcinoma, uterine rupture, or as a sterilising procedure [59]. Peripartum hysterectomy (PH) remains one of the obstetric catastrophes. It is associated with increased maternal mortality, considerable morbidity and it brings an abrupt, and usually unwelcome, end to a woman's reproductive potential [60–62].

PH complicates about 1 in 1000 deliveries [60]. The incidence, however, can vary from 1 in 442 in a Nigerian series compared with 1 in 1243 in a North American series, and 1 in 6967 in an Asian study [61–63]. The incidence varies over time, depends on the healthcare setting, and is strongly influenced by caesarean delivery rates [64]. The incidence of this procedure is lower in the United Kingdom than the United States as elective hysterectomy is usually postponed until after the puerperium when it is less hazardous. A study comparing outcomes of caesarean section showed that hysterectomy was uncommon in the vaginal birth reference group (0.05%) but was over 4 time more common among women who experienced both elective, and emergency caesarean delivery [65, 66].

18.24 Indications

Massive maternal haemorrhage is the commonest cause for postpartum hysterectomy. However, the underlying causes include uterine atony, uterine rupture and placental bed pathology [64]. There is a rising indication to undertake postpartum hysterectomy in cases of placenta accreta/percreta [67, 68]. An increase in PH for placenta accreta/percreta has also been reported and is associated with the rising caesarean delivery rate [69]. The risk of caesarean hysterectomy rises with the increasing number of prior caesareans [70].

Women with a prior caesarean should ideally have an ultrasound examination for placental localisation before the third trimester. The diagnosis of placental bed pathology and/or praevia may be suspected on ultrasound and, if the resources are available, other imaging technologies such as Doppler may be helpful diagnostically [71]. If the possibility of PH for placenta accreta/percreta is anticipated, the mother, her family and her medical team can prepare. The caesarean delivery should be performed under the supervision of an experienced obstetrician and anaesthetist. If a hysterectomy, particularly a total procedure, becomes necessary, assistance from a gynaecological oncologist should be considered if the obstetrician is not experienced in performing difficult hysterectomies. Total hysterectomies for placental bed pathology can be anticipated, whereas hysterectomy for atony usually cannot. An in-depth discussion about the management of patients with placenta accreta or percreta is beyond the scope of this chapter. Suffice to say that it requires multiprofessional management.

The rising rate of repeat elective caesarean delivery has conflicting effects on the incidence of PH. On the one hand, repeat elective caesarean delivery should, in the short-term, decrease the number of PHs for haemorrhage associated with either uterine rupture or traumatic intrapartum vaginal delivery because of the association between haemorrhage and caesarean in labour [69]. On the other hand, repeat caesareans are associated, in the long-term, with an increase in PH for pathological placental localisation, particularly as the number of repeat elective caesareans increases [70]. A woman with a prior caesarean whose family is complete may minimise her risk of hysterectomy by opting for a repeat elective caesarean [64].

The maternal death rate associated with caesarean hysterectomy from all causes is 0.7% [72] compared to 0.05% for all caesarean sections. Complication of caesarean hysterectomy is similar but higher than caesarean delivery. If hysterectomy is performed for uncontrolled uterine bleeding after delivery, the risk of the patient having disseminated intravascular coagulation (DIC) is high. Caesarean hysterectomy should not be left too late as the risk of uncontrollable haemorrhage is increased. Pelvic tissue in pregnancy is lax with increased oedema and vascularity, therefore, care is needed especially in tying pedicles, and the uterine side of the pedicle may also need to be ligated as back bleeding may be considerable [48]. There may be difficulty in identifying the lower margin of the cervix and a subtotal hysterectomy may be performed either deliberately or in error. This can be corrected either at the time of hysterectomy or as a second procedure. Prerequisites for peripartum hysterectomy are good understanding and anticipation of associated risks, focused and timely decision-making, experienced and confident surgical skill and a well-trained team, this decreases maternal morbidity and mortality and optimises patient outcome [73].

18.25 Infections

Recognised complications of the caesarean section are infections. These include endometritis, wound infection, urinary tract infections and postoperative chest infections. The infectious morbidity rates quoted vary from 18% to 83% [31]. The Royal College of Obstetricians and Gynaecologists has recommended the use of perioperative prophylactic antibiotics to reduce the risks of infections. A recent systematic review has shown that preoperative administration of antibiotics was associated with a significant 41% reduction in the rate of endometritis compared with intraoperative administration [74]. Similarly, a hospital in a developing country, compared the effect of antibiotics prophylaxis within 1 h before skin incision and after skin incision on the incidence of postoperative infections in patients undergoing caesarean section and found the risk of overall postoperative infection was significantly lower when prophylaxis was given preoperatively as opposed to intraoperatively [75]. Contrastingly, a recent multi-centre RCT found no difference in maternal infectious morbidity pre incision or after umbilical cord clamping in patients undergoing elective caesarean section. Likewise, the timing of antibiotics did not have an impact on neonatal outcomes, including neonatal sepsis, sepsis workup and NICU admission [76]. We need to be careful to extrapolate their result to emergency caesarean delivery.

18.26 Urinary Tract Infection

Catheterisation is known to have a major effect on the risk of developing a urinary tract infection. Urinary tract infection is a risk of caesarean section, as most women are catheterised pre-operatively with indwelling catheters. The risk of infection from a single catheterisation has been quoted as less than 2% [77], although Cardozo et al. [78] found that in and out catheterisation did not significantly increase the incidence of postpartum urinary tract infection, provided the catheter is introduced under aseptic techniques. It is advisable that urinary catheters should be inserted immediately prior to caesarean section in the operating theatre, as this reduces the time a catheter remains in situ and the risk of infection. The catheter should be left in women with regional anaesthesia until the anaesthetic effect wears off.

18.27 Chest Infection

Postoperative chest infection occurs in up to 10% of patients following abdominal surgery. There are no figures for the risk of infection following caesarean section but it is probably considerably lower than this. Predisposing factors include obesity, smoking and pre-existing upper respiratory tract infection [79]. It is more common following general anaesthesia than epidural anaesthesia.

Postoperative pain may cause the patient to reduce inspiration and adequate postoperative analgesia should minimise this risk. Physiotherapy and breathing exercises should be encouraged in the postoperative period.

Patients with a chest infection usually present with a cough, pyrexia and purulent sputum. There may be localised chest signs and the disease process may progress to bronchopneumonia. Treatment of postoperative chest infection includes the use of antibiotics and chest physiotherapy.

18.28 Endometritis

Endometritis is an infection of the endometrium or decidua with extension into the myometrium and parametrial tissues. It is the most common cause of fever during the postpartum period. The incidence after a vaginal delivery is 1–3% and following caesarean delivery, the incidence ranges from 13% to 90% depending on the risk factors present and whether perioperative antibiotic prophylaxis had been given [80]. Endometritis is a polymicrobial disease involving on average 2–3 organisms with the commonest organisms being group B streptococcus, *Escherichia coli* and anaerobes. The risk of endometritis is increased with the length of labour, number of vaginal examinations performed in labour [81] and the presence of chorioamnionitis [82]. The diagnosis of endometritis is made on clinical history and examination. Ultrasound scan will exclude the presence of retained products and may show the presence of a phlegmon [83].

Management of endometritis is conservative with antibiotic therapy. Isolation of the infecting organisms is usually not possible as endometrial aspirates usually contain bacteria that are not relevant to the infection. Ampicillin and cephalosporins appear to have the same efficacy in reducing postoperative endometritis. Cefuroxime is commonly used because of its long half-life (1.7 h) and suitability as a single dose regime.

18.29 Wound Infection

The incidence of wound infection after caesarean section has been quoted from 1% to 9%. These are European figures; the figures from the developing world are expected to be a lot higher. The risk is higher with prolonged rupture of membranes, prolonged labour and inadequate aseptic techniques [84]. The risk is also directly proportional to the duration of ruptured membranes and the number of vaginal examinations performed in labour.

The use of prophylactic antibiotics is controversial [85]. The Cochrane database quotes a reduction in endometritis by 75% when prophylactic antibiotics are used. The most common organisms involved are *Staphylococcus aureus*, anaerobes and gram-negative organisms such as *Streptococcus faecalis*. Staphylococci are sensitive to cloxacillin or flucloxacillin. The most appropriate antibiotics to use are broad-spectrum penicillin or cephalosporins. There is no evidence of a reduced infection rate with metronidazole. Short courses are less effective than long courses of antibiotics [86]. The extra cost of antibiotic prophylaxis may be a hindrance in poor and developing countries. However, a study showed that the cost was balanced by a reduction of length of admission with wound infections [85]. It has been said that infection increases the possibility of uterine scar rupture in future pregnancies [87]. However, there is no evidence to support this unless the uterine wound is involved and a history of a wound infection is not an indication for a repeat caesarean section [88].

18.30 Urinary Complications

The risk of bladder or ureteric injury at caesarean section is less than 1% [89]. The bladder is most commonly injured during downward dissection before entry to the uterus particularly in a repeat caesarean section. The ureters may be damaged if the uterine excision extends laterally. This is particularly likely if uterine closure is difficult and entails blind suturing. Ectopic ureters are rare; about 1:1900, and 80% of cases are associated with duplex collecting systems. They are more likely to be damaged because of their abnormal position. Pressure necrosis of the bladder following obstructed labour is rare in the developed but common in developing countries.

Management of damage to the urinary tract depends on the type of injury and when recognised. If the bladder is noted to be injured at the time of operation, it should be repaired in two layers with a suture such as Vicryl sutures and the bladder should be drained continuously with a catheter for 7–10 days. Ureteric injuries are usually best managed with the assistance of a urologist and treatment depends on the site and type of the injury. If the ureter has been tied but not cut, it is usually sufficient to remove the ligature, pass a ureteric catheter and drain the site of injury. Ureteric anastomosis is required if the ureter has been cut or crushed. A low ureteric injury may require re-implantation. A psoas hitch or Boari-Ockerblad flap is required to obtain more ureteric length and prevent tension on the repair sites [90].

A bladder or ureteric injury that is not recognised at the time of operation may present as urine draining vaginally or through the incision. Any case of unexplained fever, loin pain or haematuria occurring postoperatively should alert the obstetrician to the possibility of damage to the urinary tract. Any suspected case of injury should have intravenous urograms, micturating cystograms or cystoscopy with retrograde pyelograms done to determine the exact site and type of injury. Once this is suspected, the bladder should be drained continuously with a catheter. Surgical repair is usually needed and is performed immediately for ureteric injuries. As bladder injuries usually arise after an obstructed labour, it is necessary to allow tissue oedema to settle prior to undertaking a repair of a vesico-vaginal fistula. This repair may take place up to 3 months of the birth injury. A successful repair is usually an indication for subsequent elective caesarean section.

18.31 Impact on Future Fertility

In recent times, studies are observing the effect of caesarean section on a woman's future reproductive life. A meta-analysis suggests that patients who had undergone a caesarean section had a 9% lower subsequent pregnancy rate and 11% lower birth rate compared with patients who had delivered vaginally [91]. Further, Gurol-Urganci et al. in their study among low-risk primigravidae who were delivered by caesarean section, their subsequent birth rates compared to those who had vaginal birth were marginally lower after elective caesarean for breech with larger effects observed after elective caesarean for other indications and emergency caesarean delivery. However, the effect was smallest for elective caesarean for breech, and this was not statistically significant in women younger than 30 years of age. More studies are needed to know the full impact on fertility as well as the possible cause for this, so that we can prevent effect [92].

18.32 Management of a Previous Caesarean Section Scar

The management of a patient with a previous caesarean section scar is primarily a decision on the mode of delivery. This depends to a great extent on whether the reason for the previous caesarean section is recurrent or not. For example, pelvic contracture is a recurrent cause but some situations such as cervical dystocia are not as clear-cut. A management plan must be decided in women with a previous caesarean section. It used to be said that 'once a caesarean section always a caesarean section'. This adage has been challenged and women with a caesarean section scar are now considered for vaginal births. Absolute exceptions to this include women with a previous classical uterine incision, as this is associated with a uterine rupture rate of up to 12%. Low transverse uterine incisions with vertical T-extensions are also associated with a greater risk of uterine rupture. Relative contraindications for vaginal births after caesarean (VBAC) include multiple gestation and breech presentation. However, insufficient data exists to determine the efficacy and risks of VBAC in this group. In Britain, the majority of patients are allowed a trial of labour in the absence of cephalopelvic disproportion.

18.33 The Role of Pelvimetry

It was common practice to perform X-ray pelvimetry in women who had undergone a caesarean section. Lateral X-ray pelvimetry was used in the diagnosis of cephalopelvic disproportion, although its validity in a primigravid vertex presentation is disputed [93]. Current evidence suggests that pelvimetry should not be used after a caesarean section to decide on the mode of delivery in the next pregnancy, as it is a poor predictor of future obstetric outcome [94]. Similarly, there is no need for computerised axial tomography (CAT scanning) or magnetic resonance scanning (MRI) as alternatives to conventional X-ray pelvimetry. Shoe size, maternal height and estimations of foetal size (ultrasound or clinical examination) do not accurately predict cephalopelvic disproportion and must not be used to predict 'failure to progress' during labour [26].

18.34 Management of a Trial of Scar

Ideally the onset of labour should be spontaneous as the use of prostaglandin for induction of labour may entail a higher risk of uterine rupture and spontaneous onset of labour is associated with a higher incidence of vaginal delivery. Personnel and facilities for performing an emergency caesarean section should be readily available for women undergoing a trial of scar and as such should always be looked after in a fully equipped labour ward with facilities for caesarean section. Intrapartum electronic foetal heart surveillance is recommended because a non-reassuring foetal heart rate pattern is the most common presenting sign of uterine rupture. The only reported predictable feature of foetal heart rate patterns in response to uterine rupture is the sudden onset of foetal bradycardia.

Epidural analgesia is not contraindicated in trial of scar patients as the block does not mask the signs of uterine rupture [95, 96]. The use of syntocinon in trial of scars is also controversial and, in the past, has been discouraged both to induce and augment labour. Recent studies have found no increased risk of uterine scar rupture with the judicious use of syntocinon [97]. Syntocinon may, however, be used with more confidence in the presence of intrauterine pressure catheters and these are advocated to allow augmentation of labour to achieve optimum uterine activity [69].

The major risk associated with labouring subsequent to caesarean section is uterine rupture. Benign dehiscence, asymptomatic separation of uterine scar is considered to be 1.5% [98], many of which are only discovered after the birth and which do not influence the course of event or require any treatment. However, in those rare occurrences of catastrophic rupture, the major complication is profound foetal distress resulting in neurological damage or foetal death. It must be kept in mind that unpredictable uterine rupture can occur and that uterine rupture necessitates emergency intervention. Most women with one previous lower segment caesarean delivery can be safely offered a trial of labour and should be adequately counselled. In developed countries women who have had up to four caesarean section could be offered a trial of labour [26].

In developing countries, trial of scar could be safe if the patients are well selected, counselled, monitored and deliver in a hospital able to perform a caesarean section if indicated. Gupta et al. noted a vaginal birth (VBAC) success rate of 59% in an Indian hospital; the incidence of uterine rupture was 0.7% and that of uterine dehiscence was 10%. However, the incidence of birth asphyxia was 4%. Repeat CS rate was high (61%) because 87% of patient were from rural area and 65% of their patient were unbooked and came to hospital in labour, hence attending obstetrician felt more comfortable performing a repeat CS rather than attempting trial of labour [99].

18.35 Risks of Scar Rupture

The risk of scar rupture varies with the type of uterine scar. The commonest used estimated risk is of an overall risk of 2.2% for a classical scar and 0.5% for a lower uterine scar [100]. Studies that are more recent show similar risks [101]. The maternal mortality associated with classical scar rupture is in the order of 5% with a foetal mortality of 73%. There is no significant maternal mortality associated with a lower segment scar but there is a foetal mortality of 12.5%. The risk of scar rupture with a de Lee's incision (low vertical incision) is estimated to lie somewhere between the two, but with the increasing use of this incision to deliver pre-term infants, further evaluation is needed of the exact risks [27].

18.36 Recognition of the Ruptured Uterus

Scar rupture is classically associated with an acute onset of abdominal pain that is continuous and does not remit between contractions. However, this may not be the case with lower uterine scars, which, as they are fibrous, usually rupture painlessly. Scar rupture may also present as acute foetal distress as shown on the cardiotocograph or as an acute cessation of labour. Once the diagnosis is made, resuscitation of the mother must be commenced and preparation must be made for immediate laparotomy and delivery of the foetus. Full resuscitation may not be possible until the foetus is delivered and the bleeding margins of the tear can be sutured or damped.

Following the delivery of the baby, a decision is made as to whether repair of the rupture or a caesarean hysterectomy is more appropriate. This choice depends upon the type and extent of the rupture, the patient's general condition, in particular the presence of uncontrollable haemorrhage, and to some extent on a woman's previous obstetric history. If the patient is in a poor condition, repair of the tear has been advocated as less traumatic to the patient than hysterectomy [83]. Tears in the upper part of the uterus are more difficult to repair and hysterectomy is usually the operation of choice. Repair of the tear, if possible, along with tubal ligation has been proposed for women with large families who for cultural reasons wish to retain a uterus [102]. It would be expected that the risk of rupture in a subsequent pregnancy following repair of a tear would be high. However, no maternal morbidity was associated with this in patients delivered by elective caesarean section at 38 weeks [103]. A previous ruptured uterus is therefore an indication for an elective caesarean section. Some obstetricians advise examination of the uterine scar after delivery [105]. There is no clinical benefit in treating asymptomatic scars and scars may even be extended by the examining finger [22]. This practice is no longer carried out and must not.

18.37 Alternatives to Caesarean Section

This section takes into consideration the poor access to facilities that provide caesarean section in the developing countries. This dearth of facilities has contributed to the high incidence of perinatal and maternal morbidity and mortality. In such circumstances, delivery of the baby may have to be affected through symphysiotomy. Symphysiotomy is advocated as an alternative to caesarean section when there is mechanical difficulty during labour and the foetus is still alive [104]. This procedure is no longer practiced in the developing world and legal action is being pursued in Ireland where this practice has been branded as being barbaric [105]. However, there is a strong case for the continuation of this procedure in centres where facilities for caesarean section do not exist, as this may be the only available method of preventing a foetal and/or maternal death.

The method of delivery of a dead foetus following an obstructed labour creates a management dilemma. To deliver a dead baby by caesarean section creates potential problems. The need to have an alternative to caesarean section for delivering the dead foetus is discussed by Giwa-Osagie and Azzan [106]. The arguments in favour of destructive operations are the great dangers of caesarean section after prolonged and neglected labour in women who already have pelvic infection. The socio-cultural needs of women to have a vaginal delivery, often making the woman or her relatives refuse consent for caesarean section and the risks of scar rupture in an unattended subsequent pregnancy at home strengthens the case for embryotomy in such settings.

18.38 Court-Ordered Caesarean Section

Situations have arisen where women refuse to provide consent for a caesarean section when doctors think it is in the best interest of the foetus to do so. Compulsory surgical or invasive treatment of a male or female patient is illegal in Britain. Court rulings on these situations are that it is illegal to force a woman to submit to caesarean section. It is not just the courts that have warned against forcing medical treatment on a pregnant woman. The Royal College of Obstetricians and Gynaecologists [107] in 1994 issued ethical guidelines on the subject. These guidelines state as follows:

1. Although obligations to the foetus increase with its growth in utero, UK law does not grant it any legal status. This comes from the moment of birth.
2. The law does not limit a woman's freedom because she is pregnant. Her bodily integrity cannot be invaded on behalf of her foetus without her consent. The foetus has no remedy against injuries caused by her decision.
3. A doctor must respect the competent pregnant woman's right to choose or refuse any particular recommended course of action whilst optimising care for both mother and foetus to the best of his or her ability. A doctor would not then be culpable if these endeavours were unsuccessful.
4. The RCOG concludes that it is inappropriate and unlikely to be helpful or necessary to invoke judicial intervention to overrule an informed and competent woman's refusal of a proposed medical treatment, even though her refusal might place her life and that of her foetus at risk. A mentally competent pregnant woman cannot be forced to attend a hospital, or accept treatment, against her will and the Mental Health Act cannot be used to detain an individual against her will [107].

These legal representations should be taken on board in developing countries in the absence of any local judicial rulings.

18.39 Risk Management Issues in Caesarean Section

18.39.1 Timing of Elective Caesarean Section

The recommendation is that elective caesarean sections should take place between 39 and 40 weeks gestation unless there are obstetrics or medical reasons not to do so. It is essential to ascertain the correct gestational age before performing an elective caesarean section. Not to do so may result in an infant that is premature and that may suffer the accompanying sequelae of prematurity. It is good practice to use the first trimester dating scan for the determination of the expected date of delivery as this is the most accurate time with regard to gestational assessment.

18.39.2 Safety Practices

The WHO Surgical Safety Checklist was developed after extensive consultation aiming to decrease errors and adverse events, and increase teamwork and communication in surgery. The 19-item checklist has gone on to show significant reduction in both morbidity and mortality and is now used by a majority of surgical providers around the world [108]. It is essential that the WHO Surgical Safety checklist in performed in its true spirit. This will minimise errors such surgery on the wrong patient and the retention of swabs or surgical instruments within the patient.

18.39.3 Perimortem Caesarean Section (PMCS)

Perimortem Caesarean Section (PMCS) are not commonly done. However, when a pregnant mother arrives in the Emergency Department following cardiac arrest, PMCS is a resuscitative intervention for the mother and not for the baby as the aim is to save the mother first and foremost. Gestational age becomes irrelevant in these situations. The exception to a PMCS is during the first trimester as the uterus does not compress the inferior vena cava [109].

18.40 Conclusion

Caesarean section will always remain as an option of the mode of delivery for mothers. It is now a much safer operation than previously, hence the increase uptake will continue in developed nations despite all efforts to curtail it due to many factors, none the least the fear of litigation. Ironically, more caesarean sections need to be performed in developing countries to reduce the needless and avoidable maternal and perinatal death that occurs in these countries. There is need to provide trained personnel, facilities where caesarean delivery can safely take place as well as access to these facilities. This is necessary to lower the maternal and perinatal morbidity and mortality in low resource nations. A strong political will from the governments as well as help from charities will help see this happen.

Perioperative antibiotics, thromboprophylaxis and access to blood transfusion facilities are essential requirements in reducing the morbidity and mortality associated with caesarean sections. There is need to ensure that financial gains in the private sector do not drive the need for caesarean sections. Every age brings new challenges. The age of the rising caesarean delivery rate now brings obstetricians—with increasing frequency—the challenge of caesarean hysterectomy for placental accreta/percreta. When a decision is made to deliver a woman by caesarean, short-term considerations usually dominate. Obstetricians, however, also have a responsibility to take a woman's long-term reproductive outcomes into consideration when they are considering primary caesarean delivery in the absence of sound medical indications [64]. It is essential that adequate measures are put in place to ensure the delivery of a healthy baby and well-being of the mother.

18.41 Summary

Caesarean section is now a much safer operation than it has previously been. The increase in uptake will continue in developed nations despite all efforts to curtail it due to many factors, none the least the fear of litigation. There are needs for more uptake of caesarean section in developing countries to reduce the needless and avoidable maternal and perinatal death that occurs in these countries. There is need to provide trained personnel, facilities where caesarean delivery can safely take place as well as access to these facilities. This is a necessity to lower the maternal and perinatal morbidity and mortality in low resource nations. Perioperative antibiotics, thromboprophylaxis and access to blood transfusion facilities are essential requirements in reducing the morbidity and mortality associated with caesarean sections.

Rising caesarean delivery rate now brings obstetricians—with increasing frequency—the challenge of caesarean hysterectomy for placental accreta/percreta. When a decision is made to deliver a woman by caesarean, short-term considerations usually dominate. Obstetricians, however, also have a responsibility to take a woman's long-term reproductive outcomes into consideration when they are considering primary caesarean delivery in the absence of sound medical indications. It is essential that adequate measures are put in place to ensure the delivery of a healthy baby and well-being of the mother.

References

1. Souza JP, Betran AP, Dumont A, de Mucio B, et al. A global reference for caesarean section rates (C-Model): a multicountry cross-sectional study. BJOG. 2016;123:427–36.
2. Peel J. Caesarean section in modem obstetric practice. J Obstet Gynaecol India. 1962;125:535–48.
3. Esteves-Pereira AP, Deneux-Tharaux C, Nakamura-Pereira M, Saucedo M, Bouvier-Colle M-H, et al. Caesarean delivery and postpartum maternal mortality: a population-based case control study in Brazil. PLoS One. 2016;11(4):e0153396. https://doi.org/10.1371/journal.pone.0153396.
4. Betrán AP, Ye J, Moller A-B, Zhang J, Gülmezoglu AM, Torloni MR. The increasing trend in caesarean section rates: global, regional and national estimates: 1990–2014. PLoS One. 2016;11(2):e0148343. https://doi.org/10.1371/journal.pone.0148343.

5. Ye J, Zhang J, Mikolajczyk R, Torloni MR, Gülmezoglu AM, Betran AP. Association between rates of caesarean section and maternal and neonatal mortality in the 21st century: a worldwide population-based ecological study with longitudinal data. BJOG. 2016;123:745–53.
6. Dumont A, de Bemis L, Bouvier-Colle MH, et al. Caesarean section rate for maternal indication in sub-Saharan Africa: a systematic review. Lancet. 2001;358:1328–33.
7. Feldman GB, Freiman JA. Occasional notes: prophylactic caesarean section at term? N Engl J Med. 1985;312(19):1264–7.
8. Gifford DS, Keeler E, Kahn KL. Reductions in cost and caesarean rate by routine use of external cephalic version: a decision analysis. Obstet Gynecol. 1995;85(6):930–6.
9. Cavallaro FL, Cresswell JA, Ronsmans C. Obstetricians' opinions of the optimal caesarean rate: a global survey. PLoS One. 2016;11(3):e0152779. https://doi.org/10.1371/journal.pone.0152779.
10. WHO statement on caesarean section rates, WHO, Human reproductive programme, WHO/RHR/15.02. 2015.
11. Shearer EL. Caesarean section: medical benefits and costs. Soc Sci Med. 1993;37(10):1223–31.
12. Notzon FC, Placek PJ, Taffel SM. Comparisons of national caesarean section rates. N Eng J Med. 1987;316(7):386–9.
13. Shiono PH, Fielden JG, McNellis D, Rhoads GG. and. Pearse W H. Recent trends in caesarean birth and trial of labor rates in the United States. J Amer Med Assoc. 1987;257(4):494–7.
14. Stafford RS. The impact of non-clinical factors on repeat caesarean section. J Amer Med Assoc. 1991;265(1):59–63.
15. King DE, Lahiri K. Socioeconomic factors and the odds of vaginal birth after caesarean delivery. J Amer Med Assoc. 1994;272(7):524–9.
16. Gifford D. Caesarean delivery. http://www.rand.org/publications/fyfR/MR1284/mr1284.ch6.pdf
17. Lees DH, Singer A. Caesarean section. In: Surgery of conditions complicating pregnancy. London: Wolfe Medical; 1982. p. 111–30.
18. Jongen VH, Halfwerk MG, Brouwer WK. Vaginal delivery after previous caesarean section for failure of second stage of labour. Br J Obstet Gynaecol. 1998;105(10):1079–81.
19. Peter J, Martaille A, Roynay HD, et al. Les indications de la cesarienne. A pro pas de 1000 cas. Rev F Gynaecol Obstet. 1982;77:175–82.
20. Sykes GS, Molloy PM, Johnson P, et al. Do Apgar scores indicate asphyxia? Lancet. 1982;1(8270):494–6.
21. Nielsen TF, Ljungblad U, Hagberg H. Rupture and dehiscence of caesarean section scar during pregnancy and delivery. Am J Obstet Gynaccol. 1989;160(3):569–73.
22. Ayromlooi J, Garfinkel R. Impact of fetal scalp blood pH on incidence of caesarean section performed for fetal distress. Int J Obstet Gynaecol. 1980;17:391–2.
23. MacDonald D, Grant A, Pereira M, Boylan P, Chalmers I. The Dublin randomised controlled trial of intrapartum electronic fetal heart rate monitoring. Am J Obstet Gynaecol. 1985;154:524–39.
24. Kubli F, Boss W, Ruttgers H. Caesarean section in the management of singleton breech presentation. In: Rooth G, Bratteby LE, editors. Perinatal medicine. Stockholm Almqvist and Wiksell; 1976. p. 69–75.
25. Hannah ME, Hannah WJ, Hewson SA, et al. Planned caesarean section versus planned vaginal birth for breech presentation at term: a randomised multicentre trial. Lancet. 2000;21:356.
26. Caesarean section. NICE guidelines [CG132] Published date: November 2011 last updated: August 2012.
27. Paul RH, Phelan JP, Yen S. Trial of Labour in the patient with a prior caesarean section. Am J Obstet Gynaecol. 1985;151:297–304.
28. O'Driscoll K, Foley M. Correlation of decrease in perinatal mortality and increase in caesarean section rates. Obstet Gynaecol. 1983;61:1–5.
29. Schutte MF, Vanttemel OJC, van de Berg C, van de Pol A. Perinatal mortality in breech presentations as compared to vertex presentations in Singleton pregnancies : an analysis based upon 57819 computer registered pregnancies in the Netherlands. Eur J Obstet Gynaecol Reprod Biol. 1985;19:391–400.
30. Hofmeyr, J, Hannah M, Lawrie TA. Planned caesarean section for term breech delivery. First published: 21 July 2015, Assessed as up-to-date: 31 March 2015. Editorial Group: Cochrane Pregnancy and Childbirth Group. https://doi.org/10.1002/14651858.CD000166.pub2.
31. Enkin M. Antibiotic and caesarean section. In: Chalmers I, Enkin M, Keirse MJNC, editors. Effective care in pregnancy and childbirth. Oxford: Oxford University Press; 1994. p. 322–7.
32. Crowther CA. Effect of caesarean delivery of the second twin. Cochrane Database Syst Rev. 1997;(2):CD000047.
33. Strong TH, Phelan JP, Ahn MO, Samo AP Jr. Vaginal birth after caesarean delivery in the twin gestation. Am J Obstet Gynaecol. 1989;161:29–32.
34. Hofmeyr GJ, Barrett JF, Crowther CA. Planned caesarean section for women with a twin pregnancy: First published: 19 December 2015, Assessed as up-to-date: 18 November 2015. Editorial Group: Cochrane Pregnancy and Childbirth Group. https://doi.org/10.1002/14651858.CD006553.pub3.
35. Barrett JF, Hannah ME, Hutton EK, et al. A randomised trial of planned caesarean or vaginal delivery for twin pregnancy. N Engl J Med. 2013;369:1295–305. https://doi.org/10.1056/NEJMoa1214939.
36. Jonas HA, Khalid N, Schwartz SM. The relationship between caesarean section and neonatal mortality in very-low-birthweight infants born in Washington State, USA. Paediatr Perinat Epidemiol. 1999;13(2):170–89.
37. Lamont RF, Dunlop POM, Crowley P, Elder MG. Spontaneous pre-term labour and delivery under 34 weeks gestation. Br Med J. 1983;286:454–7.
38. National Institute for Health and Care Excellence Guideline – Caesarean section (QS32), National Institute for Health and Care Excellence (NICE).
39. Suthit Khunpradit, Emma Tavender, Pisake Lumbiganon, Malinee Laopaiboon, Jason Wasiak, Russell L Gruen. Non-clinical interventions for reducing unnecessary caesarean section: First published: 15 June 2011 Assessed as up-to-date: 28 March 2010. Editorial Group: Cochrane Effective Practice and Organisation of Care Group. https://doi.org/10.1002/14651858.CD005528.pub2.
40. Sydsjö G, Möller L, Lilliecreutz C, Bladh M, Andolf E, Josefsson A. Psychiatric illness in women requesting caesarean section. BJOG. 2015 Feb;122(3):351–8. https://doi.org/10.1111/1471-0528.12714.
41. Onah HE, Ibeziako N, Umezulike AC, Effetie ER, Ogbuokiri CM. Decision – delivery interval and perinatal outcome in emergency caesarean sections. J Obstet Gynaecol. 2005 May;25(4):342–6.
42. Adewunmi AA, Rabiu KA, Tayo TA, Ottun TA, Kehinde OA, Akinlusi FM, Orekoya OO. Decision-delivery interval and perinatal outcome in emergency caesarean section: a university teaching hospital experience. West Afr J Med. 2014;33(4):252–7.
43. Chukwudi OE, Okonkwo CA. Decision – delivery interval and perinatal outcome of emergency caesarean sections at a tertiary institution. Pak J Med Sci. 2014;30(5):946–50. https://doi.org/10.12669/pjms.305.5470.
44. Roberge S, Chaillet N, Boutin A, Moore L, Jastrow N, Brassard N, Gauthier RJ, Hudic I, Shipp TD, Weimar CH, Fatusic Z, Demers S, Bujold E. Single versus double layer closure of the hysterotomy incision during caesarean delivery and risk of uterine rupture. Int J Gynaecol Obstet. 2011;115(1):5–10.
45. Tulandi T, Hum HS, Gelfand MM. Closure of laparotomy incisions with or without peritoneal suturing and second look laparoscopy. Am J Obstet Gynaecol. 1988;158:536–7.

46. Anthony A Bamigboye, G Justus Hofmeyr. Closure versus non-closure of the peritoneum at caesarean section: short- and long-term outcomes: First published: 11 August 2014, Assessed as up-to-date: 1 November 2013. Editorial Group: Cochrane Pregnancy and Childbirth Group. https://doi.org/10.1002/14651858.CD000163.pub2.
47. Laopaiboon M, Lumbiganon P, Martis R, Vatanasapt P, Somjaivong B. Music during caesarean section under regional anaesthesia for improving maternal and infant outcomes. Cochrane Database Syst Rev. 2009;(2):CD006914. https://doi.org/10.1002/14651858.CD006914.pub2.
48. Ormezzano X, Francois TP, Viaud JY, Bukowski JG, Bourgeonneau MC, Cottron D, Ganansia MF, Gregoire FM, Grinand MR, Wessel PE. Aspiration pneumonitis prophylaxis in obstetric anaesthesia: comparison of effervescent cimetidine-sodium citrate mixture and sodium citrate. Br J Anaest. 1990;64(4):503–6.
49. Rosalie M, et al. Short- and long-term outcomes after caesarean section. Expert Rev Obstet Gynecol. 2011;6(2):205–15.
50. Caesarean Section (Consent Advice No. 7). Published: 01/10/2009.
51. Oja VA, et al. Characteristics of maternal deaths following caesarean section in a developing country. Int J Gynaecol Obstet. 1988;27:171–6.
52. Fortney JA, Susanti I, Gadalla S, Saleh S, Feldblum PJ, Potts M. Maternal mortality in Indonesia and Egypt. Int J Gynaecol Obstet. 1988;26:21–32.
53. Zwart JJ, Richters JM, Ory F, de Vries JI, Bloemenkamp KW, van Roosmalen J. Severe maternal morbidity during pregnancy, delivery and puerperium in The Netherlands: a nationwide population-based study of 371,000 pregnancies. BJOG. 2008;115(7):842–50.
54. B-Lynch C, Coker A, Lawal AH, Abu J, Cowen MJ. The B-Lynch surgical technique for the control of massive postpartum haemorrhage: an alternative to hysterectomy? Five cases reported. Br J Obstet Gynaecol. 1997;104(3):372–5.
55. Burchell CR, Olson G. Internal iliac ligation; aortogrарns. Am J Obstet Gynecol. 1966;94:117–24.
56. MBRRACE-UK. Saving Lives, Improving Mothers' Care. Lessons learned to inform future maternity care from the UK and Ireland Confidential Enquiries into Maternal Deaths and Morbidity 2009–2012.
57. Royal College of Obstetricians and Gynaecologists. Prophylaxis and management against thromboembolism in gynaecology and obstetrics. Report of the RCOG Working Party. London: Royal College of Obstetricians and Gynaecologists, 1995, 15.
58. Romero R, et al. A fetal systemic inflammatory response is followed by the spontaneous onset of pre-term parturition. Am J Obstet Gynecol. 1998;179:186–93.
59. Britton JJ. Sterilization by caesarean hysterectomy. Am J Obstet Gynaecol. 1980;137:887–90.
60. Shellhaus CS, Gilbert S, Landon MB, Varner MW, Leveno KJ, Hauth JC, et al. The frequency and complication rates of hysterectomy accompanying caesarean delivery. Obstet Gynecol. 2009;114(2 Pt 1):224–9.
61. Okogbenin SA, Gharoro EP, Otoide VO, Okonta PI. Obstetric hysterectomy: fifteen years' experience in a Nigerian tertiary centre. J Obstet Gynaecol. 2003;23(4):356–9.
62. Glaze S, Ekwalanga P, Roberts G, Lange I, Birch C, Rosengarten A, et al. Peripartum hysterectomy: 1999 to 2006. Obstet Gynecol. 2008;111(3):732–8.
63. Wingprawat S, Chittacharoen A. Suthutvoravut, Risk factors for emerging peripartum caesarean hysterectomy. Int J Gynecol Obstet. 2005;90(2):136–7.
64. Turner MJ. Peripartum hysterectomy: an evolving picture. Int J Gynaecol Obstet. 2010;109(1):9–11.
65. Lumbiganon P, Laopaiboon M, Gulmezoglu AM, et al. Method of delivery and pregnancy outcomes in Asia: the WHO global survey on maternal and perinatal health 2007–08. Lancet. 2010;375(9713):490–9.
66. Villar J, Carroli G, Zavaleta N, et al. Maternal and neonatal individual risks and benefits associated with caesarean delivery: multicentre prospective study. BMJ. 2007;335(7628):1025.
67. Flood KM, Said S, Geary M, Robson M, Fitzpatrick C, Malone FD. Changing trends in peripartum hysterectomy over the last 4 decades. Am J Obstet Gynecol. 2009;200(6):632.e1–6.
68. Knight M. Peripartum hysterectomy in the UK: management and outcomes of the associated haemorrhage. BJOG. 2007;114(11):1380–7.
69. Wen SW, Huang L, Liston R, Heaman M, Baskett T, Rusen ID, et al. Severe maternal morbidity in Canada 1991–2001. CMAJ. 2005;173(7):759–64.
70. Silver RM, Landon MB, Rouse DJ, Levano KJ, Spong CY, Thom EA, et al. Maternal morbidity associated with multiple repeat caesarean deliveries. Obstet Gynecol. 2006;107(6):1226–32.
71. Oyelese Y, Scorza WE, Mastrolia R, Smulian JC. Postpartum haemorrhage. Obstet Gynecol Clin N Am. 2007;34(3):421–41.
72. Park RC, Duff WP. Role of caesarean hysterectomy in modern obstetric practice. Clin Obstet Gynaecol. 1980;23:601–20.
73. Matthews, Rebarber. Grand rounds: practical perspective on caesarean hysterectomy: when, why, and how. Contemporary OB/GYN.
74. Baaqeel H, Baaqeel R. Timing of administration of prophylactic antibiotics for caesarean section: a systematic review and meta-analysis. BJOG. 2013;120(6):661–9. https://doi.org/10.1111/1471-0528.12036.
75. Dlamini LD, Sekikubo M, Tumukunde J, Kojjo C, Ocen D, Wabule A, Kwizera A. Antibiotic prophylaxis for caesarean section at a Ugandan hospital: a randomised clinical trial evaluating the effect of administration time on the incidence of postoperative infections. BMC Pregnancy Childbirth. 2015 Apr 12;15:91. https://doi.org/10.1186/s12884-015-0514-3.
76. Zhang C, Zhang L, Liu X, Zhang L, Zeng Z, Li L, Liu G, Jiang H. Timing of antibiotic prophylaxis in elective caesarean delivery: a multi-centre randomised controlled trial and meta-analysis. PLoS One. 2015;10(7):e0129434. https://doi.org/10.1371/journal.pone.0129434.
77. Walter S, Vejlsgaard R. Diagnostic catheterisation and bacteria in women with urinary incontinence. Br J Urol. 1978;50:106–8.
78. Cardozo LO, Barwick C, Beness C. Postpartum voiding dysfunction. Int Urogynaecol J. 1989;1:2.
79. Marshall A. Postoperative respiratory problems. In: Taylor TH, Major E, editors. Hazards and complications of anaesthesia. Edinburgh: Churchill Livingstone; 1987. p. 188–96.
80. Simmons GT, Bammel B. Endometritis. http://www.emedicine.com/med/topic676.htm
81. Apuzzio JJ, Reyelt C, Pelosi, et al. Prophylactic antibiotics for caesarean section: comparison of high risk and low risk patients for endomyometritis. Obstet Gynaecol. 1982;59:693–8.
82. Koh KS, Chan FH, Monfared AH, Ledger WJ, Paul RH. The changing perinatal and maternal outcome in chorioamnionitis. Obstet Gynaecol. 1979;53:730–4.
83. Lavery JP, Howell RS, Shaw L. Ultrasonic demonstration of a phlegmon following caesarean section. J Clin Ultrasound. 1985;132(2):134–6.
84. Rehu M, Nilsson CG. Risk factors for febrile morbidity associated with caesarean section. Obstet Gynaecol. 1980;56:259–64.
85. Mugford M, Kingston J, Chalmers I. Reducing the incidence of infection after caesarean section implication of prophylaxis with antibiotics for hospital resources. Br Med J. 1989;299:1003–6.
86. Scarpignato C, Caltabiano M, Condemi V, Mansam FE. Short-term vs. long-term cefuroxime prophylaxis in patients undergoing emergency caesarean section. Clin Thet. 1982;5:186–92.

87. Case BD, Corcoran R, Jeffcote M, Randle GH. Caesarean section and its place in modem obstetric practice. Obstet Gynaecol Commun Wealth. 1971;78:203–14.
88. Neuhoff D, Burke MS, Porreca RP. Caesarean birth for failed progress in labour. Obstet Gynaecol. 1989;73:915–20.
89. Evrad JR, Gold EM, Cahill TF. Caesarean section: a contemporary assessment. J Reprod Med. 1980;24:147–9.
90. Hendry WF. Urinary tract injuries during gynaecological surgery. In: Studd J, editor. Progress in obstetrics and gynaecology, vol. 5. Edinburgh: Churchill Livingstone; 1985. p. 36277.
91. Gurol-Urganci I, Bou-Antoun S, Lim CP, Cromwell DA, Mahmood TA, Templeton A, van der Meulen JH. Impact of Caesarean section on subsequent fertility: a systematic review and meta-analysis. Hum Reprod. 2013 Jul;28(7):1943–52. https://doi.org/10.1093/humrep/det130.
92. Gurol-Urganci I, Cromwell DA, Mahmood TA, van der Meulen JH, Templeton A. A population-based cohort study of the effect of Caesarean section on subsequent fertility. Hum Reprod. 2014;29(6):1320–6. https://doi.org/10.1093/humrep/deu057.
93. Barton JJ, Garbaciak JA Jr, Ryan GM Jr. The efficacy of x-ray pelvimetry. Am J Obstet Gynaecol. 1982;143(3):304–11.
94. Royal College of Obstetricians and Gynaecologists. Clinical Green Top Guidelines, Peritoneal Closure (15). www.rcog.org.uk. 1998.
95. Bardaracco MA, Vessey M. Recurrence of venous thromboembolic disease and the use of oral contraceptives. Br Med J. 1974;1:215–7.
96. Centres for Disease Control. US caesarean rate for 2002. http://www.cdc.gov/nchs/releases/03news/lowbirth.htm
97. Cox ML. Symphysiotomy in Nigeria. J Obstet Gynaecol Br Commun Wealth. 1966;73:237–43.
98. HMSO. DHSS report on confidential enquiries into maternal death in England and Wales 1982–84. Rep Health Soc Subj (Lond). 1989;34:87–95.
99. Gupta P, Jahan I, Jograjiya GR. Is vaginal delivery safe after previous lower segment caesarean section in developing country? Niger Med J. 2014;55:260–5.
100. Enkin M, Keirse MJNC, Renfrew M, Neilson J. A guide to effective care in pregnancy and childbirth. 2nd ed. Oxford: Oxford University Press; 1995. p. 108.
101. Molloy BG. Shiel 0 and Duignan NM. Delivery after caesarean section: a review of 2176 consecutive cases. Br Med J. 1987;294:1645–7.
102. Sheth SS. Suturing of the tear as treatment in uterine rupture. Am J Obstet Gynaecol. 1969;105(3):440–3.
103. Reyes-Ceja L, Cabrera R, Lnsfran E, Herrera-Lasso F. Pregnancy following previous uterine rupture. Study of 19 patients. Obstet Gynaecol. 1969;34(3):387–J89.
104. van Roosmalen J. Symphysiotomy as an alternative to caesarean section. Int J Gynaecol Obstet. 1987;25:451–8.
105. Payne G. Ireland orders inquiry into "barbaric" obstetric practices. BMJ. 2001;322:1200.
106. Giwa-Osagie OF, Azzan BB. Destructive operations. In: Studd J, editor. Progress in obstetrics and gynaecology, vol. 6. Edinburgh: Churchill Livingstone; 1987. p. 211–21.
107. Royal College of Obstetricians and Gynaecologists. Ethical Guidelines. 1994.
108. The Safe Surgery Saves Lives Study Group. A surgical safety checklist to reduce morbidity and mortality in a global population. N Engl J Med. 2009;360:491–9. https://doi.org/10.1056/NEJMsa0810119.
109. Press G. Perimortem cesarean section in the emergency department, Emergency Medicine updates October 22nd, 2013. Accessed 16 Jul 2016 – http://emupdates.com/2013/10/22/perimortem-cesarean-section-in-the-emergency-departmen

Obstetrical Analgesia and Anaesthesia

19

Charles Imarengiaye

Learning Objectives

At the end of a careful reading of this chapter, the reader should be able to:

- Differentiate the obstetric patient from the other patients as being unique
- Identify the physiological changes in pregnancy and implications on the anaesthetic care
- Understand the mechanisms for the pain of labour and delivery
- Articulate the need for the relief of the pain of labour
- Critically evaluate the features of an ideal labour analgesic and the various methods for pain relief during labour and delivery
- Delineate the issues with epidural analgesia in labour and the accompanying consensus
- Explain the need for adequate preoperative preparation for caesarean section and effective communication between the obstetrician, midwife and anaesthetist
- Discuss the anaesthetic options for caesarean section and the associated complications
- Identify the best anaesthetic technique for the individualised care of the patient

19.1 Introduction

Obstetric anaesthesia is a subspecialty of anaesthesia dedicated to the care of women at childbirth. Traditionally, this care is often provided in the form of labour analgesia, anaesthesia for instrumental delivery or caesarean section and the care of the critically ill woman. However, some other aspects of care may be required in anaesthesia consult clinic for the obstetric patient while attending the antenatal clinic.

The practice of obstetric anaesthesia includes the care for the lives and well-being of at least two individuals particularly at caesarean section, instrumental delivery or in labour. This burden of care, sometimes, may be a reason for concern to the anaesthetist. This trepidation associated with obstetric anaesthesia and analgesia is further accentuated by the remarkable changes in the maternal anatomy and physiology. Furthermore, the pharmacokinetics and pharmacodynamics of anaesthetic and analgesic medications are altered by the changes in the mother. There is also the worry of the drugs administered to the mother getting to the unborn infant. These peculiarities of obstetric analgesia and anaesthesia occur on daily basis in most hospitals that offer care to the pregnant woman.

The challenges of obstetric anaesthesia notwithstanding, the maternal joy accompanying the delivery of an infant may be rewarding to the efforts of the obstetric anaesthetist. This satisfaction by the mother can also be perceived by the entire multidisciplinary team involved in the care. The care of the mother by the anaesthetist at caesarean section or in the delivery room demands a clear understanding of anatomy, physiology and pharmacology.

19.2 Physiological Changes in Pregnancy and Their Implications

Pregnancy is associated with a number of changes with significant implications on obstetric analgesia and anaesthesia. These changes affect different organs and systems. The physiological changes in pregnancy may mimic a disease state and it is important to differentiate the normal physiological changes from pathological processes. Multiple pregnancies often exaggerate the physiological changes in the mother. The current

C. Imarengiaye (✉)
School of Medicine, University of Benin, University of Benin Teaching Hospital, Benin City, Nigeria
e-mail: osalumese.imarengiaye@uniben.edu

F. Okonofua et al. (eds.), *Contemporary Obstetrics and Gynecology for Developing Countries*,
https://doi.org/10.1007/978-3-030-75385-6_19

development in assisted reproduction may mean greater responsibility for the obstetric anaesthetist in the management of women with multiple gestations. Basically, changes in early pregnancy are hormonally mediated, e.g. progesterone, oestrogen, human chorionic gonadotropin and prostaglandins. As pregnancy progresses, the later changes are due to mechanical distortions resulting from the enlarging uterus.

19.3 Hormonal Changes

Progesterone remains the most important physiological change in the pregnant woman. Progesterone is secreted in the second half of the menstrual cycle in preparation for pregnancy. The corpus luteum maintains adequate secretion of progesterone until placental secretion becomes sufficient. The major function of progesterone is the capacity to induce smooth muscle relaxation and other physiological changes are dependent on this critical role.

Airway There is capillary engorgement in the entire respiratory tract including nose, pharynx larynx and trachea. Thus, the mucosa is friable and prone to easy bruising and bleeding with any airway manipulation. The bleeding may make airway control to be difficult by obscuring visibility of the larynx and increasing the risk of aspiration of the blood. All pregnant women are considered as potential difficult airway leading to difficult intubation/failed intubation/regurgitation/aspiration – a major cause of anaesthesia-related maternal morbidity and mortality worldwide.

19.4 Respiratory System

Oxygen consumption increases by 20% at rest and there is a 15% increase in metabolic rate resulting in significant increase in oxygen demand during normal pregnancy. This may increase further during painful contractions. The minute ventilation increases early in pregnancy with 30% increase by the 7th week and 50% increase at term (hyperventilation). These changes are mostly due to increase in tidal volume rather than any increase in respiratory rate. An altered sensitivity to carbon dioxide mediated by progesterone, and increased metabolic rate are thought to account for these changes in ventilation. The maternal hyperventilation increases the arterial pO_2 and the arterial carbon dioxide drops significantly with a compensatory fall in serum bicarbonate (compensatory metabolic alkalosis).

The enlarging uterus results in upward displacement of the diaphragm with a 15–20% decrease in functional residual capacity (FRC), commencing around 5 months. In the supine position, the closing volume (the volume during expiration at which airway closure begins to occur in dependent lung zones) may exceed FRC leading to hypoxaemia. The decreased FRC, increased airway closure and elevated oxygen consumption will result in early desaturation in the pregnant woman, especially during the induction of general anaesthesia.

19.5 Cardiovascular System

Blood volume increases from 65–70 to 80–85 mL/kg preferentially by the expansion of the plasma volume. Although the red blood volume increases linearly, it remains behind the relative increase in plasma volume. Consequently, the haematocrit decreases causing the physiological anaemia of pregnancy. This has implications for oxygen carriage under anaesthesia.

Cardiac output: 30–40% rise in cardiac output in the first trimester. Cardiac output continues to rise in the second trimester until it reaches a point 50% greater than the non-pregnant state. During labour, further changes due to increased stroke volume and heart rate include a 15%, 30% and 45% with latent phase contractions, active phase contractions and expulsive phase, respectively. Thus, labour could be a cardiac stress and women with pre-existing cardiac disease may decompensate in pregnancy and delivery.

Aortocaval compression: In the supine position, the gravid uterus can compress major vessel as from the 20th week. Compression of the inferior vena cava decreases venous return, decreases cardiac output and consequently causes symptomatic maternal hypotension. The compensatory mechanism for the aortocaval compression is through the sympathetic stimulation and collateral venous circulation via the azygos and the vertebral plexus. Spinal or epidural blocks may impair the compensatory mechanisms leading to exaggerated maternal hypotension. The effect of the aortocaval compression may vary from mild hypotension to cardiovascular collapse. Left uterine displacement is the major preventive measure against the symptomatic aortocaval compression. This can be accomplished by the placement of Crawford wedge under the right buttock, left lateral tilt of the operating table or manual displacement of the uterus in extreme situations.

Blood pressure: Generally, blood pressure changes occur with maternal age and parity. The nulliparous women have higher mean arterial blood pressure than parous women for a given age. However, the blood pressure increases with maternal age. The mean arterial pressure decreases by 15% during pregnancy, with 21% decrease in systemic vascular resistance and 35% reduction in pulmonary vascular resistance. The reduced systemic vascular resistance is thought to result from low resistance intervillous bed, and vasodilatation caused by prostacyclin, oestrogen and progesterone.

19.6 Gastrointestinal System

The enlarging uterus causes the stomach to assume more horizontal position. This mechanical displacement of the uterus decreases the effectiveness of the lower oesophageal sphincter, predisposing to reflux oesophagitis. Gastrin, elaborated by the placenta, increases the gastric acidity. Similarly, the gastric emptying time is increased, probably due to progesterone effect. During labour and delivery, the gastric emptying time is slowed further by the pain, anxiety and narcotic medications associated with labour. All pregnant women after 14 weeks of gestation must be treated as full stomach. This implies antacid prophylaxis and rapid sequence induction of anaesthesia.

19.7 Haematological Changes

There are major changes in the coagulation system in normal pregnancy. Plasma fibrinogen concentration increases and similar increases in all coagulation factors except V, IX and XIII. Thus, pregnancy induces a hypercoagulable state. The platelet count is moderately reduced but the function remains normal.

Fibrinolytic activity is low until an hour after placental delivery. At delivery, placental expulsion releases thromboplastic substances and this results in an increase in clotting activity. This increased clotting activity moderates the blood loss at vaginal delivery or by caesarean section. There is a return to normal coagulation and fibrinolysis to levels prior to pregnancy at about 3–4 weeks in the puerperal period.

19.8 Pain Pathway in Labour and Caesarean Section

The pain of labour can be characterised to include visceral and somatic components. The visceral component involves the cervix, lower uterine segment and the adnexa. During the first stage of labour, the presenting part stretches and distends the cervix and lower uterine segments. These noxious impulses are transmitted by sensory nerves that accompany sympathetic nerves terminating in the dorsal horn of the spinal cord. The afferent nerves pass through the paracervical region, the pelvis lumbar sympathetic chain and the white rami communicantes associated with the T10-L1 spinal nerves, and then pass through the posterior roots of these nerves to the dorsal horn.

The somatic pain results from the distention of the pelvic floor, vagina and perineum during the second stage of labour. The noxious impulses are transmitted through branches of the pudendal nerve (S2–4). The pudendal nerve innervates the posterior two-thirds of the labia majora, the vagina, vulva, perineum, and supplies motor fibres to various skeletal muscles of the pelvic floor and the perineum. It is important that central neuraxial block for caesarean section should cover sensory level to T_4.

19.9 Pain Relief in Labour

The nature of labour pain varies from one parturient to another. Characteristically, the pain of labour comprises three qualitatively distinct kinds of pain. These types of pain have been described in relation to the location of the pain: abdominal contraction pain, low-back contraction pain and continuous low-back pain.

The severity of pain experienced by parturients varies and may be affected by several factors including parity and the position of the foetus. Melzack and colleagues found that labour pain was more severe in nullipara than multipara (61% vs. 46%). In addition, none of the nulliparous women and only 6% of the parous women rated the pain of labour as minimal. Similarly, other maternal and fetal factors modify the mother's experience of pain at childbirth. The occipito-posterior position, maternal age and fetal weight are central to the nature and severity of labour pain experienced by parturients.

19.10 Why Pain Relief in Labour?

Pain and suffering wherever present should be relieved! The pain of labour, even without the specific aggravating factors, is comparatively severe, as it is only surpassed by amputation of the small digit. Besides the compassionate concerns, the pain of labour may result in physiological changes with maternal and fetal consequences. Most major systems in the body are affected by the pain of labour. The maternal and fetal consequences of the pain at parturition will be related to its severity. In labour, pain may result in maternal hyperventilation leading to marked hypocarbia. This results in uteroplacental and foetoplacental vasoconstriction, a leftward shift in oxyhaemoglobin dissociation curve and consequently fetal hypoxaemia. Maternal oxygen consumption is also increased. Pain, stress and anxiety induce elevated maternal plasma concentrations of catecholamines during labour. The pain of labour is also a major stress on the cardiovascular system. Labour results in progressive increase in maternal cardiac output from an increased stroke volume. These untoward effects of labour have been reversed with adequate pain control. In addition, severe and unrelieved labour pain has been associated with poor maternal satisfaction, postpartum depression and post-traumatic stress disorder.

19.11 Methods of Pain Relief in Labour

Several methods are available for the relief of the pain of labour. These methods are classified as pharmacological and non-pharmacological methods. The non-pharmacological methods include psychological preparation of the women, emotional support at delivery, transcutaneous electrical nerve stimulation (TENS), acupuncture and hydrotherapy. This discourse shall be limited to the pharmacological options as practiced by most anaesthetists. The utilisation of the various methods varies and requires a considerable level of training for the obstetric anaesthetist. Pethidine has long been licensed for use by midwives for the control of the pain of labour.

19.11.1 Parenteral Analgesia

Parenteral opioids are the most commonly administered alternative to epidural analgesia. This includes the use of pethidine, fentanyl, morphine, nalbuphine and remifentanil. None of these opioids meet the ideal analgesic for the management of labour pains (Box 19.1). The use of pethidine was initially limited to the intramuscular route of administration and has long been licensed for independent use by midwives in the United Kingdom. Pethidine stands out as a drug of choice for parenteral labour analgesia. It is highly lipid soluble and flexible for intramuscular or intravenous routes of administration. This may be of benefit in developing economies where the luxury of drug infusion pumps may for now, be unavailable. However, advancements in technology for drug administration have led to improved methods of the intravenous use of these agents.

Many other opioids have been used in patient-controlled analgesia (PCA) for labour. Remifentanil, because of its unique pharmacokinetics, is quite appropriate for patient-controlled labour analgesia. It has rapid onset and offset, short duration and esterase metabolised, thus independent of liver or renal functions. It crosses the placenta (mean uterine vein: maternal artery ratio = 0.88), rapidly metabolised by both mother and neonate, indicating lack of risk of prolonged respiratory depression at birth. Remifentanil provides superior analgesia when compared with intramuscular or intravenous patient-controlled pethidine as well as nitrous oxide. The potential benefits of remifentanil for obstetric analgesia may be achieved with a regime with a background infusion with rescue analgesia at peak of contraction.

Fentanyl, is equally lipid soluble, but not amenable to intramuscular administration. Like remifentanil, it is best used with facilities for intravenous patient-controlled analgesia. Morphine is used with caution due to its propensity for delayed maternal as well as fetal respiratory depression. Other opioids of interest in labour analgesia include nalbuphine, butorphanol and pentazocine. Pentazocine has both agonist and antagonist (weak) properties. Its prescription for labour analgesia may still be a feature in developing countries. Nevertheless, the problems of maternal drowsiness, nausea and vomiting as well as fetal respiratory depression with the use of the parenteral analgesics remain a major concern to the anaesthesiologist, obstetrician and neonatologist.

Parenteral analgesics for pain relief in labour appears to be limited to clinical states when lumbar epidural analgesia remains contraindicated such as the presence of coagulopathy, sepsis, previous spinal surgery, difficult back or patient's refusal of epidural analgesia (Box 19.1).

19.11.2 Inhaled Analgesia

Self-administered inhalational analgesia has been used for the relief of the pain of labour for years. The agent in common use is nitrous oxide (50%) premixed in oxygen (50%), entonox®. The administration of entonox relieves the pain of labour reasonably and could be safely used by unsupervised midwives. Several attempts have been made to improve the quality of analgesia provided to the parturient with entonox. Increasing the concentration of nitrous oxide resulted in higher number of mothers who lost consciousness during labour. Furthermore, inhalational anaesthetic vapour has been added to entonox to improve the quality of analgesic available to the parturient. Isoflurane has been most involved. The wide acceptance of entonox is probably related to its safe use even in the hands of midwives during self-administration by women in labour. Isoflurane/entonox may be safer than increasing the concentration of nitrous oxide beyond 50%, which has been shown to induce unconsciousness.

19.12 Regional Analgesia for Labour

Regional analgesia for labour can be provided in various ways. These include spinal analgesia, epidural analgesia and combined spinal epidural (CSE) analgesia and other local nerve blocks.

Box 19.1 The ideal labour analgesic

Features of the Ideal Labour Analgesic

- Rapid onset and short duration of action
- Minimal placental transfer
- Minimal effects on foetus and the newborn
- Minimal maternal central nervous system depression
- No tocolytic or oxytocic effects
- No adverse effects on uteroplacental circulation
- Maternal composure during 1st and 2nd stages of labour

The epidural technique is believed to be the most effective regional technique for pain relief in labour. However, some patients may not be good candidates for labour epidural analgesia because of contraindications to the technique, technical reasons, delayed onset of analgesia or increased pain intensity with advanced labour. The combined spinal epidural technique has gained widespread use in labour analgesia due to its rapid, reliable analgesia with minimal haemodynamic changes and motor block. The CSE is mainly employed for analgesia in late labour and some women have delivered with the spinal components only. This has led to the evolution of spinal analgesia in labour.

19.12.1 Spinal Analgesia

Spinal analgesia is an emerging and innovative technique in labour analgesia. It combines the injection of low dose bupivacaine with lipophilic opioids into the spinal space using pencil-point needle. The spinal space is usually accessed through any one of these intervertebral spaces L2/L3, L3/L4 or L4/L5 with a pencil-point spinal needle. Specifically, a combination of 1 mL of 0.25% bupivacaine with fentanyl 25 μg has been found to provide significant analgesia for 73% of multiparous women. It has rapid onset of action, provides good analgesia for the first and second stages of labour and is useful for the repair of episiotomy or perineal lacerations. Besides fentanyl, other adjuvants like clonidine, morphine have been used successfully to provide single shot spinal analgesia for labour. Maternal satisfaction with single shot spinal analgesia has been reported widely. In addition, single shot spinal analgesia does not cause impairment of maternal mobility and balance during labour.

The duration of analgesia provided by single shot spinal analgesia in labour appears to be a major limitation to its widespread application. Thus, this technique has been restricted largely to the multiparous women in whom labour is expected to be short. However, some practitioners have included the continuous spinal analgesia with a catheter in the subarachnoid space. Again, the cost of the specialised packs and catheter is a hindrance to the general application of this method. In addition, some practitioners have suggested that the single shot spinal analgesia could be repeated a number of times to accommodate the duration of labour. This is yet to become a widely accepted technique but offers a ray of hope particularly for nulliparous women with long duration of labour.

19.13 Labour Epidural Analgesia

Epidural analgesia is the most effective method of pain relief of labour in contemporary practice. It provides significant analgesia in majority of women in labour. The overall maternal experience of the birthing process was superior with epidural analgesia when compared with other pharmacological and non-pharmacological methods. Besides pain relief, epidural analgesia reduces maternal plasma concentration of catecholamine, improves uteroplacental perfusion, and blunts the hyperventilation/hypoventilation cycle associated with painful contractions. This method of pain relief in labour has undergone the most radical modification, evaluation and application.

The earliest application of lumbar epidural analgesia was as a single shot via the needle. The advent of the epidural catheter has given this technique the desired flexibility in the administration of the local anaesthetic agent. Dosing of the local anaesthetic agent could be done to achieve the desired dermatomal sensory analgesia on demand or at a determined interval. This section of the review would be restricted to the contemporary practice of Patient-Controlled Epidural Analgesia (PCEA), low dose epidural local anaesthetic and opioid administration and the combined spinal epidural analgesia.

19.14 Choice of Local Anaesthetic and Initiation of Labour Epidural Analgesia

The goal of epidural analgesia is adequate pain relief, not anaesthesia! An appreciation of this would result in better outcome with fewer side effects. During labour, the aim is to achieve rapid onset of effective analgesia, negligible motor blockade, minimal risk of materno-fetal toxicity, limited effect on uterine activity and an appreciable duration of action. There is no such ideal agent as at now.

Bupivacaine, an amide, is the most used local anaesthetic for labour epidural analgesia. Early studies with this agent indicate that the patient experiences some pain relief in 8–10 min and peak effect in 20 min. Current methods of administration of dilute solutions of bupivacaine with lipid soluble opioids have improved further the maternal experience and expectations.

Ropivacaine, a single-levorotatory isomer of bupivacaine, has emerged as a regular alternative in lumbar epidural analgesia. Studies have shown ropivacaine to be less cardiodepressant and arrhythmogenic than bupivacaine. It has also been speculated that ropivacaine has less propensity to block muscle fibres. The rather wider safety margin and minimal effect on motor blockade make it attractive to anaesthetists. In our experience, however, the motor sparing effect is not quite evident. This observation may be related to the use of dilute solutions of these agents and/or the addition of lipid soluble opioids as against the earlier administration of high concentrations of bupivacaine.

Other local anaesthetics of interest include lidocaine and 2-Chloroprocaine. These agents have limited usefulness for the initiation and maintenance of epidural analgesia for labour.

19.15 Other Adjuvants

Opioids have been used epidurally or intrathecally in combination with local anaesthetics for the relief of the pain of labour. This frequent use of epidural opioids is attributable to the synergistic interaction between opioids and local anaesthetics. The extremely lipid soluble opioids like fentanyl or sufentanil are more commonly employed as against alfentanil and meperidine. The addition of opioid allows the anaesthetist to use high volume and low concentration of local anaesthetics due to the bupivacaine sparing effect of epidural sufentanil or fentanyl. The dose-dependent decrease in epidural requirement offers a number of benefits including decreased risk of abnormally high blocks, decreased risk of local anaesthetic toxicity and minimal motor block.

Epinephrine is one of the adjuvant medications commonly added to local anaesthetic for epidural analgesia. The addition of epinephrine is thought to enhance the onset of epidural bupivacaine analgesia but may also be associated with increase in the intensity of motor block. The increased motor block is undesirable during labour and delivery. In addition, systemic absorption of epinephrine may induce maternal tachycardia and transient decrease in uterine activity as a result of stimulation of beta-adrenergic receptors. The onset of tachycardia may precipitate undue interventions by the unwary obstetrician. These factors have led to the cautious use of epidural epinephrine.

19.16 Maintenance of Lumbar Epidural Analgesia (Box 19.2)

Intermittent Bolus Injection

This is the traditional method of administration of epidural analgesia for labour. It involves administration of local anaesthetic solution at intervals. In our experience, it is best to give the local anaesthetic at specified intervals rather than on demand when patients have breakthrough pain. It is often difficult getting the patient to be as comfortable as desirable. The usual precautions of blood pressure check and the use of a titrated dose of the local anaesthetics is recommended.

Continuous Epidural Infusion

Continuous infusion of local anaesthetics involves the use of an infusion pump. The pump delivers a set volume of the local anaesthetic agent. It has been shown to result in fewer top-ups and improved maternal satisfaction. There are fears that continuous infusion may result in increased administration of greater doses of bupivacaine. However, busier centres have shifted to the use of patient-controlled analgesic devices.

Patient-Controlled Epidural Analgesia

This is largely dependent on technology. A galaxy of infusion regimens have been described for PCEA. The major advantage of this technique is that it offers a willing parturient the psychological benefit of a sense of autonomy and control. In addition, it provides the patient the opportunity of finding an acceptable threshold of comfort, which may vary from one parturient to another. The use of equipment does not preclude catheter migration. Thus, close monitoring of the patient remains vitally important.

The technique of PCEA has been refined to further improve analgesia, reduce motor block, increase maternal satisfaction and minimise intervention by the anaesthetist. One of such improvements has been the use of PCEA with continuous background infusion. The PCEA has a computer integrated continuous bolus doses. The background infusion should be about a third to half of the hourly doses.

Timed Intermittent Bolus Injection (Programmed Intermittent Epidural Bolus)

The evolution of the maintenance of labour epidural analgesia is currently on timed intermittent bolus injection or the Programmed Intermittent Epidural Bolus (PIEB). The automated systems are designed to deliver small dose of anaesthetics at programmed intervals. The programmed pump delivers about 5–10 mL of local anaesthetic at 30–60 min. The PIEB has been found to provide better analgesia, lower local anaesthetic consumption when compared with PCEA or Continuous Epidural Infusion (Box 19.2).

19.16.1 Combined Spinal Epidural Analgesia

The popularity of combined spinal epidural for pain relief in labour has soared in recent times. CSE technique has the flexibility of epidural analgesia and the rapidity and reliabil-

Box 19.2 Initiation and maintenance of labour epidural analgesia

Local anaesthetic	Concentration
Bupivacaine	0.0625–0.125%
Ropivacaine	0.08–0.2%
Levobupivacaine	0.0625–0.125%
Opioids	
Fentanyl	1.5–3 μg/mL
Sufentanil	0.2–0.33 μg/mL

ity of spinal analgesia with minimal local anaesthetic dosage. The needle through needle, single space technique is the widely used method of establishing CSE. This involves locating the lumbar epidural space and identification of the subarachnoid space with a spinal needle.

Combined spinal epidural analgesia for pain relief in labour can be achieved with short acting opioids such as fentanyl, sufentanil or pethidine. Spinal injection of fentanyl, sufentanil or pethidine provides effective analgesia for 2–3 h. If in early labour, the parturient may ambulate since there is no motor block. However, in late labour, the deposition of fentanyl/sufentanil with local anaesthetic provides immediate pain relief. Ambulation may not be advisable in such situation because of the possible motor effect of local anaesthetic agent, even if negligible. The time of activation of the epidural component of the technique is at the discretion of the attending anaesthetist. Some anaesthetists may be reluctant to dose an untested epidural catheter. It is, however, pertinent to be cautious with an untested catheter in the epidural space. The side effect profile of CSE is acceptable and includes pruritus, nausea, vomiting, hypotension, respiratory depression and postdural puncture headache. Sufentanil is more associated with fetal bradycardia than fentanyl.

19.17 Epidural Analgesia: Progress and Outcome of Labour

The very strong concerns with the effects of epidural analgesia on labour are well expressed and debated. It is important to note the current consensus opinion on these issues. Labour epidural analgesia does not increase caesarean section rate. It, however, prolongs the second stage of labour and is not associated with higher incidence of instrumental delivery. These observations have some far-reaching implications. First, more active monitoring is required especially in the second stage of labour. Second, experience and training in instrumental delivery will be emphasised for the current trainee obstetricians. This factor has actually been speculated as reason for the increased rate of instrumental delivery in the presence of epidural analgesia. Third, the principles of active management of labour should be encouraged, whenever, labour epidural analgesia is used. Furthermore, the epidural administration of dilute solutions of local anaesthetic may minimise these effects. It is salutary that labour epidural analgesia provides superior pain relief when compared to other methods of labour analgesia.

19.17.1 Anaesthesia for Caesarean Section

Caesarean section is an integral part of modern obstetrics. Therefore, anaesthesia becomes very necessary for the abdominal delivery of the newborn, forceps delivery, retained placenta or repair of trauma to the birth canal. Consequently, the anaesthetic options include general anaesthesia, regional anaesthesia or infiltration with local anaesthetics. The choice of anaesthesia is determined by the maternal health status, indication for the caesarean section, urgency of the surgical intervention and the desires of the mother. Whatever the choice of anaesthesia for the caesarean section, the clinical management begins with history taking, physical examination, relevant laboratory works and preoperative preparations and optimisation of any intercurrent medical condition.

Conduct of Anaesthesia

It is essential that all patients for caesarean section are visited by the anaesthetist to perform a preoperative assessment and develop an anaesthetic plan suitable to the parturient. The link between poor preoperative evaluation and morbidity underscores the relevance of preoperative care of the surgical patient. Beyond the establishment of rapport and gaining patient's trust, the preoperative history must inquire into the indication for caesarean section, previous exposure to anaesthesia, previous medical history, allergies, current medications, presence of dental prosthesis and the time of the last meal. A history of adverse outcomes with previous anaesthetic care would provoke the design of an anaesthetic plan to avoid such event in the planned surgery. The presence of intercurrent medical diseases means a good evaluation and control of the medical condition in other to enhance good postoperative outcome. The duration of illness, level of care, current medications for treatment and the presence or absence of related complications may provide insight into the control of the disease. It is important to identify the presence of loose tooth, dentures, false teeth and removable bridges/crowns. Failure to acknowledge these dental interventions may result in catastrophic outcome at airway control. Nevertheless, irrespective of the gestational age, the time of the last meal or drink should be documented.

The physical examination should be focused to identify the cardiorespiratory state and the ease of tracheal intubation. Good blood pressure control and absence of respiratory difficulty may indicate a stable cardiopulmonary status. However, the airway examination must be detailed enough to allow for good laryngoscopy and tracheal intubation. These predictive tests include mouth opening, neck movement, the thyromental distance and the pharyngeal view (Mallampati assessment). A combination of two or more of these tests is recommended.

The laboratory investigations include urinalysis, full blood count, electrolytes, urea and creatinine estimation. The blood group of the patient is determined and two units of donor blood cross-matched. The number of units of blood to be screened depends on the local protocols and challenges. In developing countries without a central blood donation centre, ready access to banked blood may be difficult. It may be necessary therefore to keep screened blood in the bank for women scheduled for caesarean section. Other laboratory investigations would be dependent on the health status of the mother. Coagulation profile of the parturient becomes expedient in patients with preeclampsia.

There are specific preoperative preparations of the parturient for surgery due to the physiological changes attributable to pregnancy. The preparations are many but should adhere to institutional preoperative fasting guidelines, address the volume and acidity of residual gastric volume, prophylaxis against nausea and vomiting and others as may be necessary. Parturients are expected to remain nil per os for upward of 6 h and above since the pregnant woman has a full stomach! The fasting prevents further increases in the residual gastric volume. The acidity of the gastric content is best addressed with antacids. Sodium citrate 0.3 M (30 mL) just at the induction of general anaesthesia remains the preferred choice because of its non-particulate state. However, particulate solutions like magnesium trisilicate (30 mL) would be helpful especially when freshly prepared. Others have administered ranitidine, a H_2-reeceptor blocker, for the preparation of the parturient for caesarean section. Ranitidine stops further production of acids by the oxyntic cells in the gastric mucosa but does little to the acidity of the residual gastric contents. In order to achieve the reduction of the acidity of the gastric content, ranitidine 50 mg should be given the night before surgery and repeated on the day of surgery.

19.18 General Anaesthesia for Caesarean Section

In the days past, general anaesthesia was the technique of choice because of its quick induction more than the safety. At a point, concerns about the safety and efficacy of general anaesthesia outweighed the potential benefits of its speed. Specifically, general anaesthesia was one of the leading causes of maternal mortality in the UK. Difficulties with tracheal intubation, aspiration of stomach contents were the main anaesthesia-related factors in such maternal deaths. The conduct of anaesthesia with minimal doses of induction agents and inhalation agent so as to reduce the trans-placental transfer culminated in the development of awareness under anaesthesia in the obstetric population more than the other surgical patients. A complication of general anaesthesia that provokes both patient and public concerns! The factors responsible for the loss of status of general anaesthesia for caesarean section are shown in Box 19.3:

The risks of general anaesthesia for caesarean section notwithstanding, there are clinical scenarios where regional anaesthesia is not an option. Whenever there is significant threat to foetus like fetal distress, general anaesthesia becomes the only option. Acute maternal hypovolaemia, significant coagulopathy, fixed cardiac output states, inadequate regional anaesthesia and maternal refusal of inadequate analgesia indicate general anaesthesia for the delivery of the foetus.

The induction of general anaesthesia poses a great risk to the mother and foetus. Appropriate position of the mother is key to smooth and effective induction. A small pillow should be placed beneath the occiput so as to allow for the eyes to look downward at the nipples. Rapid sequence induction with cricoid pressure is the standard of care. A predetermined dose of thiopentone (3–5 mg/kg) or propofol (1–2 mg/kg) is administered as a bolus while cricoid pressure is maintained. Laryngoscopy is facilitated with succinylcholine (1–1.5 mg/kg). A pre-selected cuffed endotracheal tube is gently passed into the tracheal through the glottis. Correct placement of the tube is confirmed by direct visualisation of the tube through the glottis, minimum of 6 traces of capnography and auscultation of adequate air entry to the lungs. The tracheal tube is then connected to the breathing system for mechanical ventilation. The sequence of events for general anaesthesia is shown in Box 19.4.

Box 19.3 Problems of general anaesthesia for caesarean section

- Risk of regurgitation and aspiration of gastric content
- Difficult laryngoscopy and tracheal intubation
- Hypoxaemia
- Supine hypotensive syndrome
- Haemorrhage
- Risk of postoperative deep vein thrombosis
- Awareness under general anaesthesia
- Death!

Box 19.4 General anaesthesia for caesarean section

- H2-receptor blocker iv/PPI/Metoclopramide
- Antacid: 0.3M sodium citrate/freshly prepared MMT
- LUD: Crawford wedge/left lateral tilt
- Baseline monitoring: HR, BP, SpO_2, ECG, $ETCO_2$, Temp
- Preoxygenation: 100% O_2 × 3–5 min/4 vital capacity breaths
- Cricoid pressure
- Rapid sequence Induction
- Laryngoscopy + Tracheal intubation
- Maintenance: 30–50% nitrous oxide in oxygen + 0.5MAC volatile agent
- Delivery: oxytocic for 3rd stage/ opioid + paracetamol ± NSAIDs
- Awake Extubation with good airway reflexes

General anaesthesia is maintained with 50% oxygen in nitrous oxide, an inhalation vapour like halothane, isoflurane or sevoflurane and neuromuscular block sustained with any of the non-depolarising neuromuscular blocker (rocuronium, atracurium, vecuronium, pancuronium etc.). Any of the inhalation vapour is useful provided that the concentration is not beyond 0.5MAC. Higher vaporiser setting may result in uterine relaxation and consequent haemorrhage. This complication is particularly dangerous and should be avoided. Specifically, the ventilation should achieve normocapnia. Following the delivery of the foetus, the nitrous oxide fraction may be increased and analgesia augmented with opioid or in its absence, infusion of paracetamol 1G over 15 min. Additional analgesics may include diclofenac suppository.

Monitoring: Standard monitoring to include heart rate, non-invasive blood pressure, electrocardiography, capnography, pulse oximetry and temperature

At the end of surgery, the airway is suctioned and the residual non-depolarising neuromuscular blocker is antagonised with neostigmine. An anticholinergic agent (atropine or glycopyrrolate) is given prior to or with the neostigmine to blunt the muscarinic side effects. The patient is allowed to continue to breathe 100% oxygen and the trachea is extubated when the patient responds well to verbal commands and the airway reflexes are active.

19.19 Regional Anaesthesia for Caesarean Section

There has been a shift from general anaesthesia to regional techniques. Indeed, regional anaesthesia precedes general anaesthesia in discussions on the anaesthetic options for caesarean section. This migration has favoured single shot spinal anaesthesia than epidural or combined spinal epidural technique. Epidural technique is not as appealing as spinal because of the slower onset and higher failure rate.

19.19.1 Spinal Anaesthesia

Single shot spinal anaesthesia is simple to conduct with rapid onset and predictable dense neural blockade. It is the preferred regional anaesthesia for elective caesarean section and some emergency cases (non-reassuring fetal heart tracing).

Technique: The conduct of spinal anaesthesia commences with antacid prophylaxis (Box 19.5). Intravenous ranitidine 50 mg diluted to 20 mL and metochlopramide10 mg is almost routine. A bolus intravenous fluid loading with 15–20 mL/kg of balanced salt solution (0.9% saline or Ringer's lactate) is mandatory. However, lack of time for preloading is no excuse for failure to offer spinal anaesthesia to the parturient. Intramuscular ephedrine 25–50 mg may suffice in such difficult moments. Supplemental oxygen is encouraged for all mothers particularly those parturients with compromised foetus.

The sitting position is preferred. The patient sits on the operating table with the feet resting on a stool such that the flexed knees are higher than the flexed hips and the head looking at the abdomen. After the aseptic preparation of the skin overlying the lumbar area, the lumbar puncture is done at the L3/4 or L2/3 interspace. The pencil-point needle, Whitacre needle, is passed gently until a loss-of-resistance is felt. Clear and free flow of cerebrospinal fluid indicates a correct identification of the subarachnoid space. Hyperbaric bupivacaine is the preferred drug for spinal anaesthesia. However, other local anaesthetic agents commonly utilised for spinal anaesthesia include lidocaine, tetracaine and procaine. The duration of action for lidocaine is short and may be useful for the very fast obstetrician. The duration and quality of anaesthesia may be improved further with the addition of adjuvants like epinephrine, morphine, diamorphine, pethidine or fentanyl.

Following the administration of the spinal medications, the needle is removed and patient is placed supine with left uterine displacement (LUD). The desired sensory level for caesarean section is T6 but T4 becomes mandatory for the obstetrician who exteriorises the uterus for repair.

Spinal induced maternal hypotension remains one of the main perioperative complications during caesarean section. It is imperative that vasopressors should be available to the anaesthetist involved in the care of women undergoing caesarean section under spinal anaesthesia. Ephedrine was considered the vasopressor of choice some decades ago. Phenylephrine has assumed the primal position. The consensus is to provide intravenous fluid preloading when feasible and maintain the systolic blood pressure above 100 mmHg. These measures could prevent the deleterious consequences of prolonged spinal induced maternal hypotension on the foetus (Box 19.5).

Box 19.5 Spinal anaesthesia for caesarean section

- H2-receptor blocker iv/PPI/Metochlopramide
- Antacid: 0.3M sodium citrate/freshly prepared MMT
- LUD: Crawford wedge/left lateral tilt
- Baseline monitoring: HR, BP, SpO_2, ECG, $ETCO_2$, Temp
- Preloading: 15–20 mL/kg 0.9% saline or Ringer Lactate
- Sitting Position: Lumbar puncture @ L2/3, L3/4
- 25G or 26G Whitacre needle
- Hyperbaric bupivacaine 10 mg + pethidine7.7–10 mg
  - Left Uterine Displacement (LUD)
- Prompt treatment of hypotension
  - Phenylephrine/ephedrine

19.20 Epidural Anaesthesia

Epidural anaesthesia is particularly popular because of the flexibility of its administration. The local anaesthetic agent can be given in incremental doses to achieve the desired sensory level. The use of the continuous technique enables the anaesthetist to maintain anaesthesia irrespective of the duration of surgery. Epidural anaesthesia as a primary technique for caesarean section should be for a reason. Quite often labour epidural analgesia is extended for surgical delivery. This is achieved by the administration of carbonated 2% lidocaine or the addition of 1 mEq of 8.4% sodium bicarbonate to each 10 mL of lidocaine. Details of the conduct and management of epidural is shown in Box 19.6.

19.21 Combined Spinal Epidural

This technique allows for the rapidity of spinal anaesthesia and the flexibility of epidural. CSE may be a preferred choice in major placental praevia, previous uterine surgeries with adhesions, possible difficult surgery and morbid obesity. In these situations, the epidural anaesthesia is activated if the caesarean section goes beyond the spinal component.

19.22 Local Anaesthesia

The use of local infiltration of anaesthesia appears to be of historical relevance in more developed countries. As a primary technique, local infiltration may be necessary when the anaesthetic personnel are unavailable. Furthermore, it may be necessary to do a local infiltration for the delivery of the foetus if the mother is severely compromised or grossly unstable. It is pertinent to understand the limitations inherent with this technique. The administration of the local anaesthetic is at different layers to the uterus. See Box 19.7 for details.

Box 19.6 Epidural anaesthesia for caesarean section

- H2-receptor blocker iv/PPI/Metochlopramide
- Antacid: 0.3M sodium citrate/freshly prepared MMT
- LUD: Crawford wedge/left lateral tilt
- Baseline monitoring: HR, BP, SpO_2, ECG, $ETCO_2$, Temp
- Preloading: 0.9% saline or Ringer Lactate
- Sitting Position: Epidural catheter @ L2/3, L3/4
- Left Uterine Displacement
- Test dose
- Epidural medications in aliquots of 3–5 mL
- 15–20 mL of 0.5% Bupivacaine ± fentanyl 50 mcg
- OR 10 mL 2% lignocaine + 5 mL 0.5% bupivacaine ± 50 mcg fentanyl
- Prompt treatment of hypotension
  - Phenylephrine/ephedrine

Box 19.7 Local infiltration for caesarean section

- Intracutaneous
- Subcutaneous injection
- Intrarectus
- Parietal peritoneal
- Visceral peritoneal
- Paracervical

19.23 Conclusion

Pain relief is indicated whenever pain exists! It is unacceptable to watch women go through labour and delivery without adequate control of the associated pain. The American College of Obstetricians and Gynaecologists and the American College of Anesthesiologists issued a joint statement on labour pain which included the following statement: "Labour results in severe pain for many women. There is no other circumstance where it is considered acceptable for a person to experience severe pain amenable to safe intervention, while under a physician's care." Most of the available methods are safe and should be offered to all parturients to make an informed choice. Anticipation, preparation and effective communication between the anaesthetist, obstetrician and midwife will lead to a better maternal experience of the birthing process.

19.24 Summary

The obstetric patient is a unique patient due to the physiological changes of pregnancy. These changes also have varying implications on the anaesthetic care. The obstetric patient is often admitted to the hospital for labour and delivery.

The labour may terminate in spontaneous vaginal delivery, assisted vaginal delivery or by caesarean section. Pain accompanies labour and delivery and the anaesthetist is often called upon to provide pain relief. The available methods could be classified as pharmacological and non-pharmacological. The pharmacological options include the use of parenteral analgesics, inhaled analgesic or regional analgesia. Epidural analgesia remains the most effective method of regional technique because of its flexibility. However, spinal analgesia is becoming a veritable option for labour analgesia due to the ease of insertion and cost-effectiveness. The duration of analgesia provided by single shot spinal analgesia in labour is a major limitation to its widespread application thus, restricting its use largely to the multiparous women in whom labour is expected to be short.

When labour terminates in caesarean section or abdominal delivery has been electively decided, the anaesthetist remains a member of the multidisciplinary care of the patient. The choice of anaesthesia is influenced by the maternal health status, indication for the caesarean section, urgency of the surgical intervention and the desires of the mother. Spinal anaesthesia is the preferred technique to general anaesthesia for caesarean delivery in the absence of contraindication. Most of the available methods labour analgesia are safe and should be offered to all parturients to make an informed choice. Anticipation, preparation and effective communication between the anaesthetist, obstetrician and midwife will lead to a better maternal experience at parturition.

Aetiology and Management of Obstetric Haemorrhage

20

Rosemary N. Ogu and Joseph Ifeanyi Brian-D Adinma

Learning Objectives

At the end of this chapter, the learner will be able to:

- Define obstetric haemorrhage, postpartum haemorrhage and antepartum haemorrhage.
- Explain the need for the prevention and early diagnosis of postpartum haemorrhage.
- Identify the components of the active management of third stage of labour.
- Critically evaluate pregnant women with obstetric haemorrhage and initiate management.
- Differentiate between prevention and management of postpartum haemorrhage.

20.1 Introduction

Obstetric haemorrhage, especially postpartum haemorrhage (PPH), continues to be a very important cause of maternal mortality and morbidity both in the developed and developing countries. Although several regional and hospital-based studies report various rates and causes of maternal mortality, obstetric haemorrhage in most cases accounts for more than 25% of maternal deaths [1, 2] with postpartum haemorrhage (PPH) being the primary cause of approximately 25% of global maternal deaths [2]. It is equally the leading cause of maternal death in low-income countries [3–5]. Obstetric haemorrhage, also the most common reason postpartum women are admitted to intensive care units, is arguably the most preventable cause of maternal mortality [2, 4, 5]. Most deaths resulting from PPH occur during the first 24 hours after birth: Improving health care for women during childbirth in order to prevent and treat PPH is an essential step towards the achievement of the Sustainable Development Goals.

Obstetric haemorrhage is defined as blood loss related to pregnancy/childbirth occurring after the 28th week of pregnancy and up to 6 weeks after delivery. Massive obstetric haemorrhage refers to acute blood loss of more than 1500 mL (25–30%) of the blood volume in pregnancy; a decrease in haemoglobin >4 g dl^{-1}; or acute transfusion requirement >4 units [6].

In this chapter, the causes of obstetric haemorrhage are elucidated and the clinical features and management of the haemorrhaging patient are reviewed.

20.2 Causes of Obstetric Haemorrhage

The causes of obstetric haemorrhage occur before or after delivery of the baby, thus antepartum haemorrhage (APH; 0.2–3.5%) or postpartum haemorrhage (PPH; 5–15%). Coagulation failure (0.2%) is rare but can occur before or after delivery. A comprehensive classification of causes of obstetric haemorrhage is shown in Fig. 20.1.

20.3 Antepartum Haemorrhage

This is conventionally defined as bleeding from the genital tract after the 28th week of pregnancy and before labour. The 28th week is related to the British legal limit of fetal viability and registration of stillbirth. Because foetuses can be salvaged at much lower gestational age, FIGO has recommended that peri-

R. N. Ogu (✉)
University of Port Harcourt Teaching Hospital, University of Port Harcourt, Port Harcourt, Nigeria
e-mail: rosemary.ogu@uniport.edu.ng

J. I. B.-D. Adinma
College of Health Sciences, Nnamdi Azikiwe University and Teaching Hospital, Nnewi, Nigeria

Ekwueme Centre for Multidisciplinary Research/Centre for Health and Allied Legal Demographical Development, Research and Training (CHALADDRAT), Nnamdi Azikiwe University, Awka, Nigeria

F. Okonofua et al. (eds.), *Contemporary Obstetrics and Gynecology for Developing Countries*,
https://doi.org/10.1007/978-3-030-75385-6_20

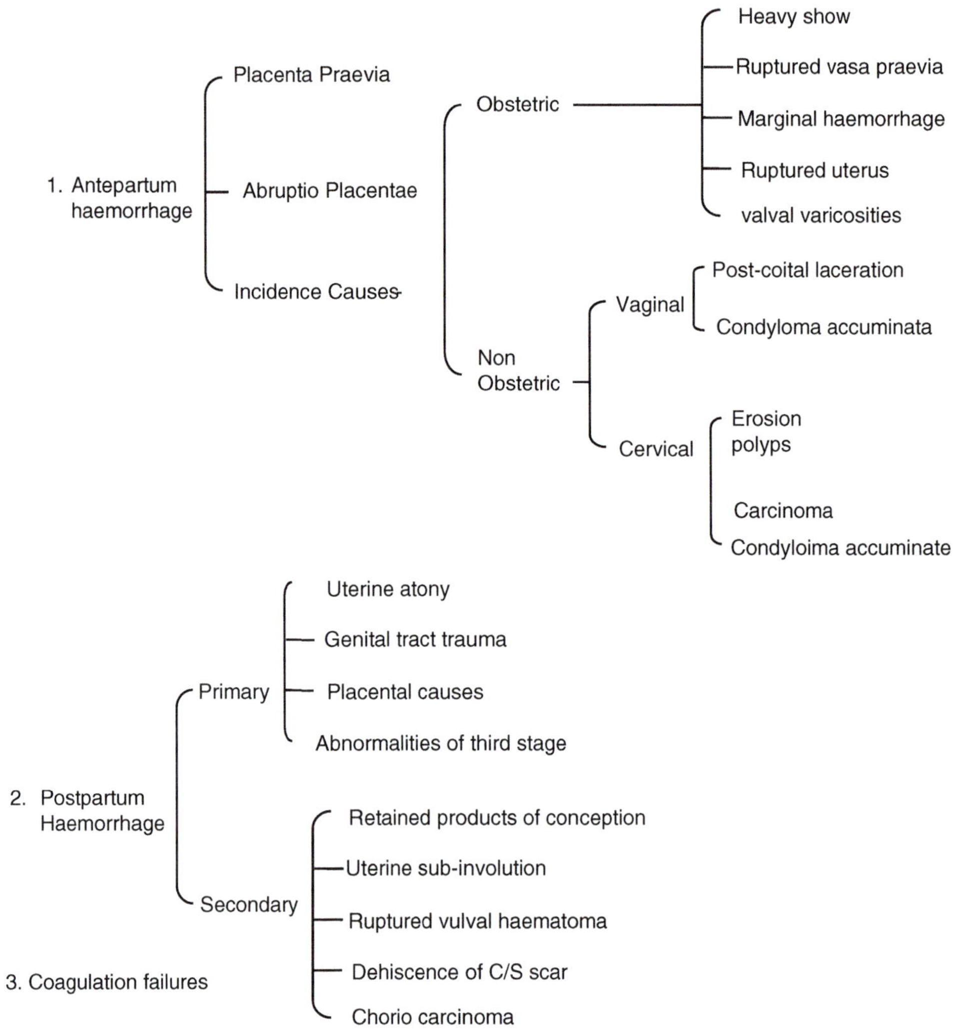

Fig. 20.1 Classification of causes of obstetric haemorrhage

natal death statistics should include foetuses born after 22 weeks or weighing 500 g or more in the definition [7]. From a reasonable point of view, 22 weeks should therefore be regarded as the dividing line between the definition of APH and abortion. Twenty-eight weeks are however still used in Nigeria. Three broad groups of antepartum haemorrhage are identified:

1. Abruptio placentae in which genital bleeding occurs following separation of a normally sited placenta.
2. Placenta praevia in which bleeding occurs from a placenta sited in the lower segment.
3. Incidental (indeterminate) haemorrhage due to other causes (see Fig. 20.1).

20.3.1 Placenta Praevia

Placenta praevia occurs when the placenta is wholly or partially inserted into the lower segment of the uterus, i.e. covering or within 20 mm of the internal os. The incidence varies between 0.2% and 1.2% [8, 9]. The incidence increases with maternal age and parity, and is more prevalent following previous caesarean section, abortions, multiple gestation and among women who smoke during pregnancy [8, 9]. Placenta praevia is also significantly associated with abnormalities of placental formation and umbilical cord insertion. There are four grades of placenta praevia:

- Grade I (Lateral) – The placenta encroaches on the lower segment of the uterus.
- Grade II (Marginal) – The placenta reaches the margin of the cervical os.
- Grade III (Partial) – The placenta covers part of the cervical os.
- Grade IV (Complete) – The placenta is centrally placed in the lower uterine segment.

Grades I and IIA are also called minor placenta praevia, while grades 11B to IV are called major placenta praevia. The A and B refers to anterior or posterior site.

20.3.1.1 Clinical Features and Diagnosis

Placenta praevia is characterised by painless, unprovoked vaginal bleeding, usually occurring in the third trimester. A warning bleed may precede actual bleeding. As pregnancy advances, cervical effacement causes separation of the abnormally sited placenta from the decidua provoking bleeding. Coitus and digital examination can also provoke bleeding. The abdomen is soft and non-tender. Fetal parts are easily palpable and the fetal heart sound is heard. These are its main distinguishing features from abruptio placentae. Often, and in particular when the placenta is posteriorly placed, the presenting part is shifted from the midline or the fetal lie remains unstable. Vaginal examination is contraindicated, since this will provoke severe bleeding. It should be undertaken only when an examination under anaesthesia (EUA) involving a 'double set-up' is arranged in the theatre with instruments and personnel ready for emergency caesarean section.

20.3.1.2 Diagnosis Is Clinical but Confirmed by Placental Localisation

Ultrasonography is nowadays the most common and convenient method of localising the placenta. The incidence of low-lying placenta from ultrasonography is high at lower gestational age. By term, the incidence had fallen to 3%. This reduction in incidence of placenta praevia with increasing gestational age is due to upward 'migration' of the placenta, as the lower segment gets formed and the upper segment enlarges upwards.

Placental localisation by radiography or by radioisotope, used in the past, has become unpopular following the advent of ultrasound. Recently, magnetic resonance imaging (MRI) has been acclaimed to be a very accurate method of diagnosing placenta praevia, but it is available only in very few centres in developing countries. It is an expensive investigation and its current use in obstetric haemorrhage is probably limited to the diagnosis of placenta accreta.

20.3.1.3 Clinical Management of Placenta Praevia

The diagnosis of placenta praevia is based on history of painless unprovoked vaginal bleeding. The fetal status is uncompromised. The patient should be properly assessed for the extent of blood loss and appropriate replacement arranged. If not already done, placental localisation is then performed and further management depends on the gestational age.

20.3.1.4 Expectant Management

The aim of expectant management is to prolong the pregnancy to an age that fetal survival is ensured, usually 36 weeks and above. This policy, which was introduced by Macafee in 1962, at the Royal Maternity Hospital, Belfast [10], involves the admission of the patient following diagnosis into a fully equipped and staffed maternity unit, in which blood is immediately available for transfusion, and full facilities for emergency caesarean section and obstetric staff are available to perform the operation on 24-hour basis. Cotton [11] in 1980, further described an 'aggressive' form of Macafee's regime using antenatal blood transfusion and tocolytic drugs to inhibit premature labour, and steroids to ripen the fetal lungs; he reported significant reduction in perinatal mortality. Silver et al. [12] in 1984 suggested a modified more flexible form of Macafee regime in which properly selected and counselled patients are managed on an outpatient basis particularly in the light of modern technological advances in perinatal care, ultrasonography and hospital organisation. Advances in perinatology and improved fetal salvage rate have led to changing views on the duration of conservative management for placenta praevia. If haemorrhage occurs after 37 weeks of pregnancy, it is best to deliver the baby. In minor grades of placenta praevia, vaginal delivery may be allowed if the head is engaged or is capable of engaging within the pelvis. Following vaginal amniotomy, the head may press on the placental edge and by a tamponade effect allow labour to proceed without reasonable bleeding. In major grades of placenta praevia, abdominal delivery is recommended.

20.3.1.5 Examination Under Anaesthesia (EUA)

If the decision to deliver the baby is taken, opinion differs as to whether to perform examination under anaesthesia, followed by caesarean section if major grade of placenta praevia is encountered, or whether to go ahead and perform caesarean section without vaginal examination under anaesthesia in the light of available clinical and ultrasound evidence. EUA is particularly useful when ultrasound results are equivocal or suggest anterior grade II placenta praevia, which may require vaginal delivery. It is performed at 37–38 weeks in the theatre with blood available and instruments and personnel for caesarean section ready should the procedure provoke torrential haemorrhage.

20.3.1.6 Caesarean Section for Placenta Praevia

Caesarean section for placenta praevia is hazardous and requires expert handling. Three or four pints of blood are provided. The Pfannenstiel incision is more commonly used, although the sub-umbilical midline(vertical) incision can also be used. Unless strong contra-indications occur, the lower segment incision is preferable to a classical caesarean section. Large vessels are occasionally encountered coursing across the potential site of the lower segment incision. Care with the incision to avoid cutting through the large veins will in most cases suffice. Otherwise, the vessels may be ligated before making the lower segment incision, or a low vertical incision can be made between the veins when they are too numerous to avoid or ligate. Following the lower segment incision, the placenta is then either incised or separated to reach the baby. Speed is important to avert exsanguination of the foetus following incision of the placenta. Placenta accreta is not an infrequently encountered fatal condition associated with placenta praevia and can cause severe haemorrhage requiring hysterectomy [13].

Caesarean section for placenta praevia should therefore be performed by a senior obstetrician and patients, especially those with previous caesarean section should be counselled on the possibility of severe haemorrhage with placenta accrete that will necessitate hysterectomy.

20.3.2 Abruptio Placentae

Abruption (Latin word meaning breaking away from a mass) describes the process of placental detachment from its site. It presents clinically in three forms:

1. External or revealed, in which vaginal bleeding is evident.
2. Internal or concealed, in which blood is trapped between the detached placenta and the uterine wall without visible vaginal bleeding.
3. Combined or mixed, in which the bleeding is partly revealed and partly concealed.

Sher [14] proposed a classification of the severity of abruptio placentae using a system of clinical grading:

Grade 1 – The cause of antepartum haemorrhage is not certain; the uterus is soft and non-tender and the diagnosis of abruption placentae is made retrospectively.

Grade 2 – Cases in which APH is accompanied by tenseness and tenderness of the uterus on abdominal palpation and the foetus is alive.

Grade 3 – Similar cases as in Grade 2 but the foetus is dead.

Grade 3A – Not associated with haemorrhagic diathesis.

Grade 3B – Associated with haemorrhagic diathesis.

This grading is useful towards an objective management of abruptio placentae. The incidence of abruptio placentae is given as 0.5–3.5% of pregnancy [15].

20.3.2.1 Aetiology

The aetiology is unclear in most cases of abruptio placentae. The condition tends to recur in subsequent pregnancy in 6% of cases [15]. Some factors associated with abruptio placentae include maternal hypertension [16], abdominal trauma [17], maternal poverty and malnutrition [18], maternal age, parity, social class and folic acid deficiency, cigarette smoking [19], drugs such as nicotine, cocaine and anticoagulants [20, 21]. Others include sudden uterine decompression as in membrane rupture in the presence of polyhydramnios and abnormalities of the uterus and placenta.

20.3.2.2 Pathology and Mechanism of Abruptio Placentae

In the mechanism of abruptio placentae [15], there is initially uterine vasospasm. Following relaxation of these vessels, vascular engorgement occurs, followed by arteriolar rupture into the decidua basalis. A decidual haematoma is formed with eventual decidual necrosis at the edge of the placenta. As blood escapes under the decidua basalis, it can dissect under the membranes ultimately escaping through the vagina as revealed bleeding, or can break through the membrane into the amniotic cavity causing blood staining of the amniotic fluid. It can also dissect under the placenta, large volumes being concealed separating the placenta from the maternal surface, or it can infiltrate the myometrium causing tetanic contraction, which can be localised or diffuse. Uteroplacental circulation is invariably impaired leading to fetal hypoxia and fetal death. Decidual necrosis and degeneration may release thromboplastin into the maternal circulation and initiate disseminated intravascular coagulation (DIC).

20.3.2.3 Clinical Presentation

Vaginal bleeding is the most common presentation. Vaginal bleeding may be minimal in spite of the fact that most of the placenta is separated, the foetus is dead and the mother is in shock. Abdominal pain that is acute and constant is the second most common form of presentation and occurs in 35% of cases [22]. With posterior uterine wall abruption, there is marked woody rigidity of the abdomen due to uterine hypertonus often associated with Couvelaire's uterus. The fetal parts are not palpable and the fetal heart sounds are inaudible. Ultrasonography helps to identify foetuses still alive. It can also localise the placenta as well as identify retroplacental clots or intraperitoneal bleeding. Severe vasospasm can cause a normal or even elevated blood pressure in great disparity to the degree of hypovolaemia and blood loss, thereby deceiving the unsuspecting practitioner as to the degree of the clinical problem.

20.3.2.4 Complications of Abruptio Placentae

The major complications include renal failure, coagulopathy, postpartum haemorrhage and hypertension with or without proteinuria. Renal failure results from prolonged hypovolemia and is a major cause of maternal mortality. The kidneys show bilateral cortical necrosis. It is preventable by adequate and appropriate fluid replacement and by the use of central venous pressure (CVP) monitoring. Coagulation failure results from the release of thromboplastin from the decidua. DIC is almost invariably followed by fibrinolysis in a few cases with the formation of fibrin degradation products (FDPs). Postpartum haemorrhage will result from increased levels of FDPs and is not related to the degree of hypofibrinogenemia. Severe hypertension with or without albuminuria may follow placental abruption in one third of cases and may be a result of the vasospasm following maternal hypovolemia.

20.3.2.5 Management of Abruptio Placentae

Prompt diagnosis and swift management are necessary to avert maternal and perinatal death. Treatment should aim at the restoration of effective circulation, delivery of a healthy non-acidotic foetus and continued monitoring of the fluid and coagulation status of the mother. Pulse and blood pressure are false assessments of the degree of blood loss, since normal values have been recorded where blood volume loss of 40–50% has occurred [23]. Revealed vaginal bleeding may be minimal while most of the blood is lost retroplacentally. An in-dwelling urinary catheter is left to monitor urine output. Normal output should exceed 30 ml/hour. If it is less than this, pulmonary artery (Swan-Ganz) catheter or central venous pressure line is recommended. CVP monitors the ability of the cardiovascular system to handle intravenous infusion. It should be maintained at about +10 cm water. Cross-matched blood or Ringer's lactate solution is usually given enough to maintain the urine output at 30 mL/hour or the haematocrit at 30%.

Grade 1 abruptio placentae is managed expectantly. The abruptio is usually minor or the diagnosis is in doubt. The patient may present with mild vaginal bleeding or with mild abdominal pain, which may be localised. Ultrasonography may have diagnosed a retroplacental clot. Conservative management should be carried out to allow fetal maturity. Delivery by induction should be performed at or before term.

Cardiotocographic surveillance is useful in determining the optimum time of intervention in grades I and II abruptio placentae and should be commenced once abruption is suspected and the foetus is alive [24]. Grade II placental abruption in the past was almost always managed by caesarean section. This is changing now with the advent of electronic fetal monitoring. Oxytocin infusion is set up to stimulate good contractions; the membranes are ruptured and prompt delivery carried out. A good perinatal outcome and reduced caesarean section rate invariably results. The decision to operate is not always easy because of the risk of haemorrhage from hypofibrinogenemia. In addition, 15% of live-born infants die during the neonatal period [24]. In grade Ill abruptio placentae, the foetus is dead and conservative management using oxytocin infusion and amniotomy is the best delivery option. When conservative management fails or vaginal delivery is contraindicated, caesarean section is recommended.

20.3.3 Incidental Causes of Antepartum Haemorrhage

The term incidental causes is used here to include a wide range of factors that can cause antepartum obstetric haemorrhage, which cannot be classified under placenta praevia or abruptio placentae (Fig. 20.1). Uterine rupture is the most important in this group and is therefore treated in greater detail.

20.3.3.1 Uterine Rupture

Uterine rupture can occur in an intact or scarred uterus and can be spontaneous or traumatic [25]. It can also be complete or incomplete depending on whether or not the peritoneal coat is involved. Rupture more commonly involves the anterior wall of the uterus.

The common causes of uterine rupture include obstructed labour, injudicious use of oxytocin in labour, injudicious use of obstetric instruments and careless obstetric manipulations such as external cephalic version. It is more common following caesarean section especially classical caesarean operation and also following hysterotomy or dilatation and curettage. Dewhurst [26] reported an incidence of scar rupture following lower segment caesarean section of 0.8–1.2%, and 8.9% following classical caesarean section. Uterine rupture is more common in the multigravida and in the unbooked patient [27, 28].

The danger of uterine rupture lies in the likelihood of delayed diagnosis since the bleeding is usually occult. A high index of suspicion is therefore required especially when any of the predisposing factors mentioned above exists, or in cases of intrapartum or postpartum collapse.

Clinical features include signs of haemorrhagic shock or evidence of collapse. The uterus may be pushed to the contralateral side by a broad ligament haematoma and fluid may be detected in the abdominal cavity.

The management of uterine rupture involves patient resuscitation, followed by surgical laparotomy. The fate of the uterus depends on the site of uterine rupture and the patient's desire for future childbearing and conservation of her uterus. Where it is necessary to conserve the uterus, and especially when uterine rupture is fundal, or involves just the dehiscence of previous scar, repair is recommended. Subsequent delivery should be by elective caesarean section. If, however, uterine rupture extends laterally to poorly accessible areas of the broad ligament, repair will be technically difficult and may cause damage to the ureters and vessels in the neighbourhood. Hysterectomy (usually a sub-total) is recommended. If the woman has strong aversion to the removal of her uterus and runs a great risk of uterine rupture if pregnancy occurs again, repair is carried out, accompanied with bilateral tubal ligation.

20.3.3.2 Marginal Haemorrhage

This refers to bleeding from the edge of a normally implanted placenta. It commonly occurs in circumvallate or extrachorial placenta and was referred to in the past as marginal sinus haemorrhage. The fibrous ring around the edge of the chorionic plate retracts and causes intermittent bleeding. There may be associated exudation of serum from the ring clots, called hydrorrhoea gravidarum. Maternal and fetal well-being are rarely affected.

20.3.3.3 Vasa Praevia

This occurs when the placental blood vessel lies in front of the presenting part of the foetus, usually in association with a velamentous insertion of the cord. The vessel can rupture and cause severe bleeding and fetal exsanguination unless a prompt caesarean section is performed. Testing the blood for fetal origin using the alkaline denaturation test is an important prerequisite to prompt diagnosis and immediate intervention. Other incidental causes of obstetric haemorrhage are of importance depending on the extent of blood loss. Exclusion of vaginal and cervical causes is made from speculum examination carried out only after placenta praevia has been ruled out by ultrasonography. Replacement of blood loss and appropriate management of the pathology is then carried out.

20.4 Postpartum Haemorrhage

Postpartum haemorrhage may be primary or secondary. Primary postpartum haemorrhage (PPH) is commonly defined as bleeding from the genital tract of 500 mL or more within 24 hours after birth. Secondary postpartum haemorrhage is bleeding from the genital tract occurring after the first 24 hours and within 6 weeks of delivery of any volume enough to compromise the cardiovascular system.

20.4.1 Incidence

The incidence of postpartum haemorrhage varies widely between 5 and 15%. The incidence of PPH is related to the management of the third stage of labour. This is the period from the completed delivery of the baby until the completed delivery of the placenta.

20.4.2 Causes of Primary Postpartum Haemorrhage

The main cause of postpartum haemorrhage is uterine atony (90% of cases). Other causes include genital tract trauma, retained placenta, placenta praevia and accreta and coagulation disorders. As a way of remembering the causes of PPH, using the '4 *T*' s' as a mnemonic is suggested: tone, tissue, trauma and thrombosis [29].

20.4.2.1 Uterine Atony

This is by far the most common cause of primary postpartum haemorrhage. Predisposing factors to uterine atony include:

1. Grandmultiparity.
2. Uterine over-distension, as may result from multiple pregnancy, polyhydramnios or fetal macrosomia.
3. Past history of postpartum haemorrhage.
4. Antepartum haemorrhage (placenta praevia and placental abruption).
5. Multiple fibromyomata.
6. Operative deliveries such as caesarean section, especially if halothane is employed for anaesthesia.
7. Prolonged labour.
8. Mismanagement of third stage of labour such as following injudicious cord traction or delivery of placenta by Crede's method.
9. Retention of products of conception – placental cotyledon or membranes.

20.4.2.2 Methods of Prevention of Postpartum Haemorrhage Due to Uterine Atony

High-quality evidence suggests that active management of the third stage of labour reduces the incidence and severity of PPH [2–5, 30–38]. Active management is the combination of (1) uterotonic administration (preferably oxytocin) immediately upon delivery of the baby, (2) early cord clamping and cutting and (3) gentle cord traction with uterine countertraction when the uterus is well contracted (i.e. Brandt-Andrews manoeuvre). Active management of the third stage of labour is considered the 'gold standard' strategy for reducing the incidence of PPH. It traditionally combines nondrug interventions (controlled cord traction and cord clamping) with the administration of a uterotonic drug, the preferred uterotonic being oxytocin. Recent recommendations [2] deemphasises the non-drug aspect of active management of third stage for prevention of PPH.

The WHO recommends that all women giving birth should be offered a uterotonic during the third stage of labour for the prevention of PPH; oxytocin 10iu (IM/IV) is the drug of choice. Other injectable uterotonics and misoprostol are recommended as alternatives in settings where oxytocin is unavailable. Current evidence reveals that the combined use of oxytocin and misoprostol gives better results for the prevention and treatment of primary PPH. The intervention; controlled cord traction, is now recommended as optional, in settings with available skilled birth attendant, and contraindicated, in settings where skilled birth attendants do not assist births. Early cord clamping is now generally contraindicated. Continuous uterine massage is not recommended as an intervention to prevent PPH in women who have received prophylactic oxytocin, as it may cause maternal discomfort, require a dedicated health professional and may not lead to a reduction in blood loss. However, surveillance of the uterine tonus through abdominal palpation is recommended in all women for early identification of postpartum uterine atony. In summary, the main intervention in the active management of third stage of labour package is the use of uterotonics. Misoprostol is thus recommended for use by community health workers and lay health workers. Following caesarean sections, oxytocin with misoprostol is the preferred oxytocic, while controlled cord traction is recommended in preference to manual removal when assisting placenta delivery.

20.4.2.3 Vulval Haematomas

This results from rupture of vulval varicosities, poor haemostasis following episiotomy repair or from bruising and damage to vessels underlying the vulval skin during passage of the fetal head in normal parturition. Two types have been identified – infralevator and the supralevator. The bleeding is usually insidious and may manifest quite late following delivery. The woman complains of perineal pain and dizziness. She is pale and develops signs of haemorrhagic shock. The patient is resuscitated with fluid and blood transfusion prior to surgery. The usual obvious infralevator haematoma is incised and evacuated. Haemostatic sutures are applied to the dead space, which may then be packed with gauze or a corrugated drain may be left in situ. Supralevator and broad ligament haematoma are best managed conservatively using blood transfusion and antibiotic to prevent infection.

20.4.2.4 Third-Stage Abnormalities

Retained Placenta

With the present-day active management of third stage of labour, placental separation and delivery are expected to follow almost immediately after the delivery of the foetus. When this does not occur 30 minutes after delivery, manual removal of the placenta is advisable. If, however, bleeding starts as a consequence of incomplete separation of the placenta, manual removal can be performed earlier than this. Placental retention can occur following poor uterine contraction or rarely when the placenta is morbidly stuck to the uterine. A full bladder may compound the retention of placenta; therefore, emptying the bladder using a sterile catheter may aid release of the retained placenta. When considerable bleeding has occurred, resuscitation of the patient who is invariably in shock is mandatory and an oxytocic given once more followed by another attempt at delivery by controlled cord traction. If this fails, the patient is taken to the operating theatre where manual removal is carried out under anaesthesia.

Morbid Adhesion of the Placenta

Morbid adherence of the placenta to the uterus is called placenta accreta. If it extends beyond the endometrium to the myometrium, it is termed placenta increta, and if it extends beyond this to the serous coat, it is termed placenta percreta. It is discovered when following retained placenta, difficulty is encountered during manual removal. If bleeding is not active, the adherent portion is left and the patient observed is covered with antibiotics. A risk of secondary postpartum haemorrhage 10–14 days later exists. If bleeding is still active and the patient desires to have more children, she is managed conservatively with oxytocics and antibiotics. When this fails, internal iliac artery ligation, angiographic embolisation or otherwise hysterectomy is advisable. If the patient has completed childbearing, hysterectomy is the treatment of choice.

Acute Uterine Inversion

This occurs when traction of the cord is attempted before uterine contraction and placental separation are established. The inversion is then induced; otherwise it can occur spontaneously in association with adherent fundal placenta. There are three degrees of acute uterine inversion:

1. Inversion of the uterine fundus up to the cervical os.
2. Inversion of the whole uterine body up to the cervical os.
3. Complete inversion of the uterine body, cervix and vagina.

The patient presents with acute abdominal pain followed by postpartum collapse and bleeding. Acute inversion occurring at the time of delivery is managed by immediate replacement. A shot of oxytocic is administered and the patient taken to the theatre for manual removal of the placenta under anaesthesia. When shock follows inversion, the patient is resuscitated with intravenous fluids. Analgesic is administered prior to manual removal of the placenta. Inversion can also be corrected using hydrostatic pressure technique described by 0' Sullivan [39].

20.4.3 Treatment of Primary Postpartum Haemorrhage

Rapid recognition and diagnosis of PPH are essential to successful management. Resuscitative measures and the diagnosis and treatment of the underlying cause must occur quickly before sequelae of severe hypovolemia develop. The major factor in the adverse outcomes associated with severe haemorrhage is a delay in initiating appropriate management.

Immediately commence resuscitation. Call for help. Raising the legs improves venous return and is consistent with the positioning used to diagnose and treat the underlying causes of bleeding. Administer oxygen and obtain intravenous access. All intravenous lines started on the labour ward for other reasons must be placed with cannulas of sufficient gauge. Samples are collected for urgent packed cell volume and grouping and crossmatching of blood. Uterine massage is recommended for the treatment of PPH as soon as it is diagnosed, and initial fluid resuscitation with isotonic crystalloids is mandatory. Intravenous access should be established with two wide bore cannulae and isotonic crystalloid using normal saline or Ringers lactate should be rushed in. Dextrose-containing solutions, such as 5% dextrose in water or diluted Normal Saline in 5% dextrose in water, have no role in the management of PPH. Remember that the loss of 1 L of blood requires replacement with 3–4 L of crystalloid because most of the infused fluid is not retained in the intravascular space but instead shifts to the interstitial space. This shift, along with oxytocin use, may result in peripheral edema in the days following PPH. Healthy kidneys easily excrete this excess fluid. Use wide-open initial infusion rates, with the goal of infusing the required replacement volume over minutes rather than hours. PPH of up to 1500 mL in a healthy pregnant woman can usually be managed by crystalloid infusion alone if the cause of bleeding is arrested. Blood loss in excess of this usually requires the addition of blood transfusion. The goal is to rapidly transfuse 2–4 units of packed red blood cells to replace lost oxygen-carrying capacity and to restore circulating volume.

Urethral catheter is passed and urine output is monitored. Pay close attention to the patient's level of consciousness, pulse, blood pressure and urine output during the course of the management of massive haemorrhage. A urine output of 30 mL/h or more likely indicates adequate renal perfusion. Closely monitor the full blood count, coagulation and blood gas values in addition to acid-base status. Pulse oximetry is useful for evaluating tissue perfusion and oxygen saturation. Frequent auscultation of the lung fields helps detect pulmonary edema or the development of adult respiratory distress syndrome. The use of tranexamic acid is advised in cases of refractory atonic bleeding or persistent trauma-related bleeding.

The use of intrauterine balloon tamponade is recommended for refractory bleeding or if uterotonics are unavailable. Bimanual uterine compression, external aortic compression and the use of non-pneumatic anti-shock garments are recommended as temporising measures until substantive care is available. If there is persistent bleeding and the relevant resources are available, uterine artery embolisation should be considered. If unavailable, surgical intervention should be used without further delay. If the third stage of labour lasts more than 30 minutes, controlled cord traction and parenteral oxytocin (10 IU) should be used to manage the retained placenta. If the placenta is retained and bleeding occurs, the manual removal of the placenta should be expedited. Whenever the manual removal of the placenta is undertaken, a single dose of prophylactic antibiotics is recommended. Other surgical options include uterine tamponade, uterine artery ligation, internal iliac arterial ligation, exploratory laparotomy and the various brace sutures; b lynch suture and hysterectomy.

20.4.4 Secondary Postpartum Haemorrhage

This is bleeding from the genital tract occurring after 24 hours and up to 6 weeks post-delivery. The incidence is between 0.3% and 1.5% [42, 43]. It results from the retention of products of conception or from uterine sub-involution. Infection invariably complicates the condition. Other causes include rupture of vulval haematoma, dehiscence of caesarean section scar and choriocarcinoma. Severe secondary PPH usually follows retained morbidly adherent placenta, and the patient may present with shock and infection. Treatment involves resuscitation with blood and fluid together with antibiotics followed by uterine exploration and evacuation in the theatre. Evacuated specimen is sent for histological analysis to rule out choriocarcinoma. Caesarean section scar dehiscence is treated by hysterectomy.

20.4.4.1 Coagulation Failure

Haemostatic Changes in Pregnancy

During pregnancy, some coagulation factors, notably fibrinogen, show increased blood level, and together with increased blood volume, increase the overall susceptibility to intravascular coagulation during pregnancy while also constituting an effective haemostatic shock following normal parturition.

The integrity of the vasculature is maintained in pregnancy by a local platelet response, which involves the formation of small fibrin clots and removal of unwanted fibrin by fibrinolysis. Apart from this, the coagulation system basically consists of the extrinsic mechanism, which involves the activation of factor VII by thromboplastin from damaged tissue, and the intrinsic mechanism in which factor XII is activated by collagen from injured blood vessel. The fibrinolytic system maintains an essential balance of the haemostatic process and involves the digestion of fibrin and fibrinogen by plasmin derived from plasminogen.

Disseminated Intravascular Coagulation (DIC)

This involves the formation of clots throughout the circulation, usually secondary to the stimulation of the coagulation system by procoagulant substances released in the blood following certain disorders of pregnancy. These disorders include abruptio placentae, amniotic fluid embolism, retention of dead foetus, placenta accreta, hydatidiform mole, septic abortion especially when induced with hypertonic saline, intrauterine sepsis, pre-eclampsia/eclampsia, acute fatty liver of pregnancy, purpura fulminans and prolonged shock. Others include thrombocytopenia, which may occur from severe megaloblastic anaemia, systemic lupus erythematosus and haemolytic uraemic syndrome (HUS); autoimmune thrombocytopenic purpura; and congenital coagulation disorders such as Von Willebrand's disease, factors VIII deficiency (haemophilia A) and factor XI deficiency (haemophilia B) and to a lesser degree factors XI and XIII deficiency. DIC results in consumption of clotting factors causing severe bleeding. In addition, fibrinolysis is stimulated with the formation of fibrin degradation products (FDPs), which also causes severe haemorrhage. FDPs in addition inhibit myometrial contractility and may affect cardiac function thereby aggravating haemorrhage and shock. A summary of the trigger mechanism of DIC is shown in Fig. 20.2, while the possible outcome is shown in Fig. 20.3.

Management

Although it may be necessary to ascertain the degree of haemostatic failure, this is not as important as taking urgent steps to replenish volume loss through judicious fluid management to avoid kidney failure. When adequate circulation is restored, fibrin degradation products are cleared from the system and normal haemostasis is reestablished. Blood is taken for the screening of platelet count, partial thrombin time or accelerated whole blood clotting time (which tests for intrinsic coagulation mechanism), prothrombin time (which tests for extrinsic clotting mechanism) and for the immunological assay of fibrin degradation products (FDPs) (which assesses the fibrinolytic system). Thrombin time is the most valuable screening test in haemostatic failure and it assesses the thrombin-clottable fibrinogen in citrated plasma sample. Normal thrombin time is 10–15 seconds accompanied with the formation of firm and stable clot.

Drugs for the Treatment of Disseminate Intravascular Coagulation (DIC)

Heparin is useful in the management of DIC when circulation is intact. When haemostasis is already defective, its use will only aggravate haemorrhage. It is therefore useful in the treatment of DIC due to conditions other than abruptio placentae.

Anti-fibrinolytic agents, aprotonin (Trasylol) and tranexamic acid (Cyclokapron) can precipitate the blockage of small organ vessels with fibrin especially vessels of the kidney and brain. This constitutes a major drawback to their use. They have, however, been recommended where severe bleeding occurs from the placental site several hours after delivery, particularly when other measures prove unsuccessful. Aprotinin has been recommended in cases of placental abruption where uterine inertia occurs in association with high levels of FDPs. Aprotinin, unlike tranexamic acid, is believed to have anti-coagulant activity in addition to anti-fibrinolytic property. This reduces its predisposition to the deposition of fibrin in vital organs, thereby making it more useful in the treatment of DIC, although high doses of the drug are necessary to achieve any substantial anti-coagulant effect. A recent WHO recommendation now strongly recommends early use of IV tranexamic acid (within 3 hours of birth) in addition to standard care for women with clinically-diagnosed PPH following vaginal birth or caesarean section. Tranexamic acid should be used in all cases of PPH, regardless of whether the bleeding is thought to be due to genital tract trauma or other causes, including uterine atony [40].

20.4.5 Evaluation of the Bleeding Patient

A thorough and accurate evaluation of the haemorrhaging patient is essential towards her effective management. Assessment should be conducted by an experienced obstetrician, anaesthetist and also a haematologist. Every obstetric unit should at all times strive to make this type of assessment possible on an emergency 24-hour basis, should ensure that facilities (including laboratory assistance) necessary for a reasonable assessment are available at all times, and that the necessary resuscitative machinery can be put in place simultaneously with the assessment. A well-outlined management protocol for the haemorrhaging patient is advisable in any obstetric unit and should be studied by every obstetric staff.

It is not easy to assess on clinical grounds the volume of blood loss particularly when bleeding is continuing. A continuous assessment is now possible, thanks to the introduction of central venous pressure (CVP) monitor and the Swan-Ganz catheter, which measures pulmonary capillary wedge pressure (PCWP). Both act as a guide towards fluid volume replacement even following special conditions such as sepsis, severe PET/eclampsia and adult respiratory distress syndrome. CVPs can only measure colloid overloads while the Swan-Ganz catheter can measure overloads of both colloids and crystalloids. Fluid replacement therapy should aim at maintaining the CVP at approximately 10 cm of water. Provided the uterus is empty, adequate and appropriate fluid replacement based on accurate monitors will blend with the body homeostatic response and achieve complete recovery from shock.

20.4.6 Resuscitation of the Bleeding Patient

Adequate and urgent fluid replacement is necessary to prevent kidney damage. Fresh whole blood is the ideal solution for the treatment of most obstetric haemorrhages [41]. It will restore circulatory volume, maintain appropriate osmotic and oncotic pressure, transport oxygen and carbon dioxide and reinstate the integrity of the homeostatic system by replenishing the depleted coagulation factors.1 Fresh whole

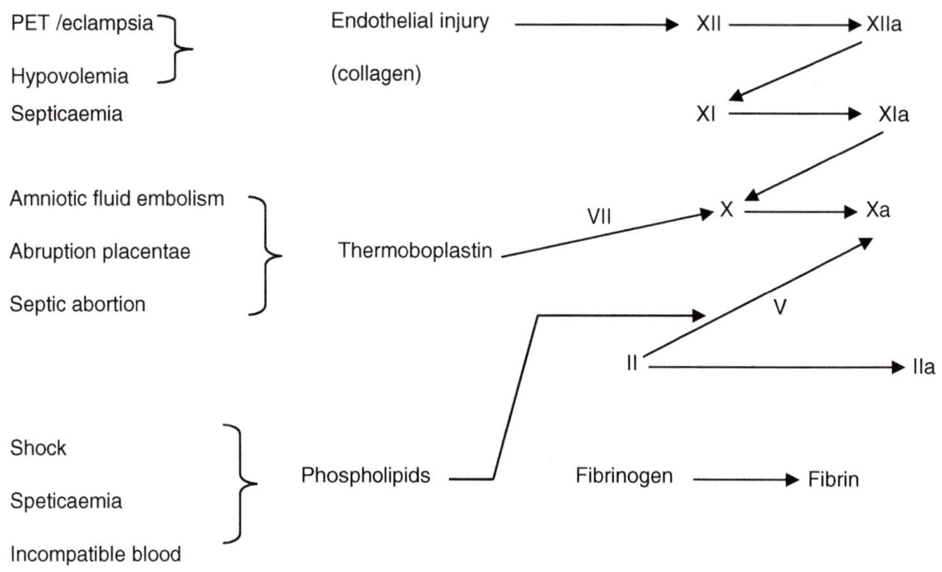

Fig. 20.2 Trigger mechanism of DIC in pregnancy

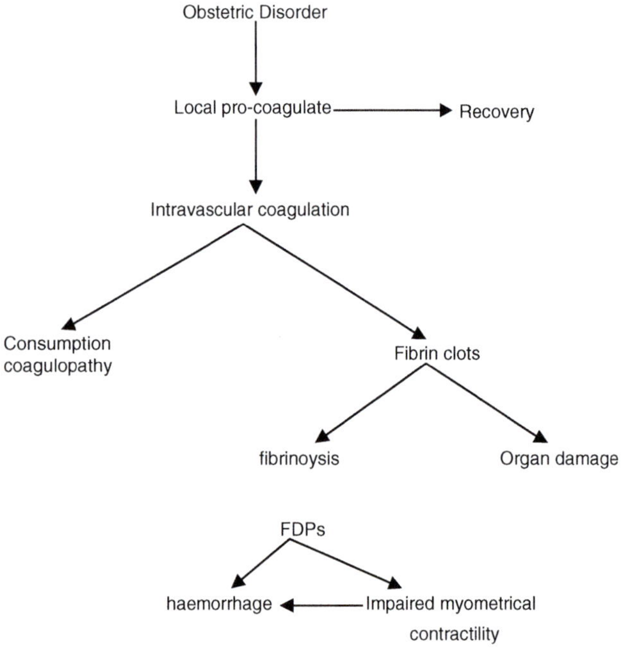

Fig. 20.3 Possible outcome in DIC

blood, unfortunately, is rarely available nowadays. Products that can be used for fluid replacement therapy are given in Table 20.1.

Both crystalloids (e.g. Hartman's solution) and colloids (e.g. haemacele) can be used for initial volume replacement, following which circulation is maintained with blood component therapy such as packed cells and fresh frozen plasma. Colloids, unlike crystalloids, remain the vascular compartment for a longer time and are therefore believed to have a better effect on the preservation and restoration of kidney function. This could be advantageous if blood replacement is not quickly available, provided the patient is no longer bleeding. Dextran has an adverse effect on platelet activity, interferes with grouping and cross-matching and induces anaphylactic reaction. These constitute drawbacks to its use in obstetric haemorrhage.

By the time 1500–2000 m1 (25–30% of blood volume) plasma substitute is infused, blood would have become available for transfusion. If this is not so and the patient is still bleeding, she should be transfused of uncross-matched blood of her group (if her blood group is known). Otherwise, she should be given 0 rhesus negative blood. Blood components are nowadays available in good blood transfusion service centres and include fresh frozen plasma (FFP), packed red cells, platelet concentrates and SAG-M blood (whole blood with the plasma component removed, while the remaining packed cell component is re-suspended into 100 mL sodium chloride, adenine, glucose and mannitol). SAG-M blood is deplete of protein and clotting factors and is unsuitable for massive obstetric haemorrhage unless it is given along with fresh frozen plasma in proportion of 8(SAG-M) to 1(FFP).

Fluosol-DA (20%) is a blood substitute with oxygen and carbon dioxide-carrying properties. It is useful in severe obstetric haemorrhage where blood is not available or is not acceptable, say on religious grounds. Some problems associated with blood transfusion include risk of transmission of infection especially HIV and hepatitis B, transfusion reactions, hypocalcaemia and even adult respiratory distress syndrome from stored blood. In recent times, the use of cell saver autologous blood transfusion (ABT) has come into focus as a safe and useful procedure, greatly reducing the

Table 20.1 Products used for fluid replacement therapy

Fresh whole blood
Plasma substitutes
a. Crystalloids
0.9% saline solution
Ringer's lactate
Darrow's solution
5% dextrose
Hartman's solution
b. Colloids
Dextrans
Hydroxyethyl starch
Gelatin solutions
Albuminoids
Gelatin derivatives (haemacele, gelofusine)
Plasma components
Fresh frozen plasma (FFP)
Frozen stored plasma (FSP)
Freeze-dried plasma (FDP)
Concentrated fibrinogen
Cryoprecipitate (Cryo)
Cryoprecipitate poor plasma
Platelet concentrate
Red cell
Sodium chloride, adenine, glucose and mannitol (SAG-M) blood

need for homologous blood transfusion and its associated risks in patients undergoing surgery [41, 42].

20.5 Control of Obstetric Haemorrhage

Meaningful stabilisation of the haemorrhaging patient can be claimed only if the bleeding is controlled. Control measures already discussed include the use of drugs, bi-manual compression and packing of the uterus, and the repair of genital tract lacerations. Other methods of control include the MAST & NASG suit, angiographic embolisation of bleeding vessels, obstetric hysterectomy and ligation of the internal iliac artery.

20.5.1 The NASG Suit

This simply means Non Pneumatic Anti-Shock Garment suit. It is a modification of the pneumatic suit developed during the Vietnam war to stabilise an injured patient during transportation. It is made from a double-layered polyvinyl material and has three chambers, one abdominal and two leg compartments, which are inflated by a foot pump. When applied and inflated, it increases systemic vascular resistance and elevates blood pressure. It can also cause auto transfusion of 300 mL of blood as well as slow down active bleeding while improving the perfusion of vital organs [43]. The NASG is a very cost-effective intervention for women in severe hypovolemic shock [44].

20.5.2 Angiographic Embolisation of Bleeding Vessels

This involves the intra-arterial injection with gelatin sponge shavings (Gelfoam-Upjohn) to arrest bleeding in postpartum haemorrhage when conservative and minor surgical procedures prove ineffective. It is usually performed through the femoral artery. Aortography is performed to identify the bleeding vessel, which is then catheterised prior to the injection of gel foam. The advantage of this procedure lies not only in the fact that it will avert the need for a major surgery following intractable obstetric haemorrhage, but also in its capacity to preserve reproductive function while saving life. Vasoconstrictive agents such as dopamine hydrochloride and vasopressin infusions administered intra-arterially have been used successfully in the management of obstetric haemorrhage.

20.5.3 Obstetric Hysterectomy

This is believed to be the most effective method of dealing with intractable haemorrhage due to uterine rupture, persistent uterine atony and morbidly adherent placenta. It should be performed as a last resort when other conservative methods of control of obstetric haemorrhage have failed. Subtotal hysterectomy is easier and faster to perform and is therefore recommended especially for haemorrhage due to uterine atony and some cases of morbid adhesion of the placenta [1]. The decision to perform hysterectomy must be taken early otherwise the patient dies on the theatre table.

20.5.4 Internal Iliac Artery Ligation

This method of controlling intractable obstetric haemorrhage is believed to be more effective for uterine atony and midline uterine perforation but less so for morbid adhesion of the placenta and uterine laceration. It involves the insertion of two ligatures, 0.5 cm apart around the anterior division of the internal iliac artery using either absorbable or non-absorbable suture material. The procedure can be performed unilaterally or bilaterally. It may not be successful in arresting haemorrhage and hysterectomy or angiographic embolisation may be required.

20.6 Conclusion

Obstetric haemorrhage clearly makes a very significant contribution to the maternal mortality rate in developed and developing countries. Reducing this high maternal mortality rate requires a collective commitment to an honest address of the diverse socio-political and economic issues involved by both the governments and people alike. The need to increase overall government spending on health services to provide adequate facilities for health institutions cannot be over emphasised. Prevention and blood replacement play a primary role in the management of obstetric haemorrhage. Every maternity unit should have laid down protocol for the prevention and management of obstetric haemorrhage and ensures the availability of blood and other resuscitative facilities together with trained personnel capable of diagnosing and adequately handling obstetric haemorrhage. Health education on pre-pregnancy child spacing, proper nutritional habits as well as painstaking monitor of the haemoglobin status in pregnancy with correction of anaemia will reduce overall fatalities associated with anaemia in pregnancy and obstetric haemorrhage.

Health facilities delivering maternity services should adopt formal protocols for the prevention and treatment of PPH and for early patient referral. The use of PPH treatment simulations for pre-service and in-service training programmes is recommended. Finally, the use of uterotonics for the prevention of PPH should be monitored and regarded as an indicator for obstetric haemorrhage prevention evaluation.

References

1. Global Burden of Disease Study 2013, Collaborators (22 August 2015). Global, regional, and national incidence, prevalence, and years lived with disability for 301 acute and chronic diseases and injuries in 188 countries, 1990–2013: a systematic analysis for the Global Burden of Disease Study 2013. Lancet (London, England). 2015;386(9995):743–800. PMID 26063472.
2. Department of Reproductive Health and research, World Health Organization (WHO). WHO recommendations for the prevention and treatment of postpartum haemorrhage. Geneva: WHO; 2012.
3. Hogan MC, et al. Maternal mortality for 181 countries, 1980-2008: a systematic analysis of progress made towards millennium development goal 5. Lancet. 2010;375(9726):1609–23.
4. World Health Organization, United Nations Children's Fund, United Nations Fund for Population Activities, The World Bank. Trends in maternal mortality: 1990–2010. Geneva, Switzerland; 2012.
5. World Health Organization. World Health Organization multicountry survey on maternal and newborn health. Geneva: WHO; 2012.
6. Shevell T, Malone FD. Management of Obstetric Haemorrhage. Semin Perinatol. 2003;27:86–104.
7. World Health Organisation WHO: Recommended Definitions, Terminology and Format for Statistical Tables Related to The Perinatal Period And Use of A New Certificate For Cause of Perinatal Deaths. Modifications recommended by FIGO as amended October 14, 1976. Acta Obstetricia et Gynaecologica Scandinavica. 1977;56:247–253.https://doi.org/10.3109/00016347709162009. PMID: 560099.
8. Kollmann M, Gaulhofer J, Lang U, Klaritsch P. Placenta praevia: incidence, risk factors and outcome. J Matern Fetal Neonatal Med. 2016;29(9):1395–8. https://doi.org/10.3109/14767058.2015.1049152.
9. Cresswell JA, Ronsmans C, Calvert C, Filippi V. Prevalence of placenta praevia by world region: a systematic review and meta-analysis. Tropical Med Int Health. 2013;18:712–24. https://doi.org/10.1111/tmi.12100.
10. Macafee CHG, Millar WG, Harley G. Maternal and fetal mortality in placenta preavia. J Obstet Gynaecol Br Comwlth. 1962;69:203–12.
11. Cotton DB, Read JA, Poul RH, Quilligan EJ. The conservative aggressive management of placenta praevia. Am I Obstet Gynaecol. 1980;137:687–95.
12. Silver R, Depp R, Sabbagha RE, Dooley SL, Socol ML, Tamura RK. Placenta praevia: aggressive expectant management. Am I Obstet Gynaecol. 1984;150:15–22.
13. Clark SL, Koonings PP, Phelan JP. Placenta previa/accreta and prior caesarean section. Obstet Gynaecol. 1986;66:89–92.
14. Sher G. A rational basis for the management of abruptio placentae. I Reprod Med. 1978;21:123–9.
15. Egley C, Cefalo RC. Abruptio placenta. In: Studd J, editor. Progress in obstetrics and gynaecology, vol. 5. Churchill Livingstone; 1985. p. 108–12.
16. Abdella TN, Sibai BM, Hays TM, Anderson GD. Relationship of hypertensive disease to abruptio placentae. Obstet Gynaecol. 1984;63:365–70.
17. Crosby WM, Costilve JP. Safety of lap-belt restraint for pregnant victims of automobile collision. New Eng J Med. 1971;284:632–5.
18. Naeye RL, Tafari N, Marboe CC. Perinatal death due to abruption placentae in an African City. Acta Obstet Gynaecol Scand. 1979;58:37–40.
19. Lehtovirta P, Forss M. The acute effect of smoking on intervillous blood flow of the placenta. Br I Obset Gynaecol. 1978;85:729.
20. Adler D, Sachs BJ, Tracey KJ, Wise WE. Abruptio placentae associated with cocaine use. Am J Obstet Gynaecol. 1983;146:220–1.
21. Howell R, Fidler J, Letsky E, De Swiet M. The risks of antenatal subcutaneous heparin prophylaxis in controlled trial. Br I Obstet Gynaecol. 1983;90:1124–8.
22. Hurd WW, Miodovnik M, Hertzberg V, Lavin JP. Selective management of abruptio placentae; a prospective study. Obstet Gynaecol. 1983;61:467–73.
23. Barry A. Accidental haemorrhage or abruption placentae: clinical features. I Obstet Gynaecol Br Commwlth. 1963;70:708–10.
24. Manolitsas T, Wein P, Beischer NA, Sheedy MT, Ratten VJ. Value of cardiotocography in women with antepartum haemorrhage — is it too late for caesarean section when the cardiotocography shows ominous features? Aust NZ J Obstet Gynaecol. 1994;34:403.
25. Helirnan IM, Pritchard JA. William's obstetrics. 14th ed. New York: Appleton Century Crofts; 1971. p. 937.
26. Dewhurst CJ. The ruptured caesarean section scar. I Obstet Gynaecol Br Commwlth. 1957;64:113–8.
27. Ozumba BC, Mbagwu SC. Emergency obstetric hysterectomy in Eastern Nigeria. Jut Surg. 1991;76:109–11.
28. Gambacorti-Passerini Z, Gimovsky AC, Locatelli A, Berghella V. Trial of labor after myomectomy and uterine rupture: a systematic review. Acta Obstet Gynecol Scand. 2016;95(7):724–34. Epub 2016 May 7
29. Smith JR, Brennan BG. Postpartum haemorrhage. In Ramus RM, editor. Medscape Obstetric diseases & conditions. 2018. Available online at http://emedicine.medscape.com/article/275038.
30. World Health Organisation. WHO. 2012. Priority life-saving medicines for women and children. Available at http://apps.who.int/iris/bitstream/10665/75154/1/WHO_EMP_MAR_2012.1_eng.pdf. Assessed 17/04/2019.
31. Udofia I, Okonofua F. Preventing primary postpartum haemorrhage in unskilled births in Africa. Afr J Reprod Health. 2008;12(2):7–9.

32. Potts M, Gerdts C, Prata N, Okonofua F, Hodoglugil N, Hosang N, Weidert K, Fraser A, Bell S. Criticism of misguided Chu et al article. J R Soc Med. 2012;105(11):454. https://doi.org/10.1258/jrsm.2012.12k080.
33. Okonofua FE, Ogu RN, Akuse JT, Ujah IAO, Galadanci HS, Fabamwo AO. Assessment of sublingual misoprostol as first-line treatment for primary post-partum haemorrhage: results of a multicentre trial. J Obstet Gynaecol Res. 2013; https://doi.org/10.1111/jog.12257.
34. Prata N, Bell S, Weidert K. Prevention of postpartum haemorrhage in low-resource settings: current perspectives. Int J Women's Health. 2013;5:737–52. https://doi.org/10.2147/IJWH.S51661.
35. Stanton CK, Newton S, Mullany LC, Cofie P, Tawiah Agyemang C, et al. Effect on postpartum Haemorrhage of prophylactic oxytocin (10 IU) by injection by community health officers in Ghana: a community-based, cluster-randomised trial. PLoS Med. 2013;10(10):e1001524. https://doi.org/10.1371/journal.pmed.1001524.
36. Jadesimi A, Okonofua FE. Tackling the unacceptable: Nigeria approves misoprostol for postpartum haemorrhage. J Fam Plann Reprod Health Care. 2006;32(4):213–4.
37. Hundley V, Avan B, Sullivan C, Graham W. Should oral misoprostol be used to prevent postpartum haemorrhage in home-birth settings in low-resource countries? A systematic review of the evidence. BJOG. 2013;120:277–87.
38. Hofmeyr GJ, Gülmezoglu AM, Novikova N, Lawrie TA. Postpartum misoprostol for preventing maternal mortality and morbidity. Cochrane Database Syst Rev 2013;7:Art. No.: CD008982. https://doi.org/10.1002/14651858.CD008982.pub2.
39. O'sullivan JV. Simple method of correcting puerperal uterine inversion. Brit Med J. 1945;2:282.
40. Vogel JP, Oladapo OT, Dowswell T, Gülmezoglu AM. Updated WHO recommendation on intravenous tranexamic acid for the treatment of post-partum haemorrhage. Lancet Global Health. 2018;6(1):PE18–9. https://doi.org/10.1016/S2214-109X(17)30428-X.
41. Meniru GI, Ugona CF. A review of secondary postpartum haemorrhage at Enugu, Nigeria, 1984—1989. Orient I Med. 1991;3:163–7.
42. Baischer NA, Mackay EV. Obstetrics and the newborn. London: WB Saunders; 1986. p. 510–8.
43. Ojengbede OA, Morhason-Bello IO, Galadanci H, Meyer C, Nsima D, Camlin C, Butrick E, Miller S. Assessing the role of the non-pneumatic anti-shock garment in reducing mortality from postpartum haemorrhage in Nigeria. Gynecol Obstet Invest. 2011;71(1):66–72. Epub 2010 Dec 15
44. Sutherland T, Downing J, Miller S, Bishai DM, Butrick E, Fathalla MMF, Mourad-Youssif M, Ojengbede O, Nsima D, Kahn JG. Use of the non-pneumatic anti-shock garment (NASG) for life-threatening obstetric haemorrhage: a cost-effectiveness analysis in Egypt and Nigeria. PLoS One. 2013;8(4):e62282. Epub 2013 Apr 30

Preterm Birth

21

Abdulmalik Bako

Learning Objectives

At the conclusion of this chapter, the learner will be able to:

- Explain the concept of preterm birth
- Distinguish between threatened, diagnosed and established preterm labour
- Evaluate the risk factors of preterm birth
- Describe the diagnostic strategy for preterm birth
- Discuss the treatment of preterm birth
- Critically justify offering antenatal corticosteroids, tocolytic, magnesium sulphate to women in preterm labour

21.1 Introduction

Preterm birth (PTB) is defined as delivery before 37 completed weeks of gestation [1]. It is a significant cause of morbidity and mortality in the newborn and childhood [2]. PTB may or may not be preceded by preterm labour (PTL), preterm premature rupture of membranes (PPROM) or cervical dysfunction. Sometimes, PTB may be iatrogenic or indicated. PTB can be defined by gestational age, birth weight (Tables 21.1 and 21.2) and initiating factor (e.g. spontaneous preterm birth versus medically indicated preterm birth). Majority of preterm births are spontaneous (70–80%).

The lower age limit of preterm birth is 20^{+0} weeks of gestation in the United States; a birth at less than 20 weeks of gestation is called a pregnancy loss, miscarriage or spontaneous abortion.

Table 21.1 PTB categorised based on the gestational age at birth [1]

Classification	Gestational age at delivery
Late preterm	34^{+0}–36^{+6} weeks
Moderately preterm	32–33^{+6} weeks
Very preterm	28–31^{+6} weeks
Extremely preterm	<28 weeks

Table 21.2 PTB categorised based on birth weight

Birth weight criteria	
Low birth weight (LBW)	<2.5 kg
Very low birth weight (VLBW)	<1.5 kg
Extremely low birth weight (ELBW)	<1.0 kg

Various risk factors for PTB have been reported including maternal, foetal and iatrogenic. This chapter will explore the magnitude of the problem of PTB, risk factors for PTB, diagnosis, management and prevention of PTB.

21.2 Epidemiology and Impact of PTB

Worldwide the rate of PTB is about 11%; the PTB rate varies from 5% in some European countries to 18% in some African countries [3]. About 15 million preterm births occur every year [4] with over 60% of preterm births occurring in Africa and South Asia [3]. The incidence of preterm birth has however been rising [3]. This is due in part to increasing rates of multiple pregnancies. Indeed, there was no decline in the rate of PTB over a 10-year period in the United Kingdom [5].

The World Health Organization (WHO) reported that complications from PTB are the leading cause of mortality in children below 5 years of age; preterm birth complications result in the death of over 1 million babies [3]. Besides, PTB remains a significant contributor to morbidity in childhood. Premature babies are at risk of admission to special care units, respiratory

A. Bako (✉)
Women's Wellness and Research Centre, Hamad Medical Corporation, Doha, Qatar

Weill Cornell Medicine-Qatar, Doha, Qatar

F. Okonofua et al. (eds.), *Contemporary Obstetrics and Gynecology for Developing Countries*,
https://doi.org/10.1007/978-3-030-75385-6_21

distress syndrome, intraventricular bleed, necrotising enterocolitis, sepsis and neurodevelopmental delay [3]. Babies born extremely preterm are at very high risk of serious illnesses that may be life-long such as cerebral palsy and learning disabilities. In the United Kingdom, PTB is the most significant cause of morbidity and mortality in the neonatal period. In England and Wales in 2012, over 52,000 infants were born prematurely (approximately 7.3% of live births) [5].

Across the world, there are stack differences in the survival of babies born preterm [3]. In low-income countries, 50% of the babies delivered at 32 weeks die as a result of deficient cost-effective care, such as temperature control, adequate breastfeeding and treatment of breathing difficulties and infection [3]. Most preterm babies survive in high-income countries; however, babies who survive the neonatal period in middle-income countries are burdened by disability due to inadequate use of technology [6].

21.3 Causes and Risk Factors

There are several risk factors for PTB; some are reversible, while some are permanent. However, no recognisable risk factor can be identified in the majority of women who deliver preterm. Risk factors for preterm delivery include history of previous preterm birth, short cervix, short interpregnancy interval (less than 18 months), history of surgery on the uterus or cervix and behavioural or lifestyle characteristics, for example, smoking and substance abuse in pregnancy. Other risk factors include obesity, low pre-pregnancy weight and maternal and foetal complications (e.g. multiple pregnancy, preterm spontaneous rupture of membranes, antepartum haemorrhage, hypertensive disease, urinary tract infection, congenital disease, etc.) (Table 21.3). Maternal and foetal complications can result in iatrogenic or indicated preterm birth because continuing with the pregnancy would pose a significant hazard to the mother or foetus.

Table 21.3 Risk factors for preterm birth

Maternal	Foetal
Previous preterm delivery	Multiple gestation
Urinary tract infection	Polyhydramnios
Antepartum haemorrhage, vaginal bleeding, especially in more than one trimester	Foetal anomaly
Premature cervical dilatation or effacement (short cervical length), history of cervical surgery	Preterm premature rupture of membranes
Systemic infection, pyelonephritis, appendicitis, pneumonia	Foetal growth restriction
Anxiety, stress	IUFD
Smoking	
Depression, use of selective serotonin inhibitors	
Abdominal surgery during pregnancy	
Substance abuse	
Occupational issues (upright posture, use of industrial machines, physical exertion, mental or environmental stress related to work or working conditions)	
Uterine anomaly and leiomyomas	
History of second-trimester miscarriage	
African American race	
Maternal age (<18 or >40)	
Sexually transmitted infections	
Low socioeconomic level	
Anaemia (haemoglobin <10 g/dL)	
Periodontal disease	
Maternal first-degree family history of spontaneous	
Preterm birth, especially if the pregnant woman herself was born preterm	
Poor nutrition and low body mass index	
Inadequate antenatal care	
Excessive uterine contractility	
Environmental factors (e.g. heat, air pollution)	

21.3.1 Maternal

21.3.1.1 Previous Spontaneous Preterm Birth (sPTB)

A key risk factor for PTB is prior preterm delivery. Recurrence of PTB tends to occur at the similar gestation [7]. Women at highest risk of PTB include those with a history of no term pregnancy between the previous sPTB and the current pregnancy and those with a history of multiple sPTB. Following one PTB, the incidence of recurrence of PTB is 15–30% and up to 60% after two previous PTBs [8].

21.3.1.2 History of Miscarriage

In a 2016 systematic review of 36 studies of outcome of pregnancy in over a million women who had surgical evacuation of the uterus (31 studies involving induced termination of pregnancy and 5 studies involving spontaneous miscarriage), women who have had surgical evacuation of the uterus had a small but statistically significant increased risk of PTB in a subsequent pregnancy when compared with controls [9].

21.3.1.3 Short Interbirth Interval

A short interbirth interval significantly increases the risk of early PTB [10]. However, short interbirth interval does not appear to affect late PTB [10]. Avoiding an interbirth interval of less than 6 months, and ideally less than 12 months, may reduce a woman's risk for PTB.

21.3.1.4 Genetic Factors

There is some evidence that PTB appears to be more frequent in women who were themselves born prematurely, have a first-degree sibling with a history of PTB and in some racial groups [11].

21.3.1.5 Race

In the United States, non-Hispanic Blacks have a higher rate of PTB than non-Hispanic Whites [12]. A woman's race/ethnicity seems to influence her microbiome and the impact of vaginal bacteria on PTB [13].

21.3.1.6 Age

There is a higher prevalence of PTB at the extremes of maternal age [14]. Obesity and chronic medical disease in older women, behavioural and socioeconomic condition and physiologic immaturity of adolescent girls may increase the risk of PTB in these women [14].

21.3.1.7 Cervical Injury and Surgery

Women with a history of injury to the cervix including cold knife or laser cone biopsy, large loop excision of the transformation zone (LLETZ) or radical diathermy are at increased risk of PTB and late miscarriage [5, 15]. Loss of cervical stroma tensile and increased susceptibility to infection from loss of cervical glands may be the reason for the association of cervical injury/surgery and PTB.

21.3.1.8 Uterine Malformation

Congenital

The increased risk for PTB depends on the specificity of the malformation of the uterus. Uterine congenital abnormality may be associated with cervical dysfunction.

Acquired

Women with uterine fibroids are at slightly increased risk for miscarriage and PTB. A large fibroid (i.e. ≥5–6 cm) or multiple fibroids appear to be an important risk factor; a submucosal location is a significant risk factor for pregnancy loss [16].

21.3.1.9 Smoking

There appears to be a dose-related influence of smoking on risk of PTB. The effect may be a direct one after adjusting for confounding factors including premature rupture of membranes, placental abruption, placenta previa and intrauterine growth restriction which are smoking-related complications [17].

21.3.1.10 Infection

Maternal systemic infections are risk factors for PTB. Malaria infection in pregnancy is a significant cause of maternal morbidity including preterm birth [18]. Wing et al. reported a higher rate of PTB in women with pyelonephritis when compared to those without pyelonephritis in an 18-year retrospective study of over 500,000 singleton pregnancies [19].

21.3.2 Foetal

21.3.2.1 Multiple Pregnancy

Multiple pregnancy contributes significantly to both spontaneous and indicated PTB [20]. Multiple pregnancy accounts for about 23% of deliveries before 32 weeks and about 17% before 37 weeks.

21.3.2.2 Vaginal Bleeding in Early Pregnancy

Women with persistent vaginal bleeding in early pregnancy and bleeding in the second trimester of pregnancy have a higher risk of having PTB than those with an isolated first-trimester bleeding [21]. The associated risk is stronger for PTB before 34 weeks than late PTB.

21.3.2.3 Prediction of Preterm Birth

PTB is difficult to predict; while about 10% of women with suspected preterm labour would go on to have PTB within the next 7 days, PTL stops on its own in about 30% of women [22].

21.4 Diagnosis

The diagnosis of PTL can be made based on uterine contractions that are painful and regular, associated with cervical dilation and effacement. The occurrence of vaginal bleeding and/or ruptured membranes increases diagnostic certainty [23]. PTL should be suspected in women reporting symptoms of abdominal pain, contractions and in whom vaginal examination including a speculum or digital vaginal examination confirms cervical length of less than 15 mm but no cervical dilatation [5]. PTL is diagnosed in women with suspected preterm labour and cervical dilatation of up to 3 cm [5]. Established PTL is diagnosed in women with cervical dilatation of at least 4 cm and regular contractions with or without ruptured foetal membranes. Because the clinical findings of early PTL are poorly predictive, suspected PTL should be considered until labour is well established. Chao et al. [24] used the following criteria to diagnose PTL:

Uterine contractions of ≥4 every 20 min or ≥8 in 60 min plus
Cervical dilation of ≥3 cm
Cervical length of <20 mm on transvaginal ultrasound
Cervical length of 20 mm to <30 mm on transvaginal ultrasound and positive foetal fibronectin [24].

Frequently women who were diagnosed with false PTL when these criteria were not met went on to have a late PTB or term delivery [24].

21.5 Triage

The initial assessment of women with suspected PTL could be in the triage unit or on the labour ward. Occasionally, women may present with symptoms suggestive of preterm labour when they attend for their planned antenatal care visit. Diagnosis of PTL includes obtaining a detailed relevant history, physical examination and laboratory investigations.

Initial assessment includes:

- Ascertaining the gestational age based on the estimated delivery date from first trimester USS
- Review of the present pregnancy, previous pregnancies and medical history including assessing the risks factors for PTL (Table 21.3)
- Recording maternal body mass index, temperature, pulse rate, blood pressure, respiratory rate and oxygen saturation
- Abdominal examination to assess for tenderness, uterine contraction (frequency, duration), foetal size, presentation and foetal heart pulsations
- A review of the antenatal notes and USS reports (if available), determining the location of the placenta

A speculum examination is performed with a wet speculum avoiding the use of gel lubricant that can interfere with the fibronectin test. The presence of liquor, discharge and bleeding should be noted, and an estimate of cervical dilation is noted. Cord prolapse should be excluded in the presence of ruptured membranes and cervical dilatation. Assessing the risk for PTB is performed by obtaining a sample of cervicovaginal secretion from the posterior fornix. The swab stick is rotated in the posterior fornix for 10 s. Techniques for obtaining a sample for foetal fibronectin without speculum examination have been described [25, 26]. Digital assessment of the cervix could be performed after excluding placenta previa and ruptured membranes. Cervical dilatation and effacement are noted.

Cardiotocograph (CTG)

A triage CTG can be offered to women in suspected PTL. A normal foetal heart rate monitoring indicates that the foetus is coping well. There is limited evidence about the specificity of the features of CTG that suggest hypoxia or acidosis in preterm foetus. The clinical decision about whether to monitor the foetus of between 23^{+0} and 25^{+0} gestational age should involve a senior obstetrician.

21.6 Transabdominal Obstetrics USS (TAUSS)

Transabdominal obstetrics ultrasound examination confirming foetal number and viability, foetal presentation, placenta localisation, foetal well-being including assessment of amniotic fluid volume and umbilical artery Doppler, foetal abnormality, estimated foetal weight and uterine abnormality provides useful clinical information. The information from USS can be used to counsel the woman and her family about prognosis and treatment plan including determining the time, route, place and mode of delivery.

21.7 Transvaginal Ultrasound (TVS)

Because the early features of PTL can be nonspecific, transvaginal measurement of the cervical length can aid management. A long cervix on TVS before 34 weeks has a high negative predictive value for PTB, while a cervical length less than 25 mm before 34 weeks is predictive of preterm labour [23].

21.8 Other Investigations

The following laboratory investigations are recommended:

- Urine culture: It is essential to request urine culture in women with suspected or diagnosed PTL because asymptomatic bacteriuria and UTI are associated with an increased risk of PTL and PTB.
- Foetal fibronectin test as described earlier in women <34 weeks of gestation.
- A rectovaginal group B streptococcal culture should be done if not performed in the last 5 weeks in settings where this is offered routinely to antenatal women.
- A high vaginal swab is recommended. Testing for sexually transmitted infections (e.g. chlamydia, gonorrhoea) depending on the woman's risk for these infections can be offered.

21.9 Treatment of Threatened and Diagnosed PTL

The treatment of threatened and diagnosed preterm labour includes:

- Admission
- Attempt to stop progression to established preterm labour
- Antenatal corticosteroids and foetal neuroprotection

Women with threatened PTL should be counselled and admitted for management. Women less than 34 weeks pregnant should be offered a course of corticosteroid and tocolytic drug [27].

21.10 Maternal Corticosteroids

The benefits of a course of corticosteroids should be explained to the woman including the reduction of risks of neonatal morbidity and mortality. The WHO (2015) recommends a course of steroids to women between 24 and 34 weeks of gestation [27]. NICE in the United Kingdom recommends that maternal corticosteroids can be considered between 23^{+0} and 23^{+6} weeks and between 24^{+0} and 25^{+6} weeks of gestation [5]. NICE also recommends that corticosteroids should be offered between 26^{+0} and 33^{+6} weeks of gestation and considered for women between 34^{+0} and 35^{+6} weeks with suspected, diagnosed or established PTL or women having an indicated PTB or those with P-PROM [5].

21.11 Tocolysis

Tocolysis for deferral of birth for 48 h is indicated to permit time for maternal administration of corticosteroids, magnesium sulphate or transfer of the woman to a facility with adequate neonatal resources to care for preterm babies. Tocolysis is recommended for women <34 weeks gestation. The choice of tocolysis depends on gestation and available tocolytic agent. Nifedipine can be considered in women admitted with threatened or suspected PTL between 24 and 25 weeks gestation and should be offered to women with intact membrane between 26 and 33 weeks gestation with threatened or diagnosed PTL [5]. The suggested dose of nifedipine is a stat oral dose of 20 mg, followed by 10–20 mg 3–4 times daily adjusted according to uterine activity (BNF, 2018) [28]. Oxytocin receptor antagonist such as atosiban can be prescribed if nifedipine is contraindicated. Beta sympathomimetic (such as ritodrine, salbutamol) may be offered if it is the only available tocolytic. However, they have significant maternal side effects that preclude their routine use including tachycardia, nausea, hypotension, tremor, pulmonary oedema and myocardial ischaemia. Foetal side effects of beta sympathomimetic include tachycardia, hypoglycaemia, hypocalcaemia, hypotension and ileus. Beta sympathomimetic drugs are contraindicated in women with cardiac disease, hyperthyroidism and poorly controlled diabetes [29]. Indomethacin is a nonspecific COX inhibitor and can be offered to women between 24 and 32 weeks of gestation. It can be given orally or per rectum as a 50-mg to 100-mg stat followed by oral 25 mg every 4 or 6 h. Indomethacin is discontinued 48 h after administration of the first corticosteroid dose. Side effects of indomethacin include premature narrowing or closure of the ductus arteriosus, which appears to depend on both duration of therapy and gestation [30].

Tocolysis should be avoided when continuation of pregnancy may be harmful to the woman or the foetus such as in women with preeclampsia with severe features, chorioamnionitis and antepartum haemorrhage. Other contraindications to tocolysis include IUFD, none reassuring foetal status, major foetal anomaly or chromosome abnormality (especially if lethal) and other maternal medical and foetal conditions that make continuing the pregnancy inadvisable.

21.12 Magnesium Sulphate for Neuroprotection

Magnesium sulphate has a role in protecting against cerebral palsy [27]; it also has some tocolytic action. The NICE recommends offering intravenous magnesium sulphate for neuroprotection of the baby to women between 24^{+0} and 29^{+6} weeks gestation and considering it in women who are in established PTL or having an indicated PTB within 24 h between 30^{+0} and 33^{+6} gestation [5]. Intravenous magnesium sulphate (4 g) is given as a bolus over 15 min, followed by an IV infusion of 1 g per hour until the delivery of the baby or for 24 h (whichever is sooner) [5]. Women on magnesium sulphate should be monitored for toxicity; their pulse rate, blood pressure, respiratory rate, deep tendon reflexes (e.g. patellar) and urinary output should be recorded every 4 h. Magnesium sulphate should be discontinued if toxicity is suspected and serum level obtained. The antidote of toxicity is 10% calcium gluconate administered IV stat, 10 ml over 3 min.

21.13 Progesterone

Progesterone supplementation reduces the odds of PTB by about one-third in women with a singleton pregnancy, one prior spontaneous singleton preterm birth and a short cervix (<25 mm) on ultrasound examination in the current pregnancy. Progesterone can be offered as a daily vaginal 100 mg suppository or weekly IM 250 mg injection [31].

21.14 Antibiotics

There is no place for routine antibiotics therapy in threatened or established preterm labour except in the treatment of suspected or diagnosed maternal infection such as urinary tract infection, chorioamnionitis or in neonatal GBS chemoprophylaxis (WHO 2015) [27].

21.15 Antimalarial Therapy

Malaria is a significant cause of maternal morbidity including spontaneous abortion, preterm labour and birth, IUGR/LBW, stillbirth, congenital infection and mortality in pregnancy [32]. Women in regions of unstable transmission, and therefore unlikely to have a sustained protective antibodies, are more at risk of PTL and PTB [32]. The treatment of malaria consists of antimalarial drugs and supportive care. The choice of antimalarial therapy will depend on the local drug resistance pattern, severity of infection and coexistence of other infections such as HIV [33].

21.16 Neonatology Review

It is essential that the woman and her family have a discussion with a neonatologist regarding the care of the neonate, prognosis and expectations. In utero transfer to an appropriate facility is easier, less expensive and safer than neonatal transfer; in utero transfer is associated with reduced neonatal morbidity and mortality.

21.17 Management of Established Preterm Labour

21.17.1 Delivery

Whenever possible, delivery of preterm foetus should be planned in a facility with appropriate resources for the care of preterm babies. In a Cochrane systematic review of caesarean section versus vaginal birth for preterm singleton pregnancies, Alfirevic et al. concluded that there was insufficient evidence to show that planned immediate caesarean delivery was better than planned vaginal birth [34]. The systematic review found that inadequate sample of women were recruited into the trials and, therefore, the decision on how best to deliver a preterm baby that is either in cephalic or breech presentation, remains the opinion and current practice within a particular hospital setting, rather than being evidence based [34]. Women and their family need to be aware that planned caesarean section of women in PTL may be protective for baby, however, it could be quite traumatic for both mother and baby [34].

21.17.2 Foetal Monitoring

Women with no other risk factors in preterm labour can be offered the choice of either CTG or intermittent auscultation. These options should be discussed with the woman and her family. Continuous intrapartum CTG can be offered if a non-reassuring foetal heart rate pattern would prompt intervention. There is limited evidence about specific CTG features which suggest hypoxia or acidosis in preterm babies; a normal GTG trace is reassuring and indicates that the baby is coping satisfactorily with labour at the time of assessment. An abnormal CTG does not necessarily indicate that foetal hypoxia or acidosis is present [5]. A senior obstetrician should lead the discussion and decision about foetal heart rate monitoring at the verge of viability ($23+^0$ and $25+^6$ weeks) [5].

21.17.3 Foetal Scalp Electrode

Foetal scalp electrode (FSE) can be used between 34 and 36 weeks of gestation if external CTG or intermittent auscultation is not possible. FSE should not be used to monitor the foetus if the gestation is less than 34 weeks unless it is not possible to monitor the foetus with either external CTG or intermittent auscultation, and the benefits outweigh the potential hazards, and the alternative of no monitoring is unacceptable to the woman [5].

21.17.4 Foetal Blood Sampling (FBS)

CTG changes and scalp pH measurements carry the same significance in PTL as in term labour. However, deterioration of foetal condition may occur more rapidly in preterm foetus. FBS is used to compliment the CTG in assessing the risk of foetal acidosis in labour. Foetal scalp pH measurement is indicated when there is suspected foetal compromise and delivery is not imminent between $34+^0$ and $36+^6$ weeks gestation and if there are no contraindications; FBS is not recommended when the foetus is less than 34^{+0} weeks. The contraindications to FBS include maternal infections such as HIV, hepatitis and herpes simplex virus and foetal bleeding disorders such as haemophilia.

21.17.5 Analgesia

Analgesia should be discussed and offered to women in PTL. Epidural neuroaxial analgesia is ideal in preventing early or inappropriate pushing. Neuroaxial analgesia is relatively contraindicated in women with coagulopathy, skin infection of the lower back and increased intracranial pressure. Patient-controlled analgesia provides a more effective option in women in whom neuraxial analgesia is not desired or contraindicated or not available. Systemic analgesia is an alternative in settings where regional analgesia is not available or in women who prefer a less invasive pain therapy or in whom regional techniques are contraindicated. Agents for systemic analgesia include opioids, for example, morphine, mixed opioid agonists-antagonists, for example, pentazocine, and inhaled nitrous oxide. Vaginal (e.g. pudendal block) and perineal infiltration with local analgesic agents such as lidocaine, levobupivacaine can be offered for episiotomy and instrumental delivery in women with no neuroaxial analgesia.

21.17.6 Mode of Delivery

There is limited evidence regarding planned caesarean birth versus planned vaginal birth [27, 34]. Performing preterm caesarean section may be difficult; there is an increased likelihood of vertical uterine incisions with implication for future pregnancies and risks of trauma to the foetus at extraction. However, caesarean section can be considered in women with breech presentation at 26^{+0} and 36^{+6} weeks.

21.17.7 Timing of Umbilical Cord Clamping

Waiting for between 30 s and 3 min before cord clamping can be performed in women in stable condition and with a vigorous baby at the time of delivery [35]. There are associated significant benefits with delayed cord clamping in preterm infants including improved transitional circulation, better establishment of red blood cell volume, decreased need for blood transfusion, lower occurrence of intraventricular haemorrhage and necrotising enterocolitis [36].

21.17.8 Post-Delivery Follow-Up and Preconception Clinic

Women who have had preterm birth should be seen in the postpartum or preconception clinic where general advice such as preconception folic acid intake and strategies to improve general health, for example, smoking cessation in addition to discussion of screening for PTL and interventions such as cervical length assessment, vaginal progesterone and cervical cerclage are discussed. Women with a history of PTB should be advised to book early in subsequent pregnancy. Early dating USS will facilitate timing of some interventions.

21.17.9 Prevention

Strategies to prevent PTB include interventions in the preconception, antenatal and intrapartum period [3]. Interventions in the preconception period include health and nutrition education (maintenance of a normal body mass index), STI prevention, better access to contraceptives and family planning and increased empowerment. WHO (2012) also recommend counselling on smoking cessation, treatment of substance use, confirmation of gestational age and detection of multiple pregnancy with USS, a minimum of eight antenatal contacts with health care professionals to identify and manage other risk factors, such as treatment of asymptomatic bacteriuria [3].

Interventions against some of the reported risk factors of PTB could help prevent the problems of PTB. In a systematic review of interventions aimed at preventing PTB, Medley et al. reported that only four interventions had clear benefits [37]. These are (1) midwife-led continuity models of care versus other models of care for all women; (2) screening for lower genital tract infections; (3) zinc supplementation for pregnant women without systemic illness and (4) cervical cerclage only for women with singleton pregnancy at high risk of PTB. The authors also reported another four interventions that may have possible benefit including group antenatal care, antibiotics for women with asymptomatic bacteriuria, pharmacological interventions for smoking cessation and vitamin D supplementation alone for women without health problems. The review did not report any intervention with clear harm to women. It is essential for healthcare providers and women at risk of PTB to carefully consider whether specific strategies to prevent PTB will be of benefit for the individual woman [37]. There is lack of good evidence for interventions relevant to women at high risk of PTB due to multiple pregnancy [37]. Bed rest, cervical cerclage or beta sympathomimetics have not been shown to have convincing benefit in preventing preterm labour in multiple pregnancy [37]. However, prevention and reduction of high-order multifoetal gestations can reduce the risk of preterm birth.

21.18 Conclusion

PTB remains a significant cause of perinatal death and disability. The rates of preterm birth have not remarkably reduced despite improvements in medical care. No biomarker performs well as a screening test for predicting PTB in asymptomatic low-risk women. It is essential to attempt to delay PTB with the administration of corticosteroid, tocolytic agent and magnesium sulphate if there are no contraindications. Delivery of women in PTL should be in a facility with appropriate resources to care for preterm infants. Interventions to prevent PTB in subsequent pregnancies should be discussed and offered to the women.

References

1. World Health Statistics. Monitoring health for the SDGs, sustainable development goals. Geneva: World Health Organization; 2018. Licence: CC BY-NC-SA 3.0 IGO. http://apps.who.int/iris/bitstream/handle/10665/44864/9789241503433_eng.pdf;jsessionid=08BF66035CAF3648BA021426748B8A5F?sequence=1. Accessed 1 Dec 2018.

2. Liu L, Oza S, Hogan D, Chu Y, Perin J, Zhu J, et al. Global, regional, and national causes of under-5 mortality in 2000-15: an updated systematic analysis with implications for the Sustainable Development Goals. Lancet. 2016;388(10063):3027–35.
3. WHO, March of Dimes, Partnership for Maternal, Newborn & Child Health, Save the Children. Born too soon: the global action report on preterm birth. 2012. www.who.int/maternal_child_adolescent/documents/born_too_soon/en/. Accessed 1 Dec 2018.
4. Blencowe H, Cousens S, Oestergaard MZ, et al. National, regional, and worldwide estimates of preterm birth rates in the year 2010 with time trends since 1990 for selected countries: a systematic analysis and implications. Lancet. 2012;379:2162.
5. National Collaborating Centre for Women's and Children's Health, 2015. https://www.nice.org.uk/guidance/ng25/evidence/full-guideline-pdf-2176838029. Accessed 1 Dec 2018.
6. http://www.who.int/news-room/fact-sheets/detail/preterm-birth
7. Esplin MS, O'Brien E, Fraser A, et al. Estimating recurrence of spontaneous preterm delivery. Obstet Gynecol. 2008;112:516.
8. Lykke JA, Paidas MJ, Langhoff-Roos J. Recurring complications in second pregnancy. Obstet Gynecol. 2009;113:1217.
9. Saccone G, Perriera L, Berghella V. Prior uterine evacuation of pregnancy as independent risk factor for preterm birth: a systematic review and metaanalysis. Am J Obstet Gynecol. 2016;214(5):572.
10. Rodrigues T, Barros H. Short interpregnancy interval and risk of spontaneous preterm delivery. Eur J Obstet Gynecol Reprod Biol. 2008;136:184.
11. Boivin A, Luo ZC, Audibert F, et al. Risk for preterm and very preterm delivery in women who were born preterm. Obstet Gynecol. 2015;125:1177.
12. Centres for Disease Control and Prevention. Preterm birth. http://www.cdc.gov/reproductivehealth/maternalinfanthealth/pretermbirth.htm. Accessed 7 Dec 2018.
13. Fettweis JM, Brooks JP, Serrano MG, et al. Differences in vaginal microbiome in African American women versus women of European ancestry. Microbiology. 2014;160:2272.
14. Fuchs F, Monet B, Ducruet T, et al. Effect of maternal age on the risk of preterm birth: a large cohort study. PLoS One. 2018;13:e0191002.
15. Castanon A, Brocklehurst P, Evans H, et al. Risk of preterm birth after treatment for cervical intraepithelial neoplasia among women attending colposcopy in England: retrospective-prospective cohort study. BMJ. 2012;345:e5174.
16. Rice JP, Kay HH, Mahony BS. The clinical significance of uterine leiomyomas in pregnancy. Am J Obstet Gynecol. 1989;160:1212.
17. Kyrklund-Blomberg NB, Cnattingius S. Preterm birth and maternal smoking: risks related to gestational age and onset of delivery. Am J Obstet Gynecol. 1998;179:1051.
18. Maternal Health Task Force. Malaria in pregnancy. https://www.mhtf.org/topics/malaria-in-pregnancy/. Accessed 6 Dec 2018.
19. Wing DA, Fassett MJ, Getahun D. Acute pyelonephritis in pregnancy: an 18-year retrospective analysis. Am J Obstet Gynecol. 2014;210:219, e1.
20. Kiely JL. What is the population-based risk of preterm birth among twins and other multiples? Clin Obstet Gynecol. 1998;41:3.
21. Szymusik I, Bartnik P, Wypych K, et al. The association of first trimester bleeding with preterm delivery. J Perinat Med. 2015;43:525.
22. ACOG, 2016.https://www.acog.org/Patients/FAQs/Preterm-Premature-Labor-and-Birth
23. Iams JD. Prediction and early detection of preterm labor. Obstet Gynecol. 2003;101:402.
24. Chao TT, Bloom SL, Mitchell JS, et al. The diagnosis and natural history of false preterm labor. Obstet Gynecol. 2011;118:1301.
25. Stafford IP, Garite TJ, Dildy GA, et al. A comparison of speculum and nonspeculum collection of cervicovaginal specimens for fetal fibronectin testing. Am J Obstet Gynecol. 2008;199:131, e1.
26. Roman AS, Koklanaris N, Paidas MJ, et al. "Blind" vaginal fetal fibronectin as a predictor of spontaneous preterm delivery. Obstet Gynecol. 2005;105:285.
27. WHO, 2015. www.who.int/reproductivehealth/publications/maternal_perinatal_health/ preterm-birth-guideline. Accessed 8 Dec 2018.
28. BNF, 2018 http://www.academia.edu/37410496/BNF_76_British_National_Formulary_September_2018_Sep_30_2018=27. Accessed 20 Dec 2018.
29. Practice Bulletin No. 159: management of preterm labor. Obstet Gynecol 2016; 127:e29.
30. Vermillion ST, Scardo JA, Lashus AG, Wiles HB. The effect of indomethacin tocolysis on fetal ductus arteriosus constriction with advancing gestational age. Am J Obstet Gynecol. 1997;177:256.
31. Society for Maternal-Fetal Medicine (SMFM) Publications Committee. The choice of progestogen for the prevention of preterm birth in women with singleton pregnancy and prior preterm birth. Am J Obstet Gynecol. 2017;216:B11.
32. Desai M, ter Kuile FO, Nosten F, et al. Epidemiology and burden of malaria in pregnancy. Lancet Infect Dis. 2007;7:93.
33. WHO. Guidelines for the treatment of malaria. 3rd ed. Geneva: World Health Organization; 2015. http://apps.who.int/iris/bitstream/10665/162441/1/9789241549127_eng.pdf?ua=1&ua=1. Accessed 20 Dec 2018.
34. Alfirevic Z, Milan SJ, Livio S. Caesarean section versus vaginal delivery for preterm birth in singletons. Cochrane Database Syst Rev. 2013;(9):CD000078. https://doi.org/10.1002/14651858.CD000078.pub3.
35. Fogarty M, Osborn DA, Askie L, et al. Delayed vs early umbilical cord clamping for preterm infants: a systematic review and meta-analysis. Am J Obstet Gynecol. 2018;218:1.
36. ACOG. Committee opinion no. 684: delayed umbilical cord clamping after birth. Obstet Gynecol. 2017;129(1):e5. https://doi.org/10.1097/AOG.0000000000001860.
37. Medley N, Vogel JP, Care A, Alfirevic Z. Interventions during pregnancy to prevent preterm birth: an overview of Cochrane systematic reviews. Cochrane Database Syst Rev. 2018;11:CD012505. https://doi.org/10.1002/14651858.CD012505.pub2.

22 The Puerperium

Aderemi O. Aisien

Learning Objectives

After studying this chapter, you should be able to:

- Define the puerperium
- Explain the implication of not providing critical care during the puerperium
- Understand the anatomical and physiological changes of pregnancy and puerperium
- Manage normal puerperium
- Recognise and manage some abnormal puerperal conditions

22.1 Introduction

The puerperium is defined as the period of 6 weeks or 42 days following delivery [1–5]. During the puerperium, the pelvic organs return to the non-gravid state and the metabolic changes of pregnancy are reversed and lactation is established [6]. In non-lactating women, the mean time to ovulation is approximately 70–75 days [7, 8]. Menstruation is reported to resume by 12 weeks postpartum in about 70% of women who are not breastfeeding. The average time to see the first menstruation is 7–9 weeks. The potential for fertility returns and in the absence of effective contraception, the woman may become pregnant.

Among women who breastfeed their infants the mean time to ovulation is about 190 days. In breastfeeding women, the length of anovulation is directly related to the frequency of breastfeeding, the length of each feed and the number of supplements that the baby is given [9]. The risk of ovulation within the first 6 months of the postpartum period in a woman exclusively breastfeeding is about 1–5% [10]. The persistent elevation of serum prolactin level in the puerperium appears to be the basis for ovulation suppression in lactating women.

The postpartum period has been increasingly important because of the recognition that maternal deaths due to complications such as infection, haemorrhage and eclampsia still occur during this period [11]. It is therefore important that health professionals pay attention to providing critical care to women during this period.

22.2 Anatomical and Physiological Changes

22.2.1 The Uterus

The weight of the pregnant uterus at term without the foetus, placenta and amniotic fluid is about 1 kg [12]. The size is roughly that of a 20-week size pregnancy and measures between 25 and 30 cm from the cervix to the fundus. The weight of the non-pregnant uterus is between 50 and 100 g. The immediate postpartum uterus has a smooth cavity with a narrow apposition of the anterior and posterior wall each with a thickness of about 4–5 cm [5]. It undergoes involution as a consequence of autolysis. The uterine muscle cells diminish in size as a result of enzymatic digestion of the cytoplasm. The excess protein produced from autolysis is absorbed into the blood stream and excreted in the urine. Involution is accelerated by the release of oxytocin in women who breastfeed. By the sixth day of delivery, the uterus is halfway between the umbilicus and the superior border of the symphysis pubis. At the end of the first postpartum week, the uterine size is about 12 weeks of gestation weighing 500 g. At the end of the second week, the uterus weighs about 300 g. It subsequently weighs 100 g or less. Within 2 weeks, the uterus can no longer be felt above the symphysis pubis. It eventually regains its non-pregnant size within about 4 weeks [5].

The superficial layer of the decidua within the endometrial cavity is sloughed off as a result of ischaemia and discharged as

A. O. Aisien (✉)
University of Benin, Benin City, Nigeria
e-mail: olabisi.aisien@uniben.edu

F. Okonofua et al. (eds.), *Contemporary Obstetrics and Gynecology for Developing Countries*,
https://doi.org/10.1007/978-3-030-75385-6_22

the lochia. The basal layer next to the myometrium is involved in the regeneration of the new endometrium. The colour of the lochia is red (lochia rubra) in the first few days after delivery. It gradually changes to pink colour (lochia serosa) in the next 3–4 days as the endometrium is formed. By the second week, it becomes a yellowish white discharge (lochia alba) [1, 5, 10]. Persistent red lochia could be an indication of delay in involution that may be associated with retained placenta tissue or infection. The height of the fundus of the uterus is measured daily as a guide to uterine involution [4].

22.2.2 The Cervix

The cervical epithelium increases in thickness and the cervical glands show both hypertrophy and hyperplasia during pregnancy. During labour and delivery, oedema and interstitial haemorrhage occur in the cervix [10]. Immediately after delivery, the cervix and the lower uterine segment become flaccid. Regression of the cervical epithelium begins within the first 4 days after delivery. As the cervix narrows, it thickens and a canal is reformed. By the end of the first week, the cervical os is a little more than 1 cm dilated. The internal os is closed by 12 day postpartum. When the uterine involution is complete, the external os does not assume its pre-gravid appearance but becomes slit like in appearance.

22.2.3 The Vagina

In the first 6 weeks following delivery, the vagina forms a spacious smooth-walled passage that gradually diminishes in size. Anatomical folds re-appear by the third week of the puerperium. Tears or episiotomies of the vagina and perineum usually heal well provided adequate suturing has been done and infection and haematoma formation do not occur [1–5].

22.2.4 Urinary System

The bladder is usually distended in labour and relatively insensitive to intra-vesical fluid pressure. Over-distension, incomplete emptying and excessive residual urine are common in the first few hours after delivery, especially when spinal or epidural anaesthesia is used. Retention of urine can also occur as a result of perineal pain following lacerations, episiotomies and caesarean section. In all cases of retention of urine, it is advisable to catheterize the patient under aseptic condition to prevent cystitis.

The bladder and urethra may show evidence of minor trauma sustained at delivery. This may further prevent micturition. In cases of prolonged obstructed labour where the bladder becomes oedematous and traumatised, petechial haemorrhages may occur in the bladder leading to haematuria after delivery.

The ureters and the calyceal systems are dilated in pregnancy. This dilatation gradually passes off and the ureters regain their pre-pregnancy size at about 6–8 weeks after delivery. The importance of this information is that intravenous urography to investigate renal disorders should not be done until 6–8 weeks after delivery to avoid incorrect result.

In the first 48 hours of delivery, diuresis may be observed. Some of the excess fluid retained during pregnancy is excreted [1, 4, 5].

22.2.5 Abdominal Wall

The muscles of the anterior abdominal are stretched in pregnancy because of the prolonged distension caused by the gravid uterus. The abdominal wall becomes soft and flabby. The abdominal wall gradually returns to the normal size in the first few weeks of the puerperium. The return is also aided by postnatal exercises [1, 5].

22.2.6 Cardiovascular System

During pregnancy the heart volume increases by about 70 and 80 ml (about 12%). The cardiac output rises within the first 10 weeks of pregnancy by about 1.5 litres/min. The rise is due to an increase in the stroke volume from about 64 ml to 71 ml with an increase in heart rate of 15 beats/min. This increases the heart rate from about 70–85 beats/min. The uterine blood flow increases during pregnancy to about 700 ml/min at term. Blood flow also increases in other organs, the largest being in the kidneys (up to 400 ml/min). Plasma volume increases until it reaches a plateau at about 32–34 weeks. The increase is 1250 ml in the first pregnancy and 1500 ml in subsequent pregnancies. The red cell mass increases by 240–400 ml. The increased red cell production is probably stimulated by a rise in erythropoietin and is associated with an increase in the proportion of foetal haemoglobin (HBF).

Plasma levels of factors VII, VIII, IX, X, XIII, fibrinogen and fibrin degradation products increase during pregnancy (fibrinogen from about 2.5 to 4 g/litre to as high as 6 g/litre). These changes are consistent with a general increase in coagulopathy. Most of these major circulatory alterations during pregnancy return to baseline by 6–8 weeks postpartum. Immediately after delivery, plasma volume is diminished by about 1000 ml because of the blood loss. However, by the third postpartum day, plasma volume increases by 900–1200 ml because of the shift of extracellular fluid into the vascular space. Oestrogen-induced elevation of the vitamin K-dependent coagulation factors return to normal within 3 weeks postpartum. The increase in coagulopathy persists for about 2 weeks after delivery. The changes in the coagulation system in addition to vessel trauma and immobility account for the increased risk of thromboembolism seen in the puerperium, especially when operative delivery is performed. Hormonal contraception should be avoided during this period [10, 13, 14].

22.2.7 Breast and Lactation

The mature breast consists of 15–25 lobes that arose from secondary buds. The lobes are arranged radially and separated from one another by fat. Each lobe consists of several lobules. The lobules are made up of large numbers of alveoli. Each alveolus has a duct that joins others to form a single larger duct for each lobe. The lactiferous ducts open separately on the nipple where they may be identified as minute but distinct orifices. The alveoli secretory epithelium synthesises the milk [5, 13, 14].

The control of the breast growth and development is not fully understood and many hormones contribute to the process. Oestrogens stimulate the proliferation of the lactiferous ducts (possibly with adrenal steroids and growth hormones), while progesterone is responsible for the development of breast lobules [3, 13].

During pregnancy, the effects of the lactogenic hormones – prolactin and human placental lactogen – are inhibited by the high levels of oestrogen and progesterone from the placenta. With their removal at delivery, milk secretion is induced and well established by the third to the fourth day after delivery. The establishment of a successful lactation is mediated by two pathways activated by suckling, an action which sent sensory impulse through the neural arc to the anterior pituitary. The impulse prevents the release of prolactin inhibitory factor (PIF) from the hypothalamus, thereby initiating prolactin production from the anterior pituitary. The action of prolactin on the secretory cells of the breasts leads to milk production. Further suckling by the infant sends sensory impulses to the posterior pituitary gland which responds by pulsatile release of oxytocin into the circulation. Oxytocin causes contraction of the myoepithelial cells surrounding the ducts and the alveoli. The action causes the milk from the nipple to be ejected into the baby's mouth. This is the 'milk let-down reflex'. The release of oxytocin into the circulation also causes contraction of the uterus which aids in the process of involution in the puerperium. Failure to place the baby on the breast early can lead to engorgement of the breasts about the third and the fourth day after delivery [1, 4, 5].

22.2.8 Colostrum and Milk

The colostrum is the deep lemon yellow coloured liquid secreted by the breasts for the first few days after delivery. It contains more minerals and protein much of which is globulin but less sugar and fat.

It persists for about 5 days before it is converted to mature milk during the following 4 weeks. It contains immunoglobulin A which may offer protection for the newborn against enteric pathogens. Human milk is a suspension of fat and protein in a carbohydrate–mineral solution. A nursing mother makes about 600 ml of milk per day [5].

22.3 Management of the Puerperium

22.3.1 Immediate Postpartum Care

After delivery, the patient remains in the labour ward for about 1–2 hours. Her vital signs are monitored every 15 minutes or more frequently as dictated by the condition of the patient. The patient is made comfortable and allowed to eat. If her vital signs remain within normal, she is transferred to the postnatal ward.

The baby is weighed. The length and head circumference are measured. The placenta is examined for completeness and weighed. The umbilical cord is examined and measured. Clinical examination of the baby is performed to rule out abnormality. He/she is thereafter cleaned dressed and handed over to the mother for exclusive breastfeeding.

22.3.2 Postnatal Ward

On the ward, the patient's pulse, blood pressure, respiratory rate, temperature are taken and charted. The vital signs are subsequently checked every 6 hours. The patient is allowed to rest. This is followed with early ambulation. Other routine care of the patient includes measurement of the fundal height after the patient might have emptied her bladder. The lochia is examined. The episiotomy site is inspected and patient encouraged to do daily sit bath. Pain relief is given and antibiotics where necessary. The mother is placed on her routine haematinics which she takes up to 6 weeks of the puerperal period. Packed cell volume is done 48 hours after delivery. Breastfeeding is encouraged. The baby is given BCG at birth. The mother receives health talk and counsel on family planning. The mother and the baby are usually discharged about 48–72 hours after delivery and given a 6-week postnatal appointment.

22.3.3 Postnatal Clinic

The mother is encouraged to discuss her complaints. Her vital signs are taken and she is examined. The baby is also examined. His/her weight is recorded. A poor weight gain of the baby may need referral to the paediatrician. If all is well with both mother and baby, they are discharged from the postnatal clinic. The baby is followed up at the infant welfare clinic and given the scheduled immunisation.

22.4 Postpartum Complications

Complications do occur during the postpartum period. Unfortunately the excitement of childbirth tends to down play the medical importance and care of the puerperium. Such complications include puerperal infections, postpartum hypertension and anaemia.

Bacterial infections around the time of delivery are among the leading causes of maternal mortality and account for about one tenth of the global maternal mortality [15, 16]. The most common is puerperal sepsis which could result in puerperal pyrexia. Risk factors include premature rupture of membranes, multiple vaginal examinations, manual removal of placenta, prolonged labour, presence of bacteria such as group B *Streptococcus* in the vagina, and caesarean section, among others [17]. Signs and symptoms include a fever greater than 38°C (100.4°F), chills, lower abdominal pain and offensive vaginal discharge.

22.4.1 Puerperal Pyrexia

This is fever in a woman in whom the temperature of 38°C or more has occurred twice in 24 hours and within 14 days after childbirth or miscarriage, excluding the first 24 hours. Causes include puerperal infection, urinary tract infection, malaria, respiratory infection, gastrointestinal infection, thrombophlebitis, phlebothrombosis, breast engorgement and mastitis with abscess.

Puerperal sepsis is a genital infection resulting from bacterial invasion during or after labour.

22.4.1.1 Causative Organisms

Aerobic Gram-Positive Organisms

- Haemolytic *Streptococcus*
- Non haemolytic streptococci
- *Staphylococcus aureus*
  Gonococci

Aerobic Gram-Negative Organisms

- *Escherichia coli*
- *Proteus*
- *Pseudomonas*
  Klebsiella

Anaerobic Gram-Positive Organisms

Anaerobic streptococci

Anaerobic Gram-Negative Organisms

- *Clostridium welchii*
  Bacteroids

22.4.1.2 Mode of Infection

This could be from exogenous origin, from infected birth attendants, instruments, etc., or endogenous origin in which the organisms may be present in the genital tract as anaerobic streptococci which are normal non-pathogenic commensals that become pathogenic in the presence of devitalised tissues.

22.4.1.3 Predisposing Factors

Improper aseptic techniques introducing large number of bacteria into the genital tract

Medical condition in the patient such as diabetes mellitus and anaemia

Intrapartum factors such as:

- Prolonged labour
- Premature rupture of membranes
- Instrumental delivery
- Manual removal of placenta
- Exploration of uterus

22.4.1.4 Features of puerperal sepsis

- Fever
- Tachycardia
- Vomiting
- Lower abdominal pain
- Tender adnexa with pain on moving the cervix from side to side
- Bogginess felt in the pouch of Douglas if pelvic abscess is formed
- Rectal symptoms include diarrhoea and tenesmus
- If septicaemia develops, patient may become jaundiced and lose consciousness
- Diagnosis is made from history and clinical examination

22.4.1.5 Investigations

- Full blood count
- Electrolyte, urea and creatinine
- Blood culture, midstream urine for microscopy, culture and sensitivity
- Endocervical swab for microscopy, culture and sensitivity Liver function test

22.4.1.6 Recommendation Practices to Prevent and Treat Maternal Peripartum Infections

Identify and correct predisposing factors to infection: treat nutritional deficiencies, anaemia, maternal medical conditions, for example, diabetes during antenatal care.

Aseptic surgical practices (e.g. use of antiseptic agents for surgical site preparation).

Routine antibiotics for women with preterm pre-labour rupture of membranes.

During labour: Digital examination every 4 hours for assessment of labour progress in active first stage.

Intrapartum antibiotics for women with group B *Streptococcus* (GBS) colonisation to prevent newborn infection.

Antibiotics, for example, ampicillin and gentamicin, are used as first-line treatment for chorioamnionitis.

At childbirth: vaginal cleansing with povidone-iodine immediately before caesarean section.

Routine antibiotics for women with the following problems:

- Manual removal of placenta
- Prophylactically, before incision for caesarean section (single dose of first-generation cephalosporin or penicillin)
- In case of third or fourth degree perineal tear
- Ampicillin and gentamicin as first-line treatment for chorioamnionitis

During the postnatal period: combination of clindamycin and gentamicin are used as first-line drugs for postpartum endometritis.

22.4.2 Hypertensive Disorders of Pregnancy

Hypertensive disorders are the most common complications of pregnancy. They complicate up to 10% of pregnancies [18]. They are classified into four categories as recommended by the National High Blood Pressure Education program working group on high blood pressure in pregnancy [19]:

- Chronic hypertension
- Preeclampsia/eclampsia
- Chronic hypertension with superimposed preeclampsia
- Gestational hypertension

Hypertensive disorders of pregnancy rank among the leading causes of maternal morbidity and mortality. The diagnosis of preeclampsia is made after 20 weeks of gestation in a woman with a systolic blood pressure of ≥140 mm Hg or a diastolic blood pressure of ≥90 mmHg measured at least 4 hours apart and associated with a proteinuria of ≥300 mg/24 hours (equivalent to ≥1+ on dipstick urinalysis). It is considered severe when the systolic blood pressure is ≥160 mmHg with a diastolic blood pressure of ≥110 mmHg while the patient is at rest and proteinuria of ≥5 g in a 24 hours urine sample or ≥2+ proteinuria on urine sample.

Recently, the American College of Obstetrics and Gynaecology (ACOG) updated management guideline in view of studies that indicated a minimal relationship between the quantity of urinary protein and pregnancy outcome in preeclampsia. Massive proteinuria has been eliminated from the consideration of preeclampsia as severe. It is submitted that diagnosis can be made in the absence of proteinuria in a pregnant woman with hypertension plus any of the following:

- New onset thrombocytopenia (<100,000/ml).
- Impaired liver function: Elevated blood concentration of liver transaminases to twice normal concentration.
- Renal insufficiency: Serum creatinine concentrations greater than 1.1 mg/dl or a doubling of the serum creatinine concentration in the absence of other renal disease.
- Pulmonary oedema.
- Visual or cerebral symptoms.

In normal pregnancy, blood pressure falls immediately post-delivery and peaks 3–6 days after delivery. In hypertensive women, this is also the case and women experience a further spike in their blood pressure several days postpartum. Of all eclampsia, 32–44% are reported to occur postpartum [20]. Blood pressure should therefore continue to be part of full postnatal check for all women, regardless of their history in pregnancy.

Factors that can cause or exacerbate hypertension postpartum are pain, anxiety, use of non-steroidal anti-inflammatory drugs [NSAIDS], ergometrine and fluid overload in labour. These factors should be assessed and antihypertensive management instituted.

Eclampsia is defined as the presence of new onset grand mal seizures in a woman with preeclampsia and can occur antepartum, intrapartum and postpartum. Some clinical symptoms are helpful in predicting impending eclampsia such as persistent occipital or frontal headaches, blurred vision, photophobia, epigastric or right upper quadrant pain or both. Magnesium sulphate is used to prevent or treat eclamptic seizures with a loading dose of 4–6 g followed by a maintenance dose of 1–2 g/hour and continue for at least 24 hours. In addition, the patient receives antihypertensive drugs to lower the blood pressure.

22.4.3 Postpartum Anaemia

Following delivery, a woman may develop postpartum anaemia (PPA) either because of postpartum bleeding (PPH) or pre-existing conditions during pregnancy. Severe postpartum anaemia is linked to about 40% maternal deaths worldwide [21]. Postpartum anaemia is associated with many symptoms such as palpitations, tiredness and breathlessness. All these may have impact on the inability of the women to care for her baby [22].

The WHO cut off for anaemia is a haemoglobin of 12 g/dl. Anaemia is classified as mild with a haemoglobin of 9–11 g/dl, moderate with a haemoglobin of 7–9 g/dl and severe at <7 g/dl.

The major causes of postpartum anaemia are postpartum iron deficiency anaemia in combination with blood loss at delivery [22].

Normal blood loss at delivery is about 250–300 ml, but PPH of 500 ml occurs in about 5–6% of women.

The best way to avoid postpartum anaemia is to implement an effective iron prophylaxis during pregnancy and reduce PPH with the use of oxytocic such as oxytocin and misoprostol.

22.5 Conclusion

The puerperium is an important period following delivery which requires monitoring because complications can occur and if appropriate measure is not taken such complications can result in maternal morbidity and mortality.

References

1. Kyari O, Otubu JAM. Normal puerperium. In: Agboola A, editor. Text book of obstetrics and gynaecology for medical students. 2nd ed. Heinemann Nigeria; 2006. p. 303–8.
2. Kwawukume EY, Acquaah-Arhin R. Puerperium. In: Kwawukume EY, Emuveyan EE, editors. Comprehensive obstetrics in the tropics. 1st ed. Asate & Hittscher Ghana; 2002. p. 356–62.
3. Campbell S, Lees C. Puerperium in obstetrics by ten teachers. 17th ed. ELST Arnold London; 2001. p. 141–55.
4. Aisien AO. Management of the puerperium. In: Okpere E, editor. Clinical obstetrics revised edition. Uniben Press Nigeria; 2003. p. 345–9.
5. Cunningham FG, MacDonald PC, Gant NF, Leveno KJ, Gilstrap LC, Hankins GDV, Clark SL. The puerperium in Williams Obstetrics. 20th ed. Appleton & Lange USA; 1997. p. 533–46.
6. Howie PW. The puerperium. In: Edmonds DK, editor. Dewhurst's Textbook of Obstetrics and Gynaecology for postgraduates. 6th ed. Blackwell Science Ltd. UK; 1999. p. 342–53.
7. Cronin TJ. Influence of lactation upon ovulation. Lancet. 1968;2(7565):422–4.
8. Perez A, Vela P, Masnick GS, Potter RG. First ovulation after child birth: the effect of breast feeding. Am J Obstet Gynecol. 1972;114(8):1041–7.
9. Gray RH, Campbell ON, Apel R, Eslami SS, Zacur H, Ramos RM, Gehret JC, Laok MH. Risk of ovulation during lactation. Lancet. 1990;335(8680):25–9.
10. Bowes WA Jr. Postpartum care. In: Gabbe SG, Niebyl JR, Simpson JL, editors. Obstetrics normal & problem pregnancies. 2nd ed. Churchill Livingstone New York; p. 753–79.
11. Varner MW. Medical conditions of the puerperium. Clin Perinatol. 1998;25(2):403–16.
12. Hytten FE, Chyne GA. The size and composition of the human pregnant uterus. J Obstet Gynecol Br Commonw. 1969;76(5):400–3.
13. Chard T and Lilford R., editors. General physiology, biochemistry and endocrinology. In basic sciences for obstetrics and gynaecology 1st ed. Springer-Verlag New York;. 1983. p. 55–116.
14. de Swiet M, Letsky E. The cardiovascular and haematological systems. In: Hytten FE, Leitch I, editors. The physiology of human pregnancy. 2nd ed. Blackwell UK; 1971. p. 3–72.
15. Khan KS, Wojdyla D, Say L, Gulmezoglu AM, Van Look PF. WHO analysis of maternal death: a systematic review. Lancet. 2006;367(9516):1066–107.
16. Say L, Chou D, Gemmill A, Tuncalp O, Moller AB, Daniel J, et al. Global causes of maternal death: a WHO systematic analysis. Lancet Global Health. 2014;2(6):e323–33.
17. WHO Recommendations for prevention and treatment of maternal and peripartum infections. September 2015 (www.who.int/reproductive health/publications/maternalperinatalhealth/peripartum-infections-guidelines).
18. The Task Force on Hypertension in Pregnancy. Hypertension in Pregnancy. ACOG; 2013.
19. Report of the National High Blood Pressure Education Program Working Group on High Blood Pressure in Pregnancy. Am J Obstet Gynecol. 2000;183(1):S1–S22.
20. Bramham K, Nelson-Piercy C, Brown MJ, Chappell LC. Postpartum management of hypertension. BMJ. 2013;346:f894.
21. World Health Organization. Iron deficiency anaemia- assessment, prevention and control. WHO/NHD/−01.3 2–01. Geneva: WHO, 2001.
22. Milman N. Postpartum anaemia I: definition, prevalence, causes and consequences. Ann Heamatol. 2011;90(11):1247–53.

Part III

Medical and Surgical Disorders in Pregnancy

Intensive Care Management of Trauma During Pregnancy

23

Pius E. Iribhogbe and Kingsley Ufuoma Tobi

Learning Objectives

After reading this chapter, the learner should be able to discuss:

- Prevalence and hospitalisation rates of trauma during pregnancy
- The common types of trauma associated with pregnancy
- Evaluation of a pregnant woman with trauma
- Management of an injured pregnant woman

23.1 Introduction

In general, 6–7% of pregnancies are complicated by trauma and 0.4% of all pregnant patients require hospitalisation for the treatment of injuries. However, these figures are probably underestimated due to poor reporting, especially in developing countries where trauma registries barely exist. A pregnant woman who suffers trauma often requires admission to the intensive care unit. The care of this patient is complicated by the pregnancy state and the systemic effects of trauma. In addition, it must always be borne in mind that two patients are being managed here, the woman and her unborn child! Special care and a multidisciplinary approach are needed to optimise outcome both for the mother and the foetus. The trauma surgeon, obstetrician and intensivist cooperate for an optimal outcome.

P. E. Iribhogbe (✉)
University of Benin, Benin City, Nigeria
e-mail: pius.iribhogbe@uniben.edu

K. U. Tobi
Department of Surgery and Anaesthesiology, University of Namibia, Windhoek, Namibia

University of Benin Teaching Hospital, Benin City, Nigeria

23.2 Types of Trauma

The types of trauma seen often among pregnant patients vary widely and it includes motor vehicle crashes, motorcycle crashes, pedestrians hit by a vehicle, falls, partner violence and penetrating trauma from stabs and gunshot injuries. Management of this group of patients, therefore, depends on the nature and severity of trauma.

23.3 Evaluation and Management

The initial management in the ED is similar to the management of the injured non-pregnant female, but recognition of the changes in pregnancy and the presence of the foetus is essential. The initial focus during resuscitation is on the mother because the optimisation of the mother improves outcome in the foetus.

In the initial management the steps are as follows: assess and resuscitate the mother first, then assess the foetus and thereafter perform a secondary survey on the mother with interventions as appropriate. The pre-hospital history focuses on the mechanism of the injury, the injuries sustained, pre-hospital signs, and initial treatment received. The primary survey involves assessment and searches for life-threatening injuries in the airway, breathing such as haemothorax and pneumothorax, circulation with particular emphasis on shock, disability and neurology with GCS determination. Effort must be made to avoid hypothermia by keeping the room and patient warm. Central venous pressure, oxygen saturation and arterial blood gases need monitoring in the pregnant patient.

The obstetric and gynaecological history should include the last menstrual period and estimated gestational age. The

F. Okonofua et al. (eds.), *Contemporary Obstetrics and Gynecology for Developing Countries*,
https://doi.org/10.1007/978-3-030-75385-6_23

fundal height and foetal heart rate should be assessed. The normal range is 120–160 beats/minute. Cardiac tocodynamometer can be used to assess the foetus after 20–24 weeks of gestation. Cardiotocographic monitoring is recommended for patients with frequent uterine activity more than 6/hour, abdominal tenderness, bleeding per vaginam or hypotension. Ultrasonographic examination of the abdomen may also be done to assess the placenta, foetus and the abdominal viscera for injuries and haemoperitoneum.

The secondary survey in the mother includes a short history of allergies, medications, past medical history, pregnancy, last meal and events of the trauma coupled with a head to toe examination. In the second and third trimester, it is important not to examine the woman supine but tilted 15 degrees to the left to avoid the supine hypotensive syndrome. This syndrome occurs when in the supine position the gravid uterus compresses the inferior vena cava leading to reduced venous return cardiac output and hypotension. It is marked by tachycardia, pallor, sweating and dizziness.

In order to appreciate the critical care of the injured pregnant patient, it is essential to review the anatomical and physiological changes in pregnancy (Fig. 23.1).

Following are the common causes of admission into the intensive care unit of the injured pregnant patient: abruptio placenta, ruptured uterus and disseminated intravascular coagulation with massive haemorrhage. Others are due to pregnancy-induced hypertension-related complications and severe trauma itself often with traumatic brain injury.

Abruptio placenta is marked by vaginal bleeding, abdominal pain and tenderness with uterine contractions. In ruptured uterus, there is a severe shock, the uterus is small for date and foetal parts may be freely palpated outside the uterus. The triad of hypertension, oedema and proteinuria heralds preeclampsia.

These patients often need close monitoring and ventilatory, inotropic and renal support.

- Close monitoring: trauma patients admitted to the ICU for close monitoring are those with injuries without immediate threat to life but have the potential to deteriorate clinically. The care of these patients involves intensive monitoring such as pulse rate (PR), non-invasive blood pressure (NIBP), mean arterial pressure (MAP) and arterial oxygen saturation (SPO_2). In addition, there is a need to institute continuous foetal heart rate monitoring in the ICU.

Nurse to patient ratio for patients requiring close monitoring is 1:2 and this can be effectively done in the high-dependency unit (HDU). However, while close monitoring is on-going, equipment and drugs for immediate intervention should be readily available such as airway control and ventilatory support. Also, obstetric coverage should be available round the clock to take decisions based on gestation age and foetal heart rate measurement.

- Ventilatory support: trauma patients when pregnant may require ventilatory assistance when they are unable to meet their oxygenation and ventilatory needs. Patients with fractured ribs from trauma or those with severe traumatic brain injury will require to be on mechanical ventilators in the ICU.

System	Changes	Potential Implication
Cardiovascular	Decreased total peripheral resistance, venous return, and blood pressure	Supine hypotensive syndrome
Blood volume	Increased plasma and total red cell volume	Hypotension from hemorrhagic shock may be masked. Almost 35% of maternal blood volume may be lost before the manifestation of maternal shock.
Coagulation	Hypercoagulable; increase in factors VII, VIII, IX, X and XII	Prone to thromboembolic phenomenon
Respiratory	Widened subcostal angle, Increased excursion of the diaphragm	Care in the passage of chest tube
Gastrointestinal	Decreased intestinal motility and secretion	Prone to vomiting and aspiration
Renal	Increased GFR and plasma blood flow	Increased calcium absorption
Musculoskeletal	Softening of ligaments Lordotic posture	Prone to falls
Endocrines	Pituitary enlarges	Shock can lead to pituitary insufficiency (Sheehan's syndrome)

Fig. 23.1 Anatomical and physiological changes in pregnancy and their clinical correlates

There are different ventilatory modes in the ICU such as to assist control ventilation (AC mode), synchronised intermittent mandatory ventilation (SIMV) and pressure support ventilation (PSV). The commonest ventilatory modes in the ICU are the AC and SIMV modes.

Patients to be ventilated will require some form of sedation and/or muscle relaxant drugs to enable them to tolerate positive pressure ventilation. The commonest sedation regimen employed at the University of Benin Teaching Hospital is the fentanyl-midazolam combination. This combination allows for adequate sedation with opioid analgesic coverage. Other sedatives that are commonly used include propofol, dexmedetomidine and diazepam.

It must be noted that, before instituting mechanical ventilation, it is essential to have an arterial blood gas analysis (ABG) done. This will enable us to determine the fractional inspired oxygen concentration to be set on the ventilator, the ventilatory frequency, the tidal volume and the inspiration pressure. Serial ABG analysis is advised to monitor patients' acid-base status. Mechanical ventilation is discontinued, that is, weaning off the ventilator when the underlying condition has resolved, there is acceptable ABG result and the patient is able to take over the work of breathing.

- Inotropic support: trauma depending on the severity can lead to varying degrees of cardiovascular collapse. This will require some forms of inotropic support to ensure adequate perfusion to vital organs in the body. For patients who have lost some amount of their blood volume, adequate fluid/blood resuscitation is paramount before placing on inotropes.

The common inotropes used for cardiovascular support include dopamine, dobutamine, epinephrine (adrenaline) and norepinephrine (noradrenaline). Others are isoprenaline, milrinone, etc. Dopamine acts in a dose-dependent manner on the kidneys, the heart and the blood vessels. Commonly, dopamine for cardiac support is given at a dose of 5–10 μg/kg.

Dobutamine has both inotropic and vasodilatory effects. It has the advantage of increasing heart contractility and rate while at the same time acting on the peripheral circulation to reduce afterload.

Norepinephrine (noradrenaline) is the drug of choice in cases of severe vasodilatation such as in severe sepsis and anaphylaxis. It produces profound vasoconstriction to increase systemic vascular resistance which in turn raises blood pressure.

Inotropic support is indicated to maintain MAP at 65–70 mmHg and a urine output of 0.5–1 ml/kg/hour. Central venous catheterisation is indicated in all patients requiring vasoactive drugs such as inotropes. Furthermore, invasive blood pressure measurement must be performed for patients on inotropes.

- Renal support: Acute kidney injury (AKI) is a common finding both in obstetrics and trauma patients. The RIFLE criteria for the diagnosis of AKI has simplified the care of patients with acute renal insult. One of the causes of AKI in trauma patients is hypovolaemia following massive blood loss. Adequate fluid resuscitation as measured by central venous pressure (CVP) of >8–10 cmH_2O and urine output >0.5 ml/kg/hour is key to renal support.

Other forms of renal support in the ICU are the use of low-dose continuous furosemide infusion and haemofiltration. Low-dose continuous furosemide infusion has been found to improve outcome in patients with AKI. Adequate cardiac output must be maintained to ensure renal perfusion for patients on low-dose continuous furosemide infusion.

Haemofiltration is best for patients in the ICU because it minimises the haemodynamic effects of dialysis. Every ICU should have a haemofiltration unit to avoid moving very unstable patients out of the unit to a dialysis ward.

23.4 Conclusion

Pregnant patients are exposed to trauma just like the other members of society. Therefore, concerted efforts are needed to provide the highest level of care for them.

Further Reading

ICU pocketbook by K U Tobi, UNIBEN Press 2016.
The ICU book 3rd edition by Paul L Marino.
Oh's Intensive care manual edited by Andrew D Bersten and Neil Soni.
Textbook of critical care. Jean-Loius Vincent, Edward Abraham, Fredrick A. More Patrick M. Kpchanek, Mitchell. P Fink.

Cardiovascular Diseases in Pregnancy

24

Obasohan Austine and Aiwuyo O. Henry

Learning Objectives

After reading this chapter, the reader should be able to identify the physiological changes associated with normal pregnancy, explain its development at the stages of pregnancy and its effects in masking or accentuating cardiac symptoms.

He should be able to differentiate between true cardiac disease and physiological changes associated mimicking cardiac disease and then invite the cardiac specialist to review and comanage the patient.

He should be able to enumerate the cardiovascular diseases commonly encountered in pregnancy in the tropics and explain the differences that exist in the epidemiology. He should be able to discuss in detail the clinical presentation of these cardiovascular diseases and differentiate between them.

He should know the details of the management of the conditions and critically differentiate between the drugs that can be used in the various conditions as well as those that are contraindicated in various stages of pregnancy.

24.1 Introduction

Pregnancy tends to be well tolerated and significantly uneventful in most women with heart disease for both mother and baby, except for those with a cardiac outflow obstruction in either the pulmonary or the systemic circulation. In the pulmonary circulation patients with Eisenmenger syndrome, pulmonary vascular obstructive disease is at a very high risk of maternal and fetal death, while aortic and mitral valve stenosis poses a significant threat to the fetus. A high risk to the mother and baby also exists in Marfan's syndrome and associated aortopathies because of the likelihood of rupture or dissection due to the markedly increased cardiac output (CO) of pregnancy. In other situations, maternal death during pregnancy in women with heart disease is unusual. However, pregnant women with heart disease do remain at risk for other complications including heart failure (HF), arrhythmia, and stroke. Cardiovascular disease covers a wide range of conditions, including hypertensive diseases, congenital heart disease, other acquired diseases such as rheumatic valvular disease, and coronary disease, cardiomyopathy, and heart failure.

Pregnancy changes mimic cardiac disease, presenting with symptoms like breathlessness, weakness, edema, syncope, and tachycardia and the patients may be wrongly diagnosed as having cardiac disease. Alternatively, the physiological changes and increased hemodynamic load of pregnancy might exacerbate the underlying cardiac disease, precipitating the manifestations of cardiac disease or complications during pregnancy. About1% to 3% of women either have cardiac disease entering pregnancy or are diagnosed with cardiac disease while they are pregnant [1]. The frequency of specific types depends on the patient population and local conditions.

Apart from the effect of pregnancy on the underlying heart disease, the effect of heart disease on the development of the fetus during pregnancy and the outcome of pregnancy are important considerations, as the cardiac output and blood flow to the uterus are affected by some heart diseases. In addition, the effect of some of the drugs used in the management of the cardiac disease may affect the development of pregnancy if it crosses the placental barrier, causing developmental abnormalities in various proportions and various degrees.

The physiological changes of pregnancy also affect absorption, excretion, and pharmacokinetics of drugs used, such that different doses of drugs are required in pregnancy in some cases.

O. Austine (✉)
College of Medicine Science, University of Benin, Benin City, Nigeria

University of Benin Teaching Hospital, Benin City, Nigeria

A. O. Henry
Delog Nigerian Limited, Lagos, Nigeria

F. Okonofua et al. (eds.), *Contemporary Obstetrics and Gynecology for Developing Countries*,
https://doi.org/10.1007/978-3-030-75385-6_24

The heritability of the cardiac condition presenting in pregnancy is often a matter of serious consideration to the mother and genetic counseling becomes an important part of management.

The physiological changes associated with pregnancy may also affect or change the presentation of existing cardiac conditions just as it may induce changes in the intensity, loudness or respiratory changes in some cardiac murmurs.

24.2 Epidemiology

The pattern of a cardiovascular disease in pregnancy varies in different parts of the world and changes with epidemiological transition. As more females adopt education to higher levels and postpone bearing children till after, the age of first pregnancy increases. This coupled with increased prevalence of cardiovascular risk factors like hypertension (HTN), diabetes mellitus, and obesity, there are an increased number of persons presenting with cardiovascular diseases in pregnancy [1]. There is also the issue of change in the pattern of cardiac diseases they present with. With enhanced survival due to improved management of congenital heart diseases, those reaching pregnancy with cardiac diseases increase, such that in the Western world, congenital heart disease now constitutes the greatest cause of maternal death [1]. Approximately 10% of all maternal deaths in the United States can be attributed to cardiac disease.

Of the women with prior cardiac disease entering pregnancy or are diagnosed with cardiac disease while they are pregnant hypertensive disorders are the most frequent cardiovascular events, occurring in 6–8% in the Western world but reaching as high as 10–25% of all pregnancies in African studies [2–4] depending on the results from population or hospital studies. In the Western world, congenital heart disease is the most frequent cardiovascular disease present during pregnancy (75–82%), with shunt lesions predominating (20–65%). Congenital heart disease represents just 9–19% outside Europe and North America. Rheumatic valvular disease dominates in non-Western countries, especially in sub-Saharan African countries [5], comprising 56–89% of all cardiovascular diseases in pregnancy. Anemia in pregnancy is unusual now in Western countries, but it still occurs in developing countries. Congestive cardiac failure (CCF) occurs from any of the usual causes but cardiomyopathies are rare, except peripartum cardiomyopathy which has a high prevalence in some parts of the world including some areas in Northern Nigeria [6]. In a study by Avila et al. in Brazil [7] involving 1000 pregnant women who had various types of cardiac diseases and were followed by the same health-care team over a 10-year period, more than 75% of the women had no complications during pregnancy. Among the remaining 25%, the following complications were seen most often: Congestive heart failure, including pulmonary edema (12.3%), cardiac arrhythmias (6%), thromboembolism (1.9%), angina (1.4%), hypoxemia (0.7%), and infective endocarditis (0.5%). The overall maternal mortality rate in this group was 2.7%, and the stillbirth and spontaneous abortion rate was 7.7%.

24.2.1 Physiological Changes in Pregnancy

24.2.1.1 Cardiovascular Physiology of Pregnancy

Normal pregnancy is associated with of 30 to 50% in blood volume and a corresponding increase in cardiac output. These increases begin during the first trimester; peak by 20 to 24 weeks of pregnancy and are either sustained until term or decrease in the last trimester. The heart rate increases by 10 to 20 beats per minute, the stroke volume increases, and there is a substantial reduction in systemic vascular resistance, with decreases in blood pressure (BP) [8].

During labor, the cardiac output increases; the blood pressure increases with uterine contractions. Immediately after delivery, the cardiac filling pressure may rise dramatically due to the decompression of the vena cava and the return of uterine blood into the systemic circulation.

The cardiovascular adaptations associated with pregnancy regress by approximately 6 weeks after delivery.

24.2.1.2 Hemodynamic Changes in Normal Pregnancy

A noticeable rise in plasma volume occurs in the sixth week of pregnancy which almost doubles by the end of the second trimester. The increased plasma volume is not accompanied by a corresponding rise in red cell mass, which increases much less resulting in the relative anemia of pregnancy. There is a peripheral vasodilatation with a fall in peripheral resistance, but uterine blood flow increases with placental growth. This decreased peripheral resistance may result in a slight fall in blood pressure most markedly in the second trimester and tends to normalize to prepregnancy levels toward the end of the third trimester. The heart size may increase in size up to 30%, partly due to dilatation to accommodate the increase in cardiac output and partly due to elevation of the diaphragm with increasing abdomen. The venous pressure in the lower extremities rises, resulting in pedal edema, which is a common finding in 80% of pregnancies [9].

During labor and delivery, about 500 mL of blood is released into the circulation, with each uterine contraction resulting in a rapid increase in cardiac output, blood pressure, and as such blood loss. During a normal vaginal delivery, approximately 400 mL of blood is lost. After delivery of the baby, there is an abrupt increase in venous return, in part not only because of autotransfusion from the uterus but also because the baby no longer compresses the inferior vena cava. This continues for about 24 to 72 hours after delivery and poses the risk of occurrence of pulmonary edema [10].

24.2.2 Critical Periods

These periods include changes that start from 6 weeks and peak at around 30 weeks, during the intrapartum period, just after delivery, and second week of puerperium.

24.2.3 Cardiac Findings in Normal Pregnancy

As the normal physiology of the body changes during pregnancy, the cardiovascular system examination shows an elevated jugular venous pressure (JVP) resulting from an increased plasma volume, loud S1, tachycardia, S2 wide split which is accentuated because of P2 delayed, occasional S3, and flow murmur in the aortic, pulmonary; ejection systolic murmur (ESM) grade 3 at the Left Lower sternal border; cervical venous hum; mammary souffle at the Left Lower sternal border of the cardiac apex (slightly down and out), prominent impulse, active precordium, low diastolic blood pressure, increased pulse pressure with bounding pulses, pulsatile fingertips, warm hands, and pedal edema (in about 60% of women). The respiratory system shows increased respiratory rate with a peak effect in about 30 weeks .This may cause hyperapnea or dyspnea. Auscultation often shows reduced breath sounds at lung bases [11].

24.2.4 Cardiovascular Diagnosis in Pregnancy

A careful medical history including personal and family history is crucial in the diagnosis. Many disorders, for example, cardiomyopathy, Marfan's syndrome, inherited arrhythmias like long QT syndromes, Brugada syndrome (catecholaminergic polymorphic ventricular tachycardia (CPVT)) can be obtained from a family history. Enquiries on sudden death in the family are important. Assessment of dyspnea is important for the evaluation of heart failure or valvular diseases. A good physical examination taking note of the physiological hemodynamic changes of pregnancy should reveal the problems. The development of dyspnea or auscultating a new murmur in pregnancy is an indication for echocardiography [12].

Electrocardiography and variants of it like the 24-hour Holter monitoring and exercise electrocardiogram (ECG) as well as echocardiography are safe in pregnancy, as they involve no radiation hazards. The latter is the mainstay of diagnosis. A chest X-ray provides radiation exposure, but the fetal load from it is about 0.01 mGy which is much less than above 50–100 mGy which has been associated with the risk of causing congenital abnormalities [13]. However, a chest X-ray is indicated only when other modalities of investigation fail to clarify the cause of dyspnea or other cardiac symptoms. Similarly, computed tomography (CT) scan and magnetic resonance imaging (MRI) are best avoided during pregnancy, though MRI has less ionizing radiation (Table 24.1).

Table 24.1 Hemodynamic changes in pregnancy

Parameter	Change	Peak Effect	Potential signs/ Symptoms
Cardiac output	Increased	24–26 wks	S3, Tachycardia
Heart Rate	Increased	3rd Trimester	Palpitations, Tachy
Stroke Volume	Increased	26wks	Nocturia, Oedema
			Cardiac enlargement
Periph Resist	Decreased	20wks	Low BP. Oedema, Syncope
Red Cell Vol	Incr but < Plasma Vol	26wks	Anaemia
Blood Viscosity	Increased	34wks	DVT/PE

Mendelson [30]

24.2.5 Pregnancy and Heart Murmurs

The altered hemodynamics of pregnancy increases in systemic blood flow and the cardiac output may bring out heart murmurs not previously heard or may bring the pregnant patient to medical attention for the first time. The increased blood flow across the valves often causes innocent systolic ejection murmurs not more than grade 1/6 or 2/6 and not accompanied by thrills. Diastolic murmurs almost never occur. If any, it suggests real cardiac disease and further investigations.

A mammary soufflé is a soft hum heard along the left sternum or breast area and is due to an increased blood flow to the breast in late pregnancy and postpartum period.

The murmurs of mitral regurgitation (MR) and aortic regurgitation (AR) are reduced in intensity in pregnancy in many cases due to the reduced peripheral resistance in pregnancy with better forward flow and less regurgitation in MR and AR. These may lead to underdiagnosis which may be important if the patient requires prophylactic antibiotic in labor which many of the patients with valvular heart disease may require [12].

24.3 Pathological Conditions and Pregnancy

24.3.1 Hypertensive Disorders

24.3.1.1 Objective

The reader should be able to know the prevalence of hypertensive disorders in pregnancy and the complications that can arise from them. He/she should be able to define exactly the hypertensive syndromes encountered in pregnancy, recognize them, know how to manage them, and be able to contrast the management of the various syndromes.

Hypertensive disorders in pregnancy are the commonest cardiovascular disease in pregnancy occurring in about 15% of all pregnancies and about 25% of all antenatal admissions. This figure is even more in developing countries [2–4], as the relative proportion of hypertensive disorders is far higher than it is in the Western world where congenital heart disease predominates. It is recognized as an important cause of maternal, fetal, and neonatal morbidity and mortality, especially in developing countries. It is a risk factor for CVD, strokes, abruptio placentae, and disseminated intravascular coagulopathy in women (Table 24.2).

The diagnosis of hypertension requires high readings on two separate occasions. A blood pressure reading of ≥140/90 mm Hg to 159/109 mm Hg is graded as mild hypertension, while that of 160/110 mm Hg and above is severe hypertension. Preexisting hypertension is defined as a blood pressure of ≥140/90 mm Hg, which either precedes pregnancy or develops <20 weeks POG. Gestational hypertension is a blood pressure of ≥140/90 mm Hg that develops >20 weeks, preeclampsia is gestational hypertension combined with proteinuria ≥0.3 g/day or ≥30 mg/mmol urea. Eclampsia is preeclampsia combined with seizures, preexisting HTN combined with superimposed gestational hypertension with proteinuria is defined as preexisting hypertension combined with further worsening of BP and proteinuria ≥0.3 g/day after 20 weeks, and antenatally unclassifiable hypertension is defined as BP first recorded after 20 wks.

Table 24.2 Hypertensive disorders in pregnancy

Preexisting hypertension	Blood pressure ≥140/90 mm Hg preceding pregnancy or develops before 20 weeks. It tends to persist after pregnancy.
Gestational hypertension	Blood pressure ≥140/90 mm Hg developing after 20 weeks. Resolves.
Preeclampsia	>140/90 mm Hg with proteinuria above 0.3 grams/day or creatinine above 30 mg/mmol.
Eclampsia	Preeclamptic toxemia (PET) + seizures. Pregnancy termination immediately.
Worsening existing hypertension with increasing proteinuria more than 0.3 grams/day	Pregnancy termination.

Preeclampsia is a much more worrisome development and tends to occur more commonly in primiparous women and those with multiple gestations. They do not usually develop frank hypertension, until the second half of gestation. The cause is not entirely clear but may relate to endothelial dysfunction causing an abnormal remodeling of the placental spiral arteries.

Although antihypertensive medications are effective in treating chronic hypertension that has worsened during pregnancy, they are not effective in preventing preeclampsia.

The management of essential hypertension in pregnancy with a good renal function is largely uneventful for mother and fetus. The use of antihypertensive medications remains the mainstay for the treatment of hypertension in pregnancy, but it is proper to observe nonpharmacological interventions as well.

Some of the considerations recommended for nonpharmacological treatment are listed as follows. Salt restriction is generally not advised, particularly close to delivery, as it may induce low intravascular volume; however, some authors advocate salt restriction in the management of preeclampsia. Calcium supplementation of at least 1 g daily during pregnancy can reduce the risk of preeclampsia by 50% without causing any harm. The effect is greatest for high-risk mothers. However, there seems to be conflicting evidence for the use of calcium supplements in pregnancy. Fish oil supplementation as well as vitamin and nutrient supplements have no role in the prevention of hypertensive disorders [1]. Weight reduction is generally not recommended, as it may lead to reduced neonatal weight. A close supervision, limitation of activities, and some bed rest in the left lateral position are also recommended.

Antihypertensive drugs are used for the treatment of all categories of hypertensive disorders in pregnancy. They have not been found to be effective in the prevention of preeclampsia. Optimal blood pressure control should be pursued, as an elevated blood pressure puts baby and mother at risk of hypertensive crisis and too low blood pressure will compromise uteroplacental circulation leading to increased fetal events.

The drug of choice for long-term management is alphamethyldopa, while others include alpha- and beta-adrenoceptor blockers such as labetalol and β-blockers like metoprolol or propranolol. The cardioselective B1 blocker, metoprolol, is preferable due to the possibility of bradycardia and respiratory depression and hypoglycemia in the newborn which have been observed with atenolol. Where others are used, the newborn should be monitored for up to 48 hours postpartum for these. The second-line medications are calcium channel blockers (CCBs) (nifedipine), but caution is advised to avoid them in the first trimester during organogenesis, as there is evidence of interference in mice though none in humans. The experience is limited. Angiotensin-converting inhibitors (ACEIs), angiotensin receptor blockers, and direct renin inhibitors are absolutely contraindicated, especially in the second and third trimester. Intravenous (IV) labetalol is preferable to IV hydralazine for emergencies due to observed increase in perinatal morbidity with hydralazine [14]. In the event that preeclampsia develops, bed rest, salt restriction, close monitoring, and magnesium sulfate often is administered in an effort to prevent eclamptic seizures and to prolong the pregnancy, thereby facilitating fetal maturity. Urgent delivery is expedient, after which the blood pressure usually normalizes [15].

24.3.2 Valvular Heart Disease

Objective To know the spectrum of cardiac valvular diseases encountered in pregnancy and the epidemiological transition occasioned by modern improved cardiac surgical treatment.

To be able to differentiate the hemodynamic effects of the various valvular heart diseases on pregnancy with their complications and the effect of pregnancy and labor on the presentation of the various valvular lesions; and their management during labor.

To prescribe an appropriate treatment for the condition including pregnancy termination or prevention.

To be able to recognize the occurrence of heart failure and invite the cardiologist to jointly manage the patient.

24.3.3 Valvular Heart Disease

Although the most common valvular lesions encountered are mitral and aortic regurgitations due to multiple causations, regurgitant lesions are generally well tolerated in pregnancy, so the most common problems encountered are due to bicuspid aortic and mitral stenosis, which tends to worsen during pregnancy because of the increase in cardiac output coupled with the increase in heart rate; this shortens the diastolic filling time and exaggerates the mitral valve gradient. Any decrease in stroke volume causes a further reflex tachycardia, which contributes to an elevated left atrial (LA) pressure. The onset of atrial fibrillation (AF) may precipitate acute pulmonary edema.

The risk posed by stenotic lesions in pregnancy is greater than that posed by regurgitant lesions. Increased cardiac output results in an increased transvalvular gradient, which in turn results in increased upstream pressures *vs.* reduced stroke volume (SV) and finally reduces the regurgitant volume.

Mitral and aortic regurgitations are fairly well tolerated in pregnancy, provided the regurgitation is no more than moderate, the mother is symptom free before pregnancy, and ventricular function is well preserved.

Mitral stenosis is usually poorly tolerated in pregnancy. Tachycardia, increased plasma volume pulmonary hypertension, transvalvular gradients, and pulmonary artery pressure measurements are less reliable markers of severity. Maternal risks include pulmonary edema in second and third trimesters. Atrial fibrillation increases the risk of thromboembolism and pulmonary edema. Fetal risks include prematurity (20–30%) and intrauterine growth retardation (IUGR) (5–20%). Persons with moderate and severe mitral stenosis should be counseled against pregnancy without prior intervention.

Mitral valve prolapse is a common condition that usually does not cause symptoms or require treatment. Most patients with mitral valve prolapse (MVP) tolerate pregnancy well. If the prolapse causes severe leak, it may require treatment before pregnancy.

Pharmacological Management of Symptoms

In mitral stenosis (MS) patients with symptoms or with pulmonary arterial hypertension (PAH), restricted activities and B1-selective blockers are recommended. Diuretics are recommended when congestive symptoms persist, despite β-blockers. Balloon mitral valvuloplasty is recommended for NYHA (New York Heart Association) class 3 or 4 or systolic pulmonary artery pressure (PAP) >50 mm hg, preferably after 20 weeks (contraindicated in asymptomatic women).

Anticoagulation is required for paroxysmal or permanent atrial fibrillation, LA thrombus, prior embolism. It should be considered in moderate to severe MS with spontaneous ECHO contrast, LA > 40 ml/m^2, low CO, and CCF. Vaginal delivery is recommended in mild MS, NYHA classes 1 and 2, and no PAH. Lower segment Cesarean section (LSCS) is accepted in moderate to severe MS, NYHA classes 3 and 4 [16].

24.3.3.1 Aortic Stenosis

Aortic stenosis (AS), though a stenotic lesion is usually well tolerated in pregnancy. Even severe AS may be asymptomatic. Maternal risk includes arrhythmias (3–25%), while fetal risks include preterm labor, intrauterine growth retardation (IUGR), and low birth weight. Patients may go into heart failure and should be managed with low-dose diuretics. Arrhythmias like AF can be managed with β-blockers or calcium channel blockers (CCBs) to control the heart rate. Digoxin may also be used.

Prior to pregnancy, patients with severe or symptomatic aortic stenosis with left ventricle (LV) ejection fraction (EF) less than 50%, or a fall in blood pressure with exercise or a recent progression in the stenosis should have their condition treated either by valvuloplasty or by surgical correction.

Women with bicuspid aortic valve disease or any type of aortic valve stenosis need to be evaluated by a cardiologist before planning a pregnancy. In some cases, surgery is recommended to correct the valve before pregnancy.

During pregnancy, severe symptomatic aortic stenosis, which is refractory to medical therapy or associated with life-threatening symptoms, may be subjected to balloon aortic valvuloplasty in a noncalcified valve or emergency aortic valve replacement (AVR).

Delivery should be by vaginal delivery with regional anesthesia in non-severe AS. And by LSCS (lower segment Cesarean section) in severe aortic stenosis.

24.3.3.2 Aortic Artery Disease and Pregnancy

Pregnancy because of its hyperdynamic state increases the risk of aortic dissection in patients with aortic diseases like aortic aneurysm, dilated aorta or Marfan's syndrome, or other connective tissue diseases. Pressure in the aorta increases during pregnancy and when bearing down or pushing during delivery. These factors should be assessed prior to pregnancy and counseling done. In Marfan's syndrome, genetic counseling is appropriate.

Pharmacological Management of Symptoms

HF should be treated with diuretics. Atrial fibrillation should be managed by β-blockers, while CCBs are given to control the heart rate. Digoxin may also be used. Prepregnancy intervention is indicated for symptomatic severe AS, left ventricular ejection fraction (LVEF) <50%, severe left ventricular hypertrophy (LVH) (PW > 15 mm), treadmill test (TMT) with symptoms or falling BP, recent progression of AS, and ascending aortic dimension >50 mm. BAV or emergency AVR is recommended for severe symptomatic AS which is refractory to medical therapy or in the presence of life-threatening symptoms. Vaginal delivery is recommended for non-severe AS, but LSCS is the rule for severe AS [17].

Pulmonary stenosis (PS) is generally well tolerated. Complications of severe PS include right ventricular (RV) failure and arrhythmias. Prepregnancy balloon valvuloplasty is considered in patients with severe PS and in NYHA class 3/4, despite medical therapy and bed rest, on whom percutaneous pulmonary valvotomy cannot be performed or has failed. Severe PR with impaired RV function prepregnancy pulmonary valve replacement (preferably bioprosthesis) should be considered.

Mechanical prosthetic valves show excellent performances, long-term durability but are thrombogenic. However, bioprosthetic valves also show good performances, they are much less thrombogenic but have a high risk of valve degeneration.

24.3.3.3 Prosthetic Cardiac Valves

In pregnancy, anticoagulation for prosthetic heart valves should be modified because of the recognized risk of warfarin embryopathy in the first trimester, thus warfarin must be discontinued.

The approaches are that a pregnant woman with a prosthetic valve could be given either low molecular weight heparin (LMWH) or unfractionated heparin twice daily throughout pregnancy or any of the heparins till the 13th week and then put on warfarin from weeks 13 to 35, to be followed by a return to heparin for delivery (Braunwald) [12]. Aspirin for bioprostheses is safe and need not be adjusted. Antibiotic prophylaxis for delivery is not recommended by the 2008 American Association guidelines [15, 16].

24.3.3.4 Congestive Cardiac Failure

Most cardiac diseases end up in heart failure, especially with the hemodynamic load imposed on preexisting heart disease by pregnancy, and congestive heart failure is a common observation in developing countries, as in many cases preexisting cardiac conditions are undiagnosed before presentation during pregnancy.

The usual management guidelines of cardiac failure are applied, but the use of diuretics is restricted, as it might cause hypoperfusion to the placenta with fetal compromise. Diuretics should only be used if there is pulmonary congestion. Frusemide and hydrochlorothiazide are safe. Aldosterone antagonists like spironolactone should not be used, as they are associated with antiandrogenic features, especially in the first trimester. There are no data for eplerenone.

Inotropes generally can be used as in heart failure generally. Dopamine and levosimendan can be used if intravenous inotropes are required. ACEIs, angiotensin receptor blockers (ARBs), and even rennin antagonists are contraindicated in pregnancy, due to established fetotoxicity and should not be used. β-blockers are indicated in most cases of heart failure and should be used where tolerable. The B1 cardioselective blocker metoprolol is preferable. Atenolol should not be used, due to reports of hypoglycemia and bradycardia in the newborn. Fetal monitoring for 24 to 48 hours postpartum should be done for neonatal bradycardia, hypoglycemia, and respiratory depression.

Anticoagulation should be used in heart failure with reduced ejection fraction, especially as pregnancy is a procoagulant state as the coagulation activity is increased. Oral anticoagulants are recommended in patients with intracardiac thrombus or spontaneous ECHO contrast on imaging or evidence of embolization or heart failure with atrial fibrillation. Oral anticoagulants may be reversed with appropriate antagonists before delivery or preferably switched to low molecular heparin (LMWH) after 36 weeks and fractionated heparin 36 hours before delivery. When LMWH is used, anti factor Xa levels should be monitored [18].

Planned vaginal delivery with epidural analgesia is preferable in stable patients, unless there are obstetric indications to the contrary. Urgent delivery should be considered in advanced heart failure or unstable cases and Cesarean section (C/S) with combined spinal and epidural anesthesia is recommended in line with the European Society of Cardiology (ESC) Committee guidelines [1].

ACEI may be resumed after delivery and captopril, enalapril, and benazepril are safe in breast feeding women. There are views to suggest that due to the high demands of breast feeding and lactation, they should be avoided in severe heart failure cases. A recent randomized pilot study suggests that the addition of bromocryptine to standard heart failure treatment leads to an improved ventricular function and outcome in women with advanced heart failure from peripartum cardiomyopathy (PPCM) [19] (Fig. 24.1).

24.3.4 Cardiomyopathy

Dilated Cardiomyopathy (DCM) Dilated cardiomyopathy is a heart muscle disease of unknown cause associated with global dilatation of the heart chambers with reduced or impaired systolic contractility. It presents with the typical symptoms of heart failure, left ventricular (LV) dilatation without significant hypertrophy. It can be differentiated from peripartal cardiomyopathy (PPCM)by the "time of manifestation.". If undiagnosed before conception, the condition is unmasked during the first and second trimester when hemodynamic load is increasing. Secondary cardiomyopathies, such as infiltrative, toxic, and storage diseases, manifest themselves in pregnancy. A reduced left ventricular ejection fraction less than 40% is a predictor of high risk. As there is a risk of deterioration of DCM during gestation and peripartum period, it often resembles PPCM. A family history of heart failure is in favor of DCM.

Patients with idiopathic dilated cardiomyopathy are usually counseled not to have a pregnancy, if the ejection fraction is lower than 40%. This is largely because angiotensin-converting enzyme inhibitors (ACEIs), which is their mainstay of management, are contraindicated in pregnancy and their use in maintaining ventricular function is very essential. Where pregnancy is considered, a prior echocardiographic assessment must be done and the progress of pregnancy monitored. Symptomatic patients who proceed with a pregnancy without prior counseling may need hydralazine for afterload reduction, bed rest, and low-dose diuretics for heart failure. Early delivery is advised for such patients.

Peripartum Cardiomyopathy Peripartum cardiomyopathy (PPCM) is a dilated cardiomyopathy documented with echocardiographic left ventricular dysfunction occurring in the last month of pregnancy or within 5 months of delivery. The common risk factors include multiparity, being black or of African descent, older maternal age, and preeclampsia. Most patients present in the first month postpartum [20].

PPCM presents with diastolic dysfunction due to hypertrophied noncompliant myocardium heart failure with subsequent pulmonary congestion, severe syncope, and cardiac arrhythmias.

PPCM patients generally tolerate pregnancy well. There is increased risk in patients who were symptomatic before pregnancy.

Management is done with hydralazine and nitrates, β1-selective blockers. Diuretics may be used with caution, with the exception of aldosterone antagonists which must be avoided. Anticoagulation is also recommended to prevent thromboembolic event and AF.

24.3.4.1 Hypertrophic Cardiomyopathy: (HCM)

It is characterized by diastolic dysfunction due to hypertrophied noncompliant myocardium. There is asymmetric hypertrophy of the left ventricle usually with the septum more heavily hypertrophied, such that the ratio of LV septal thickness to the LV posterior wall thickness is more than 1.5. There may be severe left ventricular outflow tract obstruction

Fig. 24.1 Anticoagulation Strategies

Anticoagulation Strategies

- OAC throughout pregnancy best strategy [esp. if warf<5 mg, Acitrom (acenocoumar) <2 mg]
- Discontinuation of OAC b/w 6 &12 wks and replacement by UFH (a PTT≥2x control; infusjon in high risk pts) or LMWH twice daily (according to weight and target anti-Xa level-6 hours post-dose 0.8-1.2U/mL in patients with a warfar in dose requ·redo >5 mg/ day
- OAC discontinued and UFH (a PTT≥2xcontrol) or adjusted-dose LMWH (anti Xa level -6 hourspost-dose 0.8-1.2 U/ mL) started at the 36th week
- LMWH replaced by i.v. UFH at least 36 hours before planned delivery. UFH should be continued untill4-6 hours bofore planned delivery and restarted 4-6 hours after delivery if there are nobleeding complications
- If delivery starts while on OACs, caesarean delivery is indicated to prevent fetal bleed

(LVOTO) and arrhythmias ((supraventricular (SVT) and ventricular (VT), both of which contribute to syncopal attacks and heart failure.

Patients with hypertrophic cardiomyopathy usually present with palpitation, angina, and breathlessness. The findings at presentation show left ventricular outflow tract obstruction, mitral regurgitation, arrhythmias, and diastolic dysfunction. However, some patients are asymptomatic. HCM has an autosomal dominant inheritance pattern with variable penetrance.

Most women with hypertrophic cardiomyopathy tolerate pregnancy well. The decrease in afterload that might exacerbate the outflow gradient is largely offset by the maternal increase in plasma volume. Medications such as β-blockers, which alleviate the outflow tract obstruction, may be continued throughout pregnancy. Patients who have significant symptoms before pregnancy may not do well [12].

Low-dose diuretics may be helpful to treat heart failure in pregnancy, but care must be taken not to cause volume depletion of the patient and exacerbate the left ventricular outflow gradient. β-blockers are useful in cases with mild LVOTO and/or wall thickness more than 15 mm to prevent a sudden pulmonary congestion. Delivery under β-blockers is also recommended.

- β-blockers- help to control the heart rate in AF and to suppress ventricular arrhythmias. Verapamil is a second choice, but there is the fear of atrioventricular (AV) block in the fetus. Cardioversion may be required for persistent arrhythmias because AF is poorly tolerated in pregnancy. Therapeutic anticoagulation is given as indicated.
- For cases with severe left ventricular outflow tract obstruction, IV fluids are only given judiciously in view of diastolic dysfunction. Syntocinon slow infusion may be used with caution. (hypotension, arrhythmias, and tachycardia).
- Epidural anesthesia and spinal block should be avoided in cases of hypotension, blood loss should be promptly replaced, and valsalva maneuver should be avoided. Epidural anesthesia where used must be with caution. For majority of cases, Cesarean section is indicated, although purely for obstetric. reasons only [12].

24.3.5 Congenital Heart Disease

Coarctation of aorta (COA) Unrepaired native COA and those repaired with residual HTN, residual coarctation, or aortic aneurysms have an increased risk of aortic rupture and rupture of a cerebral aneurysm during pregnancy and delivery. Risk factors to be screened for include aortic dilatation which may result in rupture, endoaortitis, LV failure, and bicuspid aortic valve. Aggressive treatment of hypertension is advocated to avoid placental hypoperfusion. If uncorrected, it is a very dangerous lesion in pregnancy, as it causes increased afterload in the heart and decreased perfusion for uterus. Percutaneous intervention for re-coarctation is associated with a higher risk of aortic dissection than outside pregnancy. However, covered stents may lower the risk of dissection. Vaginal delivery with epidural analgesia is preferred.

24.3.5.1 Cyanotic Congenital Heart Disease

Tetralogy of Fallot (TOF)

This is a congenital heart disease associated with four components of a ventricular septal defect, overriding aorta over both ventricles, infundibular pulmonary stenosis and right ventricular hypertrophy. Without repair, survival is shortened and many women do not reach pregnancy. If they get to the age, repair is indicated before pregnancy, lest complications will compromise both mother and fetus. If repaired, TOF patients usually tolerate pregnancy well. Anticipated cardiac complications during pregnancy include arrhythmias, heart failure, thromboembolism, progressive aortic root dilatation, and infective endocarditis. Risk factors include right ventricular dysfunction and pregnancy associated with persisting increase in RV size. In repaired symptomatic TOF, RV dilatation takes place due to severe PR, prepregnancy PVR (homograft).

Ebstein's Anomaly

In Ebstein's anomaly without cyanosis and heart failure, pregnancy is often tolerated well. If symptomatic with cyanosis and/or heart failure, it should be treated before pregnancy or the patient counseled against pregnancy. Hemodynamic status depends on the severity of tricuspid regurgitation (TR) and RV function. When associated with atrial septal defect (ASD) and Wolff-Parkinson-White (WPW) syndrome, the incidence of arrhythmias is increased. Other complications include shunt reversal and cyanosis; and paradoxical emboli.

Transposition of the Great Arteries

Surgical repair [atrial switch operation (Senning or Mustard repair)] is indicated. There is increased risk of arrhythmias and heart failure. For patients with underlying bradycardia or junctional rhythm, B-blocker therapy should be used with caution. There is an irreversible decline in the right ventricular function in 10% of cases. Patients with a moderate impairment of RV function or severe TR should be advised against pregnancy.

Congenitally Corrected Transposition of Great Artery

Risk depends on the functional status, ventricular function, presence of arrhythmias, and associated lesions. Complications associated with this condition include arrhythmias and HF. Patients are predisposed to developing AV block. Hence, β-blockers are to be used with caution. There is an irreversible decline in the RV function in 10% of the cases. Patients with a NYHA functional class III or IV, and those with ejection fraction (EF) <40% or severe TR should be counseled against pregnancy.

Pulmonary Hypertension and Eisenmenger

Low pregnancy-independent exercise capacity, superimposed on the gestational CV demands, insufficient adaptation of the right heart and poorly compliant pulmonary vasculature [21, 22] and even moderate PAH can worsen during pregnancy – due to a decrease in SVR and overload of RV.

High maternal mortality risk is reported (30–50% in older series and 17–33% in more recent studies) in patients with severe pulmonary hypertension and Eisenmenger syndrome [23]. Maternal death occurs in "the last trimester of pregnancy & in the first months after delivery." The major causes of maternal deaths include pulmonary hypertensive crises, pulmonary thrombosis, and refractory right heart failure. This occurs even in patients with little or no disability before or during pregnancy. The risk factors for maternal death are: late hospitalization, severity of PAH, and GA. Neonatal survival rates are reported to be 87–89%.

Management plans include the avoidance of multiple pregnancies, maintenance of circulating **V**olume, and avoidance of systemic **H**ypotension, **H**ypoxia, and **A**cidosis which may precipitate refractory heart failure. Supplemental oxygen therapy if there is hypoxemia; hemodynamic monitoring by the Swan–Ganz catheter is no longer indicated. Diuretics must be used judiciously and at the lowest dose to avoid hemoconcentration and intravascular volume depletion. Microcytosis and iron deficiency should be treated with supplemental oral or intravenous iron therapy. Anticoagulation should be continued in patients where there is indication for use outside pregnancy. However, it must be used with caution in Eisenmenger syndrome because patients are prone to hemoptysis and thrombocytopenia. Prostacyclin or aerosolized iloprost is also advocated to improve hemodynamics during delivery. Planned lower segment Cesarean section and vaginal delivery with incremental regional anesthesia are favored over emergency LSCS delivery.

24.3.5.2 Management of Cyanotic Mothers

Medical

Restriction of physical activity and supplemental oxygen are recommended and because of the increased risk of paradoxical embolism, the prevention of venous stasis (use of compression stockings and avoiding the supine position) is important. For prolonged bed rest, administration of prophylactic heparin should be considered. Hematocrit and hemoglobin (Hb) levels are not reliable indicators of hypoxemia. Diuretics and iron therapy are indicated in patients with Eisenmenger syndrome.

Vaginal delivery is advised in most cases (timely hospital admission, planned elective delivery, and incremental regional anesthesia). If the maternal or fetal condition deteriorates, an early Cesarean delivery should be planned because of the risks of anesthesia.

Aortic Diseases

On account of susceptibility to dissection, hormonal changes during pregnancy (most often in the last trimester of pregnancy (50%) or during the early postpartum period), an enlarged aortic root diameter [Marfan >45 mm; bicuspid AoV >50 mm (>27 mm/m^2)] is observed.

Previous Aortic Dissection

Imaging of the entire aorta is performed before pregnancy. Vaginal delivery when the aortic dimension is <40 mm, vaginal delivery with epidural anesthesia in 40–45 mm, and LSCS when>45 mm (In non-marfan, >40 mm).

Arrhythmia

Premature extra beats and sustained tachyarrhythmias become more frequent and may even manifest for the first time during pregnancy. Paroxysmal supraventricular tachycardia (PSVT) is observed in 20–44% of pregnancies [24]. Immediate electrical cardioversion is recommended for acute treatment of any tachycardia with hemodynamic instability. For acute conversion of PSVT, vagal maneuver followed by IV adenosine is recommended. IV metoprolol or propranolol can also be considered. For long-term management of SVT, oral digoxin or metoprolol/propranolol is recommended. If not successful, oral sotalol or flecainide may be used.

Immediate electrical cardioversion of VT is recommended for sustained, unstable, and stable VT. IV sotalol or procainamide may be considered for a/c conversion of sustained, hemodynamically stable, and monomorphic VT. Amiodarone should be avoided because it crosses the placental barrier and can have toxic effects on the fetus. Oral metoprolol, propranolol, or verapamil is recommended in idiopathic sustained ventricular tachycardia (VT). If unsuccessful, use oral sotalol, flecainide, or propafenone. β-blockers are recommended during pregnancy and also postpartum in congenital long QT syndrome.

Implantable cardioverter defibrillator (ICD) implantation, if clinically indicated, is recommended prior to pregnancy but if required, during pregnancy also. Implantation of proton pump inhibitor (PPI) or ICDs (preferably one chamber) should be considered with ECHO guidance, especially if the fetus is beyond 8 weeks' gestation.

Coronary Artery Disease

Acute coronary syndromes are rare in pregnancy [25], but can occur at any stage. However they are rarer in the Nigerian or African series where coronary artery disease is still relatively uncommon [26]. The risk factors are the same outside pregnancy, hypertension, hyperlipidemia, cigarette smoking, family history of premature coronary artery disease, diabetes, sedentary lifestyle, and obesity, but additional risk factors in pregnancy include advanced maternal age, preeclampsia, blood transfusion, and thrombocytosis [25]. Coronary dissection (left anterior discending (LAD)) is a cause for MI. ECG and troponin measurements are conducted in all patients with chest pain. Aortic dissection must be ruled out in all pregnant women with chest pain. Percutaneous coronary intervention (PCI) is the treatment of choice in ST segment elevation myocardial infarction (STEMI). Streptokinase does not cross the placenta but can lead to increased bleeding risk in the mother.

24.3.5.3 Venous Thromboembolism

Learning Objective

The reader should be able to understand the pathophysiological basis of venous thromboembolism (VTE) and enumerate the risk factors in pregnancy.

He should be able to distinguish between the two syndromes of VTE and be able to recognize them and anticipate their occurrence toward their prevention.

He should also be able to list the investigations necessary to confirm the diagnosis with the limitations of each. He should be able to initiate appropriate treatment while inviting the necessary specialists to comanage with him.

Venous thromboembolism (VTE) occurs commonly in pregnancy with a 4–5-fold risk compared with nonpregnant women and is the leading cause of maternal deaths in the USA, being responsible for about 10% of maternal deaths. It involves two related syndromes, deep vein thrombosis (DVT) and pulmonary embolism (PE). Pregnancy is a risk factor for VTE in many ways. In fact, all the components of the Virchoff triad of VTE occur in pregnancy: hypercoagulation, venous stasis, and vascular damage. The effect of the enlarging uterus compresses the veins, especially the inferior vena cava (IVC), leading to stasis and reduced flow. The pressure is more prominent in the lower limbs leading to peripheral varicosities. Also in pregnancy, there is increased production of fibrinogen and other procoagulant factors like factor VII, factor VIII, von Willebrand factor, and factor X and diminished level of protein S, which has anticoagulant activity. There is also dimunition of fibrinolysis with an increase in the levels of plasminogen activity inhibitors I and II, which all lead to an enhanced coagulability of blood in pregnancy. There are also vascular wall changes with increased carotid media and intimal thickness in pregnancy [27]. Thrombophilias occur in as much as 50% of pregnancies, unlike in just 10% of the general population.

A major factor of risk for VTE in pregnancy is a personal or family history of thrombosis or thrombophilia. Thrombophilia may either be genetic, of which factor V Leiden (FVL) and prothrombin G20210A are the commonest inherited thrombophilias, or it may be acquired, of which the antiphospholipid syndrome is the commonest acquired thrombophilia [12]. Antiphospholipid antibody syndrome is defined by the presence of one or more antiphospholipid antibodies; and one or more clinical manifestations most commonly thrombosis or recurrent miscarriages. For example, a positive test for lupus anticoagulant or medium to high levels of anticardiolipin immunoglobulin G (IgG) or immunoglobulin M (IgM) antibodies provides evidence if found twice at least 6 weeks apart. Thrombophilias are associated with pregnancy complications including early or late pregnancy loss, intrauterine growth restriction (IUGR), and abruption placentae.

Other factors leading to an increased risk of VTE in pregnancy include age above 35 years, obesity body mass index (BMI) >30 kg/m^2, grande multiparity, bed rest, and immobilization for more than 4 days. The presence of hyperemesis gravidarum or dehydration and occurrence of medical problems (e.g., CCF, nephrotic syndrome), PET, surgery, especially Cesarean section and trauma, are high-risk factors [12].

DVT is usually associated with symptoms of unilateral leg swelling and pain more proximally in pregnancy than outside it. It results commonly from thrombosis of the pelvic veins or deep iliac vein. It occurs more commonly on the left leg, due to the anatomy of the right artery crossing the left iliac vein. The risk for DVT is increased throughout pregnancy, but it is the highest in the last trimester. Homan's sign, that is, pain with dorsiflexion is neither sensitive nor specific. A swelling of diameter 2 cm or more in midcalf than the other side is suggestive. Diagnosis is made by Doppler ultrasonography or venography where the result of ultrasound is equivocal.

Pulmonary embolism(PE) occurs more in the postpartum period than during pregnancy. Over 60% of it occurs after a C/S, especially when complicated by postpartum hemorrhage or infection. Symptoms can vary from a mild dyspnea and tachycardia to chest pain, cyanosis, and cardiopulmonary collapse. ECG usually will show evidence of right ventricular strain (T wave inversion or the right ventricular leads), but the often-described pathognomonic S1Q3T3 pattern is infrequently found. The D dimer test is helpful to exclude pulmonary embolism (PE) when negative, as it has a high negative predictive value. Diagnosis is confirmed by a spiral CT examination. Where this is not available, a ventilation perfusion (V/Q) scan is performed, along with ultrasonography. Chest X-ray and pulmonary angiography are avoided in pregnancy because of the radiation hazards.

Treatment

Due to the prevalence and severity of VTE, special consideration is given to the management like the treatment of acute thrombotic events or appropriate prophylaxis in high-risk individuals.

Antcoagulants are used. Oral anticoagulants, Vitamin K antagonists like warfarin, are avoided, especially in early pregnancy (up to 13 weeks) due to embryopathy causing nasal bridge and central nervous system (CNS) abnormalities in the fetus. Heparin (low molecular weight) and unfractionated heparin are safe, but low molecular weight heparin is preferred because of its reliability and ease of administration. Cases are individualized, depending on the risk as outlined above for treatment and prophylaxis. Once therapy is started in pregnancy, it is usually continued through pregnancy until 6 weeks postpartum. Even outside pregnancy once indicated, it is given for 3–6 months.

Where prosthetic cardiac valves are concerned, due to the reported thrombotic episodes with heparins, warfarin may still be used after the 13th week and changed again to heparin before delivery. Heparins should be stopped about 6–12 hours before induction of labor or 12–24 hours before planned C/S and resumed 4–6 hours after normal delivery or 6–12 hours after C/S. Where anticoagulants will continue for more than 6 weeks postpartum due to the indication, it is worth the while to go to warfarin about 1 to 2 weeks after delivery, rather than heparins.

Active treatment with heparin is usually monitored with activated partial thromboplastin time (APTT) though more reliable with unfractionated heparin, while prophylactic dose is usually fixed depending on the agent used.

The NOAC (**N**on-**V**itamin K Antagonist **O**ral **A**nti**c**oagulants) should not be used in pregnancy**,** as there is no sufficient experience with their use in pregnancy.

Effect of Pregnancy on Heart Disease

Pregnancy causes worsening of cardiac status, CCF, bacterial endocarditis, pulmonary edema, pulmonary embolism, and rupture of aneurism. But there is no long-term effect on the basic defect.

Effect of Heart Disease on Pregnancy

Heart disease can cause abortion, preterm labor, IUGR, congenital heart disease in the fetus, and intrauterine fetal demise.

Risk Stratification

Several risk scores have been developed, of which the CARPREG (Cardiac Disease in Pregnancy Study) [1] risk score is most widely known and used. As regards women with congenital heart disease, the CARPREG score of 12 may also be associated with a higher risk of late cardiovascular events postpregnancy [28].

General Management

Management requires a high index of suspicion, timely diagnosis, and effective management team approach (obstetrician, cardiologist, anesthetist, neonatologist, cardiothoracic and vascular (CTV) surgeon, and nursing staff).

Preventive Concepts in Managing Cardiovascular Diseases in Pregnancy

General Preventive Measures

Patients with heart disease in pregnancy should be advised to book their pregnancy much earlier and ensure regular antenatal visit until term. It is necessary for the attending physician to identify risk factors for cardiovascular disease in the patients and stratify them to effectively manage them. Women with heart disease in pregnancy should be advised to rest adequately and avoid strenuous activities. Patients with pregestational hypertension should have their blood pressure control optimized, and those with diabetes should also have their blood sugar controlled. They should be advised on the need to avoid high-risk behaviors like smoking or alcohol consumption. Those with mechanical heart valves should be advised to adhere strictly to anticoagulant use in order to prevent thromboembolic phenomenon.

Preconceptional Counseling

Patients with heart disease who wish to be pregnant should be advised on the risks to the mother and the fetus. They should be seen in high-risk pregnancy units where detailed investigations are carried out to include ECG and echocardiogram. A functional capacity assessment by exercise ECG testing is also important, as those who cannot achieve 70% of their expected may have difficulties with carrying the pregnancy through.

Pregnancy Onset

When pregnancy results in a patient with heart disease, she should report as early as possible to the multidisciplinary team, such that drugs used in her treatment are reviewed as quickly as possible. Such drugs include warfarin which causes embryopathy especially in the first trimester, spironolactone and ACEI which cause renal defects in the fetus.

Medical Termination of Pregnancy

Termination is advised in early pregnancy in very few high-risk groups only like primary pulmonary hypertension, Eisenmenger syndrome, coarctation of aorta, and Marfan's syndrome with dilated aortic root above 4.5 cm. Suction evacuation is preferred only in the first trimester better before 8-weeks' gestation.

Antenatal Care

Antenatal care (ANC) must involve a counseling of risk and prognosis with routine visits every 2 weeks up to 30 weeks then weekly. On each visit, ask for the presence of cough, dyspnea, and other cardiac symptoms, note the pulse rate, BP, weight, anemia, auscultate lung bases, and reevaluate the functional grade. Ensure treatment compliance and exclude fetal congenital anomaly by ultrasonography and fetal ECHO at 20 weeks in maternal congenital heart disease. A proper contraceptive advice at the time of discharge must be given.

24.4 Future Prospects

The potential to use pregnancy history as a marker to determine women at risk of cardiovascular disease appears exciting, and in 2011, the American Heart Association guidelines for the prevention of cardiovascular diseases in women identified pregnancy complications as risk factors for the development of cardiovascular diseases [29] 2011.

References

1. ESC Guidelines on the management of cardiovascular diseases during pregnancy: the Task Force on the Management of Cardiovascular Diseases during Pregnancy of the European Society of Cardiology (ESC). Eur Heart J. 2011;32(24):3147–97.
2. Samuel A, Ibrahim D. Hypertension in pregnancy among rural women in Katsina State, Nigeria. J Basic Clin Reprod Sci. 2017;6(1) https://doi.org/10.4103/2278-960.194500.
3. John S, Olukayode D. 2016, The hypertensive disorders of pregnancy in Ogun State Nigeria. Preeclampsia in low and middle income countries. Pregnancy Hyper. 2018;6(3):209.
4. Singh S, Ekele BA, Egondu SC, Ikechukwu NE. Hypertensive disorders in pregnancy among pregnant women in a nigerian teaching hospital. J Nigeria Med Assoc. 2014;55(5):384–8.
5. Joshi G, Joshi S, Jha S, Joshi A, Singh Y. Maternal heart disease and pregnancy outcome: Findings from a retrospective cohort in a tertiary care government hospital in Haldwani, Nainital. India. Nigerian J Cardiol. 2015;12(2):120.
6. Karaye KM, Henein MY. Peripartum cardiomyopathy. A review article. Int J Cardiol. 2013;164:33–8.
7. Avila WS, Rossi EG, Ramires JA, Grinberg M, Bortolloto MR, Zugalia M da Luz PL. 2003. Hypertension in patients with heart disease. Experience with 1000 cases. Clin Cardiol. 2003;26(3):135–42.
8. Cardiovasculae disease and pregnancy. https://medscape.com.
9. Akinwusi PO, Oboro VO, Adebayo PA, Akintunde AA, Adeniji AO, Isawumi IA, et al. Cardiovascular and electrocardiographic changes in Nigerians with a normal pregnancy. Cardiovasc J Afr. 2010;21:71–5.
10. Thornburg KL, Jacobson S-L, Giraud GG, Morton MJ. Haemodynamic changes in pregnancy. Semin Perinatol. 2000;24(1):11–4.
11. Hall ME, George EM, Granger JP. The heart during pregnancy. Revista Española dCardiología (English Edition). 2011;64(11):1045–50.
12. Braunwald's Heart Disease: A Textbook Of Cardiovascular Medicine, 10th Edition. Eds Zipes DP, Libby P, Bonow RO, Mann DL and Tomaselli GF. IN Carole Waynes: Pregnancy and heart disease. p 1755.
13. Sanghavi M, Rutherford JD. Cardiovascular physiology of pregnancy; Circulation. 2014;130(12);1003–8.
14. Brent RL. The effect of embryonic and fetal exposure to x-ray, microwaves, and ultrasound: counseling the pregnant and nonpregnant patient about these risks. Semin Oncol. 1989;16:347–68.
15. Sihai BM. Treatment of hypertension in pregnancy. N Engl J Med. 1996;335:257–65.
16. Nithin PG. Pregnancy and Heart disease. https://slideplayer.com/slide/2320848/.
17. Warnes CA, Williams RG, Ashore TM, Child JS, Connolly HM, Dearani JA, et al. ACC/AHA 2008 Guidelines for management of adults with Cong Heart disease. Executive summary. Cirulation. 2008;118(23):2395–451.
18. Bowater SE, Thorne SA. Management of pregnancy in women with acquired and congenital heart disease. Postgrad Med J. 2010;86(1012):100–5.
19. Friedrich E, Hameed AB. Fluctuations in anti-factor Xa levels with therapeuticenoxaparin anticoagulation in pregnancy. J Perinatol. 2010;30:253–7.
20. Sliwa K, Hilfiker-Kleiner D, Petrie MC, Mebazaa A, Pieske B, Buchmann E,Regitz-Zagrosek V, Schaufelberger M, Tavazzi L, van Veldhuisen DJ,Watkins H, Shah AJ, Seferovic PM, Elkayam U, Pankuweit S, Papp Z,Mouquet F, McMurray JJ. Current state of knowledge on aetiology, diagnosis,management, and therapy of peripartum cardiomyopathy: a position statementfrom the Heart Failure Association of the European Society of CardiologyESC Guidelines 2011Working Group on peripartum cardiomyopathy. Eur J Heart Fail 2010;12:767–78.
21. Franklin W, Benton MK, Parekh D. Cardiac disease in pregnancy. Tex Heart Inst J. 2011;38(2):151–3.
22. Weiss BM, Zemp L, Seifert B, Hess OM. Outcome of pulmonary vascular disease in pregnancy: a systematic overview from 1978 through 1996. JACC. 1998;31(7):1650–7.
23. Bédard E, Dimopoulos K, Gatzoulis MA. Has there been any progress made on pregnancy outcomes among women with pulmonary arterial hypertension. Eur Heart J. 2009;30:256–65.
24. Silversides CK, Harris L, Haberer K, Sermer M, Colman JM, Siu SC. Recurrence rates of arrhythmias during pregnancy in women with previous tachyarrhythmia and impact on fetal and neonatal outcomes. Am J Cardiol. 2006;97(8):1206–12.
25. Roth Elkayam U. Acute myocardial infarction associated with pregnancy. L Am Coll Cardiol. 2008;52(3):171–80.
26. Nkoke C, Luchuo E. Coronary heart disease in sub-saharan Africa: still rare, misdiagnosed or underdiagnosed? Cardiovasc Diagn Ther. 2015; https://doi.org/10.3978/j.issn.2223-3652.2015.08.01.
27. Niemczyk NA, Bertolet M, Catov JM, Desai M, McClure C, Roberts JM, Sekikawa A, Tepper PG, Barinas-Mitchell EJ. Common carotid artery thickness increases throughout the pregnancy cycle: a prospective cohort study. BMC Pregnancy Childbirth. 2018;18:195.
28. Balint OH, Siu SC, Mason J, Grewal J, Wald R, Oechslin EN, et al. Cardiac outcomes after pregnancy in women with congenital heart disease. Heart. 2010;96:1656–61.
29. Mosca L, Benjamin EJ, Berra K, et al. Effectiveness-based guidelines for the prevention of cardiovascular disease in women-2011 update: a guideline from the American Heart Association. Circulation. 2011;123:1243.
30. Mendelson AM. Acquired heart disease in pregnancy [Internet]. Chap. 10. In: Sciarra JJ, editor. Gynaecology and obstetric: medical complications, vol. Vol 3. Haggerstown: Lippincott Williams and Wilkins; 2004. Available from: https://www.glowm.com/resources/glowm/cd/pages/about.html.

Respiratory Disorders in Pregnancy

25

Obasohan Austine and Aiwuyo O. Henry

Learning Objectives

After reading this chapter, the reader should be able to:

- Identify the physiological changes associated with healthy pregnancy, explain its development at the stages of pregnancy and its effects in masking or accentuating respiratory symptoms.
- Enumerate the respiratory diseases commonly encountered in pregnancy in the tropics and explain the differences that exist in the epidemiology.
- Discuss in detail the clinical presentation of these respiratory diseases and differentiate between them.
- Discuss the management of the conditions and critically differentiate between the drugs that can be used in the various diseases as well as those that are contraindicated in various stages of pregnancy.
- Understand the risks associated with asthma in pregnancy to mother and child.
- Understand the guidelines for management of asthma in pregnancy, the principles involved and to list the probable risks associated with the drugs used in its management.

25.1 Introduction

The respiratory system can be adversely affected by the structural and functional changes that accompany normal pregnancy (from early pregnancy to early postpartum). A pre-existing pulmonary problem can significantly be worsened by pregnancy and also normal pregnancy can be compromised by pre-existing respiratory disease. In a healthy pregnant woman, the level of stress from the respiratory system on the pregnancy is minimal compared to the cardiovascular system-induced stress. This is partly due to the fact that both minute ventilation and cardiac output increase by about 40% in pregnancy (from 7.5 L/min to 10.5 and 4.5 to 12 L/ min respectively), the minute ventilation can increase up to 1000 times with exercise while cardiac output can only increase about 300–400 times (12–16 L/min); thus, the 40% increase in cardiac output represents a greater proportion of cardiac reserve than that of minute ventilation in relation to respiratory reserve capability [1]. Also troublesome chronic respiratory diseases tend to become problematic after childbearing age unlike congenital heart disease and rheumatic heart diseases, so they tend to complicate pregnancy more [2].

O. Austine (✉)
College of Medicine Science, University of Benin, Benin City, Nigeria

University of Benin Teaching Hospital, Benin City, Nigeria

A. O. Henry
Delog Nigerian Limited, Lagos, Nigeria

25.2 Anatomic Changes in Normal Pregnancy

Basic structural changes occur in the upper and lower airways, thoracic cage and the respiratory muscles, most notably the diaphragm.

In the upper airways, there is hyperaemia, friability, mucosal oedema and hypersecretion of the airway mucus. Nasal obstruction, epistaxis, sneezing episodes, and vocal changes may occur. Nasal and sinusoidal polyposis is often seen and tends to recur in women with each pregnancy [3–5]. Nasal obstruction may contribute to upper airway obstruction during sleep, leading to snoring and even obstructive sleep apnoea.

In the lower airway, the anatomic changes are not characteristic. But some of the mucosal changes that affect the upper airways may also occur in the central portion of the airway, such as the larynx and trachea. Non-specific complaints of airway irritation, such as irritant cough or sputum production, may be intensified during pregnancy, often in association with functional changes in airway reactivity and/ or coexistent pulmonary conditions.

F. Okonofua et al. (eds.), *Contemporary Obstetrics and Gynecology for Developing Countries*,
https://doi.org/10.1007/978-3-030-75385-6_25

The physiological causes of nasal mucosal changes appear to be predominantly mediated by oestrogens [3].

The enlarging uterus produces upward displacement of the diaphragm. Although the diaphragm may be elevated up to 4 cm cephalic, diaphragmatic function is not impaired. There is increase in the antero-posterior and transverse diameters of the thoracic cage and diminished tone and activity of the abdominal muscles [3, 4]. There is also progressive relaxation of the ligamentous attachments of the ribs which broadens the subcostal angle by approximately 50%. There is a 5 to 7 cm increase in chest circumference and an upward and lateral displacement of the cardiac apex on chest radiography [6].

Both respiratory and cardiovascular changes ensure the delivery of necessary oxygenated blood and other nutrients required for this process.

25.3 Respiratory Physiology and Pregnancy

There are marked changes in lung volumes. The expiratory reserve volume (ERV) decreases by 8% to 40% and the residual volume (RV) by 7% to 22%. There is a 10% to 25% decrease in functional residual capacity (FRC) after the fifth or sixth month of pregnancy. Inspiratory capacity (IC) increases during pregnancy. Vital capacity (VC) and total lung capacity (TLC) are not substantially changed in normal healthy pregnant women, although total lung capacity does minimally decrease in the third trimester. Residual volume-to-total lung capacity ratio is low in the third trimester [3, 7, 8].

Tidal volume increases considerably, 30–35%, as a result of increased ventilatory drive thought to be related to increased progesterone levels. This leads to a 30–50% increase in minute volume which occurs towards the end of the first trimester and remains constant throughout pregnancy [6]. Maximum voluntary ventilation does not change greatly during pregnancy. Values of FEV1 throughout pregnancy are not significantly different from the non-pregnant condition. Increased gastric and oesophageal pressure occurring in late pregnancy has been considered major factors that produce a decrease in trans-pulmonary pressure leading to peripheral airway collapse [6].

There is an increase in lung water, resulting in a change in the elastic properties of the lungs. Progressive increases in airway conductance have been reported to occur between 6 months of pregnancy and term along with a decrease in airway resistance. Total pulmonary resistance, consisting of both airway and tissue resistance, is reduced by approximately 50% in pregnancy [1]. However, lung compliance does not change. The compliance of the thoracic cage decreases, as the anatomic changes in chest wall and the decrease in tone and activity of the abdominal musculature. In early pregnancy, the diffusing capacity is either unchanged or slightly increased. Throughout the rest of the pregnancy, the diffusing capacity decreases, returning to normal or slightly lower than normal values [6].

Arterial pCO2 falls to levels of 32 to 28 mmHg, plasma bicarbonate decreases to 21 to 18 mEq and arterial pH is, however, maintained in the range of 7.40 to 7.45. Values for arterial PO2 are generally greater than 100 mmHg during pregnancy [6].

With the supine position, the alveolar-arterial oxygen gradient may widen, and mild arterial hypoxemia may develop. Respiratory responses during parturition are greatly affected by stage of labour and the response to pain and anxiety [6].

During labour, tidal volumes ranging from 350 to 2250 ml and minute ventilations from 7 to 90 L/min have been recorded. The possibility of relative hypoventilation between contractions coupled with the grave implications of foetal hypoxaemia makes it reasonable to be liberal in the use of oxygen [1, 9].

Sleep quality is often poor in pregnancy. Sleep disruption can be due to leg cramps, low back pain, urinary frequency or responsibilities relating to child care. Total sleep time and daytime sleepiness increase during the first trimester, whereas sleep time decreases and complaints of an increase in the number of nocturnal arousals increase in the third trimester [10]. Polysomnographic studies have shown an increase in sleep latency, an increase in the amount of stage I sleep and a decrease in rapid eye movement (REM) sleep and delta sleep, as well as an increase in the number of awakenings (Tables 25.1 and 25.2).

Table 25.1 Respiratory parameters in pregnant* versus non-pregnant** women

Respiratory parameter	Non-pregnant**	Pregnant*
Minute ventilation	Normal 7.5 L/min	Increased to 10.5 L/min
O2 consumption	30 ml/min	Increased to 40 ml/min
Minute volume	Normal	Increased
Tidal volume	Normal	Increased
Functional residual capacity	Normal	Decreased
Respiratory rate	Normal	Normal
PaO2		104–108 mmHg (13.8–14.3 kPa
PaCO2	35–42 mm hg (4.6–5.3 KPa)	27–32 mmHg (3.6–4.2 KPa)
Plasma HCO3	20–30 mmol/L	18–21 mmol/L
Arterial pH		7.4–7.45

This state of respiratory alkalosis leads to a compensatory metabolic acidosis

25.4 Dyspnoea of Pregnancy

Incidence of dyspnoea in pregnancy ranges from 60% to 70% [9]. It commonly occurs during the first and second trimester and remains stable or improves near term. Increased ventilatory drive (stimulation of the respiratory centre in the brain) due to increased levels of progesterone in pregnancy, and increased mechanical load with excessive chemoreceptor sensitivity to carbon dioxide or hypoxemia are the usual causes [11]. The increasing size of the uterus presses on the diaphragm making it more difficult for the lungs to fully expand causing shallow breathing and breathlessness [11].

A chest radiograph with shielding of the foetus should be performed in any patient being evaluated for unexplained dyspnoea in pregnancy when other cardiac modalities of investigation are negative [9].

Distinguishing between physiological and pathological causes of dyspnoea in pregnancy can be quite challenging diagnostically and the outline in the following table modified from Niharika et al. [12] outlines the clinical characteristics, helpful investigations and necessary intervention to aid diagnosis, which is quite helpful (Table 25.3).

The common respiratory diseases encountered in pregnancy include bronchial asthma, pulmonary thromboembolism from deep vein thrombosis and pulmonary hypertension from cardiac disease; and in developing or low-resource countries, infections like pulmonary tuberculosis and pneumonias occur commonly. Less commonly sleep disorders and obesity cause problems.

Table 25.2 Rate of pregnancy changes in respiratory parameters[a]

Functional residual capacity	Decreased by 10–25%
Total pulmonary resistance	Decreased by 50%
Expiratory reserve volume	Decreased by 8–40%
Reserve volume	Decreased by 7–20%
Tidal volume	Increased (30–35%)
Minute volume	Increased 20–50%

Functional residual capacity (FRC) = reserve volume + expiratory reserve volume (ERV)

[a]Modified from Leighton and Fish [9]

25.5 Effect of Respiratory Diseases on the Respiratory System During Pregnancy

25.5.1 Bronchial Asthma

Bronchial asthma is one of the commonly encountered diseases in pregnancy occurring in about 5–10% of pregnancies and increasing in prevalence [13]. The course of asthma in pregnancy is variable as the effect of pregnancy might have variable effects on it. While the stress of pregnancy might be enough to trigger increased occurrences in some individuals, the increased levels of steroid hormones in pregnancy do ameliorate the features and reduce the occurrence of attacks. In general, one third of patients improve, one third remains undisturbed and stable while a third tend to worsen [14]. The picture tends to be the same through subsequent pregnancies. Those who get symptomatic during pregnancy often have the greatest difficulty during 24–36 weeks of gestation either triggered by lack of adherence to medications or have infections, viral or bacterial, consequent upon reduced immunity in pregnancy. Severe exacerbation and inadequate control in pregnancy are associated with low ventilation which is associated with increased gestational hypertension and premature delivery and low birth weight [15].

The risks of poorly controlled asthma to the mother and foetus are greater than those posed by most medications (including oral corticosteroids) [16]. No association exists between mild asthma and preterm delivery or adverse perinatal outcomes. However, moderate or severe asthma tends to be associated with an increased maternal caesarean secion rate and neonatal sepsis. Conversely prematurity and neonatal sepsis tends to be associated with development of bronchial asthma in later life.

The clinical features of asthma is similar in and out of pregnancy and the pharmacologic management is quite similar utilising inhaled short-acting beta2 agonists, inhaled corticosteroids, inhaled long-acting beta2 agonists and systemic corticosteroids. Leukotriene receptor antagonists and theophylline are safe. Oral corticosteroid

Table 25.3 Causes of dyspnoea[a]

Causes of dyspnoea	Clinical characteristics/investigations/intervention
Dyspnoea of pregnancy	Need deep breath intermittently/inability to breath deep enough. None. Reassurance
Asthma/airway disease	Dyspnoea with chest tightness or wheezing. Spirometry Pre- and post-bronchodilation inhaled B agonists + = – inhaled steroids
Cardiac disease	Myocardial/valvular dysfunction. Orthopnoea/PND second tri end/PP Echocardiogram. Diuretics, B blockers
Arrhythmias	Sudden onset/cessation. Assoc. palpitations/chest discomfort ECG, Holter/event monitor. B blockers, Ca channel blockers
Venous thromboembolism	Sudden onset, any trimester. Associated DVT features CT, PulmAngio, V/Q scan, Doppler study. Anti-coagulation heparin in pregnancy, warfarin postpartum

[a]Modified from Niharika et al. [12]

Table 25.4 Asthma management in pregnancy

	Symptoms	Medications
Step 1	Mild/intermittent	No daily medication. Short-acting inhaled B2 agonist, for example, salbutamol
Step 2	Mild but persistent.	Low-dose inhaled corticosteroids
Step 3	Moderate, persistent daily	Low-dose steroids + long-acting B2 agonists, for example, salmeterol or medium-dose inhaled corticosteroids
Step 4	Severe persistent continuously/frequent nocturnal symptoms	High-dose inhaled corticosteroids + long-acting B2 agonist and systemic steroids

Adapted from Niharita et al. [12]

use in the first trimester is associated with a small increased risk of isolated cleft lip with or without cleft palate (0.1–0.3%), and may be associated with increased risks of pregnancy-induced hypertension, preeclampsia, preterm delivery and low birth weight [17, 18]. Budesonide has the best safety record in pregnancy. Because of the risks associated with poor control and exacerbations, guidelines recommend managing asthma actively during pregnancy with regular review, provision of a written action plan, use of prevention medications as indicated for other adults with asthma and management of co-morbid conditions such as rhinitis. Use of short-acting B agonists (SABA) as reliever medication and inhaled corticosteroids (IHC) for women with persistent asthma is recommended [19]. The use of an algorithm that adjusted inhaled corticosteroids (IHC) using a marker of eosinophilic lung inflammation, the exhaled nitric oxide fraction (FeNO) and added long-acting B2 agonists when symptoms remained uncontrolled resulted in fewer exacerbations and improved infant respiratory health at 12 months (Table 25.4).

25.6 Pneumonias

Community-acquired pneumonias occur with particularly high incidence among pregnant women with certain predisposing factors like smoking or respiratory disorders. This is due to the physiologic adaptations in the respiratory and immunologic systems as well as the anatomic changes in pregnancy, increasing susceptibility. In addition, the effect of the disease on the foetus as well as the risks associated with the use of the requisite anti-chemotherapeutic agents to the foetus are of immense concern.

The changes in pregnancy include alterations in cellular immunity with a reduction in lymphocyte proliferative response especially in the second and third trimesters. These are meant to protect the foetus from the mother immunologically. There is decreased natural killer cell activity, decrease in number of T-helper cell populations and reduced lymphocyte cytotoxic activity. The hormones prevalent in pregnancy including progesterone, human chorionic gonadotrophin (HCG), alpha foetoprotein and cortisol contribute to inhibit cell-mediated immunity. These changes could increase the risk from infection especially viral and fungal infections [20–24].

Anatomically, the enlarged uterus of pregnancy leads to diaphragmatic elevation by up to 4 cm and splaying of the thoracic carina. There is also an increase in the transverse diameter of the thoracic cage. These changes can lead to an impairment of the ability to clear secretions. The decrease in functional capacity described earlier, increased oxygen consumption and increase in lung water occurring in pregnancy all add to the vulnerability to lung injury in pregnancy [1]. Obstetric and anaesthetic intervention including intubation pose added hazards especially with aspiration pneumonia [25].

Although pneumonias are the commonest causes of non-obstetric infections in the pregnant woman, the incidence has reduced from the early days of antibiotics, prior to 1965 (6–9 per 1000 deliveries) to similar incidence outside pregnancy (less than 1 per 1000 deliveries) ostensibly due to antibiotic use and better obstetric care but this is expected to rise due to a relatively higher proportion of patients with chronic medical problems reaching pregnancy [1] as it is one of the risk factors for pneumonia in pregnancy. Other risk factors include anaemia, cigarette smoking, diminished immunity, having asthma, including other prolonged or chronic medical illnesses, having a job that involves working with children and spending prolonged time in hospital or nursing homes.

Tocolytic drugs used to induce labour have been associated with pneumonia through the promotion of pulmonary oedema and increasing respiratory insufficiency and pneumonia [26]. The use of antepartum corticosteroids to enhance foetal lung maturity is also associated with high risk for pneumonia [27].

25.6.1 Pathogens

The commonest causes of community- acquired pneumonias are typically the same as in non-pregnant people, which being mainly Streptococcus pneumonia , then followed by haemophilus influenza and the atypical organisms Mycoplasma pneumonia. Other organisms that have been documented include Legionella species and Coxiella burnetti but these are rare. The common viruses are influenza viruses A, B and C. Type A is typically associated with epidemic disease, can cross the placenta and has been associated with description of CNS abnormalities in the foetus. Other viruses include varicella virus and less commonly rubella, infectious mononucleosis and hantavirus infection. Fungi may rarely complicate pregnancy but can occur in those with depressed immunity (cell mediated). The organism tends to be coccidioidomycosis. Cryptococcus usually causes meningitis, and presentation as isolated pneumonia is unusual [1].

With HIV infection most pneumonias are still bacterial, mainly Streptococcus, but there is a higher proportion of atypical bacteria like Pneumocystis carina pneumonia (PCP), less commonly *Pseudomonas aeruginosa*.

The clinical features are usually the same as in non-pregnant women with cough, which worsens with sputum, fever, chills and dyspnoea except that the dyspnoea is often underreported because it is a usual feature of many pregnancies, thus requiring a high index of suspicion. Common symptoms include cold and flu-like symptoms such as sore throat, headache and body pains. Postpartum pneumonia is also well described especially with aspiration which may occur during labour or unprepared emergency Caesarean section [25].

Although the clinical diagnosis of pneumonia should be straightforward, evidence of misdiagnosis and especially delayed diagnosis is abound. Delayed diagnosis is dangerous as it leads to abortions, prematurity, and low birth weight [26]. As the definite diagnosis of pneumonia is by a chest X-ray, this should not be delayed because of the little hazard posed by a chest X-ray. The baby could be screened off and a plain chest X-ray alone done. A lateral chest X-ray causes more exposure to irradiation and so should be avoided. Almost all pneumonias can be diagnosed by a straight chest X-ray alone. The differential diagnosis of alveolar shadowing in pregnancy include non-cardiogenic pulmonary oedema in eclampsia and PET, pulmonary oedema secondary to tocolytic drugs, aspiration pneumonias and rarely chorion carcinoma with pulmonary metastasis which may mimic pneumonia [1].

Mothers with pneumonia are more likely to deliver early prematurely and have infants with low birth weight. Prostaglandin synthesis or the host's inflammatory response to infection is thought to be responsible [26].

Treatment of pneumonia in pregnancy is with same antibiotics having considered the usual features of possibility of foetal toxicity, teratogenicity and expression of the drug in breast milk. The penicillins, cephalosporins and macrolides except erythromycin are safe. Erythromycin is associated with hepatotoxicity. Quinolones, tetracyclines, chloramphenicol and sulpha drugs are contraindicated in pregnancy and should be avoided. Pneumococcal vaccine is not recommended for pregnant women and those who are breastfeeding [28].

Antiviral agents especially the neuraminidase inhibitors are useful in viral pneumonias but for non-availability of safety records are best avoided. Oseltamivir has been recently associated with good effects in the treatment of influenza in pregnancy because of its systemic absorption while varicella pneumonia is treated with intravenous acyclovir [12]. Influenza vaccine is not recommended in pregnancy but in epidemics where immunisation is required in the first trimester should be avoided [28].

25.7 Tuberculosis

Every year worldwide over 1 billion tuberculosis (TB) infections, 9 million new cases and approximately 1.7 million deaths are estimated to occur [29].

Tuberculosis was harmful during pregnancy, and termination of pregnancy was recommended. However, in recent times, tuberculosis during pregnancy is rarely an indication for a therapeutic abortion. Pulmonary tuberculosis is fortunately now a rare complication of pregnancy. Although patients used to deteriorate very rapidly in the puerperium, this is now not so [30]. The incidence of tuberculosis increased in recent years because of increased HIV infection, increased immigrant population and reduced public health services.

The problems in the management of tuberculosis depend on which drugs might be used safely in pregnancy. Streptomycin causes damage to the vestibular and auditory parts of the eighth cranial nerve, but this fact has been disputed [31]. Para-amino salicylic acid (PAS) has several the disadvantages: it is bulky and difficult to swallow, may cause gastrointestinal side effects, and is not particularly potent as an anti-tuberculous drug; but none of these problems is specific to pregnancy. Isoniazid is a potent anti-tuberculous drug and may cause peripheral neuritis. However, its use has been studied extensively in pregnancy [32] and found not to cause a rise in perinatal mortality. Ethambutol has come to replace PAS, although it may cause retrobulbar neuritis. However, there is no evidence that this occurs [33, 34].

The drug of first choice for the treatment of tuberculosis appears to be rifampicin. However, it is teratogenic in mice and so at present cannot be recommended in the early stages of pregnancy.

25.7.1 Diagnosing Tuberculosis in Pregnancy

Symptoms like malaise and fatigue may be ignored in pregnancy as they indicate late diagnosis. Sputum examination and culture, same as for non-pregnant, must be done. Occasionally bronchoscopy might be necessary to obtain samples. Maternal prognosis depends on site and the timing of diagnosis. Morbidity increases as much as fourfold in late diagnosis. Perinatal outcome is also bad with late diagnosis as it may increase incidence of prematurity and low birth weight.

Tuberculin skin testing is necessary. The guidelines developed by the American Thoracic Society/CDC [35] are helpful and the following are considered positive:

1. 5 mm or greater induration is positive in HIV patients, those with close contact with TB patient or those with CXR of healed old TB.
2. 10 mm or greater induration in immigrants from endemic areas, homeless, who live in nursing home or correctional facilities, inject drugs, are part of high-risk minority or have another medical disease which increases TB risk.
3. 15 mm or greater in all other patients.

Patients who have had prior BCG vaccination should be interpreted similarly. Once a patient is determined positive, she should have a chest x-ray CXR with shielding of the foetus.

25.7.1.1 Anti-Tuberculous Therapy

The standard treatment for TB in the non-pregnant state is a combination of four drugs: Rifampicin, Isoniazid (INH), Ethambutol and Pyrazinamide for 6 months; the first four drugs for 2 months and Rifampicins and INH for a further 4 months making a total of 6 months. In pregnancy, however, TB patients should be treated with Rifampicin, INH and Ethambutol for 9 months; the three drugs for first 2 months and then Rifampicin and INH continued for another 7 months totalling 9 months. Latent TB is treated with INH daily or twice weekly for 9 months with pyridoxine supplementation [9, 12].

No increase in congenital malformations or foetal damage have been shown by studies when rifampicin, isoniazid and ethambutol are used in combination.

25.7.1.2 Breast Feeding and TB

Breast feeding appears to be safe when the mother is taking standard anti-tuberculous medication. If the mother is taking isoniazid, pyridoxine supplementation should be given to the child as a small amount of isoniazid is present in breast milk. It is usually unnecessary for the child to receive treatment unless the mother is diagnosed with open (infectious) at the time of delivery. For mothers with open tuberculosis. Breast feeding can be done with isoniazid prophylaxis. Mother can use a face mask. For neonates, INAH prophylaxis is given for 3 months, and check for mantoux. If mantoux is negative, give BCG vaccination

25.7.1.3 Contraception

Oral contraceptives can be used but its effectiveness is reduced because of induction of liver enzymes, which metabolise the drug fast to ineffective levels.

25.8 Pulmonary Venous Thromboembolism

This has been more extensively treated in the section on cardiovascular disease in pregnancy as it is more related to cardiovascular and haematological problems but a few guides are given below.

Venous thromboembolism (VTE) occurs in 0.5 to 3.0 per 1000 pregnancies in those without a history of thromboembolism [36]. Prior thromboembolic disease, smoking, prior venous thrombosis and thrombophilia are risk factors for deep venous thrombosis or pulmonary embolism (PE) during pregnancy.

The risk of venous thromboembolism is greatest in the postpartum period. Evaluation with venous ultrasound of the lower limbs to assess patency or thrombus blockage is essential. If negative, a ventilation-perfusion (V-P) scan or echocardiography should be performed. A D-dimer test which is useful for its high negative predictive value outside pregnancy is less useful because of its lower sensitivity as the value of D-dimer rises throughout pregnancy. Computed tomography examination is associated with some radiation hazards but may be performed with caution [36]. Confirmed cases of venous thromboembolism during pregnancy should be managed with unfractionated or low molecular weight heparins.

Warfarin should be avoided due to the risk of embryopathy. The novel oral anti-coagulants (NOACs), for example, rivaroxaban are not recommended in pregnancy.

25.9 Pulmonary Hypertension

Pulmonary hypertension poses one of the highest risks for maternal mortality [4]. The cardiovascular and haemodynamic changes associated with pregnancy, anaesthesia and delivery pose a severe risk to women with primary pulmonary hypertension, Eisenmenger's syndrome and secondary pulmonary hypertension. Studies have documented maternal mortalities in these groups from 30 to 56%, although most of these studies evaluated patients who did not receive current vasodilator therapy. Women with primary pulmonary hypertension are advised against pregnancy and if patients found in early pregnancy, termination is considered [37]. However, recent case reports have documented successful use of intravenous or inhaled epoprostenol, and sildenafil in pregnant women with pulmonary hypertension; however, their long-term effect on overall pregnancy-related mortality is unknown [37, 38]. Nitric oxide (NO), a pulmonary vasodilator, has been used successfully in a number of reports in women with pulmonary hypertension without complications [38–40].

25.9.1 Pulmonary Oedema

Obstetric causes of pulmonary oedema include aspiration pneumonia, sepsis, transfusion reactions, allergic reactions, disseminated intravascular coagulation, amniotic fluid embolism, toxaemia of pregnancy, tocolytic therapy and eclampsia, the latter being the most common cause of pulmonary oedema. Bromocriptine therapy to suppress lactation can also cause postpartum pulmonary oedema. Decreased venous tone and venous resistance lead to iatrogenic pulmonary oedema. Treatment is with a short course of intravenous furosemide and specific treatment of the underlying condition. Diuretics are generally avoided because of placental hypoperfusion.

25.9.2 Pleural Effusion

Pleural effusions occur with toxaemia of pregnancy, preeclampsia, pulmonary oedema, pulmonary embolism, choriocarcinoma and amniotic fluid embolism. Small pleural effusions are common in the postpartum period in normal pregnancy.

25.9.3 Sleep-Disordered Breathing

Hormonal changes of increased oestrogen result in hyperaemia and upper airway narrowing. Increased progesterone results in increased respiratory drive. Other physiologic changes in sleep (decreased FRC and respiratory system compliance) predispose to alterations in sleep during pregnancy. While snoring is increased in pregnancy, sleep-disordered breathing may worsen during pregnancy, the incidence and prevalence of sleep-disordered breathing during pregnancy are unknown. Symptoms of sleep-disordered breathing should be reviewed with women who develop pregnancy-induced hypertension or preeclampsia, and all pregnant women with symptoms of sleep-disordered breathing should be evaluated with a polysomnogram and treated with nasal continuous positive airway pressure as indicated.

25.10 Nitric Oxide (NO) in Pregnancy and Disease

NO also known as Nitrogen Monoxide was discovered by Joseph Priestley, a theologian in 1772, but later found in 1987 to have endothelial vasodilatory properties. It is commonly the air pollutant produced by vehicle emissions and plant machinery. It is one of the gases signalling molecules which enable communication between the cells and involved in regulation of physiological and pathological events like cell growth, differentiation and functioning [41]. As it has a limited biologic life, its effects are limited to the lungs where it works as a pulmonary vasodilator.

Inhalation of the gas leads to a diffusion through the alveolar capillary membrane and pulmonary arterial muscles leading to muscle relaxation, reduced pulmonary vascular resistance and more blood flow to the lungs. One of the mechanisms is due to the close affinity of NO for haem. By this process, NO activates a haem-containing enzyme called soluble guanylyl cyclase, which is activated a 1000-fold to produce the signalling molecule cyclic GMP (3,5 cyclic guanosine monophosphate) leading to vascular relaxation. There are other pathways by which NO influences the activities of cells; for example, the action of NO with other free radicals such as oxygen and superoxide anions to produce reactive oxidants [41]. It may, thus, also have adverse effects as it can also produce cytotoxic oxygen radicals which exert anti-platelet and cytotoxic effects. The balance between the protective and adverse effects of NO is determined by the relative amount of NO and reactive radicals, so administration of the gas should be monitored with an electrochemical analysis machine.

Recent case reports have documented successful use of intravenous or inhaled epoprostenol, and sildenafil in pregnant women with pulmonary hypertension; however, their long-term effect on overall pregnancy-related mortality is unknown.

Also it is known [42] that uterine arteries have increased endothelial nitric oxide synthase (NOS) activity, which produces NO. Nitric oxide (NO) has close interaction with iron-containing particles and binds with haem and proteins expressed during pregnancy. However, whether these mediate vasodilatation during pregnancy remains to be established. There are controversies over the studies of placental NOS in preeclampsia, although an abnormality is likely (above). NOS activity decreases towards the end of gestation and administration of exogenous NO relaxes the myometrium, but whether endogenous NO contributes to uterine quiescence in pregnancy is yet unconfirmed.

Some researchers from the University of Warwick Medical School [43] have postulated that there is reduced level of NO or its activity in the placenta in preeclampsia, stating that this leads to a release of a stress hormone called CRH (corticotrophin releasing hormone), which directly influences NO production and that in preeclampsia there is an abnormality in this mechanism. The abnormality then causes a cascade of signalling errors through a number of protein receptors called G-protein-coupled receptors (GPCRs) that prevent activation of the enzymes responsible for NO production. It is hoped that targeting the protein receptors would activate the enzyme that releases NO.

References

1. De Swift M. Respiratory disease in pregnancy. Postgrad Med J. 1979;55:325–8.
2. Lomaro A, Aliverti A. Respiratory physiology of pregnancy. Breathe. 2015;11:297–301.
3. Weinberger SE, Weiss ST, Cohen WR, Jw W, Johnson TS. Pregnancy and the lung. Am Rev Respir Dis. 1980;121:559–81.
4. Contreras G, Gutiérrez M, Beroíza T, Fantin A, Oddo H, Villarroel L, et al. Ventilatory drive and respiratory muscle function in pregnancy. Am Rev Respir Dis. 1991;144:837–41.
5. Gilroy RJ, Mangura BT, Lavietes MH. Rib cage and abdominal volume displacements during breathing in pregnancy. Am Rev Respir Dis. 1988;137:668–72.
6. Tarun M, Sharma S. Pulmonary disease and pregnancy. [online, 6 screens] Medscape available from https://emedicine.medscape.com/article/303852-overview#a1.
7. McAuliffe F, Kametas N, Costello J, et al. Respiratory function in singleton and twin pregnancy. BJOG. 2002;109:765–9.
8. Jensen D, Webb KA, Davies GA, O'Donnel DE. Mechanical ventilatory constraints during incremental cycle exercise in human pregnancy: implications for respiratory sensation. J Physiol. 2008;586:4735–50.
9. Leighton B, Fish J. Pulmonary disease in pregnancy. Glob Libr Women's Med. 2008:1756–2228.
10. Xialonglong X, Dongguan L, Zhangyi Z, Manoj S, Yong Z. Sleep duration and quality in pregnancy. Int J Environ Res Public Health. 2017;14(7):817.
11. Garcia-Rio F, Pino JM, Gomez L, Alvarez-Sala R, Villasante C, Villmor J. Regulation of breathing and perception of dyspnea in healthy pregnant women. Chest. 1996;110(2):446–53.
12. Niharika M, Chen K, Hardy E, Powrie R. Respiratory disease in pregnancy. Best Pract Res Clin Obstet Gynaecol. 2015;29(5):598–611.
13. Kwon HL, Belanger K, Bracken MB. Asthma prevalence among pregnant and childbearing aged women in the US. Estimates from national health surveys. Ann Epidemiol. 2003;13:317–24.
14. Murphy EV. Managing asthma in pregnancy. Breathe. 2015;11:258–67.
15. Schatz M, Dombrowski MP, Wise R, Momirova V, Landom M, Mabie W. Spirometry is related to prenatal outcomes in pregnant women with asthma. Am J Of ObstetGynaecol. 2006;194(1):120–6.
16. [Guideline] National Asthma education and Prevention Program. Managing asthma during pregnancy: recommendations for pharmacologic treatment. National Guideline Clearing House. Jan, 2005.
17. Garne E, Vinkel Hansen A, Morris J, Jordan S, Klungsoyr K, Engeland A, et al. Risk of congenital anomalies after exposure to asthma medication in first trimester of pregnancy- a cohort linkage study. BJOG. 2016;123(10):1609–18.
18. Bakhirevia LN, Jones KL, Schatz M, Johnson D, Chambers CD. Asthma medication use in pregnancy and fetal growth. J Allergy ClinImmunol. 2005;116(3):503–9.
19. National Heart, Lung and Blood Institute, National Asthma Education and Prevention program Asthma and Pregnancy Working Group. Managing asthma in pregnancy: recommendations for pharmacologic therapy 2004 update. J Allergy ClinImmunol. 2005;115:34–46.
20. Lim WS, Marcfarlane JT, Colthorpe CL. Pneumonia and pregnancy. Thorax. 2001;56(5):398–405.
21. Baley JE, Schater BZ. Mechanisms of diminished natural killer cell activity in pregnant women and neonates. J Immunol. 1985;14:3042–8.
22. Bulmer R, Hancock W. Depletion of circulating T lymphocytes in pregnancy. ClinExpImmunol. 1977;28:302–5.
23. Lederman MM. Cell mediated immunity and pregnancy. Chest. 1984;86:6–95.
24. Sridama V, Pacini F, Yang SL, Moawad A, Reily M, DeGroot LJ. Decreased level of T helper cells, a possible cause of immunodeficiency in pregnancy. N Engl J Med. 1982;307:352–6.
25. Maclenan FM. Maternal mortality from Mendelsons syndrome: an explanation. Lancet. 1986;1:587–9.
26. Munn MB, Groome LJ, Atterbury JL, Baker SL, Hoff C. Pneumonia as a complication of pregnancy. J Matern Fetal Med. 1999;8:151–4.
27. Rothmensch S, Vishne TH, Celentano C, Dan M, Ben-Rafael Z. Maternal infectious morbidity following courses of Betamathasone. J Infect. 1999;39:49–54.
28. Salisbury DM, Begg NT, Department of Health 1996. Influenza. In: Salisbury DN, Begg NT, editors. Immunisation against infectious disease. London: HMSO. p. 167–72.
29. Mehta N, Chen KK. Respiratory disease in pregnancy. Best Pract Res Clin Obstetr Gynaecol. 2015;29:598–611.
30. de March AP. Tuberculosis and pregnancy. Five- to ten-year review of 215 patients in their fertile age. Chest. 1975;68(6):800–4.
31. Conway N, Birt BD. Streptomycin in pregnancy: effect on the fetal ear. Br Med J. 1965;2(5456):260–3.
32. Hammond EC, Selikoff IJ, Robitzek EH. Isoniazid therapy in relation to later occurrence of cancer in adults and infants. Br Med J. 1967;2(5555):792–5.
33. Lewitt T, Nebel L, Terracina S, Karaman S. Ethambutol in pregnancy: observations on embryogenesis. Chest. 1974;66:25.
34. Brobowitz ID. Ethambutol in pregnancy. Chest. 1974;66:20.
35. American Thoracic Society/CDC. American Thoracic Society 1990: diagnostic standards and treatment of tuberculosis. Am Rev Resp Dis. 1990;142:725–35.
36. European Society of G, Association for European Paediatric C, German Society for Gender M, Regitz-Zagrosek V, Blomstrom Lundqvist C, Borghi C, et al. ESC guidelines on the management of cardiovascular diseases during pregnancy: the task force on the Management of Cardiovascular Diseases during pregnancy of the European Society of Cardiology (ESC). Eur Heart J. 2011;32(24):3147–97.
37. Weiss BM, Zemp L, Seifert B, Hess OM. Outcome of pulmonary vascular disease in pregnancy: a systematic overview from 1978 through 1996. JACC. 1998;31(7):1650–7.
38. Monnery L, Nanson J, Charlton G. Primary Pulmonary hypertension in pregnancy. A role for novel vasodilators. Br J Anaesth. 2001;87(2):295–8.
39. Robinson JN, Banerjee R, Landzberg MJ, Thiet MP, et al. Inhaled Nitric Oxide therapy in pregnancy complicated by pulmonary hypertension. Am J of Obst and Gynecol 1999. 1999;180(4):1045–6.
40. Goodwin TM , Gherman RB, Hameed A, Uri E. Favourable response of Eisenmenger syndrome to inhaled nitric oxide during pregnancy. Am J Obstetr Gynecol. 1999;180(1 Pt.1):64–7.
41. Bruckdorfer R. The basics about Nitric Oxide. Mol Aspects Med. 2005;26(1–2):3–31.
42. Hart CM. Nitric Oxide in adult lung disease. Chest. 1999;115:1407–17.
43. University of Warwick 2006. Researchers Reveal How NO Helps Pregnant Women with Hypertension. www.sciencedaily.com/releases/2006/09/080920092244htm.

Hypertension in Pregnancy

26

Michael Olumide Gbala and Adedokun Isaac Adegoke

Learning Objectives

After studying this chapter, the reader should be able to:

- Define hypertension in pregnancy.
- Classify hypertension in pregnancy.
- Enumerate the risk factors for hypertension in pregnancy.
- Describe various pathogenesis of hypertension in pregnancy.
- Critically evaluate patients with hypertension in pregnancy.
- Discuss treatment options in patients with hypertension in pregnancy.
- Discuss the use of antihypertensive in pregnancy.
- Recall the use and monitoring of magnesium sulphate as an anticonvulsant in severe hypertension in pregnancy.
- Enumerate the various preventive options for preeclampsia.

26.1 Introduction

Normal human pregnancy is characterised by initial fall in blood pressure due to physiologic decrease in the systemic vascular resistance [1]. The 30% decrease in systemic vascular resistance that normally occurs early in pregnancy typically generates a 10% decrease in blood pressure as early as 7 weeks of gestation and even more by mid-pregnancy [1]. The decrease in blood pressure in early pregnancy reaches its nadir at 16–18 weeks of gestation, followed by return to pre-pregnancy levels by the third trimester. The hypertensive disorder of pregnancy remains the leading cause of maternal and perinatal morbidity and mortality [2–7]. Hypertension in pregnancy affects about 1–35% of pregnancies worldwide [2]. The observed wide variation in the incidence of hypertensive disorder of pregnancy across the globe is due to differences in the definition of the condition and the diagnostic methods. Preeclampsia and eclampsia seem to create more concern than others; however, any form of hypertension in pregnancy increases the risk of adverse pregnancy outcomes [3–6].

26.2 Definition

Hypertension in pregnancy is defined as systolic blood pressure greater than or equal to 140 mmHg and/or diastolic blood pressure greater than or equal to 90 mmHg (Korotkoff [5]). These measurements should be taken on two occasions at least 4 hours apart [1, 3]. Although during emergency, when faced with severe hypertension, the diagnosis of hypertension in pregnancy can be confirmed within a shorter interval (even within minutes) to facilitate timely therapy [1]. Elevations of both systolic and diastolic blood pressures are important as both have been associated with adverse maternal and foetal outcome [4].

Detecting a rise in booking or preconception blood pressure (>30/15 mmHg), rather than relying on an absolute value has in the past been considered useful in diagnosing preeclampsia in women whose blood pressures are less or equal to 140/90 mmHg. Available evidence does not support the notion that these women have an increased risk of adverse outcomes [8]. However, such a rise may be significant in some pregnant women, particularly in the presence of proteinuria, hyperuricaemia, or a small for gestational age (SGA) infant, and these women need closer monitoring.

Severe hypertension in pregnancy is defined as systolic blood pressure ≥160 mmHg or diastolic blood pressure

M. O. Gbala (✉)
University of Medical Sciences (UNIMED) Teaching Hospital, Ondo, Nigeria

UNIMED, Ondo, Nigeria

A. I. Adegoke
Department of Obstetrics and Gynaecology, University of Medical Sciences Teaching Hospital, Ondo, Nigeria

F. Okonofua et al. (eds.), *Contemporary Obstetrics and Gynecology for Developing Countries*,
https://doi.org/10.1007/978-3-030-75385-6_26

≥110 mmHg or both. Severe hypertension in pregnancy is considered to be a hypertensive emergency that requires urgent intervention. The American Congress of Obstetricians and Gynaecologists (ACOG) Committee Opinion on "Emergent Therapy for Acute Onset, Severe Hypertension with Preeclampsia or Eclampsia" recommends that severe hypertension that persists for 15 minutes or more in the setting of preeclampsia or eclampsia is a hypertensive emergency that requires immediate intervention [9].

Appropriate blood pressure measurement technique is essential for identifying and monitoring hypertension in pregnancy. Blood pressure is highly variable within subjects; appropriate care must be taken to standardise practice in order to minimise various factors that affect clinic blood pressure measurement, especially choice of cuff size, degree of stimulation, posture, and talking.

26.3 Proteinuria

Significant proteinuria is present when 24-hour urine protein collection is equal to or exceeds 300 mg of protein. The presence of ≥5 grams of protein in a 24-hour urine collection upstages preeclampsia from mild to severe. The spot urine protein:creatinine ratio has also been used to define significant proteinuria in the identification of preeclampsia. The ACOG practice bulletin "Chronic Hypertension in Pregnancy" notes that a protein:creatinine ratio in the range of 0.15–0 0.3 g protein/g creatinine can be used to identify women who should be further evaluated [10].

The presence of 2+ or 3+ proteinuria or repeated +1 dipstick testing increases both sensitivity and specificity and, therefore, should be assumed to represent significant proteinuria until proven otherwise by confirmatory tests. Twenty-four-hour urine protein remains the gold standard for quantifying proteinuria in pregnancy.

26.4 Classification

Hypertension in pregnancy can be described as chronic, gestational, preeclampsia, or eclampsia depending on the gestational period, tendency for post-partum resolution, presence of proteinuria, or convulsion. The National High Blood Pressure Education Program Working Group on High Blood Pressure in Pregnancy classified hypertensive disorder in pregnancy into four categories [5]:

- Chronic hypertension
- Preeclampsia-eclampsia
- Preeclampsia superimposed on chronic hypertension
- Gestational hypertension (This class has replaced the old term "pregnancy-induced hypertension" (PIH) because of its precision.)

The recommended classification for hypertensive disorders of pregnancy by The International Society for the Study of Hypertension in Pregnancy is as shown below [6, 7].

Hypertension known before pregnancy or present in the first 20 weeks:

1. Chronic hypertension
   (a) Essential
   (b) Secondary
2. White-coat hypertension
3. Masked hypertension

Hypertension arising de novo at or after 20 weeks:

1. Transient gestational hypertension
2. Gestational hypertension
3. Preeclampsia* – de novo or superimposed on chronic hypertension

*Preeclampsia can deteriorate rapidly and without warning; ISSHP classification does not recommend classifying it as "mild" or "severe".

26.5 Chronic Hypertension

Chronic hypertension is diagnosed when hypertension is detected prior to the onset of pregnancy or diagnosed before 20th week of gestation or in a patient who has been using antihypertensive drugs before pregnancy. Hypertension that persists beyond 42 days post-partum is also classified as chronic hypertension. The complications associated with chronic hypertension include abruptio placenta, intrauterine growth restriction, mid-trimester pregnancy losses and preterm delivery.

26.6 White-Coat Hypertension

This refers to elevated office/clinic (≥140/90 mmHg) blood pressure but normal blood pressure measured at home or work (<135/85 mmHg); it is not an entirely benign condition and conveys an increased risk for preeclampsia [6, 7].

26.7 Masked Hypertension

This form of hypertension is characterised by blood pressure that is normal at a clinic or office visit but elevated at other times. It is difficult to diagnose. However, it is most typically diagnosed by 24-hour ambulatory BP monitoring (ABPM) or automated home blood pressure monitoring (HBPM) [7].

26.8 Transient Gestational Hypertension

This hypertension is usually detected in the clinic but then settles with repeated BP readings, such as those taken over the course of several hours during observation in a Day Assessment Unit. This type of hypertension occurs in the 2nd or 3rd trimester. It is very important to monitor this group of women because this condition is associated with about 40% risk of developing true gestational hypertension or preeclampsia in the index pregnancy [7].

26.9 Gestational Hypertension

Gestational hypertension (hypertension of pregnancy or chronic hypertension identified in the latter half of pregnancy) has replaced the old term "pregnancy-induced hypertension" (PIH) because of its precision. Gestational hypertension is characterised by new onset of elevated blood pressure during the second half of pregnancy or in the first 24 hours post-partum, without accompanying proteinuria or abnormal blood tests (elevated liver enzymes, low platelets, or elevated serum creatinine), and in the absence of symptoms blood pressure normalises in the post-partum period, usually within 10 days. The diagnosis changes to chronic hypertension if BP does not normalise during this period.

Gestational hypertension has little effect on maternal and perinatal morbidity and mortality when it develops at term. However, these pregnancies may be complicated by abruptio placenta and intrauterine foetal growth restriction.

26.10 Preeclampsia-Eclampsia

Preeclampsia is unique to human pregnancy. It is a multisystemic disorder characterised by hypertension and involvement of one or multiple organs. Proteinuria is no longer not mandatory to diagnose preeclampsia but it is the most commonly recognised additional clinical feature especially in developing countries where the resources for immediate identification of other features may not be available. It is difficult to diagnose preeclampsia superimposed on underlying renal disease because these patients commonly have impaired glomerular filtration rate and/or proteinuria.

Preeclampsia is diagnosed by hypertension and the coexistence of one or more of the following new-onset conditions [6]:

1. Proteinuria (spot urine protein/creatinine >30 mg/mmol or >300 mg/day or at least 1 g/L["2 +"] on dipstick testing)
2. Other maternal organ dysfunction:
   - Renal insufficiency (creatinine >90 umol/L; 1.02 mg/dL)
   - Liver involvement (elevated transaminases – at least twice upper limit of normal ± right upper quadrant or epigastric abdominal pain)
   - Neurological complications (examples include eclampsia, altered mental status, blindness, stroke, or more commonly hyperreflexia when accompanied by clonus, severe headaches when accompanied by persistent visual scotomata)
   - haematological complications (thrombocytopenia – platelet count below 150,000/dL, DIC, haemolysis)
3. Uteroplacental dysfunction
   - Foetal growth restriction

It is therefore good practice that all asymptomatic women with less than severe hypertension and no dipstick proteinuria should have the appropriate laboratory investigations done to exclude maternal organ dysfunction. Without these investigations, appropriate exclusion of preeclampsia cannot be done.

26.11 Risk Factors

- Nulliparity
- New partner/paternity
- Age <18 years or >35 years
- History of preeclampsia
- Family history of preeclampsia in a first-degree relative
- Black race
- Obesity
- Interpregnancy interval <2 years or >10 years
- Maternal chronic hypertension
- Pre-existing diabetes
- Thrombophilia
- Renal disease
- Systemic lupus erythematosus
- History of migraine [11]
- Multiple gestations
- Hydrops foetalis
- Triploidy
- Gestational trophoblastic disease
- Oocyte donation or donor insemination
- Collagen vascular disease

The increased prevalence of chronic medical conditions including chronic hypertension in women older than 35 years may be responsible for increased frequency of preeclampsia in older gravidas. Higher incidence of preeclampsia in black women compared to other races has been linked to greater prevalence of chronic hypertension in blacks. Increased risk of recurrent preeclampsia in subsequent pregnancies is found in women who develop preeclampsia during pregnancy (about 18% overall risk). The risk almost triples (about 50%) in women who develop severe preeclampsia before 27 weeks gestation. Women in this category also have increased risk of developing cardiovascular disease later in life [12].

26.12 Theories of Preeclampsia

The aetiology of preeclampsia is elusive and theories abound to describe its pathogenesis. Acceptable theories on the pathogenesis of preeclampsia account for the observation that hypertensive disorders due to pregnancy are very much more likely to develop in the woman who is exposed to the chorionic villi for the first time; is exposed to a superabundance of chorionic villi as with multiple gestation or hydatidiform mole; has preexisting vascular disease and is genetically predisposed to hypertension developing during pregnancy. The physiologic endpoint in women with preeclampsia is endothelial damage. Vasospasm is central to the aetiopathogenesis of preeclampsia and eclampsia.

26.12.1 Increased Response to Pressor Agents

Women with early preeclampsia show increased vascular reactivity to pressors. These substances include norepinephrine, angiotensin II and vasopressin. As early as 1973, Gant and co-workers [13] described increased sensitivity to angiotensin II long before the onset of pregnancy-induced hypertension. Nulliparas who remained normotensive were refractory to the pressor effect of the administered angiotensin II. Women who became hypertensive lost this refractoriness before the onset of hypertension similar to what was observed in women with chronic hypertension.

26.12.2 Abnormal Invasion of the Trophoblast

Conversion of the maternal spiral arteries within the decidua to larger competent vessels is one of the important steps in the development of a normal placenta. The spiral arteries are invaded by the cytotrophoblastic cells in the first trimester leading to destruction of the muscular and elastic tissues in the arterial wall. These tissues are subsequently replaced with fibrinoid material. This transformation results in spiral arteries with increased blood flow and decreased responsiveness to vasoconstrictor stimuli. This initial invasion by trophoblastic cells is known as "primary wave of trophoblastic invasion".

Between 12 and 16 weeks gestation, the second wave of cytotrophoblastic invasion occurs which affects the myometrial segments of the spiral arteries with a further increase in choriodecidual blood flow. In a normal pregnancy, by the 22nd week, the trophoblast has invaded the spiral arteries supplying the intervillous space. The endothelium is replaced by trophoblast, and the internal elastic lamina is replaced by trophoblast and a fibrin containing amorphous matrix. The diameter of the spiral arteries is increased to 4–6 times than in the pre-pregnancy state. There is unimpeded blood flow into the intervillous space, and over the villous tree containing foetal vessels. This ensures easy exchange of nutrients, oxygen and metabolic wastes.

Preeclampsia is characterised by shallow trophoblast invasion and unconverted narrow spiral arteries. The myometrial segments maintain their smooth muscle coats which are sensitive to pressor agents. There is also reduction in choriodecidual blood flow. Similar abnormalities were also observed in normotensive patients with intrauterine growth restriction (IUGR) and found to be absent in some cases of preeclampsia [14].

26.12.3 Prostaglandins

The exact mechanism by which prostaglandins and other related substances mediate vascular reactions during pregnancy remains unclear. It is known that in normal pregnancy, there is increased production of prostacyclin and thromboxane with the balance in favour of prostacyclin production [15]. Prostacyclin is produced by vascular endothelium and the renal cortex while thromboxane is produced by platelets and trophoblast. Prostacyclin is a potent vasodilator while thromboxane is a potent vasoconstrictor. The disruption in the delicate balance between the prostaglandins, in which there is increased prostacyclin-thromboxane ratio, may play an important role in the aetiology of preeclampsia [15].

26.12.4 Vascular Endothelial Injury

In preeclampsia, the vascular endothelium of the mother appears to be an important target of factors that are triggered by placental ischaemia and/or hypoxia. A critical balance exists between endothelium-derived relaxing and contracting substances that maintain vascular homeostasis. Disruption of this balance results in the vasculature being predisposed to vasoconstriction, leucocyte adherence, mitogenesis, prooxidation, and vascular inflammation [16]. Many markers of endothelial dysfunction are elevated before the clinical features of preeclampsia are noticed; therefore, they may serve as predictors of the condition. The roles of nitric oxide, endothelin-1(ET-1), and vascular endothelial growth factor have been studied extensively [17–20].

Nitric oxide appears to play an important role in the renal vasodilation in normal pregnancy but its role remains unclear in preeclampsia. Studies have shown that chronic nitric oxide synthase inhibition in pregnant rats causes hypertension associated with peripheral and renal vasoconstriction, proteinuria, intrauterine growth restriction, and increased foetal morbidity [17]. Endothelin-1 is a vasoconstrictor stimulated by endothelial damage. It also increases oxidative stress in placenta villi. Increased production of ET-1 may play an important role in the pathogenesis of preeclampsia [21].

Elevated serum levels of vascular endothelial growth factor (VEGF), associated with vascular permeability and endothelial activation have been reported in patients with preeclampsia [22].

26.12.5 Genetic and Immunological Factors

About three decades ago, Chesley and Cooper described the tendency for genetic susceptibility in the aetiology of preeclampsia and eclampsia. Certain HLA types are more common in the mothers and the foetuses that are products of preeclamptic pregnancies. They observed that some medical conditions that have genetic predisposition (e.g. hypertension and diabetes) also predispose to preeclampsia. A multifactorial inheritance was considered [23].

Dekker and Sibai studied the role of immune maladaptation in the pathophysiology of preeclampsia. It was observed that women at risk of developing preeclampsia have lower T-helper cells compared with women who remain normotensive starting from early second trimester. Antibodies against endothelial cells were found in 50% of women with preeclampsia as against 15% prevalence in normotensive controls [24]. The immunisation concept is supported by the observation that preeclampsia develops more frequently in multipara impregnated by a new partner.

26.12.6 Coagulation Abnormalities

Preeclampsia is characterised by activation of the coagulation cascade. Although consumption of procoagulants sufficient to be detected by standard testing is found in only about 10% of cases of preeclampsia, sensitive tests of activation of the cascade can be detected in most preeclamptic women. Other coagulation abnormalities include vasospasm and haemostatic abnormalities. Laboratory markers of platelet and endothelial activation are early increase in fibronectin levels, worsening thrombocytopenia, and raised platelet turnover. The elevated levels of fibronectin predates the clinical onset of preeclampsia and may be used for diagnosing superimposed preeclampsia in women with chronic hypertension [25]. Other coagulation abnormalities include increased thrombin–antithrombin III complex, reduced protein C (normal protein S), and elevated levels of α-thromboglobulin [26].

26.13 Clinical Features and Multisystem Involvement in Preeclampsia

Patients are usually asymptomatic at the onset of the disease. Symptoms of preeclampsia include new-onset headache (frontal and throbbing), scintillations and scotomata (presumed to be due to cerebral vasospasm), new-onset constant epigastric pain (due to hepatic swelling and inflammation) with or without oedema.

26.13.1 Cardiovascular Findings

Hypertension is usually the earliest clinical sign in preeclampsia. The elevated blood pressure in preeclampsia is due to increased total peripheral resistance as cardiac output is normal or slightly reduced. There is general arteriolar narrowing in which humoral factors such as angiotensin II, endothelins, and catecholamines have been implicated [13, 21]. Hypertension, defined as repeat blood pressure measurements ≥140/90 mmHg, results from abnormal vasoconstriction. The blood pressure usually rises gradually and may not reach the hypertensive range until third trimester [27].

Preeclampsia does not affect the myocardium directly; however, the heart responds to the physiological changes caused by preeclampsia. There is reduction in longitudinal, circumferential, and radial systolic strain [28], but the left ventricular ejection fraction is usually normal [29]. Physiologic response to increase afterload is believed to be responsible for the decreased left ventricular performance in preeclampsia [28–30].

Pulmonary oedema may be present in severe preeclampsia. Increased pulmonary vascular hydrostatic pressure compared with plasma oncotic pressure, capillary leak, iatrogenic volume overload are possible causes of pulmonary oedema in preeclampsia.

26.13.2 Gastrointestinal Findings

Epigastric or right upper quadrant abdominal tenderness due to hepatic swelling and capsular stretch. Changes in hepatic function are usually seen in severe forms of preeclampsia. Peripartal haemorrhagic necrosis, subcapsular haematoma, hepatic rupture, elevated aspartate aminotransferase and increased alkaline phosphatase levels are other gastrointestinal findings in preeclampsia. Histologic findings include periportal and sinusoidal fibrin deposition and microvesicular fat deposition [31, 32].

26.13.3 Renal Findings

Glomerular endotheliosis, which is characterised by glomerular capillary endothelial swelling with sub-endothelial deposits of protein material, is seen in preeclampsia [33]. Proteinuria is invariably present in preeclampsia and preeclampsia is the most common cause of severe proteinuria in pregnant women. Podocyturia which is shedding of live podocytes is seen in patients with preeclampsia and it predates the onset of proteinuria in preeclampsia [34]. It was discovered that podocyturia in the second trimester had a significantly higher sensitivity and specificity for the subsequent diagnosis of preeclampsia than any single angiogenic marker or their combination. Screening for podocyturia may therefore allow for accurate identification of pregnancy at risk for preeclampsia [34].

The glomerular filtration rate decreases by about 40 percent in preeclampsia compared to pregnant normotensive controls. There is reduced renal plasma flow with normal or slightly elevated creatinine. Oliguria with rising creatinine is seen in severe preeclampsia. Other findings include hyperuricaemia and hypocalciuria [35].

26.13.4 Haematologic Findings

Thrombocytopenia is the most common coagulation abnormality in preeclampsia. Thrombocytopenia in preeclampsia is believed to be due to microangiopathic endothelial injury and activation resulting in the formation of platelet and fibrin thrombi in the microvasculature. The resultant accelerated platelet consumption (and possible immunological interplay) leads to thrombocytopenia. A platelet count less than 100,000/μL is seen in severe preeclampsia [36].

About 10% of patients with severe preeclampsia have coagulation abnormalities consistent with disseminated intravascular coagulopathy (DIC) [37]. The underlying aetiology of DIC in severe preeclampsia is not known, but it has been suggested that it could be due to vascular damage resulting from vasospasm [38]. Reduced antithrombin III levels [39], and reduction in the ratio of factor VIII bioactivity to factor VIII antigen [40] are some of the features of coagulation derangement seen in mild preeclampsia.

26.13.5 Central Nervous System

The central nervous system (CNS) symptoms include headache and visual symptoms. Examination findings are generalised hyperreflexia with or without ankle clonus. Visual symptoms include blurred vision, flashing lights, diplopia, and amaurosis fugax (blindness in one eye). Rarely, there may be cortical blindness which is transient. However, blindness may be permanent following retinal conditions such as retinal detachment, retinal artery or venous thrombosis, optic nerve damage, and retinal ischaemia [41].

Presence of seizures in preeclampsia changes the diagnosis to eclampsia. One in 400 cases of mild preeclampsia and 1 in 50 cases of severe preeclampsia will develop eclampsia. Histopathological findings include cerebral oedema, haemorrhage, microinfarcts, vasculopathy, and fibrinoid necrosis [42, 43].

26.14 Prevention of Preeclampsia

Preeclampsia remains a major cause of maternal and perinatal morbidity and mortality in both developed and developing countries. Therefore, any intervention that could prevent or minimise the risk of developing preeclampsia will go a long way in improving maternal and neonatal outcome globally. Any effective prevention requires identification of the at-risk group, together with an intervention that will mitigate or eliminate the development of the condition. In the last three decades, obstetricians have relied on medical, obstetric, and family history to identify women at risk of developing preeclampsia and eclampsia [6]. The screening method unfortunately identifies only about 30% of cases with a high false-positive rate [44].

Based on the experience gained from the multi-parameter Bayesian risk assessment algorithms used in first trimester aneuploidy screening, pregnant women at increased risk of developing early onset preeclampsia can now be identified on the basis of a combination of maternal demographic and historical features, biophysical parameters (body mass index, mean arterial blood pressure, Doppler assessment of placental vascular resistance at 12–14 weeks gestation-uterine artery pulsatility index), and maternal serum analytes (mainly pregnancy-associated plasma protein A, PAPP-A and placental growth factor, PIGF). About 90% of women at risk of developing preeclampsia prior to 34 weeks with a false-positive rate of 10% can be identified when these parameters are combined in a validated algorithm (Foetal Medicine Foundation, London) [44, 45].

In 2011, WHO put forward recommendations for prevention and treatment of preeclampsia and eclampsia [46] as stated below:

1. In areas where dietary calcium intake is low, calcium supplementation during pregnancy (at doses of 1.5–2.0 g elemental calcium/day) is recommended for the prevention of preeclampsia in all women, but especially those at high risk of developing preeclampsia. Quality of evidence (QE)-Moderate, Strength of Recommendation (SR)-Strong.
2. Low-dose acetylsalicylic acid (aspirin, 75 mg) is recommended for the prevention of preeclampsia in women at

high risk of developing the condition. QE-Moderate, SR-Strong.

3. Low-dose acetylsalicylic acid (aspirin, 75 mg) for the prevention of preeclampsia and its related complications should be initiated before 20 weeks of pregnancy. QE-Low, SR-Weak.
4. Women with severe hypertension during pregnancy should receive treatment with antihypertensive drugs. QE-Very low, SR-Strong.
5. The choice and route of administration of an antihypertensive drug for severe hypertension during pregnancy, in preference to others, should be based primarily on the prescribing clinician's experience with that particular drug, its cost and local availability. QE-Very low, SR-Weak.
6. Magnesium sulphate is recommended for the prevention of eclampsia in women with severe preeclampsia in preference to other anticonvulsants. QE-High, SR-Strong.
7. Magnesium sulphate is recommended for the treatment of women with eclampsia in preference to other anticonvulsants. QE-Moderate, SR-Strong.
8. The full intravenous or intramuscular magnesium sulphate regimens are recommended for the prevention and treatment of eclampsia. QE-Moderate, SR-Strong.
9. For settings where it is not possible to administer the full magnesium sulphate regimen, the use of magnesium sulphate loading dose followed by immediate transfer to a higher level healthcare facility is recommended for women with severe preeclampsia and eclampsia. QE-Very low, SR-Weak.
10. Induction of labour is recommended for women with severe preeclampsia at a gestational age when the foetus is not viable or unlikely to achieve viability within 1 or 2 weeks. QE-Very low, SR-Strong.
11. In women with severe preeclampsia, a viable foetus and before 34 weeks of gestation, a policy of expectant management is recommended, provided that uncontrolled maternal hypertension, increasing maternal organ dysfunction or foetal distress are absent and can be monitored. QE-Very low, SR-Weak.
12. In women with severe preeclampsia, a viable foetus and between 34 and 36 (plus 6 days) weeks of gestation, a policy of expectant management may be recommended, provided that uncontrolled maternal hypertension, increasing maternal organ dysfunction or foetal distress are absent and can be monitored. QE-Very low, SR-Weak.
13. In women with severe preeclampsia at term, early delivery is recommended. QE-Low, SR-Strong.
14. In women with mild preeclampsia or mild gestational hypertension at term, induction of labour is recommended. QE-Moderate, SR-Weak.
15. In women treated with antihypertensive drugs antenatally, continued antihypertensive treatment post-partum is recommended. QE-Very low, SR-Strong.
16. Treatment with antihypertensive drugs is recommended for severe post-partum hypertension. QE-Very low, SR-Strong.
17. Advice to rest at home is not recommended as an intervention for the primary prevention of preeclampsia and hypertensive disorders of pregnancy in women considered to be at risk of developing those conditions. QE-Low, SR-Weak.
18. Strict bed rest is not recommended for improving pregnancy outcomes in women with hypertension (with or without proteinuria) in pregnancy. QE-Low, SR-Weak.
19. Restriction in dietary salt intake during pregnancy with the aim of preventing the development of preeclampsia and its complications is not recommended. QE-Moderate, SR-Weak.
20. Vitamin D supplementation during pregnancy is not recommended to prevent the development of preeclampsia and its complications. QE-Very low, SR-Strong.
21. Individual or combined vitamin C and vitamin E supplementation during pregnancy is not recommended to prevent the development of preeclampsia and its complications. QE-High, SR-Strong.
22. Diuretics, particularly thiazides, are not recommended for the prevention of preeclampsia and its complications. QE-Low, SR-Strong.
23. The use of corticosteroids for the specific purpose of treating women with HELLP syndrome is not recommended. QE-Very low, SR-Weak.

Investigations

- Urinalysis: send for microscopy, culture, and sensitivities if proteinuria is present.
- Frequent monitoring of FBC, LFTs, renal function, electrolytes, and serum urate: to identify rising values to help guide the decision as to when to deliver:

Table 26.1 Rating scheme for the strength of the evidence

Quality of evidence	
Grade	Definition
High	Further research is very unlikely to change confidence in the estimate of effect
Moderate	Further research is likely to have an important impact on confidence in the estimate of effect and may change the estimate
Low	Further research is very likely to have an important impact on confidence in the estimate of effect and is likely to change the estimate
Very low	Any estimate of effect is very uncertain

- HELLP syndrome (Haemolysis, Elevated Liver Enzymes, Low Platelet count): platelet count falling below 100 × 10^9/L, abnormal liver enzymes (ALT or AST >70 IU/L).

- Clotting profile studies is indicated in severe preeclampsia or thrombocytopenia.
- Twenty-four-hour urine collections for protein quantification and creatinine clearance.
- For the assessment of foetus: – ultrasound assessment of foetal growth and the volume of amniotic fluid, and Doppler velocimetry of umbilical arteries are done.
- Cerebral imaging (MRI or CT) is not indicated in uncomplicated eclampsia. However, imaging is necessary to exclude haemorrhage and other serious abnormalities in women with focal neurological deficits or prolonged coma.
- Other tests that that can be informative include blood smear, serum lactate dehydrogenase (LDH), and serum bilirubin concentrations. Elevated LDH, indirect bilirubin levels, and red cell fragmentation are seen in microangiopathic haemolysis.

26.15 Management of Preeclampsia

Despite the axiom that delivery is the only cure for preeclampsia, clinicians must try to minimise maternal risk while maximising foetal maturity. The optimal management of a woman with preeclampsia depends on gestational age and severity of the condition. Management in the hospital is multidisciplinary involving the obstetric team, anaesthetist, haematologist, and paediatrician [47–49].

Usually, patients with mild preeclampsia are managed conservatively, that is, without delivery of the baby, until at least 34 weeks, as long as they are haemodynamically stable, without coagulation abnormalities and in the absence of HELLP syndrome. However, placenta delivery remains the cure for preeclampsia.

To carry out a conservative management, there is need for a comprehensive management plan to monitor maternal and foetal conditions. This includes monitoring of blood pressure, documenting signs and symptoms of severe preeclampsia (such as headache, visual symptoms, and epigastric pain), daily maternal weights, laboratory investigations (e.g. platelet count, liver function test), and 24-hour urine protein weekly. Non stress test, biophysical profile, Doppler studies and ultrasonic growth assessment should be used to monitor foetal condition. In essence, patients are managed based on the severity of their condition.

If the blood pressure is mildly elevated, that is, 140–149/90–99 mmHg, monitor blood pressure at least four times a day with twice-weekly blood tests for FBC, electrolytes, renal function test, and LFT.

If the blood pressure is moderate, that is, 150–159/100–109 mmHg, monitor blood pressure at least four times a day. Give antihypertensive labetalol (alternatives are methyldopa or nifedipine) to keep systolic blood pressure < 150 mmHg and diastolic blood pressure between 80 and 100 mmHg. Blood tests are done three times per week.

Intravenous labetalol, hydralazine, or oral nifedipine can be used in the treatment of acute severe hypertension [7]. All Obstetric units saddled with management of hypertension in pregnancy are expected to develop and maintain a uniform management protocol to be used by everyone in such units or departments. This uniform protocol can be reviewed as deemed fit by the department or units. In our centre, University of Medical Sciences Teaching Hospital Ondo state, intravenous Labetalol is our first line in the management of acute severe hypertension in pregnancy.

Generally, in severe preeclampsia delivery is indicated as delivery of the foetus and placenta is the only cure. However, preterm delivery may adversely affect neonatal outcome therefore the management plan for delivery, including thresholds for early delivery should be discussed with the woman on an individual basis and properly documented. Prenatal corticosteroids should be given to help foetal maturity if pregnancy is less than 34 weeks. Antihypertensives should be given and continued after delivery based on blood pressure. Angiotensin-converting enzyme (ACE) inhibitors, angiotensin II receptor antagonists and diuretics should be avoided although may be indicated post-partum. Magnesium sulphate should be considered when there is concern about the risk of eclampsia as it reduces the risk by >50% [46, 50].

Magnesium sulphate is the drug of choice in controlling seizures [46]. This position is supported by Magpie trial as well. Using the Pritchard regimen, magnesium sulphate is initiated by giving 4 g bolus magnesium sulphate intravenously over 5–10 minutes and simultaneously administering 10 g intramuscularly (5 g each buttock), that is, 14 g loading dose. This is then followed by 5 g intramuscularly at 4-h intervals into alternate buttocks for 24 hours [51]. Recurrent seizures should be treated with a further bolus of 2 g $MgSO_4$. Some researchers have modified this regimen by limiting the maintenance doses to 12 hours instead of 24 hours with encouraging results [52]. The Pritchard regimen is now popular in low-resource settings. The Federal Ministry of Health in Nigeria recommends Pritchard regimen [53]. There is need for fluid restriction to avoid fluid overload in the intrapartum and post-partum periods. Total fluid should not be more than 80 ml/hour or 1 ml/kg/hour.

The decision to deliver is made once the patient is stable. If the gestational age is less than 34 weeks and delivery can be deferred, corticosteroids should be administered, but it is very important to reassess the benefits of conservative management after 24 hours. The decision on the mode of delivery depends on the foetal presentation and condition, together with favourability of the cervix for induction of labour [54].

While in labour, there is need for continuous blood pressure monitoring. Ergometrine and Syntometrine should be avoided in the management of third stage of labour.

26.16 Eclampsia

Eclampsia refers to the occurrence of new onset, generalised, tonic-clonic seizures or coma in a woman with preeclampsia. The incidence of eclampsia in the western world is 1 in 2000 to 1 in 3000 pregnancies, but the incidence is tenfold higher in tertiary centres, developing countries and in cases of multiple gestation [55, 56]. Eclampsia is associated with high maternal and foetal morbidity and mortality. Globally, about 2% of women with eclampsia die as do about 7% of their offspring with much higher mortality rates in developing countries [57–59].

Eclampsia is a multisystemic disorder involving the central nervous, hepatic, cardiovascular, renal, and haematologic systems. In the central nervous system, seizure can lead to stroke, oedema, brain herniation (with its attendant sequelae), stroke and predisposes to cognitive impairment and epilepsy later in life [60]. Preeclampsia is believed to be a prodrome for eclampsia; however, eclamptics present with a broad spectrum of symptoms and signs ranging from severe hypertension and proteinuria to mild or absent hypertension with no proteinuria. Therefore, eclampsia is not always a progression from severe preeclampsia to seizure [57].

Prolonged eclamptic seizure can cause maternal acidosis, hypoxia, and brain trauma. Abruptio placenta complicates about 20–50% of eclampsia after prolonged seizure [61]. Seizures also result in foetal hypoxia.

The diagnosis of eclampsia in low-resource settings relies mainly on clinical features. However, CT or MRI should be used to show evidence of oedema or haemorrhage (intracerebral or cerebellar). The differential diagnoses of eclampsia include epilepsy, trauma, neoplasms, drug toxicity, and meningitis.

The principle of management of eclampsia is stabilisation and delivery by the most expedient (fastest and safest) route. Stabilisation involves administration of $MgSO_4$ in preference to other anticonvulsants [46]. Mean arterial blood pressure should be lowered in patients with severe hypertension by 15–20% using labetalol, hydralazine or nifedipine. Sodium nitroprusside and nitroglycerin should be avoided because they contain cyanide which can cause foetal toxicity. Angiotensin-converting enzyme (ACE) inhibitors are contraindicated in pregnancy. Fluid therapy should be monitored closely as in severe preeclampsia.

26.17 Conclusion

Hypertension in pregnancy is common. It causes significant maternal and perinatal morbidity and mortality if not promptly and properly managed. However, effective implementation of the prediction and prevention strategies coupled with early diagnosis and appropriate treatments are very germane in curtailing the debilitating effects of hypertension on pregnancy outcomes. Maintenance and regular review of uniform departmental management protocols for hypertension in pregnancy and regular audits of maternal and foetal outcomes are strongly indicated in all obstetric units saddled with management of hypertension in pregnancy.

References

1. American College of Obstetricians and Gynaecologists. ACOG Practice Bulletin No. 203. Chronic hypertension in pregnancy. Obstet Gynecol. 2019;133:e26–50.
2. Chesley LC. Hypertensive disorders in pregnancy. New York: Appleton-Century-Crofts; 1978.
3. Itam IH, Ekabule JE. A review of pregnancy outcome in women with eclampsia at the University of Calabar Teaching Hospital, Calabar. Trop J Obstet Gynaecol. 2002;18:66–8.
4. Seligman S. Which blood pressure? Br J Obstet. Gynaecol. 1987;94(6):497–8.
5. Report of the National High Blood Pressure Education Program Working Group on High Blood Pressure in Pregnancy. Am J Obstet Gynecol. 2000;183(1):S1–22.
6. Tranquilli AL, Dekker G, Magee L, Roberts J, Sibai BM, Steyne W, et al. The classification, diagnosis and management of the hypertensive disorders of pregnancy: a revised statement from ISSHP. Pregnancy Hypertens. 2014;4:97–104.
7. Brown MA, Laura AM, Louise CK, Karumanchie SA, McCarthyf FP, Shigeru S, et al. The hypertensive disorders of pregnancy: ISSHP classification, diagnosis & management recommendations for international practice. Pregnancy Hypertens. 2018;13:291–310.
8. Levine RJ, Ewell MG, Hauth JC, Curet LB, Catalano PM, Morris CD, et al. Should the definition of preeclampsia include a rise in diastolic blood pressure of >/=15 mm Hg to a level <90 mm Hg in association with proteinuria? Am J Obstet Gynecol. 2000;183(4):787–92.
9. Menzies J, Magee LA, Li J, et al. Instituting surveillance guidelines and adverse outcomes in preeclampsia. Obstet Gynecol. 2007;110:121–7.
10. American College of Obstetricians and Gynaecologists (ACOG). Practice Bulletin No.125. Chronic hypertension in pregnancy. Obstet Gynaecol. 2012;119:396–407.
11. Facchinetti F, Allais G, Nappi RE, D'Amico R, Marozio L, Bertozzi L, et al. Migraine is a risk factor for hypertensive disorders in pregnancy: a prospective cohort study. Cephalalgia. 2009;29(3):286–92.
12. Craici I, Wagner S, Garovic VD. Preeclampsia and future cardiovascular risk: formal risk factor or failed stress test? Ther Adv Cardiovasc Dis. 2008;2(4):249–59.
13. Gant HF, Daley GL, Chand S, Whalley PJ, MacDonald PC. A study of angiotensin II pressor response throughout primigravid pregnancy. J Clin Invest. 1973;52:2682.
14. Shepard BL, Bonnar J. An ultrastructural study of uteroplacental spiral arteries in hypertensive and normotensive pregnancies and fetal growth retardation. Br J Obstet Gynaecol. 1987;157:331.

15. Friedman SA. Preeclampsia: a review of the role of prostaglandins. Obstet Gynecol. 1988;71:122.
16. Taylor RN, de Groot CJ, Cho YK, Lim KH. Circulating factors as markers and mediators of endothelial cell dysfunction in preeclampsia. Semin Reprod Endocrinol. 1998;16:17–31.
17. Conrad KP. Animal models of pre-eclampsia: do they exist? Fetal Med Rev. 1990;2:67–88.
18. Conrad KP, Kerchner LJ, Mosher MD. Plasma and 24-h NOx and cGMP during normal pregnancy and preeclampsia in women on a reduced NOx diet. Am J Physiol Renal Physiol. 1999;277:F48–57.
19. Mastrogiannis DS, O'Brien WF, Krammer J, Benoit R. Potential role of endothelin-1 in normal and hypertensive pregnancies. Am J Obstet Gynecol. 1991;165:1711–6.
20. Clark DE, Smith SK, He Y, Day KA, Licence DR, Corps AN, Lammoglia R, Charnock-Jones DS. A vascular endothelial growth factor antagonist is produced by the human placenta and released into the maternal circulation. Biol Reprod. 1998;59:1540–8.
21. August P, Lindheimer M. Pathophysiology of preeclampsia. In: Laragh J, Brenner BM, editors. Hypertension. New York: Raven; 1995. p. 2407–26.
22. Baker PN, Krasnow J, Roberts JM, Yeo K. Elevated serum levels of vascular endothelial growth factor in patients with preeclampsia. Obstet Gynecol. 1995;86:815.
23. Chesley LC, Cooper DW. Genetics of hypertension in pregnancy: possible single gene control of preeclampsia and eclampsia in the descendants of eclamptic women. Br J Obstet Gynaecol. 1986;93:898.
24. Dekker GA, Sibai BM. Etiology and pathogenesis of preeclampsia: current concepts. Am J Obstet Gynecol. 1998;179(5):1359–75.
25. Lockwood CJ, Peters JH. Increased plasma levels of EDI+ cellular fibronectin levels predict clinical signs of preeclampsia. Am J Obstet Gynecol. 1990;162:358.
26. Socol MI, Weiner CP, Louis G. Platelet activation in preeclampsia. Am J Obstet Gynecol. 1985;151:494.
27. Cunningham FG, Lindheimer MD. Hypertension in pregnancy. N Engl J Med. 1992;326:927.
28. Shahul S, Rhee J, Hacker MR. Subclinical left ventricular dysfunction in preeclamptic women with preserved left ventricular ejection fraction: a 2D speckle-tracking imaging study. Circ Cardiovasc Imaging. 2012;5:734.
29. Rafik Hamad R, Larsson A, Pernow J. Assessment of left ventricular structure and function in preeclampsia by echocardiography and cardiovascular biomarkers. J Hypertens. 2009;27:2257.
30. Hankins GD, Wendel GD Jr, Cunningham FG, Leveno KJ. Longitudinal evaluation of hemodynamic changes in eclampsia. Am J Obstet Gynecol. 1984;150:506.
31. Minakami H, Oka N, Sato T. Preeclampsia: a microvesicular fat disease of the liver? Am J Obstet Gynecol. 1988;159:1043.
32. Dani R, Mendes GS, Mediros JL. Study of the liver changes occurring in preeclampsia and their possible pathogenic connection with acute fatty liver of pregnancy. Am J Gastroenterol. 1996;91:292.
33. Spargo B, McCartney CP, Winemitter R. Glomerular capillary endotheliosis in toxemia of pregnancy. Arch Pathol. 1959;68:593.
34. Craici IM, Wagner SJ, Bailey KR, Fitz-Gibbon PD, Wood-Wentz CM, Turner ST, et al. Podocyturia predates proteinuria and clinical features of preeclampsia. Hypertension. 2013;61:1289–96.
35. Taufield PA, Ales KL, Resnick LM. Hypocalciuria in preeclampsia. N Engl J Med. 1987;316:715.
36. Burrows RF, Hunter DJ, Andrew M, Kelton JG. A prospective study in investigating the mechanism of thrombocytopenia in preeclampsia. Obstet Gynecol. 1987;70:334.
37. Roberts JM, May WJ. Consumptive coagulopathy in severe preeclampsia. Obstet Gynecol. 1976;48:163.
38. Pritchard JA, Cunningham FG, Mason RA. Coagulation changes in eclampsia: their frequency and pathogenesis. Am J Obstet Gynecol. 1976;124:855.
39. Weiner CP, Brandt J. Plasma antithrombin III activity: an aid in the diagnosis of preeclampsia-eclampsia. Am J Obstet Gynecol. 1982;142:275.
40. Redman CWG, Denson KWE, Beilin LJ. Factor VIII consumption in preeclampsia. Lancet. 1977;2:1249.
41. Carpenter F, Kava HL, Plotkin D. The development of total blindness as a complication of pregnancy. Am J Obstet Gynecol. 1953;66:641.
42. Sheehan HL, Lynch JB. Pathology of toxaemia of pregnancy. London: Chuchill and Livingston; 1973.
43. Richards A, Graham D, Bullock R. Clinicopathological study of neurological complications due to hypertensive disorders of pregnancy. J Neurol Neurosurg Psychiatry. 1988;51:416.
44. Poon LC, Kametas NA, Chelemen T, Leal A, Nicolaides KH. Maternal risk factors for hypertensive disorders in pregnancy: a multivariate approach. J Hum Hypertens. 2010;24:104–10.
45. Akolekar R, Syngelaki A, Poon L, Wright D, Nicolaides KH. Competing risks model in early screening for preeclampsia by biophysical and biochemical markers. Fetal Diagn Ther. 2013;34(1):43.
46. World Health Organization (WHO). WHO recommendations for prevention and treatment of pre-eclampsia and eclampsia. Geneva: World Health Organization (WHO); 2011. p. 38.
47. Barton JR, Stanziano GJ, Sibai BM. Monitored outpatient management of mild gestational hypertension remote from term. Am J Obstet Gynecol. 1994;170:765.
48. Management of severe preeclampsia and eclampsia. 2012 Guidelines and Audit Implementation Network.
49. Hypertension in pregnancy. Nice clinical guideline (March 2008).
50. Duley L, Gulmezoglu AM, Henderson-Smart DJ, et al. Magnesium sulphate and other anticonvulsants for women with pre-eclampsia. Cochrane Database Syst Rev. 2010;(11):CD000025. https://doi.org/10.1002/14651858.CD000025.pub2.
51. Pritchard JA, Cunningham FG, Pritchard SA. The Parkland Memorial Hospital protocol for treatment of eclampsia: evaluation of 245 cases. Am J Obstet Gynecol. 1984;148:951–63.
52. Ekele BA, Ahmed Y. Magnesium sulphate regimens for eclampsia. Int J Gynaecol Obstet. 2004;87:149–50.
53. FMOH. National Clinical Service Protocol for Obstetrics and Neonatal Care; 2006.
54. Johnson DD. Induced labour for pre-eclampsia and gestational hypertension. Lancet. 2009;374(9694):951–2.
55. Mattar F, Sibai BM. Eclampsia VIII. Risk factors for maternal morbidity. Am J Obstet Gynecol. 2000;182(2):307–12.
56. Makhseed M, Musini VM. Eclampsia in Kuwait 1981–1993. Aust N Z J Obstet Gynaecol. 1996;36(3):258–63.
57. Douglas KA, Redman CWG. Eclampsia in the United Kingdom. BMJ. 1994;309:1395–400.
58. Duley L. The global impact of pre-eclampsia and eclampsia. Semin Perinatol. 2009;33(3):130–7.
59. Katz VL, Farmer R, Kuller JA. Preeclampsia into eclampsia: toward a new paradigm. Am J Obstet Gynecol. 2000;182:1389–96.
60. Vezzani A, Granata T. Brain inflammation in epilepsy: experimental and clinical evidence. Epilepsia. 2005;46(11):1724–43.
61. Shaner MD. Neurological problems of pregnancy. In: Bradley WG, Daroff RB, Fenichel GM, Marsden CD, editors. Neurology in clinical practice. 85. II. Boston: Butterworth-Heinemann; 2000. p. 2257–67.

Critical Care Management of Severe Preeclampsia-Eclampsia and Obstetric Hypertensive Crisis

27

Jacob Aghomon Unuigbe

Learning Objectives

This chapter brings to the reader vast clinical information in respect of severe preeclampsia-eclampsia and obstetric hypertensive crisis (SP-EOHC):

- Epidemiological, aetiological and pathophysiological background on SP-EOHC
- Focus on evidence-based approach to critical maternal and perinatal care
- Team approach to patient management
- Management of seizures and hypertensive crisis with emphasis on careful choice of drug medication
- Obstetric management with emphasis on surveillance aimed at assuring maternal and perinatal safety
- Critical intrapartum and postnatal maternal care
- Puerperal and later-life obstetric and medical surveillance of mothers

27.1 Introduction

Despite the worldwide decline in maternal mortality rates in the last two decades, high rates still exist, notably in impoverished communities, with over 85% living in sub-Saharan Africa and Southern Asia [1]. At the country level, in 2008, Nigeria (with 50,000 maternal deaths) was second only to India (with 63,000 maternal deaths) out of a global total of 358,000 maternal deaths [2]. And, according to a UNFPA report, India (19% or 56,000) and Nigeria (14% or 40,000) accounted for roughly one-third of the global maternal deaths in 2010 [3].

Latest figures in 2012 show a decreasing global trend with an annual total of 287,000 deaths in 2010 from a total of 543,000 deaths in 1990 [4]. Nigeria does not appear to benefit from this global trend. Nigeria is one of the 10 most unsafe countries for a woman giving birth and is reportedly responsible for 14% of the world's maternal deaths [5]. Nigeria's maternal mortality ratio (MMR) is estimated to be 576 deaths per 100,000 live births, with a lifetime risk of 1 in 30 women [5]. Health facility MMRs in different regions in Nigeria covering specific periods of time over the past three decades from 1988 include the following:

Olatunji et al. from Shagamu (1696/100,000 live births); Alabi et al. from Federal Medical Centre, Kogi State (463/100,000 live births); Onakewhor and Gharoro, UBTH, Edo State (454/100,000 live births); Igberase and Ebeigbe, Baptist Medical Centre, Eku, Delta State (2232/100,000 live births); Kullima et al. Federal Medical Centre, Nguru (2849/100,000 live births); and Oladapo et al. OOUTH, Shagamu, (2989/100,000 live births) [6].

Sadly, severe preeclampsia-eclampsia and obstetric hypertensive crisis (SP-EOHC) contributes an increasing prominent quota to these uncontrolled deaths. Preeclampsia and eclampsia are the leading causes of maternal mortality and are responsible for 28% of maternal deaths, followed by haemorrhage (24%) and pregnancy-related infection/sepsis (14.2%) [7]. The proportion of MMR that is attributable to preeclampsia/eclampsia ranges from 12.4% of 97 maternal deaths in South Eastern [8] to 42.2% of 277 maternal deaths in North Western Nigeria [9].

The industrialised countries present a totally different picture. Successive UK triennial Confidential Enquiry into Maternal Deaths (CEMD) reports over the past two decades show a decreasing trend in the contribution of hypertensive crisis to maternal morbidity and mortality [9–11]. In the most recent CEMD report (2009–2012) [12], deaths from SP-EOHC are now at the lowest ever recorded rate; the rate

J. A. Unuigbe (✉)
College of Health Sciences, Igbinedion University, Okada, Nigeria
e-mail: unuigbe.jacob@iuokada.edu.ng

F. Okonofua et al. (eds.), *Contemporary Obstetrics and Gynecology for Developing Countries*,
https://doi.org/10.1007/978-3-030-75385-6_27

decreased significantly between 2006–2008 (19 deaths – 0.83/100,000 maternities) and 2010–2012 (9 deaths – 0.38/100,000 maternities). This follows the introduction of NICE guidelines on hypertension in pregnancy in 2010 [13].

It is pertinent to note that in the 2006–2008 UK triennial report (2011) [14], 9 of the 19 maternal deaths resulting from SP-EOHC occurred among black women, six of whom were black Africans. Black African women seem particularly susceptible to aggressive forms of preeclampsia. In Nigeria, preeclampsia and eclampsia are responsible for about 8000 of the estimated 57,000 maternal deaths that occur annually.

This chapter focuses on evidence-based approach to the *critical care management of severe preeclampsia and obstetric hypertensive crisis (SP-EOHC)*. The aim is to increase the safety and stability of the woman and constantly monitor foetal well-being as an integral part of management protocol.

27.2 Aetiology of Preeclampsia: Abnormal Placentation

Figure 27.1 [15] presents a graphic representation of events at the placental site with explanation provided on the aetiological sequence of preeclampsia.

The net result is impaired trophoblast invasion and the spiral arteries remain as small calibre resistance vessels resulting in reduced placental perfusion and ischaemia.

Brosens et al. have painstakingly studied the disorders of deep placentation and provided evidence to implicate this pathology as an important background to major negative obstetric and perinatal outcomes 'Major Obstetric Syndromes' in affected women [16] (Table 27.1 below).

Figure 27.2 graphically shows the 'cascade mechanisms' of events that finally result in severe preeclampsia and eclampsia and the numerous serious systemic complications. These complications affect the haematological, hepatic, cardiovascular, renal, and central nervous (including the eyes) systems, and the placenta [17].

27.2.1 Mechanism of Seizures Complicating Preeclampsia

Two hypotheses are propounded regarding the mechanism of seizures complicating preeclampsia [18].

Table 27.1 Brosens classification of defective deep placentation: Association with adverse pregnancy outcomes [16]

Type of myometrial (junctional zone) spiral artery remodelling	Phenotype (pregnancy outcome)
1. Partial	Preterm labour Preterm prelabour rupture of membranes Intra uterine growth restriction without Hypertension
2. Absent	Preeclampsia
3. Absent with obstructive lesions	Preeclampsia with intra uterine growth restriction Abruptio placentae Placental infarcts with foetal death Late spontaneous miscarriage

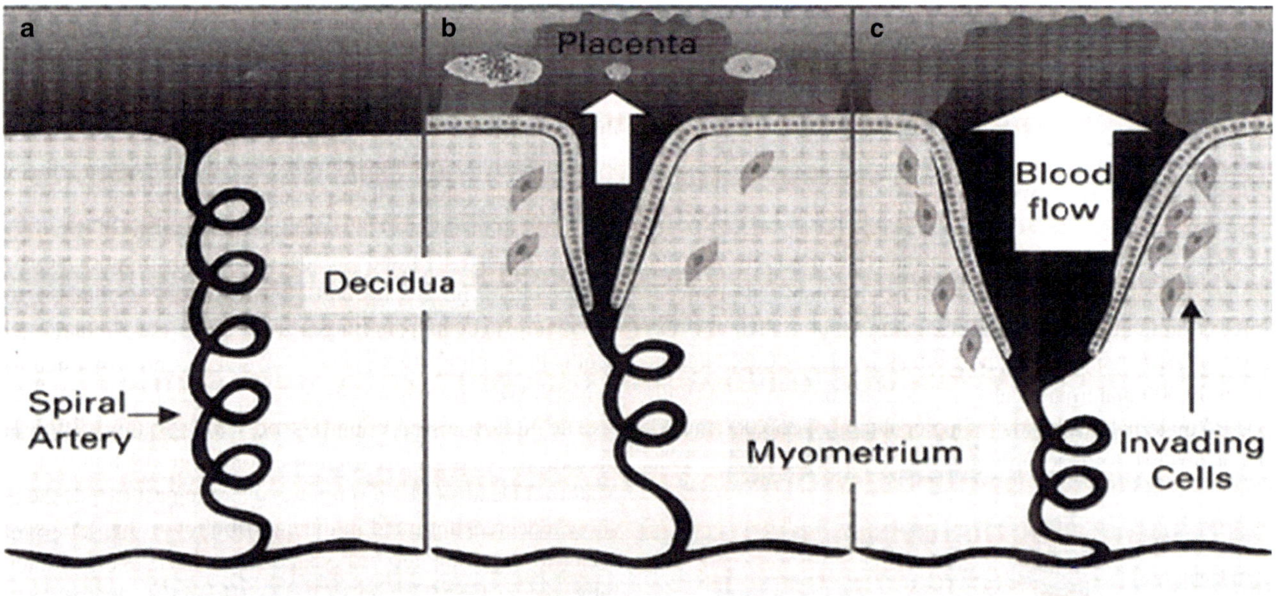

Fig. 27.1 In normal placental development, invasive cells of placental origin (trophoblast) invade maternal uterine spiral arteries (**a**) transforming them from smallcalibre resistance vessels (**b**) at the myometrial JZ, to high-calibre capacitance vessels, providing adequate perfusion to sustain foetal development (c). (Courtesy Crocker and Heazell [15])

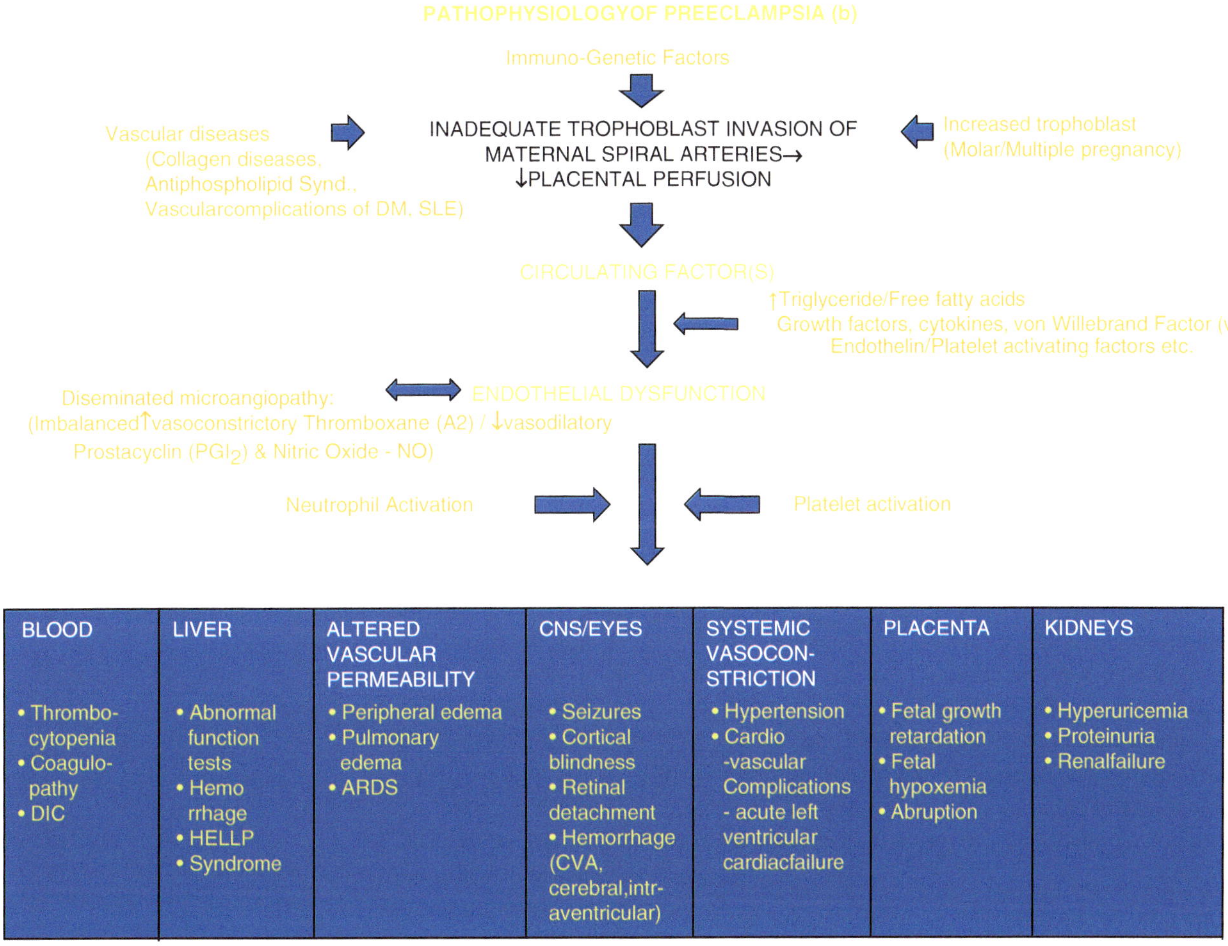

Fig. 27.2 Pathophysiology of Preeclampsia. (Unuigbe, JA)

1. The cerebral circulation is in a state of 'over-autoregulation' during preeclampsia in response to elevated cerebral perfusion pressure causing transient ischaemia complicated by vasogenic oedema (and reversible clinical course). This pathological process does not progress to ischaemic necrosis that would be complicated by cytotoxic oedema (and irreversible cerebral cortical lesion).
2. This is a form of hypertensive encephalopathy during which a rapid BP rise overcomes the myogenic cerebral arterial (and arteriolar) vasoconstriction, causing the loss of autoregulatory capacity and blood-brain barrier (BBB) disruption with subsequent vasogenic oedema. The unexplained propensity for hyperperfusion and oedema formation in the posterior cerebral cortex is termed *the posterior reversible encephalopathy syndrome (PRES)*. Suggested possible explanation is the decreased sympathetic innervations of the posterior cerebral arteries.

27.3 Principles of Management of Severe Preeclampsia and Eclampsia

The WHO Technical Consultation [14, 19] made a total of 23 recommendations on interventions in the management of women with severe preeclampsia and eclampsia. Ten of these interventions have strong supporting evidence, and four strongly lack supporting evidence. These recommended interventions need to be adopted, with local adaptations where necessary, in the protocol for patient management.

27.4 Team Approach

Success with comprehensive emergency obstetric care (CEmOC), especially with respect to SP-EOHC, is very much tied to team approach that relies on active timely full participation of all team members. Specifically, emphasis is now tilted in the direction of meticulous team approach to maternity care based on the concept of a 24-hour health institutional combat readiness (24H-HICR). The ACOG identifies the continued development of the Obstetric Gynaecologic Hospitalist (Labourist) Model as the potential approach to achieving professional and patient satisfaction while maintaining safe and effective care across delivery settings [20–24]. An expert review by Olson et al. [25] addresses the advantages, challenges, and variety of hospitalist models, focusing on what may be considered an emerging trend and a sustainable model for improved patient care and safety. The RCOG in collaboration with the National Health Service (NHS) has adopted a policy of increased senior medical staff participation in emergency obstetric care with specific injunction on 'increased consultant presence in delivery suites'. [26–28] The team approach to CEmOC constitutes the main focus for the SP-EOHC management protocol.

The key personnel required for sustainable '24-HICR' obstetric team include the following:

1. Obstetric Registrar on call.
2. Anaesthetic Registrar on call.
3. Senior labour ward midwife.
4. Consultant Obstetrician on call.
5. Consultant Anaesthetist/Intensivist [22] on call.
6. Haematology and clinical chemistry laboratory staff need to be aware of case.
7. Hospital administrative officer-on-duty needs to be aware of case.

Criteria for patient inclusion in the management protocol [14]

Any woman with severe proteinuric hypertension where the decision has been made to deliver and with one of the following criteria (1–3, or):

1. Hypertension (>140/90 mm Hg) with proteinuria (>0.3 g/day or >2+) and at least one of the following:
   (a) Headache, visual disturbance, epigastric pain.
   (b) Clonus (>3 beats).
   (c) Platelet count less than 100 × 10^9/L, ALT (Alanine aminotransferase) >50 iu/l.
   (d) Creatinine greater than 100 or creatinine clearance less than 80.
2. Severe hypertension (systolic ≥160 mm Hg or diastolic ≥110 mm Hg) with proteinuria (>0.5 g/day or >2+).
3. Eclampsia.
4. Clinical discretion should be used to include women who present with atypical symptoms.

Identifying life-threatening severe preeclampsia

- Severe HTN in association with proteinuria.
- HTN in association with severe proteinuria (≥5 g/24 hours).
- Clinical evidence of multi-organ involvement:
  - Pulmonary oedema
  - Seizures
  - Oliguria (<500 ml/24 hours)
  - Thrombocytopenia (<10^5/mm^3)
  - Abnormal liver enzymes/epigastric pain/right upper quadrant pain
  - Persistent severe neurological symptoms (altered mental status, headaches, blurred vision or sudden blindness)
- Oedema not a mandatory diagnostic feature but a warning presentation when present.
- The HELLP syndrome represents a peculiar presentation of severe preeclampsia.

Differential Diagnoses of Eclampsia

It is vitally important that any medical staff summoned to see an obstetric patient presenting with convulsions has the following in mind:

1. Eclampsia
2. Epilepsy
3. Cerebral malaria
4. A. Meningitis
   B. Encephalitis
5. Diabetes mellitus
   - Hyperglycaemia
   - Hypoglycaemia
6. Drug intoxication
7. SS disease – Cerebral vascular ischaemia
8. Raised intracranial pressure/intracranial vasculopathy:
   - Abscess
   - Tumour
   - Ruptured aneurysm
   - Haemorrhage from other sources

Maternal Observations and Investigations

1. Monitoring requires a one-to-one expert nursing care.
2. All maternal observations should be recorded on a specialised pregnancy-induced hypertension chart or an ICU chart.
3. Oxygen saturation should be continuously monitored when possible.
4. Blood pressure recordings should be made every 15–20 minutes.
5. Maternal temperature should be recorded hourly.
6. A Foley catheter should be in situ and hourly urinary output measured.
7. Routine blood samples should be taken every 12–24 hours, including full blood count, urea and electrolytes, creatinine and liver function tests.

Foetal monitoring
Minimum assessment of foetal well-being should include the following:

1. Growth assessment scans by medical staff.
2. Liquor volume assessment.
3. Continuous external foetal monitoring (CTG).
4. Umbilical cord Doppler if the woman's condition allows, when possible.

27.5 Management of Seizures [29]

27.5.1 Management of Seizures: The +MAGPIE Study

The Eclampsia Trial Collaborative Group (ETCG), co-ordinated by the Perinatal Trials Service in Oxford, conducted a landmark multicentre study on 1687 women with eclampsia from 28 centres in South America, India and Africa comparing Magnesium sulphate[1] with phenytoin on one hand, and magnesium sulphate with Valium on the other. The 'MAGPIE Study'[2] (1995) established that magnesium sulphate is more effective in preventing recurrent seizures following eclampsia than either phenytoin or diazepam [30–34]. Unfortunately, difficulties still exist regarding acceptance and use of $MgSO_4$ in many developing countries, including Nigeria [35].

27.5.2 Mechanisms of Magnesium Sulphate for Seizure Prevention [18]

The mechanisms by which magnesium sulphate ($MgSO_4$) is effective at preventing eclamptic convulsions are likely multifactorial and have been reviewed in many publications and will only be summarised here. $MgSO_4$ is a calcium antagonist and as such could inhibit vascular smooth muscle contraction. $MgSO_4$ is a potent vasodilator, however, its effects in the cerebral circulation are considerably less effective than systemic vasculature. In addition, the sensitivity to $MgSO_4$ is decreased in cerebral arteries from late-pregnant and postpartum animals, suggesting $MgSO_4$ is not acting as a vasodilator in the cerebral circulation. $MgSO_4$ has been shown to protect the blood-brain barrier (BBB), likely through its calcium antagonistic effects in the cerebral endothelium. When pregnant rats were treated with clinically relevant doses of $MgSO_4$, they had significantly less BBB permeability during acute hypertension. Thus, $MgSO_4$ could prevent recurrent seizures by protecting the BBB. Lastly, $MgSO_4$ is an N-Methyl-D-aspartate (NMDA) receptor antagonist and thus would act as an anticonvulsant if it were in high enough concentration in the brain.

[1] ($MgSO_4 \cdot 7H_2O$ = Epsom Salt).

[2] MAGPIE = MAGnesium for PreventIon of Eclampsia.

27.5.3 Management of Seizures

1. General measures [36] valid for all types of seizures: Securing airway, oxygenation circulation:
   - Turn patient to side.
   - Protect patient from injury but do not restrain patient.
   - Maintain airway (insert airway if possible) + give 100% O_2 by tight face mask once seizures stop.
   - Suction mouth if necessary.
   - Establish IV access for medication, hydration, blood work.
2. All women with eclampsia should be treated with magnesium sulphate as the first-line drug of choice. The intravenous (IV) route is preferable.
3. A loading dose of 4 g magnesium sulphate should be given (IV) over 5–10 minutes. With this bolus dose as an immediate protection, a second (intramuscular) loading dose 10 g (*Not favoured by many clinicians*) is given as two injections of 5 g in each buttock, followed by a maintenance infusion of 1–2 g/hour IV per hour, continued for at least 24 hours after the last seizure. Recurrent seizures should be treated by a further I.V. bolus of 2 g magnesium sulphate.
4. Use of diazepam on mothers, especially in late pregnancy, is generally discouraged; may be administered in single doses if fits continue, at the discretion of the consultant/neurologist. Prolonged use of diazepam is associated with increased incidence of maternal mortality.
5. Magnesium levels (normal value 0.7–1.0 mmol/litre) should be monitored when repeat fits occur or renal compromise is evident (therapeutic range 2–4 mmol/litre).
6. Deep tendon reflexes should be monitored hourly when magnesium therapy is commenced. If reflexes are absent, or respirations are less than 14 per minute, or SaO_2 less than 95%, magnesium therapy should be stopped.
7. Monitor urinary output – should not be less than 25 ml/hour.
8. If the fits continue, it is important to exclude other causes of fits and a CT scan should be considered.
9. Reversal of the depressant effects of $MgSO_4$: Give 10 ml of 10% calcium gluconate (1 g IV) over 10 minutes.
10. Prophylactic H_2 antagonists (antacids) should be given until the woman is transferred to normal postnatal care.

27.6 Use of Magnesium Sulphate: Maternal, Perinatal, Infant and Late Childhood Effects [37–41]

A country-wide multicentre, placebo-controlled, double-blind randomised trial was conducted by Rouse et al. [37] in the USA in 2008, involving 2241 expectant mothers at imminent risk for delivery between 24 and 31 weeks' gestation. Women assigned to receive $MgSO_4$ were given a 6-g bolus intravenously followed by a constant infusion of 2 g per hour, or matching placebo, for about 3 hours. Maternal effects of $MgSO_4$ treatment, significant but tolerable included flushing, sweating, pain/burning at intravenous site, nausea or vomiting and respiratory depression. Foetal exposure to magnesium sulphate before anticipated preterm delivery did not reduce the combined risk of moderate/severe cerebral palsy or death (stillbirth/infant death) However, the rate of cerebral palsy was reduced among child survivors. Other publications [38–40] essentially confirm the foetal neuroprotective effect of $MgSO_4$. A more recent meta-analysis and Cochrane review by Sana Usman et al. [41] from London, UK, on the use of $MgSO_4$ in preterm deliveries provides further evidence in favour of modest neuroprotective effect which is greater the earlier the gestational age at delivery. The authors recommend its use in preterm deliveries less than 30–32 weeks of gestation, guided by local policy.

Specifically, the effects of magnesium sulphate on intrapartum foetal CTG and perinatal outcome have been scrutinised in a study by Duffy et al. [42] In a 4-year retrospective cohort study (from Washington University, St Louis, MO, USA) of 5387 consecutive term deliveries, of whom 248 (4.6%) had prenatal $MgSO_4$ for severe preeclampsia/eclampsia, women exposed were compared to women not exposed to magnesium. The results show that maternal exposure to magnesium is associated with lower fetal heart rate (FHR) baseline within the accepted normal range, decreased variability, and fewer prolonged decelerations without evidence of adverse effect on neonatal outcome. These findings suggest that magnesium minimally blunts foetal response towards tachycardia, marked variability and prolonged decelerations, thus implying an overall minimal masking effect of magnesium on signs of foetal distress, not severe enough to influence the overall perinatal outcome.

27.7 Management of Hypertension

Women with acute severe late pregnancy and intrapartum hypertension have significantly higher risk of severe maternal morbidity than women without severe hypertension [43]. Severe hypertension is defined as greater than 160/110 mm Hg or mean arterial pressure (MAP) greater than 125 mm Hg. Significantly, while diastolic BP is a useful index of severity of preeclampsia, elevated systolic BP (≥160) carries the serious risk of intracranial (intracerebral) haemorrhage [10, 12]. Cerebrovascular accident accounts for 15–20% of deaths from eclampsia. The risk of haemorrhagic stroke correlates directly with the degree of elevation in systolic blood pressure and is less related to, but not independent of, the diastolic blood pressure [17].

Aggressive antihypertensive therapy is recommended at sustained systolic and diastolic blood pressures of 160 and 110 mm Hg, respectively. The commonly used drugs for obstetric hypertensive crisis are hydralazine, immediate release oral nifedipine and labetalol. *Protocols that include additional requirements in order to provide urgent IV hypertension therapy lead to unnecessary and dangerous delays (that can be fatal) in reducing time to treatment for severe hypertension for pregnant and post-partum patients* [29].

It is pertinent to consider the danger attendant in induction of general anaesthesia in the midst of uncontrolled hypertension. Induction of anaesthesia and endotracheal intubation carry the grave risk of dangerously increasing an already high blood pressure to a catastrophic level that imperils the brain (cerebral haemorrhage), the heart (myocardial ischaemia) and the lungs (pulmonary oedema), all important causes of maternal death. Blood pressure must be brought down to safe levels before induction of general anaesthesia [29, 44, 45].

27.8 Hydralazine

Hydralazine was until recently considered the first-line drug of choice for management of severe hypertension titrated against blood pressure, except in the presence of tachycardia (greater than 120 bpm). The agreed dose is 5 mg IV repeated every 20 minutes, to a maximum cumulative dose of 20 mg (Fig. 27.3).

27.8.1 Obstetric Side Effects of Hydralazine

Hydralazine is still considered useful and effective for treatment of acute hypertensive crisis by advocates but many obstetricians now shy away from its adoption as a first-line drug of choice. The adverse effects are considered grave and include severe maternal 'overshoot' hypotension and considerably reduced placental blood flow that may be disproportional to administered doses, with resulting adverse effects on foetal heart rates – maternal and foetal tachycardia. The attendant increased caesarean section rates may occasionally be secondary to the foetal distress caused by these side effects. Other recorded side effects include increased incidence of placental abruption and maternal oliguria [45–47].

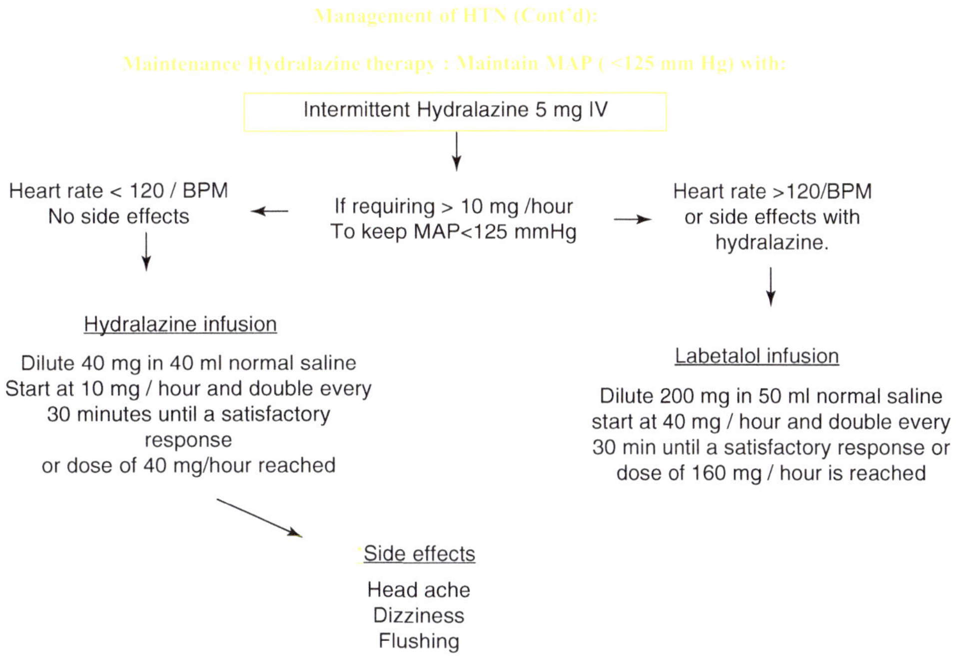

Fig. 27.3 Parenteral treatment of HTN with hydralazine

These side effects are considered sufficiently serious to warrant discontinuation of hydralazine use as a first-line drug in increasing number of obstetric units [45].

27.9 Adalat (Nifedipine)

Nifedipine notably in the form of *immediate release oral nifedipine* has now found a favourable place as a useful first-line antihypertensive medication. Oral nifedipine and intravenous labetalol regimes were found to be similarly effective, or nifedipine more effective in the control of acute hypertensive crisis [48, 49]. The ACOG has now added nifedipine as a first-line treatment option in the management of obstetric hypertensive crisis [29].

When sustained severe obstetric hypertension is established, the common regimen of oral nifedipine administered is 10 mg, repeated every 20 minutes with patient's vital signs under surveillance. Usually, a cumulative maximum dose of 50 mg is required to bring the blood pressure to safe level – 140–150/90–100. Maintenance dose of nifedipine, 10 mg 8-hourly or long-acting nifedipine (Adalat-Retard), 20 mg 12-hourly, is administered. Other regimens include additional use of hydralazine or labetalol in combination with nifedipine [29].

Caution needs to be exercised in its use, notably when $MgSO_4$ is in use because of the synergistic Ca++ – blocking effect, which can lead to profound hypotension and shock [29]. Sublingual nifedipine must be avoided at all cost because of possible irreversible severe hypotension with consequent severe maternal and perinatal morbidity and mortality.

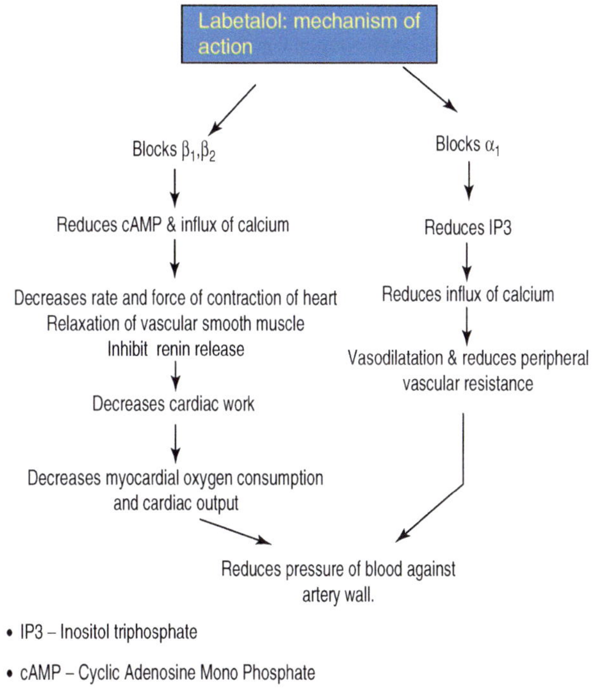

Fig. 27.4 Labetalol: mechanism of action

27.10 Labetalol (Fig. 27.4)

27.10.1 Labetalol: Clinical Pharmacology

Labetalol combines both selective, competitive α_1 – adrenergic blocking and non-selective, competitive β – adrenergic blocking activity in a single substance. In man, the ratio of α- to β-blockade are about 1:3 and 1:7 following oral and IV administration respectively. Labetalol produces dose-related falls in blood pressure without reflex tachycardia and without significant reduction in heart rate, through a mixture of its α- and β-blocking effects. Haemodynamic effects are variable with small non-significant changes in cardiac output.

Doses of labetalol that control hypertension do not affect renal function in mild-to-severe hypertensive patients with normal renal function.

Due to the α_1-receptor blocking activity of labetalol, BP is lowered more in the standing than in the supine position, and symptoms of postural hypotension can occur. This should be considered during IV administration and positioning of patients. Such patients should not be allowed to move to an erect position unmonitored until their ability to do so is established.

Labetalol is now considered by increasing number of physicians as the first-line drug of choice for management of acute hypertensive crisis. Labetalol is considered to be at least as effective, more predictable, more acceptable, and produces no change in heart rate compared to hydralazine [45, 50]. Indeed, some studies suggest possible advantages and no apparent disadvantages for the foetus during its use in pregnancy [51]. The protocol of combined use of magnesium sulphate and Labetalol (Labet) adopted in Benin City, Nigeria was found to be beneficial in the plan to reduce mortality complicating severe preeclampsia, eclampsia and severe hypertensive crisis in pregnancy [52].

Treatment is commenced with parenteral labetalol (*Trandate, Labet, Normodyne)*, 20 mg bolus, followed at 10–20 minute intervals by 40 mg, 80 mg, 80 mg and 80 mg boluses till the desired BP (140–150/85–95 mm Hg) is achieved. The maximum cumulative dose that can be given is 300 mg. This is followed up with oral labetalol, through nasogastric tube if necessary, commencing with a dose of 200 mg 8-hourly. The usual maintenance dosage of labetalol is between 200 and 400 mg twice daily (the maximum daily dose of 2400 mg is hardly applicable to obstetric patients).

27.11 Intravenous Use of Labetalol for Hypertensive Crisis

Two methods recommended:

1. *Repeated IV injections*:
   Initial dose of 20 mg by slow injection for 2 minutes; repeat injection of 40 mg after 10–20 minutes; and then repeated doses of 80 mg given at 10–20-minute intervals till the desired BP (130–150/85–95) is achieved. The maximum cumulative dose of labetalol that can be administered is 300 mg. The maximum effect on BP usually occurs within 5 minutes of administration. Continue antihypertensive treatment with oral Trandate (usually 200 mg 8-hourly).
2. *Slow continuous infusion:*

Effective IV dose is usually in the range of 50–200 mg given at infusion rate of 2 mg minute. A total of 300 mg may be required. Monitor BP during infusion, and continuous infusion till satisfactory response is obtained. After discontinuation, oral labetalol is initiated.

Method: The contents of 2 vials[3] (40 ml) are added to 160 ml of compatible IV fluids. The resultant 200 ml of solution will contain 200 mg labetalol (1 mg/1 ml). The diluted solution should be administered (using an *Ivac* or a *Cardiff* infusion pump at a rate of 2 ml/min) to deliver 2 mg/minute.

27.11.1 Side Effects

1. Postural hypotension and scalp tingling.
2. Bradycardia (Severe bradycardia controlled with atropine 1–2 mg intravenously).
3. Nausea, vomiting, headache and epigastric pain.
4. Foetal bradycardia and distress (caused by severe maternal bradycardia).

27.11.2 Precautions [29, 50]

1. Patient should be kept in the supine position during IV administration.
2. Labetalol injection should not normally be given to patients with digitalis resistant *heart failure or atrio ventricular block.*
3. Caution with *asthmatic* patients or individuals prone to bronchospasm. Resulting bronchospasm is controlled by using selective – acting bronchodilator, for example, salbutamol, or atropine 1 mg IV.
4. Caution with *diabetics*, as it may prevent appearance of features (e.g. tachycardia) of acute hypoglycaemia. Betablockade also reduces release of insulin in response to hyperglycaemia. Therefore, necessity for adjustment of diabetes treatment arises.
5. Anaesthesia – With labetalol therapy, patient requires IV atropine prior to induction of GA; the effect of halothane on BP may be enhanced by labetalol.
6. Caution with women with history of impaired *hepatic* function. Severe hepatocellular injury is a recorded very rare complication.

[3]Two vials (20 ml/vial) of Trandate and Normodyne brands and four vials (10 ml/vial) of *Labet* brand.

7. Paradoxical hypertensive responses have been recorded with treatment of pheochromocytoma. Chung et al. reported intraoperative dramatic elevation of blood pressure during resection of a pheochromocytoma [53] This was caused by elevated systemic vascular resistance index (SVRI) and decreased cardiac index (CI), secondary to β-adrenergic blockade with labetalol. A suggestion is made for prompt replacement of labetalol with β-adrenergic blockers or other vasodilators when such a condition arises.

27.12 Treatment of Resistant Hypertension [29]

On the rare occasion when IV labetalol, hydralazine, or immediate release oral nifedipine fails to relieve severe hypertension, urgent consultation with an anaesthesiologist, intensivist, or maternal-foetal medicine specialist to discuss second-line intervention is recommended. Second-line alternatives include nicardipine or esmolol by infusion pump and sodium nitroprusside. Sodium nitroprusside should be reserved for extreme cases, and used for the shortest time, because of potential for maternal, foetal, and neonatal cyanide and thiocyanate toxicity, and increased maternal intracranial pressure and worsening of cerebral oedema.

27.13 Fluid Balance Management

The following guidelines need to be strictly adhered to in order to maintain safe fluid and electrolyte balance.

1. Fluid intake should be restricted to 85 ml/hour because of the risk of renal and respiratory sequelae; the risk of grave respiratory complications, notably pulmonary oedema, is greater than renal dysfunction or failure [54].
2. Urinary output should be measured hourly.
3. 500 ml human albumin solution (HAS) should be considered:
   - prior to antihypertensive therapy
   - prior to caesarean section
   - if oliguria is evident (defined as urinary output less than 100 ml in a consecutive 4-hour period)
   - prior to administration of regional anaesthesia.
4. If HAS has previously been administered, the insertion of a central venous pressure (CVP) line should be considered. If further complications occur, especially oliguria, after the administration of HAS, a line is recommended. Although the success rate of the subclavian-vein route is greater than the antecubital-fossa route, clinicians should use the route with which they are more familiar.
5. If the central venous pressure value is greater than 10 mm Hg, 20 mg furosemide should be considered.
6. If the central venous pressure value is less than 10 mm Hg, HAS 500 ml should be considered.
7. A further dose of 20–40 mg furosemide should be considered if there is persistent oliguria.

27.14 Obstetric Management

In the obstetric management of the patients, the choice lies between expectant and interventionist options. Expectant management [55, 56] includes in-patient care with steroids (with gestations remote from term), magnesium sulphate (as required), antihypertensive drugs and close maternal and foetal monitoring to identify indications for delivery. Also to be considered is in-utero transfer to centres with facility for intensive neonatal care for preterm babies. Figure 27.5 provides a clinical algorithm for the proposed management of severe preeclampsia remote from term. Table 27.2 provides a summary of indications for interventionist option in management [56, 57].

27.15 Eclampsia: Mode of Delivery

Caesarean section should no longer be considered a better option for women with eclampsia; indeed, abdominal surgery can place both mother and foetus at increased risk of adverse events, notably, if the mother is unstable and general endotracheal anaesthesia is used. Immediate delivery does not necessarily imply caesarean section; a properly managed and successful vaginal delivery is less haemodynamically stressful to the mother while providing additional advantages to term or late preterm neonate [57, 58]. A number of studies, including a randomised controlled pilot study by Seal et al. [59] provide evidence that a policy of early caesarean section delivery with ≥34 weeks' gestation, is not associated with better maternal or perinatal outcomes.

The decision to proceed with delivery through abdominal or vaginal route should be individualised based on such factors as parity, gestational age, Bishop's score, foetal status and maternal desire for vaginal birth. Prolonged inductions/labour must be avoided [60].

27.16 Post-partum SP-OHC [61]

The following need to be considered in the immediate postpartum surveillance of the woman with SP-OHC during the puerperium, notably in the first week:

1. New-onset HTN-preeclampsia
2. Persistent gestational HT N – preeclampsia

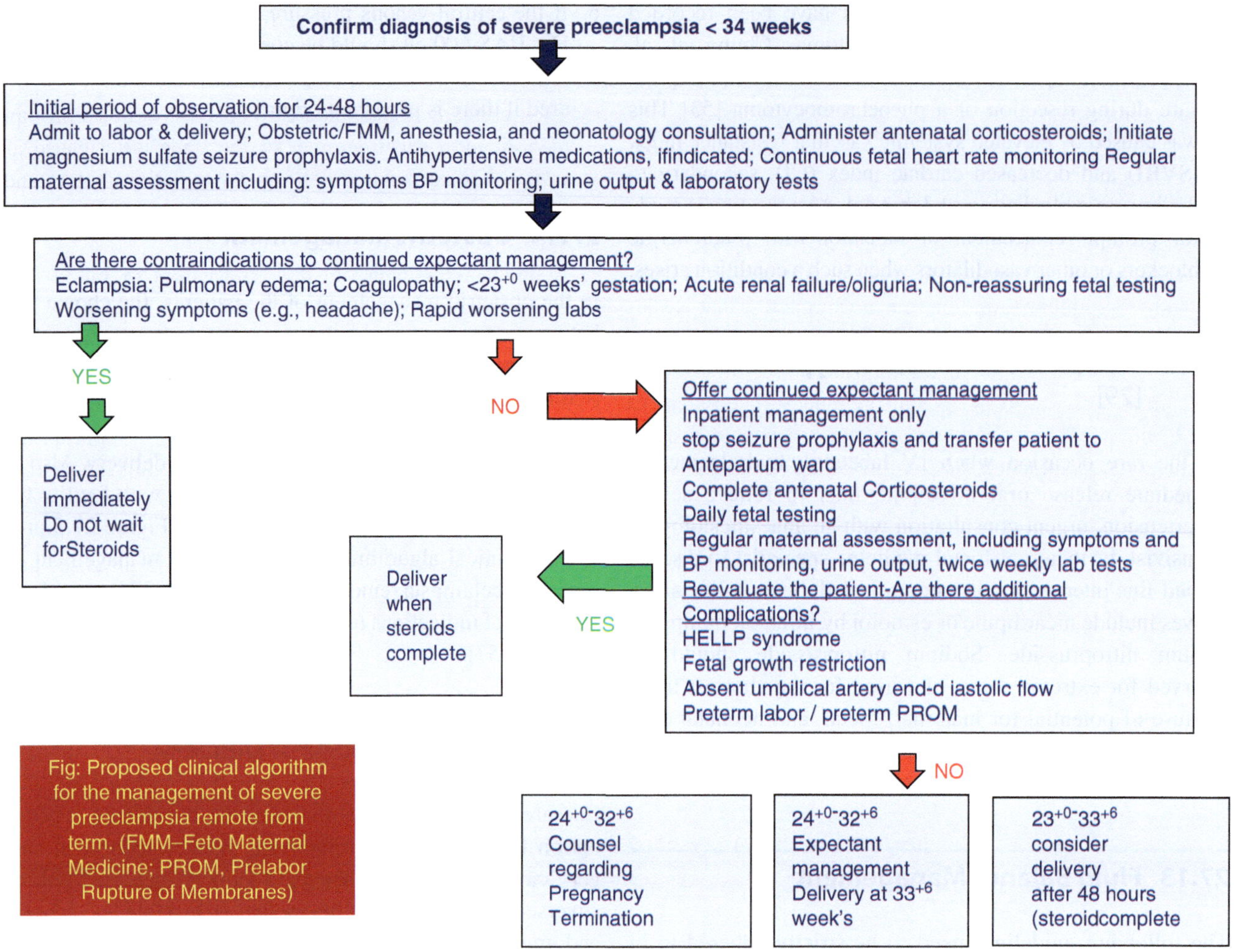

Fig. 27.5 Proposal for management of severe preeclampsia remote from term. (Courtesy Sibai and Norwitz [55])

Table 27.2 Indications for immediate delivery during expectant management of severe preeclampsia [56–58]

Foetal Indications	≥34 weeks gestation 33–34 weeks with documented foetal lung maturity Estimated foetal weight ˂5 percentile by ultrasound Abnormal foetal testing Repetitive variable or late decelerations Biophysical profiles (BPP) ≤4 on 2 occasions at least 4 hours apart Persistent reverse end-diastolic flow on umbilical artery Doppler velocimetry Rupture of membranes
Maternal indications	Preterm labour or vaginal bleeding Eclampsia or encephalopathy Pulmonary oedema or despite therapy Persistent thrombocytopenia Severe epigastric pain or cerebral symptoms Maternal request Severe hypertension unresponsive to maximum drug

3. Late-onset eclampsia
4. HELLP syndrome
5. Pre-existing/undiagnosed HTN – renal, adrenal, thyroid diseases
6. Cerebral vasoconstriction syndrome
7. Cerebral venous thrombosis/stroke
8. TTP/haemolytic uraemic syndrome

Increased awareness of differential diagnosis constitutes a cornerstone in the management of the patient. Team approach with a stepwise multidisciplinary approach makes for timely accurate diagnosis and successful management. Ideally, post-partum surveillance, including monitoring of the woman's blood pressure, requires an interval postnatal visit before the traditional 6 weeks postnatal visit. Thereafter women with persistent residual medical (cardiovascular, renal, neurological) challenges should be referred for appropriate medical consultation and follow-up.

27.17 SP-EOHC: Later-Life Medical Diseases

SP-EOHC may well represent a 'milestone' or an 'eye-opener' event that reflects a woman's lifetime syndrome of medical disability that will, in later life, culminate in serious medical conditions such as chronic hypertension [62, 63], diabetes mellitus [64], kidney [65] and cardiovascular diseases and death [66]. A spectacular systematic review and meta-analysis by Bellamy et al. [67] on long-term consequences of preeclampsia revealed that the relative risks (RRs) for hypertension were 3.70 after 14 years follow-up, for ischaemic heart disease 2.16 after 12 years, for stroke 1.81 after 10 years, and for venous thromboembolism 1.87 after 5 years. Overall mortality after preeclampsia was increased 1.5-fold after 14 years. Long-term follow-up studies also reveal that babies born preterm or growth-restricted are at increased risk of developing hypertension, coronary artery disease, and diabetes mellitus, and for growth-restricted female neonates, preeclampsia in later life [68, 69].

27.18 Summary and Recommendation

This chapter has explored the severe morbidity and mortality attending SP-EOHC and the important criteria that determine the successful outcome of obstetric and perinatal care of patients. Team approach, attention to timely emergency care of mothers, and use of appropriate anticonvulsant and antihypertensive medication are crucial to successful outcome in obstetric and perinatal management. Careful postnatal and puerperal care and later-life meticulous multidisciplinary surveillance, in alliance with internists, is an essential follow-up component of patients' care.

References

1. Trends in Maternal Mortality 1990–2015. Estimates developed by WHO, UNICEF, UNFPA, World Bank Group and the United Nations Population Division. Geneva: WHO; 2015. p. 1–100.
2. Trends in Maternal Mortality 1990–2008. Estimates developed by WHO, UNICEF, UNFPA, and The World Bank. Geneva: WHO; 2010. Assessed 7 Sept 2010. www.who.int/en/reproductivehealth.
3. Trends in Maternal Mortality: 1990 to 2010. WHO, UNICEF, UNFPA, and The World Bank estimates. Geneva: WHO; 2012.
4. Department of Health. Why mothers die, 1997–1999: the confidential enquiries into maternal deaths in the UK. London: RCOG; 2001.
5. NPC & ICF International. Nigeria demographic and health survey 2013; 2014.
6. Kirk K, Chattopadhyay I. A systematic review of the treatment and management of preeclampsia and eclampsia in Nigeria. Washington, DC: Population Council, USAID; 2015. p. 13.
7. Oladapo O, Adetoro O, Ekele B, Chama C, Etuk S, Aboyej A, Gulmezoglu A. When getting there is not enough: a nationwide cross-sectional study of 998 maternal deaths and 1451 near-misses in public tertiary hospitals in a low-income country. Br J Obstet Gynaecol. 2015. https://doi.org/10.1111/1471-0528.13450.
8. Nwagha UI, Nwachukwu D, Dim C, Ibekwe PCP, Onyebuchi A. Maternal mortality trend in South East Nigeria: less than a decade to the millennium development goals. J Womens Health. 2002;19(2):323–7.
9. Nwobodo E, Ahmed Y. Maternal mortality associated with eclampsia in Sokoto, Nigeria. Orient J Med. 2011;23:1–4.
10. The confidential enquiry into maternal and child health (CEMACH). Why mothers die, 2000–2002. Report on confidential enquiries into maternal deaths in the United Kingdom. London: RCOG; 2004.
11. The confidential enquiry into maternal health (CEMACH): saving mothers' lives. Reviewing maternal deaths to make motherhood safer, 2003–2005. CEMD in the UK. London: RCOG; 2007.
12. Knight M, Kenyon S, Brocklehurst P, Neilson J, Shakespeare J, Kurinczuk JJ, editors. Saving lives, improving mothers' care: lessons learned to inform future maternity care from the UK and Ireland confidential enquiries into maternal deaths and morbidity 2009–2012. Oxford: National Perinatal Epidemiology Unit, University of Oxford; 2014. p. 1–97.
13. NICE – National Institute for Health and Care Excellence. CG107 hypertension in pregnancy. 2010. From http://www.nice.org.uk/guidance/CG107.
14. The confidential enquiry into maternal and child health (CMACE). Saving mothers' lives. Reviewing maternal deaths to make motherhood safer: 2006–2008. 8th report of the CEMD in the UK. BJOG, An Int J Obstet Gynaecol. 2011;118(Suppl. 1):1–205.
15. Crocker I, Heazell A. Chapter 2: The pathophysiology of hypertension. In: Heazell A, Norwitz ER, Kenny LC, Baker P, editors. Hypertension in pregnancy. 1st ed. Cambridge: Cambridge University Press; 2010. p. 19–33.
16. Brosens I, Pijnenborg R, Vercruysse L, Romero R. "The great obstetrical syndromes" are associated with disorders of deep placentation. Am J Obstet Gynecol. 2011;204(3):193–201.
17. Norwitz ER, Chaur-Gong H, Repke JT. Acute complications of preeclampsia. Clin Obstet Gynecol. 2002;45(2):308–29.
18. Cipolla MJ, Kraig RP. Seizures in women with preeclampsia: mechanisms and management. Fetal Matern Med Rev. 2011;22(2):91–108.
19. World Health Organization. WHO Recommendations for prevention and treatment of preeclampsia and eclampsia. Geneva: WHO Press; 2011.
20. McCue B. What is an obstetrics/gynecology hospitalist? Obstet Gynecol Clin N Am. 2015;14(3):457–61.
21. Stevens TA, Swaim LS, Clark SL. The role of obstetrics/gynecology hospitalists in reducing maternal mortality. Obstet Gynecol Clin N Am. 2015;42(3):463–75.
22. American College of Obstetricians and Gynecologists. Committee opinion no. 459: the obstetric-gynecologic hospitalist. Obstet Gynecol. 2010;116:237–9.
23. Garite TJ, Levine L, Olson R. Business and organizational models of obstetric and gynecologic hospitalist groups. Obstet Gynecol Clin N Am. 2015;42(3):533–40.
24. American College of Obstetricians and Gynecologists (ACOG) Committee Opinion Number 657. The Obstetric and Gynecologic Hospitalist. ACOG Committee on patient safety, quality improvement and obstetric practice. Obstet Gynecol. 2016;127(2):419.
25. Olson R, Garite TJ, Fishman A, Andress IF. Obstetrician/gynecologist hospitalists: can we improve safety and outcomes for patients and hospitals and improve lifestyle for physicians? Am J Obstet Gynecol. 2012;207(2):81–6.
26. Edmonds S, Allenby K. Experiences of a 24-hour resident consultant service. TOG: Obstet Gynaecol. 2008;10:107–11.
27. Royal College of Obstetricians and Gynaecologists (RCOG). The future workforce in obstetrics and gynaecology in England and Wales: overview summary. London: RCOG; 2009.

28. Royal College of Obstetricians and Gynaecologists (RCOG). Labour ward solutions. RCOG Good Practice No. 10, January 2010.
29. American College of Obstetricians and Gynecologists (ACOG) Committee Opinion Number 692. Emergent therapy for acute-onset, severe hypertension during pregnancy and the postpartum period. J Obstet Gynaecol. 2017;129:769–70.
30. Eclampsia Trial Collaborative Group. Which anticonvulsant for women with Eclampsia? Evidence from the Collaborative Eclampsia Trial. Lancet. 1995;345:1455–63.
31. Atallah. The Eclampsia Trial, a model of international collaborative study with worldwide benefits. Sao Paulo Med J. 1995;113(4):927–8.
32. Duley L, Henderson-Smart DJ, Chou D. Magnesium versus Phenytoin for Eclampsia. Cochrane Database Syst Rev. 2010;(10):CD000128.
33. Duley L, Henderson-Smart DJ, Walker GJ, Chou D. Magnesium sulphate versus diazepam for eclampsia. Cochrane Database Syst Rev. 2010;12:CD000127.
34. Fawcett WJ, Haxby EJ, Male DA. Magnesium: physiology and pharmacology (Review Article). Br J Anaesth. 1999;83:302–20. (pp 304–307).
35. Ekele BA. Use of magnesium sulphate to manage preeclampsia and eclampsia in Nigeria: overcoming the odds. Ann Afr Med. 2009;8(2):73–5.
36. Anthony J. Chapter 78: Critical care of the obstetric patient. In: James DK, Steer PJ, Weiner CP, Gonik B, Crowther CA, Robson SC, editors. High risk pregnancy, management options. 4th ed. St Louis: Elsevier Saunders; 2011. p. 1347–60.
37. Rouse DJ, Hirtz DG, Thom E, et al. A randomized, controlled trial of magnesium sulphate for the prevention of cerebral palsy. N Engl J Med. 2008;359(9):895–905.
38. Stanley FJ, Crowther C. Antenatal magnesium sulfate for neuroprotection before preterm birth? N Engl J Med. 2008;359(9):962–4.
39. Doyle LW, Crowther CA, Middleton P, Marret S. Magnesium sulphate for women at risk of preterm birth for neuroprotection of the fetus. Cochrane Database Syst Rev. 2007;3:CD000025.
40. Royal College of Obstetricians and Gynaecologists (RCOG). The management of severe preeclampsia/eclampsia. Guideline No. 10(A). London: RCOG; 2006.
41. Usman S, Foo L, Tay J, Bennett PR, Lee C. Use of magnesium sulfate in preterm deliveries for neuroprotection of the neonate. RCOG – Obstet Gynaecol. 2017;19(1):21–8.
42. Duffy RC, Odibo AO, Roehl KA, Macones GA. Effect of magnesium sulfate on fetal heart rate patterns in the second stage of labor. Obstet Gynecol. 2012;119(6):1129–36.
43. Kilpatrick SJ, Abreo A, Greene N, Melsop K, Peterson N, Shields LE, Main EK. Severe maternal morbidity in a large cohort of women with acute severe intrapartum hypertension. Am J Obstet Gynecol. 2016;215(1):91.e1–7.
44. Unit of Perinatal and Paediatric Epidemiology, University of Liverpool. Regional audit of the management of severe pre eclampsia and eclampsia. Mersey perinatal annual report. Liverpool: University of Liverpool; 1996.
45. Dekker G. Chapter 35: Hypertension. In: James DK, Steer PJ, Weiner CP, Gonik B, et al., editors. High risk pregnancy, management options. 4th ed. St Louis: Elsevier Saunders; 2011. p. 599–626.
46. American College of Obstetricians and Gynecologists – Practice Bulletin # 125. Chronic hypertension in pregnancy. Obstet Gynecol. 2012;119(2):396–407.
47. Magee LA, Cham C, Waterman EJ, et al. Hydralazine for the management of hypertension in pregnancy: meta analysis. Br Med J. 2003;327:955–60.
48. Raheem IA, Saaid R, Omar SZ, Tan PC. Oral nifedipine versus intravenous labetalol for acute blood pressure control in hypertensive emergencies of pregnancy: a randomized trial. Br J Obstet Gynaecol. 2012;119(1):78–85.
49. Shekhar S, Sharma C, Thakur S, Verma S. Oral nifedipine or intravenous labetalol for hypertensive emergency in pregnancy: a randomized controlled trial. Obstet Gynecol. 2013;122(5):1057–63.
50. Walker JJ, Greer I, Calder AA. Treatment of acute pregnancy-related hypertension: labetalol and hydralazine compared. Postgrad Med J. 1983;59(Suppl 3):168–70.
51. Pickles CJ, Symonds EM, Broughton PF. The fetal outcome in a randomized double-blind control trial of labetalol versus placebo in pregnancy-induced hypertension. Br J Obstet Gynaecol. 1989;96(1):38–43.
52. Unuigbe JA, Ebomwonyi IO, Sule Z, Agbon-Ojeme GE, Uwaifo JO, Omorogbe SO. Management of severe pre-eclampsia, eclampsia, and severe obstetric hypertensive crisis using a combination protocol of Magnesium Sulphate and Labetalol (Labet). Presented at the 9th RCOG International Conference in Athens, Greece, September 27–29, 2011.
53. Chung PCH, Li AH, Lin CC, Yang MW. Elevated vascular resistance after labetalol during resection of a pheocromocytoma. Can J Anesth. 2002;49(2):148–50.
54. Tuffnell DJ, Jankowicz D, Lindlow SW, et al. Outcome of severe preeclampsia/eclampsia in Yorkshire, 1999–2003. Br J Obstet Gynecol. 2005;112:875–80.
55. Sibai BM, Norwitz ER. Chapter 9: Management of severe pre-eclampsia. In: Heazell H, Norwitz ER, Kenny LC, et al., editors. Hypertension in pregnancy. 1st ed. Cambridge: Cambridge University Press; 2010. p. 129–40.
56. Sibai BM, Barton JR. Expectant management of severe preeclampsia remote from term: patient selection, treatment and delivery indications. Am J Obstet Gynecol. 2007;196:514.el–9.
57. Repke JT, Norwitz ER. Management of eclampsia. In: Heazell A, Norwitz ER, Kenny LC, Baker PN, editors. Hypertension in pregnancy. 1st ed. Cambridge: Cambridge University Press; 2010. p. 141–58.
58. Churchill D, Duley L. Interventionist versus expectant care for preeclampsia before term. Cochrane Database Syst Rev. 2002;(3):CD003106.
59. Seal SL, Gosh D, Kamilya G, et al. Does route of delivery affect maternal and perinatal outcome in women with eclampsia? A randomized controlled pilot study. Am J Obstet Gynecol. 2012;206(6):484.e1–7.
60. Nassar AH, Adra AAM, Chakhtoura N. Severe preeclampsia remote from term: labor induction or elective caesarean delivery? Am J Obstet Gynecol. 1998;179:1210–3.
61. Sibai BM. Etiology and management of postpartum hypertension-preeclampsia. Am J Obstet Gynecol. 2012;206(6):470–5.
62. Chelsey LC, Annitto JE, Cosgrove RA. The remote prognosis of eclamptic women. Am J Obstet Gynecol. 1976;124:446–59.
63. Sibai BM, Sarinoglu C, Mercer BM. Eclampsia V11. Pregnancy after eclampsia and long-term prognosis. Am J Obstet Gynecol. 1992;166:1757–61.
64. Sibai BM, el Nazer A, Gonzalez-Ruiz A. Severe preeclampsia-eclampsia in young primigravid women: subsequent pregnancy outcome and remote prognosis. Am J Obstet Gynecol. 1986;155:1011–6.
65. Vikse BE, Irgens LM, Leivestad T, Skjaerven R, Iversen BM. Preeclampsia and the risk of end-stage renal disease. N Engl J Med. 2008;359:800–8009.
66. Funai EF, Friedlander Y, Paltiel O, et al. Long-term mortality after preeclampsia. Epidemiology. 2005;16:206–15.
67. Bellamy L, Casas JP, Hingorani AD, Williams DJ. Preeclampsia and the risk of cardiovascular disease and cancer in later life: systematic review and meta-analysis. Br Med J. 2007;335:974–85.
68. Barker DJ. The developmental origins of well-being. Philos Trans R Soc Lond B Biol Sci. 2004;359:1359–66.
69. Innes KE, Marshall JA, Byers TE, Calonge N. A woman's own birth weight and gestational age predict her later risk of developing preeclampsia, a precursor of chronic disease. Epidemiology. 1999;10:153–60.

28 Haemoglobinopathies in Pregnancy

Hadiza Shehu Galadanci and Aisha Amal Galadanci

Learning Objectives

After reading this chapter, the reader will be able to:

- Discuss the epidemiology of sickle cell disease in pregnancy.
- Describe the pathophysiology of sickle cell disease.
- Explain the effect of sickle cell disease on pregnancy.
- Explain the effect of pregnancy on sickle cell disease.
- Discuss the management of sickle cell disease in pregnancy.
- Discuss the management of complications of sickle cell disease in pregnancy.
- Discuss the methods of reducing the impact of morbidity and mortality of sickle cell disease in pregnancy.

28.1 Introduction

Haemoglobinopathies is a collective term used for inherited disorders of haemoglobin synthesis. There could be disorders of the globin synthesis with impaired α and β chains as in thalassemia. There could also be structural haemoglobin variants as in sickle cell anaemia (HbS), or HbC, HbD or HbE and O-Arab. Individuals with sickle cell disease (SCD) can be homozygote SS (HbSS), heterozygotes SC (HbSC) and heterozygotes S-beta thalassaemia (HbS beta thalassaemia). The homozygous state (HbSS) is referred to as sickle cell anaemia (SCA).

Five beta-S globin haplotypes (β^S haplotypes) have been identified at specific restriction sites and named according to their region of origin and prevalence: Bantu, Benin, Senegal, Arabic-Indian (Saudi) and Cameroon. They are important in the comprehension of the clinical diversity of SCA patients [1]. Benin, Senegal and Bantu haplotypes respectively include: Nigeria, Morocco, Benin, countries right of Benin, the Mediterranean, North and Central West Africa; regions of Senegal, Atlantic West Africa, up the Niger River, Central and South African countries. Cameroon haplotypes come from the central area of Cameroon. Saudi, the fifth haplotype, is found in the eastern province of Saudi Arabia and in Central India [2–5].

Substantial proportion of children with SCD survive to adulthood as a result of advances in technology and medical care that they receive. In the USA and other high-resource settings, universal newborn screening (NBS) and comprehensive care for SCD has directly contributed to a dramatic reduction (3–0.13 per 100 person years) in SCD-related mortality, and approximately 99% of children with SCD born in the USA are expected to survive into adulthood [6, 7]. As such, more women with SCD are reaching child-bearing age and therefore presenting with pregnancy. Pregnancy in SCD is a high-risk pregnancy especially in homozygous HbSS which may be associated with adverse maternal and foetal outcome. On the other hand, women with HbC trait or even HbS trait may go through a pregnancy with no complication. Active prenatal management of women with SCD involving simple cost-effective interventions even in an African setting can go a long way in reducing the morbidity and mortality associated with SCD in pregnancy.

28.2 Prevalence

Worldwide, SCD is one of the most common inherited single gene autosomal recessive genetic disorders. Yearly, it has been estimated that about 300,000 babies are born with SCD [8]. People with SCD are more predominant in Africa, and in the

H. S. Galadanci (✉)
College of Health Sciences, Africa Centre of Excellence for Population Health and Policy, Bayero University, Kano, Nigeria

A. A. Galadanci
Aminu Kano Teaching Hospital, Bayero University, Kano, Nigeria

F. Okonofua et al. (eds.), *Contemporary Obstetrics and Gynecology for Developing Countries*,
https://doi.org/10.1007/978-3-030-75385-6_28

Middle East, the Mediterranean, the Caribbean, Central and South America, even though its origin is linked to Middle East and sub-Saharan Africa [9]. Sub-Saharan Africa has the greatest burden with over 200,000 babies born every year with the disease [10]. Approximately, 150,000 Nigerian babies with HbSS are born yearly, one of the highest in the world [11, 12]. UK records an estimated 12,000–15,000 individuals with SCD and 300 children delivered with HbSS [9], whereas in the USA, approximately 2000 babies are born with the disease every year. [13] However, women with haemoglobinopathies in pregnancy are now seen all over the world as a result of increased mobility of individual and inter-ethnic marriages.

28.3 The Pathophysiology of Sickle Cell Disease

The pathogenesis of sickle cell disease (SCD) lies in a point mutation in the sixth codon of the beta (β) globin chain where thymine substitutes adenine (GAG-GTG). As a result, valine replaces glutamic acid. Thus, the sixth amino acid in normal adult haemoglobin (HbA) is glutamic acid; however, in sickle haemoglobin (HbS), it is valine [14]. This minor change in the structure is responsible for profound changes in molecular stability and solubility of the haemoglobin molecule [15].

Deoxy HbS is less soluble than deoxy HbA and tends to crystallise out of solution inside erythrocytes when oxygen concentration is low in tissues. The single HbS molecules (monomers) cross-link with each other to form polymers via the valine residues in position six [14]. This polymerisation of HbS inside the red cells is responsible for the sickling of the red cells, that is, the characteristic half-moon appearance that resembles the curved knife used for harvesting wheat. This may result in blockage of different areas of microcirculation or large vessels causing infarcts of various organs [14, 16, 17]. When examined ultrastructurally, sickled cells show bundles of fibres aligned along the long axis of the cell or of the pointed projections. Each fibre consists of filaments arranged in pairs. Each filament is made up of HbS molecules stacked in a helical manner.

Polymerisation is a time-dependent process and occurs only on deoxygenation where HbS molecules aggregate to form a polymer of critical size. Once a critical polymer is formed, aggregation of additional HbS molecules occurs to form well-aligned fibres. The time between deoxygenation and formation of polymer of critical time is known as delay time or lag phase. This has significance when sickling and unsickling occur due to deoxygenation and oxygenation, respectively, in circulation [10]. The sickling of red cells induced by hypoxia is initially reversible if oxygen concentration increases as may happen when the red cell returns to the lung [8]. Repeated sickling and unsickling of red cells lead to membrane damage and the shape of the red cells become permanently altered leading to the formation of irreversibly sickled cells which does not return to normal even with reoxygenation. These cells appear on air-dried blood films as elongated cells one or both ends of which are pointed. They have rigid cell membranes and are trapped and destroyed in the spleen. The severity of haemolysis correlates with the number of these cells in circulation [10].

Factors which influence sickling include the following:

1. Temperature: Cold induces vasoconstriction and increase sickling.
2. Decreased oxygen tension: This is the most important determinant affecting sickling.
3. Intracellular concentration of HbS and other haemoglobins: There is a direct relationship between the amount of HbS in the red cell and propensity of red cells to sickle. In sickle-cell trait due to the predominance of HbA in the cell, sickling is prevented unless the oxygen tension is considerably low. In contrast, in red cells of patients with sickle cell anaemia (SCA), HbS is the predominant form of haemoglobin (80–90%) and sickling occurs readily. HbF does not participate with HbS in sickling process and therefore infants do not develop manifestation till the time HbF declines to adult values.
4. Mean corpuscular haemoglobin concentration (MCHC): Increased MCHC due to cellular dehydration favours the intermolecular contact between HbS and enhances polymerisation.
5. Association with thalassaemias: In sickle cell β+ thalassaemia, due to the presence of HbA, the disease is milder.
6. Interaction with other abnormal haemoglobins: HbS interacts less readily with HbC or HbD than with other HbS molecules and therefore, persons with HbSD or HbSC disease have milder manifestation compared to those with HbSS disease.
7. Low pH: Decrease in pH increases sickling by inducing the deoxygenated state of haemoglobin.

28.4 Effect of Pregnancy on Sickle Cell Disease

Nowadays, children with SCD survive to adulthood as a result of advances in technology and medical care that they receive. As such, more women with SCD are reaching child-bearing age and therefore presenting with pregnancy. Pregnancy which is a stressful condition further adds strain on the already stressed physiological reserve of a patient with sickle cell disease, thus leading to increased risk of crises especially the haemolytic and vaso-occlusive crises. These can become worse towards end of pregnancy. The vaso-occlusive crises can lead to severe painful crises with organs such as bone, kidney, lungs, liver, spleen and brain being affected.

28.5 Effect of Sickle Cell Disease on Pregnancy

Generally, pregnancy in SCD patient is a high-risk pregnancy associated with increased maternal and perinatal complications. Complications affecting the mother and the foetus are premature rupture of membranes, increased risk of antenatal admission, premature labour, pre-eclampsia, eclampsia, anaemia, urinary tract infection and thromboembolic complications. Other complications include pulmonary complications, postpartum complications, intra-uterine growth restriction, foetal distress in labour, low birth weight (LBW) and intra-uterine foetal death leading to high perinatal and maternal mortality [18–22].

All studies comparing the maternal complications and foetal complications in pregnant women with and without SCD were recently studied using systematic review as well as meta-analysis [23]. It showed a three times higher risks of growth restriction (pooled OR 2.79, 95% CI 1.85–4.21, $P < 0.001$), double the risk of prematurity (pooled OR 2.14, 95% CI 1.56–2.95, $P < 0.001$) and twice the chance of LBW (pooled OR 2.00, 95% CI 1.42–2.83, $P < 0.001$) in SCD patients in pregnancy as compared to controls. Overall perinatal mortality, stillbirths and neonatal mortality were significantly higher irrespective of country of residence. The same study revealed a higher risk of pre-eclampsia (overall pooled OR 2.05, 95% CI 1.47–2.85, $P < 0.001$), eclampsia (pooled OR: 3.02, 95% CI: 1.20–7.58, $P = 0.019$), caesarean section delivery and bacterial infection (pooled OR: 2.48, 95% CI: 1.23–5.01, $P = 0.011$) in women with SCD as compared to women without SCD. In addition, women with SCD in low income countries had a higher risk of maternal deaths as compared to women without SCD. Some studies have also shown increased risk of antepartum haemorrhage [24]. It is important to state here that with intensive prenatal care in conjunction with haematologist, use of blood transfusion services, foetal surveillance and optimal timing of delivery, there has been decreased maternal and perinatal morbidity and mortality associated with SCD in pregnancy. In addition, studies have demonstrated that even in developing countries, pregnancy can be without complications in SCD patients when given adequate quality care [25].

28.6 Management of Sickle Cell Disease in Pregnancy

28.6.1 Clinical Presentations

Patients may present with different symptoms of SCD. Those patients with HbSS present with more severe form of the disease as compared with those with HbSC or HbS/B+ thalassaemia, whilst those with persistence of HbF present with less severe form of the disease. Usually, clinical symptom does not manifest until the age of 3–4 months. Splenic sequestration and sepsis that occur in the first 3 years of life are usually the cause of high mortality in countries that have the challenge of providing high quality health care services. This is different in developed countries with SCD patients having over 45 years life expectancy and living a normal life with intermittent episodes of vaso-occlusive crisis [9].

1. Painful Vaso-occlusive Crisis

The commonest crisis is the vaso-occlusive crisis, which is usually triggered by violent exercise, dehydration, deoxygenation, exposure to cold, obstetric delivery, surgical operation, etc. [13]. The spleen, bones and lungs are the common organs that are susceptible to infarct formation. In majority of the cases, the first clinical presentation of SCD is the "hand-foot" syndrome, which present as painful dactylitis because of infarcts of the small bones. Vaso-occlusive crisis of the spinal cord and that of the brain (where 7% of the patients develop stroke) are the most serious complications. Abnormal blood flow depicting arterial stenosis can be detected using transcranial doppler (TCD) and this can predict strokes in children which can be averted in majority of cases by regular blood transfusion [14].

2. Sequestration Crisis

This is one of the most important causes of SCD-related death within the first 2 years of life. It is caused by trapping of large numbers of erythrocytes in the spleen or sometimes in the liver. Since a large proportion of blood is pooled in these organs, there is a fall in Hb level. It is more common in children than adults. It is in fact rare in adult HbSS patients whose spleen would have been destroyed by repeated infarction (auto splenectomy). Reduced or absent splenic function makes people with SCD susceptible to infection. This is the reason why they routinely take prophylactic antimicrobials or anti-malarials in malaria endemic regions. Features of sequestration crisis include marked pallor and progressive enlargement of spleen or liver. Reticulocytosis and/or presence of nucleated red blood cells in the peripheral film are important features that help to differentiate it from aplastic crisis in which there is reticulocytopenia.

3. Aplastic Crisis

This occurs as a result of infection with parvo virus B19 in which it multiplies in and destroys erythrocyte precursors in bone marrow leading to severe anaemia. B19 infection causes maturation arrest of marrow erythroid precursors at the stage of pronormoblasts early normoblasts [14]. The natural course of the infection is 10–14 days. The fall in Hb level does not get severe before infection resolves because the normal erythrocyte life span is 100–120 days. The features of aplastic crisis include weakness, headache, facial erythema and gradual progression of anaemia usually over 3–5 days unlike in sequestration crisis that occurs within hours (6 hours) and low reticulocyte count in the presence of reduced Hb level [6, 8].

4. Skin

Chronic leg ulcers are common around ankles on the medial aspect. They don't heal readily and have a tendency to recur. Recurrent chronic leg ulcers are commonly seen in SCD patients. These occur mainly around the ankles and usually don't heal easily.

5. Skeletal System

Other skeletal changes apart from vaso-occlusive crisis in bone are avascular necrosis of the head of the femur and humerus, osteomyelitis and widening of medullary cavity as a result of marrow hyperplasia.

6. Respiratory System

Cough with associated chest pain (pleuritic type) and sudden onset of acute fever is termed "acute chest syndrome (ACS)." It may be caused by infarction or infection, but the differentiation is difficult. Repeated occurrences of acute chest syndrome can cause chronic lung disease. Pulmonary hypertension and corpulmonale can also occur [16].

7. Other Clinical Features

Chronic damage to the liver may occur through microinfarcts. Pigment (bilirubin) gall stones are frequent. The kidneys are vulnerable to infarctions of the medulla with papillary necrosis. Failure to concentrate urine aggravates the tendency to dehydration and crisis. Nocturnal enuresis is common. A proliferative retinopathy and priapism are the other clinical complications.

28.6.2 Laboratory Investigations

1. Full blood count – This is done to estimate the haemoglobin level. The Hb is usually between 6 and 9 g/dl.
2. Peripheral blood film – Sickle cells (crescent shape) and codocytes will be seen in the blood film. Likewise, Howell-jolly bodies may also be seen, suggesting features of splenic atrophy.
3. Screening tests for HbS include:
   (a) Sickling test – This test is used to detect for the presence of haemoglobin S. It is performed by adding certain reducing agents such as 2% sodium metabisulphite or sodium dithionite to red cells to induce deoxygenation. If the red cells contain HbS, they become sickle shaped when they are deprived of oxygen while cells that do not contain HbS remain normal.
   (b) Solubility test – This is a screening test used to detect the presence of haemoglobin S. The principle of the test is based on insolubility of haemoglobin S in a solution that contains solution that contain high phosphate buffer, a reducing agent (sodium dithionate and saponin). Small amount of blood is added to the solution. Red cells are haemolysed and HbS if present is reduced by dithionite, forming insoluble polymers which refract light and solution becomes turbid [14].
4. Haemoglobin electrophoresis – This is done to detect abnormal HbS, HbC or variant bands.
5. High performance liquid chromatography (HPLC) – This has largely replaced traditional electrophoresis because it reliably quantifies the fraction of HbA2, F and S.
6. Other investigations that could inform clinical management include:
   (a) Transcranial doppler (TCD) measurement of velocity of blood flow in carotid and cerebral vessels to identify those at increased risk of stroke
   (b) Abdominal ultrasonography to detect gall bladder stones in patients with right hypochondrial pain
   (c) Echocardiography to detect pulmonary hypertension
   (d) Urinalysis – A 24-hour urine protein quantification and renal USS to detect sickle cell nephropathy
   (e) Chest X-ray to detect acute chest syndrome

28.7 Treatment

28.7.1 Preconception Care

One of the aims of preconception care is for a woman to start a pregnancy in an optimal condition. Therefore, a woman with sickle cell disease planning to get pregnant should receive preconception care so that she can start the pregnancy in an optimal condition.

She should receive information on how to avoid risk factors that trigger crisis and how dehydration from early pregnancy nausea and vomiting can also trigger crisis. She should understand her increased risk of getting anaemia and having crisis in pregnancy, as well as her risk of having foetal complications such as intra-uterine growth restriction [9]. She should have renal and liver function test to screen for renal and hepatic derangement, respectively, and also echocardiography to screen for pulmonary hypertension. Likewise, she should have retinal screening and screening for iron overload and red cell antibodies [9]. Folic acid prophylaxis as well as antimalarial prophylaxis in malaria endemic area are continued before pregnancy and throughout the pregnancy. Women on hydroxyurea should be discontinued 3 months before they embark on a pregnancy because of the risk of teratogenesis [9].

28.7.2 Prenatal Diagnosis

Pregnant women from high-risk ethnic group such as in sub-Saharan Africa should be routinely screened for HbS carrier state. Those with HbSS and with carrier state (HbAS) should have their partners also screened. If both parents are found to be positive, they should be offered adequate counselling on the risk of having sickle cell affected baby. Prenatal diagnosis and an option pregnancy termination should be discussed with the couple [26]. There are two methods of prenatal diagnosis of sickle cell disease:

1. Chorionic Villus Sampling (CVS)

   This is carried out transcervical at 10–12 weeks or transabdominal from 10 weeks, where few villi are collected from the chorion frondosum under ultrasound guidance using long malleable polyethylene catheter. The chorionic villi are then subjected to foetal DNA analysis. This is a preferred method [16]. Possible complications from the procedure are foetal loss, limb deformities and vaginal bleeding.
2. Foetal Blood Analysis

This is done at 18 weeks and 0.5–2 ml of foetal blood is obtained from the umbilical vein using a spinal needle under ultrasound guidance. The foetal blood obtained is then subjected to analysis which involves globin chain synthesis using carboxymethyl (CM)-cellulose chromatography, and the complication of foetal loss is comparatively greater [16].

28.7.3 Antenatal Care

Pregnancy in sickle cell disease is considered a high-risk pregnancy which should be managed by a multidisciplinary team approach, consisting of an experienced obstetrician, midwife and a haematologist who has a special interest in SCD. Early booking is recommended during which prenatal diagnosis can be offered. It is also important to ensure that the woman is well educated on good compliance with prophylactic drugs, avoidance of extreme of temperature, dehydration, overexertion and other precipitating factors. Adequate rest and nutrition are also essential. As a high-risk pregnancy, they should be seen fortnightly till 30 weeks and weekly till delivery. Where sickle cell disease centres exist, they are managed in such centres, as studies have shown that such centres are associated with reduced risk of spontaneous miscarriages, preterm labour and perinatal death [27]. Women with HbSC should be managed and monitored as women with HbSS, since some can develop complications like postpartum infections, antenatal hospital admission intra-uterine growth restriction [28] and painful crisis [29].

Women with early pregnancy symptoms of nausea and vomiting should be adequately treated to avoid dehydration that can precipitate sickle cell crisis. During each antenatal visit, urinalysis should be performed and blood pressure should be measured since pregnant women with SCD have increased risk of pre-eclampsia and eclampsia [16]. Clinical as well as ultrasound assessment of foetal growth should be offered as they have a high risk of intra-uterine growth restriction and pre-eclampsia [16]. Four-weekly ultrasound will allow early detection of foetal growth restriction for early institution of management. When indicated, a Doppler ultrasound and/or a biophysical profile can be done for proper management of intra-uterine growth restriction. Another aim of antenatal care is to prevent anaemia especially in Malaria endemic zone such as Nigeria. Therefore, clinical as well as laboratory assessment to prevent anaemia is done in each visit.

28.7.4 Drug Use in SCD Women in Pregnancy

Daily folic acid, which should have been started during the preconception care is continued throughout the pregnancy. However, iron supplementation is only recommended for women with demonstrable iron deficiency as some have been shown to have iron overload [30]. Prophylactic antimalarials with proguanil is also continued throughout pregnancy. This is very important as one of the risk factors for sickling crisis is malarial parasitaemia. It is pertinent to mention here that women with HbAS (sickle cell trait, SCT) are known to be less susceptible to malaria caused by *Plasmodium falciparum*. At any time, if malaria infection is confirmed, complete treatment of malaria with artesunate combined therapy (ACT) should be given even though the woman may be on antimalarial prophylaxis. As pregnant women with SCD are at a higher risk of pre-eclampsia, they are recommended to take daily 75 mg of aspirin starting at 12 weeks till 34 weeks after ensuring the patient has no sensitivity to low dose Aspirin.

Routine prophylactic blood transfusion is not recommended even though studies have shown that prophylactic blood transfusion reduced the incidence of maternal painful crisis but did not have any effect on foetal and maternal outcome [9]. Blood transfusion is also not without complication including alloimmunisation. Therefore, blood transfusion (top-up transfusion) is only indicated when there is severe anaemia with Hb of 6 g/dl, in repeated crises, twin pregnancies, after a caesarean delivery or in the event of postpartum haemorrhage (PPH) [9]. In patients with acute chest syndrome or acute stroke, exchange blood transfusion is recommended. Low-molecular-weight heparin is recommended for all pregnant women with SCD during hospital admission due to the increased risk of thromboembolism [9].

28.7.5 Sickle Cell Disease Crises in Pregnancy

Vaso-occlusive crisis is usually the commonest indication for hospital admission and the most common complication of SCD in pregnancy [27]. The patient usually presents with severe pains and management should be by the multidisciplinary team. A detailed history is obtained and clinical examination is done to identity risk factors or precipitating factors such as malaria or infections. Investigation should include renal function test, complete blood count, reticulocyte count and malarial parasite. Other tests such as liver function test, chest X ray and urine culture will be as indicated. Ultrasound scan should be done to assess the well-being of the foetus.

Intravenous fluid is commenced once adequate oral fluid intake is not assured. Oxygen therapy may be indicated when the oxygen saturation falls and referral to ICU may be necessary. Treatment with analgesics should start with paracetamol for mild pain, NSAID for mild-to-moderate pain, weak opiates can be given for moderate pain and stronger opiates given for cases presenting with severe pain. As a result of pethidine-related seizures in patients with SCD, pethidine is avoided [9]. In endemic malaria zones, antimalarials (ACT) should be given. Broad-spectrum antibiotics are indicated in cases of high suspicion of infection or in women with febrile illness. As stated above, thromboprophylaxis should be provided for women with vaso-occlusive crisis on admission. Other supportive treatment, include laxatives, antihistamine and antiemetics [9].

28.7.6 Acute Chest Syndrome (ACS) in Pregnancy

Patient with ACS should be managed by a multidisciplinary team which should include critical care specialist apart from the obstetrician, midwife and haematologist. They usually present with dyspnoea tachypnoea, chest pain and cough. These symptoms mimic those of pneumonia and therefore treated similarly. Chest X-ray should be requested with abdominal shield, which may show presence of infiltrate. Early recognition and institution of therapy is essential and critical care team should be involved early for possible admission to ICU if required. Treatment involves oxygen therapy, intravenous antibiotics and blood transfusion. The blood transfusion may be top-up when the Hb is <6.5 g/dl or as exchange blood transfusion in severe hypoxia [9].

28.7.7 Acute Stroke in Pregnancy

Women with SCD could also present with the complication of acute stroke which could be as a result of both infarction and haemorrhage. Usually, they present with acute neurological impairment. Such a patient should be treated as an emergency and an urgent brain imaging investigation should be carried out to confirm the diagnosis. An urgent exchange blood transfusion should then be carried out by the haematologist to reduce the risk of long-term neurological damage [9].

28.7.8 Pulmonary Embolism in Pregnancy

Another complication could be pulmonary embolism and in which case patient usually present with acute hypoxia. This is also a medical emergency and requires treatment with the critical care team. Definitive investigation and treatment should be commenced including administration of therapeutic low-molecular-weight heparin once diagnosis is made.

28.7.9 Acute Anaemia in Pregnancy

A pregnant woman with SCD may present with acute anaemia as a complication. This could be as a result of malaria especially in malaria endemic zone as in Nigeria. It could also be as a result of infection with parvovirus B19 (erythrovirus) which lead to aplastic crisis and splenic sequestration [9]. Blood film for malaria parasite and reticulocyte should be carried out. A low reticulocyte count suggests infection with the erythrovirus. Treatment will include transfusion of blood and definitive treatment of the cause of the anaemia. Anti-malaria and antibiotics may be indicated. Patients with erythrovirus should be isolated and treated by foeto-maternal specialist as vertical transmission can occur leading to hydrops fetalis [9]

28.7.10 Intrapartum Care

The risk of perinatal mortality and maternal morbidity is increased in women with SCD in pregnancy and complications like pre-eclampsia and eclampsia are also increased [23]. Therefore, it has been suggested that pregnancy should not be allowed to go beyond 40 weeks so as to prevent late pregnancy-associated complications and harmful perinatal events [9].

Vaginal delivery is not contraindicated in SCD and hence women with SCD should be allowed normal vaginal delivery in the absence of any complication. Dehydration should be avoided in labour as this can trigger crisis. As such adequate oral fluid intake should be encouraged and intravenous fluid given when necessary. An input/output chart should be maintained to prevent fluid overload. Broad-spectrum antibiotics should be given especially in developed countries where the risk of infection is high.

Oxygen therapy may be instituted when required and pulse oximeter can be used to monitor the oxygen saturation. Women with SCD in labour should be given adequate analgesia such as opiates but avoiding pethidine [9]. Epidural anaesthesia can be offered where indicated and regional anaesthesia is the recommended anaesthesia for caesarean section.

Close foetal monitoring is required and if possible electronic foetal heart rate monitoring as a result of the higher risk of perinatal death and foetal distress. Clinical examination of the patient should be carried out 4 hourly assessing for pallor, jaundice, oedema, pyrexia, hypertension, tachycardia, raised pulse pressure, pulmonary oedema and hepatosplenomegaly. Haemoglobin estimation is done 6 hourly and urine also tested for proteinuria.

The second stage of labour can be shortened using operative vaginal delivery. The third stage of labour should be managed adequately using oxytocics and blood loss minimised. Any blood loss should be assessed and possibilities of replacement with blood transfusion considered.

28.7.11 Postpartum Care

In pregnant women with SCD, the postpartum period is very critical. Acute massive sickling can occur at this period leading to acute sequestration crisis. Therefore, close clinical monitoring is required in order to identify it early and institute treatment early. The liver and spleen span should be monitored as well as the haemoglobin level. Early mobilisation is encouraged and adequate hydration and oxygenation maintained. In case of bone pain crisis, analgesia should be added. Antibiotics (prophylactic) to prevent infection should be continued. Heparinization using low-molecular-weight heparin should be given for up to 7 days after discharge from the hospital in normal delivery and for 6 weeks after a caesarean delivery [9]. Women should be encouraged to start breast feeding early.

There is the need to counsel women with SCD to limit their family size in view of the fact that each pregnancy is an added stress to their already stressful clinical state. Barrier methods are safe and can be used. Progestogens have been demonstrated to be effective and safe in SCD [31]; hence, women can be encouraged to use the injectables such as depo provera, progestogen only pill and the progesterone-impregnated intra-uterine device.

In view of the increased risk of infection, the use of IUCD should be approached with caution likewise because of the increase of thromboembolism in SCD, the use of oral contraceptive pills should also be with caution. Bilateral tubal ligation can be offered if the woman desires to have a permanent method of contraception.

28.8 Challenges of Managing Sickle Cell Disease in Pregnancy in Low and Middle Income Countries (LMICs)

Management of sickle cell disease in pregnancy in low and middle resource countries is saddled with a lot of challenges, because of which it is associated with high morbidity and mortality for both the mother and the foetus. Challenges include those of late presentation, high parity, lack of or inadequate diagnostic facilities as well as lack of quality blood transfusion services. Other challenges are lack of multidisciplinary teams in health facilities and lack of intensive care facilities, which may be required for sickle disease patients with complications in pregnancy. Sickle cell disease pregnant women may also be required to be delivered before term and therefore the availability of special care baby units (SCBU) is essential in such cases, which may not be adequate or available in low and middle income countries (LMICs).

28.9 Prevention

SCD during pregnancy and postpartum is associated with several complications. Prevention involves early detection through newborn screening and treatment of complications Preconception care, quality antenatal care, intrapartum care and postpartum care are all essential in ensuring good outcome for SCD in pregnancy. Multidisciplinary team approach in managing SCD in pregnancy cannot be overemphasised. The general measures of prevention of burden of SCD includes:

28.9.1 Health Education

Health education involves creating awareness of the disease, its complications and economic load through mass media.

28.9.2 Vaccinations

Patients with SCD are at a high risk of infection with encapsulated bacteria such as *Neisseria meningitides, Streptococcus pneumonia and Haemophilus influenza* because of hyposplenism. Therefore young children with SCD are recommended to have penicillin prophylaxis. However, there is no randomised trial evidence in older patients or pregnant women [32]. According to the UK guidelines, daily penicillin prophylaxis should be given to all patients with SCD [33, 34]. In addition, women should also be given *H. influenza* type b and the conjugated meningococcal C vaccine as a single dose if they have not received it previously, as part of their primary immunisations.

28.9.3 Genetic Counselling

Genetic counselling to both partners will improve the awareness of SCD and sickle cell trait (SCT). Given SCD is a genetic disorder, knowledge of haemoglobin genotype is important at a very young age, and genetic counselling will provide unbiased information about reproductive health.

28.9.4 Newborn Screening

Identification of SCD through newborn screening (NBS) will help in the education of the disease and how to manage it. NBS will also dramatically reduce SCD-related mortality and awareness of being a heterozygote (SCT) and will ensure correct antenatal counselling for the family, and in the future for the patient [35]. However, despite the high load of SCD in sub-Saharan Africa, few medical centres have newborn SCD screening programmes.

28.10 Summary

Nigeria has the most burden of SCD in the world with an estimated 150,000 babies delivered yearly with SCD compared to 2400 children in the USA and 300 in the UK. A pregnancy in a patient with SCD is a high-risk pregnancy, especially in patients with more severe SCD (HbSS), a history of cerebral vasculopathy or with acute chest syndrome. Preconception care, quality antenatal, intrapartum, postpartum and family planning services, using a multidisciplinary approach are all essential in ensuring improved outcomes for both mother and baby.

References

1. Nagel RL. The origin of the Haemoglobin S gene: clinical, genetic and anthropological consequences. Einstein Q J Biol Med. 1984;2(1):53–62.
2. Adorno EV, et al. Clinical and molecular characteristics of sickle cell anaemia in the northeast of Brazil. Genet Mol Biol. 2008;31(3):621–5.
3. Auricchio MTBM. Frequency and origins of Haemoglobin S mutation in African-derived Brazilian populations. Hum Biol. 2007;79(6):667–77.
4. Cabral CHK, et al. Determination of βs haplotypes in patients with sickle-cell anaemia in the state of Rio Grande do Norte, Brazil. Genet Mol Biol. 2011;34(3):421–4.
5. Desai DV, Hanani H. Sickle cell disease: history and origin. Internet J Haematol. 2004;1(2):1–4.
6. Odame I, Kulkarni R, Ohene-Frempong K. Concerted global effort to combat sickle cell disease: the first global congress on sickle cell disease in Accra, Ghana. Am J Prev Med. 2011;41(6 Suppl 4):S417–21.
7. Makani J, Komba AN, Cox SE, et al. Malaria in patients with sickle cell anaemia: burden, risk factors, and outcome at the outpatient clinic and during hospitalisation. Blood. 2010;115(2):215–20.
8. Serjeant GR. Sickle-cell disease. Lancet. 1997;350:725–30.
9. Royal College of Obstetricians and Gynaecologists. Management of sickle cell disease in pregnancy. Green-top Guideline No. 61. London: RCOG; 2011.
10. Serjeant GR. The emerging understanding of sickle cell disease. Br J Haematol. 2001;112:3–18.
11. Anie KA, Egunjobi FE, Akinyanju OO. Psychosocial impact of sickle cell disorder: perspectives from a Nigerian setting. Glob Health. 2010;6:1.
12. World Health Organization. Report by the Secretariat of the Fifty-ninth World Health Assembly A59/9; 2006.
13. Therrell BL Jr, Lloyed-Puyear MA, Eckman JR, Mann MY. Newborn screening for sickle cell disease in the United States: a review of data spanning 2 decades. Semin Perinatol. 2015;39:238–51.
14. Okpala I. Sickle cell disease & thalassaemias. In: Okpala I, Johnson C, editors. Synopsis of haematology including blood disease in the tropics. 1st ed; Blackwell Publishers, United Kingdom, 2010. p. 47–70.
15. Lal A, Vichinsky EP. Sickle cell disease. In: Hoffbrand AV, Catovsky D, Tuddenham EGD, editors. Postgraduate haematology. 6th ed. Massachusetts: Blackwell; 2011. p. 125–18.
16. Kawthalkar SM. Essentials of haematology. 2nd ed. New Delhi: Jaypee Brothers Medical Publishers; 2013. p. 171–84.
17. Hoffbrand AV, Moss PAH. Genetic disorders of haemoglobin. In: Essential haematology. 6th ed. Oxford: Blackwell Publishing; 2006. p. 44–57.
18. Wilson NO, Ceesay FK, Hibbert JM, et al. Pregnancy outcomes among patients with sickle cell disease at Korle-Bu Teaching Hospital, Accra, Ghana: retrospective cohort study. Am J Trop Med Hyg. 2012;86:936–42.
19. Dare FO, Makinde OO, Fasuba OB. The obstetric performance of sickle cell disease patients and homozygous Haemoglobin C disease patients in Ile-Ife, Nigeria. Int J Gynaecol Obstet. 1992;37:163–8.
20. Odum CU, Anorlu RI, Dim SI, Oyekan TO. Pregnancy outcome in HbSS-sickle cell disease in Lagos, Nigeria. West Afr J Med. 2002;21:19–23.
21. Boulet SL, Okoroh EM, Azonobi I, Grant A, Craig Hooper W. Sickle cell disease in pregnancy: maternal complications in a Medicaid enrolled population. Matern Child Health J. 2013;17:200–7.
22. Barfield WD, Barradas DT, Manning SE, Kotelchuck M, Shapiro-Mendoza CK. Sickle cell disease and pregnancy outcomes: women of African descent. Am J Prev Med. 2010;38:S542–9.
23. Boafor TK, Olayemi E, Galadanci N, Hayfron-Benjamin C, Dei-Adomakoh Y, Segbefia C. Pregnancy outcomes in women with sickle-cell disease in low and high income countries: a systematic review and meta-analysis. BJOG. 2015;23:691–8. https://doi.org/10.1111/1471-0528.13786.
24. Kassim AA, Aliyu MH, Galadanci H, Tuuli MG, Rodeghier M, DeBaun MR, Oppong SA, Villers MS, Jamison MG, De Castro

LM, James AH. Morbidity associated with sickle cell disease in pregnancy. Am J Obstet Gynecol. 2008;199:125.e1–5.
25. Rahimy MC, Gangbo A, Adjou R, Deguenon C, Goussanou S, Alihonou E. Effect of active prenatal management on pregnancy outcome in sickle cell disease in an African setting. J Am Soc Hematol. 2000;96(5):1685–9.
26. Royal College of Obstetricians and Gynaecologists. Amniocentesis and chorionic villus sampling. Green-top Guideline No. 8. London: RCOG; 2010.
27. Powars DR, Sandhu M, Niland-Weiss J, Johnson C, Bruce S, Manning PR. Pregnancy in sickle cell disease. Obstet Gynecol. 1986;67:217–28.
28. Sun PM, Wilburn W, Raynor BD, Jamieson D. Sickle cell disease in pregnancy: twenty years of experience at Grady Memorial Hospital, Atlanta, Georgia. Am J Obstet Gynecol. 2001;184:1127–30.
29. Serjeant GR, Hambleton I, Thame M. Fecundity and pregnancy outcome in a cohort with sickle cell–haemoglobin C disease followed from birth. BJOG. 2005;112:1308–14.
30. Aken'Ova YA, Adeyefa I, Okunade M. Ferritin and serum iron levels in adult patients with sickle cell anaemia at Ibadun, Nigeria. Afr J Med Med Sci. 1997;26:39–41.
31. Legardy JK, Curtis KM. Progestogen-only contraceptive use among women with sickle cell anaemia: a systematic review. Contraception. 2006;73:195–204.
32. Gaston MH, Verter JI, Woods G, Pegelow C, Kelleher J, Presbury G, et al. Prophylaxis with oral penicillin in children with sickle cell anaemia. A randomised trial. N Engl J Med. 1986;314:1593–9.
33. Sickle Cell Society. Standards for the clinical care of adults with sickle cell disease in the UK. London: Sickle Cell Society; 2008.
34. Working Party of the British Committee for Standards in Haematology Clinical Haematology Task Force. Guidelines for the prevention and treatment of infection in patients with an absent or dysfunctional spleen. BMJ. 1996;312:430–4.
35. Yang YM, Andrews S, Peterson R, et al. Prenatal sickle cell screening education effect on the follow up rates of infants with sickle cell trait. Patient Educ Couns. 2000;39:185–9.

Anaemia in Pregnancy

29

Olayinka Ogunbode and Olatoye Ogunbode

29.1 Introduction and Definition

Anaemia occurs globally and is a major public health problem in women of reproductive age, especially in developing countries. It is a major direct and indirect cause of maternal mortality and is associated with high foetal wastage [1, 2]. Despite various interventions over the past four decades, it continues to acquire greater magnitude as a result of impoverishment of the population, arising from conflicts, wars, and global economic recession [3]. Although iron deficiency is considered as the commonest cause, anaemia in the tropics may also result from non-nutritional causes such as malaria, acute and chronic infection, acute and chronic inflammation and haemoglobinopathies. Human immunodeficiency virus (HIV) infections have also contributed significantly to the increased prevalence of anaemia [4].

Anaemia can be defined as diminution below normal of the total circulating red blood cells or haemoglobin (HB) mass for an individual's age, sex and population. The normal haemoglobin range between 12 and 14 g/dl, with men having higher haemoglobin levels than women. In the non-pregnant woman, haemoglobin of 12 g/dl or below is suggestive of anaemia; however, in recognition of the physiological changes affecting haemopoiesis during pregnancy, a lower level of haemoglobin (11 g/dl) is customarily accepted for the definition of anaemia.

Globally, 56 million pregnant women are estimated to be anaemic by the World Health Organization with the developing countries contributing over 80% [5–7]. In Africa, the prevalence is estimated to be 35–75% accounting for 2–12% of direct maternal deaths [8]. In Nigeria, the prevalence is between 17% and 88% [6, 9, 10].

In general, deficiency anaemias are prevalent in developing countries as a result of poverty and its accompanied under-nutrition [11]; however, this can be masked by anaemia caused by red cell haemolysis from infective conditions such as malaria (Table 29.1). In West Africa where malaria is endemic, haemolytic anaemia is common in contrast to East Africa, where iron deficiency is the commonest form [12]. Thus, the order in which the major causes of anaemia exist is strongly determined by the environmental parasitic profile [13]. In Nigeria the main causes are malaria infection, folic acid and iron deficiency, antepartum and post-partum haemorrhage.

With the World Health Organization definition of anaemia in pregnancy (level of haemoglobin 11 g/dl or less), one-third of antenatal patients would be classified as anaemic [13]. In practice, many hospitals in Nigeria use a lower level of haemoglobin (10 g/dl or less) as indicating anaemia, based on the work of Lawson which showed that no serious maternal or foetal harm occurs until haemoglobin value was below 10 g/dl [14]. In developing countries, it is, however, advisable to apply the WHO definition for diagnosing anaemia for the benefit of standardization and meaningful comparison whenever data are being presented or discussed globally. Additionally, unless we start to adopt the World Health Organization's definition, there will not be adequate awareness of the magnitude of the problem of anaemia in our community. Only then will there be prompt and adequate efforts to improve the haematological status of our expectant women.

O. Ogunbode · O. Ogunbode (✉)
Department of Obstetrics and Gynaecology, University of Ibadan, Ibadan, Nigeria

F. Okonofua et al. (eds.), *Contemporary Obstetrics and Gynecology for Developing Countries*,
https://doi.org/10.1007/978-3-030-75385-6_29

Table 29.1 Environmental influence on order of frequency of different types of anaemia

A. General cause of anaemia in the developing countries is malnutrition. Therefore, deficiency anaemias top the list.

Iron deficiency	–	very high
Folic acid deficiency	–	very high
Vit. B_{12} deficiency	–	rare

B. When endemic infections are prevalent (e.g. malaria), anaemia associated with infections tends to overshadow the nutritional anaemias. Accordingly, the nutritional anaemias will be less frequently seen. Thus,the pattern of anaemia in Nigeria before 1976 was:

Megaloblastic anaemia (because of red cell haemolysis)	–	very high
Folic acid deficiency	–	high
Iron deficiency	–	low.
Vit. B_{12} deficiency	–	rare

C. With infections substantially controlled (a situation that now exists in Nigeria, 1985), severe anaemias become rare and the deficiency anaemias attain nearly the same frequency as megalobastic anaemia which is still caused by malaria infection.

Megaloblastic anaemia	}	common in nearly equal frequency
Folic acid deficiency	}	
Iron deficiency	}	
Vit. B_{12} deficiency	–	rare

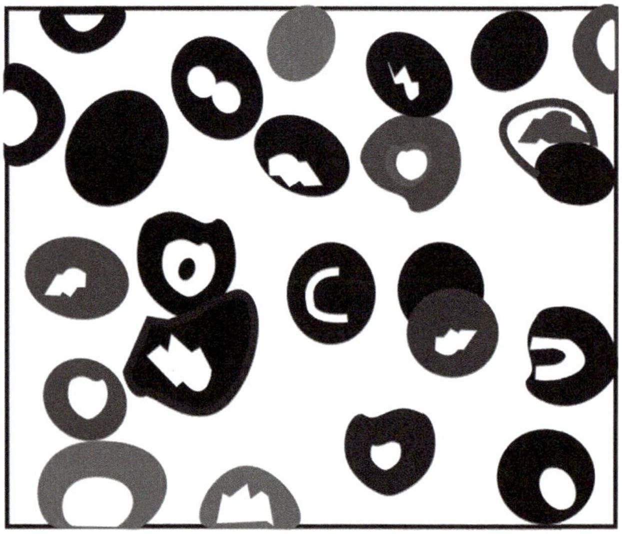

Fig. 29.1 Peripheral blood film showing target cells visible in the upper half of the film

29.2 Environmental Factors and Pattern of Anaemia

Malaria infection was and perhaps is still the most important factor responsible for causing anaemia in Nigeria and in other areas where the parasite is endemic. The incidence and severity of malaria are increased in pregnancy due to the decreased immunity and increased parasitaemia. However, severe anaemias, which used to account for about 15% of all anaemias are now considerably less common, present in only about 4% of patients currently seen with anaemia [3]. The main reason for this significant reduction is the various initiatives over the past years such as the Safe Motherhood Initiative (SMI), Roll Back Malaria (RBM) and Millennium Development Goals (MDG). This can be attributed to improved prevention of malaria infection through the distribution of free insecticide-treated nets (ITN) to pregnant women and the increased use of intermittent preventive treatment of malaria using sulphadoxine-pyrimethamine (IPTp-SP) combination of anti-malarial medication [15].

The second factor is the prompt diagnosis and treatment of malaria infection. The average Nigerian now knows that malaria infection must be considered whenever a febrile illness develops. Anti-malarial drugs are therefore first administered and medical attention sought only when significant improvement does not occur after a few days. Furthermore, the practice of primary health care in the past decade has ensured that anti-malarial drugs are the commonly prescribed drugs in rural areas. There is thus an increased global prophylactic use of anti-malarials and this has led to a reduction in patients who have the potential of developing acute malarial infection. With adequate control of severe malarial infection, the underlying deficiencies of folic acid and iron have become apparent in the now predominantly mild-to-moderate degrees of anaemia (packed cell volume (PCV), 19–33%).

Studies have shown that iron deficiency amongst pregnant Nigeria women is of dietary origin [16]. Although staple foods in Nigeria are rich in iron (the available daily range in a balanced diet being 26–40 mg), many of our patients who belong to the low socio-economic group are unable to afford a diet that provides adequate iron. In fact, the average daily iron consumption of many of these patients is less than 10 mg. The situation, therefore, is that mild-to-moderate anaemia is now more commonly seen. Iron deficiency is nearly as common as folic acid deficiency, as some degree of iron deficiency is present in at least 90% expectant women seen with dimorphic anaemia. The implication of the foregoing is that iron supplement has become as desirable as antimalarials and folic acid in the management of anaemia in pregnancy.

Nigeria because of its large population has the highest number of HIV-positive pregnant women in Africa and the prevalence of anaemia has been documented to be higher amongst this group of women. This may be attributed to the disease or medications given for the treatment of the condition [4, 17].

29.3 Physiological and Other Considerations

Blood volume is usually increased during pregnancy. The increase in the plasma component of about 50% is much is higher than in the red cells of about 30% and the haemoglobin is consequently reduced to a varying extent, occasionally resulting in anaemia. This phenomenon is termed physiological anaemia and occurs in varying proportions. The increased blood volume can also pose a positive danger. For example, in the cardiac patient, the increased circulatory volume could lead to heart failure and because of the reduced oxygen-carrying capacity of diluted blood, the foetus, in severe anaemia, may be insufficiently oxygenated.

There is also an increased demand for haemopoietic factors, the best known of which is iron. The pregnancy demand of iron is approximately 900 mg, of which about 500–600 mg go to the uterus and its contents. Between 150 and 200 mg of iron is lost from a normal delivery and a similar amount is required for lactation. In addition to the above requirements, about 500 mg of iron is needed for the increased maternal haemoglobin mass; this iron is returned to the store after delivery. On the credit side some iron, about 250 mg, is saved as a result of amenorrhoea throughout pregnancy. This still leaves a total likely ultimate iron deficit of about 600–700 mg. Thus, pregnancy creates a state of negative iron balance.

It may take 6–12 months after delivery to recover from the iron deficit of pregnancy from a good diet. Therefore, anaemia is relatively more common in grandmultiparous women, particularly those in whom pregnancies succeed each other rapidly. In environments where the diet is poor in iron or where poverty does not permit adequate dietary iron intake, it will take a much longer period to regain the iron loss resulting from pregnancy. To meet the iron needs of pregnancy, a woman requires about 2.5–6 mg of elemental iron daily with much of this requirement in the second and third trimester.

A common cause of anaemia in pregnancy is inadequate absorption of iron. This may be an important factor in developing countries where malabsorption syndromes are prevalent. Even in patients with normal absorptive capacity, certain factors predispose to deficiency anaemia. The first is inadequate dietary iron. In the developing countries, the average daily dietary iron intake of the great majority of expectant women in around 9 mg, whereas the normal daily requirement for pregnant women is about 20 mg. Of the total amount of iron in food, only a fraction (10–15%) is available for absorption [18, 19]. Natural foods such as liver, meat, egg and certain fruits are good sources of iron, but they are generally outside the reach of an average person in developing countries.

Phytic acid, present in brown bread, which also contains iron, tends to interfere with iron absorption by combining with iron to form insoluble salts. Intestinal disorders such as chronic diarrhoea also adversely affect iron absorption. By contrast, iron absorption is favourably enhanced by the presence of hydrochloric acid in the stomach. As is well known the ferrous salts are more readily absorbed than the ferric salts, hence the dietary value of fresh vegetables and fruits that are rich in vitamin C.

A lot has been said of iron but other substances are also necessary for the formation of red cells by an active bone marrow. These include folic acid and vitamin B12 (the haemopoietic principle) in the synthesis of nucleic acid and subsequently nucleoprotein. Folate requirement is increased in pregnancy and since the storage of folate in the body is small, this need cannot be met without a supplemented diet. Malaria infection also adds to the increased requirement.

Women, whether in the rich or poor communities of the world, are potentially prone to varying degrees of anaemia during pregnancy. Three of the reasons evident from the physiological considerations are:

1. *Physiologic Haemodilution*: This occurs particularly in the second trimester of pregnancy. The increase in plasma volume outstrips the increase in red cell volume and therefore anaemia tends to result.
2. *Increase Demands of Blood-Forming Substances*: There are increased demands by the developing foetus, the placenta and the increase in the body weight of the expectant woman.
3. *Failure to take Haematinics*: This predisposes to anaemia in pregnancy through inadequate intake of haematinics either from foods or by medication. The cause of inadequate intake of haematinics is often ascribed to nausea and vomiting which are common features of early pregnancy. This phenomenon is a more common feature of early pregnancy. This phenomenon is more common in the primigravida but there would appear to be some hereditary elements in its frequency. For example, it is known to be more common in women whose mothers had suffered from this complication of pregnancy.

29.4 Main Types of Anaemia

In order to give a panoramic view of the causes of anaemia, it is sometimes good to present the main groups with examples, as follows:

1. *Deficiency Anaemias*: The main examples are folic acid and iron deficiency, more rarely vitamin B12 deficiency may occur. Other micro or macronutrients needed for the production of haemoglobin may also be contributory factors.
2. *Haemolytic Anaemias*: There are two main categories in this group:
   (a) *Hereditary Cause of Red Cell Haemolysis*: Examples include abnormal haemoglobins [haemoglobin sickle cell (HbSC), HbSS, thalassaemia), red cell membrane defects (spherocytosis) and enzyme disorders [glucose-6-phosphate dehydrogenase (G6PD) deficiency].
   (b) *Acquired Causes of Red Cell Haemolysis*: In the developing countries, at least equally important examples are malaria, severe chest infection, urinary tract infection and septicaemia from any cause.
3. *Haemorrhagic Anaemias*: Blood loss can occur in two forms. Frank blood loss is seen in patients with threatened abortion, antepartum or postpartum haemorrhage. On the other hand, the blood loss could be from heavy hookworm infestation.
4. *Anaemias of Bone Marrow Pathology*: In this situation, every other factor is present normally, but there is failure of adequate formation of new red blood cells. Factors that can be responsible are bone marrow destruction (aplastic), infiltration (e.g. leukemias, metastases from malignancies) and chronic medical disorders (e.g. kidneys, liver, bowels) also contribute to this group of anaemias.

29.5 Management of Anaemia in Pregnancy

The principles underlying the management of anaemia in pregnancy are as follows:

(a) *Identification and Treatment of the Cause*: From a good history, clinical examination and investigations.
(b) *Correction of Anaemia*: By the most appropriate method (depending on the severity of the anaemia and how much time one has on hand – in other words, the gestational age of the pregnancy at the time of diagnosis). It must be remembered that the objective is to correct the anaemia before the onset of labour or term.

29.6 Diagnosis

To reach a diagnosis the history must be detailed, the clinical examination must be thorough and appropriate investigations must be carried out to confirm the diagnosis. The history must include age, ethnicity, occupation, use of social or recreational drugs, medications, dietary habits and known familial diseases. Others include the obstetrics, gynaecology and medical and travel history. Investigations can also be used to monitor response to definitive treatment.

The classical symptoms of tiredness, weakness and dizziness are present in only a small percentage of patients with anaemia. In fact, it is common for patients with haemoglobin of less than 6.8 g/dl (PCV, 18%) to walk into the clinic without any complaint. Many patients with anaemia (over 80% of them) are picked up from the routine estimation of the haematocrit level during visits to the antenatal clinic. This fact underscores the importance of routine haemoglobin estimation in pregnant women at each visit to the antenatal clinic. In severe cases, however, the classical symptoms may exist with dyspnoea and generalized oedema.

29.7 Clinical Examination

The clinical examination must be systematic. From a careful general examination, one may suspect a likely cause of the anaemia. For example, patients with abnormal haemoglobins are generally slender in stature, with long and thin limbs. Another feature is the prominence of the forehead (bossing). An important sign often missed in these patients is scarification marks at the joints particularly the elbow and knee joints representing traditional treatment for bone pains. Sometimes scarification marks may be seen in the splenic area.

The central sign of anaemia is pallor and the areas to examine for pallor are the tongue and the mucous membranes (conjunctivae, the tongue and the buccal mucosa). Anaemia can also be detected by examining the palms of the hand and the fingernail beds. The nails may show the existence of koilonichia, which is a feature of severe iron deficiency. Jaundice should be excluded, as its presence suggests a haemolytic cause. The other aspects of general examination of the patient should be carried out such as examining for lymphadenopathy, oedema, etc. after the general features, the systems should be examined for the purpose of further evaluation of the anaemia.

The respiratory system is examined for gross pathology such as tuberculosis or chronic chest infection and a particular search must be made for basal crepitation, which are present in patients with anaemia complicated by heart failure.

The next system is the cardiovascular system. In many patients with anaemia, there is some degree of cardiac hypertrophy probably caused by the increase in workload on the heart in its efforts to adequately oxygenate the body tissues. It is therefore not unusual for the apex beat to be slightly displaced laterally from the mid-clavicular line. In patients with moderate-to-severe anaemia, a pan-systolic murmur (ejection or haemic murmur) may be heard. With adequate treatment of the anaemia the murmur normally disappears.

On the abdomen, a general examination is made but particular attention should be paid to the spleen. Splenic enlargement coexisting with anaemia suggests a haemolytic aetiology. It should be emphasized that splenic size is both of diagnostic and prognostic importance. The size of the spleen in patients with haemolytic anaemia varies inversely with the control of underlying haemolytic process. While it is recognized that in tropical countries splenic enlargement may be present in the non-anaemic patient as in the tropical splenomegaly syndrome its existence in an anaemic patient should raise the suspicion of red cell haemolysis until proven otherwise.

29.8 Investigations

Investigations vary from simple side room test to sophisticated laboratory procedure. The packed cell volume (PCV) using capillary blood is most usually done; however, a full blood count (FBC) is preferable because it estimates the Hb concentration and other indices such as the total and differential white cell counts, mean corpuscular volume (MCV), mean corpuscular haemoglobin (MCH), mean corpuscular haemoglobin concentration (MCHC) and platelets count. Peripheral blood film is useful in identifying the type of anaemia as microcytic, hypochromic, macrocytic, megaloblastic or dimorphic varieties.

In the diagnosis of iron deficiency anaemia, the iron status is usually assessed by the measurement of haemoglobin (HB), serum iron (SI), total iron-binding capacity (TBC), transferrin saturation (TS) pr T1 percentage, serum ferritin and erythrocyte protoporphyrin. Values diagnostic of iron deficiency are as follows:

Serum iron: mean 102 ± 42 μg/dl	– Low in iron deficiency
Total iron binding capacity: mean 444 ± 94 μg/dl	– High in iron deficiency
Serum transferrin below 12 μg/l (normal 14.2–120 μg/l)	

It should be noted that these indices (measurements) of iron deficiency anaemia can be affected by both inflammation and iron deficiency. For example, both iron deficiency and inflammation are associated with a decrease in HB, SI and with an increase in erythrocyte protoporphyrin.

Thus, transferrin saturation is affected by inflammation and infection because they decrease serum iron levels. Increase in serum iron caused by iron supplements haemolytic diseases and liver diseases such as hepatitis B virus infection will also lead to higher transferrin saturation.

Inflammation due to subclinical malaria or other parasites had been associated with a rise in the level of serum ferritin. Therefore, in Africa, serum ferritin is not a reliable indicator of iron status unless inflammation is also taken into consideration.

Malaria parasite can be easily identified by microscopic examination of the thin and thick films of the peripheral blood sample. Newer rapid diagnostics kits are also available for easy diagnosis of malaria especially in areas with shortage of laboratory scientists.

Stool microscopy may help in detecting occult blood and ova of parasites (hookworm) while urine microscopy, culture and sensitivity is useful in identifying infections of the urinary system. Coombs' test will help in detecting autoimmune causes.

With the increased embracement of voluntary counselling and confidential testing (VCCT) for HIV infection and prevention of mother-to-child transmission (PMTCT) of HIV services, many pregnant women are now aware of their HIV status. Rapid testing kits for HIV are available for testing women with unknown status.

29.9 Clinical Approach to the Management of Anaemia in Pregnancy

When the diagnosis of anaemia in pregnancy is made, particularly in the asymptomatic patient, questions relevant to the establishment of a possible cause should be asked – such as a history of any febrile illness preceding the event (malaria), dietary status, blood loss, recurrent bone pains in childhood (common in patients with abnormal haemoglobins).

Questions should also be directed to relevant systems such as the chest or urinary tract. After this, the appropriate investigations should be carried out.

(i) For patients with mild-to-moderate degrees of anaemia, the following investigations are suggested:
  - Mild anaemia, Hb 9–11 g/dl (PCV, 27–33%)
  - Moderate anaemia, Hb 6.6–9 g/dl (PCV, 19–26%)
    (a) Estimation of the PCV to confirm the severity of the anaemia
    (b) Full blood count and differentials
    (c) Blood films – a *thick film* for malaria parasites; a *thin film* for red cell morphology
    (d) Haemoglobin electrophoresis
    (e) Urinalysis including culture and sensitivity
    (f) Liver function tests
    (g) Stool for hookworm ova

(h) Blood grouping and Rhesus factor in preparation for possible blood transfusion
(i) Where relevant and where facilities exist, serum iron, total iron-binding capacity, serum folate and serum ferritin

(ii) For patients with severe anaemia, Hb 6.8 g/dl or less (PCV, 18% or less), the following additional investigations are required:
(a) Chest radiography to exclude chronic chest infection, for example, tuberculosis
(b) Bone marrow biopsy for a clearer cause/type of existing anaemia (because the peripheral blood picture is always several weeks behind the bone marrow state)

From the history, a careful clinical examination and the above investigations, it should be possible to arrive at a diagnosis in the majority of patients with anaemia.

29.10 Treatment

All anaemic patients in areas where malaria is endemic should receive anti-malarials. If malaria parasitaemia is found, a full course of anti-malarials should be given. The specific anti-malarial depends on the trimester of pregnancy. Although Quinine is safe throughout all trimesters, artemisinin-based combination therapy (artemether/lumefantrine) is the recommended first-line treatment for uncomplicated malaria in the second and third trimester. The oral route is preferred except in situations where there is severe vomiting.

Any other identifiable cause should be treated (e.g. urinary tract infection, hookworm infestation, dietary deficiencies such as iron, folic acid and very rarely vitamin B_{12}).

29.10.1 Correction of Anaemia

1. Oral haematinics.
2. Parenteral haematinics.
3. Blood transfusion (usually packed red cells). A potent diuretic, for example, frusemide 40 g, given intramuscularly or by the intravenous routine may occasionally be administered along with the blood transfusion.
4. Exchange blood transfusion.

29.10.2 Choice of Method for Correcting Anaemia

General guidelines are given because each case must be assessed individually, the objective being to correct the anaemia before term or before onset of labour, whichever is earlier.

29.10.3 Mild Anaemia

For patients with mild anaemia, oral haematinics such as fersolate 200 mg or other equivalent iron preparations plus folic acid 5 mg daily is administered. The former practice of increased dosage of haematinics, for example, ferrous sulphate 200 mg thrice daily, was found from recent studies to be of no significant advantage [12]. However, if a mildly anaemic patient is seen late in pregnancy from the Week 37 onwards, blood transfusion with packed cells should be given, 500 ml transfused slowly over a period of 8 hours at a time and given only to those at serious carefully considered risks.

29.10.4 Moderate Anaemia

The same principle for the management of mild anaemia should operate, but because of the higher risks in these patients resort to blood transfusion would be earlier, from about the Week 32 of pregnancy.

29.10.5 Severe Anaemia

Irrespective of the gestational age of the pregnancy, caution should be exercised in the use of blood transfusion to correct the anaemia. In patients with severe anaemia alone and deserving transfusion, a slow blood transfusion in the form of packed cells is appropriate and this can be repeated every third day until the haematocrit gestation of the pregnancy. A haematocrit level of 28% is acceptable before the Week 34 of pregnancy. After the Week 36, the objective should be to correct the anaemia to a PCV minimum level of 33%.

For patients with imminent heart failure, usually patients with haematocrit level of 15% or less, or patients with established heart failure (irrespective of the haematocrit level), a potent diuretic should be added to each 500 ml of packed cells. Again, transfusion is repeated on alternate days as often as desirable. One important point about transfusion in severe anaemia is that blood transfusion should be slowly administered – 500 ml being given over a period of approximately 4 hours, but faster and less than 4 hours when the anaemia is due to acute blood loss.

In addition, in the majority of cases a broad-spectrum antibiotic (amoxicillin/clavulanic acid, 1 g, 12 hourly for 1 week) should be given to patients with severe anaemia, as prophylaxis against infection. In patients with severe anaemia, the body resistance to infection is very low and this explains the justification for antibiotic prophylaxis. In a few of them, an infection would have already been in existence. In such situation, efforts must be made to identify the site and type of infection. Appropriate antibiotics should be commenced as soon as possible.

29.11 Exchange Blood Transfusion

This is the most rapid method of correcting anaemia but it is also the most expensive and laborious. Its advantage over packed cell transfusion is only marginal and greatest within the first 12 hours following transfusion. Therefore, it is a method now rarely used. The only indication for exchange blood transfusion in anaemia in pregnancy is when correction of the anaemia must be made very quickly, a situation which exists in a patient with *severe anaemia in early labour.*

29.12 Parenteral Iron Therapy

This approach is relevant because of the prevailing circumstances in many developing countries. First, for economic, socio-cultural, educational reasons and because of the high endemicity of parasitic infections, the prevalence of anaemias including iron deficiency remains high. Second, most antenatal patients cannot be relied upon to take drugs strictly according to prescriptions once outside medical supervision. Third, many women book late in pregnancy resulting in a short time for the correction of anaemia by oral medications. Another compounding factor is the lack of blood bank facilities due to unpreparedness of the public to donate blood to match the high demand.

The overall situation thus favours parenteral iron therapy provided the clinical picture is that of iron deficiency, there is no previous history of hypersensitivity to parenteral iron and there is ability to monitor the infusion as for blood transfusion. Although with time, the haemoglobin response to oral and parenteral therapy should be the same, experience from controlled clinical studies has shown that parenteral therapy is often more effective principally because of poor compliance by patients on oral therapy. There is also the psychological satisfaction among our patients that a good treatment is that which includes injection. This has led to a very high acceptance rate for parenteral therapy.

The appropriateness of the widespread use of parenteral iron in our practice has been reinforced by evidence of satisfactory haematological responses to treatment of a large number of patients with anaemias associated with iron deficiency. The routes of administration are:

(a) *Intravenous iron preparation*: The simplest is imferon total dose infusion (TDI). The dose required is related to the body weight of the patient and the haematocrit level (deficit from normal values) as shown in Table 29.2. The procedure for TDI is as shown in Table 29.3.

(b) *Intramuscular iron*: The common preparations are iron dextran (imferon), iron polysorbitol gluconic acid complex (ferastral) and iron sorbitol (jectofer). Most experience is limited to imferon and ferastral. The advantage of ferastral is that it can be given in a higher dose. The manufacturers advocate the administration of 10 ml, in two divided doses. However, from experience, it is more acceptable and much less painful to give not more than 4 ml imferon and 5 ml ferastral at a time. A serious disadvantage of intramuscular iron is the staining of the overlying skin, which is more obvious in fair-skinned people. It is possible to reduce the incidence of staining by a skilful technique such as the Z-technique which involves pulling the tissues laterally while the needle is being inserted so

Table 29.2 Dosage of imferon

Patient's	Weight	Observed haemoglobin						
		3.0G	4.4G	5.9G	7.4G	8.9G	10.4G	11.8G
Kg	lb.	20%	30%	40%	50%	60%	70%	80%
		Total dose of imferon in ml						
5	10	5	5	4	3	3	2	2
9	20	10	9	8	6	5	4	3
14	30	14	13	11	9	8	6	4
18	40	19	17	15	12	10	7	5
23	50	24	21	18	15	12	9	6
27	60	29	25	22	18	15	11	8
32	70	34	30	25	21	17	13	9
36	80	38	34	29	24	19	15	10
41	90	42	38	32	27	22	16	11
45	100	48	42	36	30	24	18	12
50	110	53	46	39	33	26	20	14
55	120	58	51	43	36	29	22	15
59	130	62	53	47	39	31	23	16
64	140	67	59	50	42	34	25	17
68	150	72	63	54	45	36	27	18
73	160	77	68	57	48	38	29	20
77	170	82	72	61	51	41	31	21
82	180	86	76	64	54	43	32	22
86	190	91	80	68	57	45	34	23
91	200	96	84	72	60	48	36	24

1 m. Imferon 1 = 50 mg Fe
This formula makes an allowance for the replenishment of body iron stores. In pregnancy, add 10 ml (500 mg Fe) to the calculated dose

Table 29.3 Procedure of administration of imferon total dose infusion (TDI)

1. Determine the patient's total requirements from the dosage table including the additional requirements for pregnancy, if applicable
2. Add the total calculated volume of imferon aseptically to one pint of sterile normal saline or 5% dextrose solution in the absence of normal saline
3. A test dose should be given at a rate not exceeding five drops per minute for 10 minutes under strict medical supervision. If this test dose is well tolerated, the rate of infusion may be increased to 45–6 drops per minute
4. If there are any signs of intolerance (urticarial rash, loin pains, chest pain, respiratory discomfort or any significant change from the pre-infusion general feeling, acute hypersensitivity) to the test dose, the infusion should be stopped at once

Symptoms frequently subside on ceasing the infusion but treatment for shock may be necessary in patients with severe reaction

One contraindication to the use of iron dextran apart from a history of hypersensitivity is overwhelming sepsis

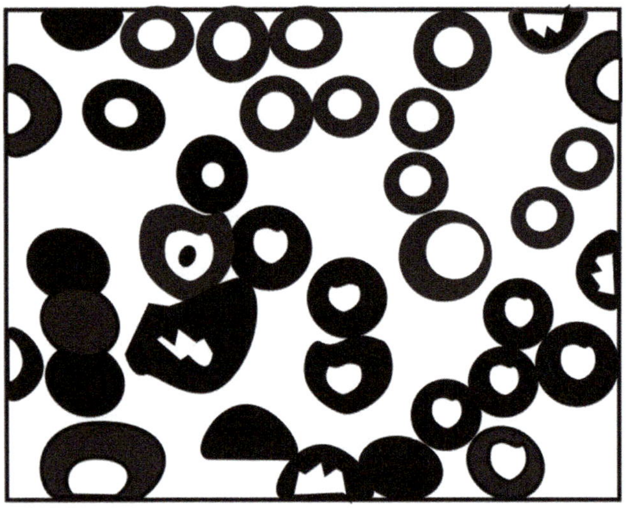

Fig. 29.2 Peripheral blood films a patient with anaemia in pregnancy. Note the polymorphic appearance of the red cells, microcytic, macrocytic, normocytic cells, with varying degrees of hypochromia

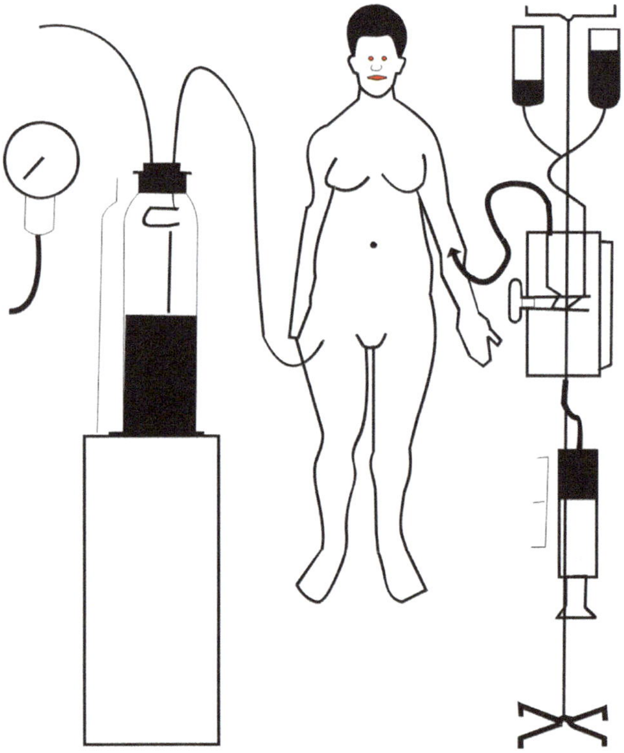

Fig. 29.3 Exchange blood transfusion

that the needle track and therefore the track of the leakage is zig-zagged.

In summary, the choice of parenteral iron would depend on the practitioner who has to take into account the facilities available to him for a safe therapy. A constraint to imferon infusion in the developing countries is inadequate medical manpower for supervision during the infusion. This constraint is not a serious one since if many of those patients are not given parenteral iron, they would have to be given blood which would require equal supervision by medical or paramedical personnel. On the other hand, with the single-handed practitioner or in most parts of the rural areas, the intramuscular therapy would seem to be more applicable. The advantages of parenteral iron therapy are listed in Table 29.4.

Table 29.4 Advantages of imferon (TDI) in the developing countries

1. Certainty of dosage and administration
2. Avoidance of repeated injections
3. Economy in time for the patient and hospital staff
4. Saving of blood, particularly in obstetrics and elective surgery
5. Reliable haematological response when time is short before delivery or surgery

A rare complication of correction of anaemia is iron overload. First, it results from the treatment of refractory anaemia with multiple blood transfusions and also due to an abnormal increased absorption, when iron is given orally. It rarely follows massive or repeated parenteral iron administration because of the predominantly reticulo-endothelial localization of parenterally injected iron complexes. Second, following TDI infusion, for days and even weeks after a large injection, plasma iron concentrations may remain high, but virtually all of the iron remains attached to dextran. From the plasma it is gradually taken up by the reticulo-endothelial system and only when needed, iron is split off and transported by transferrin to the marrow for haemoglobin synthesis.

The advocation of a liberal use of imferon to conserve the relatively little available blood for use in case of severe anaemias or dire emergencies should be seen as an interim measure dictated by prevailing circumstance. The long-term improvement in problems associated with anaemia will come from an improved socio-economic state of the population.

Furthermore, through education, the following will emerge:

(a) The development of an awareness to utilize maximally existing medical facilities, inadequate as they are
(b) An increased willingness and appreciation of the need to donate blood for obstetric and other emergency use
(c) The encouragement of a higher compliance rate with oral medication
(d) An early report for booking during pregnancy

29.12.1 Malaria Chemoprophylaxis

Some epidemiologists argue that by administering malaria chemoprophylaxis, the natural immune system will be interfered. Removal of the protection after delivery theoretically places the subject under a greater threat of severe malaria infection. Also, the patient is prevented from improving her immune status. Furthermore, some anti-malarials, particularly the 4-aminoquinoline drugs, have been reported to cross the placenta and to cause foetal abnormalities, including loss of vision, ototoxicity and cochleovestibular disturbances.

There is no question that malaria, even in the non-pregnancy state, can lead to severe morbidity and death from cerebral malaria. However, few the deaths may be, if even one death per 100,000 subjects, it is justifiable to protect all those at risk of infection, particularly in an endemic region. Therefore, the potential benefits of chemoprophylaxis outweigh the possible immunological derangement that may follow such practices.

Thus, there is today a general agreement among obstetricians, many epidemiologists and pharmacological scientists on the regular use of malaria chemoprophylaxis during pregnancy and the puerperium. The main factors dictating this practice are as follows:

1. Prevention/reduction of malaria attacks in the pregnant woman in view of the maternal and perinatal morbidity or mortality that may occur following such infection.
2. Protection of the lowered acquired immunity to malaria reckoned to occur during pregnancy particularly in the primigravidae.
3. Malaria is endemic in the tropics; therefore, pregnant as well as non-pregnant women are susceptible to malaria infection.

29.12.2 What Drug(s) to Give as Malaria Chemoprophylaxis?

The approach to malaria prophylaxis varies from one region to the other and sometimes from one practitioner to another in the same centre. The choice of drug is usually dictated by the regional experience of the practitioner with respect to the drug resistance profile of malaria parasites or outcome of research on malaria chemoprophylaxis conducted by or known to the prescriber.

Currently, intermittent preventive treatment of malaria in pregnancy (IPTp) with sulphadoxine/pyrimethamine (SP) is the recommended regimen. This involves the administration of three tablets of sulphadoxine/pyrimethamine (500 mg/25 mg) given twice or thrice during pregnancy at 4 weeks interval and started after quickening which is about the 16–18 week of gestation. Two doses are recommended for low-risk patients while patients with immunosuppression in HIV infection are given three doses. The IPT-Sp is avoided during the first trimester because of risk of teratogenicity and after 34 weeks of gestation because of the risk of hyperbilirubinaemia and kernicterus in the newborn since sulphonamides and bilirubin competes together for binding site on serum albumin, thereby increasing the free circulating levels of bilirubin. However, recent recommendations from WHO allows its continued use at 4 weekly intervals till delivery in malaria endemic area. The previously used weekly administration of pyrimethamine 25 mg (daraprin) has been found to be non-effective and no longer recommended. Other previous practices of the administration of 600 mg base chloroquine to expectant mothers at the first antenatal visit was found to be non-effective and promoted the development of resistance strains of plasmodium species.

Considerable space has been devoted to malaria prevention because of its importance in the causation of anaemia in the tropics and the contemporary issues surrounding the subject.

Other methods of preventing anaemia that must be mentioned are prophylactic haematinics, health education on nutritional supplementation, treatment of hookworm infestations when diagnosed and birth spacing which is assisted by the knowledge and practice of family planning. One preventive method that requires further discussion is haematinic supplementation. All patients now require iron 200 mg daily and folic acid 5 mg. The practice of some health institutions to administer iron 200 mg thrice daily has been found to be of no advantage over the single dose regimen for prophylaxis.

29.13 Adverse Effects of Anaemia in Pregnancy

Anaemia has adverse effects on the expectant woman as well as the foetus. In the mother these include loss of work and home care through weakness by incapacitation and easy fatigue, cardiac failure in severe cases and occasionally, maternal death may be the result of anaemia. Deaths are common in neglected cases and where prompt treatment cannot be given. There is predisposition to infections and aggravation of other complications of pregnancy such as pre-eclampsia. After delivery, some of the patients are prone to postpartum haemorrhage and infections.

In the foetus, abortion, intra-uterine growth restriction (IUGR), intra-uterine death and preterm delivery are recognized complications during pregnancy. Babies that survive delivery are prone to perinatal complications and are also liable to anaemia later in life since their development will be governed by similar environmental factors to which the mothers had been exposed.

29.14 Prevention of Anaemia

The prevalence of anaemia is strongly influenced by the level of education and socio-economic status. It is therefore clear that prevention is difficult in many developing countries, but certain measures, as stated below, will lead to a reduction.

(a) A vigorous campaign for early booking for antenatal care
(b) Dietary advice during the counselling class at antenatal clinics
(c) The administration of anti-malarial and haematinics throughout pregnancy and the puerperium
(d) Through education, early marriage will be reduced and by extension, diminished complications of pregnancy
(e) Health education in secondary schools, with references to pregnancy

29.15 Summary

Anaemia, as elsewhere, is the commonest complication of pregnancy. Its prevalence in the developing countries is high, of the order of 60%. The main causes are dietary deficiencies caused by poverty and environmental endemic parasitic infections. The high frequency of abnormal haemoglobins further aggravates the problems of anaemia in the tropics.

The principles of management are identification of the cause to enable correct treatment and correction of the anaemia by the most appropriate methods. The overall objective is to make sure that the patient is not anaemic by term or onset of labour, whichever occurs earlier.

Attention has been drawn to the place of parenteral iron in the developing countries and the need for measures that will lead to a reduction in the unacceptably high prevalence of the condition in obstetric practice.

References

1. Abe E, Omo-Aghoja LO. Maternal mortality at the central hospital, Benin city Nigeria: a ten year review. Afr J Reprod Health. 2008;12(3):17–26.
2. Ujah I, Aisien O, Mutihir J, Vanderjagt D, Glew R, Uguru V. Factors contributing to maternal mortality in north-Central Nigeria: a seventeen-year review. Afr J Reprod Health. 2005;9(3):27–40.
3. Ogunbode O. Anaemia in pregnancy. In: Ogunbode O, editor. Medical disorders in tropical obstetrics. 1st ed. Ibadan: Evan Brothers Nigeria Publishers Ltd; 1997. p. 1–20.
4. Uneke CJ, Duhlinska DD, Igbinedion EB. Prevalence and public-health significance of HIV infection and anaemia among pregnant women attending antenatal clinics in south-eastern Nigeria. J Health Popul Nutr. 2007;25(3):328–35.
5. Adesina O, Akinyemi O, Oladokun A. Anemia in pregnancy at two levels of health care in Ibadan, south west Nigeria. Ann Afr Med. 2011;10(4):272–7.
6. Oladipo A, Falana A, Adegoke F, Sambo A, Kungu J. Prevalence of anemia among pregnant women and its determinants in Northern Nigeria. Eur J Nutr Food Saf. 2015;5(5):865–6.
7. De Benoist B, McLean E, Egli I, Cogswell M. Worldwide prevalence of anaemia 1993–2005. WHO Global Database Anaemia; 2008. p. 1–40.
8. Obed SA, Ekem I. Anaemia in pregnancy. In: Kwawukume EY, Ekele BA, Danso KA, Emuveyan E, editors. Comprehensive obstetrics in the tropics. 2nd ed. Accra: AGLC Press; 2015. p. 332–7.
9. Obasi I, Nwachukwu N. Comparative iron related anaemia in pregnancy in Ebonyi state, South-east Nigeria. J Med Sci. 2013;13(6):425–31.
10. Nwizu E, Iliyasu Z, Ibrahim S, Galadanci H. Socio-demographic and maternal factors in anaemia in pregnancy at booking in Kano, Northern Nigeria. Afr J Reprod Health. 2011;15(4):33–41.
11. World Health Organization. Haemoglobin concentrations for the diagnosis of anaemia and assessment of severity. Vitamin and Mineral Nutrition Information System. Geneva: World Health Organization; 2011. (WHO/NMH/NHD/MNM/11.1). http://www.who.int/vmnis/indicators/haemoglobin.Pdf. Accessed 5 May 2016.
12. Letsky EA. Maternal anaemia in pregnancy. Iron and pregnancy – a haematologist's view. Fetal Mater Med Rev. 2001;12(3):159–75.
13. Guyatt HL, Snow RW. The epidemiology and burden of plasmodium falciparum -related anemia among pregnant women in sub-saharan Africa. Am J Trop Med Hyg. 2001;64(1):36–44.
14. Lawson JB, Stewart DB. Anaemia in pregnancy. In: Lawson J, Stewart D, editors. Obstetrics and gynaecology in the tropics and developing countries. London: Edward Arnold Publishers; 1969. p. 73.
15. Asa O, Onayade A, Fatusi A, Ijadunola K, Abiona T. Efficacy of intermittent preventive treatment of malaria with sulphadoxine-pyrimethamine in preventing anaemia in pregnancy among Nigerian women. Matern Child Health J. 2008;12(6):692–8.
16. Vanderjagt DJ, Brock HS, Melah GS, El-Nafaty AU, Crossey MJ, Glew RH. Nutritional factors associated with anaemia in pregnant women in Northern Nigeria. J Health Popul Nutr. 2007;25(1):75–81.
17. Olatunbosun OA, Abasiattai AM, Bassey EA, James RS, Ibanga G, Morgan A. Prevalence of anaemia among pregnant women at booking in the university of Uyo teaching hospital, Uyo, Nigeria. Biomed Res Int. Hindawi Publishing Corporation. 2014;2014:1–8.
18. Stoltzfus R, Dreyfuss M. Guidelines for the use of iron supplements to prevent and treat iron deficiency anemia. International Nutritional Anaemia Consultative Group (INACG); 1998. p. 1–46.
19. Milman N. Oral iron prophylaxis in pregnancy: not too little and not too much! J Pregnancy. 2012;2012:1–8.

30 Diabetes in Pregnancy

Rosemary N. Ogu and Biodun Olagbuji

Learning Objectives

At the conclusion of this chapter, the reader will be able to:

- Define hyperglycaemia in pregnancy, gestational diabetes mellitus, and diabetes in pregnancy.
- Explain the need for early detection of hyperglycaemia in pregnancy.
- Identify the methods for screening for hyperglycaemia in pregnancy.
- Critically evaluate pregnant women with hyperglycaemia and initiate a review by ophthalmologists, endocrinologists, and dieticians.
- Differentiate between medical nutrition therapy, insulin therapy, oral hypoglycaemic agents, and lifestyle modification.

30.1 Introduction

Hyperglycaemia in pregnancy is one of the most frequent medical disorders encountered during pregnancy and is of principal concern because of the increased risk of maternal and fetal complications in both well- and less-resourced settings. Hyperglycaemia first diagnosed during index pregnancy increases maternal risk for future diabetes and cardiovascular disorders as well as the vulnerability to diabetes and cardiometabolic disorders in offsprings exposed to hyperglycaemia in utero [1]. Long-term metabolic and cardiovascular implications of hyperglycaemia during pregnancy for mother and child are now generally recognised with major implications for public health. To prevent adverse pregnancy outcomes and to prevent or delay the future onset of type 2 diabetes in mother and the offspring, timely detection, optimum treatment, and preventive postpartum care and follow-up are necessary [1–3].

This chapter reviews the prevalence, pathophysiology, clinical presentation, testing and diagnosis, management, and prevention of hyperglycaemia in pregnancy. The controversies are also discussed. Lastly, each section considers how the condition compares and contrasts between well- and less-resourced settings.

30.2 Definitions and Classification of Hyperglycaemia in Pregnancy

The definition and classification of hyperglycaemia in pregnancy has evolved over time, and continues to be debated [4, 5]. Hyperglycaemia first detected at any time during pregnancy should be classified as either: diabetes mellitus in pregnancy or gestational diabetes mellitus [1, 4]. As previously defined, gestational diabetes mellitus refers to "any degree of glucose intolerance with onset or first recognition during pregnancy" [6–8]. This definition included women with diabetes or impaired glucose tolerance as described in non-pregnant adults [4]. The inclusion of such a broad range of glucose abnormalities in one definition raised concerns because of the special considerations about management during pregnancy and postpartum follow-up in women with more severe hyperglycaemia. Drawing conclusions about this group is particularly difficult because of the lack of good quality data at higher levels of hyperglycaemia since these women are excluded from epidemiological studies and randomised trials of GDM treatment [1, 4]. These efforts are also spurred by the increasing prevalence of diabetes and GDM and of greater

R. N. Ogu (✉)
University of Port Harcourt Teaching Hospital, University of Port Harcourt, Port Harcourt, Nigeria

Gestational DM Study Group, WHARC WHO FMOH MNCH Study Team, Abuja, Nigeria
e-mail: rosemary.ogu@uniport.edu.ng

B. Olagbuji
Ekiti State University Teaching Hospital, Ado-Ekiti, Nigeria

F. Okonofua et al. (eds.), *Contemporary Obstetrics and Gynecology for Developing Countries*,
https://doi.org/10.1007/978-3-030-75385-6_30

prevalence of maternal and fetal complications resulting from diabetes mellitus antedating pregnancy [1]. Therefore, these concerns have informed the current classification of hyperglycaemia first detected in pregnancy into (1) gestational diabetes, and (2) diabetes first detected during pregnancy or overt diabetes in pregnancy [1, 2, 4, 5, 9]. Based on the new WHO 2013 report and as recommended by FIGO in the 2015 FIGO guidelines, gestational diabetes can now be defined as any degree of glucose intolerance or hyperglycaemia first detected at any time during pregnancy that is not diagnostic of diabetes in the non-pregnant adults. Diabetes first detected in pregnancy or overt diabetes in pregnancy refers to hyperglycaemia first detected in pregnancy that is diagnostic of diabetes in the non-pregnant adult population. A third category of hyperglycaemia in pregnancy is 'diabetes detected prior to pregnancy' (either type 1 or 2 diabetes).

Summary classification of hyperglycaemia in pregnancy:

1. Gestational diabetes mellitus (GDM)
2. Diabetes in pregnancy/overt diabetes in pregnancy
3. Diabetes detected prior to pregnancy (Type 1 or 2)

This modified classification is of international standards, objectively reproducible, and facilitates a worldwide uniform strategy for detection and classification. GDM makes up about 84% of hyperglycaemia in pregnancy.

30.3 Epidemiology of Hyperglycaemia in Pregnancy

The International Diabetes Federation estimates that 20.9 million (16.2%) live births to women aged 20–49 years are affected by some form of hyperglycaemia in pregnancy. In essence, approximately one in six live births are affected by hyperglycaemia in pregnancy. Moreover, one in seven births is to women with gestational diabetes [2]. The majority (84%) of hyperglycaemia in pregnancy is gestational diabetes [1], and the proportions due to diabetes in pregnancy/overt diabetes in pregnancy and diabetes predating pregnancy are 7.4% and 7.5% respectively [2]. Worldwide, the number of women with diabetes is projected to rise from 199.5 million in 2015 to 313.3 million in 2040 [2]. Applying the percentage increase (57%) in a number of women with diabetes between 2015 and 2040, an estimated 32 million live births will be affected by maternal hyperglycaemia in 2040. As there are an estimated 318 million adults with prediabetes or impaired glucose tolerance (IDF Atlas) the projected number of live births that will be affected by maternal hyperglycaemia in 2040 is expected to be higher [2].

The global prevalence of hyperglycaemia in pregnancy ranges from 1% to 28% [1]. However, these global estimates as well as regional and national estimates show wide variations and are related to study setting, population studied, screening methods, or diagnostic thresholds and criteria [10]. Regardless of these factors, the prevalence of hyperglycaemia in pregnancy is increasing with time [10]. The increasing prevalence of hyperglycaemia in pregnancy is related to ageing population of pregnant women, increasing prevalence of obesity in women of reproductive age, and increasing prevalence of type 2 diabetes worldwide [11]. In terms of regional burden, estimates of hyperglycaemia in pregnancy in women within the age group 20–49 years range from as low as 10.5% in sub-Saharan Africa, translating to 3.3 million live births affected by this condition, to as high as 24.2% in South East Asia, translating to 6.7 million live births affected (IDF Atlas 2015) (Table 30.1).

Table 30.1 Hyperglycaemia in pregnancy in women aged 20–49 years by IDF region, 2015

IDF region	Raw prevalence	Age-adjusted prevalence	Number of live births affected
Africa	10.5%	9.5%	3.3 million
Europe	15.8%	13.7%	1.7 million
Middle East and North Africa	21.8%	17.7%	3.7 million
North America and Caribbean	14.9%	11.9%	1.0 million
South and Central America	13.2%	11.5%	0.9 million
South-East Asia	24.2%	26.3%	6.7 million
Western Pacific	12.4%	12.1%	3.7 million

Source: IDF Diabetes Atlas [2]

According to a recent systematic review, the prevalence of hyperglycaemia first detected in pregnancy ranges from 0.4% to 24.3% in low and middle-income countries, and the prevalence of diabetes first detected in pregnancy (including type 1 and 2 diabetes mellitus) ranges from 0.2% to 0.7% [12]. The prevalence rates of hyperglycaemia first detected in pregnancy are highest in India, Vietnam, and Cuba [12]. In sub-Saharan Africa, the prevalence of hyperglycaemia first detected in pregnancy (both GDM and DIP) in women of African origin ranges from 0% in Tanzania to 15.2% in Nigeria. In Nigeria, the prevalence of gestational diabetes ranges from 1.01% to 15.2% [13–15]. Using the universal screening-based approach, recent studies suggest that gestational diabetes occurs in up to 15.2% of pregnancies in Nigeria with the new WHO criteria whilst lower prevalence are seen with the old diagnostic criteria. Although the prevalence rates of gestational diabetes are higher in women with one or more risk factors (4.5–9.4%) for this disorder compared to women with no risk factors (1.8–6.4%) [13], the absence of risk factors is not protective against GDM [1, 16].

Table 30.2 Risk factors for GDM

Ethnicity
Older age
High parity
Overweight and obesity
Excessive weight gain in index pregnancy
Short stature
Polycystic ovarian syndrome (PCOS)
History of diabetes mellitus in first degree relatives
History of poor pregnancy outcome (e.g. fetal loss, miscarriage, congenital abnormalities)
Macrosomia in previous and/or index pregnancy
GDM in a previous pregnancy
Pre-eclampsia
Multifetal pregnancy

Adapted from "The International of Federation of Gynaecology and Obstetrics (FIGO) Initiative on Gestational Diabetes Mellitus: A pragmatic guide for Diagnosis, Management, and Care" [1]

30.4 Risk Factors for Hyperglycaemia in Pregnancy

There are several risk factors for gestational diabetes mellitus suggested in the literature (Table 30.2). It has been shown that not all women with GDM in index pregnancy have risk factors for this disorder. A study from Sweden has shown that less than half of women diagnosed with GDM in index pregnancy have one or more of the associated risk factors [17]. Olagbuji and colleagues reported that the prevalence rates of gestational diabetes are comparable in women with- and without risk factors for GDM [13]. Given the likelihood of the missed opportunities for detecting gestational diabetes in women with no risk factors, it seems logical that the identification of women with GDM requires subjecting all pregnant women to testing for this condition.

30.5 Pathophysiology and Clinical Presentation

Before insulin discovery, only 2% of successful pregnancies were seen in diabetes. Late menarche (hypothalamic anovulation), premature menopause (by up to 10 years compared to non-diabetic siblings), oocyte dysfunction (due to oxidative stress from hyperglycaemia), and sperm abnormalities from high percentage of spermatocytes with nuclear DNA damage due to oxidative stress lead to an increased miscarriage rate and erectile dysfunction. GDM is associated with increased perinatal morbidity, the characteristics of which are the same as for infants of mothers with overt diabetes (e.g. macrosomia, neonatal hypoglycaemia, hyperbilirubinaemia, and respiratory distress syndrome).

Pregnancy induces changes in maternal metabolism to accommodate and nurture the growth of the fetus in the womb from conception until term birth. Even though the mother eats intermittently, the fetus must be nourished continuously. This is achieved by complex interactions of the feto-placental-maternal unit, through secretion of hormones and metabolic mediators that create insulin resistance and modify maternal carbohydrate, lipid, and amino acid metabolism to ensure adequate nutrient supply to the fetus. These interactions are geared to create a harmonious balance between the needs of the mother, those of the fetus, and the mother's ability to provide for these needs. In response to increasing insulin resistance, maternal insulin secretion increases and euglycaemia is maintained. This is achieved at the cost of higher maternal insulin level and lower than normal non-pregnant fasting glucose levels.

Insulin resistance continues to increase as pregnancy advances and is well established by the 24th week. As long as the maternal pancreas continues to increase insulin production and secretion, hyperglycaemia is prevented. When this capacity is overwhelmed by rising insulin resistance, maternal hyperglycaemia ensues. Maternal insulin production capacity is thus put under immense stress during pregnancy. This explains why women with pre-existing insulin resistance (e.g. overweight, obese, or excessive weight gain during pregnancy, PCOS, impaired glucose tolerance (IGT), or metabolic syndrome) or those with lower ability to produce insulin (e.g. short stature, stunted) are more prone to GDM.

The underlying pathophysiologic process responsible for the clinical features seen in pregnancies complicated by hyperglycaemia is tabulated in Table 30.3.

Notwithstanding its severity, hyperglycaemia that is already present at conception and embryogenesis increases the women's vulnerability and risk of complications. A woman with undiagnosed diabetes antedating pregnancy may also have undiagnosed complications including retinopathy and nephropathy, which markedly increase pregnancy risks [5]. Furthermore, hyperglycaemia during the critical period of organogenesis may lead to a high risk of spontaneous abortions and congenital anomalies. Diabetes in pregnancy, because of the attendant greater risk of hyperglycaemia, may also result in aberrations in fetal growth and macrosomia. This can lead to additional short-term complications, for example, obstructed labour, shoulder dystocia, neonatal hypoglycaemia, or the risk of neurological damage. Moreover, there is a risk of onset or exacerbation of microvascular complications, such as retinopathy or nephropathy during pregnancy. For these reasons, ensuring meticulous glucose control before conception and throughout pregnancy is recommended.

Table 30.3 Underlying pathophysiologic process responsible for the clinical features seen in pregnancies complicated by hyperglycaemia

Stage	Underlying process	Sequalae/clinical features
All stages	Increased insulin resistance and reduced sensitivity to insulin action → HPL, progesterone, prolactin, cortisol, oestrogen	Nausea and vomiting → & maternal hypoglycaemia
1st trimester	Maternal hyperglycaemia → damage to embryonic DNA by generating excess free radicals and modifying key regulatory genes During organogenesis glycaemic control is critical	Congenital malformations
2nd trimester	Maternal hyperglycaemia → facilitated diffusion of glucose across the placenta →↑ fetal pancreatic cells → fetal hyperinsulinaemia	Insulin is the major fetal GH and produces excessive growth particularly in fat. Others include HPGH, fetal IGF, and TNFα → asymmetric macrosomia
3rd trimester	Maternal and fetal hyperglycaemia → metabolic milieu	Hypoxia acidosis and still birth
At birth	Fetal hyperglycaemia	Transient neonatal hypoglycaemia
Childhood and Adolescence	Insulin resistance	Obesity

Table 30.4 Complications of Gestational Diabetes Mellitus and Diabetes in Pregnancy

Gestational diabetes mellitus[a]	
Maternal morbidity	Fetal/neonatal/child morbidity
Pregnancy	Stillbirth
Spontaneous abortion	Neonatal death
Preeclampsia	Congenital malformation
Gestational hypertension	Shoulder dystocia
Excessive fetal growth (macrosomia, large for gestational age)	Respiratory distress syndrome
Hydramnios	Cardiomyopathy
Urinary tract infections	Neonatal hypoglycaemia
Delivery	Neonatal polycythaemia
Preterm labour	Neonatal hyperbilirubinaemia
Traumatic labour	Neonatal hypocalcaemia
Instrumental delivery	Erb's palsy
Caesarean section	*Fetal origins of disease*:
Postoperative/postpartum infection	Diabetes
Postoperative/postpartum haemorrhage	Obesity
Thromboembolism	Hypertension
Puerperium	Metabolic syndrome
Failure to initiate and/or maintain breastfeeding	
Infection	
Long-term postpartum	
Weight retention	
GDM in subsequent pregnancy	
Future overt diabetes	
Future cardiovascular disease	
Diabetes detected prior to pregnancy/diabetes in pregnancy	
Retinopathy	
Nephropathy	
Chronic hypertension	
Cardiovascular disease – atherosclerotic heart disease	
Diabetic ketoacidosis	

[a]Adapted from "The International Federation of Gynaecology and Obstetrics (FIGO) Initiative on Gestational Diabetes Mellitus: A pragmatic guide for Diagnosis, Management, and Care" [1]

30.6 Clinical Presentation

Gestational diabetes usually is asymptomatic, whilst diabetes first detected in pregnancy may present with overt symptoms of hyperglycaemia as in diabetes (types 1 and 2 diabetes) predating pregnancy. Overt symptoms of hyperglycaemia during pregnancy can include excessive thirst, a dry mouth, fatigue, frequent urination, weight loss and blurred vision, but these symptoms are rare and are often masked by normal pregnancy symptoms [2]. Many women with gestational diabetes lack clinical signs and symptoms because of the association of this disorder with slightly elevated blood glucose levels. In settings with sub-optimal screening strategy for gestational diabetes, many cases may be detected only at the time when maternal and fetal complications are identified (see Table 30.4).

30.7 Consequences of Hyperglycaemia in Pregnancy

Women with gestational diabetes mellitus have a heightened risk for perinatal and long-term postpartum complications (Table 30.4). In addition to the perinatal complications associated with gestational diabetes mellitus, women with diabetes detected prior to pregnancy or diabetes in pregnancy are at increased risk of retinopathy, nephropathy, chronic hypertension, and cardiovascular disease (e.g. atherosclerotic heart disease) [18–20].

30.8 Diagnosing Hyperglycaemia in Pregnancy

Biochemical testing is critical for the diagnosis of GDM and Diabetes in Pregnancy because these conditions are often asymptomatic. Based on the evidence from the landmark multinational Hyperglycaemia and Adverse Pregnancy Outcome (HAPO) study [21], the International Association of Diabetes in Pregnancy Study Groups (IADPSG) (2010) [9]and World Health Organization (2013) [4] proposed diagnostic thresholds for gestational diabetes and diabetes in pregnancy. Currently, these diagnostic cut-off values are widely accepted and preferred by other several international organisations including the American Diabetes Association

Table 30.5 Diagnostic cut-off values for blood glucose

Glucose measure	Glucose concentration threshold	
Gestational diabetes mellitus	mmol/l	mg/dl
FPG Fasting Blood Glucose	5.1–6.9	92–125
1-h plasma glucose	10.0	180
2-h plasma glucose	8.5–11	153–199
Diabetes in pregnancy/overt diabetes		
FPG Fasting Blood Glucose	7.0	126
HbA1c Glycated Haemoglobin	6.5%	
RPG Random Plasma Glucose	11.1	200

Adapted from IADPSG 2010 and WHO 2013; Recommended by FIGO 2015

and the International Federation of Gynaecology and Obstetrics (FIGO) [1, 2]. Various studies have shown that, hyperglycaemia that is less severe than that of diabetes in pregnancy (overt diabetes) is associated with increased risks of adverse perinatal consequences [21–24].

Tests for detecting hyperglycaemic disorders in pregnancy include fasting plasma glucose (FPG), random plasma glucose (RPG), glycosylated haemoglobin (Hb A1c), 50-g oral glucose challenge test, and 75-g 2-hour oral glucose tolerance test (fasting or non-fasting) [1, 4, 9, 25]. Two strategies (one-step and two-step) of the glucose load test are often used in the detection of hyperglycaemic disorder of pregnancy [25]. In the two-step approach, a 50-g glucose challenge test is followed by a 75-g glucose load test if the glucose threshold meets or exceeds 7.2 mmol/l (130 mg/dl), 7.5 mmol/l (135 mg/dl), or 7.8 mmol/l (140 mg/dl). In the one-step approach, a 75 g glucose load is administered either in the fasting or non-fasting state (FIGO guide). On the basis of IADPSG (2010) and WHO (2013) recommendations and as adopted by FIGO and published in 2015, the diagnosis of hyperglycaemic disorder at any time during pregnancy is made from one or more of the following cut-off values for blood glucose (Table 30.5) [1, 4, 9].

When the level of hyperglycaemia first detected by testing at any time during the course of pregnancy meets the criteria for diagnosis of diabetes in the non-pregnant state, the condition is called DIP. Those criteria as shown in Table 30.5 are as follows: fasting plasma glucose (FPG) $\geq$7.0 mmol/l or 126 mg/dl, and/or 2-hour 75-g oral glucose tolerance test (OGTT) value $\geq$11.1 mmol/l or 200 mg/dl, or random plasma glucose (RPG) $\geq$11.1 mmol/l or 200 mg/dl associated with signs and symptoms of diabetes.

30.9 Management

The main goal of treatment of pregnancies complicated by hyperglycaemic disorders is to maintain normoglycaemia as much as possible for the purpose of preventing maternal and fetal/neonatal complications during antepartum, intrapartum, and postpartum periods [1]

30.9.1 Prenatal Care

Care of women with pregnancies complicated by hyperglycaemia can be delivered via the multidisciplinary/shared or standard antenatal- model of care depending on the available resources and infrastructure in a particular setting. A multidisciplinary team approach that includes a specialist endocrinologist, specialist obstetrician, diabetes nurse/midwife specialist, and dietician in a dedicated Obstetric-Endocrine Clinic is ideal [26]. The management of HIP can be individualised depending on the severity of hyperglycaemia.

30.9.2 Counselling/Health Promotion

When HIP is diagnosed, it is important for healthcare providers to explain the following to women

(i) Implications of HIP for both herself and baby
(ii) Role of a healthy lifestyle (healthy diet and exercise)
(iii) Role of blood glucose monitoring (including self-monitoring)
(iv) Possible need for pharmacological therapy (oral hypoglycaemic agents and insulin)
(v) Need for maternal and fetal monitoring
(vi) Timing and mode of delivery

30.10 Blood Glucose Monitoring

All pregnant women with hyperglycaemia should be counselled on the importance of self-monitoring of capillary blood glucose using a handheld glucometer [1]. As with diagnostic recommendations, glycaemic targets, and frequency of glucose monitoring in women with HIP differ across guidelines (Table 30.6 below). Generally, fasting (<95 mg/dl), 1-hour postprandial (<140 mg/dl), and 2-hour postprandial (<120 mg/dl) glycaemic targets are recommended [1, 4, 27, 28]. It is important to highlight that women with HIP who are on insulin or glibenclamide should maintain their glucose levels above 72 mg/dl (4 mmol/l). The frequency of self-monitoring of plasma glucose remains unresolved as there is no RCT to justify any specific recommendation [1]. A general recommendation is to check the capillary glucose four times daily at fasting and either at 1-hour or 2-hour following each meal [1]. The issue of timing of glucose monitoring in relation to a meal is also controversial [1]. A randomised control trial by De Veciana et al. found that postprandial blood glucose monitoring in women with GDM was associated with better pregnancy outcomes and glycaemic control compared to a preprandial glucose monitoring approach [29].

Table 30.6 Treatment targets and frequency of blood glucose monitoring

	FIGO 2015	ACOG	ADA	NICE	CDA	IDF
Frequency of glucose monitoring	*All resource setting: 3–4 times daily [fasting, 2–3 daily after each meal (either 1- or 2-hours)]* Low resource setting: At least once (after a meal) daily	Generally recommend testing four times daily (fasting, after each meal)	*Generally recommends fasting and pre- and postprandial monitoring of blood glucose; but no specific testing frequency*	Multiple insulin injections daily: monitor fasting, pre-meal, 1-hour postprandial, and bedtime All others: monitor fasting and 1-hour postprandial	Monitor fasting and postprandial glucose daily	Monitor fasting and postprandial glucose daily, preferably 1 hour after eating
Treatment targets	*FPG < 5.3 mmol/l (95 mg/dl)* *1-hour postprandial < 7.8 mmol/l (140 mg/dl)* *2-hour postprandial < 6.7 mmol/l (120 mg/dl)*	Postprandial glucose goals (mg/dl): 1-hour <140 2-hour <120	Fasting 95 mg/dl (5.3 mmol/l) and either One-hour post meal: 140 mg/dl (7.8 mmol/l) or Two-hour post meal: 120 mg/dl (6.7 mmol/l)	Capillary glucose goals (mg/dl): Fasting <95 1-hour <140 2-hour <115	Goals (mg/dl): Fasting <95 1-hour PP <140 2-hour PP <120	Capillary glucose goals (mg/dl): Fasting 90–99 1-hour PP <140 2-hour PP <120–127 Target as low as possible ensuring patient comfort and safety

30.11 Lifestyle Management

Following HIP diagnosis, individualised first-line therapy including nutritional/dietary and exercise therapies should be commenced and continued for 1–2 weeks before considering pharmacological therapy. However, women with severe forms of overt diabetes/DIP may be commenced on lifestyle and pharmacological therapies simultaneously. Nutritional therapy for GDM focuses on restricting calories with emphasis on low-glycaemic index foods, fibre-rich diets and total amount, quality and distribution of carbohydrate as strategies for achieving appropriate weight gain, target blood glucose, successful pregnancy outcomes, and absence of ketones [1, 20, 30]. It is beneficial for diets to include carbohydrates from fruit, vegetables, legumes (beans, peas, soybeans, etc.), whole grain, and low-fat milk [20]. Recommendations for physical activity in women with HIP include planned activity (e.g. walking for 30mins after a meal), and brisk walking or arm exercises (while seated in a chair) for 10 minutes following each meal [1, 28]. Reduction in blood glucose levels by up to 23 mg/dl has been reported among women with HIP [31]. Existing RCT data suggest that lifestyle change is sufficient to achieve target blood glucose (i.e. normoglycaemia) in 80–90% of women with HIP [22, 32].

The ADA recommends nutrition counselling (with a registered dietitian, if possible) and a diet that adequately meets the needs of pregnancy but restricts carbohydrates to 35–40% of daily calories [33].

30.12 Pharmacological Therapy

Pharmacological therapy including oral hypoglycaemic drugs (metformin or glyburides) and insulin is introduced when glycaemic control is not achieved with diet and exercise for a period of 1–2 weeks. Oral hypoglycaemic drugs can be used as a second-line therapy, and can be replaced with insulin if glycaemic control is achieved. Data from RCTs demonstrate the effectiveness and short-term safety of both glyburide and metformin for the treatment of hyperglycaemia detected in index pregnancy [34–36]. If oral hypoglycaemic therapy is insufficient in achieving optimal glycaemic control, insulin therapy is required. Offer insulin instead of metformin to women with gestational diabetes if metformin is contraindicated or unacceptable to the woman [28].

30.12.1 Monitoring Maternal Well-Being

In addition to continuous glucose monitoring, women with pre-exiting diabetes in pregnancy should be offered retinal assessment at booking, 16–20 gestational weeks (in women with diabetic retinopathy at first prenatal clinic visit), and at 28 weeks [1, 20, 28]. Renal assessment (serum creatinine, urinary albumin/creatinine ratio, and total protein excretion) should also be undertaken at prenatal booking visit in women with pre-existing diabetes. Because DIP/overt diabetes detected for the first time in index pregnancy is most likely due to pre-existing diabetes, both retinal and renal evaluations can be considered in women with this severity of hyperglycaemia detected in index pregnancy.

30.12.2 Monitoring Fetal Well-Being

Fetal well-being surveillance can be carried out via:

1. Fetal kick count
2. Cardiotocography (nonstress test)
3. Biophysical profile

NICE recommendations [28] for well-being surveillance include:

1. Ultrasound: (a) at 20 weeks for detecting structural abnormalities (including cardiac anomaly), and (b) at 28, 32, 36 for assessing fetal growth and amniotic volume
2. Cardiocotography at 38 and 39 weeks for assessing fetal well-being

30.13 Intrapartum Care

30.13.1 Timing and Mode of Delivery

It is recommended that timing and mode delivery should be discussed during prenatal appointments, notably the third trimester, and women with uncomplicated pre-existing diabetes or any form of hyperglycaemia first detected in pregnancy should be advised to have elective delivery (either by induction of labour or caesarean section if indicated) prior to 40 completed weeks of gestation, especially between 37^{+0} and 38^{+6} weeks, to prevent stillbirth [28]. For women with any form of hyperglycaemia and any complication, elective delivery is advised before 37 weeks [28]. Published NICE guideline recommends maintaining maternal capillary blood glucose between 4 and 7 mmol/l for all women in labour. The guideline also recommends the use of intravenous dextrose and insulin infusion for all women with type 1 DM at the onset of established labour and also for women with other forms of hyperglycaemia whose antenatal blood glucose profiles are not maintained between 4 and 7 mmol/l. A generally recommended standardised intravenous insulin therapy during the intrapartum period is as follows:

- Nil by mouth until after the birth of the baby
- Start intravenous dextrose 10% in 500 ml, 100 ml/hour preferably via IMED® pump
- Hourly blood glucose estimation by glucose meter
- Insulin infusion by an intravenous pump mounted onto the intravenous line, initially at 2 U/hour when blood glucose more than 7 mmol/l (50 U human soluble insulin in 50 ml, 0.9% saline, 2 ml/hour)
  - Adjust insulin infusion rate to maintain blood glucose 4.0–7.0 mmol/l according to glucose meter:
  - If less than 4.0 mmol/l and not rising, then decrease by 1 U/hour to a minimum of 0.5 U/hour
  - If more than 7.0 mmol/l and not falling, then increase by 0.5 U/hour
- After delivery of the placenta:
  - Halve the rate of insulin infusion, to a minimum of 0.5 U/hour
  - Adjust as before to maintain blood glucose 4.0–7.0 mmol/l
  - Refer to medical record or contact diabetes team for advice about subcutaneous insulin dose before next main meal

With the use of insulin and therapeutic management, treatment of gestational diabetes (GDM) is effective in reducing adverse outcomes such as macrosomia, large for gestational age, shoulder dystocia, and pre-eclampsia/hypertensive disorders in pregnancy. The risk reduction for these outcomes is in general large, the number need to treat is low, and the quality of evidence is adequate to justify the treatment of GDM [1].

30.14 Postpartum Care and Long-Term Follow-Up

Disclosure: This section is derived from the FIGO 2015 Guide

The postpartum period is crucial, not only in terms of addressing the immediate perinatal problems, but also in the long term for establishing the basis for early preventive health for both mother and child, who are at an increased risk for future obesity, metabolic syndrome, diabetes, hypertension, and cardiovascular disorders.

30.14.1 Immediate Postpartum Period

Infections: Mothers with diabetes have an increased risk of infection and thus require extra attention in order to detect early signs of genitourinary, uterine, and surgical site infections (episiotomy and caesarean delivery), particularly if the delivery has been prolonged or required operative intervention. Women with diabetes in pregnancy are at a higher risk compared with women with GDM. The large-sized offspring of diabetic mothers do not suckle well; this may lead to milk retention and a higher risk of breast abscess.

Except for neonates with infant respiratory distress syndrome or those with aspiration during birth, the risk of infection in the offspring of mothers with diabetes is no higher than in the offspring of women without diabetes [1, 37].

Breastfeeding: The advantages of breastfeeding remain incontrovertible and mothers with GDM and diabetes in pregnancy should be encouraged and supported to initiate and maintain breastfeeding [38–42]. Breastfeeding is protective against the occurrence of infant and maternal complications including reduction in childhood obesity, T2DM, and even T1DM and helps postpartum weight loss. Treatment with insulin or commonly used OADs, such as glyburide and metformin, is not a contraindication to breastfeeding as levels of OAD medications in breast milk are negligible and do not cause hypoglycaemia in the baby.

30.14.2 Contraception

Women with GDM and diabetes should be encouraged to space their pregnancies in order to maintain and achieve optimal health between pregnancies. This also helps reduce the risk of GDM or diabetes in a subsequent pregnancy. In women with diabetes, pregnancy planning helps ensure that conception can occur when the mother's metabolic health is optimal to reduce risks of spontaneous abortions or congenital malformations. These women must have access to and should receive advice about safe and effective methods of contraception. With advances in contraceptive technology, clinicians can now offer their patients a relatively large range of options ensuring efficacy, efficiency, and satisfaction with regard to individual preferences.

30.14.3 Postpartum Glucose Testing

For all women diagnosed with hyperglycaemia for the first time during pregnancy (GDM and diabetes in pregnancy), the glycaemic status should be re-evaluated with a 75-g oral OGTT at 6–12 weeks after delivery. Diagnosis during this period should be based on the currently recommended 2013 WHO criteria for diabetes, impaired fasting glucose (IFG), and impaired glucose tolerance (IGT) in the non-pregnant state. Women who do not have diabetes or pre-diabetes, according to these definitions, are still at risk of progression to diabetes and other cardiovascular problems and require ongoing surveillance. The EBCOG advises that women with a history of GDM should have lifelong screening for the development of diabetes or prediabetes, at least every 3 years. As currently there is insufficient evidence to recommend one test over the other; HbA1C, FPG, or 75-g 2-hour OGTT are all considered appropriate to test for diabetes and prediabetes in the postpartum period. Women with a history of GDM found to have prediabetes should receive specific lifestyle interventions with or without metformin to prevent diabetes [43]. In Nigeria, and sub-Saharan Africa as a whole, there is however no clear guidance about the type of tests (should these women undergo annual OGTTs, or can fasting plasma glucose or HbA1c measurement suffice?) or the frequency and duration for ongoing surveillance. When guidance exists, it is often poorly implemented (Nigeria Obstetric Centre's Survey 2016).

30.14.4 Reducing Long-Term Risk of T2DM and Cardiovascular Disease

Irrespective of the glycaemic status on early postpartum testing, it should be assumed that women with GDM have the same or a higher level of future risk of diabetes and cardiovascular disease as people with pre-diabetes and they should be advised to maintain a healthy lifestyle with an appropriate diet, regular exercise, and normal body weight. Furthermore, to ensure optimal health before attempting their next pregnancy, that is, prior to trying for another pregnancy or discontinuation of contraception, consultation with healthcare providers knowledgeable about diabetes prevention should be instituted.

Progression to diabetes is more common in women with a history of GDM compared with those without a GDM history. Both "intensive lifestyle" and metformin have been shown to be highly effective in delaying or preventing diabetes in women with IGT and a history of GDM. Data from the Diabetes Prevention Program Outcomes Study (DPPOS) show that the benefits of lifestyle intervention and metformin seen in the DPP study continue over a longer period. Among women without a history of GDM, "intensive lifestyle" reduced the progression to diabetes by 30% [44]. As part of the ongoing Diabetes and Women's Health Study, women who increased their total physical activity levels by equivalent to 150 minutes per week of moderate intensity physical activity had a 47% lower risk of T2DM (RR 0.53; 95% CI, 0.38–0.75); the association remained significant after additional adjustment for BMI [45]. Increasing physical activity is believed to lower the risk of progression from GDM to T2DM.

Postpartum care is a critical area that should not be overlooked because of the long-term and intergenerational consequences [46]. Aside from the 6 weeks postnatal visit, and routine yearly checks with the obstetricians/physicians, women with GDM do visit health services focused on the well-being of their babies (for instance, for the child's vaccination program and to monitor the child's growth and development) and are likely to do so at regular intervals for at least 5 years. Healthcare providers, obstetricians, family physicians, internists, and paediatricians must therefore link postpartum follow-up of a GDM mother with the child's vaccination and routine paediatric care program, to ensure continued follow-up and engagement of the high-risk mother-child pair.

30.15 Controversies

30.15.1 GDM Screening: Selective Versus Universal Testing

Successful screening tests require that the condition is prevalent in the target population, that treatment improves the prognosis and that the treatment is cost-effective. Gestational diabetes mellitus meets all these criteria [1, 43]. Diabetes is a growing non-communicable disease (NCD) epidemic. The ongoing epidemic of obesity and diabetes has led to more type 2 diabetes in women of childbearing age, with an increase in the number of pregnant women with undiagnosed type 2 diabetes. In pregnancy, early detection is essential to improve feto-maternal outcomes and mitigate future type 2 diabetes and co-morbidities associated with gestational diabetes mellitus (GDM). It is thus reasonable to test women for hyperglycaemia at their initial prenatal visit. Pregnancy provides a unique opportunity to screen for, identify and manage diabetes and potential diabetes whilst at the same time, halt the escalation of diabetes that emerges as a result of the offspring born to a woman with gestational diabetes and ensuring the next generations born to women with gestational diabetes are spared from this medical condition. Thus, GDM screening must be done for all pregnant women if effective early therapeutic interventions are to be instituted. It is, therefore, crucial for health workers to understand that the absence of GDM risk factors is not protective against GDM and so risk-based screening is not acceptable for the current management of gestational diabetes mellitus.

30.15.2 Timing of Testing: Early Pregnancy Testing or Testing at 24 to 28 Weeks of Gestation?

Twenty-four to 28 weeks of gestation was the period routinely advocated for screening for GDM. However, with the age at onset of T2DM decreasing globally; many women with previously unknown T2DM become pregnant and their diabetes is first detected during routine testing in pregnancy. Similarly, with women at high risk of diabetes unable to withstand the metabolic stress of pregnancy and develop diabetes for the first time during pregnancy, their diabetes is first detected during routine testing in pregnancy. Compared with gestational diabetes, DIP is more likely to be detected as early as the first trimester provided appropriate testing is undertaken. Thus in the new FIGO Guidelines, a call is made for testing for hyperglycaemia in pregnancy early in the first trimester.

30.16 Summary

Hyperglycaemia in pregnancy(HIP) is one of the most frequent medical disorders encountered during pregnancy. HIP is of utmost concern because of the increased risk of adverse feto-maternal outcomes and long-term risk for future diabetes and cardiovascular disorders for mother and child. To prevent these adverse pregnancy outcomes and delay/prevent future onset of diabetes/metabolic syndrome in mother and offspring, timely detection, optimum treatment, and preventive postpartum care and follow-up are crucial. Medical students, doctors and indeed all healthcare providers must first be knowledgeable to initiate this timely detection by screening all pregnant women and instituting optimum treatment and care. This chapter provides the necessary knowledge.

References

1. Hod M, Kapur A, Sacks DA, Hadar E, Agarwal M, Di Renzo GC, et al. The International Federation of Gynaecology and Obstetrics (FIGO) initiative on gestational diabetes mellitus: a pragmatic guide for diagnosis, management, and care. Int J Gynaecol Obstet. 2015;131(3):173–211.
2. IDF Diabetes Atlas – Home [Internet]. 2015 [cited 2016 Mar 6]. Available from: http://www.diabetesatlas.org/.
3. Nielsen KK, Kapur A, Damm P, de Courten M, Bygbjerg IC. From screening to postpartum follow-up – the determinants and barriers for gestational diabetes mellitus (GDM) services, a systematic review. BMC Pregnancy Childbirth. 2014;14(1):41.
4. WHO I Diagnostic criteria and classification of hyperglycaemia first detected in pregnancy [Internet]. [cited 2016 Mar 6]. Available from: http://www.who.int/diabetes/publications/Hyperglycaemia_In_Pregnancy/en/.
5. Colagiuri S, Falavigna M, Agarwal MM, Boulvain M, Coetzee E, Hod M, et al. Strategies for implementing the WHO diagnostic criteria and classification of hyperglycaemia first detected in pregnancy. Diabetes Res Clin Pract. 2014;103(3):364–72.
6. Metzger BE, Coustan DR. Summary and recommendations of the Fourth International Workshop-Conference on Gestational Diabetes Mellitus. The Organizing Committee. Diabetes Care. 1998;21(2):161–7.
7. Surveillance WHOD of ND. Definition, diagnosis and classification of diabetes mellitus and its complications: report of a WHO consultation. Part 1: Diagnosis and classification of diabetes mellitus. 1999 [cited 2016 Aug 29]; Available from: http://www.who.int/iris/handle/10665/66040.
8. American Diabetes Association. Diagnosis and classification of diabetes mellitus. Diabetes Care. 2009;32(1):62–7.

9. International Association of Diabetes and Pregnancy Study Groups Consensus Panel. International Association of Diabetes and Pregnancy Study Groups recommendations on the diagnosis and classification of hyperglycaemia in pregnancy. Diabetes Care. 2010;33(3):676–82.
10. Mwanri AW, Kinabo J, Ramaiya K, Feskens EJM. Gestational diabetes mellitus in sub-Saharan Africa: systematic review and metaregression on prevalence and risk factors. Trop Med Int Health. 2015;20(8):983–1002.
11. Standards of medical care in diabetes—2016: summary of revisions. Diabetes Care. 2016;39(1):4–5.
12. Kanguru L, Bezawada N, Hussein J, Bell J. The burden of diabetes mellitus during pregnancy in low- and middle-income countries: a systematic review. Glob Health Action. 2014;7:23987.
13. Olagbuji BN, Atiba AS, Olofinbiyi BA, Akintayo AA, Awoleke JO, Ade-Ojo IP, et al. Prevalence of and risk factors for gestational diabetes using 1999, 2013 WHO and IADPSG criteria upon implementation of a universal one-step screening and diagnostic strategy in a sub-Saharan African population. Eur J Obstet Gynecol Reprod Biol. 2015;189(1):27–32.
14. Akhidue K, Ogu R, Chinenye S. Diabetes in pregnancy: the Nigerian perspectives using the new WHO criteria. 0823P. [Internet]. International Diabetes Federation; 2015. [cited 2016 Feb 23]. Available from: https://www.idf.org/sites/default/files/045_2015-progrbook_scientific-part3P-29-10-15.pdf.
15. Mbanya JCN, Motala AA, Sobngwi E, Assah FK, Enoru ST. Diabetes in sub-Saharan Africa. Lancet. 2010;375(9733):2254–66.
16. Chinenye S, Ogu R, Korubo I. Diabetes advocacy and care in Nigeria: a review. Niger Health J. 2016;15(4):145–50.
17. Ostlund I, Hanson U. Occurrence of gestational diabetes mellitus and the value of different screening indicators for the oral glucose tolerance test. Acta Obstet Gynecol Scand. 2003;82(2):103–8.
18. Schaefer UM, Songster G, Xiang A, Berkowitz K, Buchanan TA, Kjos SL. Congenital malformations in offspring of women with hyperglycaemia first detected during pregnancy. Am J Obstet Gynecol. 1997;177(5):1165–71.
19. Omori Y, Jovanovic L. Proposal for the reconsideration of the definition of gestational diabetes. Diabetes Care. 2005;28(10):2592–3.
20. Kitzmiller JL, Block JM, Brown FM, Catalano PM, Conway DL, Coustan DR, et al. Managing preexisting diabetes for pregnancy: summary of evidence and consensus recommendations for care. Diabetes Care. 2008;31(5):1060–79.
21. HAPO Study Cooperative Research Group, Metzger BE, Lowe LP, Dyer AR, Trimble ER, Chaovarindr U, et al. Hyperglycaemia and adverse pregnancy outcomes. N Engl J Med. 2008;358(19):1991–2002.
22. Landon MB, Spong CY, Thom E, Carpenter MW, Ramin SM, Casey B, et al. A multicentre, randomised trial of treatment for mild gestational diabetes. N Engl J Med. 2009;361(14):1339–48.
23. Diouf I, Charles MA, Thiebaugeorges O, Forhan A, Kaminski M, Heude B, et al. Maternal weight change before pregnancy in relation to birthweight and risks of adverse pregnancy outcomes. Eur J Epidemiol. 2011;26(10):789–96.
24. Durnwald C. Gestational diabetes: linking epidemiology, excessive gestational weight gain, adverse pregnancy outcomes, and future metabolic syndrome. Semin Perinatol. 2015;39(4):254–8.
25. Donovan LE, Savu A, Edwards AL, Johnson JA, Kaul P. Prevalence and timing of Screening and diagnostic testing for gestational diabetes mellitus: a population-based study in Alberta, Canada. Diabetes Care. 2016;39(1):55–60.
26. American Diabetes Association. Preconception care of women with diabetes. Diabetes Care. 2004;27(1):s76–8.
27. Canadian Diabetes Association Clinical Practice Guidelines Expert Committee, Thompson D, Berger H, Feig D, Gagnon R, Kader T, et al. Diabetes and pregnancy. Can J Diabetes. 2013;37(1):S168–83.
28. Diabetes in pregnancy: management from preconception to the postnatal period | Key-priorities-for-implementation | Guidance and guidelines | NICE [Internet]. [cited 2016 Jul 6]. Available from: https://www.nice.org.uk/guidance/ng3/chapter/Key-priorities-for-implementation.
29. de Veciana M, Major CA, Morgan MA, Asrat T, Toohey JS, Lien JM, et al. Postprandial versus preprandial blood glucose monitoring in women with gestational diabetes mellitus requiring insulin therapy. N Engl J Med. 1995;333(19):1237–41.
30. Jovanovic-Peterson L, Peterson CM, Reed GF, Metzger BE, Mills JL, Knopp RH, et al. Maternal postprandial glucose levels and infant birth weight: the Diabetes in Early Pregnancy Study. The National Institute of Child Health and Human Development--Diabetes in Early Pregnancy Study. Am J Obstet Gynecol. 1991;164(1):103–11.
31. Avery MD, Walker AJ. Acute effect of exercise on blood glucose and insulin levels in women with gestational diabetes. J Matern Fetal Med. 2001;10(1):52–8.
32. Crowther CA, Hiller JE, Moss JR, McPhee AJ, Jeffries WS, Robinson JS, et al. Effect of treatment of gestational diabetes mellitus on pregnancy outcomes. N Engl J Med. 2005;352(24):2477–86.
33. Committee on Practice Bulletins--Obstetrics. Practice Bulletin No. 137: Gestational diabetes mellitus. Obstet Gynecol. 2013;122(2 Pt 1):406–16.
34. Langer O, Conway DL, Berkus MD, Xenakis EM-J, Gonzales O. A comparison of glyburide and insulin in women with gestational diabetes mellitus. N Engl J Med. 2000;343(16):1134–8.
35. Rowan JA, Hague WM, Gao W, Battin MR, Moore MP. Metformin versus insulin for the treatment of gestational diabetes. N Engl J Med. 2008;358(19):2003–15.
36. Gui J, Liu Q, Feng L. Metformin vs insulin in the management of gestational diabetes: a meta-analysis. PLoS One. 2013;8(5):e64585.
37. Linder N, Lahat Y, Kogan A, Fridman E, Kouadio F, Melamed N, et al. Macrosomic newborns of non-diabetic mothers: anthropometric measurements and neonatal complications. Arch Dis Child Fetal Neonatal Ed. 2014;99(5):F353–8.
38. Owen CG, Martin RM, Whincup PH, Smith GD, Cook DG. Does breastfeeding influence risk of type 2 diabetes in later life? A quantitative analysis of published evidence. Am J Clin Nutr. 2006;84(5):1043–54.
39. O'Reilly M, Avalos G, Dennedy MC, O'Sullivan EP, Dunne FP. Breast-feeding is associated with reduced postpartum maternal glucose intolerance after gestational diabetes. Ir Med J. 2012;105(5):31–6.
40. Plagemann A, Harder T, Franke K, Kohlhoff R. Long-term impact of neonatal breast-feeding on body weight and glucose tolerance in children of diabetic mothers. Diabetes Care. 2002;25(1):16–22.
41. Mayer-Davis EJ, Rifas-Shiman SL, Zhou L, Hu FB, Colditz GA, Gillman MW. Breast-feeding and risk for childhood obesity: does maternal diabetes or obesity status matter? Diabetes Care. 2006;29(10):2231–7.
42. Gunderson EP. Impact of breastfeeding on maternal metabolism: implications for women with gestational diabetes. Curr Diab Rep. 2014;14(2):460. Available from: http://link.springer.com/10.1007/s11892-013-0460-2.
43. Benhalima K, Damm P, Assche AV, Mathieu C, Devlieger R, Mahmood T, et al. Screening for gestational diabetes in Europe: where do we stand and how to move forward? Eur J Obstet Gynecol Reprod Biol. 2016;201:192–6.
44. Aroda VR, Christophi CA, Edelstein SL, Zhang P, Herman WH, Barrett-Connor E, et al. The effect of lifestyle intervention and metformin on preventing or delaying diabetes among women with and without gestational diabetes: the Diabetes Prevention Program Outcomes Study 10-year follow-up. J Clin Endocrinol Metab. 2015;100(4):1646–53.
45. Bao W, Tobias DK, Bowers K, Chavarro J, Vaag A, Grunnet LG, et al. Physical activity and sedentary behaviours associated with risk of progression from gestational diabetes mellitus to type 2 diabetes mellitus: a prospective cohort study. JAMA Intern Med. 2014;174(7):1047–55.
46. Kapur A. Pregnancy: a window of opportunity for improving current and future health. Int J Gynaecol Obstet. 2011;115(1):50–1.

Venous Thromboembolism in Pregnancy

31

Omolade Awodu

Learning Objectives

At the conclusion of this chapter, the reader should be able to:

- Identify the various risk factors that are associated with venous thromboembolism in pregnancy.
- Critically evaluate pregnant women who are at risk of developing venous thromboembolism.
- Recall the various symptoms and signs of venous thromboembolism and their peculiarities in pregnancy.
- Have an appropriate knowledge and understanding of the diagnostic algorithm of venous thromboembolism in pregnancy.
- Appreciate the role of imaging studies in the diagnosis of venous thromboembolism in pregnancy.
- Understand the indications for the use of different anticoagulants in pregnancy.
- Critically evaluate and treat pregnant women with venous thromboembolism.
- Critically evaluate and manage adverse effects of anticoagulation during pregnancy and the puerperium.

31.1 Introduction

Venous thromboembolism (VTE) comprises deep venous thrombosis (DVT) and pulmonary embolism (PE). In pregnancy, a 4–5-fold increase in VTE incidences has been reported over the non-pregnant state [1]. Pregnancy-related venous thromboembolism is over 10 times more common than in non-pregnant women of the same age. Venous thromboembolism is a major cause of direct maternal mortality in the developed world despite improvements in diagnosis and treatment; mortality as high as 8.5–14 per million life births have been reported in some European studies [2, 3]. Pulmonary embolism constitutes about 10–20% of VTE and it accounts for most of VTE mortality which is about 9% of maternal deaths making it the seventh leading cause of maternal mortality [4, 5]. Elevated levels of procoagulant clotting factors and decreased fibrinolysis accompany normal pregnancy thus making pregnancy a hypercoagulable condition. The hypercoagulability results from increased fibrin generation occasioned by an increase in the levels of coagulation factors VIII, fibrinogen, X, VII, von Willebrand's factor (VWF) and decreased levels of physiologic anticoagulants protein C, protein S and acquired resistance to activated protein C [1, 6]. In addition, there is reduced fibrinolysis from increased activities of plasminogen activator inhibitors 1 and 2(PAI-I and PAI-2) as well as decreased tissue plasminogen activators (tPA) [6]. Other factors contributing to increased risk of VTE in pregnancy includes inherited and acquired thrombophilia, smoking, obesity, immobility and infection [4, 5].

The diagnosis and treatment of VTE are more complex than in the non-pregnant state as many of the symptoms and signs of VTE such as leg swelling, pain and dyspnoea are commonly found in normal pregnancy. This limits the accuracy of clinical diagnosis to about 5% for DVT and 8% for PE. In addition, most diagnostic tests for VTE involve exposure to radiation. A substantial fear of foetal irradiation may limit objective diagnostic testing to confirm or exclude DVT or PE in pregnant women even though studies have shown that radiation doses of 15 rads or less do not appear to increase the risk of foetal malformations [5, 7, 8].

The treatment of VTE in pregnancy is heparin. Low molecular weight heparin (LMWH) is the preferred pharmacological agent in most cases. Vitamin K antagonists are rarely used because of the likelihood of causing foetal malformation [2, 9–10]. Induction of labour is preferred to cae-

O. Awodu (✉)
University of Benin/University of Benin Teaching Hospital, Benin Cityy, Nigeria
e-mail: omolade.awodu@uniben.edu

F. Okonofua et al. (eds.), *Contemporary Obstetrics and Gynecology for Developing Countries*, https://doi.org/10.1007/978-3-030-75385-6_31

sarean section in women on therapeutic anticoagulation except there is an obstetric indication for caesarean section. Therapeutic anticoagulation should be continued throughout pregnancy and for 6 weeks post-delivery with at least 3 months of anticoagulant therapy in total.

31.2 Epidemiology of VTE in Pregnancy

Pulmonary embolism is a leading cause of maternal mortality in the Western world [11]. The reported incidence of VTE in pregnancy ranges from 0.6 to 1.7 episodes per 1000 deliveries [4, 12]. The risk of VTE was 38% higher in women who are 35 years or older and 64% higher in black women. It accounts for 1.1 deaths per 100,000 pregnancies [12]. There is a paucity of data on the prevalence of VTE among pregnant women in Africa. This may not be unconnected with diagnostic challenges. In a case-control study, an incidence of 448/100,000 births/year was reported among Sudanese women [13]. At a glance, the VTE rates in pregnancy may appear low; they, however, represent about 4–10 folds increased risk compared with rates observed in the non-pregnant women of comparable age [1, 14]. The left leg is favoured in pregnancy-related VTE; the predilection for the left leg is presumably due to the pressure of the gravid uterus, and the May–Thurner's syndrome in which the left iliac vein is compressed by the right iliac artery (compression of the left iliac vein by the right iliac and ovarian arteries which cross the vein on the left side). Almost 90% of DVT occur in the left leg in pregnancy compared to 55% in non-pregnant women [15]. DVT in pregnancy also occurs more in the iliac and femoral veins than in non-pregnant women. This is of clinical importance in that iliofemoral DVT; being more proximal has a higher chance of resulting in pulmonary embolism. About 12% of DVTs in pregnancy are in the pelvic veins compared to only 1% in the general population. This should be taken into consideration when investigating suspected DVT in pregnancy.

VTE can occur at any time during pregnancy; however, there are conflicting reports regarding the timing, whist some studies suggest a higher incidence in the first trimester, others have not confirmed any association between gestational age and occurrence of VTE. Ginsberg et al. reported isolated left leg thrombosis in 58 of 60 women with first episodes of venous thrombosis in pregnancy, 13 (21.7%) of the patients had VTE in the first trimester, 28 (46.7%) in the second trimester and 19 (31.7%) during the third trimester [16, 17]. In a meta-analysis study, two-thirds of cases of DVT occurred in the antepartum period with equal distribution across the trimesters, whilst 43–68% of pregnancy-related episodes of pulmonary embolism were seen in the puerperium [18].

31.3 Pathophysiology of DVT in Pregnancy

Normal haemostasis represents a balance between pro- and anti-coagulant processes. A change in this balance determines the clinical outcome of thrombosis or haemorrhage. In pregnancy, there is disequilibrium between the anticoagulants and the procoagulants in favour of the procoagulants. The physiological changes of pregnancy result in a hypercoagulable and hypofibrinolytic state that helps to protect the mother from haemorrhagic complications at the time of delivery.

All the three components of the Virchow's triad (hypercoagulability, venous stasis and vascular endothelial injury) are affected in pregnancy. Also, physiological changes during and immediately after pregnancy favour thrombosis. The increased levels of factors II, VII, VIII and X and decreased levels of free protein S and an acquired protein C resistance which lead to an increase in fibrin generation create a hypercoagulable condition. In addition, progesterone and other pregnancy-related hormones induced vasodilatation, this, and the compression of the pelvic veins by the gravid uterus, lead to stasis of blood in the lower limb veins. In addition, at delivery, there is injury to the pelvic vessels thus completing the Virchow's triad. Studies, using Doppler ultrasonography of the lower limb veins have shown a reduction of up to 50% in blood flow velocity in the lower limb veins between the 25th and 29th week of gestation till about 6 weeks postpartum [19].· Furthermore, a number of additional risk factors may superimpose on the background prothrombotic environment.

31.4 Risk Factors for Venous Thromboembolism in Pregnancy

The predisposition of pregnancy to thrombosis is related to the elevated levels of procoagulant clotting factors as stated above, which may be a physiological mechanism of securing haemostasis postpartum. Inherited and/or acquired risk factors may superimpose on the background prothrombotic state of pregnancy. Inherited thrombophilia, previous thrombosis as well as the antiphospholipid syndrome increase the chances of developing VTE. Pregnant women must therefore be risk assessed at the first visit. Assessment should be done whenever there is a change in clinical condition or there is hospitalisation. History should include previous and family history of VTE. In women with thrombophilia, a family history of VTE is an important determinant of VTE risk in pregnancy. Table 31.1 summarises the risk factors of DVT.

Table 31.1 Risk factors of VTE in pregnancy [20]

Heritable thrombophilia
Antithrombin deficiency
Protein C deficiency
Protein S deficiency
FVG1691A(factor V Leiden)Sickle cell disease
Hyperhomocysteinaemia
Dysfibrinogenaemia
Acquired thrombophilia
Antiphospholipid antibodies
Pre-pregnancy
Age >35 years
Obesity (pre-pregnancy or early pregnancy BMI > 30 kg/m [2])
Parity > 3
Smoking
Gross symptomatic varicose veins
Paraplegia
Medical conditions, for example,
Systemic lupus erythematosus
Nephrotic syndrome
Heart disease
Myeloproliferative disorders
Other malignancies
Inflammatory conditions
Previous VTE
Single
Oestrogen-related
Thrombophilia-related
Unprovoked
Related to temporary risk factor
Recurrent events
Family history of VTE
Transient
Hyperemesis
Ovarian hyperstimulation syndrome (OHS)
Long distance travel (>4 h)
Immobility (>4 days bed rest)
Dehydration
Severe infection (e.g. pyelonephritis)
Pregnancy-related
Multiple pregnancy
Pre-eclampsia
Prolonged labour
Assisted reproduction therapy
Post-natal
Post-partum haemorrhage
Blood transfusion
Mid cavity instrumental delivery
Immobility after delivery

31.5 Clinical Features of VTE in Pregnancy

Clinical features of both DVT and PE in pregnancy are not specific and are similar to the non-pregnant state. Clinical diagnosis of DVT outside pregnancy requires a high index of suspicion; only about 20–30% of cases are confirmed by objective testing. In pregnancy, the diagnosis is more unreliable because symptoms and signs of DVT such as leg swelling, chest pain and dyspnoea (Table 31.2) are also commonly found in normal pregnancy thereby reducing the accuracy of clinical diagnosis to about 8% for DVT and 5% for suspected PE [9, 21].

Table 31.2 Symptoms and signs of VTE in pregnancy

Deep vein thrombosis
Leg pain or discomfort (left leg more commonly affected)
Leg swelling (swelling of entire limb is suggestive of iliac veins thrombosis)
Tenderness
Fever
Lower abdominal pain (if pelvic veins are affected)
Elevated white cell count
Pulmonary embolism
Pleuritic chest pain
Cough
Fainting
Haemoptysis
Tachypnoea
Tachycardia
Raised jugular venous pressure (JVP)
ECG changes (S1Q3T3) may be present
Hypoxaemia
Respiratory alkalosis
There may be symptoms and signs of DVT
Differential diagnosis of DVT in pregnancy
Ruptured Barker's cyst
Cellulitis
Superficial thrombophlebitis
Muscle strain
Trauma
Pulmonary embolism
Chest infections
Atelectasis

31.6 Diagnosis of VTE in Pregnancy

The diagnosis of VTE in pregnancy requires a high index of suspicion on the part of the attending obstetrician. This is because symptoms and signs that may mimic features of VTE in pregnancy often accompany normal pregnancy. Objective tests have to put into consideration maternal and foetal safety. There are few studies on the diagnosis and treatment of VTE in pregnancy. Decisions are often made based on the extrapolations from studies conducted in the non-pregnant state. D-dimer testing and pretest probability assessment which have been found to be very useful in the non-pregnant state have not been embraced in the diagnosis of VTE in pregnancy because D-dimer levels are usually elevated in pregnancy. During pregnancy, there is a progressive increase in the levels of D-dimer, and by term, and the immediate postpartum period, the levels are often abnormal. In addition, other factors like multiple pregnancy, caesarean delivery and post-partum haemorrhage further increase the levels, thereby reducing the specificity of the test in pregnancy. Though a study has suggested using a higher cut off in pregnancy this has not been clinically validated [23]. In an attempt to identify a pretest prediction variable for VTE in pregnancy, Chan WS et al. classify pregnant women with DVT into low-risk and high-risk categories. In a multicentre study involving 194 pregnant women, they developed a pregnancy-specific model (Table 31.3) using three criteria: left leg symptoms, a difference in calf circumference of at least 2 cm and first-trimester presentation (LEFt) [22]. All the 17 women with objectively confirmed DVT met at least one criterion, DVT was not diagnosed in women that did not meet any of the criteria (0%; 95% CI, 0–4.2%) and in 16.4% of cases (95% CI, 10.5–24.7%) that met one criterion, while thrombosis was found in 58.3% (95% CI, 35.8–75.5%) of cases that met 2 or 3 criteria [22]. Whenever there is a clinical suspicion of DVT, a compression ultrasound scan (CUS) of the limbs should be requested immediately. Anticoagulation should be commenced if the clinical suspicion is high. If DVT is confirmed, anticoagulation should be continued. If CUS is negative and the clinical suspicion is low, anticoagulation should be discontinued. If the clinical suspicion remains high magnetic resonance imaging should be considered to rule out iliac vein thrombosis which may be associated with swelling of the entire limb and back pain [15]. Figure 31.1 shows the algorithm for the diagnosis and treatment of DVT in pregnancy.

31.7 Diagnosis of PE

Investigations to rule out PE in pregnancy are equally challenging due to concerns about foetal radiation exposure as well as exposure of the maternal breasts to radiation.

Table 31.3 Calculation of initial dose of drugs by early pregnancy weight [9]

Initial dose	Early pregnancy weight in (Kg)					
	<50	50–69	70–89	90–109	110–125	>125[a]
Enoxaparin (mg; b.d)	40	60	80	100	120	
	5000	6000	8000	10,000	12,000	
Dalteparin (i.u.; bud)	175 units/kg once daily all weights					
Tinzaparin						

Once daily doses of enoxaparin can be given as 60 mg, 90 mg, 120 mg, 150 mg and 180 mg for early pregnancy weights of <50, 50–69, 70–89, 90–109 and 110–125 kg, respectively

[a]Haematologist's input required

However, studies have shown that radiation doses of 5 rads or less do not appear to be associated with risk of foetal loss [7, 8].

Once there is a clinical suspicion of acute PE, a chest X-ray should be ordered, this may show features of PE (like atelectasis, effusion, pulmonary oedema) or show an underlying pathology like pneumothorax or pneumonia. A normal chest X-ray does not exclude PE as normal findings are found in about 50% of objectively confirmed PE [2, 21]. A useful approach is to do bilateral lower limb duplex ultrasonography scanning; if DVT is confirmed, no further investigation will be necessary as both conditions have the same treatment modality. A second advantage is that further exposure of the foetus to radiation is avoided.

If chest X-ray is normal, and lower limb imaging is negative and the clinical suspicion is still high, a computed tomography pulmonary angiogram (CTPA) or ventilation/perfusion (V/Q) lung scan should be performed.

Other investigations include: arterial blood gases which show reduced PaO_2 and normal or low $PaCO_2$. ECG helps in excluding other diagnosis such as myocardial infarction and pericardial disease, it may also show sinus tachycardia. The choice between CTPA and V/Q scanning for the diagnosis of PE in pregnancy is controversial. Both have been reported to have high negative predictive value [24]. However, an advantage of CTPA is the lower radiation dose to the foetus when compared to a V/Q scan. Some authors have recommended V/Q scan as the first line in pregnancy because of lower radiation dose to the breast, which is particularly sensitive to radiation because of hormones-induced increase in glandular activity of the breast [20, 21] and that V/Q scan is preferred when the chest radiograph is normal [25]. The final choice of lung imaging will depend on local availability and expertise, considerations for family history of breast cancer and previous chest CT scan which may post an additional risk to the mother. Newer imaging techniques like magnetic resonance pulmonary angiogram and ventilation and perfusion single-photon emission computed tomography (V/QSPECT) may also be considered but these are not yet available in most developing countries.

31.8 Screening for Thrombophilia

Screening for inherited thrombophilia (Table 31.1) is not necessary prior to therapy because both the physiological changes of pregnancy and the pathophysiology of acute thrombus will not make the diagnosis conclusive. For example, massive thrombi are associated with decreased levels of antithrombin and protein C, and pregnancy itself causes a fall in protein S levels as well as an acquired activated protein C resistance which is found in about 40% of

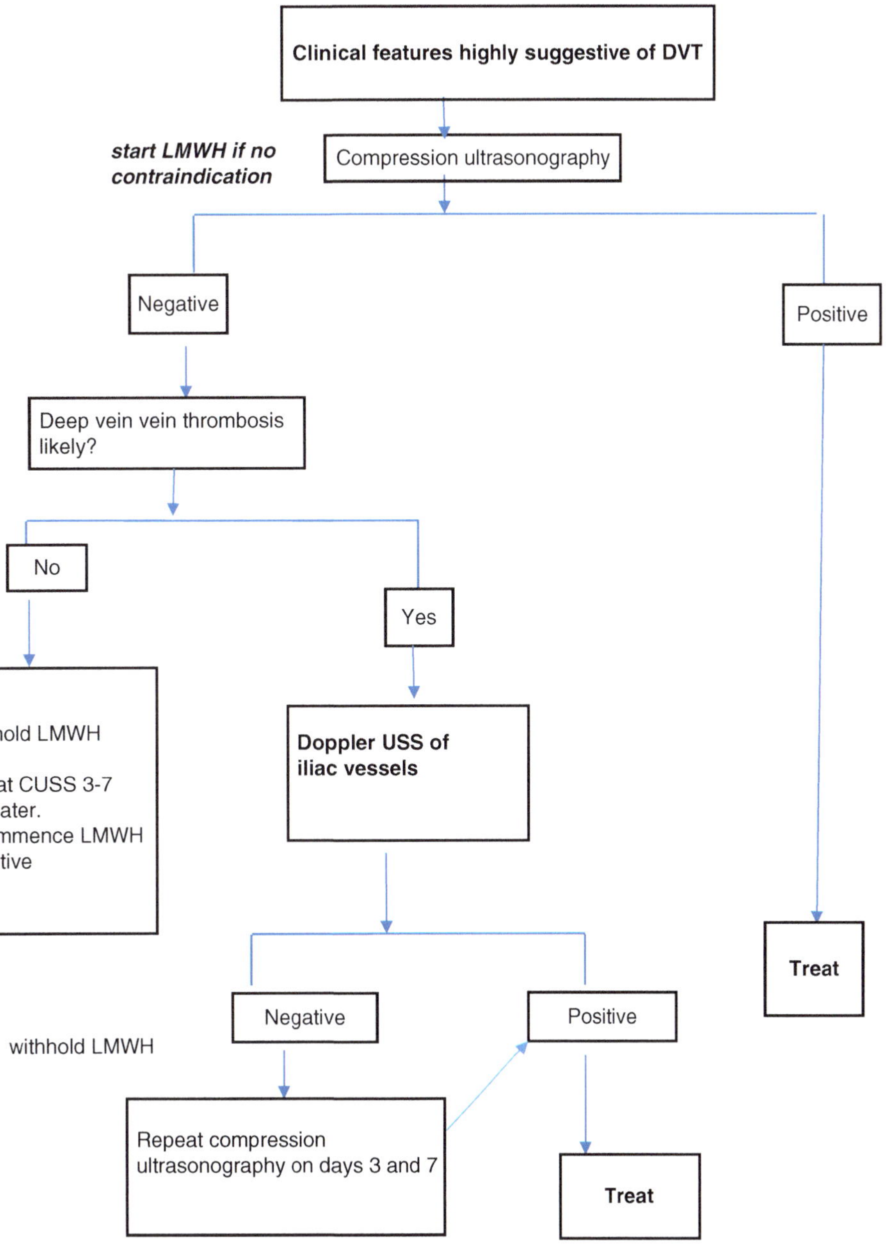

Fig. 31.1 Algorithm for the diagnosis of suspected deep vein thrombosis (DVT) during pregnancy. Abbreviation: DVT deep venous thrombosis, LMWH low molecular weight heparin, CUSS compression ultrasonography

pregnancies [9]. Moreover, thrombophilia does not change the treatment of acute VTE, making screening unnecessary [26]

31.9 Management of Acute VTE

Baseline blood investigations must be performed before the commencement of anticoagulant therapy. This is because the use of anticoagulant is dependent on the platelet count, liver and renal functions. *Blood* should be taken for full blood count, liver function test, electrolyte urea and creatinine.

The goal of therapy is to prevent extension and reduce the recurrence of DVT and to limit extension and prevent death from PE. Low molecular weight heparin (LMWH) is the anticoagulant of choice in pregnancy. It can be used for both the initial management and maintenance therapy. Coumarin derivatives like warfarin cross the placenta when used early in pregnancy (6–12 weeks). They are potentially teratogenic and are associated with adverse pregnancy outcomes such as prematurity, miscarriages and a risk of foetal/ maternal intracerebral haemorrhages if taken close to term. Unfractionated heparin (UFH) does not cross the placenta; it is therefore safe in pregnancy. However, LMWH has been shown to be more effective and associated with a lower risk of haemorrhagic complications and lower mortality than UFH in non-pregnant women.

The optimal management of acute VTE requires a multidisciplinary approach involving the obstetrician, haematologist, anaesthetist, respiratory physician and a cardiologist.

31.10 Treatment of VTE in Pregnancy

Once there is a high clinical suspicion of DVT or PE, treatment should be commenced unless there is a strong contraindication to anticoagulant therapy. Safety of the mother and the foetus must be taken into consideration when making decisions on therapy. LMWH has a more favourable safety profile than UFH, more convenient once or twice daily dosing, and absence of the need for regular laboratory monitoring with the activated partial thromboplastin time (APTT) which is less reliable in pregnancy. However, monitoring using anti-Xa activity may be considered in individuals with extremes of body weight (weight <50 kg or >90 kg).

The weight adjusted twice daily dosing regimen of LMWH is preferred over the once daily dosing in order to compensate for the increase glomerular filtration rate that occurs in the second trimester of pregnancy.

The incidence of heparin-induced thrombocytopenia is low following LMWH use in pregnancy; unless there is a history of previous HIT from UFH, platelet count monitoring is not necessary.

31.11 Management of the Limb in Acute DVT

Initial measures in the management of lower limb DVT should include elevation of the legs and wearing of graduated compression stockings (GCS) on the affected limb; this has the benefit of reducing pain and swelling. Pregnant women with DVT must be duly informed on self-administration of LMWH as well as safe disposal of syringes and needles. Early mobilisation is encouraged as it has not been found to be associated with an increased risk of PE but rather pain and swelling were relieved faster compared to those who have restricted mobility [27]. Movements can start as soon as the patient is stable after commencement of anticoagulation.

31.12 Use of Inferior Vena Cava Filters

Retrievable inferior vena cava (IVC) filters can be considered in women who had contraindications to pharmacological anticoagulants such as active bleeding, extensive DVT close to the time of delivery or recurrent PE despite adequate anticoagulation. Delivery should be delayed whenever possible to allow for pharmacological anticoagulation rather than the use of IVC filters. Complications such as perforation of IVC during filter insertion, filter migration, filter tilt, increased risk of lower limb DVT, cava thrombosis and rarely infections can occur following IVC insertion [14, 15]. It should therefore be considered only when there is an absolute contraindication to pharmacological anticoagulation.

31.13 Treatment of Acute Massive PE in Pregnancy

Massive PE associated with haemodynamic compromise (low blood pressure, tachycardia) is a medical emergency and should be managed in the intensive care unit. Thrombolytic therapy should be considered in such patients because of the advantage of reducing the clot burden. UFH is preferred to LMWH in managing massive PE because of its more rapid onset of action and shorter half-life. Loading dose of 80 units/kg followed by a continuous intravenous infusion of 18 units/kg/hour should be given. In patients who have received thrombolysis, the loading dose of heparin should be omitted and an infusion started at 18 units/kg/hour. The activated partial thromboplastin time (APTT) is used to determine the efficacy of UFH. The APTT is done 4–6 hours after the loading dose, 6 hours after any dose change and then at least daily when in the therapeutic range [9]. Management should involve a multidisciplinary team including a haematologist. The APTT ratio should be in the therapeutic range of 1.5–2.5 the control plasma (Fig. 31.2).

31.14 Maintenance Therapy

Therapeutic dose of LMWH should be continued all through pregnancy and at least 6 weeks postpartum. Treatment should last for at least 3 months in total.

31.15 Complications of Heparin Therapy

Allergic skin reactions, bleeding and heparin-induced thrombocytopaenia (HIT) may complicate heparin therapy. Patient should be properly counselled prior to commencement of therapy whenever possible. HIT is more common with UFH, platelet counts should be monitored every 2–3 days till day 14 of treatment. Prolonged use of UFH during pregnancy could also cause osteoporosis and fractures. In situations where heparin could not be administered either due to HIT or allergic skin reactions, alternatives like danaparoid, a low molecular weight heparinoid, fondaparinux, or argatroban can be considered [15, 27].

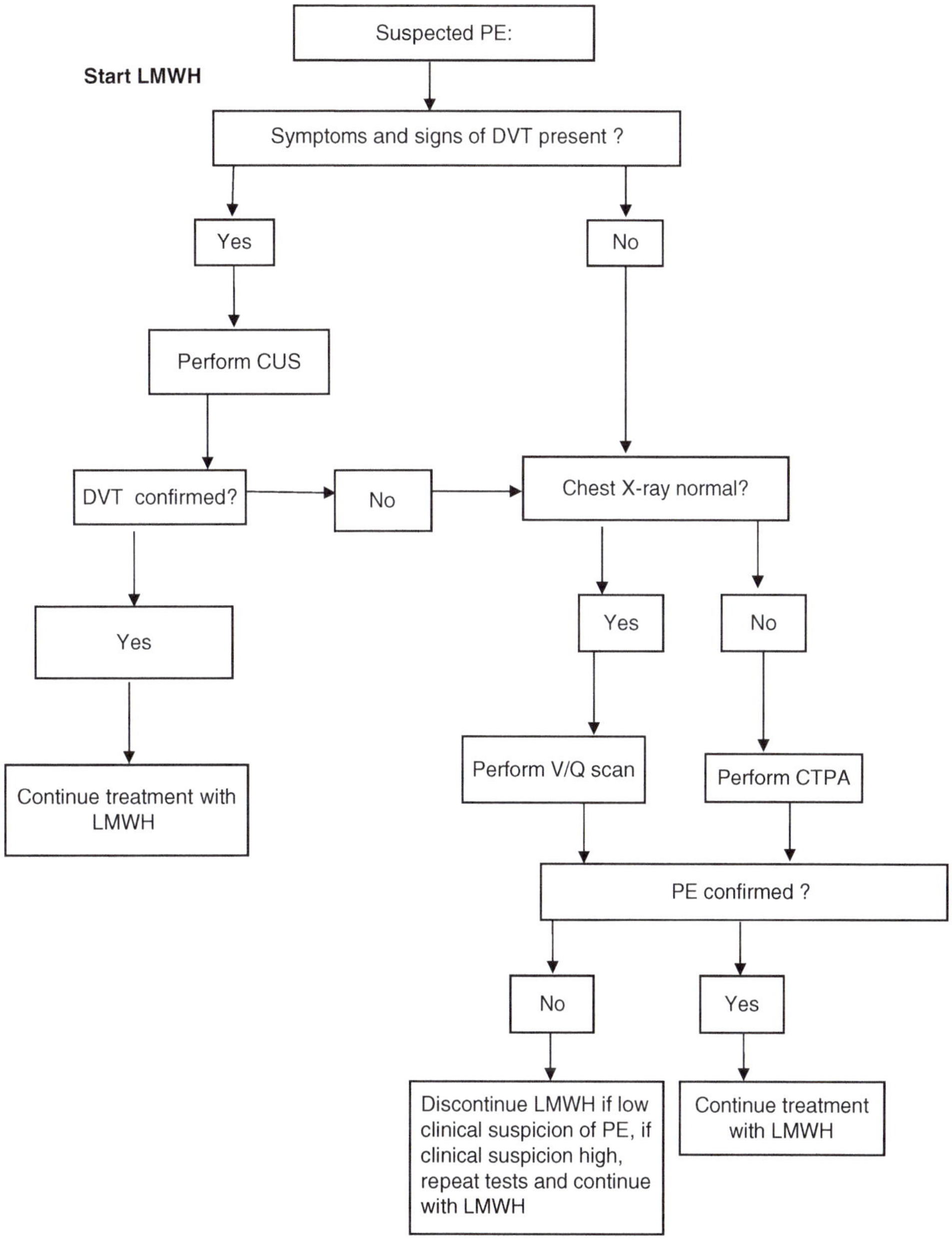

Fig. 31.2 Diagnostic algorithm for suspected pulmonary embolism in pregnancy adapted from Royal College of Obstetricians and Gynaecologists green top guidelines 37 b, 2015. Abbreviations: PE pulmonary embolism, LMWH low molecular weight heparin, DVT:deep vein thrombosis, CUS compression ultrasonography, V/Qscan ventilation/perfusion scan, CTPA computed tomography pulmonary angiogram

31.16 Management of Labour and Delivery

Labour and delivery can further increase haemorrhage in a fully anticoagulated woman; therefore, the goal of management should be to minimise blood loss as well as preventing thrombosis due to interruption of anticoagulant therapy in the peripartum period. Patient should be counselled to discontinue LMWH at the first sign of labour during the antenatal period if vagina delivery is anticipated.

Proper hydration must be maintained, the use of anti-embolism stockings should be encouraged. Following an uneventful delivery with no unusual bleeds, prophylactic dose of LMWH should be started 6 hours after delivery; treatment dose based on the calculated postpartum body weight can be commenced on the second-day postpartum [9, 15]. Where elective caesarean section is planned, the last therapeutic dose should be given 24 hours before surgery. The first prophylactic dose after delivery by caesarean section can be given 6 hours later provided there is no unusual bleed. LMWH should not be given for at least 24 hours after an epidural or spinal catheter has been removed.

31.17 Induction of Labour

Full blood count, basic coagulation profile and blood grouping and cross-matching should be performed as soon the woman presents for induction of labour.

In a primigravida with an unfavourable cervix, the last therapeutic dose of LMWH could be given 12 hours before the first inducing agent is administered while a multiparous woman with a favourable cervix could get the last therapeutic dose of LMWH 24 hours prior to commencement of induction [15]. Women at high risk of bleeding who require anticoagulation should be given UFH because of its shorter half-life and its complete reversal by protamine sulphate compared to LMWH. Women on LMWH with bleeding complications should be referred to the haematologist. Protamine sulphate could be used to reverse some of the anti-Xa effects of LMWH [28].

31.18 Postpartum Management

Immediately after delivery, the woman should be clinically assessed for bleeding risks or active bleeding. In the actively bleeding patients, haematologist should be consulted while local and surgical measures of combating haemorrhage are instituted. Anticoagulation should be withheld until the woman is haemostatically stable. Women without contraindication to anticoagulation should be commenced on therapeutic anticoagulation. LMWH or VKAs can be used post-delivery as neither is contraindicated in breastfeeding [29]. The choice, duration of postpartum anticoagulation and the need for regular blood tests (if VKAs) should be discussed with the patient. Therapeutic anticoagulation should be given for at least 6 weeks postpartum until at least 3 months of anticoagulation has been given in total. Longer period of anticoagulation will be determined by the risk of recurrence [9, 15]. Doses of LMWH should be recalculated based on the post-delivery weight. In women who prefer warfarin, warfarin should not be started until the 5th day after delivery and the INR should be tested daily during the period of overlap with LMWH, the dose of warfarin should be adjusted to keep the INR at 2–3. LMWH should not be discontinued until therapeutic INR has been maintained for at least 24 hours [9, 15].

31.19 Prevention of Post-thrombotic Syndrome (PTS)

Post-thrombotic syndrome is a common complication of DVT with a reported prevalence of 42% [30]. Persistent leg swelling, pain, dermatitis, dependent cyanosis, chronic pigmentation and venous ulceration in severe cases are the prominent features. The clinical benefits of compression stockings in the prevention of PTS are not clear; while some studies have reported a reduction in leg pain with the use of compression stockings, others did not find any clinical benefit [31, 32]. Prolong use of LMWH (>12 weeks) has been reported to significantly lower the risk of developing PTS. The Royal College of Obstetricians and Gynaecologists recommends the use of graduated compression stockings on the affected leg only to reduce the pain and swelling of DVT in pregnancy.

31.20 Summary

Venous thromboembolism is an important and preventable cause of maternal mortality. Diagnosis is difficult because symptoms and signs are often not specific especially in pregnancy. A high index of clinical suspicion is of the essence. D-dimer testing which has a negative prediction value in the non-pregnancy state is often elevated in normal pregnancy and therefore not useful for exclusion of VTE in pregnancy. Compression ultrasonography scan should be ordered whenever there is a clinical suspicion of DVT in pregnancy. Considerations should be given to maternal and foetal safety when investigating VTE in pregnancy. Imaging is essential to avoid inappropriate treatment and can be performed without exposing the foetus to any specific risks. A chest X-ray should always be performed to exclude other causes and should be ordered when there is a clinical suspicion of PE. Patients with normal chest X-ray should have a V/Q scan while those with abnormal chest X-ray should have a CTPA. A patient with suspected PE with positive lower limbs CUS requires no further investigation and should be treated. LMWH is the pharmacological anticoagulant of choice in pregnancy. However, thrombolysis should be considered in patients with haemodynamic instability. UFH is preferred in acute massive PE because of its quicker onset of action and shorter half-life. UFH is monitored with the APTT, levels should be between 1.5 and 2.5 the control normal pooled plasma. IVC filters should be considered in women with absolute contraindication to pharmacological anticoagulation. Both LMWH and VKA can be used postpartum. Treatment should last till at least 6 weeks postpartum for at least 3 months duration of total anticoagulation. Graduated compression stockings reduce pain and swelling of the affected leg.

References

1. Pomp ER, Lesenlelink AM, Rosendaal FR, Doggen CJ. Pregnancy postpartum period and prothrombotic defects:risk of venous thrombosis in the MEGA study. J Thromb Haemost. 2008;6(4):632–7.

2. Bates SM, Ginsberg JS. How we manage venous thromboembolism during pregnancy. Blood. 2002;100:3470–8.
3. Bates SM, Greer IA, Palbinger I, Sofaer S, Hirsh J. Venous thromboembolism, thrombophilia, antithrombotic therapy and pregnancy. American College of Chest Physicians Evidence-Based Clinical Practice Guidelines(8th edition). Chest. 2008;133:844S–86S.
4. Chang J, Elam-Evans LD, Berg CJ, Herndon J, Flowers L, Seed KA, Syverson CJ. Pregnancy-related mortality surveillance--United States 1991-1999 NMWR. Surveil Summ. 2003;52(2):1–8.
5. Rodger M. Evidence base for the management of venous thromboembolism in pregnancy. Haematology Am Soc Haematol Educ. 2010;2010:173–80.
6. Brenner B. Haemostatic changes in pregnancy. Thromb Res. 2004;114:409–14.
7. Ratnapalan S, Bentur Y, Koren G. Doctor, will that X-ray harm my unborn child? CMAJ. 2008;179:1293–6.
8. Prenatal radiation exposure: a fact sheet for physicians, Atlanta: Centre for Disease Control, 2005.
9. Royal college of Obstetrician and Gynaecologists. Thromboembolic disease of pregnancy and puerperium: acute management. Green top guideline no 37b London: RCOG; 2015 available at https://www.rcog.org.uk/guidelines
10. Bates SM, Middeldorp S, Rodger M, James AH. Guidance for the treatment and prevention of obstetric-associated venous thromboembolism. J Thromb Thrombolysis. 2016;41:92–128.
11. Lewis G, editor. Confidential enquiry into maternal and child health: saving mothers' lives-reviewing maternal deaths to make motherhood safer 2003–2005. London: CEMACH; 2007.
12. James AH, Jamison MG, Brancazio LR, Myers ER. Venous thromboembolism during pregnancy and the postpartum period:incidence, risk factors, and mortality. Am J Obstet Gynecol. 2006;194(5):1311–5.
13. Gader AA, Haggaaz AE, Adam I. Epidemiology of venous thrombosis during pregnancy and puerperium in Sudanese women. Vasc Health Risk Manag. 2009;5:85–7.
14. Bates SM. Thrombophilia in pregnancy. In: Kitchen, Kessler, Konkle, editors. Consultative haemostasis and thrombosis. 3rd ed. Philadelphia: Elsevier Saunders; 2013. p. 627–43.
15. Khali A, Bowles L, O'Brien P, Cohen H. Systemic thromboembolism in pregnancy: venous thromboembolism. In: Cohen H, O'Brien P, editors. Disorders of thrombosis and haemostasis in pregnancy a guide to management. 2nd ed. London: Springer-Verlag; 2015.
16. Treffers PE, Huidekoper BL, Weenink GH, Kloosterman GJ. Epidemiological observations of thrombo-embolic disease during pregnancy and in the puerperium in 56022 women. Int J Gynaecol Obstet. 1983;21:327–31.
17. Ginsberg JS, Edwards P, Burrows RF, Bona R, Prandoni P, Buler HR, Lensing A. Venous thrombosis during pregnancy: leg and timing of presentation. Thromb Haemost. 1992;67:519–20.
18. Ray JG, Chan WS. Deep vein thrombosis during pregnancy and the puerperium: a meta-analysis of the period of risk and leg presentation. Obstet Gynaecol Suiv. 1999;54:265–71.
19. Macklon NS, Greer LA, Bowman AW. An ultrasound study of gestational and postural changes in the deep venous system of the leg in pregnancy. Br J Obstet Gynaecol. 1977;104:191–7.
20. Royal college of Obstetrician and Gynaecologists. Reducing the risk of venous thromboembolism during pregnancy and the puerperium. Green top guideline no. 37a London: RCOG; 2009 available at https://www.rcog.org.uk/guidelines
21. Scarsbook AF, Evans AL, Owen AR, Gleeson FV. Diagnosis of suspected venous thromboembolic disease in pregnancy. Clin Radiol. 2006;61(1):1–12.
22. Chan W-S, Lee A, Spencer FA, Crowder M, Rodger M, Ramsay T, Ginsberg JS. Predicting deep venous thrombosis in pregnancy: out in "LEFt field?". Ann Intern Med. 2009;151:85–92.
23. Kovac M, Mikovic Z, Rakicevic L, Srzentic S, Mandic V, Djordjevic V, Radojkovic D, Elezocovic I. The use of D-dimer with new cutoff can be useful in diagnosis of venous thromboembolism in pregnancy. Eur J Obstet Gynecol Reprod Biol. 2010;148(1):27–30.
24. Moriarty JM, Bolster F, O'Connor C, Fitzpatrick P, Lawler LP, Kavanagh EC, et al. Frequency of nonthromboembolic imaging abnormalities in pregnant women referred for computed tomography pulmonary arteriography. Can Assoc Radiol J. 2015;66(1):24–9. (Level III evidence).
25. Bordeleau S. Towards evidence based emergency medicine: best BETs from the Manchester Royal Infirmary. BET 2: imaging for the diagnosis of pulmonary embolism in pregnant women. Emerg Med J. 2013;30(3):251–2.
26. Said JM, Ignjatovic V, Monagle PT, Walker SP, Higgins JR, Brennecke SP. Altered reference ranges for protein C and protein S during early pregnancy: implications for the diagnosis of protein C ad protein S deficiency during pregnancy. Thromb Haemost. 2010;103:984–8.
27. Magnani HN. An analysis of clinical outcomes of 91 pregnancies in 83 women treated with danaparoid (orgaran R). Throm Res. 2010;125:297–302.
28. Van Veen JJ, Maclean RM, Hampton KK, Laidlaw S, Kitchen S, Toth P, Makris M. Protamine reversal of low molecular weight heparin: clinically effective? Blood Coagul Fibrinolysis. 2011;22:565–70.
29. Clark SL, Porter TF, West FG. Coumarin derivatives and breast feeding. Obstet Gynecol. 2000;95:938–40.
30. Mccoll MD, Ellison J, Greer IA, Trait RC, Walker ID. Prevalence of the post thrombotic syndrome in young women with previous venous thromboembolism. Br J Haematol. 2000;108:72–4.
31. Brandjes DP, Buller HR, Heijboer H, Huisman MV, de Rijk M, Jagt H, Cate J. Randomised trial of effect of compression stockings in patients with symptomatic proximal-vein thrombosis. Lancet. 1997;349:759–62.
32. Kahn SR, Shapiro S, Ducruet T, Wells PS, Rodger MA, Kovacs MJ, Anderson D, Tagalaski V, Morrison DR, Solymoss S, et al. Graduated compression stockings to treat acute leg pain associated with proximal DVT. A randomised controlled trial. Thromb Haemost. 2014;112(6):1137–41.

Inherited Bleeding Disorders in Pregnancy

32

Omolade Awodu

Learning Objectives

At the conclusion of this chapter, the reader should be able to:

- Identify the diverse inherited bleeding disorders in pregnancy.
- Understand the diverse acquired bleeding disorders in pregnancy.
- Critically evaluate haematological management of obstetric haemorrhage (OH) and post-haemorrhage care.
- Have a deep understanding of disseminated intravascular coagulation (DIC) in pregnancy.

32.1 Introduction

Pregnancy is characterised by an alteration in the haemostatic mechanism with a tendency towards hypercoagulability which is geared towards protecting the mother and the foetus from excess bleeding at delivery. The concentrations of coagulation factors II, VII, VIII, X and von willebrand factor (VWF) have all been widely reported to be elevated in pregnancy; these together with impaired fibrinolysis make pregnancy a hypercoagulable condition [1, 2]. This level of increase in procoagulant clotting factors is not seen in women with inherited bleeding disorders; they are therefore at increased risk of bleeding complications during pregnancy. There are a variety of inherited and acquired disorders that may tilt the balance towards hypocoagulability during pregnancy and puerperium with a greater risk of bleeding with any haemostatic challenge.

O. Awodu (✉)
University of Benin/University of Benin Teaching Hospital, Benin City, Nigeria
e-mail: omolade.awodu@uniben.edu

Inherited bleeding disorders (IBDs) are not common with a prevalence of 0.01–1% for von Willebrand disease (VWD) and 1:5000 live male births for haemophilia A and less commonly FXI and FXIII deficiencies [3]. When present, however, they could pose significant haemostatic challenge to both the foetus and the mother during pregnancy as well as at the time of delivery in women who are otherwise asymptomatic. The possibility of carrying an affected foetus who may suffer significant haemostatic disturbances during labour and delivery is a major source of worry for women with IBDs. Severely affected foetuses are at risk of intracranial haemorrhage during labour. Therefore, women with IBD require individualised care during pregnancy and the peri-partum period.

IBD may result from any heritable abnormality of primary and secondary haemostasis which include platelet disorders, von Willebrand disease (VWD), Haemophilia A and B and other rare clotting factors deficiencies. VWD is the most common IBD affecting about 1% of the population, with a prevalence of 10–20% in women with menorrhagia and delayed postpartum haemorrhage [4, 5]. The risk of miscarriage and antepartum haemorrhage in women with VWD and carriers of haemophilia A or B is not clear [4–6]; however, it has been demonstrated that these women are at increased risk of primary and secondary postpartum haemorrhage, and the underlying condition may be overlooked by clinicians. Pregnant women with inherited bleeding disorders have increased risk of postpartum haemorrhage which usually occurs over 2–3 weeks after delivery [5]. The median duration of bleeding after delivery is 21–27 days in normal pregnancy while the elevated clotting factors return to basal levels within 14–21 days [7]. Postpartum bleeding may last longer in women with IBDs. Acquired causes of bleeding during pregnancy may be due to maternal or placental related factors, or non-pregnancy related conditions that result in thrombocytopaenia or coagulopathy. The management of obstetrics haemorrhage involves identifying and treating the underlying cause/causes as well as replacing deficient blood constituents. Here lies the challenge as blood components supply is still grossly inadequate in low-income countries.

F. Okonofua et al. (eds.), *Contemporary Obstetrics and Gynecology for Developing Countries*,
https://doi.org/10.1007/978-3-030-75385-6_32

Therefore, focus should be on averting haemorrhage. Management of women with bleeding disorders during pregnancy should involve a multidisciplinary team of obstetricians, haematologists, paediatricians, anaesthetist as well as other relevant health care professionals. The haematologist should be involved at all stages from pregnancy, during delivery and the immediate postpartum period. This chapter focuses on inherited and acquired disorders of primary and secondary haemostasis. Specifically, this chapter highlights management of pregnant women with vWD and haemophilia carrier states which together constitute about 90% of IBD. This chapter focuses on acquired causes of bleeding in pregnancy, specifically immune thrombocytopaenia in pregnancy, disseminated intravascular coagulation in pregnancy and haematological management of obstetric haemorrhage. Some of these conditions are rare and often overlooked by the attending clinicians; their importance rests on the propensity to cause significant postpartum haemorrhage (PPH).

32.2 Inherited Bleeding Disorders

32.2.1 von Willebrand Disease (VWD)

vWD results from a qualitative or quantitative defect in von Willebrand factor (VWF), a large multimeric glycoprotein that plays a major role in the formation of primary platelet plug by mediating adhesion and aggregation of platelets at the sites of vascular injury. VWF also serves as the carrier molecule for coagulation FVIII in plasma, protecting it from proteolytic degradation, thereby prolonging its half-life in the circulation [8]. VWF level increases progressively during pregnancy, starting from the sixth week, and rising up to 3–4 times baseline levels [9]. In women with type 1 VWD, this increase is beneficial because normal values of VWF would have been achieved before delivery. However, patients with baseline levels <15 IU/dl may fail to reach normal levels. In type 2B, the increase in dysfunctional VWF protein enhances abnormal platelet binding leading to thrombocytopaenia in affected individuals. Type 2 N VWD is characterised by low factor VIII levels, while patients with type 3 disease have severe deficiency of VWF with little or no rise in its level in pregnancy [6] (Table 32.1).

32.2.2 Epidemiology

VWD is the most common inherited bleeding disorder with a prevalence of 1% in the general population. The presentation is variable depending on the type. Type 3 has the most clinically severe bleeding and occurs in 0.02% of the population [6, 10]. The prevalence of rare clotting factors disorders ranges between 1:500,000 and 1:2,000,000 [10].

32.2.3 Clinical Features

Despite the physiological increase in VWF in pregnancy, women with VWD have increased risk of bleeding events and even deaths during childbirth. The clinical features of VWD are a reflection of its dual roles in normal haemostasis, which are mediating platelet plug formation and protecting FVIII from clearance in plasma. Severe disease presents both as mucocutaneous haemorrhages as well as typical haemophilic bleeds such as subcutaneous haematomas, joint and muscle bleeds.

Milder forms may not present until after significant haemostatic challenge such as childbirth.

Abortions or miscarriages in the first or second trimester are accompanied with significant bleeding because the increase in VWF and FVIII levels at this period is not sufficient to withstand the haemostatic challenge.

A detailed bleeding history should be taken to identify cases that present first time during pregnancy.

Type 2B VWD is associated with progressive thrombocytopaenia in pregnancy and should be considered in the differential diagnosis of thrombocytopenia in pregnancy.

The diagnosis of type 3 disease is often made in childhood in affected patients.

Approximately, 30% of women with VWD will bleed during the first trimester, primary postpartum haemorrhage occurs in 15–30% while delayed postpartum haemorrhage is

Table 32.1 Characteristics of common IBD

Disorder	Defect	Plasma concentration	Prevalence
vWD Type 1	Quantitative deficiency of vWF. Autosomal dominant inheritance	vWF level – 15–40 IU/l	85% of cases
Type 2	Qualitative (functional defect) subclassified into: 2A, 2B, 2M and 2N, based on their pathophysiology		15% of cases
Type 3	Severe quantitative deficiency. Almost undetectable levels of vWF	vWF <1 IU/L, FVIII <20 IU/dl	Very rare (1 in 1,000,000)
Haemophilia A and B	X-linked recessive inheritance; males are sufferers while females are carriers	Carriers have 50% of normal values. Levels range from 22 to 116 IU/dl	Haemophilia A affects 1 in 5000 live male births; haemophilia B affects 1 in 30,000 live male births
Factor XI deficiency (haemophilia C)	Autosomal recessive inheritance		Prevalence in heterozygotes is about 8% in Ashkenazi Jews

seen 20–25%, perineal haematoma and significant bleeding may also be seen after miscarriages [4–6].

32.2.4 Diagnosis

The physiologic increase in VWF and FVIII levels in pregnancy may hinder the diagnosis of milder forms of the disease during pregnancy. Women in whom there is a clinical suspicion of VWD should have platelet count as well as basic coagulation screening tests (prothrombin time (PT) and activated partial thromboplastin time (APTT)) done. These, however, do not routinely detect VWD except in type 2B where FVIII is equally low with a subsequent prolongation of the APTT. Specific assays for VWF-Ag and FVIII-C are available for confirmation of diagnosis.

The platelet count will be normal except in type 2B disease. The prothrombin time is also normal and the APTT will be normal except in types 2B or type 3 disease. The bleeding time is no longer favoured routinely due to the lack of standardisation. It is still useful in developing countries when properly carried out. It is usually prolonged in vWD.

32.2.5 Antenatal Management

Once a diagnosis of VWD in pregnancy is made, antenatal management and delivery should be planned in conjunction with the haematologist, the anaesthetist and neonatologist.

Pregnant women with VWD should be fully informed about their condition and potential bleeding risks during pregnancy, delivery and in the puerperium should be discussed. This is particularly important in patients with type 2 or 3 VWD. The possibility of having an affected child should be discussed with the woman and the husband and genetic counselling should be offered [11].

Regular monitoring of VWF:AC (von Willebrand factor antigen) together with FVIII C (factor VIII activity) is recommended at booking, 28 weeks, 34 weeks gestation and prior to any invasive procedure. The platelet count should be monitored in patients with type 2B VWD; platelet transfusion and VWF-containing products may be needed for bleeding and to cover surgical and invasive procedures and spontaneous miscarriages [11, 12]. Availability of blood components should be confirmed prior to delivery in centres where these are not readily available.

32.2.6 Delivery

Women with VWD can have a normal vaginal delivery if the VWF level is up to 50 IU/dl and FVIII level is >40 IU/dl and can have a caesarean section if their FVIII level is greater than 50 IU/dl. Desmopressin (1–8-deamino-D-arginine vasopressin, DDAVP), a synthetic analogue of vasopressin, has been shown to reduce bleeding complications associated with pregnancy and childbirth in pregnant women with VWD. Though the use of DDAVP in pregnancy has not been clinically validated, no complication has been reported following its use in pregnancy [11–13]. It acts specifically through type 2 vasopressin receptors and stimulates the release of ultra-large VWF multimers from storage in the Wiebel Palade bodies of the endothelial cells. It causes a transient increase in VWF and FVIII levels. It is administered by slow intravenous infusion at a dose of 0.3 μ/kg body weight over 20 minutes. Subcutaneous routes can also be used. It is also available as a nasal spray. There is a three- to fivefold increase in both VWF and FVIII levels within 30–60 minutes of administration.

Delivery in women with type 2 and type 3 VWD or moderate to severe type 1, or a history of severe bleeding, should be at a centre where there are obstetricians, haematologists, good laboratory as well as blood bank support. Women with severe disease will require plasma-derived VWF concentrates to maintain levels above 50 IU/dl for at least 3 days after vagina delivery and 5 days after caesarean section [11]. Cryoprecipitate is rich in VWF and should be used in resource-poor countries where factor concentrates that contain vWF are not available. Complications of treatment with plasma-derived concentrates include transmission of viral infections. This is now very rare because of pre-donation screening of donors and viral inactivation of commercial concentrates. In view of the possibilities of babies being affected, instrumental deliveries should be avoided for foetuses at risk of having severe type 1, type 2 or type 3 disease.

Levels of VWF should be assayed whenever an invasive procedure is anticipated. Prophylaxis DDAVP should be given whenever VWF is less than 30-40 IU/dl. A frequent concern is the effect of DDAVP in the foetus; there is a potential danger of foetal hyponatraemia as a result of maternal antidiuretic effect [11, 13]. Fluid intake should be restricted to 1 litre for about 24 hours because of the selective effect of DDAVP on type 2 vasopressin receptors leading to fluid retention and maternal hyponatremia. The benefits of DDAVP include its wide availability, relatively low cost even in resource-poor countries, and its reduction in the use of blood products [11].

Patients should be advised to avoid products that interfere with platelet adhesion such as aspirin and other non-steroidal anti-inflammatory drugs (NSAID).

32.2.7 Tranexamic Acid

It is a fibrinolysis inhibitor. It is useful in patients with mild VWD. It is contraindicated in women with haematuria and

Table 32.2 Protocol for postpartum management

Immediately after delivery, the woman should be examined to ascertain surgical haemostasis and effective uterine contractions.
Prophylactic tranexamic acid should be administered.
Patients who have very low pre-pregnancy levels and a history of good response to DDAVP should be given the drug.
The levels of VWF activity should be maintained at >50 IU/DL for 3 days following vagina delivery or 5 days post caesarean section in patients with type 2 and type 3 or severe type 1 disease [11].
Patients should be counselled and encouraged to report any excessive blood loss after discharge.
Women who have excessive bleeding despite adequate prophylaxis should be considered for oral contraceptive pills.

Adapted from Pavord [11]

should not be used during pregnancy because it crosses the placenta.

32.2.8 Management of the Neonate

Following delivery, cord blood samples should be taken to assay for VWF. Initial levels may be unreliable because the stress of labour can cause a temporary elevation. The assay should be repeated in about 6–12 months [11]. Circumcision should be avoided till the VWF level is known.

FVIII and FWF levels begin to fall from 24 hours to 2 weeks after birth. Secondary postpartum haemorrhage may occur in spite of prophylaxis with an onset from the second to third week of delivery [6, 11, 14] (Table 32.2).

32.2.9 Haemophilia

Haemophilia is an X-linked inherited bleeding disorder characterised by deficiency of factor VIII (in haemophilia A) or factor IX (in haemophilia B).

Males are typically affected while females are carriers.

The incidence is equal across races with an estimated of 1/10000, 1/5000 live male births for haemophilia A and 1/30000 live male births for haemophilia B.

Haemophilia is very rare in females. Daughters of known male haemophiliacs are obligate carriers. Carrier mothers have a 50% chance of transferring the disease to their female offsprings and their sons have a 50% chance of having the disease. FVIII levels usually increase up to three folds normal from baseline levels from the sixth week of pregnancy. While factor IX is unaffected [12], carriers of FIX deficiency are therefore more susceptible to bleeding episodes with haemostatic challenge of early pregnancy and delivery.

The expected mean clotting factor level of carrier females is 50% of normal values. In most carriers, the increase in FVIII level in pregnancy lessens any potential bleeding risk at childbirth. However, a few carriers may have factor levels in the haemophilic range, and those with baseline values <15 IU/dl may not achieve normal values before delivery and are at a risk of excessive bleeding during childbirth and the postpartum period. The factor level should be checked at 34 weeks. The sex of the foetus should be known before delivery so as to take the necessary precautions to prevent intracranial haemorrhages which affects 1–4% of male haemophilic neonates [5, 11, 13, 15–17].

32.2.10 Management of Delivery in Pregnant Carriers (Table 32.3)

32.2.11 Prenatal Diagnosis

The foetal sex should be determined by ultrasonography before planning prenatal diagnosis. Prenatal diagnosis in a male foetus helps in instituting appropriate management during labour and delivery.

32.3 Acquired Bleeding Disorders in Pregnancy

Obstetrics haemorrhage may result from pregnancy-related factors or primary haematological disorders in pregnancy. Acquired bleeding disorders in pregnancy may be due to acquired deficiency of coagulation factors and quantitative or qualitative platelet disorders. The conditions associated with acquired bleeding disorders are listed in Table 32.5.

Table 32.3 Guidelines for the management of delivery in carriers of haemophilia

Establish a good rapport with the haematologist concerning the case.
Written delivery plan should be drawn up in advance.
Delivery should be in unit with suitable expertise and facilities including stock of concentrates in carriers carrying an affected foetus.
Determine foetal gender by ultrasound.
Foetal sex should be known to the obstetrician before delivery.
Epidural anaesthesia is permitted if FVIII level is >50 IU/dl.
Avoid foetal scalp electrodes.
Normal vaginal delivery should be the routine option, but delivery should be by the least traumatic method, and early recourse to caesarean section should be considered.
Elective caesarean section should be considered in women carrying an affected foetus to prevent intracranial haemorrhage.
Avoid vacuum(ventrose) extraction.
IM injections should be avoided until factor VIII/IX level is known.
Oral vitamin K should be given to affected neonates.
Immunisations should be given to the newborn either through the subcutaneous or intradermal route until the factor level is known.
Cranial ultrasound computed tomography scan should be carried out for all neonates with haemophilia if delivery was traumatic or there was history of prolonged labour or preterm delivery.

Adapted from UKHCDO Guidelines for Haemophilia 2006; 12: 301–336 [16]

32.3.1 Thrombocytopaenia in Pregnancy

Thrombocytopaenia is platelet count less than the lower limit of the reference range (100–400 × 10^9/l in Nigerians and 150–400 × 10^9 in Caucasians) [18]. The international working group defines thrombocytopaenia as platelet count less than 100 × 10^9/l. Thrombocytopaenia is the second most common haematological disorder in pregnancy after anaemia. The worldwide prevalence of thrombocytopaenia in pregnancy is about 7–8% [19] at platelet count <150 × 10^9/l; however, the prevalence decreases to 1% if the more stringent cut off of <100 × 10^9/l adopted by the international work group on thrombocytopaenia is used. It results from diverse causes (Table 32.5) with overlapping pathogenesis and clinical features. An absolute decrease in platelet count should be differentiated from pseudothrombocytopaenia or apparent thrombocytopaenia which commonly results from extraneous factors such as platelet clumping from the use of ethylene diamine tetra acetic acid (EDTA) as an anticoagulant, platelet satellitism which occurs when platelets form rosettes around white blood cells and as such cannot be accurately counted or the presence of large platelets in circulation which are wrongly counted as red cells by the haematology autoanalyser. A careful examination of a well-prepared blood smear by a haematologist will exclude absolute thrombocytopaenia in such cases. Pseudothrombocytopaenia or spurious thrombocytopaenia should be considered before ordering extensive laboratory tests.

32.3.2 Gestational Thrombocytopaenia (GT)

Gestational thrombocytopaenia (GT) or incidental thrombocytopaenia is a benign condition in which there is a mild reduction of platelet count in pregnancy. It is often an incidental finding, occurring in the second or third trimester of pregnancy. It is found in 5% of all pregnant women. A prevalence of 13.5% has been reported among pregnant women in Nigeria [20]. It is a leading cause of thrombocytopaenia in pregnancy accounting for about 70–75% of cases [20–23]. The pathogenesis is unclear. Haemodilution from an increase in plasma volume and platelet destruction at the placental bed may play a role [21, 23].

32.3.3 Clinical Presentation

Mostly asymptomatic, usually an incidental finding in the second or third trimester of pregnancy. The platelet counts rarely fall below 70 × 10^9/l; pregnancy and delivery are uneventful. The platelet count returns to normal within 2–12 weeks of delivery [24]. There is no association with neonatal thrombocytopaenia. The clinical significance is that it may cause a diagnostic confusion with immune thrombocytopenia especially when early pregnancy platelet counts are not available.

32.3.4 Immune Thrombocytopaenia (Idiopathic Thrombocytopaenic Purpura (ITP))

ITP is an acquired quantitative platelet disorder characterised by immune-mediated platelet destruction. Presence of antiplatelet autoantibodies against platelet surface antigens mediate an accelerated destruction of platelets as well as an impairment of megakaryocytopoiesis.

The international working group on ITP [25] proposed certain criteria for diagnosis which include: platelet count <100 × 10^9/l, isolated thrombocytopaenia in the presence of an otherwise normal full blood count, peripheral blood film and biochemical indices. In addition, there should be no pathological features suggesting an underlying disease [25, 26].

It is therefore a diagnosis of exclusion. ITP is classified into two types:

1. Primary ITP, which is an autoimmune thrombocytopaenia characterised by platelet count less than 100 × 10^9/l.
2. Secondary ITP, which includes all other forms of immune-mediated thrombocytopaenia except primary ITP. Secondary ITP may be seen in systemic lupus erythematosus, antiphospholipid antibodies, chronic lymphocytic leukaemia, *Helicobacter pylori* infection and hepatitis C virus infection.

It accounts for 1–5% of thrombocytopaenia per 10,000 pregnancies [21].

The exact pathogenesis of ITP is not clear. Antiplatelet antibodies (IgM or IgG) produced by activated B lymphocytes, impaired megakaryocyte production, and T cell mediated cytotoxicity have been implicated in its pathogenesis.

32.3.5 Clinical Features

The presentation is variable depending on the platelet count, and it is the same as the presentation outside pregnancy. It may be asymptomatic, an incidental finding in the first trimester of pregnancy, in which case it may be a diagnostic confusion with gestational thrombocytopaenia, which is rare in early pregnancy. Bleeding manifestations are unusual with platelet counts >50 × 10^9/l. Symptoms typically reflect abnormalities of primary haemostasis, and they include: mucocutaneous haemorrhages, petechial haemorrhages, epistaxis and rarely intracranial haemorrhage. Physical examination in severe cases will show widespread purpura, petechiae haemorrhages and ecchymotic patches on the skin and mucous membranes. Clinical evaluation should include detailed drug history, use of corticosteroids, family history as well as history of neonatal thrombocytopaenia in previous successful pregnancies; positive history indicates pre-existing ITP.

32.3.6 Laboratory Investigations

Full blood count shows isolated thrombocytopaenia. There is usually no anaemia unless there is excessive blood loss; other anaemic work up is often normal. Consult should be sent to the haematologist for examination of the peripheral blood smear to rule out spurious thrombocytopaenia and any underlying marrow pathology. Bone marrow examination is not necessary except to exclude haematological disorders of marrow origin. Some of the laboratory tests for ITP in pregnancy are shown in Table 32.7.

There is no single test for the confirmation of immune thrombocytopaenia. It remains a diagnosis of exclusion [25, 26].

32.3.7 Management of ITP During Pregnancy

Management of ITP during pregnancy should involve a multidisciplinary team of obstetricians, haematologists, anaesthetists and neonatologists. The aim of management is to maintain a platelet count that is sufficient to prevent bleeding episodes during pregnancy and delivery.

The platelet count should be closely monitored during pregnancy and should be done more frequently as the woman approaches term.

The underlying disease should be treated in patients with secondary ITP. Bone marrow evaluation is not necessary for confirmation of ITP in pregnancy except to rule out an underlying marrow pathology if there are clinical and laboratory indications (Tables 32.4, 32.5, 32.6, and 32.7).

32.3.8 Treatment of ITP During Pregnancy

The focus should be on prevention of bleeding manifestations and haemorrhagic complications during delivery and in the puerperium. Most women with ITP in pregnancy will not require treatment. Therapeutic decision should be based on the urgency to bring the platelet count to a level adequate to maintain haemostasis. There are no clinically validated thresholds for ITP in pregnancy. Members of the team should agree on the platelet thresholds as soon as diagnosis is made. A suggested threshold for intervention is presented in Table 32.8.

Table 32.4 Causes of thrombocytopaenia and acquired bleeding disorders in pregnancy

Condition	Mechanism	Diagnostic features
Pregnancy related		
Gestational thrombocytopaenia	Haemodilution combined with platelet destruction in the placenta bed	Normal pre-pregnancy and booking platelet count. Onset usually at second or third trimester. The platelet count is mildly reduced. It may be an incidental finding
Preeclampsia/Eclampsia	Increased destruction/consumption	Hypertension, proteinuria, neurological symptoms
HELLP syndrome	Increased destruction	Elevated liver enzymes, and evidence of haemolysis
Acute fatty liver of pregnancy	Increased destruction	Haemolysis, anaemia, prolonged PT, APTT and hypofibrinogenaemia
Non-pregnancy related		
Pseudothrombocytopaenia	Artefact from EDTA	Platelet clumping on peripheral smear
Microangiopathies (TTP, HUS, DIC)	Increased destruction	Neurological symptoms and signs, fever, renal impairment, multiple organs dysfunction, bleeding diathesis, thrombosis
SLE		
Antiphospholipid syndrome	Increased destruction	Recurrent foetal loss/miscarriages, thrombosis
Drug induced	Multifactorial	History of drug ingestion
Viral infections (HIV, HCV, CMV, EBV)	Multifactorial	Viral screening positive
Hypersplenism	Increased pooling	Splenomegaly
ITP	Antibody-mediated destruction Decreased production	Petechiae haemorrhages, ecchymosis, absence of other causes of thrombocytopaenia
Haematological conditions Aplastic anaemia Leukaemia/lymphoma Type 2B VWD	Decreased production from marrow infiltration VWF has increased affinity for platelet Gp1b	Reduction in all the cell lines Lymph nodes enlargement, hepatosplenomegaly, anaemia, blasts in peripheral and marrow smears
Liver disease	Decreased marrow production	Deranged liver function tests, prolonged PT, APTT
Nutritional deficiencies(folic acid, B/12, iron)	Decreased marrow production	Anaemia

Table 32.5 Classification of thrombocytopaenia

Thrombocytopaenia	Platelet count
Mild	100–150 × 10^9/l
Moderate	50–100 × 10^9/l
Severe	<50 × 10^9/l

Table 32.7 International consensus report on platelet thresholds for intervention [27, 28]

Intervention	Platelet count
Antenatal non-invasive procedure anticipated	≥20 × 10^9/l
Dental extraction	≥30 × 10^9/l
Vagina delivery	≥50 × 10^9/l
Caesarean section	≥50 × 10^9/l
Spinal anaesthesia	≥75 × 10^9/l
Epidural anaesthesia	≥75 × 10^9/l

Table 32.8 Treatment options for immune thrombocytopaenia in pregnancy

First-line therapy	Response
Prednisolone	3–15 days
Dexamethasone	2–15 days
High dose methylprednisolone	2–14 days
IVIG	1–3 days
Anti-RhD (Rh + women) – not licensed for this indication in many countries	1–5 days

Indications for treatment include:

- Evidence of bleeding
- Platelet count <20–30 × 10^9/l
- Imminent invasive procedure

Modalities for treatment are the same for ITP outside of pregnancy.

First-line drugs are corticosteroids and intravenous immunoglobulin (IVIG). Prednisolone is given at a dose of 0.5–2 mg /kg /day. Though prednisolone is considered safe to both foetus and mother, during pregnancy, it should be started at a dose of 10–20 mg/day and gradually increased until the lowest dose required to maintain a haemostatically effective platelet count is achieved [28]. Side effects include weight gain, hyperglycaemia, osteoporosis, hypertension and psychosis in the mother.

Intravenous immunoglobulin (IVIG) should be considered in the following situations

- Failure of response to corticosteroid.
- An excessively high dose of corticosteroid required to maintain an adequate platelet count.
- A rapid rise in platelet count is required.
- The platelet count falls below 10 × 10^9/l.
- Imminent delivery or invasive procedure.
- Thrombocytopaenia and bleeding.

Table 32.6 Evaluation of suspected ITP

Full blood count: normal red cells and white cell counts?
Peripheral blood smear
Basic coagulation screening tests (PT, APTT, D-dimers, fibrinogen normal?)
Liver function tests
Viral screen (HIV, HCV)
Antiphospholipid antibodies (LA, ACL, anti B2 glycoprotein)
Antinuclear antibodies (ANA)

HIV human immunodeficiency virus, *HCV* hepatitis C virus, *PT* prothrombin time, *APTT* activated partial thromboplastin time, *LA* lupus anticoagulant, *ACL* anticardiolipin

A single dose of 1 g/kg which shows an increment in platelet count within 24 hours is now being favoured over the traditional dose of 0.4 g/kg for 4 days [26, 27]. Side effects of IVIG include headaches, chills, myalgia, arthralgia and back pain. These are seen in about 5% of patients on IVIG. Serious side effects like acute renal failure and myocardial infarction are rare [28].

32.3.8.1 Splenectomy

Splenectomy is technically difficult in pregnancy, especially in the third trimester. It is indicated when there is failure of first-line drugs. Complications include post-splenectomy infections, increased risk of foetal loss and other risks associated with surgery.

Azathioprine may be used in refractory cases and has been reported to be safe in pregnancy [28]; however, it has a very long onset of therapeutic effect (30–180 days) which limits its use.

Rituximab, an anti-CD 20, and other immunosuppressive drugs are not recommended for use in pregnancy.

32.3.9 Disseminated Intravascular Coagulation (DIC) in Pregnancy

The International Society on Thrombosis and Haemostasis defines DIC as an acquired syndrome characterised by intravascular activation of coagulation leading to widespread fibrin deposition with failure of localisation arising from multiple causes. It can originate from or cause damage to the microvasculature and, if sufficiently severe, may result in organ dysfunction [29]. The ongoing activation of coagulation may result in depletion of platelets and coagulation factors culminating in widespread haemorrhage (consumption coagulopathy). The prevalence in all pregnancies is 0.02–007% [30, 31]. The overall prevalence of DIC is low, but it is an important cause of morbidity and mortality in pregnancy accounting for 6–24% of maternal mortality [31, 32]. The exact prevalence is not known in developing countries. It is expected that it will be higher, given the higher prevalence of

Fig. 32.1 Pathogenesis of DIC. *TNF – tumour necrosis factor alpha, IL-1 – interleukin 1, IL-2 – interleukin 2, TF – tissue factor, TM – thrombomodulin, PC – protein C, APC – activated protein C*

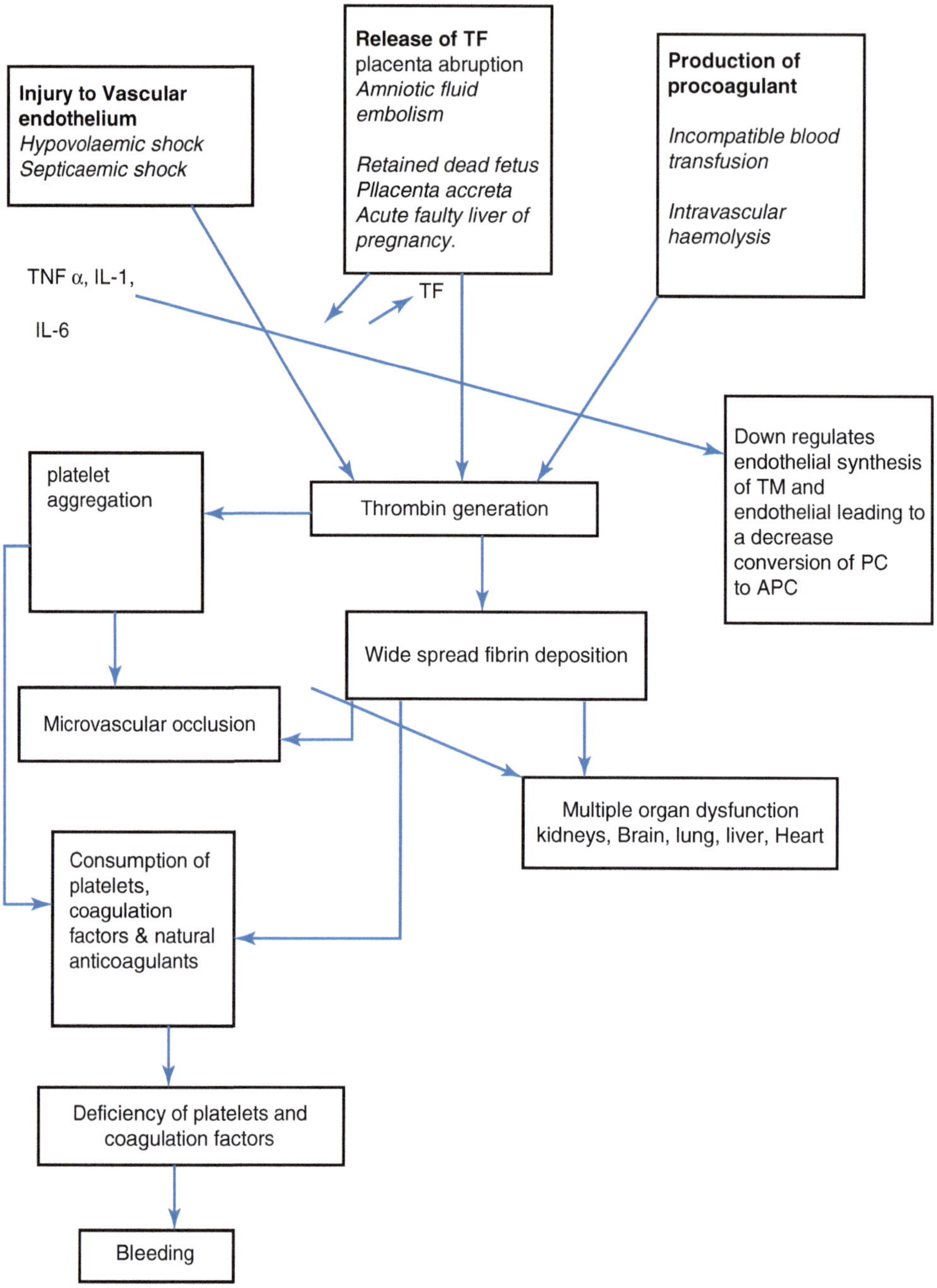

associated conditions like preeclampsia/eclampsia and postpartum haemorrhage. Placenta abruption represents about 37% of the causes of DIC in pregnancy. Others include postpartum haemorrhage 29%, severe preeclampsia/HELLP syndrome 14%, acute fatty liver of pregnancy 8%, sepsis 6% and amniotic fluid embolism 6% [30]. The aetiologies of DIC in pregnancy are diverse and mainly pregnancy related. The causes are listed in Table 32.10. The pathophysiology is triggered by different mechanisms (Fig. 32.1, Tables 32.9 and 32.10).

Pathophysiology of obstetrics DIC is complex. It is triggered by excessive activation of coagulation and downregulation of physiologic anticoagulants and dysregulation of fibrinolysis.

32.3.10 Clinical Features of DIC

DIC in pregnancy presents almost invariably with bleeding and the features of the triggering condition. Typically, there are petechiae haemorrhages, ecchymosis, prolonged bleeding from venepuncture sites, oozing from surgical incision sites, urinary tract, gastrointestinal tract and other systems in about 65% of cases. Other features include altered senso-

Table 32.9 Causes of DIC during pregnancy

Pregnancy related	Non-pregnancy related
Amniotic fluid embolism	Sepsis (Gram-positive and Gram-negative bacteria)
Preeclampsia/ eclampsia	Pancreatitis
	Malaria
Abruptio placentae	Trauma – head injury, crush injury
Placenta praevia	Extensive burns
HELLP syndrome	Malignancy
Septic abortion	Acute promyelocytic leukaemia
Intrauterine foetal death	Solid tumours
	Vascular disorders
Acute fatty liver of pregnancy	Vascular aneurysm
	Giant haemangiomas
	Acute liver failure
	Severe immunological reactions
	ABO incompatibility – acute haemolytic transfusion reactions
	Transplant rejection
	Severe allergic or toxic reactions
	Toxic shock syndrome
	Snake venom
	Spider venom

Table 32.10 Mechanisms of consumptive coagulopathy in pregnancy [23]

- Injury to vascular endothelium/release of tissue factor
  - Preeclampsia
  - Hypovolemic shock
  - Septicaemic shock
  - Abruptio placentae
  - Amniotic fluid embolism
  - Retained dead foetus
  - Placenta accreta
  - Acute fatty liver of pregnancy
- Production of procoagulants
  - Acute haemolytic transfusion reaction
  - Septicaemia
  - Intravascular haemolysis
  - Acute promyelocytic leukaemia in pregnancy

rium, acute renal failure and hypovolemic shock. There may also be thrombotic manifestations but these are not common in pregnancy.

32.3.11 Diagnosis

The diagnosis is based on clinical suspicion which is reinforced by laboratory tests. There is no single test that is specific for the diagnosis of DIC. Pregnancy is characterised by elevation of coagulation factors; furthermore, the platelet count may be reduced in normal pregnancy. The extent to which the normal physiological changes in haemostasis in pregnancy can influence the interpretation of results is not clear.

Coagulation screening tests are often prolonged in DIC; however, DIC is a very dynamic process and laboratory results only reflect the clinical situation at time of sample collection. The PT and APTT are prolonged in 50–69% of cases. Fibrinogen level has been reported to be normal in 57% of DIC cases [33]. In the majority of cases, the laboratory findings are characterised by a falling platelet count, prolonged PT (prothrombin time) and APTT (activated partial thromboplastin time), low fibrinogen level and elevated fibrin degradation products (FDPS). The International Society on Thrombosis and Haemostasis developed a scoring system based on the platelet count, PT, FDPS and fibrinogen level which can be used for the diagnosis of DIC. The scoring system has been reported to have a sensitivity of 97% and a specificity of 91% [34] (Table 32.11).

Table 32.11 Diagnostic scoring system for overt DIC (This algorithm is not recommended if there is no underlying disorder that is associated with DIC) [29]

Global coagulation test	Results	Score 0, 1 or 2 points
Platelet count	$>100 \times 10^9/l$	= 0
	50–100 × 10^9	= 1
	$<50 \times 10^9$	= 2
Elevated fibrin-related makers (soluble fibrin monomers, D-dimers, fibrin degradation products)	No increase	= 0
	Moderate increase	= 1
	Strong increase	= 3
Prolonged prothrombin time (in seconds above upper limit of normal)	<3s	= 0
	3–6s	= 1
	>6s	= 2
Fibrinogen level	>1.0 g/dl	= 0
	<1.0 g/dl	= 1

Total score >5 comparable with overt DIC (repeat score daily)
<5 suggestive for non-overt DIC (repeat scoring 1–2 days)

32.3.12 Treatment of DIC in Pregnancy

DIC is a life-threatening manifestation of a very severe underlying illness.

- The treatment of DIC should be geared towards a prompt identification and treatment of the underlying cause as well as replacement of deficient coagulation factors and platelets.
- Vital signs should be closely monitored.
- A quick assessment of site/s and extent of blood loss should be done.
- Supportive care should include adequate haemodynamic support to maintain tissue perfusion through the use of appropriate blood products. This a main challenge in resource-poor countries. Unavailability of appropriate blood products contributes to the already high morbidity and mortality associated with DI in resource-poor countries.
- The haematologist should be consulted in all cases and availability of blood products discussed.

32.3.12.1 Platelet Transfusion

The platelet count should be actively monitored in all patients with overt DIC, who are actively bleeding or at risk of bleeding, and should be transfused with platelet concentrate. The target should be to achieve a platelet count of >50 × 10^9/l. Where platelet concentrate is not available, platelet rich plasma should be given.

32.3.12.2 Fresh Frozen Plasma (FFP)

FFP contains all the coagulation factors and should be given at a volume of 15–20 ml/kg.

- Cryoprecipitate.

Cryoprecipitate is rich in fibrinogen and is indicated when the fibrinogen level is less than 1.0 g/dl.

- Packed red cells.

Red cells should be given as needed to maintain tissue perfusion.

The PT and the APTT should be maintained as close to the normal range as possible. Systemic anticoagulation is indicated in established thrombosis.

- Antifibrinolytic agent like tranexamic acid are contraindicated because they prevent the removal of fibrin clots.
- The use of anticoagulant in acute DIC with excessive bleeding is controversial.
- Recombinant FVIIa is not licensed for use in pregnancy.

32.3.13 Haematological Management of Obstetric Haemorrhage (OH)

Obstetrics haemorrhage includes antepartum and postpartum haemorrhages. It is defined by the American College of Obstetricians as either a 10% reduction in haematocrit between admission and postpartum or the need for blood transfusion. It has also been defined as any blood loss that can provoke a physiological change threatening a woman's life [35]. It is a leading cause of maternal morbidity and mortality worldwide. The prevalence of obstetrics haemorrhage in Nigeria ranges between 3.1 and 4.28% [36, 37].

The haematology team should be contacted as soon an assessment of moderate to severe obstetric haemorrhage is made or anticipated. A rapid assessment of the estimated blood loss should be made. An accurate assessment is often difficult as visual assessments are often considerably less than the actual blood loss. In clinical assessment, it should be remembered that most pregnant women are generally young and healthy, with good cardiac and respiratory reserve and can withstand losses as much as 1800–2100 ml before hypotension is noticed [38]. Blood loss in excess of 40% of the patient's blood volume (estimated blood volume is about 100 ml/kg body weight at term) is potentially life threatening, and the woman will require urgent blood transfusion [39]. The initial assessment should include, whenever possible, an evaluation of possible haematologic aetiological factors like von Willebrand disease and other inherited coagulation factor deficiencies. Obstetric haemorrhage may be complicated by DIC due to pre-existing activation of the haemostatic system in pregnancy. The team should focus on the need for rapid and appropriate use of blood components. The hospital massive blood transfusion protocol should be activated where available.

Baseline coagulation profile – PT, APTT, fibrinogen level – as well as the full blood count should be carried out at onset of bleeding. The results should be rapidly available for it to be useful. There should be 4-hourly monitoring of tests or more frequently depending on the clinical status of the patient. Subsequent results should be interpreted with reference to baseline values.

The goals of haematological management of massive haemorrhage are to:

- Maintain tissue or organ perfusion and oxygen delivery by restoring blood volume and haemoglobin through rapid provision of red cells
- Maintain haemostasis through the use of additional blood components to correct resultant coagulopathy and thrombocytopaenia

Acidosis and hypothermia increase the risk of DIC, and the patient should be kept warm and blood components should be transfused through a blood warmer wherever possible.

32.3.14 Red Cells

Transfusion of red cells achieves the dual purpose of increasing oxygen delivery to tissues as well as helping to secure haemostasis through the effect on platelet margination and function [40].

- Transfusion with packed red cells should be commenced once the haemoglobin falls below 6–7 g/dl. The target haemoglobin should be 8 g/dl or more.

In case of emergencies, with unbooked patients, where ABO and D blood groups are not known, uncross-matched group O RH negative red cells should be given; however, blood must be collected for full crossmatch prior to transfusion. Full serological crossmatch should be carried out in patients with atypical antibodies; the least incompatible blood red cells should be transfused. A major challenge in resource-poor countries is the inadequacy of blood components supply. All at-risk women should be properly counselled on the inherent danger of OH and the need to get at least 2 units of blood either through voluntary donation or family replacement, stored prior to delivery. This approach will reduce the perennial shortage of blood in most obstetric units in these countries.

32.3.15 Fresh Frozen Plasma (FFP)

FFP contains all the coagulation factors except FVIII which depreciates to about 60% of normal values [35]. The use of crystalloids as plasma volume expanders will further dilute the coagulation factors in a woman that is bleeding severely. While it is generally believed that the use of FFP should be guided by laboratory results, in reality, there is an urgent need for coagulation factors replacement, and therefore, FFP can be given empirically based on clinical judgement or suspicion of a coagulopathy.

FFP is indicated when the PT or APTT is greater than 1.5 times the control plasma or mean normal range. It is given at a volume of 12–15 ml/kg; a unit of FFP is about 200–250 ml. There is no widely accepted ratio of red cells to FFP transfusion; however, a general guide of 4 units of FFP to 6 units of red cells can be used (red cell: FFP – 1.5:1) [35].

32.3.16 Cryoprecipitate

Cryoprecipitate is rich in fibrinogen, von Willebrand factor and FVIII. In massive obstetrics haemorrhage, fibrinogen may be depleted especially when an estimated blood volume or more has been replaced. Fibrinogen level rises as part of the normal haemostatic response in pregnancy [1], up to 5–7 g/dl at term. In OH, the fibrinogen level is low due to rapid consumption of fibrinogen as large volume of clots is formed, which implies that by the time fibrinogen level is within the normal range of 1.5–4 g/dl, a lot of fibrinogen would have been consumed [35]. The deficiency should be corrected with cryoprecipitate if the level is <2 g/dl. The recommended adult dose is one unit/5-10Kg body weight; this raises the plasma fibrinogen level by about 1 g/dl [40]. Ten bags of cryoprecipitate will raise the plasma fibrinogen level by approximately 1 g/dl.

FFP and cryoprecipitate should be transfused within 4 hours once released from the blood bank.

32.3.17 Platelets

Thrombocytopaenia in OH may result from the predisposing aetiology, haemodilution from resuscitating measures or from a superimposed coagulopathy.

The need for platelet transfusion should be anticipated early and the haematologist informed. This is very important in resource-poor countries where platelets concentrates are not routinely stocked. The target should be to keep the platelets count >75 × 10^9/l. Platelets should be RH compatible with the donor; in emergencies, RH positive platelets can be given to an RH negative woman if RH compatible platelets are not available, but 250 IU of anti-D should be administered in addition to routine prophylaxis [39].

32.3.18 Recombinant Factor VIIa (RVIIa)

RVIIa is not licensed for use in massive obstetrics haemorrhage, but it may be considered in women who refuse blood transfusion. It is available in Nigeria through the Haemophilia Foundation of Nigeria (HFN).

There is a risk of thrombosis associated with its use. This should be weighed against the potential benefits.

32.3.19 Tranexamic Acid

Tranexamic acid, which have previously been associated with reduction in mortality in trauma patients, has recently been found in the World Maternal Antifibrinolytic (WOMAN) trial to reduce death due to bleeding by 31% in women with primary postpartum haemorrhage when given within 3 hours of onset of haemorrhage [41].

32.3.20 Monitoring

Regular full blood count and coagulation profile should be done to guide management, with the goal of maintaining the haemoglobin concentration at >8 g/dl, platelet count >50 × 10^9/l and the PT and APTT less than 1.5 times the mean control levels, while fibrinogen level is kept above 1 g/dl. If bleeding persists in the absence of any identifiable cause, inherited bleeding disorders should be considered and investigated as discussed earlier in this chapter.

32.3.21 Evaluation Post Haemorrhage

Bleeding is accompanied by the release of acute phase proteins which can predispose to venous thromboembolism. Transfusion is also a risk factor for thrombosis. Therefore, once haemorrhage has been adequately controlled and coagulation tests are normal, women should be risk assessed and thromboprophylaxis commenced if there are additional risk factors. Iron tablets should be given to replenish the stores if there are no contraindications to oral iron.

References

1. Pomp ER, Lesenlelink AM, Rosendaal FR, Doggen CJ. Pregnancy postpartum period and prothrombotic defects:risk of venous thrombosis in the MEGA study. J Thromb Haemost. 2008;6(4):632–7.
2. Brenner B. Haemostatic changes in pregnancy. Thromb Res. 2004;114:409–14.
3. Rodeghiero F, Castaman G, Dini E. Epidemiological investigation of the prevalence of von Willebrand disease. Blood. 1987;69:454–9.
4. James AH, Jamison MG. Bleeding events and other complications during pregnancy and child birth in women with von Willebrand disease. J Throm Haemost. 2007;5:1165–9.
5. James AH. More than menorrhagia: a review of the obstetric and gynaecological manifestations of bleeding disorders. Haemophilia. 2005;11:295–307.
6. Kadir RA, Lee CA, Sabn CA, Pollard D, Economides DL. Pregnancy in women with von Willebrand disease or factor XI deficiency. Br J Obstet Gynaecol. 1998;105(3):314–21.
7. Dahlman T, Hellgren M, Blomback M. Changes in blood coagulation and fibrinolysis in the normal puerperium. Gynecol Obstet Investig. 1985;20:37–44.
8. Sadler JE. Biochemistry and genetics of von Willebrand factor. Annu Rev Biochem. 1998;67:395–424.
9. Giangrande PL. Management of pregnancy in carriers of haemophilia. Haemophila. 1998;4:779–84.
10. Chi C, Kadir RA. Management of women with inherited bleeding disorders in pregnancy. Obstet Gynaecol. 2007;9:27–33.
11. Pavord S. Inherited disorders of primary haemostasis. In: Pavord S, Hunt B, editors. The obstetric haematology manual. Cambridge: Cambridge University Press; 2010. p. 176–85.
12. Pavord S. Inherited coagulopathies. In: Pavord S, Hunt B, editors. The obstetric haematology manual. Cambridge: Cambridge University Press; 2010. p. 186–93.
13. Trigg DE, Stergiotou I, Peitsidis P, Kadir RA. A systematic review: the use of desmopressin for treatment and prophylaxis of bleeding disorders in pregnancy. Haemophilia. 2012;18(1):25–33.
14. Kujovich JL. Von Willebrand disease and pregnancy. J Thromb Haemost. 2005;3:246–53.
15. Roque H, Funai E, Lockwood CJ. Von Willebrand disease and pregnancy. J Maternal Fetal Med. 2000;9:257–66.
16. Lee CA, Chi C, Pavord S, Bolton-Maggs PHB, Pollard D, Hinchcliffe-Wood A, Kadir RA. The obstetric and gynaecological management of women with inherited bleeding disorders-review with guidelines produced by a task force of UK Haemophilia Centre Doctors Organisation. Haemophilia. 2006;12(4):301–36.
17. Tarantino MD, Gupta SL, Brusky RM. The incidence and outcome of intracranial haemorrhage n newborns with haemophilia: analysis of the Nationwide inpatient sample database. Haemophilia. 2007;13(4):380–2.
18. Esien EM, Usanga EA, Ayeni O. The Normal platelet count and platelet factor 3 availability in some Nigerian Population Groups. Eur J Haematol. 1973;10(5):378–83.
19. Mcrae KR. Thrombocytopaenia in pregnancy; differential diagnosis, pathogenesis and management. Blood Rev. 2003;17(1):7–14.
20. Ajibola SO, Akinbami A, Rabiu K, Adewumi A, Dosunmu A, Adewumi A, Osikomaiya B, Ismail K. Gestational thrombocytopaenia in pregnant women in Lagos, Nigeria. Niger Med J. 2014;55:139–43.
21. Mcrae KR, Samuels P, Schreiber AD. Pregnancy associated thrombocytopaenia: pathogenesis and management. Blood. 1992;80:2697–714.
22. Shehata N, Burrows RF, Kelton JG. Gestational thrombocytopaenia. Clin Obstet Gynecol. 1999;42:327–34.
23. Granchev RV, Ludlam CA. Acquired an congenital haemostatic disorders in pregnancy and the puerperium. In: B-Lynch C, Keith LG, Lalonde AB, Karoshi M, editors. A textbook of postpartum haemorrhage. Duncow UK: Sapiens; 2006. p. 209–32.
24. Sainio S, Kekomaki R, Riikonen S, Teramo K. Maternal thrombocytopaenia at term: a population based study. Acta Obstet Gynaecol Scand. 2000;79:744–9.
25. RodeghieroF, Stasi R, Gernsheimer T, Michael M, Provan D, Arnold D, BrusselJ, Cines D, Chong B, Cooper N, Godeau B, Lechner K, Mazzucconi MG, McMillan R, Sanz M, Imbach P, Blanchette V, Kuhne T, Ruggeri M, George GN. Standadisation of terminology, definitions, and outcome criteria in immune thrombocytopaenic purpura of adults and children: report from an international working group. Blood. 2009;113:2386–93.
26. Tsiara S, Nelson-Piercy C, Cooper N. Thrombocytopaenia in pregnancy:Gestational thrombocytopaenia and Immune thrombocytopaenic purpura. In: Cohen H, O'Brien P, editors. Disorders of thrombosis and hemostasis in pregnancy: a guide to management. 2nd ed. London: Springer; 2015. p. 261–77.
27. Kumar R. ITP in adults :management including recent advances. In: Sudhir M, editor. Monograph on platelet disorders. Japur: Bharat Lamination; 2015. p. 87.
28. Provan D, Stasi R, Newland AC, Blanchette VS, Bolton-Maggs P, Bussel JB, et al. International consensus report on the investigation and management of primary thrombocytopenia. Blood. 2010;115:168–86.
29. Taylor FB, Toh CH, Hoots WK, Wada H, Levi M. Towards definition, clinical and laboratory criteria and scoring system for disseminated intravascular coagulation. J Thromb Hemost. 2001;85(5):1327–30.
30. Liang BL, Hong DH. Diagnosis and management of obstetric acute disseminated intravascular coagulation. Zhonghua Fu Chan Ke Za Zhi. 1992;27(3):147–9. 188
31. Rattray DD, O'Connell CM, Baskett TF. Acute disseminated intravascular coagulation in obstetrics: a tertiary centre population review (1980 to 2009). J Obstet Gynaecol Can. 2012;34(4):341–7.
32. Kor-anantakul O, Lekhakula A. Overt disseminated intravascular coagulation in obstetric patients. J Med Assoc Thail. 2007;90(5):857–64.
33. Spero JA, Lewis JH, Hasiba U. Disseminated intravascular coagulation: findings in 246 patients. J Throm Hamost. 1980;43(1):28–33.
34. Bakhtiari K, Meijers JC, Levi M. Prospective validation of the international society on thrombosis and haemoastasis scoring system for disseminated intravascular coagulation. Crit Care Med. 2004;32(12):2416–21.
35. Lefkou E, Hunt B. Management of obstetrics haemorrhage: hemostatic management. In: Pavord S, Hunt B, editors. The Obstetric Haematology Manual. Cambridge: Cambridge University Press; 2010. p. 166–9.
36. Green KI, Ojule JD, Mmon CF. Primary post partum Haemorrhage at the University of Port Harcourt Teaching Hospital: prevalence and risk factors. Nigerian Health J. 2015;15(3):111–7.
37. Fakoya TA, Oloyede OA, Alayo AM. Review of primary postpartum haemorrhage in Sagamu, Nigeria. Nigerian Med Pract. 2007;52(30):51–4.
38. Francois KE, Foley MR. Antepartum and postpartum haemorrhage. In: Gabbes S, Niebyl J, Simpson J, editors. Obstetrics: normal and problem pregnancies. 5th ed. Philadelphia: Churchill Livingstone; 2007. p. 456–85.
39. Royal College of Obstetricians and Gynaecologists. Prevention and management of postpartum haemorrhage, Green-top guideline, vol. vol. 52. London: RCOG Press; 2009.
40. Ponnampalam S, Wilson S, Khalil A. Acquired bleeding disorders in pregnancy: obstetric haemorrhage. In: Cohen H, O'Brien P, editors. Disorders of thrombosis and hemostasis in pregnancy: a guide to management. 2nd ed. London: Springer; 2015. p. 237–59.
41. The lancet (editorial) 2017; 389(100840) available at www.thelancet.com.

Haematological Disorders in Pregnancy

33

Mathew Ebose Enosolease

Learning Objectives

At the end of this chapter, the reader is expected to be able to:

- Define anaemia in the context of pregnancy.
- Know the causes of anaemia in pregnancy, and in particular have a general overview of the common causes.
- Should be able to take adequate history and examine the pregnant woman especially at booking.
- Investigate and conduct relevant anaemia work-up in pregnancy in relation to the aetiologies.
- Institute simple antenatal micronutrient supplements such as iron and folic acid with a view to preventing maternal and foetal complications of some micronutrients' deficiency.
- Appreciate certain types of anaemia syndromes that may complicate pregnancy such as HELLP (haemolysis, elevated liver enzymes and low platelets).
- Understand the concept of multidisciplinary approach to the management of anaemia in pregnancy.

33.1 Introduction

Haemopoietic tissues adapt most profoundly to tissue/organ changes in pregnancy. Indeed, people usually noticed that the skin of the pregnant individual is fairer within the second month of pregnancy owing to haemodilution which increases disproportionately relative to expansion of the red cell mass. Haematological adaptation to pregnancy takes several forms. In particular, the metabolism of various micronutrients, vitamins, and haemostatic proteins are significantly altered to accommodate the physiological changes that take place in pregnancy. Unfortunately, some of these changes also account for various complications such as haemostatic disequilibrium resulting in thrombohaemorrhagic and thromboembolic disorders. Aside from these changes, either a number of disorders develop or previously occult ones become overt. The common ones are iron and folate deficiencies and less common are either acquired or inherited disorders of red blood cells. The haemoglobinopathies, particularly sickle cell diseases, deserve special consideration and will be discussed later (Table 33.1).

Below are some commonly requested haematologic baseline tests in pregnancy.

1. Full Blood Count (FBC)
   - Haematocrit (packed cell volume, PCV)
   - Red cell indices: Mean corpuscular volume (MCV), mean corpuscular haemoglobin (MCH), mean corpus-

Table 33.1 Some haematological disorders in pregnancy

Anaemia:	
(a) Acquired	Iron deficiency, folate, cobalamin (B12)
(b) Inherited	Haemoglobinopathies: Sickle cell disease, thalassaemia, red cell enzymopathies such as glucose-6-phosphate dehydrogenase deficiency (G6PD), pyruvate kinase deficiency (PK), red cell membrane cytoskeletal abnormalities (hereditary spherocytosis (HS)), etc.
White blood cells count and differentials	Upper reference limit in pregnancy may be as high as 16×10^9/L and up to 25×10^9/L at immediate postpartum
Platelets	Thrombocytopaenia: Immune thrombocytopaenia, thrombotic thrombocytopaenic purpura (TTP), haemolytic uraemic syndrome (HUS), haemolysis, elevated liver enzymes and low platelets (HELLP) syndrome
Transfusion	Red cells alloimmunisation: Haemolytic disease of newborn (HDN)
Haemostatic abnormalities	Thromboembolic and thrombohaemorrhagic disorders

M. E. Enosolease (✉)
Department of Haematology, University of Benin, Benin City, Nigeria

University of Benin Teaching Hospital, Benin City, Nigeria
e-mail: mathew.enosolease@uniben.edu

F. Okonofua et al. (eds.), *Contemporary Obstetrics and Gynecology for Developing Countries*,
https://doi.org/10.1007/978-3-030-75385-6_33

cular haemoglobin concentration (MCHC) and red cells count, reticulocytes count
- White blood cells count per microlitre (WBC/μl) and differentials (reported in percentage)
- Platelets count per microlitre (Plt/μl)
2. Haemoglobin electrophoresis/high-performance liquid chromatography (HPLC) where available.
3. Blood grouping usually ABO and Rhesus.
4. Haemostatic profile including prothrombin time, thrombin time, activated partial thromboplastin time and fibrinogen are only requested if indicated. Others such as protein S, protein C, antithrombin activity are rarely requested. Increased FDP (fibrinogen degradation products) and D-dimers are consequences of increased fibrinolysis (Table 33.2).

33.1.1 Anaemia in Pregnancy

This is a reduced ability of haemoglobin to deliver adequate O_2 for tissue oxygenation and may be quantitatively defined as haemoglobin (Hb) concentration less than 11 g/dl (WHO), 10.5 g (CDC), but 10 g/dl is accepted in developing countries [1, 2]. The blood picture of physiologic anaemia of pregnancy is normocytic and normochromic. Anaemia may be mild 8–11 g/dl, moderate 6–8 g/dl and severe <6 g/dl [3]. The major causes include iron and folate deficiencies and both will be briefly discussed.

33.1.2 Iron Deficiency

Iron-deficient state: The iron store is low or completely empty with transferrin fallen below 15%, increasing iron-deficient erythropoiesis, increasing red cell protoporphyrin; but red cell indices are still within reference values. Haematocrit is normal and overt symptoms/signs of anaemia are absent.

Iron deficiency anaemia. Refers to the full-blown iron deficiency state with visible decrease in red cell indices, microcytosis, hypochromia, target cells together with symptom and signs of anaemia.

33.1.3 Epidemiology

Iron deficiency anaemia is the most common cause of anaemia worldwide and is responsible for over 65% of anaemia in pregnancy in some settings. It is responsible for about 9%, 14% and 37% for first, second and third trimester cause of anaemia, respectively, in moderate- to high-income countries [4, 5]. By contrast, the prevalence ranges from 16% to 55% from first to third trimester in low-income countries including Nigeria [6–8].

33.1.4 Aetiology

1. Dietary deficiency is by far the most common cause of iron deficiency. The major source of iron is protein: meat, liver, fish dairy products in preference to plant sources whose iron is less bioavailable. For economic, cultural and religious reasons, women in poor countries may not have enough iron store before pregnancy.
2. Adolescent pregnancy. These are growing girls who would usually have poor reserve of iron.
3. Poor child spacing. Frequent pregnancies deplete iron stores. The foetus is a very effective parasite for maternal micronutrients. It is known that neonates and infants born to micronutrient-deficient mothers have normal haemoglobin levels, serum iron, serum ferritin, serum transferrin saturation, folate and B12 in both termed and preterm babies, though preterm levels are rapidly depleted because they have low but appropriate nutrient levels for their gestational age. This is because micronutrients transfer, particularly iron, occurs in the last 4 weeks of pregnancy. However, many studies have shown evidence of preterm delivery, low birth weight and increased perinatal mortality in newborn of women with iron deficiency anaemia.

33.1.5 Absorption and Iron Homeostasis

Daily iron intake is 30 mg of which only 5–10% may be absorbed but pregnancy can up this to 15–30% [5, 9]. This is because the relative hypoxia seems to downregulate hepcidin

Table 33.2 Some reference ranges in pregnancy

Haematology parameter	Non-pregnant age matched	First trimester	Second trimester	Third trimester	References
Haemoglobin g/dl	12–15.8	11–13.9	9.5–15	9.5–15	1,2
PCV (Hct)%	35.4–44.4	31–41	30–39	28–40	1,2
WBC × 10^3/ul	3.5–9.1	5.7–13.6	5.6–14.8	5.9–16.9	3
Neutrophil (%)	NS	54.15 ± 9.21	47.95 ± 17.92	55.31 ± 11.97	1,3,4
Eosinophil (%)	NS	10.51 ± 5.18	9.71 ± 3.08	10.87 ± 4.88	1,3,4
Monocytes (%)	NS	1.8 ± 0.65	0.84 ± 0.42	1.36 ± 0.74	1,3,4
Lymphocytes (%)	NS	33.07 ± 6.41	40.52 ± 1932	32.68 ± 12.51	1,3,4
Platelet × 10^3/ul	165–415	174–391	155–409	146–429	1,3,4
Serum iron ug/dl	41–141	72–143	44–178	30–193	1

(NS not significant)

secretion. Iron is maximally absorbed in the duodenum and upper jejunum.

Certain factors such as reducing agents – vitamin C – will enhance absorption while increasing pH, phytates, tannin in tea, antacids all will decrease absorption.

Iron status is dependent on the degree of absorption which is determined by a number of proteins, namely tissue ferritin and transferrin receptors. The level of these proteins are themselves regulated by certain proteins such as DMT-1 (di-metal iron transporter 1), IRP (iron responsive protein) and IRE (iron-responsive element). The amount of iron eventually absorbed, stored, transferred to macrophages (stored iron) or released to developing erythropoietic tissues is controlled by the level of hepcidin, a 25-amino acid polypeptide synthesised in the liver. Hepcidin is the major hormone controlling iron absorption and regulation. Low body iron or hypoxia downregulates hepcidin, and hence the activities of DMT-1 at the enterocytes brush border and hypoxia-inducible factor (HIF-2) at apical enterocytes and ferroportin at basal enterocytes. Ferroportin controls the entry of iron into portal vein where it is bound to transferrin for utilisation and storage [5].

33.1.5.1 Iron Balance

Total iron store in women of child bearing age is 5 mg/kg, average total is ~300 mg but a minimum of 500 mg in store is necessary for adequate iron supply in pregnancy [4, 5, 9].

Daily losses ~1.35 mg/day.

Daily requirement is 2 mg, 4 mg and 6 mg in first, second and third trimester, respectively.

Lactation: 0.5–1 mg/day.

All the above lead to iron depletion

33.1.6 Requirement in Pregnancy and Delivery [5, 9]

Increase in red cell mass	450 mg
Foetus and placenta	300 mg
Blood loss at delivery	240 mg
Basal maternal requirement	250 mg

Average requirement for normal singleton foetus up to delivery is approximately 1240 mg.

33.1.7 Clinical Features

Iron deficiency without anaemia has no obvious features; however, unexplained irritability, poor mentation, easy fatigue and poor exercise tolerance may be seen. Patients with IDA may complain of features of anaemia: tiredness, reduced exercise tolerance, shortness of breath and headache. Others include pica (unusual craving for non-food items especially clay) is common in pregnancy, dysphagia in association with koilonychias (spoon shaped nails in severe chronic IDA) and angular cheilosis (Paterson-Kelly syndrome) may occur. Pallor and signs of cardiovascular challenges may be seen. Signs of anaemic heart failure occur in severe anaemia [4–8, 10].

33.1.8 Laboratory Features

1. Full blood count (FBC), also known as complete blood count (CBC):

   Haematocrit is decreased, white cells count (WBC) may be normal, increased or slightly decreased, platelet count is usually raised. Red cells indices are low. MCV is less than 75 fentolitre. Normal MCV does not preclude IDA as it is raised by up to 4 fentolitre (fl) in normal pregnancy, and again folate deficiency commonly coexists with iron deficiency. MCH is less than 27 picogram (pg). Reduction mirrors severity. MCHC is reduced.
2. Blood picture shows microcytosis, hypochromia, anisopoikilocytosis and numerous platelets.
3. Bone marrow cytology shows micronormoblasts with ragged cytoplasmic outline. Perl stain (iron stain) demonstrates negative iron. Siderocyte is absent.
4. Serum iron low, less than 15 μg/dl.
5. Serum transferrin receptor (TFR) is raised.
6. Serum transferrin saturation is reduced.
7. Serum hepcidin is raised.
8. Red cell protoporphyrin is raised.

33.1.9 Management

Oral iron is very effective provided compliance is adequate. Ferrous sulphate is cheap, available and popular in Nigeria. Others are ferrous fumarate or gluconate all which are effective. PO ferrous sulphate 200 mg three times daily (elemental iron = 60 mg). Untoward effects are usually GIT irritations, nausea, vomiting, diarrhoea and constipation. Simply change from one to the other.

Enteric coated iron preparations, though more physically appealing, are costly for nothing as they are poorly absorbed. This is because their free iron ions are not available at duodenum and jejunum.

Parenteral iron: Iron dextran (imferon) and iron sorbitol are available intramuscular/intravenous injections. Iron may be given intramuscularly at 50 or 100 mg daily, but I prefer 250 mg deep intramuscular injection weekly. Patients appear to be happier, but local skin irritations are not infrequent.

Test dose as below must be given. Total iron dose (1–2 g) as infusion dextrose water over 6-hour period may be given with caution. Each dose must be preceded by test (10%), observe for 60 minutes before continuing. Facilities for cardiopulmonary resuscitation must be available because parenteral iron could precipitate anaphylaxis.

It is only given in severe IDA and only necessary if diagnosed late in pregnancy when rapid replenishment is desired. Patient is not compliant to oral iron or there is gastric intolerance or malabsorption such as Crohn's disease. Otherwise, no special advantage is gained over oral iron.

33.1.10 Folate, B12 and Megaloblastic Anaemia

Folate is the second commonest cause of anaemia in pregnancy. Though commoner in the poorer countries, it is by no means confined to these regions as it is a consequence of poor eating habits. Folate and B12 deficiencies are the common causes of megaloblastic anaemia.

33.1.11 Epidemiology

Prevalence in countries where most foods are fortified with folic acid is only about 5%. Deficiency is a reflection of poverty, poor cooking and eating habit. Folates are abundant in vegetables and animal sources but are heat labile and hence easily destroyed by cooking.

Daily requirement (non-pregnant women) is 100–150 μg while intake in average good diet is 200–250 μg. Daily requirement in pregnancy is 400 μg. Excessive utilisation increases the catabolism of folate coenzymes in rapidly proliferating tissues, and placenta transfer cannot be provided by normal diet alone [5, 9, 11]. Therefore, folic acid supplement is advocated.

Cobalamin deficiency is less common and may be due to antibodies against intrinsic factor, IF, (pernicious anaemia) (Table 33.3).

About 800 μg of folate would have been transferred at term and a further 100 μg daily during puerperium and 25 μg daily throughout breastfeeding.

33.1.12 Absorption

Folates are polyglutamates in foods and must be reduced to monoglutamates for absorption in the duodenum/jejunum, circulate in plasma as methyl-THF and enters cells as such where it must be re-polyglutaminated. Cobalamin is absorbed in the distal ileum and in the cell and serves as co-factor enabling folate to act as a single carbon transfer such as the conversion of homocysteine to methionine liberating THF (active folate) important in DNA synthesis.

Table 33.3 Some characteristics of folates and B12

Characteristics	Folates (μg)	B12 (μg)
Dietary intake	200–250 μg	3–7 μg
Daily utilisation	100–150 μg	1–2 μg
Daily foetal requirement	400 μg (including mother)	50 μg
Total body stores	10–12 mg	2–4 mg
Time to depletion (non-pregnant)	3–4 months	2–4 years
Sources	Vegetables, animal sources	Animal sources especially liver
Cooking	Heat labile	No effect
Site of maximum absorption	Duodenum/jejunum	Distal ileum
Daily supplementation	Necessary, folic acid 5 mg	Not necessary
Therapeutic form	Folic acid	Hydroxocobalamin
Metabolic importance	Co-enzyme	Co-factor
Deficiency	Megaloblastic anaemia, neural tube defect	Megaloblastic anaemia, neuropathies, psychosis

33.1.13 Pathogenesis

Both vitamins are required for rapidly proliferating cells, synthesising DNA which include haemopoietic cells, all epithelial surfaces such as the mouth, stomach, gastrointestinal enterocytes and genito-urinary-tracts. The gonads and foetus are severely affected by their deficiencies. Deficiency causes inhibition of thymidylate monophosphate which is a rate limiting step in the synthesis of DNA [5].

33.1.14 Clinical Features

The patient may be asymptomatic. Symptoms and signs of anaemia are insidious in onset. Jaundice – peculiarly described as lemon-yellow tint due to ineffective erythropoiesis – may be seen. Other features include epithelial abnormalities manifesting as angular glossitis, red beefy tongue and malabsorption of other nutrients which may lead to weight loss.

Purpuric spots due to thrombocytopaenia (megaloblastic is a cause of pancytopaenia); infection, particularly urinary tracts; reversible melanin hyperpigmentation (mechanism is unknown) may occur.

Neural tube defects-anencephaly, meningomyelocele, encephalocele and spina bifida (deficiency in first 12 weeks of conception especially in the first 4 weeks). The incidence of harelips and cleft palate is also reduced with folate prophylaxis.

Prophylactic folate has been associated with reduced incidence of childhood acute lymphoblastic leukaemia in the offspring of these mothers.

Neuropathies, combined degeneration of the spinal cord (posterior and pyramidal tracts), dementia visual impairment and sometimes psychosis (B12).

33.1.15 Diagnosis

1. FBC: HCT/PCV is low, MCV high >95 fl. White blood cells and platelet counts may be normal or reduced.
2. Peripheral blood film: Macrocytosis, anisopoikilocytosis, hyper-segmented neutrophils.
3. Reticulocyte count is low (for the degree of anaemia).
4. Red cell and serum folate both are low (high if megaloblastic anaemia is due to B12 deficiency).
5. Bone marrow cytology (gold standard for diagnosis) shows hyper-cellularity with numerous dying cells (ineffective erythropoiesis), megaloblasts, giant metamyelocytes. Bone marrow stainable iron is increased.

   Please note that a concomitant presence of iron deficiency could blunts all the above except HCT
6. B12 assay blood, methyl malonyl CoA in urine or blood (B12 deficiency).
7. Schilling's test is no longer popular and not suitable in pregnancy because of radiation.

33.1.16 Treatment

Oral PO folic acid 5 mg three times daily in severe anaemia, particularly near term, continue post-delivery and all through lactation.

Intramuscular hydroxocobalamin (if due to B12) 1000 μg twice or thrice weekly (6 or 7 doses), then 1000 μg two monthly throughout life in proven B12 malabsorption.

Iron must be given simultaneously.

33.1.17 Prevention

Folate supplementation must be given in pregnancy regardless of good foods. Ideally supplementation should commence at least 3 months before planned conception. This will significantly reduce neutral tube defects and reduces anaemia in pregnancy. Infertility may also be prevented. Folates also prevent or reduce foetal prematurity and recurrent abortion.

33.1.18 Haemoglobinopathies

This is a group of genetically inherited disorders characterised by defective haemoglobin synthesis. This defect may be qualitative or structural in nature, and the most studied and best known being sickle cell disease (structural) or quantitative abnormality resulting in globin chains imbalance called the thalassaemia. Until modern medicine, mortality was uniformly high, but a good number now survive into adulthood even in developing countries, and many are capable of raising their own families. Haemoglobinopathies remain the most extensively studied single gene disorders. Occurrence used to be largely restricted to the tropics, subtropics and the Mediterranean populations but modern travels and trans-Atlantic trades have redistributed the conditions and is now seen in most parts of the world.

33.1.19 Antenatal/Neonatal Screening

All women at booking should be screened for abnormal haemoglobin. This is extremely important especially in countries where abnormal haemoglobin/variants are common. In Nigeria, for instance, haemoglobin phenotype distribution at birth is typically: Hb AA 75%; Hb AS 20–25%; Hb SS 2%; Hb SC <0.5%. Hb SC is common in central West Africa such as Ghana [12]. Others such as Hb Sβ^0 or HBSβ^+ are also seen. The women who have Hb AS phenotype should have their partners checked for haemoglobin variants using haemoglobin electrophoresis, and where available HPLC to quantify haemoglobin types. This will form the basis for genetic counselling and the need for prenatal diagnosis to determine foetal haemoglobin genotype and so well-informed and preferred parents' decision for possible intervention.

33.1.20 Sickle Cell Disease and Pregnancy

Sickle diseases are a group of structural genetic abnormality of haemoglobin with varying severity. Sickle cell anaemia (SCA, Hb SS) is the commonest and most severe. Others are Hb SC, Hb SD-Punjab, Hb SD-Arab, Hb SE, etc.

SCA is characterised by variable acute presentations such as vaso-occlusive crisis (VOC), hyperhaemolytic crisis (HHP), sequestration crisis and aplastic crisis or more correctly erythroid aplasia. Other acute problems include acute chest syndrome (ACS) and stroke. A number of chronic presentations are actually complications of the disease, and virtually all organs be may be affected including the gonads [10, 12–14].

33.1.21 Pathogenesis and Pathology of Pregnant Sickle Cell Anaemia (SCA) Clients

Background The lifespan of red cells in SCD patients is markedly reduced to only few weeks, and it is further reduced if there are inflammatory processes. This means that these red cells are constantly being destroyed (usually extravascularly) due to prolonged sickling which progressively damage membrane of these cells. Such damaged cells will leak out potassium ions and water resulting in cellular dehydration and change in shape and becomes less deformable. These cells are rapidly destroyed. In an attempt to compensate for the excessive haemolysis, the bone marrow becomes hyperplastic, and expansion of diploe and extramedullary haemopoiesis may occur. There is hyperbilirubinaemia and gallstone formation from excessive haemolysis.

SCA is a hyper-coagulable state, and pregnancy is also a known hypercoagulable state. The effect of these conditions would be unarguable additive. These women would theoretically be expected to suffer more of the presentations above particularly vaso-occlusive crisis.

Vaso-occlusive crisis is the commonest acute presentation in pregnancy. Susceptibility to vaso-occlusive crisis (VOC) depends on several factors. These include environmental factors such as extremes of temperature, infections or infestation such as malaria, fever and dehydration, hypoxia and some intrinsic factor such as haemoglobin concentration, co-inheritance with abnormal haemoglobin (haemoglobin SC, haemoglobin SD), concomitant thalassaemia, level of foetal haemoglobin (HbF) and 2,3 DPG, which will all modify the occurrence and severity of vaso-occlusive crisis. When red cells are deoxygenated, haemoglobin molecules easily aggregate to form polymers which alters the shape of red cells and become less deformable. This is sickling. This tendency increases in microvasculature where these cells can become permanently sickled and occlude micro-circulation. Hypoxic environment is created with the release of several pain and pro-inflammatory cytokines. The reduced rheology enhances platelets-endothelial and granulocytes-endothelial interactions, depletion of nitric oxides, more sickling, tissue hypoxia, infarction and necrosis. All these could result in excruciating pain in any parts of the body though bones pains are more frequent. Hypercoagulability which is enhanced in pregnancy is a critical factor which contribute immensely to this pathology. It must be stated, however, that the mechanism of VOC is still evolving.

33.1.22 Maternal and Foetal Outcome

Most obstetricians regard pregnant HbSS as high risk. Other types of sickle cell disease such as HbSC have better obstetric history. Prenatal, antenatal postpartum care must be vigorous and individualised.

Complications and various crises, particularly VOC, are more frequent and often severe. VOC is reported to be as common as 50% in some places, whereas Nana O Wilson et al. reported only 8% in Ghana though this was a retrospective study. It is more frequent in labour, and it is thought to precipitate in early labour rather than the reverse [13–15].

Acute chest syndrome pulmonary embolism and pulmonary hypertension are not uncommon. Pre-eclampsia, eclampsia, premature delivery, premature rupture of membrane and premature labour are common. Others include intra-uterine growth retardation, increased rate of spontaneous abortion, stillbirth and neonatal death. There is also high caesarean section rate largely owing to failed induction of labour.

Other common effects of sickle disease in pregnancy include: pregnancy-induced hypertension and pre-eclampsia, renal diseases such as urinary tract infections, haematuria and hyposthenuria [14].

Maternal mortality is >9% in Nigeria and Ghana. But report from Republic of Benin indicated better obstetrics performance in these patients most likely because of special SCD maternal care and neonatal screening programme. This report is nearly comparable to mortality of 1–2% in the UK and the USA.

33.1.23 Management of Sickle Cell Disease in Pregnancy

The management of these patients should be multidisciplinary in approach and should involve the obstetrician who is familiar with sickle cell disease, the haematologist, the anaesthetist as well as specially trained nurses in haematology, genetic counsellors and clinical psychologists.

Pre-Conception Counselling and Screening Premarital counselling is of utmost importance. Intending couples having known their haemoglobin phenotypes (or genotype) should be informed of the options available to them should they marry and desire to have children. Opportunities for prenatal diagnosis and abortion if it is culturally and religiously acceptable to them should be discussed.

They must have folic acid supplement with or without pregnancy.

Daily hydroxyurea: Hydroxyurea is reputed to significantly ameliorate the course of the disease by a number of mechanisms: the induction of foetal haemoglobin (HbF), cyto-reduction of granulocytes and platelets and hence reduced neutrophil-endothelial as well as platelet-endothelial interactions, and increased nitric oxide thereby dilating vessels. However, this drug should be stopped at least 3 months to planned conception because of the remote possibility and yet unproven teratogenicity.

At Booking These women together with their families must be advised on all possibilities such as increased risk of crises, including acute chest syndrome, the need for blood transfusion-top or exchange, pregnancy-induced hypertension, pre-eclampsia/eclampsia, prompt presentation and treatment of infections, the effect on baby such as intrauterine growth retardation, prematurity and intrauterine death. Involve other specialists – haematologist and anaesthetist – early and throughout pregnancy, labour and puerperium [9, 13, 14].

Review all medications, stop hydroxycarbamide in the first trimester and introduce antimalarial and penicillin prophylactics. Folic acid supplementation is compulsory, and iron supplementation may also be necessary if serum iron is low. Encourage round the clock hydration. Water and or various orange/apple juices are good hydration agents. Encourage early presentation for all conditions and develop a low threshold for hospitalisation.

Screening for possible pathogens particularly hepatitis B, HCV, HIV etc. should carried out.

Blood groups: ABO, Rhesus, others (and antibody titre if necessary) must be done. Determine that there are no unusual antibodies that might complicate transfusion when it becomes necessary.

Full blood counts: Monitor the haematocrit, leucocyte (granulocytes count) and platelet count regularly and emphasise more frequent and regular antenatal visits.

Throughout Antenatal Period Continue folic acid supplementation and consider dose increase to 5 mg three times daily if blood firm is macrocytic. Other prophylaxis should be continued.

FBC must be done on every visit, and foetus should be closely monitored with pelvic ultrasonography to determine foetal wellbeing. Antenatal visits must be more regular as per protocol of local hospital where it exists.

Hospitalisation should be considered if:

- Pain: any pain not resolving with 2–4 hours on good analgesia
- Suspicion of infection whether pulmonary, upper respiratory infection or urinary tract infection
- Suspicion of any complications
- Patients who are vomiting or unable to tolerate orally
- Vaso-occlusive crisis or acute chest syndrome suspected

Once VOC is diagnosed, she must be admitted and hydrated with hypotonic solution, usually 5% dextrose water or D/S, potent analgesic (IV paracetamol) and when not adequate opioid should be given. Nonsteroidal analgesic should be avoided particularly near term. Check electrolytes, urea creatinine as well as liver functions. Treat the precipitating cause and maintain strict input and output chart to monitor fluids.

33.1.24 Acute Chest Syndrome (ACS)

ACS is characterised by hypoxia, tachycardia, chest pain, fever >38.5 °C, leucocytosis and pulmonary infiltrates. Though can arise de novo, it usually accompanies vaso-occlusive events, microembolisation of bone marrow fat or infection from chlamydia, mycoplasma, *Legionella* and *Haemophilus influenza* in children.

Hypoxia from ACS may lead wild spread sickling and vaso-occlusion leading to several multi-infarcts in the pulmonary bed with some degree of multi-organ failure. Some patients will have elements of bronchospasm. Thorough clinical examination, especially auscultation and basic investigation such as chest radiograph, FBC, E&U and blood culture should be done.

Treatment must be aggressive with oxygen, analgesia and potent broad-spectrum antibiotics. Bronchodilators are useful in some patients. Blood transfusion, whether top-up or exchange transfusion, may be necessary to reduce sickling process. In women who have had one episode of ACS, exchange transfusion or regular top-ups could prevent recurrence.

33.1.24.1 Labour

Mode of delivery must be planned ahead of time. Women with normal pelvis should be allowed to go into spontaneous labour. Every stage of labour must be managed actively. Oxygen monitoring-pulse oximeter, oxygen saturation must be monitored by anaesthetist. Oxygen should be given when necessary. Check FBC, E&U. All other specialists including the neonatologist must be available. Transfuse only when it is necessary. Labour should not exceed 12 hours, but caesarean section should be avoided whenever possible.

Regional (epidural) analgesia/anaesthesia is favoured to have less likelihood of painful crisis or ACS. At delivery, assess blood loss and need for transfusion.

Postpartum Mother should be well hydrated and as comfortable as possible. Regular monitoring of vital signs 4-hourly in the first 24 hours of delivery, daily monitoring of FBC and E&U. The neonatologist will examine and monitor the baby.

Early ambulation to prevent VTE is encouraged. The use of prophylactic low-molecular-weight heparin and graduated compression stocking may be helpful.

Breastfeeding should be allowed, but mother must be well hydrated.

Mother should regularly attend postnatal visits.

33.2 Thalassaemia

Reduced synthesis of the affected globin chains results in decreased haemoglobinisation of the affected erythroid cells and an excess of the non-affected chains which continue to be synthesised normally. The normally synthesised chains then accumulate in red cells and become harmful for the cell. This group is known under the general term "thalassemia." There are two major types: α and β, which are sub-classified according to the degree of globin chain deficiency. While α-thalassaemia is mainly due to gene deletion, β-thalassaemia is due to point mutation. Common notation is as in Table 33.4.

Beta-thalassaemia major is the most severe and will be briefly discussed. The alpha gene is duplicated. Complete deletion of all four genes (--/--) is rare and not compatible with life (hydrop fetalis). Alpha-thalassaemia is usually asymptomatic except HbH (--/-α) which, under extreme conditions such as pregnancy, may require blood transfusion.

Homozygous beta-thalassaemia major (β^0/β^0) is transfusion dependent from birth. Many are now able to live normal lives as long as they continue to have adequate blood transfusion with good iron chelation and endocrine monitoring with hormonal replacement where necessary. Some have had bone marrow/stem cells transplant and are free from the disease.

It is characterised by excessive accumulation of other haemoglobin chains mainly α which precipitate in the red cells since they cannot form viable haemoglobin tetramers. Such globin precipitations result in death of red cell precursors (ineffective erythropoiesis) and cause extramedullary erythropoiesis, hence the typical thalassaemia facie in poorly treated patients. Excess accumulation of iron in tissues, particularly heart muscles and endocrine glands can result in permanent damage. T2*MRI may be used to quantify cardiac iron and assess cardiac damage. Thyroid functions, gonadal hormones, blood glucose may be used to assess some endocrine functions.

Pregnancy is now possible in some who had good transfusion management. These women must be closely monitored for sickle disease, and in addition, bisphosphonate, iron chelators should be stopped prior to and during pregnancy [16].

Folic acid 5 mg daily and vitamin D and calcium should continue. No Vitamin C supplement.

Expected problems include cardiac abnormalities including heart failure and high rate of caesarean section.

Table 33.4 Haemoglobin chain variants: the thalassaemias

Alpha-thalassaemia		Beta-thalassaemia	
Normal	αα/αα	Normal	β/β
Silent carrier	-α/αα	Minor	β/β^0, β/β^+
Minor	-α/-α, --/αα	Intermedia	β^+/β^+, β^0/β^+
Hb H disease	--/-α	Major	β^0/β^0
Barts hydrops fetalis	--/--		

33.3 Other Causes of Anaemia in Pregnancy

33.3.1 Immune and Non-immune Haemolytic Anaemia

Immune cytopaenias are common during the second and third decades of life and coexist or predate pregnancy. Pregnancy could influence the course of immune cytopaenias such that there might be remission, relapse or new presentations. The pathogenesis is further complicated by hormonal changes in pregnancy and consequently immune modulation.

Common immune cytopaenias include autoimmune haemolytic anaemia (AIHA), immune thrombocytopaenic purpura (ITP) and autoimmune neutropenia. They are characterised by immune autoimmune antibodies against own red cells, platelets and neutrophils. Severe cytopaenia occurs only when the bone marrow is unable to compensate for the excessive and prematurely destroyed cells. Management is difficult if treatment is needed because there is no universally efficacious regimen. It depends on individual obstetrician/haematologist's clinical experience. Investigate as non-pregnant individuals who should include FBC including peripheral blood film, reticulocytes count, Coomb's tests especially direct antiglobulin test (DAT), identification of the offending antibody IgG, complements and serum haptoglobin. Haemoglobinuria and haemosiderinuria will signify intravascular haemolysis.

Steroid is the mainstay and this must be delicately balanced in pregnancy. Blood transfusion may be necessary in poorly compensated ones, particularly near term. Maternal immune antibody (IgG) may cross the placenta and cause foetal and neonatal haemolytic, and this might take 4–6 months before it disappears from the infant's blood stream.

33.3.2 Foetomaternal Alloimmunisation Syndromes

These are conditions where previously immunised mothers produce antibody or antibodies which can cross the foetomaternal barrier to cause destructions of cells in the foetus. Foetal and neonatal alloimmune thrombocytopaenia and haemolytic disease of foetus/newborn are the well-known ones.

33.3.3 Haemolytic Disease of Foetus/Newborn

HDFN is characterised by rapid haemolysis of foetal/neonatal red blood cells due to maternal red antibodies. The mother would have been previously immunised by red cell antigen(s) which are not present in her own red cells. This means that the mother must be incompatible with the foetus and she is usually Rhesus negative. Sometime ABO antigens which are paternally derived but absent in the mother may generate immune antibodies. In any normal pregnancy, there is foetal red cells trafficking into the maternal circulation which becomes apparent in the second trimester and is maximum at delivery. Thus, it is unlikely in first pregnancy.

33.3.3.1 Aetiopathogenesis

Several foetal red cells antigens (not present in the mothers) would stimulate allo-antibody in the mothers. These are immune antibodies (IgG) small enough to cross the placenta and attach to foetal and neonatal red cells resulting in rapid destructions of foetal or neonatal cells.

Several red cell antigens may stimulate immune antibodies, but Rhesus D negative is the most immunogenic. Rhesus c is second only to the absence of Rhesus D: The mother is *Rhesus D negative* and the foetus Rhesus D positive. If there was previous sensitisation, new leakage of foetal blood cells generates anamnestic reactions producing IgG1 and IgG3 in several folds of maternal antibody against previously encountered Rhesus positive red cells [11, 17]. This will continue more vigorously as pregnancy is advancing. This is now clearly visible by second trimester. The antibodies cross the placenta, bind to foetal cells, chop off their membrane and eventually haemolysed them in the reticuloendothelial system of foetus. The excess bilirubin produced is filtered by the placenta into maternal circulation and metabolised in the maternal liver. The foetal bone marrow initially tries to compensate for the excessive haemolysis, but it is soon overwhelmed; hence, extramedullary haemopoietic assistance becomes increasing important. Thus, signs of severe anaemia and anaemic heart failure characterised by extramedullary hyperactivities – hepatomegaly, splenomegaly, portal hypertension, placentomegaly and oedema – of all tissues/organs may be seen depending on the level of attempted compensation. Some foetuses will die utero of anaemic heart failure – cardiomegaly, skin oedema, pleural and pericardial effusion, ascites, polyhydramnios all features of erythroblastosis fetalis [11, 17]. Simple uterine scan can show even early development of these features and hence early intervention such as intra-uterine blood transfusions. Most children are born with mild to moderate anaemia, little or no jaundice, but the jaundice usually becomes overwhelming soon after birth and urgent measures must be taking to forestall brain damage from unconjugated hyperbilirubinaemia.

If mother and baby are ABO incompatible, there is a very high chance that the foetal red cells leaked into the mother would have undergone quick haemolysis long before they are able to initiate any immune sensitisation.

Anti-K causes mainly erythropoietic arrest of red cells precursors and haemolysis if present is negligible. Other blood group antigens such as Duffy and Kidd can also generate HDFN.

The ABO red cell antigens can cause mild to moderate HDFN. The mother in this case must be blood group O and foetus could be blood group A, B or AB. Unlike HDFN due to Rhesus-D negative, it can occur in the first pregnancy but much less severe because ABO antigens are not well developed in foetus and are found in other issues. Thus, they are easily diluted out thereby reducing the potency.

33.3.4 Management

Booking: All pregnant women must reconfirm their ABO and Rhesus blood group. If they are Rhesus negative, further history of previous pregnancies and foetal outcome must be obtained. Their husband must be ABO and Rhesus grouped even if she is re-married.

Determine antibody titre at booking. Anti-D and anti-C can now be determined accurately with flow cytometry while others still depend on old method of serial dilution. Serial dilution is available in some remote villages.

Expectant mother must be sampled for antibody titre every 4 weeks till 28 weeks, then 2 weekly till delivery and should be interpreted as in Table 33.5 [11, 17, 18].

Doppler flow velocity at middle cerebral artery (MCA) greater than 1.5 normal velocity can also be used to determine the severity of the anaemia and, thus, the need for intervention.

33.3.5 Prevention

Prophylactic anti-D has been in use for decades and has greatly reduced the risk of HDFN, and appropriate dose of anti-D has lowered the mortality from 46 to 1.6 per 100,000 births in the UK.

Anti-D should be given immediately after delivery or after procedure exceeding 12 weeks of gestation or within 72 hours. Coverage might still be possible if given within 10 days.

Dose: Estimate the approximate foetomaternal transfusion/leak using Kleihauer test (old and tedious) or flow cytometry where available. 125 IU (25 μg) is expected to counteract 1 ml of foetal blood, and about 4 ml is the

Table 33.5 Antibody titres and severity

Antibody	Mild	Moderate	Severe
Anti-D	<4 IU	4–15 IU	>15 IU
Anti-C	<7.5 IU	7–20 IU	>20 IU
Anti-K (even low titre)	Severe anaemia	Severe anaemia	Severe anaemia

average but could be much more in assisted delivery. Most centres will give 500 IU (100 µg) after delivery. Some obstetrician may give as high as 1500 IU though no real advantage is conferred [17, 18].

33.3.6 HELLP Syndrome

There is a subset of pre-eclampsia/eclampsia who develop haemolytic anaemia from microangiopathy, thrombocytopaenia and derangement of coagulation with well-recognised clinical features and established laboratory components called HELLP: *h*aemolysis, *e*levated *l*iver enzymes, *l*ow *p*latelets. HELLP occurs in about 20% of pre-eclampsia and 10% of eclampsia. The target organ is mainly the liver and occurs 2–3 times more in the second or third trimester. Platelet count is low, prothrombin time (PT) and activated partial thromboplastin time (APPT) and fibrinogen levels are normal. C-reactive protein could be normal, raised or decreased in the presence of elevated liver enzymes. ADAMTS 13 is decreased (if raised would suggest TTP) [19, 20]

33.3.7 Other Haematological Abnormalities

Other causes of maternal anaemia include pregnancy-induced haemolytic anaemia, intestinal helminths such as hookworm infestation, helminths associated haematuria (Schistosomiasis: S. haematobium) are not uncommon in poor rural settings.

Coagulation and haemostatic dysfunctions including thromboembolic conditions are discussed elsewhere in this book. Rarely, haematological malignancies may be seen in pregnancy or even predates it. The management options are challenging. Reproductive issues are daunting from infertility to depression and distress in the ever-increasing number of cancer survivors in the reproductive age group [21]. For those who are able to get pregnant, a conservative approach would mean consideration to terminate all pregnancies before 20 weeks and if beyond this period then modified regimen might be appropriate during therapy. At all times, however, the decision taken by expectant mother, family and medical team must be in the best interest of the pregnant woman.

33.4 Summary

This chapter introduced haemopoietic tissues and their necessary adaptations to the physiological changes in pregnancy. It also defined anaemia in the context of pregnancy, provided reference values to guide the reader in the diagnosis and discussed the different causes of anaemia in pregnancy. It introduced the reader to the basic mechanisms of the common causes of anaemia in pregnancy. It emphasised the role of good and adequate history taking including family history as well as basic haematologic investigations such as blood groupings and haemoglobin phenotyping at booking. It provided a systematic management plan for some haematologic conditions from booking and beyond. The role for multidisciplinary approach to ensure events-free pregnancy is also advocated.

References

1. Milman N, Bergholt T, Byg KE, Eriksen L, Hvas AM. Reference intervals for haematological variables during normal pregnancy and postpartum in 434 healthy Danish women. Eur J Haematol. 2007;79(1):39–46.
2. Viteri FE. The consequences of iron deficiency and anaemia in pregnancy on maternal health, the foetus and the infant. SCN News. 1994;(11):14–8. PMID: 12288229. (Pubmed).
3. Awodu OA, Enosolease ME, Ubaru AG, Famodu AA. Leucocytes counts in pregnant women with sickle cell trait. Afr J Reprod Health. 2002;3(6):112–6.
4. Fernando EV. The consequences of iron deficiency and anaemia in pregnancy on maternal health, the Foetus and the Infant. Assessed at http://www.unsystem.org/SCN/archives/scnnews 11/ch07.htm.
5. Hoffbrand AV, Moss PAH. Hypochromic anaemia; megaloblastic and macrocytic anaemia. In: Hoffbrand's essential haematology. 7th ed. United Kingdom: Wiley Blackwell; 2016. 20–40 and 48–59.
6. Agbola A. Anaemia in pregnancy. In: A textbook of obstetrics and gynaecology for medical students. Ibadan: Heinemann Publishers Ltd. p. 376.
7. Olubukola A, Odunayo A, Adsina O. Anaemia in pregnancy at two levels of healthcare in Ibadan, south West Nigeria. Ann Afr Med. 2011;10(4):272–7.
8. Olujimi AO, Abasiattai AM, Bassey EA, James RS, Ibanga G, Morgan A. Prevalence of anaemia among pregnant women at booking in the University of Uyo Teaching Hospital, Uyo, Nigeria. BioMed Res Inter. 2014. https://doi.org/10.1155/2014/849080. Assessed May 2016.
9. Strong J. Haematinics deficiency. In: Pasvord S, Hunt B, editors. The obstetric haematology manual. Cambridge Medicine. p. 13–27.
10. Osungbade KO, Oladunjoye AO. Preventive treatment of iron deficiency anaemia: a review of their effectiveness and implication for health system strengthening. J Pregnancy. 2012;2012:454601. https://doi.org/10.1155/2012/454601. Assessed May, 2016.
11. Lyll H, Myers B. Maternal autoimmune cytopenias. In: Pasvord S, Hunt B, editors. The obstetric haematology manual. Cambridge Medicine. p. 45–58.
12. Adu EM, Isibor CN, Ezie E. Prevalence of haemoglobin variants among Ika ethnic nationality of Delta state. Int J Med Res. 2014;3(2):6.
13. Rahimy MC, Gango A, Adjou R, Deguenon C, Gousanou S, Alihonou E. Effect of active prenatal management on pregnancy outcome in sickle cell disease in an African setting. Blood. 2000;96(95):1685–9.
14. Wilson NO, Cessay FK, Hibbert JM, Driss A, Obed SA, Adjei AA, Gyasi RK, Adeerson WA, Stiles JK. Pregnancy outcomes among patients with sickle cell disease at Korle-Bu Teaching Hospital Accra, Ghana: Reproductive Cohort Study. Am J Trop Med Hyg. 2012;86(6):936–42.

15. Enosolease ME, Awodu OA, Ejele AO. The influence of Fetal haemoglobin in sickle cell anaemia patients. AJMR. 2002;9(5):112–5.
16. Jensen CE, Tuck SM, Wonke B. Fertility in β-Thalassaemia major: a report of 16 pregnancies, preconception evaluationand review of the literature. Br J Obstet Gynaecol. 1995;102:625–9.
17. Allard S, Conteras M. Clinical blood transfusion. In: Hoffbrand AV, Higgs DR, Keeling BM, Mehta AB, editors. Postgraduate haematology. 7th ed. Wiley Blackwell. p. 214–45.
18. Delaney M, Matthews DG. Hemolytic disease of the foetus and newborn: managing the mother, foetus and newborn. In: Haematology 2015, American Society of Haematology Educational program, 57th ASH annual meeting and exposition. Orlando Florida December 5-8; 2015. p. 146–51.
19. Cunningham FG, Lindheimer MD. Hypertension in preganacy. N Engl J med. 1992;326:927–32.
20. Lattuada A, Rossi E, Calarosa C, et al. Mild to moderate reduction of a von Willebrand factor cleaving protease (ADAMSTS-13) in pregnant women with HELLP microangiopathic syndrome. Haematologica. 2003;88:1029–34.
21. Loren AW. Fertility issues in patients with haematologic malignancies. In: Haematology 2015, American Society of Haematology Educational program, 57th ASH annual meeting and exposition. Orlando Florida December 5-8; 2015. p. 138–45.

Mental Health Disorders in Pregnancy and Puerperium

34

Victor N. Chilaka and Francis Githae Muriithi

Learning Objectives

By the end of the chapter, the reader should be able to:

- Recognise the significance of mental health disorders in pregnancy and puerperium and appreciate its significant contribution to maternal mortality.
- Should be able to appreciate the signs and symptoms of mental health disorders in pregnancy and puerperium, make a diagnosis, initiate management and provide safety for the patients even in poorly resourced health services.
- Should understand the diagnostic criteria and an idea of the standard scales used for screening depression and their limitations.
- Should be able initiate simple management and counselling for the affected patient.
- Critically evaluate the different options available for the management of these patients and be able to refer appropriately for further management in difficult conditions.
- Should understand the importance of follow-up, involving the family and mental health professionals in this highly recurrent condition.

34.1 Introduction

Mental health conditions arising before, during or after pregnancy are important causes of indirect maternal morbidity and mortality mainly, in South Asia and sub-Saharan Africa [29]. The World Health Organization estimates the worldwide prevalence of mental health disorders at 10% during pregnancy and at 13% in the puerperium with even higher rates in the developing countries at 15.9% and 19.8% for antenatal and postpartum periods, respectively [12]. It has been claimed in the past that postnatal depression is uncommon in Nigeria and other developing countries because of the enormous community support during and after childbirth. However, objective studies do not seem to support this claim. Using Edinburgh Postnatal Depression Scale (EPDS) objectively on postpartum Nigerian women showed that the incidence of postpartum depression in them was 27.2% which did not differ much in developed countries [10].

Mental health problems contribute to indirect maternal deaths. In the United Kingdom, the maternal mortality rate continues to fall largely as a result of a reduction in deaths from "direct" pregnancy causes. The indirect causes such as maternal mental health problems have not reduced significantly. The confidential enquiry into maternal deaths published in the 2015 Mothers and Babies: Reducing Risk through Audits and Confidential Enquiries across the UK, MBRRACE-UK, report covering the period 2009–2013, published that "One in eleven of the women who died during or up to six weeks after pregnancy died from mental health-related causes. However, almost a quarter of all maternal deaths between six weeks and a year after birth are related to mental health problems, and one in seven of the women who died in this period died by suicide. Although severe maternal mental illness is uncommon, it can develop very quickly in women after birth; the woman, her family and mainstream mental health services may not recognise this or move fast enough to take action" [19]. Substance abuse and complex social situations were significant contributors to mental health problems.

V. N. Chilaka (✉)
Women's Wellness and Research Centre, Hamad Medical Corporation, Doha, Qatar

F. G. Muriithi
East Midlands North Deanery, Queen's Medical Centre, Nottingham University Hospitals NHS Foundation Trust, Nottingham, UK

F. Okonofua et al. (eds.), *Contemporary Obstetrics and Gynecology for Developing Countries*,
https://doi.org/10.1007/978-3-030-75385-6_34

Mental health as an indirect cause of maternal mortality has largely been unexplored in Africa as it is overshadowed by direct obstetric causes such as haemorrhage, infection, toxaemias of pregnancy, abortion complications and obstructed labour, as well as indirect causes such as anaemia, malaria and HIV [29].

Africa's cultural heterogeneity, varied cultural and societal ideologies, may have a negative impact on all aspects of mental health: care-seeking behaviour, treatment of sufferers by the society and health professionals, as well as receiving minimal attention in health budgetary allocation and health policy formulation. It is often thought that people suffer from mental health problems as a result of sorcery, witchcraft and ancestral spirits [1].

Most women who suffer from mental health problems do so in the reproductive years with the initial episode in pregnancy or the puerperium. The effects of mental health disorders in pregnancy and puerperium may be subtle or severe to the extent of suicide and affecting the children's growth and development. The majority of conditions are treatable [33]. Mental health is a huge determinant of not only pregnancy but general health as well [16].

Depression, anxiety, post-traumatic stress disorder and puerperal psychosis are the most prevalent at estimated incidence rates of 18.3%, 14%, 5.9% and 0.1%, respectively [26, 27].

The children of women affected by mental health disorders may experience developmental and psychological disturbances [28].

34.1.1 Depression

34.1.1.1 Incidence/Prevalence

Major depression is the commonest psychiatric disorder in reproductive age women. Incidence in pregnancy ranges from 7% in the first trimester to 13% and 12% in the second and third trimesters, respectively. Worldwide postpartum incidence is estimated at 13% [30].

Figure 2 shows an estimated prevalence of depression in low and middle-income countries [13].

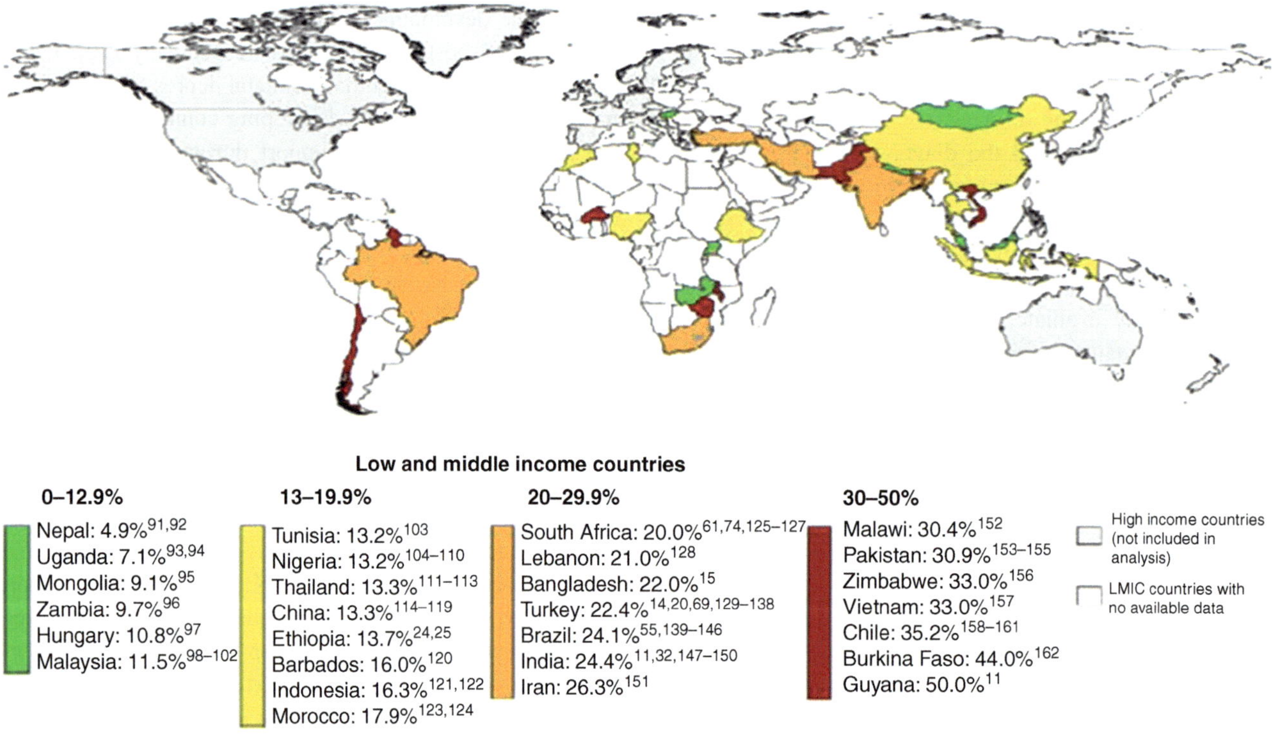

34.1.1.2 Clinical Presentation [15]

DSM-5[1]	ICD-10
Major Depression: At least five symptoms present for at least 2 weeks, for most of nearly every day **A symptom must be:** • Depressed mood • Markedly diminished interest or pleasure in all or most activities (anhedonia) **Other Symptoms:** • Substantial weight loss when not dieting or weight gain, or increase or decrease in appetite • Insomnia or hypersomnia • Psychomotor agitation or retardation • Fatigue or loss of energy • Feelings of worthlessness or excessive or inappropriate guilt • Diminished ability to think or concentrate or indecisiveness • Recurrent thoughts of death or suicidal ideation (with or without a specific plan) Symptoms cause clinically significant distress or impairment in social, occupational, or other important areas of functionality Symptoms not due to direct physiological effects of a substance or another medical condition The occurrence of a major depressive episode is not better explained by schizoaffective disorder or other psychotic disorders and there has never been a manic or hypomanic episode **Depressive episode with insufficient symptoms*** Depressed affect and at least one other of the above symptoms associated with clinically significant distress or impairment persisting for at least 2 weeks **With peripartum onset†** Onset of mood symptoms happens during pregnancy or in the 4 weeks after delivery Onset of mood symptoms happens during pregnancy or in the four weeks after delivery.	**Severe depression.** At least seven symptoms, usually present for at least 2 weeks, experienced with severe intensity for most of every day All three key symptomsassociated should be present: • Persistent sadness or low mood • Loss of interests or pleasure • Fatigue or low energy At least four associated symptoms should be present: • Disturbed sleep • Poor concentration or indecisiveness • Low self-confidence • Poor or increased appetite • Suicidal thoughts or acts • Agitation or slowing of movements • Guilt or self-blame • Individual unable to continue with social, work or domestic activities, except to a very restricted extent **Moderate depression** At least two key symptoms and three associated symptoms should be present **Minor depression** At least two key symptoms and two associated symptoms should be present, with no symptoms present to an intense degree **With postpartum onset** Disorder commencing within 6 weeks of delivery ICD=international classification of diseases (published by WHO2). DSM=diagnostic and statistical manual of mental disorders. *Changed from minor depression in DSM-4 (two to four depressive symptoms experienced for at least 2 weeks, one symptom should be depressed mood or loss of pleasure). †Changed from with postpartum onset in DSM-4 (on-set of mood symptoms within first 4 weeks after delivery).

34.1.1.3 Investigations

There are no specific investigations for depression. However, it is good clinical practice to rule out medical problems that may present with similar symptoms. This includes anaemia and thyroid disorders.

34.1.1.4 Diagnosis

Diagnosis is aided by active screening at any contact before, during or after pregnancy as most women may not actively seek treatment for depression. This is especially so in Africa, where there may be stigma associated with mental illness.

It is advisable to target women who may have known risk factors for depression for screening. These risk factors include past personal or family history of mental health illness, marital conflict, domestic violence, the very young, limited social support, illicit drug use, lower socio-economic status, lower educational status and history of crime.

There are a variety of screening tools available. The Centre for Epidemiological Study Depression Scale (CES-D) is used extensively and has recently been used in pregnant populations [23]. The Edinburgh Postnatal Depression Scale (EPDS) is validated for the screening of depression in the postpartum period [6, 20]. It is important to ensure that these scales are validated for adoption into your specific patient population.

The scales are meant for screening, not diagnosis. It is advisable to involve a trained mental health worker in the assessment and subsequent management of pregnant patients with mental health disorders.

Routine antenatal universal psychosocial assessment is so far not supported by evidence [3].

34.1.1.5 Management

Multidisciplinary care is recommended. This may include the midwife, obstetrician, mental health nurse, psychologist, psychiatrist and social worker. In limited resource settings, there is a role for the provision of mental health services through non-specialists in a task-shifting or task-sharing model [5]. This is to bridge the gap created by a lack of mental health specialists in these areas.

Management depends on the severity of depression and is a shared decision between the woman and the primary care giver.

Mild depression may benefit from psychotherapy as a first line. Medical management with antidepressants is indicated when psychotherapy is unsuccessful, moderate to severe depression or when the patient has functional impairment. The choice of medical therapy is either selective serotonin reuptake inhibitors (SSRI) or serotonin and norepinephrine reuptake inhibitors (SNRI). Tricyclic antidepressants have a higher fatal toxicity index and are less preferred than selective agents. Electroconvulsive therapy may be advised by a psychiatrist in extreme cases.

Evidence in support of non-pharmacological management, such as depression-specific acupuncture, maternal massage, bright light therapy and omega-3 fatty acids for the treatment of antenatal depression, is inconclusive [7].

34.1.1.6 Follow Up

Most depression will resolve within 1–6 months post-delivery. Follow up with a mental health specialist is advised.

34.1.1.7 Prevention

There is little research and no known way of preventing depression in the antenatal period [15]. However, psychosocial and psychological interventions significantly reduce the rates of postpartum depression. Promising interventions include the provision of intensive, professionally-based postpartum home visits, telephone-based peer support and interpersonal psychotherapy [8].

34.1.1.8 Special Considerations in Limited-Resource Settings

Mothers in limited-resource settings already face a heavy burden of everyday living. Maternal depression affects not only maternal wellbeing but also the psychological and physical development of the children [22]. Effects of maternal depression lead to negative bio-psychosocial consequences introducing inequality right from childhood [31].

The SSRI sertraline may be an appropriate first line for breastfeeding mothers. Most of the other antidepressants are secreted in breast milk and may have effects on the neonate.

Comorbidities such as HIV may co-exist with pregnancy and worsen depression in limited-resource settings.

The World Health Organization encourages the use of community health workers to integrate maternal psychosocial wellbeing with child development using a five-pillar approach: family support, empathic listening, guided discovery using pictures, behavioural activation and problem solving [32].

34.1.2 Anxiety

34.1.2.1 Incidence/Prevalence

Anxiety disorders are commonly overlooked and may coexist with depression. The estimated prevalence of anxiety disorders in pregnancy in Africa is 14% [26].

The spectrum of anxiety disorders may include generalised anxiety disorder, obsessive-compulsive disorder (OCD) and post-traumatic stress disorder (PTSD) phobias, including tocophobia.

Pregnancy and puerperium may worsen an existing disorder or trigger the onset of a new one. Generalised anxiety disorder and obsessive-compulsive disorder are more common postnatally than in the general population [25].

34.1.3 Clinical Presentation

Specific diagnostic criteria are listed in the Diagnostic and Statistical Manual of Mental Disorders: Fifth Edition [2, 4].

34.1.3.1 Further References [14, 21]

Clinical presentations for the specific disorders are summarised below:

(a) *Generalised anxiety disorder* This disorder is characterised by anxiety that is generalised and persistent. Women complain of the physical symptoms of nervousness, trembling, muscular tensions, sweating, light-headedness, palpitations, dizziness and epigastric discomfort. Women often express fears that the woman, baby or a relative will have a negative experience.
(b) *Post-traumatic stress disorder (PTSD)* Women with PTSD experience flashbacks arising from previous negative experiences and may be expressed as dreams or nightmares, avoidance and distress.
(c) *Obsessive-compulsive disorder (OCD)* Women with this disorder may have intrusive thoughts, images or ideas that the patient finds distressing but difficult to resist. These are distinguishable from psychotic delusions and are identified as irrational, with the woman retaining insight. They may perform rituals or acts as an avoidance strategy. An example may include the fear of contamination with repeated handwashing or the fear of outsiders seeing the pregnancy as it may lead to a bad omen. Coping may include seeking reassurance from others which in its most severe form, continual reassurance and OCD, can be extremely disabling.
(d) *Tocophobia* This disorder is characterised by a morbid fear of pregnancy and the birthing process. Some women with this phobia will avoid pregnancy and childbirth altogether. This fear may happen in women who have never been pregnant before or in women following a previous traumatic pregnancy or delivery. Some women may be able to overcome spontaneously while others cannot cope, leading to a termination of the pregnancy or avoidance of a vaginal delivery over a caesarean section.

34.1.3.2 Investigations/Diagnosis

A high index of suspicion and correlation of current symptoms to past obstetric history may aid in diagnosis. A mental health professional might assist in narrowing down the diagnosis following existing diagnostic aid tools such as DSM V or ICD 10.

It is essential to rule out medical conditions such as anaemia, thyroid problems or cardiac conditions that may present in a similar manner by performing the relevant clinical examination and laboratory tests.

34.1.3.3 Management
Mild anxiety may be treated by aided self-help interventions; moderate and severe forms may require psychotherapy or pharmacological treatment with SSRIs, SNRI or TCAs or a combination of both. Women with tocophobia may benefit from a review with their care provider to explore the triggers and come up with a shared care plan, as well as building trust with the team that shall eventually deliver her.

34.1.3.4 Follow-Up
Immediate debrief and a review via a birth experience clinic following an adverse event may be helpful towards the prevention of an anxiety disorder in a future pregnancy.

34.1.3.5 Prevention
Cognitive behavioural therapy, childbirth education and antenatal self-guided intervention workbook with weekly telephone guidance may prevent antenatal anxiety [15].

Evidence for other mind-body interventions such as yoga or hypnotherapy is not strong [18].

34.1.4 Psychotic Disorders

Psychotic disorders include bipolar disorder, schizophrenia, schizoaffective disorder, psychotic depression and postpartum psychosis [17].

34.1.4.1 Incidence/Prevalence
Bipolar disorder affects approximately 1% of women with, 25–50% of them suffering postpartum psychosis. Postpartum psychosis affects 1–2/1000 births in the general population [17].

34.1.4.2 Clinical Presentation
The symptoms of psychotic disorders are outlined in the DSM V and the ICD 10.

Common symptoms of common psychotic disorders are summarised below.

- *Bipolar disorder:* It may be characterised by either mania or hypomania. Mania is an abnormally and persistently elevated or irritable mood for greater than a week with associated functional impairment. It may be associated with inflated self-esteem, grandiosity, reduced need for sleep with daytime fatigue or lowered energy, talkativeness, flight of ideas, increased goal-directed activities, disinhibition, increased pleasurable activities with high potential for painful consequences. Hypomania is characterised by similar symptoms but is of shorter duration and with less functional impairment.
- *Schizophrenia:* This disorder is characterised by hallucinations and delusions. It may also be associated with disorganised speech, catatonia, lack of motivation, self-neglect, inability to experience pleasure, low attention span, inability to show facial expressions and inability to start or complete tasks.
- *Schizoaffective disorder* is a variant of schizophrenia, while *psychotic depression* is depression with delusions and hallucinations.
- *Postpartum psychosis* is a psychiatric emergency with symptoms of depression, severe confusion, loss of inhibition, paranoia, delusion and hallucinations with a sudden onset usually in the first 2 weeks after childbirth. The most severe symptoms tend to last from 2 to 12 weeks, and recovery takes 6–12 months. It is associated with an increased suicide and infanticide rate. It is potent contributor to maternal deaths.

About half of women who suffer from postpartum psychosis have no risk factors; but women who have a prior history of mental illness, especially bipolar disorder, obsessive-compulsive disorders (OCD), prior episodes of postpartum psychosis or a family history of mental health problems are at a higher risk. The prevalence of these extreme mental health disorders is about 4 per 1000 pregnancies, and differs from postpartum depression and maternity blues which are milder conditions.

34.1.4.3 Investigations/Diagnosis
Diagnostic aids utilise the DSM V and the ICD 10 criteria. Medical and pregnancy-specific conditions that may lead to similar presentation must be assessed and ruled out.

34.1.4.4 Management
Puerperal psychosis is a psychiatric emergency.

Multidisciplinary care is advised between the midwifery, obstetric, mental health and social care teams. Acute management includes assessment for self-harm or risk of infanticide and ensuring the relevant teams are informed and admission for care in a safe environment.

Specific pharmacotherapy is best guided by the mental health professional with input on drug safety by the obstetric team.

Bipolar-specific pharmacotherapy may include lithium (increases risk of foetal heart defects including Ebstein anomaly), anticonvulsants, for example carbamazepine, sodium valproate, which may stabilise mood but increase risk of neural tube defects. Severe cases may benefit from electroconvulsive therapy. Psychosis may be treated with a choice of first-, second- or third-generation antipsychotics.

34.1.4.5 Prevention

There are no known interventions that prevent psychosis in pregnancy. It is a subject with more questions than answers [11]. Identification of risk factors and flagging them up may enable early detection and intervention, which may improve outcomes [9]. Recommendations from the confidential enquiry point to the red flag signs of the following: significant changes in mental state, new thoughts or acts of violent self-harm and expressions of incompetency/estrangement from the infant. These should be triggers for consideration of admission to a special unit for closer observation and care. There should also be additional training for liaison, crisis and home treatment teams. There should be some form of support and education for families and a need for greater awareness of these conditions among mental health staff and clinical networks

34.1.4.6 Follow-Up

Puerperal psychosis has a good prognosis [9]. However, some patients may require long-term medication or follow up by a mental health specialist. It is important to link such patients with social workers who may assist with further support within the community.

Learning Points on Maternal Mental Illness

Psychiatric disorder associated with childbirth is common and involves both new episodes related to childbirth and recurrences of pre-existing conditions.

10% of new mothers will develop a depressive illness: half will be at the severe end of the spectrum. Biological factors may be the most important aspect in the severe forms of postpartum onset conditions.

4 per 1000 will develop puerperal psychosis.

Risk of developing severe mental illness is substantially elevated, particularly in the first 3 months postpartum (includes puerperal psychosis OCD and schizophrenia).

Family history of bipolar disorder increases the risk of such an illness after childbirth – 1 in 2.

34.1.5 Maternal Mental Health, Suicide and Maternal Mortality

Mental health conditions predispose mothers to suicidal ideation and eventual suicide. Suicidal behaviour is among the leading causes of injury and death worldwide and indeed a leading cause of maternal death in some countries [13].

The United Kingdom Confidential Enquiries into Maternal Death and Morbidity 2016 [19] highlighted the impact of maternal suicide on overall maternal mortality. Maternal deaths by suicide were the leading cause of direct maternal deaths up to 1 year following childbirth. Maternal deaths from suicide up to 1 year (2/100,000) matched cardiac deaths which was the commonest single cause of indirect (and direct) maternal deaths. Almost a quarter of women who died between 6 weeks and 1 year after pregnancy died from mental health–related conditions (1 in 7 by suicide). These suicide rates completely eclipsed the suicide rates in the non-pregnant female population.

A South African study estimated suicidal ideation in pregnancy among HIV-infected women at 39% [24]. This is perhaps reflective of most of Africa that has a comparable HIV burden. Maternal mental wellbeing ought to be a priority during antenatal, intrapartum and postpartum care. Apart from HIV, other vulnerable groups that are of relevance especially in the African setting are: pregnant adolescent girls, displaced and war-affected women, women with disabilities, sex workers and women from marginalised communities [32].

It is essential also to note that a detailed analysis of the suicide groups did show stark differences between peripartum suicides and when it happens or attempted outside of pregnancy. The report shows that the highest risk is within the first 12 weeks of delivery pointing towards the effects of pregnancy and childbirth. Unlike interval suicide attempts in females (which is usually from overdose of tranquillisers), peri-partum suicides were particularly violent (82%) including self-immolation hanging and intentional road traffic accidents. Such pattern of deaths did cut across all levels of social class with no particular predilection.

Focusing on early diagnosis, appropriate multidisciplinary management for mental health problems during and after pregnancy will go a long way towards a reduction in maternal mortality due to indirect causes [24].

Learning Points on Maternal Suicide

Women with a past episode of severe mental illness following delivery have a 1:2–3 chance of recurrence.

50% of women with serious mental ill-health died between 28 weeks of pregnancy and 12 weeks postpartum.

Suicide profile of child-bearing women is different in many respects to that of other women.

The risk of illness is usually not identified or managed appropriately.

Health professionals are not sharing information on mental health conditions (because of stigma)

Women requiring specialist in-patient care after delivery are not being admitted to specialist units.

Serious physical illness can present with psychological symptoms, result from or complicate mental illness. In many cases, a psychiatric diagnosis delayed the treatment of a fatal physical illness.

The following are "red flag" signs for severe maternal illness and require urgent senior psychiatric assessment:

- Recent significant change in mental state or emergence of new symptoms.
- New thoughts or acts of violent self-harm.
- New and persistent expressions of incompetency as a mother or estrangement from infant.

References

1. Aina OF. Mental illness and cultural issues in West African films: implications for orthodox psychiatric practice. Med Humanit. 2004;30(1):23–6.
2. American Psychiatric Association. Diagnostic and statistical manual of mental disorders. 5th ed. Arlington: American Psychiatric Association; 2013.
3. Austin MP, Priest SR, Sullivan EA. Antenatal psychosocial assessment for reducing perinatal mental health morbidity. Cochrane Database Syst Rev. 2008;(4):Cd005124.
4. Centres for Disease Control and Prevention (CDC). International classification of diseases, Tenth Revision (ICD-10). 2017. Retrieved 03/01/2017, 2017.
5. Chowdhary N, Sikander S, Atif N, Singh N, Ahmad I, Fuhr DC, Rahman A, Patel V. The content and delivery of psychological interventions for perinatal depression by non-specialist health workers in low and middle income countries: a systematic review. Best Pract Res Clin Obstet Gynaecol. 2014;28(1):113–33.
6. Cox JL, Holden JM, Sagovsky R. Detection of postnatal depression. Development of the 10-item Edinburgh Postnatal Depression Scale. Br J Psychiatry. 1987;150:782–6.
7. Dennis CL, Dowswell T. Interventions (other than pharmacological, psychosocial or psychological) for treating antenatal depression. Cochrane Database Syst Rev. 2013;(7):Cd006795.
8. Dennis CL, Dowswell T. Psychosocial and psychological interventions for preventing postpartum depression. Cochrane Database Syst Rev. 2013;(2):Cd001134.
9. Di Florio A, Smith S, Jones I. Postpartum psychosis. Obstet Gynaecol. 2013;15(3):145–50.
10. Ebeigbe PN, Akhigbe KO. Incidence and associated risk factors of postpartum depression in a tertiary hospital in Nigeria. Niger Postgrad Med J. 2008;15(1):15–8.
11. Essali A, Alabed S, Guul A, Essali N. Preventive interventions for postnatal psychosis. Cochrane Database Syst Rev. 2013;(6):Cd009991.
12. Fisher J, de Mello MC, Patel V, Rahman A, Tran T, Holton S, Holmes W. Prevalence and determinants of common perinatal mental disorders in women in low- and lower-middle-income countries: a systematic review. Bull World Health Organ. 2012;90(2):139g–49g.
13. Gelaye B, Kajeepeta S, Williams MA. Suicidal ideation in pregnancy: an epidemiologic review. Arch Womens Ment Health. 2016;19(5):741–51.
14. Goodman JH, Chenausky KL, Freeman MP. Anxiety disorders during pregnancy: a systematic review. J Clin Psychiatry. 2014;75(10):e1153–84.
15. Howard LM, Molyneaux E, Dennis CL, Rochat T, Stein A, Milgrom J. Non-psychotic mental disorders in the perinatal period. Lancet. 2014;384(9956):1775–88.
16. Howard LM, Piot P, Stein A. No health without perinatal mental health. Lancet. 2014;384(9956):1723–4.
17. Jones I, Chandra PS, Dazzan P, Howard LM. Bipolar disorder, affective psychosis, and schizophrenia in pregnancy and the postpartum period. Lancet. 2014;384(9956):1789–99.
18. Marc I, Toureche N, Ernst E, Hodnett ED, Blanchet C, Dodin S, Njoya MM. Mind-body interventions during pregnancy for preventing or treating women's anxiety. Cochrane Database Syst Rev. 2011;(7):Cd007559.
19. Knight M, Nair M, Tuffnell D, on behalf of MBRRACE-UK, editors. Saving lives, improving mothers' care—surveillance of maternal deaths in the UK 2012–14 and lessons learned to inform maternity care from the UK and Ireland Confidential Enquiries into Maternal Deaths and Morbidity 2009–14. National Perinatal Epidemiology Unit, Oxford: University of Oxford; 2016.
20. Murray D, Cox JL. Screening for depression during pregnancy with the Edinburgh depression scale (EDDS). J Reprod Infant Psychol. 1990;8(2):99–107.
21. O'Connell M, Leahy-Warren P, Khashan AS, Kenny LC. Tocophobia – the new hysteria? Obstet Gynaecol Reprod Med. 2015;25(6):175–7.
22. Parsons CE, Young KS, Rochat TJ, Kringelbach ML, Stein A. Postnatal depression and its effects on child development: a review of evidence from low- and middle-income countries. Br Med Bull. 2011;101(1):57–79.
23. Radloff LS. The CES-D scale. Appl Psychol Measur. 1977;1(3):385–401.
24. Rodriguez VJ, Cook RR, Peltzer K, Jones DL. Prevalence and psychosocial correlates of suicidal ideation among pregnant women living with HIV in Mpumalanga Province, South Africa. AIDS Care. 2017;29(5):593–7.
25. Ross LE, McLean LM. Anxiety disorders during pregnancy and the postpartum period: a systematic review. J Clin Psychiatry. 2006;67(8):1285–98.
26. Sawyer A, Ayers S, Smith H. Pre- and postnatal psychological wellbeing in Africa: a systematic review. J Affect Disord. 2010;123(1–3):17–29.
27. Shehu CE, Yunusa MA. Obstetric characteristics and management of patients with postpartum psychosis in a tertiary hospital setting. Obstet Gynaecol Int. 2015;2015:386409.
28. Stein A, Pearson RM, Goodman SH, Rapa E, Rahman A, McCallum M, Howard LM, Pariante CM. Effects of perinatal mental disorders on the foetus and child. Lancet. 2014;384(9956):1800–19.
29. Storm F, Agampodi S, Eddleston M, Sorensen JB, Konradsen F, Rheinlander T. Indirect causes of maternal death. Lancet Glob Health. 2014;2(10):e566.
30. Victoria Hendrick MD. Psychiatric disorders in pregnancy and the postpartum principles and treatment. Totowa New Jersey: Humana Press; 2006.
31. Walker SP, Wachs TD, Grantham-McGregor S, Black MM, Nelson CA, Huffman SL, Baker-Henningham H, Chang SM, Hamadani JD, Lozoff B, Gardner JM, Powell CA, Rahman A, Richter

L. Inequality in early childhood: risk and protective factors for early child development. Lancet. 2011;378(9799):1325–38.
32. World Health Organisation. WHO Guidelines Approved by the Guidelines Review Committee. WHO recommendations on antenatal care for a positive pregnancy experience. Geneva, World Health Organization Copyright (c) World Health Organization; 2016.
33. World Health Organisation. Maternal mental health. Retrieved 02/01/2017. 2017. from http://www.who.int/mental_health/maternal-child/maternal_mental_health/en/.

HIV in Pregnancy

35

Chris Ovoroyeguono Agboghoroma

Abbreviations

3TC	Lamivudine 300 mg OD
ART	Antiretroviral therapy
ATV/r	Atazanavir/ritonavir 300 mg + 100 mg
AZT	Azidothymidine or zidovudine – ZDV 300 mg BD
DRV/r	Darunavir + ritonavir 800 mg +100 m OD
DTG	Dolutegravir 50 mg OD
EFV	Efavirenz 600 mg OD
FTC	Emtricitabine 200 mg OD
LPV/r	Lopinavir/ritonavir 400 mg + 100 mg
NRTIs	Nucleoside reverse transcriptase inhibitors
NVP	Nevirapine 200 mg OD for 14 days, then 200 mg BD
RAL	Raltegravir 400 mg OD
TDF	Tenofovir disoproxil fumarate 300 mg OD

Learning Objectives

At the conclusion of this chapter, the reader should be able to:

- Appreciate the magnitude of the problem of HIV infection in pregnancy.
- Determine the effects of HIV infection in pregnancy.
- Discuss HIV combination prevention methods.
- Critically evaluate the determinants of HIV transmission from mother to child.
- Understand the issues involved in HIV counselling for pregnant women.
- Explain the tests used in the diagnosis and follow-up of HIV infection.
- Discuss the measures to reduce HIV transmission during antenatal, intrapartum and postpartum period.
- Recall the recommended antiretroviral drugs for treatment and prophylaxis of HIV-positive pregnant women and their HIV-exposed infants.
- Evaluate infant feeding options in the context of prevention of mother-to-child transmission of HIV.

35.1 Introduction

Acquired immunodeficiency syndrome (AIDS) was first reported in the United States in 1981 amongst homosexuals. Human immunodeficiency virus (HIV), its causative agent, was identified in 1983. Since then, HIV infection has been reported in every country, and the global epidemics has remained unabated with associated morbidity and mortality in all age groups and gender especially in sub-Saharan Africa. While sexual activity is the main source of HIV transmission in adults, mother-to-child transmission (MTCT) accounts for over 90% of all paediatric (children less than 15 years) infections.

HIV infection is a common medical condition in pregnancy. The median prevalence of HIV among antenatal clients in sub-Saharan Africa is estimated to be 4.9% [1]. The morbidity and mortality associated with paediatric HIV infection in sub-Saharan Africa is a major impediment to child survival in the continent. Some reports suggest that at

Note: Dolutegravir-based regimen should be avoided by women during preconception period and in first trimester of pregnancy due to risk of neural tube defect in their babies.

C. O. Agboghoroma (✉)
Reproductive Medicine and Endocrinology Unit, Department of Obstetrics & Gynaecology, National Hospital, Abuja, Nigeria

F. Okonofua et al. (eds.), *Contemporary Obstetrics and Gynecology for Developing Countries*,
https://doi.org/10.1007/978-3-030-75385-6_35

least one-third of HIV-infected children in Africa and other developing countries die within their first year of life [2, 3].

Although, there is yet no vaccine or cure for HIV infection, much progress has been made towards effective treatment for the infection. With the current use of combination antiretroviral therapy (ART), mortality from HIV/AIDS has been drastically reduced and HIV can now be effectively managed [4]. Also, much have been achieved in efforts to reduce paediatric HIV infections through prevention of mother-to-child transmission (PMTCT) strategies which have been successfully employed in some countries. MTCT rates in most developed nations is now below 2% compared with the background transmission rate of about 15–45% in the absence of effective interventions [5–7]. This development is regarded as one of the greatest medical achievements thus far in the twenty-first century. There are on-going global efforts to eliminate MTCT of HIV and prevent deaths from HIV infections.

35.2 Disease Description: Human Immunodeficiency Virus (HIV) and Acquired Immunodeficiency Syndrome (AIDS)

HIV-1 and less commonly HIV-2 are the viruses that cause AIDS. They belong to the family of retroviruses. Three major classes of HIV-1 have been identified – M (main), N (new) and O (outlier). Among M group viruses, which account for >90% of HIV infections worldwide, there are nine subtypes, called clades, designated by the letters A-D, F-H, J and K, as well as many recombinant forms. The most common subtype in West Africa is clade A, while clade B is the most common subtype in the Americas and Western Europe [8]. Viral diversities are greatest in sub-Saharan Africa.

HIV-2 is found primarily in West Africa. It is associated with a lower viral load and slower rate of both CD4 cell decline and clinical progression. Compared with HIV-1, HIV-2 is less transmissible (5–8-fold less efficient than HIV-1 in early -stage disease and a 20–30-fold lower rate of vertical transmission) [9].

HIV infection of a host cell begins with the binding of the virus particle (virion) to the host cell. Subsequent replication and integration into the host genome cause progressive depletion of CD4 cells, leading to increased risk for development of opportunistic infections, tumours and AIDS.

HIV has been isolated from many human bodily fluids including blood, seminal fluids, pre-ejaculate, cerebrospinal fluid, saliva, tears and breast milk. It is found in both cell-free and cell-associated fractions. The World Health Organization (WHO) has adopted clinical staging for HIV disease (Stage 1–4) ranging from asymptomatic infection to point when AIDS-defining symptoms are present [10].

35.2.1 Epidemiology of HIV/AIDS

The HIV/AIDS epidemic has been reported globally. Since the first report in 1981, over 70 million people have been infected worldwide and about 36 million people have died from AIDS-related causes. Over the last three decades, sub-Saharan Africa continued to bear the greatest burden of HIV/AIDS epidemic. While sub-Saharan Africa is about 12% of the world's population, the 2011 Joint United Nations programme on HIV/AIDS (UNAIDS) [1] report showed that it is home to 69% of the 34.0 million HIV-infected persons, 71% of the 2.5 million total new infections and 70% of 1.7 million deaths from AIDS-related causes worldwide. The UNAIDS report also showed that about 330,000 children acquired new infections (through MTCT route) in 2011. The highest number of new paediatric HIV infection was in Nigeria 69,000 (20.9%), South Africa followed with 29,000 (8.8%) and Mozambique 27,000 (8.2%). The majority of new paediatric HIV infections (over 90%) occurred in sub-Saharan Africa where most of the HIV-infected pregnant women are located. Apart from India, 21 out of 22 countries with the highest estimated numbers of HIV-infected pregnant women are in sub-Saharan Africa, with South Africa having the highest number 241,300 (19.4%), followed by Nigeria 228,800 (18.4%) and Mozambique 98,300 (7.9%).

Over time, the epidemic, which was once dominated globally by infected males, has become progressively feminised in sub-Saharan Africa with over 60% of infected population being females. This situation has been attributed to socio-cultural factors that are prevalent in Africa that made females in the society more vulnerable to HIV infection [11]. It is also estimated that about 50% of people leaving with HIV globally are unaware of their status.

Countries in sub-Saharan Africa have generalised HIV. The estimated global HIV prevalence among adults aged 15–49 years is 0.8% but that for sub-Saharan Africa is 4.9%. Some of the countries have national median HIV prevalence of over 10%, with the highest being Swaziland with a prevalence of 25.9% [12]. In Nigeria, the HIV prevalence among pregnant women was 1.8% in 1991, 4.5% in 1995, 5.8% in 2001, 5% in 20 03, 4.6% in 2008, 4.1% in 2010 and 3.0% in 2014 [13]. A 2018 national HIV/AIDS survey among adults aged 15–64 years in Nigeria revealed a prevalence of 1.5% [14].

35.2.2 Risk Factors for HIV Transmission

Currently the commonest route of HIV transmission is sexual intercourse which can be heterosexual (penile-vaginal), homosexual (penile-anal) or oral sex. Nonsexual transmission include infection with contaminated blood products; injection drug use; occupational exposures, such as accidental needle sticks; and perinatal transmission or MTCT.

The risk factors facilitating transmission can generally be categorised into infectiousness of the host (source), susceptibility of the recipient and viral properties. A host is more infectious, with more advanced stage of infection as measured by low CD4 count or high viral load as well as exposure during primary infection. Factors that reduce viral load and improve the CD4 count decrease the risk of transmission. Susceptibility of the recipient is increased in situations such as genital ulcer disease and other sexually transmitted infections, as well as trauma during sexual intercourse.

35.2.3 HIV Management

Much advances have been made in the management of persons infected with HIV. While HIV infection was invariably fatal in the early phase of the HIV epidemic, recent advances have ensured that the disease can be effectively managed with antiretroviral drugs as a chronic medical condition. However, it is yet not curable. The management of HIV should be by multidisciplinary team of experts ensuring the following:

- Early diagnosis and evaluation.
- Combination antiretroviral therapy (ART) and effective monitoring for failure and resistance development. ART is the single most important intervention, and the WHO in 2016 recommend lifelong treatment for all HIV-infected persons irrespective of the disease stage. Adherence to treatment and retention in care are essential.
- Prophylaxis and treatment for opportunistic and co-infections,
- Supportive care including nutrition, psychosocial, mental health, substance abuse and spiritual.
- Palliative care.

35.2.4 HIV Prevention

Prevention of new infections is an essential strategy in the control of HIV/AIDS. Vaccines are not yet available against HIV infections. For maximal impact on reduction of HIV transmission and acquisition, combination prevention involving biomedical, behavioural and structural approaches is presently recommended.

Biomedical Interventions that reduce HIV risk practices and/or the probability of HIV transmission per contact event include the following:

- Use of antiretroviral drugs by infected person to achieve optimal viral suppression and by people without HIV as pre-exposure prophylaxis (PrEP) or post-exposure prophylaxis (PEP).
- Effective management of sexually transmitted infections (STIs).
- Male and female condoms and condom-compatible lubricant. Use of condom is associated with 80% reduction risk in male-to-female sexual transmission and 64% reduction in transmission among men who have sex with men [10].
- Needle and syringe programme among injection drug users.
- Opioid substitution therapy – with methadone or buprenorphine.
- Blood safety measures including screening of all blood and blood products before transfusion.
- Application of universal precaution.
- Voluntary medical male circumcision (VMMC) has been associated with 60% reduction in the risk of female-to-male sexual transmission.

Behavioural interventions can reduce the frequency of potential transmission events, including the following:

- Targeted information and education, such as school-based sex education, peer counselling and community-level and interpersonal counselling including brief interventions to disseminate behavioural messages which can encourage people to reduce risk behaviour and increase behaviour that is protective (such as safer drug use, delaying sexual debut, reducing the frequency of unprotected sex with multiple partners, using condoms correctly and consistently and knowing self-HIV status and that of partner).
- Deployment of social media and mobile technology in HIV prevention programme.

Structural and supportive interventions can increase access to, uptake of and adherence to biochemical and behavioural interventions. Such interventions address the critical social, legal, political and environmental enablers that contribute to HIV transmission including legal reforms, measures to reduce stigma and discrimination. Measures to promote gender equality and prevention of gender-based violence, economic empowerment, access to schooling and supportive interventions designed to enhance referrals, adherence, retention and community mobilisation are also important.

35.2.5 HIV Infection and Pregnancy

At the early phase of the HIV epidemic when mortality from HIV was high, there were ethical issues and concerns about the welfare of the child when the parents would not be alive or be in a healthy state to cater for the child. In the present era of use of combination ART, HIV-positive couples can have a fulfilled family life with healthy children.

Higher rates of infertility have been documented among HIV-positive group compared to the general population. This has been attributed to many factors – HIV-positive females are more prone to tubo-peritoneal factors from increased susceptibility to pelvic infections. It is also reported that HIV-positive men tend to have reduced seminal parameters (including count, motility and morphology). Other factors include condom use especially in a sero-discordant couple; reduction in the frequency of sexual activity occasioned by chronic ill-health and psychological reasons. Success rates in assisted reproductive technology in HIV-positive women are also reduced compared to non-infected persons primarily due to poor ovarian response [15].

HIV is more readily transmitted and acquired during pregnancy. This has been attributed to hormonal and immunological changes in pregnancy. Also couples are less likely to use condoms consistently during pregnancy. Most studies that have examined the impact of pregnancy on HIV disease (using virologic, immunologic and clinical parameters) have shown no significant differences in HIV progression or survival between women who had been pregnant and those who had not experienced pregnancy [16]. While this is the situation in asymptomatic women or women with early-stage infection, with advanced HIV disease, maternal health may actually deteriorate in the course of pregnancy especially in the absence of ART [17]. A decline in the absolute CD4 count attributed to haemodilution in pregnancy tend to occur, but CD4 percentage remains stable. Viral load is however not affected by haemodilution of pregnancy and may increase transiently in the postpartum period.

Maternal HIV infection has been associated with adverse outcomes in pregnancy [18]. Spontaneous abortions, preterm delivery, intrauterine growth restriction (IUGR) and low-birth-weight (LBW) infants are more common in HIV-infected pregnancies. HIV-related maternal mortality is also common in Africa where it accounts for over 6% of all maternal deaths [19]. These complications are related to advanced disease states (or their treatment), presence of co-infections and poor nutritional status.

Furthermore, HIV adversely affects the frequency, natural history, presentation and treatment of many infections in pregnancy, including vulvo-vaginal candidiasis, bacterial vaginosis, genital herpes simplex, human papilloma virus (HPV), syphilis, trichomonas vaginalis, cytomegalovirus, toxoplasmosis, hepatitis B and C, malaria, urinary tract infections and bacterial pneumonia. In addition to these infections and parasitic infestations, any of the HIV-related opportunistic infections – such as tuberculosis, *Pneumocystis jirovecii* pneumonia – are more frequent during pregnancy and in the puerperium.

Another major concern about HIV infection in pregnant women is the risk of transmission of the virus to the baby, as the chance of survival in infected children is poor.

35.3 Mother-to-Child Transmission (MTCT) of HIV

Mother-to-child transmission (MTCT) or vertical transmission of HIV accounts for about 10% of all infections but over 90% of paediatric infections. HIV can be transmitted from an infected mother to her child through the placenta, breaks in the skin, mucous membrane or gastro-intestinal tract. This may occur at any time during the period of pregnancy, labour and delivery or breastfeeding.

Without interventions, the risk of MTCT is estimated to range from 15% to 25% in developed countries and 25–45% in developing countries [20, 21]. Studies have shown that in non-breastfed infants, 65% infections occur around the time of labour and delivery and 35% in utero [22]. In breastfeeding population, 30–50% of infected infants contract their infection through breastfeeding [23]. The differences in MTCT rates between the developed and developing countries is partly attributed to postnatal transmission – breastfeeding [24]. Other factors contributing to the high burden of MTCT in sub-Saharan Africa are higher prevalence of HIV in women of reproductive age, high total fertility rate and poor access to PMTCT interventions.

35.3.1 Factors That Influence Mother-to-Child Transmission (MTCT) of HIV

Factors that influence MTCT can be grouped into viral, maternal, placenta, obstetrics, mode of delivery, foetal/neonatal and breastfeeding factors. With the current recommendation and use of combination antiretroviral therapy in pregnancy, the risk of MTCT with many of the listed factors are reduced [25].

(i) **Viral Factors**
   (a) **Viral load:** This is the single most important determinant of MTCT as it correlates significantly with the risk of transmission both in women who have received treatment and those who have not. The risk of transmission is more with higher levels of HIV as in advanced diseases and at the time of seroconversion [25]. However, there is no level of maternal viral load (even when undetected) below which transmission cannot occur, and there is no limit of maternal viraemia above which MTCT will always occur [26].
   (b) **Viral genotype (strain variation):** HIV-1 is more infective than HIV-2. Different HIV-1 subtypes or clade groups also exist with different cell tropism and in turn their infectivity either in utero, through genital tract or in breast milk. Also increased strain diversity in the mother may influence the rate of

transmission. Hence, repeated exposure during pregnancy to different strain through unprotected sex increases transmission risk [20].

(c) **Viral phenotype (biological growth characteristics):** Different viral phenotypes show differing tissue tropism. Foetal blood mononuclear cells may be more susceptible to macrophage tropic, non-syncytium-inducing HIV phenotypes and thus may influence MTCT [27].

(d) **Viral resistance:** The development of resistance mutations, as may occur with prolonged antiretroviral monotherapy (e.g. nevirapine or zidovudine) in perinatal prophylaxis, increases the risk for transmission [28].

(ii) **Maternal Factors**

(a) **Maternal immunological status:** Reduced maternal immune status, reflected by low CD4 cell count, low CD4 percentage or low CD4/CD8 ratio, has been associated with increased risk of MTCT. Infection through breastfeeding has also been associated with lack of IgM and IgA in breast milk.

(b) **Maternal nutritional factors:** Vitamin A deficiency has been associated with increased genital tract HIV shedding and higher risk of transmission [29].

(c) **Maternal immune factors (including neutralising antibodies):** Conditions of reduced maternal immune factor enhances transmission.

(d) **Sexually transmitted infections (STIs):** The presence of STIs (especially those associated with ulcers such as syphilis) increases genital tract HIV shedding and plasma viraemia, both of which increases risk for MTCT.

(e) **Behavioural factors**: Some behavioural factors including cigarette smoking and maternal hard drug use have been associated with increased transmission [30, 31]. Unprotected sexual intercourses during pregnancy have also been linked to increased transmission. This has been attributed to increased concentration or viral strain diversity of HIV-1, or the effect of cervical or vaginal inflammation or abrasions.

(iii) **Placenta Factors**

Placenta disruption from effects of cigarette smoking, hard drug use, malaria (*Plasmodium falciparum*) placental parasitisation and abruptio placenta increases exposure of the foetus to maternal blood and hence increases the risk of transmission. Both clinical and histological evidence of chorioamnionitis are associated with higher risk of transmission [32].

(iv) **Obstetrics Factors**

Obstetric factors are important determinants of MTCT. Transmission may occur through direct skin and mucus membrane contact between the infant and maternal blood or cervico-vaginal secretions and blood during labour, ingestion of virus from these secretions and ascending infection to the amniotic fluid. Factors that increase the chance and duration of contact between the foetus and maternal blood/genital secretions tend to increase the risk of transmission. These include:

(a) Invasive obstetrics procedures such as chorionic villus sampling, amniocentesis, cordocentesis, amnioscopy, intrauterine pressure catheters, penetrating scalp electrodes or scalp blood sampling
(b) Episiotomy and vaginal tears
(c) Instrumental deliveries (vacuum delivery and forceps) which can cause foetal or maternal injury including micro-lacerations
(d) Prolonged labour
(e) Prolonged rupture of foetal membranes (more than 4 hours)

(v) **Mode of Delivery**

Delivery by elective caesarean section and before membrane rupture is associated with reduce risk of MTCT by about 50% compared to vaginal delivery [23]. In caesarean section, foetal contact with genital secretions is avoided and contact with maternal blood is transient.

(vi) **Foetal/Neonatal Factors**

HIV entry to the foetus may occur through the gastrointestinal tract (GIT) following ingestion of virus in utero or at birth. Generally, in neonate, there is decreased acidity, decreased mucus, lower 1gA activity and thinned mucosa in the GIT, which may facilitate transmission. The immune system in the newborn (especially in premature babies) may also be deficient in macrophage and T-cell immune response increasing the susceptibility to infection [34].

Genetic susceptibility has also been documented. Concordance between infant and maternal human leucocyte antigen (HLA) has been associated with increased risk of transmission. Mutations may also play a role. Homozygous deletion of the genetic factor for CCR-5 receptor (a co-receptor for macrophage-tropic strains of HIV) confers a high degree of natural resistance to HIV transmission [35].

In **multiple births**, the first-born has a higher risk of infection. This may be due to longer period of exposure of the first infant to infected blood and secretions within the birth canal.

(vii) **Breastfeeding**

Breastfeeding is estimated to account for 30–50% of MTCT of HIV in developing countries. Breast milk contains both cell-associated and cell-free virus, the level of which is related to the stage of maternal HIV disease, level of immune suppression (CD4 cell count) and vitamin A levels. Risk of transmission is highest in the first few months of breastfeeding, but increased duration of breastfeeding increases risk. Transmission is also more likely in mothers who become newly infected or seroconvert while breastfeeding. Other potential variables for transmission include cracked nipples, breast abscesses, mastitis, pattern of breastfeeding (especially mixed feeding) and oral thrush in the child [36].

35.4 Comprehensive Approach to Prevention of Mother-to-Child Transmission (PMTCT) of HIV

The following four-pronged approach is recommended by the World Health Organization (WHO) for the prevention of mother-to-child transmission of HIV [37]:

(i) Primary prevention of HIV infection in women of reproductive age and their partners
(ii) Prevention of unintending pregnancies among HIV positive women
(iii) Prevention of HIV transmission from infected mothers to their infants
(iv) Provision of appropriate treatment, care and support to HIV-infected mothers, their infants, partners and family

This approach has resulted in significant reduction of MTCT of HIV from the base line value of over 25–45% to less than 2% in many countries. There is good prospect of eliminating MTCT of HIV by the year 2030

35.4.1 Management of HIV in Pregnancy

The management of HIV in pregnancy is aimed at optimising the health of the mother during pregnancy, labour and delivery in order to have a healthy baby who is not HIV infected. It involves appropriate treatment including use of combination antiretroviral therapy (ART) and opportunistic infections (OIs) prophylaxis and treatment. It involves provision of well supervised and professional preconception, antenatal, delivery and postnatal care for the mother and expert care of the infant.

35.5 Preconception Care

The main goal of preconception care is to provide services for health promotion, counselling, screening and interventions for women of reproductive age before pregnancy to reduce risk factors that might affect subsequent pregnancies. In the context of HIV infection, preconception care services include the following:

- Selection of effective and appropriate contraceptive options to reduce the chance of unwanted pregnancy and until the optimal maternal health status for pregnancy is achieved.
- Ensure appropriate therapy to maximally reduce viral load and optimise immune function before pregnancy.
- Means of achieving safe conception especially in a serodiscordant relationship, minimising both horizontal (sexual) and perinatal transmission of HIV. Available options ranged from timed unprotected intercourse, pre-exposure prophylaxis, insemination with donor semen and sperm wash combined with assisted reproductive technology-intrauterine insemination (IUI), in vitro fertilisation (IVF) and intracytoplasmic sperm injection (ICSI.
- Modification of ART regimen that has potential for teratogenicity and adverse side effects.
- ART adherence promotion.
- Diagnosis, prophylaxis and treatment of opportunistic infections such as tuberculosis.
- Diagnosis and treatment of STIs.
- Optimisation of maternal nutritional status.
- Recommendation for safe sexual practices.
- A discussion of the effects of HIV infection on pregnancy and PMTCT strategies.

While preconception care is desirable in women living with HIV, this service may not be readily accessible to women in many developing countries

35.5.1 HIV Testing and Counselling in Pregnancy

The 'opt-out' approach to HIV testing and counselling has been shown to be very useful in eliciting positive response from potential clients in the antenatal setting. In this approach, HIV testing is offered to all clients as part of routine antenatal tests during the first antenatal visit, but the client reserves the right to decline the test without any sanctions from the provider. HIV testing may also be offered late in pregnancy (about 36 weeks) or in labour to women of unknown HIV status and those who had tested negative earlier in pregnancy. HIV testing and counselling should be voluntary and adhere to the principles of consent, confidentiality, counselling, correct test results and connections to care, treatment and prevention services. HIV testing and counselling involves pre-test information, HIV testing (preferably with same day result), post-test counselling and follow-up counselling [38].

35.5.2 Pre-test Information

HIV pre-test information should be provided to all antenatal clients prior to HIV test. The care provider should undertake the following as part of pre-test information:

- Introduce self and other health workers present and establish rapport.
- Gain the clients' confidence and assure them of confidentiality.
- Provide information about HIV and AIDS, transmission, HIV testing, window period and the meaning of positive and negative test results.
- Emphasise the benefits of HIV testing and PMTCT services.
- Provide information on the benefits of postpartum mother-infant pair follow-up and early infant diagnosis.
- Discuss partner testing and the issues of concordant and discordant test results.
- Discuss the services available in the case of either a negative or positive result including availability of antiretroviral drugs.
- Discuss disclosure to partner and family.
- Discuss any concern that the clients may have.

35.5.3 HIV Test

The diagnosis of HIV infection is either by direct detection of the viral particles or its components or by indirect methods of detection of antibodies against the virus. The direct methods of HIV detection include p24 antigen test, RNA polymerase chain reaction (PCR), DNA PCR and viral culture. The indirect antibody tests methods include simple or rapid tests, enzyme-linked immunosorbent assay (ELISA) tests and western blot tests. The simple or rapid test is the one commonly used in developing countries for its simplicity and low cost. It is easy to perform and can be undertaken by any trained health worker and the results are obtained in less than 30 minutes.

35.5.4 Post-test Counselling

All clients who have had HIV testing should be counselled when the test results are given, regardless of the outcome of the test. However, the issues in post-test counselling depend on the result of the test.

For clients with HIV positive result, the post-test counselling should include the following:

- Disclosure of the result immediately, simply and clearly in a neutral manner to the client.
- Allow time for her to appreciate the implication of the test result.
- Determine if she understands the meaning and implications of the test result.
- Provide support in coping with emotions arising from the test result.
- Discuss disclosure of the result to third party – when, how and to whom.
- Discuss HIV testing for partner and other family members.
- Discuss how to access essential PMTCT services including antiretroviral (ARV) prophylaxis and treatment.
- The importance of early commencement and adherence to ARV drugs.
- The need to screen for STIs, tuberculosis (TB) and cervical cancer.
- The available infant feeding options including the importance of exclusive breastfeeding (EBF) with antiretrovirals for HIV free survival.
- The mode of delivery and the need for health facility-based delivery.
- Issues of personal risk reduction plan.
- The need for family planning in the postpartum period.
- The need to access available care and support services on account of the HIV infection.
- The need for early infant diagnosis, follow-up and linkages.

Clients with HIV negative result should be counselled on the meaning and on how to remain negative including risk reduction strategies. Patients who are negative may need to be rescreened 3–6 months (after window period) and/or during labour.

35.5.5 Follow-Up Counselling

Follow-up counselling is meant to provide support for infected mother and baby. The issues in follow-up counselling include:

- Adherence to prescribed drugs
- Concerns about relationships, for example, sexual
- Risk reduction
- Referral to other care and support services for both mother and baby
- Partner involvement
- Disclosure
- Stigma, fear of isolation and discrimination
- Coping with own feelings: anger, loneliness, suicidal thoughts, hopelessness and depression
- Economic empowerment, employment and other social and spiritual supports

35.5.6 Antiretroviral Treatment for HIV-Positive Pregnant Women

The combination of three or more antiretroviral drugs (from at least two different classes of antiretroviral) in the form of highly active antiretroviral therapy (HAART) revolutionised the management of HIV. Combination antiretroviral therapy (ART) is the gold standard for treatment of HIV infections. Its use has transformed HIV infections from an inevitable fatal disease to chronic and manageable medical condition. Its use in pregnancy is associated with improvement in maternal health and better obstetric outcome. It is the single most important intervention in preventing mother-to-child transmission of HIV during pregnancy, labour and delivery and breastfeeding. HIV-positive women who are pregnant or breastfeeding are eligible for antiretroviral treatment or prophylaxis irrespective of their clinical stage or CD4 cell count.

Antiretroviral drugs act principally to reduce maternal viral load and also serve as pre-/post-exposure prophylaxis for the infant.

35.5.7 Classes of Antiretroviral Drugs

The antiretroviral drugs currently in use belong to the following main classes:

(i) Nucleoside/nucleotide reverse-transcriptase inhibitors (NRTIs/NtRTIs) – azidothymidine (AZT) or zidovudine (ZDV), lamivudine (3TC), abacavir (ABC), emtricitabine (FTC), starvudine (d4T), tenofovir (TDF) – an NtRTI
(ii) Non-nucleoside reverse-transcriptase inhibitors (NNRTIs) – efavirence (EFV), nevirapine (NVP) and etravirine (ETV)
(iii) Protease inhibitors (PIs) – lopinavir (LPV), ritonavir (RTV), atazanavir (ATV), indinavir (IDV), saquinaqvir (SQV), nelfinavir (NFV)
(iv) Integrase strand transfer inhibitors (INSTIs) – raltegravir (RAL), dolutegravir (DTG)

35.5.8 Antiretroviral Regimen in Pregnancy

The antiretroviral drug regimen applied in the management of HIV-1-infected pregnant women and for PMTCT in most developing countries is based on World Health Organization (WHO) recommendations. This has evolved over the past few years from the use of single dose nevirapine, to zidovudine monotherapy, dual therapy with zidovudine and nevirapine and currently combination drug therapy. The use of combination therapy during pregnancy, labour and breastfeeding period is associated with significant reduction in the risk of HIV transmission and improvement in the health of the mother. The 2016 WHO guideline recommended that all pregnant and breastfeeding women with HIV irrespective of CD4 count and clinical stage should initiate triple antiretroviral drugs (HAART), which should be maintained through the period of MTCT risk (pregnancy, labour, breastfeeding) and continued lifelong [39]. Prior to 2016, only persons who met treatment eligibility criteria for their own health (CD4 count ≤500cells/mm^3 or WHO clinical stage 3 and 4) were placed on lifelong therapy and those not meeting these criteria were offered antiretroviral prophylaxis during the MTCT window period and discontinued thereafter.

Though lifelong treatment is associated with increased cost of management, and tendency for increased toxicity and drug resistance development, it, however, has the potential to reduce transmission rates for future births, lower the odds of transmission to sexual partners and improve maternal survival.

The selection of antiretroviral drug depends on whether the woman is treatment naïve, or has demonstrated resistance to certain drugs, or has other toxicity considerations and co-morbidities including hepatitis B virus (HBV) and hepatitis C virus (HCV). One of the drugs should have the ability to cross the placenta well to achieve pre-exposure prophylaxis for the foetus/infant.

Table 35.1 shows the 2018 WHO-recommended regimen [40] for first-line, second-line and third-line antiretroviral drug treatment for pregnant or breastfeeding women with HIV-1 infections. Most of the regimens are available as fixed-dose combination and once daily use to reduce the number of daily pills which promote better adherence with resultant reduction in resistance development.

The first-line ART consists of two nucleotide/nucleoside reverse-transcriptase inhibitors (NRTIs) backbone plus an integrase strand transfer inhibitors (INSTIs) or non-nucleoside reverse-transcriptase inhibitor (NNRTI). The second-line ART consists of two nucleotide/nucleoside reverse-transcriptase inhibitors (NRTIs) backbone plus a ritonavir-boosted protease inhibitor (PI). The third-line regimen include newer drugs with minimal risk of cross resistance to the previous drugs used. Drugs in this category include INSTs, second-generation NNRTIs and PIs.

Table 35.1 2018 WHO-recommended antiretroviral treatment regimen for HIV-1 infections in pregnant and breastfeeding women

	Preferred regimen	Alternative regimen
First-line ART	TDF + 3TC (or FTC) + DTG	TDF + 3TC (or FTC) + EFV AZT + 3TC + DTG
Second-line ART	AZT + 3TC (or FTC) + LPV/r (or ATV/r)	TDF + 3TC (or FTC) + DTG
Third-line ART	DRV/r + DTG (or RAL) + 1–2 NRTIs	

The non-nucleoside reverse transcriptase inhibitors are ineffective in management of HIV-2 infections [9]. The PIs are therefore used in combination with the two NRTI (backbone drugs) as the first-line regimen

35.5.9 When to Commence Antiretroviral in Pregnancy

Early sustained suppression of the virus is associated with decreased risk of perinatal transmission. Women on an effective antiretroviral treatment prior to pregnancy should be allowed to continue their drugs without disruption. Following diagnosis of HIV, ARV can be started at any time in pregnancy and as soon as possible in order to achieve maximal suppression of the viral replication before delivery. The issue of nausea and vomiting in pregnancy and the potential for teratogenicity has led to consideration of delaying initiation of ARV till after the first trimester. After 12 weeks' gestation, ART should be started as soon as possible irrespective of the viral load and CD4 level to decrease the risk of perinatal transmission.

35.5.10 Discontinuation of Antiretroviral Therapy in Pregnancy and Breastfeeding Period

Discontinuation of ART containing an NNRTI such as nevirapine and efavirenz that have a long half-life, which can be detected up to 21 days or more after discontinuation, predisposes to sub-therapeutic drug levels and NNRTI-resistant mutation. In order to avoid this, it is recommended that the other two drugs – NRTIs with shorter half-life – should be continued for another 7–30 days. Discontinuation or changing ARV regimens that are effectively suppressing viral load is not recommended except if there is major contraindication or complications attributable to any of the drug components. Recent reports indicate that efavirenz is probably not associated with higher risk of neural tube defects and can be safely used in early pregnancy. It is also reported that interruption of ART is associated with loss of virological control, which can lead to increased risk of perinatal transmission [41–44].

35.5.11 Problems with Use of Antiretroviral Therapy in Pregnancy

Strict adherence to antiretroviral use is essential to avoid development of drug resistance. Vomiting in early pregnancy and interaction with other medications may affect effective antiretroviral use in pregnancy. Regular clinical, immunological (CD4 cell count) and virological (viral load) monitoring is necessary for early detection of treatment failure and the need to switch to second- or third-line antiretroviral regimen. In situations where drug resistance could be a problem especially in drug-experienced clients, drug resistance testing may become necessary.

There is also concern about potential teratogenic, mutagenic and carcinogenic effects with use of antiretroviral in pregnancy. Short-term follow-up of babies exposed to antiretroviral has not shown any significant abnormality. Long-term follow-up monitoring data are, however, necessary to confirm safety.

The development of drug toxicity – in form of anaemia, mitochondrial toxicity (lactic acidosis, pancreatitis, peripheral neuropathy, myopathy and cardiomyopathy), hyperlipidaemia, fat redistribution, insulin resistance and bone disorders – osteopenia, osteoporosis and osteonecrosis have been documented. Severe mucus membrane/skin eruptions including Steven Johnson's syndrome can result from the use of nevirapine. Haematological and clinical chemistry monitoring is therefore necessary for patients on antiretroviral.

The use of ART has also been associated with some adverse pregnancy outcomes including preterm delivery and pre-eclampsia.

35.6 Obstetrics Care

The obstetric care for HIV-infected women is not fundamentally different from non-infected women. However, additional measures are taken to reduce the risk of MTCT [45]. The care should be sensitive, supportive, non-discriminatory and not stigmatising. Where possible, a multidisciplinary team of health workers including obstetricians, general practitioners, nurses/midwives, HIV physicians, paediatricians, social workers, nutritionist and counsellors should be involved. Some specific measures are necessary to reduce the risk of HIV transmission during the antenatal, intrapartum and postpartum period.

35.6.1 Antenatal Care

A comprehensive and quality antenatal care provides the opportunity to diagnose women who are HIV positive and who would benefit from expert care to optimise their heath condition and reduction in the risk of vertical and sexual transmission of HIV. In a situation where the life of the woman is seriously threatened by the continuation of the pregnancy, termination of pregnancy should be in accordance with the provision of the prevailing laws. HIV infection is not an indication for termination of pregnancy.

When a woman is known to be HIV positive or is diagnosed as HIV positive during pregnancy, her obstetric and medical care should be strengthened and modified. The few modifications during the antenatal care for an HIV-positive woman include avoidance of invasive procedures such as chorionic villus sampling, amniocentesis or cordocentesis and external cephalic version in a breech presenting foetus. Special care would also need to be taken in situations of premature rupture of membranes and ante-partum haemorrhage.

The HIV-positive pregnant woman should be counselled to adopt behavioural changes that can reduce the risk of MTCT – including limiting or stoppage of cigarette smoking, alcohol consumption, recreational drugs use, unprotected sex to avoid reinfection with another subtype of HIV or infection of partner in a sero-discordant relationship.

In addition to the standard antenatal care, HIV-infected women should be evaluated and managed appropriately for HIV-related illnesses and opportunistic infections. Special attention should be paid to respiratory tract infections, persistent diarrhoea, urinary tract infections, oral/vaginal candidiasis, sexually transmitted infections, herpes zoster and weight loss. Where possible, laboratory investigations should include serial full blood count, screening for sexually transmitted infections (syphilis, chlamydia, gonorrhoea, hepatitis B and C), liver function test, renal function test, lipid profile, CD4 cell count and quantitative viral load assessment. Drug resistance testing may be necessary in women who are antiretroviral experienced. Repeat viral load testing in the mid third trimester to assess for viral suppression should be undertaken. Based on investigation findings, appropriate treatment should be offered.

Adequate diet should be ensured by intake of energy- and protein-rich foods, fruits and vegetables. Micronutrient supplement including iron, folic acid, calcium, zinc, magnesium, selenium and vitamins A, B6, B12, C and D are particularly necessary as anaemia is common in HIV patients. Some antiretroviral drugs such as zidovudine are associated with bone marrow suppression and can lead to severe anaemia. Multivitamin supplementation has been shown to increase maternal CD4 and CD8 counts and reduce stillbirths, severe preterm births, low birth weights and small-for-gestational age [46].

If not on ART prior to pregnancy, HIV-positive client should be commenced on ART as soon as possible in the antenatal period. Antimalarial prophylaxis in form of intermittent preventive treatment (IPTp) with sulphadoxine-pyrimethamine (SP) on at least three occasions, and at least 4 weeks apart in the second and third trimester is essential in HIV-infected pregnant women to reduce placental malaria infection, which could also increase perinatal transmission risk [47].

When the CD4 cell count is below 350 cells/mm^3 and the risk of tuberculosis and/or *Pneumocystis jirovecii* pneumonia is high, appropriate chemoprophylaxis with isoniazid and/or co-trimoxazole become necessary [38].

35.6.2 Intrapartum Care

About 50–60% of MTCT and most of accidental exposures among health care providers occur in the intrapartum period. It is, however, important that the patient is not isolated, discriminated or treated differently from other women in labour. Supportive measures, empathy and caring attitudes by the health care providers are necessary to boost her morale. Universal safety precautions are essential, and labour management should follow standard labour and delivery guidelines with a few modifications and avoiding unnecessary trauma or prolongation of the second stage.

Intrapartum treatment is dictated by the ART regimen a pregnant woman received during the antenatal period and the degree of viral suppression that has been achieved. Women who had been on an effective ART with viral load less than 1000 copies/mL should be allowed to continue their established drug regimen as much as possible during labour or prior to having an elective or scheduled caesarean section. Women who had not commenced antiretroviral should be started on combination ART in labour. Some authorities also recommend the intrapartum administration of IV zidovudine if viral load is unknown or greater than or equal 1000 copies/mL [25, 48].

35.6.3 Unbooked/Unknown HIV Status in Labour

Women who present in labour and have no documented HIV test result during pregnancy and those who have tested negative earlier in pregnancy should be tested and counselled in labour (with the right to opt-out). If this is not possible during labour; it should be offered as soon as possible in the postpartum period. Women with positive results should be offered ART in labour and continued postpartum. They should be linked to care and support in the postpartum period.

35.6.4 Mode of Delivery

With the current recommendation and use of ART in all HIV-positive pregnant women, the tendency is to undertake vaginal delivery except for obstetric indications. However, because of peculiar situations when ART has not been effectively utilised and the possibility that viral load is high (>1000 copies/mL) at about 36 weeks' gestation, caesarean section remains an option for delivery. Hence, the mode of delivery decisions to prevent HIV transmission should be individualised and take into account factors such as type and duration of ART regimen used, viral load, duration of membrane rupture, amount of time expected until vaginal delivery is accomplished and patient's preference.

When vaginal delivery is the accepted option, some modifications to standard obstetric practice (through minimising the exposure of the infant to infected maternal blood and cervico-vaginal secretions) have been associated with reduction in the risk of perinatal transmission. These include:

- Avoidance of prolonged rupture of membrane (>4 hours). Artificial rupture of membranes should be avoided as much as possible until second stage of labour.
- Avoidance of prolonged labour.
- Regular swabbing of the vagina with 0.25% chlorhexidine, especially before every vaginal examination.
- Avoidance of invasive procedures that breaks the baby's skin, such as intrauterine pressure catheters, penetrating scalp electrodes or scalp blood sampling.
- Avoidance of routine episiotomy and perineal lacerations. Episiotomy should be undertaken only when indicated.
- Avoidance of instrumental deliveries. Vacuum extraction especially is associated with micro-lacerations of the scalp.

Elective caesarean section has been associated with up to 50% reduction in the risk of MTCT [33]. Recent reports suggest that caesarean section can be avoided if effective antiretroviral therapy is used to maximally suppress maternal viral load to <1000 copies/ml near the time of delivery [48]. Mother-to-child transmission risk is significantly reduced in women who had vaginal delivery while on effective antiretroviral drugs and with low viral load. The benefits of caesarean delivery in reducing transmission in women on antiretroviral and with low viral load may still be present but would be of small magnitude. Caesarean section is also associated with several fold increased risk of postpartum infections, including uterine infections and pneumonia, anaesthesia risks and surgical complications [49]. When caesarean section is the choice, it should be undertaken at 38 weeks, before the onset of labour (elective or schedule) and prior to rupture of membranes. The use of prophylactic antibiotics is essential to prevent infections which tend to be common in situations associated with immune deficiency.

35.6.5 Postpartum Care

In the immediate postpartum period, routine physical examination with emphasis on the vital signs, detection of anaemia, breast, abdomen and perineum (e.g. for tears, bleeding, infected lochia, etc.) is recommended. HIV-infected women are more prone to postnatal infections including urinary tract infection (UTI), acute respiratory tract infection (ARI), puerperal sepsis, infected episiotomy and caesarean section wound sepsis. An organised follow-up care and referral is essential for effective management of HIV-related medical and social problems.

Issues to be addressed in the postpartum period include the following:

- Review and support for the infant feeding method chosen by the mother
- Good perineal hygiene and proper handling of body fluids
- Discussion about issues of partner testing, sexual activity and protection of sexual partners against HIV infection
- Need for contraception and use of condom
- Continuation or commencement of maternal antiretroviral therapy or prophylaxis
- Prophylaxis for opportunistic infections and TB management if indicated
- Infant ARV prophylaxis
- Infection prevention and prompt medical treatment
- Importance of early infant diagnosis at 6 weeks
- Schedule postnatal visits at 2, 4 and 6 weeks and baby immunisation
- Need for referral to adult ART clinic after postnatal period

Breast care In order to avoid cracked nipples, mastitis and breast abscess, breastfeeding mothers should be educated on the following:

- Correct breastfeeding technique with proper attachment of baby on breast
- Prompt treatment of vaginal thrush and/or infant oral thrush
- Washing the breast once daily and avoiding use of creams and lotions on the nipples

Women who do not breastfeed should wear a comfortable brassier to limit milk production and support the breast.

35.6.6 Contraception

Following appropriate counselling, review of medication, medical history and clinical assessment, HIV-infected clients can be offered an appropriate and effective contraception in the postpartum period. Apart from nonoxynol-9 (spermicides), most methods of contraception may be utilised, including lactational amenorrhea method (LAM), male and female condoms, hormonal methods, intra-uterine contraceptive devices and sterilisation. Dual contraception with concomitant use of a more effective contraceptive method and male or female condom to prevent HIV and STIs is the standard. It is therefore necessary to make provision for contraceptive service as part of comprehensive care for the HIV-infected client [50]. HIV-positive women who may be on infant formulae need special attention for contraception as they lack the contraceptive benefits of breastfeeding.

35.6.7 Cervical Screening

Due to higher risk of cervical dysplasia and cervical cancer in HIV-positive women, it is recommended that they should have cervical smear during the postnatal check-up and at least annually. Six monthly smears are advised in women with CD4 count below 200 cells/mL or those with symptoms of AIDS [11].

35.6.8 Management of HIV-Exposed Infants

35.6.8.1 Immediate Care

The immediate care of the newborn includes the following:

- Mouth and nostrils should be wiped with gauze at delivery of the head.
- Clamp cord immediately after baby is delivered and avoid milking of the cord.
- Cut cord under cover of lightly wrapped gauze swab to avoid blood spurts.
- Keep baby warm by placing infant on mother's body for skin-to-skin contact.
- Wipe dry with a towel or surgical cloth to remove maternal blood and body fluids.
- If indicated, use mechanical/electrical suction unit at a pressure below 100 mmHg or bulb suction. Mouth-operated suction should be avoided.
- Give vitamin K injection after baby has been properly cleaned, ensuring injection safety.
- Support mother to initiate her choice of infant feeding within 30 minutes of delivery.

35.6.8.2 Antiretroviral Prophylaxis

As part of measure to prevent HIV transmission to the newborn, all HIV-exposed neonates should receive post-exposure prophylaxis which should be commenced within 72 hours of birth. Nevirapine or zidovudine syrup should be given for 6 weeks or longer in situations where the mother did not receive optimal ART prior to delivery.

35.6.8.3 Prophylaxis for Opportunistic Infections

For prophylaxis against *Pneumocystis jirovecii* pneumonia (PCP), HIV-exposed infants should be offered co-trimoxazole (CTX) from 6 weeks until HIV status is determined. HIV-positive infants are continued on CTX.

Babies born to HIV-positive women with open tuberculosis (still infectious) who opt to breastfeed should receive prophylaxis against tuberculosis using isoniazid (INH) 5 mg/kg/day for 6 months. Vaccination with BCG is either delayed until INH prophylaxis is completed or repeated after completing course. INH-resistant BCG may also be given.

35.6.8.4 Infant Feeding

Breast milk is regarded as the best food for infants because of its nutrition, protective, psychological and economic values. Breastfeeding also has contraceptive benefits in women. Postnatal transmission through breast milk is a major source of paediatric infection in developing countries where breastfeeding is the norm. HIV-infected pregnant women in developed countries are requested not to breastfeed their babies, and this has contributed to the low level of MTCT in these societies.

Efforts to reduce MTCT through breast milk led to recommendation of use of replacement feeding (in form of commercial infant formula or home-prepared formula from animal sources like cow or camel) when it is acceptable, feasible, affordable, sustainable and safe (AFASS). Replacement feeding has, however, been associated with higher mortality and morbidity from diarrhoea, malnutrition and pneumonia in infants in many settings where it was used in developing countries. Recent reports also indicate that transmission through breast milk can be significantly reduced if the mother and/or baby is placed on antiretroviral drugs during the period of breastfeeding [51]. This was the basis for the current recommendation of exclusive breastfeeding for the first 6 months of life, introducing appropriate complementary foods thereafter, and continue breastfeeding till the infant reaches 12 months of age and discontinue once a nutritionally adequate and safe diet without breast milk can be provided. The mother is expected to be on lifelong antiretroviral treatment or extended antiretroviral prophylaxis until 1 week after cessation of all breast milk and the infant on nevirapine or zidovudine prophylaxis for 6 weeks [10, 51].

35.6.8.5 Early Infant Diagnosis

Early infant diagnosis (EID) using polymerase chain reaction (PCR), for example DNA PCR, to detect the presence of viral particle can be undertaken soon after birth. Current practice is to confirm diagnosis at 6 weeks. Antibody testing may not reliably confirm the true HIV status of a child until 18 months of age. Early diagnosis is necessary in tracking the effectiveness of efforts to prevent MTCT. It enables early commencement of ARV therapy in HIV-infected infants. It also serves as incentive for women to adopt measures that will ensure their babies remain HIV negative [52, 53].

35.6.9 Summary and Conclusion

HIV is more readily transmitted and acquired during pregnancy. The prevalence of HIV infection in pregnancy is high in developing countries. All pregnant women should be tested for HIV using the opt-out strategy. Those that test negative in early pregnancy should have a repeat HIV test in the third trimester or during labour. Women seen for the first time during labour should have rapid HIV test in labour or in the immediate postpartum period. HIV in pregnancy is a major concern as it is associated with adverse outcomes in pregnancy – spontaneous miscarriage, preterm delivery, intrauterine growth restriction (IUGR), low birth weight and maternal mortality. HIV adversely affects the frequency, natural history presentation and treatments of many infections in pregnancy including vulvo-vaginal candidiasis, bacterial vaginosis, genital herpes simplex, syphilis, trichomonas vaginalis, hepatitis B and C, urinary tract infections and bacterial pneumonia. HIV-related opportunistic infections – such as tuberculosis, *Pneumocystis jirovecii* pneumonia – are more frequent during pregnancy. Another major concern about HIV infection in pregnancy is the risk of transmission of the virus to the baby. Multiple strategies involving biomedical, behavioural and structural approaches should be engaged in HIV prevention.

The four-pronged WHO recommendation for prevention of mother-to-child transmission (PMTCT) of HIV are as follows: (i). primary prevention of HIV infection in women of reproductive age and their partners; (ii). prevention of unintending pregnancies among HIV-positive women; (iii). prevention of HIV transmission from infected pregnant women to their infants; (iv). provision of appropriate treatment, care and support to HIV-infected mothers, their infants, partners and family. This approach has resulted in significant reduction of MTCT of HIV from the base line value of 25–45% to less than 2% in many countries. There is good prospect of eliminating MTCT of HIV by the year 2030 in many countries. Preconception counselling for HIV-positive women is essential. Prior to pregnancy, persons living with HIV should be provided reproductive health services including contraception until her health situation is optimised and safe for pregnancy. The obstetrics and medical care for an HIV-positive woman should be strengthened and modified. In addition to the standard antenatal care, they should be evaluated and managed appropriately for HIV-related illnesses and opportunistic infections. HIV-positive pregnant women should receive appropriate antiretroviral treatment in line with current recommendations. The strategy of providing antiretroviral treatment for all HIV-positive clients irrespective of CD4 count and WHO clinical stage has potential of improving maternal health and eliminating mother-to-child transmission of HIV. Vaginal delivery should be allowed except in women with high viral load (1000 copies/mL or more) at term or when there are other indications for caesarean section. The use of invasive monitoring techniques, such as intrauterine pressure catheter or foetal scalp electrode, and operative vaginal delivery should be avoided as they can increase risk for perinatal transmission. Breast milk feeding is discouraged in settings where formula feeding is acceptable, feasible, affordable, sustainable and safe. However, exclusive breastfeeding of HIV-exposed infants is the preferred option in many developing countries. Breast milk transmission is rare if the mother and/or baby are placed on antiretroviral drugs during the period of breastfeeding. Health workers should be abreast of new research findings related to HIV in pregnancy to ensure the benefits of new scientific information are promptly translated to clinical care.

References

1. UNAIDS. Global report: UNAIDS report on the global AIDS epidemic. Geneva: UNAIDS; 2012.
2. Dabis F, Leroy V, Castetbon K, et al. Preventing mother-to-child transmission of HIV-1 in Africa in the year 2000. AIDS. 2000;14:1017–26.
3. Dabis F, Ekpini ER. HIV-1/AIDS and maternal and child health in Africa. Lancet. 2002;359:2097–104.
4. Pallela FJ, Delaney KM, Moorman AC, Loveless MO, Fuhrer J, Satten GA, et al. Declining morbidity and mortality among patients with advanced human immunodeficiency virus infection. N Engl J Med. 1998;338:853–60.
5. Townsend C, Cortina-Borja M, Peckham C, Lyall H, de Ruiter A, Tookey P. Very low risk of mother-to-child transmission of HIV in women on HAART achieving viral suppression in the UK and Ireland. AIDS. 2008;22:973–81.
6. McKenna MT, Hu X. Recent trends in the incidence and morbidity that are associated with perinatal human immunodeficiency virus infection in the United States. Am J Obstet Gynecol. 2007;197:S10–6.
7. Mahy M, Stover J, Kirigu L, Hayashi C, Akwara P, Luo C, et al. What will it take to achieve virtual elimination of mother-to-child transmission of HIV? An assessment of current progress and future needs. Sex Transm Infect. 2010;86(Suppl 2):ii48–55.
8. Bartlett, JG, Gallant JE. Medical management of HIV infection. 2004th ed. Baltimore: Johns Hopkins Medicine Health Publishing Business Group, 2004.
9. US Department of Health and Human Services, Health Resources and Services. A guide to the clinical care of women with HIV/AIDS - 2013 edition. Rockville, Maryland. Department of Health and Human Services, Health Resources and Services. 2013. Available at: http://www.hab.hrsa.gov. Accessed 5 July 2016.
10. World Health Organization. WHO case definition of HIV for surveillance and revised clinical staging and immunological classification of HIV-related disease in adults and children. Geneva, WHO. 2007. Available at: http://www.who.int/hiv/pub/guigelines/HIVstaging150307.pdf. Accessed 5 July 2016.
11. Agboghoroma OC. Gynaecological and reproductive health issues in HIV-positive women. West Afr J Med. 2010;29(3):135–42.
12. UNAIDS. Global AIDS update 2016. Global AIDS Response Progress Reporting (GARPR) 2016; UNAIDS 2016 estimates. Available at: http://wwwunaids.org. Accessed on 5 July 2016.

13. Federal Ministry of Health (FMOH). 2014. National HIV sero-prevalence sentinel survey among pregnant women attending ante-natal clinics in Nigeria. Abuja. FMOH; 2015.
14. National Agency for the Control of AIDS (NACA). Nigeria HIV/AIDS Indicator and Impart Survey (NAIIS): national summary sheet. Abuja. NACA; 2019.
15. Agboghoroma OC, Giwa-Osagie OF. Infertility management in HIV-positive clients. Afr J Reprod Health. 2012;16(4):13–20.
16. French R, Brocklehurst P. The effect of pregnancy on survival in women infected with HIV: a systematic review of the literature and meta-analysis. Br J Obstet Gynaecol. 1998;105:827–35.
17. Ryder RW, Nsa W, Hassig SE, Behets F, Rayfield M, Ekungola B, et al. Perinatal transmission of the human immunodeficiency virus type 1 to infants of seropositive woman in Zaire. N Engl J Med. 1989;320:1637–42.
18. Brocklehurst P, French R. The association between maternal HIV – infection and perinatal outcome: a systematic review of the literature and meta-analysis. Br J Obstet Gynaecol. 1998;105:836–48.
19. Khan KS, Wojdyia D, Say L, Gulmezoglu AM, Van Look PFA. WHO analysis of causes of maternal death: a systemic review. Lancet. 2006;367:1066–74.
20. The Working Group on Mother – to – Child Transmission of HIV. Rates of mother-to-child transmission of HIV I in Africa, America and Europe: result from 13 perinatal studies. J Acquir Immune Defic Syndr Hum Retrovirol. 1995;8:506–10.
21. De Cock KM, Fowler MG, Mercier E, et al. Prevention of mother-to-child HIV transmission in resource-poor countries: translating research into policy and practice. JAMA. 2000;283:1175–82.
22. Rouzious C, Costagliola D, Burgard M, et al. Estimating timing of mother-to-child human immunodeficiency virus type 1 (HIV-1) transmission by use of a Markov model: the HIV infection in Newborns French Collaboration Study Group. Am J Epidemiol. 1995;142:1330–7.
23. Dunn DT, Newell ML, Ades AE, Peckham CS. Risk of human immunodeficiency virus type 1 transmission through breast-feeding. Lancet. 1992;340:585–8.
24. Garcia PM, Kalish IA, Pitt J, et al. Maternal levels of plasma human immunodeficiency virus type I RNA and the risk of perinatal transmission. N Engl J Med. 1999;341:394–420.
25. British HIV Association. British HIV Association guidelines for the management of HIV infection in pregnant women 2012 (2014 interim review). HIV Med. 2014;15(Suppl. 4):1–77.
26. Dickover R, Garratty E, Plaeger S, Bryson Y. Perinatal transmission of major, minor, and multiple HIV-I strains in Utero and intrapartum. 7th Conf. Retroviruses Opportunistic infect (Abst 181), Jan 30 Feb. 2, 2000.
27. Reinhardt PP, Reinhardt B, Lathey JL, Spector SA. Human cord blood mononuclear cells are preferentially infected by non-syncytium-inducing, macrophage tropic human immunodeficiency virus type I isolates. J Clin Microbiol. 1995;233:292–7.
28. Kuhn L, Abrams EJ, Weedon J, et al. Disease progression and early viral dynamics in human immunodeficiency virus-infected children exposed to zidovudine during prenatal and perinatal periods. J Infect Dis. 2000;182:104–11.
29. Nimmagadda A, O'Brien WA, Goetz MB. The significance of vitamin A and carotenoid status in persons infected by the human immunodeficiency virus. Clin Infect Dis. 1998;26:711–8.
30. Turner BJ, Hauck WW, Fanning R, Markson LE. Cigarette smoking and maternal-child HIV transmission. J Acquir Immune Defic Syndr Hum Retrovirol. 1997;14:427–37.
31. Lyman WD. Perinatal AIDS: drugs of abuse and transplacental infection. Adv Exp Med Biol. 1993;335:211–7.
32. Goldenberg RI, Vermund SH, Geopfert AR, Andrews WW. Choriodecidual inflammation: a potentially preventable cause of perinatal HIV-I transmission? Lancet. 1998;352:1927–30.
33. International Perinatal HIV Group. The mode of delivery and the risk of vertical transmission of HIV-I: a meta-analysis from fifteen prospective cohort studies (the International Perinatal HIV Group). N Engl J Med. 1999;340:977–87.
34. WHO/UNAIDS. HIV in pregnancy: a review WHO/CHS/RHR/99.15 and UNAIDS/99. 35E 1999.
35. Kostrikis LG, Neumann AU, Thomson B, et al. A polymorphism in the regulatory region of the CC-chemokine receptor 5 gene influences perinatal transmission of human immunodeficiency virus type I to African – American infant. J Virol. 1999;73:10264–71.
36. UNICEF, UNAIDS, WHO. A review of HIV transmission through breast feeding. WHO/FRH/UNT/CHD 98.3 UNAIDS 98.5 UNICEF/PD/NUT (J) 98.3 Geneva 1998.
37. UNAIDS. Countdown to zero. Global plan towards the elimination of new HIV infections among children by 2015 and keeping their mothers alive. Geneva, UNAIDS; 2011.
38. Federal Ministry of Health. National guidelines for HIV prevention, treatment and care. Abuja: Federal Ministry of Health; 2016.
39. World Health Organization. Consolidated guidelines on the use of antiretroviral drugs for treating and preventing HIV infection. Recommendations for a public health approach. 2nd ed. Geneva: World Health Organization; 2016.
40. World Health Organization. Updated recommendations on first line and second line antiretroviral regimens and post-exposure prophylaxis and recommendations on early infant diagnosis of HIV: interim guidelines. Supplement to the 2016 consolidated guidelines on the use of antiretroviral drugs for treating and preventing HIV infection. Geneva: World Health Organization; 2018.
41. Cooper E, Charurar M, Burns DN, Blattner W, Hoff R. Trends in antiretroviral therapy and mother-infant transmissioin of HIV. The Women and Infants Transmission Study Group. J Acquir Immune Defic Syndr. 2000;24(1):45–7.
42. Royal College of Obstetricians and Gynaecologists. Management of HIV in pregnancy. Guideline No. 39, 2004. RCOG, London.
43. Cohen MS, et al. Prevention of HIV-1 infection with early antiretroviral therapy. N Engl J Med. 2011;365(6):496–505.
44. Galli L, Puliti D, Chiappini E, et al. Is the interruption of antiretroviral treatment during pregnancy an additional major risk factor for mother-to-child transmission of HIV type 1? Clin Infect Dis. 2009;48(9):1310–7.
45. Agboghoroma OC. Management of HIV in pregnancy: a clinical review. Trop J Obstet Gynaecol. 2005;22(1):65–73.
46. Fawzi WW, Msamanga GI, Spiegelman D, Urassa EJN, McGrath N, Mwakagile D, et al. Randomised trial of effects of vitamin supplements on pregnancy outcomes on T-cell counts in HIV-I infected women in Tanzania. Lancet. 1998;351:1477–82.
47. Ayisi JG, Van Ejik AM, Newman RD, ter Kuile FO, Shi YP, Yang C, et al. Maternal malaria and perinatal HIV transmission. Emerg Infect Dis. 2004;10(4):643–52.
48. Centres for Disease Control and Prevention. United States Public Health Service Task Force recommendations for use of antiretroviral drugs in pregnant HIV-1 infected women for maternal health and Interventions to reduce perinatal HIV-1 transmission in the United States. MMWR 2002;51 (No. RR-18).
49. van Ham MA, van Dongen PJ, Mulder J. Maternal consequences of caesarean section. A retrospective study of intra-operative and post-operative maternal complications of caesarean section during a 10-year period. Eur J Obstet Gynecol Reprod Biol. 1997;74:1–6.
50. Agboghoroma OC. Contraception in the context of HIV/AIDS. A review. Afr J Reprod Health. 2011;15(3):15–23.
51. World Health Organization. Guidelines on HIV and infant feeding 2010. Geneva: World Health Organization; 2010.
52. Agboghoroma OC. Prevention of mother-to-child transmission of HIV/AIDS. In: Okonofua FE, editor. Confronting the challenge of reproductive health in Africa: a textbook for students and development practitioners. Benin: WHARC; 2014. p. 345–66.
53. Donnelly M, Davies JK. Contemporary management of human immunodeficiency virus in pregnancy. In: Swamy GK, Rayburn WF, editors. Obstet Gynaecol Clin North Am Infect Dis Pregnancy. 2014;41(4):547–67.

Non-HIV Viral Infections in Pregnancy

36

Joseph Onakewhor, Toby Kenneth Maduako, and Friday Okonofua

Learning Objectives

At the conclusion of this chapter, the reader should be able to:

- The epidemiology, clinical features and management of hepatitis B, hepatitis C and rubella viruses in pregnancy.
- Their modes of acquisition and transmissibility.
- The prevention methods useful for reducing the burden of the infections in developing countries.
- Research gaps relating to these viral infections in pregnancy with relevance to developing countries.

36.1 Introduction

Hepatitis B virus (HBV) is an infectious virus that attacks liver cells causing their necrosis and inflammation [1, 2]. Hepatitis B virus (HBV) genome is a partially double-stranded circular DNA molecule of ~3.2 kb in length. It is ubiquitous, heterogeneous and virulent [3].

There are eight hepatitis B virus genotypes; A, B, C, D, E, F, G and H. The genotype E (HBV/E) predominates in the West and Central African crescent spanning from Senegal to Angola. Genotypes A and D are few. In Nigeria, the main HBV genotype is E (HBV/E) accounting for 96.4% and few are HBV/A3 accounting for 3.6% of cases [3].

36.1.1 Epidemiology

Though hepatitis B is a vaccine-preventable infection [4], it constitutes a major global health risk and is a silent epidemic. While the estimated global population of people who have sero-markers for current and past infection of HBV is put at about two billion [3], estimated 240 million (4–6% of the world population) are chronically infected and are carriers of the virus [1, 5].

Chronic carriers are persons infected with the virus who are unable to clear the virus within 6 months of acquiring the infection [1]. Though HBV is a vaccine-preventable infection [1, 6], efforts to achieve prevention are yet to yield the desired results. About 4.5 million new infections occur each year. The onset of acute disease is usually insidious with one out of four progressing to liver disease. Hepatitis viral infections cause approximately 1.45 million deaths each year due to chronic active hepatitis, cirrhosis and primary liver carcinoma [1, 7, 8].

The infection is transmitted via contact with or exchange of body fluids from infected person through vertical and or horizontal modes of infection. Exposed infants are at risk of infection through mother-to child transmission (MTCT) [3, 9, 10]. Chronic infection occurs in about 90% of infected infants. Children less than 5 years of age account for about 30%, while those aged 5 years and above account for less than 5% of infection. The continued viral replication in the liver and persistent viraemia accentuates the disease and the risk of infection [3].

36.1.2 Grading of the Prevalence of Hepatitis B Surface Antigen and Geographic Distribution of HBV Infection

The prevalence of hepatitis B surface (HBsAg+) is graded into three groups:

J. Onakewhor (Deceased)
University of Benin, Benin City, Nigeria

University of Benin Teaching Hospital, Benin City, Nigeria

T. K. Maduako
University of Benin Teaching Hospital, Benin City, Nigeria

F. Okonofua (✉)
Centre of Excellence in Reproductive Health Innovation, Department of Obstetrics and Gynaecology, University of Benin, Benin City, Nigeria

Women's Health and Action Research Centre, Benin City, Nigeria

University of Medical Sciences, Ondo City, Ondo State, Nigeria

F. Okonofua et al. (eds.), *Contemporary Obstetrics and Gynecology for Developing Countries*,
https://doi.org/10.1007/978-3-030-75385-6_36

(i) High ≥8%
(ii) Intermediate 2–7%
(iii) Low <2%

The prevalence of HBsAg+ is high in most sub-Saharan countries including Nigeria. The prevalence of the antigen (HBsAg+) in Nigeria is reported to be between 8% and 11% in the general population. Some studies have reported higher prevalence of up to 40% [3, 11].

At the University of Benin Teaching Hospital (UBTH) [9, 10, 12], we reported a prevalence of 4.3% among pregnant women and 6.8% among spouses of HBV-infected pregnant women (who were seropositive for the virus). This high prevalence is not unconnected with the delay in commencing routine screening and vaccination of the Nigerian population against the virus.

The vaccination of children against HBV was introduced into the Nigerian National Program on Immunization (NPI) in 1995. However, the service became available only in 2004 [3, 13, 14]. The pentavalent (five-in-one) vaccine for protection against diphtheria, tetanus, whooping cough, HBV and *H. influenza* type b (all through a single dose) [9] was introduced into the NPI on June 22, 2012 [15].

Other factors that contribute to the high prevalence of the virus in Nigeria include the lack of national HBV surveillance programme and the MTCT of HBV in utero during pregnancy, intrapartum and postnatal period [16, 17]. The initial low immunization coverage increased from about 15% in 1979 to 80% in 2007 [3].

36.1.3 Mother-to-Child Transmission of Hepatitis B Infection

The best intervention to prevent mother-to-child transmission (MTC) of hepatitis B infection is by getting the mother tested in the pre-pregnancy period and getting her immunized with HBV vaccine. This will eliminate the infection and prevent MTCT. Immunoprophylaxis with 200 IU hepatitis B immunoglobulin (HBIG) followed by standard vaccination can prevent MTCT by 95% [18]. With the combination of maternal antenatal anti-retroviral treatment with appropriate infant vaccination, the rate of MTCT and vaccine non-response can be significantly reduced [19, 20].

In the absence of post-exposure immunoprophylaxis, HBV-exposed newborns whose mothers are HBsAg+/HBeAg+ positive have 70–90% risk of having chronic infection at the age of 6 months [21] while HBsAg+/HBeAg-exposed infants have less than a 10% risk of having chronic infection in the absence of post-exposure immunoprophylaxis [22]. Among women in Sydney, Australia, the reported MTCT rate was 3% [23], while 65% was reported for Indian women with HBeAg+ and HBV DNA [24].

The presence of HBeAg in a pregnant woman is a risk factor for MTCT. The reported prevalence of this antigen among Sydney [23] and Indian women [24] was 29% and 56.8% while 12.5% was reported in Turkish for same population with anti-HBe of 77.8% [25]. We have reported HBeAg prevalence of 3.0% and anti-HBe (HBeAb) of 77.5% at the UBTH, with no infant infected [12].

36.1.4 Signs and Symptoms of HBV

The clinical signs and symptoms due to HBV infection are indistinguishable from that due to other forms of viral hepatitis. Thus, serologic testing for virus-specific diagnosis may be necessary [26]. Though HBV is a common cause of jaundice, haemolysis due to malaria in pregnancy in malaria endemic regions, haemoglobinothies and HELLP (haemolysis, elevated liver enzymes and low platelet count) syndrome due to pre-eclampsia are differential diagnoses that require evaluation. The symptoms of malaise, anorexia, fever, weakness and nausea may mimic those of malaria or urinary tract infection in pregnancy and these should be excluded by appropriate laboratory tests.

36.1.5 Diagnosis and Evaluation of HBV-Infected Pregnant Women

The diagnosis of HBV infection starts with the history of exposure to HBV which many patients may not know or remember as the infection may be insidious. History of previous jaundice may be relevant and for infants and children, history of HBV-infected mother is relevant. The most common cause of jaundice in *pregnancy is* acute viral *hepatitis* [26]:

History of multiple sexual partners and sexual intercourse with sero-discordant partners where the seronegative is not protected by immunization [9, 27], transfusion of unscreened blood or transplant of an infected organ, illicit drug use, sharing of sharp objects as in tattoos or scarifications for social or medical purposes are risk factors for HBV infection. Others are family history of liver disease and hepatocellular carcinoma (HCC).

36.1.6 Laboratory Diagnosis

Routine screening is advised for the general population especially those at risk which include health workers and those involved in risky social and sexual behaviours.

The simplest laboratory diagnosis is the detection of the hepatitis B surface antigen (HBsAg) in the clients' blood using simple rapid tests. The test is cheap and easily available and can be used at primary healthcare level when staffs are well trained to carry out the tests. Recent availability of five-panel test to detect not just the surface antigen, but in addition, the HBeAg and antibodies to the surface antigen (anti-HBsAg), HBeAb (anti-HBe) and HBcAb (IgG/IgM antibodies) has been of immense value [12].

Tests should be done to assess HBV replication by assaying for viral load (HBV DNA) using Polymerase Chain Reaction (PCR) test, where the facility is available.

Laboratory evaluation of the liver disease is essential, and these include complete blood counts with platelets and hepatic panel, total and direct serum bilirubin, alanine aminotransferase (ALT) and/or aspartate aminotransferase (AST) and alkaline phosphatase (ALP). Others are prothrombin time (PT), total protein, albumin and, in severe cases, serum ammonia. These tests are useful to diagnose hepatitis [1, 26].

Tests should also be done to exclude other differential diagnosis of HBV and viral co-infections. These include hepatitis C virus (HCV), human immunodeficiency virus (HIV), mononucleosis and Epstein-Barr virus (EBV) infections, autoimmune disease and widespread systemic infection with liver failure and HELLP syndrome [1, 12, 26]. Manteaux test for tuberculosis (TB) is required, especially when there is HIV/HBV co-infection. Screening for hepatocellular carcinoma (HCC) by assaying for Alfa fetoprotein (AFP) at baseline and in high-risk patients is essential. Ultrasound evaluation of the liver architecture and the foetus is of value. Liver biopsy can be done after delivery to grade and stage liver disease for patients who meet criteria for chronic hepatitis [1].

36.1.7 Management of HBV-Infected Pregnant Women

After confirmation of diagnosis of HBV infection, clinical and laboratory evaluation of the patient should be carried out. The HBV+ pregnant mother is co-managed with a physician (gastroenterologist) and commenced on antiretroviral drugs (ARVs) throughout the duration of the pregnancy, while the paediatrician is notified about the impending delivery of HBV-exposed baby with the intention to commence the newborn on hepatitis B immunoglobulin (HBIG) at birth and HBV vaccination following the Guidelines on National Programme on Immunization. The patient's evaluation continues throughout pregnancy and delivery, after which she should be referred to the physician for follow-up management.

36.1.8 Drug Treatment

In hepatitis B mono-infected pregnant women, the World Health Organization [1] recommends the same indications for treatment as in other adults, and Tenofovir is the drug of choice.

Those to be given priority for treatment include adults, adolescents and children with chronic hepatitis B (CHB) and when there is clinical evidence of cirrhosis (compensated or decompensated). Adults who are more than 30 years in age without clinical evidence of cirrhosis but with persistent abnormally elevated ALT levels and high viral replication (load >20,000 IU/mL) should be treated as well [1]. Also recommended for treatment are persons with only persistently abnormal levels of ALT irrespective of HBeAg status, when HBV DNA testing is unavailable (conditional recommendation, low quality evidence) [1].

Although the WHO made no recommendation for the routine use of antiretroviral drugs for PMTCT of HBV to prevent MTCT, in HIV/HBV co-infected pregnant women, treatment is recommended. In such cases, the first line of treatment is once daily fixed-dose combination of tenofovir + lamivudine (or emtricitabine) + Efaverenz. This regimen is also recommended as first line for lifelong treatment of HIV and antiretroviral therapy initiated for PMTCT [1]. The current WHO Guideline (WHO, 2016) [28] recommends lifelong treatment of all HIV-infected persons irrespective of CD4+ Cell count or viral load levels as the 'public health approach'. Optimum drug selection and monitoring are essential taking into cognizance side effects and the long-term sequelae of the drugs on both mother and foetus/infant.

At the UBTH, Benin City, Nigeria PMTCT of HBV infection programme was introduced into the antenatal care in 2005. The result of the evaluation of the programme showing the time and gestational age at diagnosis is shown in the figure below [12].

The mother is commenced on Lamivudine 150 mg, twice daily and Tenofovir 300 mg daily in the antenatal period throughout pregnancy and delivery.

Monitoring of renal function is mandatory during tenofovir therapy. After delivery, the woman is referred to the physician (Gastroenterologist) for further evaluation and follow-up management.

The baby is followed up by the paediatrician and the outcome of the prevention of MTCT of HBV is assessed. The result of the outcome of the programme at the UBTH has been very encouraging, with a recorded 100% prevention of MTCT for the HBV-exposed babies that were followed up to 12 months after birth [12]. However, exposed babies were more likely (11.3%) to be non-responders (HBsAb negative) to the standard-three-dose vaccination compared with 3.0% for non-exposed infants; $p < 0.01$ [12]. In contrast,

Schönberger et al. [29] reported antibody titres ≥10 mIU/ml were detected in 75.8% of children of HBV-carrier mothers compared with 63.6% of non-carrier mothers [29].

36.1.9 Management of Hepatitis B-Exposed Babies

The recommendation for HBV-exposed neonates is the administration of hepatitis B immunoprophylaxis with 200 IU HBV immunoglobulin (HBIG) within 12 hours of birth. In addition, a three-course vaccination with hepatitis B vaccine at birth is recommended starting first dose as soon as possible and preferably within 24 hours. The second dose is given 4–6 weeks later and the third dose is given at 6 months after birth in accordance with national programmes on immunization. The standard testing to determine immune response requires quantitative assay for anti-HBs levels. Effective immunization is expected to produce adequate immune response with antibodies>10mIU/mL [30–32]. Full response to vaccination occurs in about 85–90% of individuals and can provide protection for at least 25 years [33].

36.1.10 Vaccine Non-responders

Some vaccinated individuals may not respond adequately to the immunization with the standard three-intramuscular-dose series of the HB vaccine by failing to produce protective antibody levels (anti-Hbs antibody >10 mIU/mL) [30–33]. The incidence of non-responders is put at 5–10% among healthy individuals [30] and administration of booster doses may be indicated [34–40].

At the UBTH, we reported vaccine non-response rate of 8% among babies followed up for 12 months and had booster doses. Similar level of non-response (6.7%) was reported for among Brazilian women with HIV/HBV co-infection [41].

The risk factors for poor or non-response to HBV vaccination include current or past HBV infections, preterm neonates with birth weight <2000 g vaccinated at age <1 month [13] male gender and obesity [36], alcohol, smoking, increasing age especially age of 40 years, advanced liver disease, renal dialysis patients [42] and other immunosuppression conditions including HIV [43].

Newborns, health-care workers, renal dialysis [42] and diabetic [44] patients and others at –risk of HBV infection [19] are recommended for routine vaccinations. In HIV+ mothers, when maternal antenatal anti-retroviral treatment is combined with appropriate infant vaccination (HBIG plus HBV Vaccination), the rate of MTCT and vaccine non-response is reduced [1, 45].

36.1.11 Breastfeeding

Though some studies have reported MTCT of HBV during breastfeeding, the general recommendation is that breastfeeding is not contraindicated in HBV-infected mothers [1, 46], provided the viral load is low, no cracked nipples or other risk factors contraindicating breastfeeding are absent.

36.2 Prevention

Prevention is the most effective way of managing this infection and the steps stated below are critically essential.

36.2.1 General Awareness

General awareness is low; many persons are yet to acknowledge the reality of the virus in the population. Worldwide, hepatitis is still being largely ignored [47]. Raising the awareness of the general population of the existence and risks associated with hepatitis B infection is an important public health measure to curtail the disease. This should lead to behavioural modification, avoidance of risky behaviours and embarking on personal and general measures including vaccination to prevent the infection.

To raise awareness and understanding of viral hepatitis and the diseases that it causes, the World Health Organization (WHO) and partners mark **World Hepatitis Day** with various themes on July 28 every year. The sixth World Hepatitis Day in 2013, was marked with the overall theme 'See no evil, speak no evil, hear no evil', represented by the **three wise monkeys**, with an old proverb that is commonly used to highlight how people often deal with problems by refusing to acknowledge them' [47]. It emphasizes, '**This is hepatitis... Know it. Confront it**'. '**It is a silent killer**' [47]. In 2014, The WHD theme was 'Hepatitis: Think again' [48]. In 2015, the theme was '**Prevent *hepatitis*. Act now**' and in May 2016, the World Health Assembly adopted the theme for WHD 2016 as '**... elimination**' [49]. These captivating themes are strategies put in place to raise awareness and measures to aid 'elimination movement' for hepatitis.

36.2.2 Vaccination

Hepatitis B vaccine is 95% effective in preventing the infection. Maurice Hilleman in 1981 discovered the vaccine and vaccination was first introduced in 1982. The recombinant vaccine by Pablo DT Valenzuela in 1986 [5] replaced the earlier vaccine [12]. Efforts to achieve universal prevention are being intensified [1]. The introduction of routine HBV screening of pregnant women into antenatal care programmes should be part of the elimination plan. Uninfected (seronegative) women should be vaccinated after delivery. Exposed infants should have HBIG at birth and complete routine vaccination on schedule [22] and screened for evidence of protection or infection and managed accordingly.

Currently, 81% of world's infants are vaccinated and protected from hepatitis B infection. However, many developing countries are lagging behind in this very important prevention strategy [30]. Generally, the **three-intramuscular-dose series of the HBV vaccine fail** to produce protective antibody levels (> 10 mIU/mL) in 5%–10% of healthy individuals [30, 31]for reasons stated previously. The need for booster doses in HB vaccine programmes is controversial and the WHO has not recommended universal administration of booster doses [30]. However, under condition of non-response to HBV vaccination, booster doses have been proven to be beneficial [3–32, 50]. For co-infections such as HIV and other infections, causes of immunization failure should be investigated.

36.2.3 Antenatal and Partner screening for HBV

Where routine screening of pregnant women for HBsAg to determine HBV infection is not currently being practised and especially in developing countries of Africa and Asia where the infection is endemic and high (>8%) [1, 30], measures should be taken urgently to address and institute such interventions. Partners (spouses) should be screened, and those infected are referred for treatment and while the seronegatives persons have complete vaccination.

36.2.4 Course of *Hepatitis B* Virus (*HBV*) Infection on *Pregnancy*

It is not clear what the *effect* of chronic *hepatitis B* virus (*HBV*) infection on *pregnancy* is [51]. Similarly, the *impact* of *pregnancy* on the clinical *course* of acute *hepatitis B* is still unclear mainly because most studies have not included matched controls [52]. However, the risk of developing chronic HBV is as high as 90% in those exposed at birth without vaccination. In those exposed during childhood, the risk is much lower (20–30%). Thus, HBV infection is inversely proportional to the age at the time of exposure. Maternal screening programmes and universal vaccination of infants have significantly reduced transmission HBV rates [53].

36.3 Other Viruses in Pregnancy

Because there is no vaccine for protection for these viruses and routine screening in pregnancy is not recommended by the World Health Organization, they will not be discussed in detail in this chapter. However, prevention strategies should be upheld in all circumstances.

36.4 Hepatitis C Viral Infection in Pregnancy

With the availability of vaccine for the prevention of hepatitis B infection and its control being firmly established, other viruses are becoming important on their deleterious effects on human health. Hepatitis C viral (HCV) infection is currently a global problem, and its effects are the commonest indication for liver transplant.

36.4.1 Epidemiology

A 2013 estimate of persons with HCV-antibody positive is put at 110 million with 80 million persons being chronically infected [54, 55]. This a downward reversal from the previous estimate of over 170 million people infected with the virus worldwide, and only half of the patients treated with the current standard therapies achieve a sustained viral response [56].

Globally, HCV-related morbidity and mortality due to cirrhosis and hepatocellular carcinoma (HCC) is on the increase with approximately 700,000 deaths occurring each year [55]. In pregnancy, the global seroprevalence of HCV is 0.15–2.4% in the USA and European countries, while Egypt has a much higher prevalence of 8.6% [57, 58].

Viral replication is extremely robust, and more than 10 trillion HCV virion particles are estimated to be produced per day, even in the chronic phase of the infection [59]. Like HIV, HCV has distinct but related genotypes and multiple subtypes with geographical or regional spread. Though, a higher prevalence of 6% and 28% has been reported in the general Egyptian population [57, 58], worldwide, the prevalence of hepatitis C virus (HCV) infection in pregnant women is estimated to be between 1% and 8%, and in children between 0.05% and 5% [59]. At the UBTH, Nigeria, we found a seroprevalence of HCV antibodies in pregnancy to be 1.86% [60]. The diverse morphology and fastidiousness of HCV has made vaccines discovery elusive [58, 60].

36.4.2 Symptoms of Hepatitis C Infection

The infection may be asymptomatic and thus be unnoticed. About 60–70% of patients with acute HCV infection are asymptomatic [61]. When symptoms do occur, these may include fever, abdominal pain, nausea, jaundice, physical illness, malnutrition and increased burden on pregnancy, labour and the puerperium, thereby increasing maternal and neonatal morbidity and mortality. The quality of life, even in the absence of severe disease, can be jeopardized by hepatitis C virus (HCV) infection [62].

While some individuals are able to clear the virus on their own, others may not but harbour the viruses in the liver for more than 6 months and thus become chronic carriers. These carriers may live for many years without major health problems. However, like hepatitis B, active HCV infections can cause severe liver damage; hepatic cirrhosis and cancer [63].

36.4.3 Risk Factors and Mode of Transmission of Hepatitis C Virus

Before the availability of facilities in 1991 for screening HCV in blood meant for transfusions, this was a mode of transmission [63]. However, unscreened blood transfusion in poor health settings still poses risk for HCV infection [64]. Hepatitis C can also be spread from sharing needles by intravenous drugs users (Injection drug abuse) and for tattoos done with needles and paints that have not been properly sterilized and very rarely, and homo- and heterosexual sex are important routes of HCV transmission. Sexual intercourse among monogamous couples accounts for less than 1% infection [63, 65, 66]. Transplant of an infected donor organ is a rare mode of transmission. Intrauterine and perinatal infection can occur during pregnancy and the puerperal infection occurs from HCV-infected mother. While HBV may survive dying for more than 7 days in the dry state and still remain infectious, HCV is infectious only for hours [65].

The estimated transmission risks for needle stick injuries for HBV, HCV and HIV are 30%, 3% and 0.3%, respectively, depending on the size of the inoculum, the size of the needle and the depth of inoculation [58, 65].

36.4.4 Vertical Transmission of HCV

Like many maternal transmissible viral infections, HCV can cross the placenta during the antenatal and intrapartum periods to infect the foetus, the effect of which is increased perinatal morbidity and mortality in later life [60, 63, 65–67]. In developing countries, parenteral transmission remains a common route of paediatric infection with HCV while in developed countries, perinatal transmission is the leading cause of HCV infection in children [59].

The risk of vertical or mother-to- child transmission (MTCT) of HCV-exposed infants ranges between 3% and 5% or approximately 1 in 20 chances, if the mother is known to be anti-HCV-positive. The risk is higher with high maternal viral load and co-infection with HIV in mothers not on antiretroviral therapy [59, 63]. Co-infection with HIV increases the rate of mother-to-child transmission up to 19.4% [68]. Spontaneous clearance rate is high and ranges between 25% and 50% [59]. In other words, approximately, 1 in 4 children with hepatitis C may clear the virus on their own [69].

However, the morbidity may be delayed. In addition to these, the non-availability of vaccine and recommendation for treatment of HCV infection in pregnancy militates against effective prevention of the infection in pregnant women and their infants [6]. Delivery by elective caesarean section and withholding breastfeeding are not reliable means of reducing MTCT of HCV [59, 60].

36.4.5 Diagnosis

The diagnosis of HCV involves detection of antibodies against the virus or detection of the viral particle, HCV RNA and viral load assay using PCR test. Detection of either anti-HCV by enzyme immunoassay (EIA) or HCV RNA using the reverse transcriptase polymerase chain reaction (RT-PCR) is the standard method for HCV diagnosis. According to the Center for Disease Control and Prevention (CDC), a positive EIA should have further supplemental recombinant immunoblot assay (RIBA ™) or RT-PCR for HCV RNA [70]. In addition to other ancillary tests, Liver function test and ultrasound scan of the liver is essential to assess the degree of hepatic involvement.

For exposed infants, current guidelines require a positive anti-HCV test in infants born to infected mothers after 12 months or two positive HCV RNA tests at least 6 months apart to diagnose persistent perinatal infection [59].

36.4.6 Treatment of HCV in Pregnancy

Hepatitis C infection can be cured by antiviral treatment but awareness related to its asymptomatic nature, access to diagnosis and treatment remains low in many settings [71]. The World Health Organization is yet to make specific recommendations for treatment of HCV in pregnancy, and to prevent MTCT of the virus. In the non-pregnant state, initiating treatment in patients with HCV/HIV co-infection is a priority as the HCV-related disease could progress more rapidly [72].

A WHO new recommendation is the use of direct-acting antiviral agents (DAAS) for the treatment of HCV (Strong recommendation, moderate quality of evidence) [72]. This recommendation replaced the previous regimen where pegylated interferon plus ribavirin for non-pregnant patients was recommended [71]. The newer all-oral direct-acting antiretroviral HCV regimens (DAAs) used in treating HIV/HCV co-infection that produce sustained virological response have not been approved for use in pregnancy [71]. The fear of toxicity and their effects on pregnant mothers and their foetuses/infants is a major concern. Also, the WHO recommendation for 'specific subgroup consideration in the use of sofosbuvir/pegylated interferon and ribavirin for patients with HCV genotype 3 infection with cirrhosis and patients with genotypes 5 and 6 infection with and without cirrhosis' as an alternative treatment option [71] does not include pregnant women.

However, Ozaslan et al. [69], reported that of a total of eight infants exposed to interferon alfa and/or ribavirin during pregnancy, none showed congenital anomalies or malformations. He therefore opined that in patients with acute hepatitis C during pregnancy, the use of interferon therapy should be considered with close monitoring. This old regimen for HCV treatment provided low yield of success of viral suppression especially in HIV/HCV co-infections and for those for whom stabilization of the HIV disease should precede HCV treatment [59, 72].

36.4.7 Complications of HCV in Pregnancy

Compared with HCV-negative mothers, women with HCV-positive antibodies are at higher risk of cholestasis in pregnancy, and it tends to occur earlier in the gestation [59, 73].

36.4.8 Course of HCV on Pregnancy and Pregnancy on the Course of HCV

Apart from cholestasis, chronic HCV in pregnancy does not seem to increase the risk of pregnancy complication and does not have any adverse *effect* on the *course of pregnancy and* the birth weight of the newborn infant. In fact, some women may even have improvement as assessed by viral load and detectable elevated serum alanine aminotransferase (ALT) levels. In early pregnancy, it may become undetectable in the third trimester with returned to elevated ALT levels by 6 months post-partum. Conversely, pregnancy has no effects on the course of HCV hepatitis [68, 70, 74].

36.5 Rubella in Pregnancy

Rubella virus is among the maternally transmissible microorganisms but is not non-sexually transmittable. Outside pregnancy, it is transmitted by airborne droplets from the sneeze or cough of infected people and humans are the only known host [75, 76]. The virus was discovered in 1962 by Parkman, Beuscher and Arenstein, and independently by Weller and Neva as co-discoverers [77]. A worldwide outbreak occurred in 1964–1965. This led to the development of and first licensed vaccines in 1969. The current RA 27/3 vaccine was introduced in 1979.

Though, a viral infection with mild febrile symptoms and a rash in adults and children, neonatal manifestations of antenatal infection with rubella virus is a syndrome of severe congenital birth defects, bilateral sensorineural deafness, cataract, mental retardation, microcephaly and congenital heart defects (commonly patent ductus arteriosus or peripheral pulmonary artery stenosis), among others, known as congenital rubella syndrome (CRS). This syndrome was recognized about six decades ago [75, 78, 79].

36.5.1 Epidemiology

The incidence of new rubella infection has fallen drastically in developed countries. The WHO Region of the Americas was the first in the world to be declared free of endemic transmission of rubella in April 2015 [75]. This success was due to massive immunization campaigns across the USA, Latin America and Europe, while the year 2010 was targeted for the elimination of rubella infection and new cases of CRS across these regions [80–83].

In England and Wales, nine cases of rubella were reported in 2014. With the national uptake of antenatal screening for rubella, susceptibility fell slightly from 98.10% in 2012 to 97.79% in 2013 [84–86]. In spite of the global progress made to eliminate new infections and prevent CRS, the WHO African and South-East Asian regions are still lagging behind and have the lowest vaccine coverage with resultant highest rate of CRS [75].

In Nigeria, the reported national prevalence for rubella IgG is 54–76% [87–90]. At the UBTH, Benin City, Nigeria, we reported a prevalence of rubella IgG among pregnant women to be 53%, among which 9.7% were IgM seropositive [76].

Although, rubella has no specific treatment, it is a vaccine-preventable disease. Each year, over 100,000 babies are born with CRS worldwide [75]. In Nigeria, there is no national data on the burden of CRS.

36.5.2 Symptoms of Rubella Infection

The incubation period for rubella is 14–21 days during which period the patient is asymptomatic. The patient may remain asymptomatic after the incubation period. Sub-clinical infection occurs in 20–50% of cases. Where they exist, the symptoms in adults including pregnant women may include low-grade fever, mild conjunctivitis, lethargy and joints pains especially of the wrist and hand and coryza in the prodromal phase [75, 78]. These symptoms usually run a self-limiting course and disappear within 7–10 days. The symptoms may however be confused with malaria in malarial endemic areas or for other viral infections such as parvovirus B19 [91].

Other features of rubella infection include macular rash and posterior auricular lymphadenopathy (glands in the cheeks or neck), seizure, muscle aches and temporary low platelet count when the blood is evaluated. While adults tend to have more pronounced symptoms, the symptoms may be mild with very little malaise in children [75, 85].

A pregnant woman infected with rubella virus in early (8–10 weeks of) pregnancy, the chance of passing the virus on to her foetus is 90% and can result in miscarriage, stillbirth or severe birth defects in up to 90% of surviving infants. When there is re-infection in persons with immunity, the immune response is modified with lower risk to the foetus [75].

From 11–16 weeks of pregnancy, the risk of rubella-related foetal damage reduces to 10–20% and becomes rare after 16 weeks of gestation [12]. Infants with CRS pose further risk of infecting other susceptible persons as they may excrete the virus for a year or more [75].

36.5.3 Diagnosis of Rubella

In pregnancy, rubella has non-specific clinical symptoms. Consequently, the detection of rubella-specific antibodies, IgM in saliva sample is indicative of active infection. The test is both sensitive and specific. Serological detection of rubella IgG may suggest past or current infection, and thus not specific to confirm acute infection. The definitive or gold standard for diagnosis is the use of polymerase chain reaction (PCR) testing to detect the viral particle. There is also need to exclude other viral infections especially the **TORCH** (**TO**xoplasmosis, **R**ubella, **C**ytomegalovirus, **H**erpes simplex) group of infections [85].

36.5.4 Treatment of Rubella Infection

Rubella has no specific treatment. However, symptoms though self-limiting can be relieved with appropriate medications when necessary. Prevention is therefore the best approach to the control of rubella infection and its deleterious effects on future generation.

36.5.5 Complication of Rubella Infection

In pregnancy, rubella can cause in addition to CRS, transient intrauterine growth restriction, thrombocytopenic purpura, haemolytic anaemia, jaundice, radiolucent bone disease and meningoencephalitis [75, 80–82, 85, 91, 92].

The effect of CRS on afflicted children can lead to lifelong disabilities. Apart from hearing impairments, ocular and cardiac lesions, children with CRS may also suffer from autism, diabetes mellitus (immune-mediated and may be delayed to adolescence or adulthood) and thyroid dysfunction [75, 85, 91, 92]. Apart from microcephaly bilateral sensorineural deafness, cardiac lesions and cataracts, other ocular lesions of rubella include congenital glaucoma, pigmentary retinopathy ('salt and pepper'), severe myopia and micro-ophthalmia are other permanent lesions. Also, there may be 'late-onset' disease at 3–12 months with rash, diarrhoea, pneumonitis and associated high mortality [85].

The lesions of CRS are costly to manage and corrective surgeries and other expensive care may be out of reach of many children in poor or developing economies [75, 85, 93]. In the USA, approximately 20,000 cases of CRS were reported in the mid-1960s, during an outbreak, from 1964 to 1965 [75, 93]. The associated economic cost for medical attention was astronomical, costing at least US $220,000 per case [76, 93, 94].

36.5.6 Prevention of Rubella

The first step towards rubella prevention is raising awareness of the general population on deleterious effects of rubella infection to the unborn baby of an infected mother and embrace measures to prevent it.

The mainstay of rubella prevention is through vaccination [75, 93, 94]. Rubella vaccine is a live attenuated strain that has been in use for more than 40 years. A single dose gives more than 95% long-lasting immunity, which is similar to that induced by natural infection [75]. Therefore, awareness campaign and counselling of women and girls for rubella test and vaccinating those who are seronegative is a practical step necessary for rubella prevention.

Pregnant women should be counselled and tested in the antenatal period and vaccinated in the immediate partum period to avoid the risk of passing the virus to the foetus that may result in vaccine-associated foetal malformation [95].

The period of vaccination of children in the National Programme on Immunisation (NPI) in Nigeria is another window of opportunity for women's counselling and vaccination, as women are mostly involved in getting their children to immunization centres in Nigeria [76].

Routine vaccination of girls in early teens was a major contribution to the prevention of rubella infection in pregnancy and eradication of CRS in developed countries [75, 80, 95].

36.5.6.1 Vaccination

Vaccination is recommended for all children, women of reproductive age in the pre-pregnancy period. For children, the recommendation is that children should receive the first dose of a combined vaccine (measles-mumps-rubella (MMR) or measles-mumps-rubella-varicella (MMRV) at 12–15 months of age [95]. The second dose is given at 18 months of age or at 4–6 years of age [95]. Massive campaigns and full implementation of this measure resulted in declaring in April 2015, the WHO Region of the Americas the first in the world to be free of endemic transmission of rubella, thus, saving from the great danger associated with CRS [75, 94].

36.6 COVID-19

COVID-19 (also called coronavirus disease) is a potentially severe acute respiratory infection caused by severe acute respiratory syndrome coronavirus 2 (SARs-CoV-2) [4]. The virus was first identified as a cause of an outbreak of pneumonia of unknown cause in Wuhan province, China in December 2019, and because of its rapid global spread, it was declared a pandemic by the World Health Organization in March 2020. As of June 29, 2020, a total of 10,014,377 cases have been reported from nearly all countries, with a total number of 498,693 deaths, accounting for a case fatality rate of nearly 5%. Of these cases, 386,190 (3.9%) were reported from African countries, and 24,567 (0.24%) from a country like Nigeria. The death rates reported from African countries have so far been lower in African countries as compared to the rest of the world – 9664 (1.9% of the global death rate) in Africa and 565 (0.1%) in Nigeria.

Severe Acute Respiratory Syndrome Coronavirus 2 (SARS-CoV-2) is a member of the Coronavirus family, whose members cause a range of infectious diseases from the common cold to Severe Acute Respiratory Syndrome (SARS) and the Middle East Respiratory Syndrome (MERS) [4]. This virus appears to spread readily, through respiratory droplets in air and surfaces, fomite or faecal methods and other modes of transmission still evolving. The symptoms include fever, cough, loss to taste and smear and shortness of breath. In severe cases, it may result in more severe breathing difficulties and could lead to pneumonia, severe acute respiratory disease, kidney failure and death.

Diagnosis of COVID-19: The WHO recommends the confirmation of COVID-19 infection with nucleic acid real-time polymerase chain reaction (RT-PCR) test using respiratory samples [6]. Even in more advanced countries, the use of RT-PCR to diagnose COVID-19 suffers from a number of limitations such as the cost and expertise required to set up RT-PCR testing centres and the reported false-negatives for COVID-19 infections [14]. Furthermore, the turnover time to run a PCR test limits the amount of samples that can be tested per unit time. In addition, the non-homogenous nature of respiratory samples from different parts of the body such as throat swab, saliva or endotracheal aspirate, affect the sensitivity of COVID-19 test using RT-PCR [16]. Thus, research is currently on-going to validate the use of antibody-based rapid diagnostic test (RDTs) kits, which could present a unique opportunity to scale-up COVID-19 testing [18].

Treatment of COVID-19: To date, no specific treatment or drug treatment has been found for COVID-19. However, specific symptoms can be treated, based on an assessment of the patient's clinical condition. These include anti-viral agents, the most prominent of which has been remdesivir, which had been shown to demonstrate some beneficial effects in the USA [10]. Other methods of treatment include breathing support, such as with a mechanical ventilator [10], and steroids to reduce the associated lung swelling. Dexamethasone was recently found to have a profound effect in reducing mortality in patients with severe complications of COVID-19 and has been approved for use by the WHO [10]. In such cases, transfusion of blood plasma may also be useful.

Prevention of COVID-19: No vaccines have yet been identified for the COVID-19, but a number of candidate vaccines are currently undergoing trial in various parts of the world. Thus, efforts are being concentrated on primary prevention in order to reduce the community spread of the disease. Primary prevention measures being promoted by health systems and governments around the world include restrictions of international and local air travels, lockdowns of national economies, testing and quarantining of confirmed and suspected cases, washing of hands, the use of alcohol-based sanitizers, use of face-masks and cleaning of contaminated surfaces [5].

COVID-19 in Pregnancy: We know little about COVID-19 in pregnancy and related immunological, physiological and cardiovascular changes that naturally occur during pregnancy which can lead to worsening of respiratory infections due to systemic effects on the body. The mechanism by which this occurs is due to increased heart rate with increased oxygen consumption and stroke volume, as well as decreased pulmonary capacity and functional residual capacity which are the main physiological changes that increase the complications of COVID-19 in pregnant women compared to the non-pregnant population [2–3].

More so, pregnancy is associated with immunosuppression which makes pregnant women more susceptible to infectious diseases [2]. It is often postulated that COVID- 19 epidemic may have serious consequences for pregnant women. However, in a recent publication in NEW YORK (Reuters Health), pregnant women with COVID-19 were often asymptomatic, and nearly 9 out of 10 had mild diseases. The authors concluded that strategy including universal testing of all pregnant women admitted in labour units in addition to those who present for triage evaluation of symptomatic complaints has obvious benefits that should inform best practices to protect patients, their families and the obstetrical providers who care for them.

Furthermore, there are currently no data suggesting an increased risk of miscarriage or early pregnancy loss in relation to COVID-19 [7]. Case reports from early pregnancy studies with SARS and MERS do not demonstrate a convincing relationship between infection and increased risk of miscarriage or second trimester loss. As there is no evidence of intrauterine foetal infection with COVID-19, it is therefore currently considered unlikely that there will be congenital effects of the virus on foetal development [7]. There are case reports of preterm birth in women with COVID-19, but it is unclear whether the preterm birth was always iatrogenic, or whether some were spontaneous. At the time of writing this book, ongoing researches are to look at a possibility of vertical transmission of SARS-CoV-2 from mother to foetus and creating significant infections in foetuses and neonates [2].

Currently, the clinical attributes and vertical transmission capability of COVID-19 in pregnant patients are obscure; this raises questions about COVID-19 in pregnancy. These include the following questions: Are the symptoms of COVID-19 infection different in pregnant women compared to the general population? Are pregnant women with COVID-19 pneumonia at a higher risk of death? Are pregnant women with COVID-19 pneumonia at higher risk of obstetrics complications such as preterm labour and low birth weight? Can infection transmit vertically and cause foetal and neonatal disease? Therefore, it is crucial to find answers to these questions to gain insight and ensure a management protocol for pregnant women.

References

1. WHO. Guidelines for the prevention, care and treatment of persons with chronic hepatitis B infection. Policy Brief, March 2015. WHO/HIV/2015.5.
2. Parkin DM. The global health burden of infection-associated cancers in the year 2002. Int J Cancer. 2006;118:3030–44. [PubMed].
3. Forbi JC, Vaughan G, Purdy MA, Campo DS, Xia GL, et al. Epidemic history and evolutionary dynamics of hepatitis B virus infection in two remote communities in rural Nigeria. PLoS One. 2010;5:e11615.
4. Anna C. World Hepatitis Day: the history of the hepatitis B vaccine. Planned Parenthood Advocates of Arizona; 2012.
5. Komatsu H. Hepatitis B virus: where do we stand and what is the next step for eradication? World J Gastroenterol. 2014;20(27):8998–9016.
6. Zanetti AR, Van Damme P, Shouval D. The global impact of vaccination against hepatitis B: a historical overview. Vaccine. 2008;26:6266–73.
7. WHO. "This is Hepatitis, Know it, confront it". WHO. 2013 http://www.who.int/campaigns/hepatitis-day/2013/event/en/.
8. WHO. Prevent hepatitis: Act Now. WHO. 2015. http://www.who.int/campaigns/hepatitis-day/2015/en/. Assessed 1 July, 2016.
9. Onakewhor JU, Offor E, Okonofua FE. Maternal and neonatal seroprevalence of hepatitis B surface antigen (HBsAg) in Benin City, Nigeria. J Obstet Gynaecol. 2001;21:583–6.
10. Onakewhor JUE, Offor E, Okonofua FE. Seroprevalence of maternal and neonatal antibodies to human immunodeficiency and hepatitis B viruses in Benin City, Nigeria. J Med Biomed Res. 2002;1(1):32–8.
11. Odemuyiwa SO, Mulders MN, Oyedele OI, Ola SO, Odaibo GN, et al. Phylogenetic analysis of new hepatitis B virus isolates from Nigeria supports endemicity of genotype E in West Africa. J Med Virol. 2001;65:463–9. https://doi.org/10.1002/jmv.2058.abs. CrossRef PubMed/NCBI Google Scholar.
12. Onakewhor JUE, Charurat M, Matthew O, Osagie E, Asemota MO, Omoigberale A. Immunologic Pattern of Hepatitis B Infection among Exposed and Non- Exposed Babies in A PMTCT Program in Low Resource Setting: Does Every Exposed Newborn Require 200IU of Hepatitis B Immunoglobulin? J Vaccines Vaccin. 2013;4:7. https://doi.org/10.4172/2157-7560.1000207.
13. Sadoh AE, Eregie CO. Age at presentation for infant immunization in Nigeria: implications for hepatitis B immunization. Public Health. 2008;122:1318–20.
14. World Health Organization (WHO) vaccine preventable diseases monitoring system 2005 global summary. Immunization profile-Nigeria.
15. World Health Organization. Nigeria Launches Penta Vaccine WHO. 2012.
16. CDC. A comprehensive immunization strategy to eliminate transmission of hepatitis B virus infection in the United States. MMWR. 2006;55:16.
17. Uyar Y, Cabar C, Balci A. Seroprevalence of hepatitis B virus among pregnant women in northern Turkey. Hepat Mon. 2009;9:146–9.
18. Pan CQ, Duan ZP, Bhamidimarri KR, Zou HB, Liang XF, et al. An algorithm for risk assessment and intervention of mother to child transmission of hepatitis B virus. Clin Gastroenterol Hepatol. 2012;10:452–9.
19. EASL. Combined maternal treatment and infant vaccination effective in reducing mother-to-child HBV transmission. Medscape, 2009.
20. Centers for Disease Control and Prevention (CDC). Use of hepatitis B vaccination for adults with diabetes mellitus: recommendations of the Advisory Committee on Immunization Practices (ACIP). MMWR Morb Mortal Wkly Rep. 2011;60: 1709–11.
21. Wong VC, Ip HM, Reesink HW, Lelie PN, Reerink-Brongers EE, et al. Prevention of the HBsAg carrier state in newborn infants of mothers who are chronic carriers of HBsAg and HBeAg by administration of hepatitis-B vaccine and hepatitis-B immunoglobulin: double-blind randomised placebo-controlled study. Lancet. 1984;1:921–6.

22. Stevens CE, Toy PT, Tong MJ, Taylor PE, Vyas GN, et al. Perinatal hepatitis B virus transmission in the United States. Prevention by passive-active immunization. JAMA. 1985;253:1740–5.
23. Wiseman E, Fraser MA, Holden S, Glass A, Kidson BL, et al. Perinatal transmission of hepatitis B virus: an Australian experience. Med J Aust. 2009;190:489–92.
24. Dwivedi M, Misra SP, Misra V, Pandey A, Pant S, et al. Seroprevalence of hepatitis B infection during pregnancy and risk of perinatal transmission. Indian J Gastroenterol. 2011;30:66–71.
25. Uyar Y, Cabar C, Balci A. Seroprevalence of hepatitis B virus among pregnant women in northern Turkey. Hepat Mon. 2009;9:146–9.
26. Contag SA. Hepatitis in pregnancy. Medscape. 2016. http://emedicine.medscape.com/article/1562368-overview. Assessed 4 July, 2016.
27. Onakewhor JUE, Olagbuji BN, Okpere EE. Partners' attitude and risk factors for couple infection with hepatitis B virus in a prevention of mother-to-child transmission. West Afr J Med. 2013;32(2):110–4.
28. WHO. Consolidated Guidelines on the use of antiretroviral drugs for treating and preventing HIV infection: recommendation for a public health approach. 2nd ed. WHO; 2016.
29. Schönberger K, Riedel C, Rückinger S, Mansmann U, Jilg W, Von Kries R. Impact of maternal carrier status on immunologic markers for protection after hepatitis B vaccination in infancy: a meta-analysis. Vaccine. 2012;30(44):6314–26. https://doi.org/10.1016/j.vaccine.2012.07.080.
30. Komatsu H. Hepatitis B virus: where do we stand and what is the next step for eradication? World J Gastroenterol. 2014;20(27):8998–9016. https://doi.org/10.3748/wjg.v20.i27.8998. PMCID: PMC4112872.
31. Roukens AH, Visser LG. Hepatitis B vaccination strategy in vaccine low and non-responders: a matter of quantity of quality? Hum Vaccin. 2011;7:654–7. [PubMed].
32. Leuridan E, Van Damme P. Hepatitis B and the need for a booster dose. Clin Infect Dis. 2011;53:68–75. [PubMed].
33. Van Damme P, Van Herck K. A review of the long-term protection after hepatitis A and B vaccination. Travel Med Infect Dis. 2007;5:79–84.
34. Jan CF, Huang KC, Chien YC, Greydanus DE, Davies HD, Chiu TY, Huang LM, Chen CJ, Chen DS. Determination of immune memory to hepatitis B vaccination through early booster response in college students. Hepatology. 2010;51:1547–54. [PubMed].
35. Wu TW, Lin HH, Wang LY. Chronic hepatitis B infection in adolescents who received primary infantile vaccination. Hepatology. 2013;57:37–45. [PubMed].
36. Roukens AH, Visser LG. Hepatitis B vaccination strategy in vaccine low and non-responders: a matter of quantity of quality? Hum Vaccin. 2011;7:654–7. [PubMed].
37. Li ZK, Nie JJ, Li J, Zhuang H. The effect of HLA on immunological response to hepatitis B vaccine in healthy people: a meta-analysis. Vaccine. 2013;31:4355–61. [PubMed].
38. Lin CS, Xie SB, Liu J, Zhao ZX, Chong YT, Gao ZL. Effect of revaccination using different schemes among adults with low or undetectable anti-HBs titers after hepatitis B virus vaccination. Clin Vaccine Immunol. 2010;17:1548–51. [PubMed].
39. Heininger U, Gambon M, Gruber V, Margelli D. Successful hepatitis B immunization in non- and low responding health care workers. Hum Vaccin. 2010;6. [PubMed].
40. Boot HJ, van der Waaij LA, Schirm J, Kallenberg CG, van Steenbergen J, Wolters B. Acute hepatitis B in a healthcare worker: a case report of genuine vaccination failure. J Hepatol. 2009;50:426–31. [PubMed].
41. Abramczuk BM, Mazzola TN, Moreno YMF, Zorzeto TQ, Quintilio W, et al. Impaired humoral response to vaccines among HIV-exposed uninfected infants. Clin Vaccine Immunol. 2011;18:1406–9.
42. Pasricha N, Datta U, Chawla Y, Singh S, Arora SK, et al. Immune responses in patients with HIV infection after vaccination with recombinant hepatitis B virus vaccine. BMC Infect Dis. 2006;6:65.
43. Landrum M, Hullsiek KH, Crum-Cianflone N (2010) Hepatitis B vaccine response predicts progression to clinical AIDS or Death. 17th conference on retroviruses & opportunistic infections.
44. 55Centers for Disease Control and Prevention (CDC). Use of hepatitis B vaccination for adults with diabetes mellitus: recommendations of the advisory committee on immunization practices (ACIP). MMWR Morb Mortal Wkly Rep. 2011;60:1709–11.
45. Poorolajal J, Mahmoodi M, Majdzadeh R, Nasseri-Moghaddam S, Haghdoost A, Fotouhi A. Long-term protection provided by hepatitis B vaccine and need for booster dose: a meta-analysis. Vaccine. 2010;28:623–31. [PubMed].
46. Chen X, Chen J, Wen J, Xu C, Zhang S, et al. Breastfeeding is not a risk factor for mother-to-child transmission of hepatitis B virus. PLoS One. 2013;8:e55303.
47. WHO. "This is Hepatitis, Know it, confront it". WHO. 2013. http://www.who.int/campaigns/hepatitis-day/2013/event/en/.
48. WHO. 'Hepatitis: Think again'. http://www.who.int/campaigns/hepatitis-day/2014/en/. Assessed 5 July, 2016).
49. World Hepatitis Alliance. World Hepatitis Day 2016 theme announced.
50. http://worleuropean/. Consensus Group on Hepatitis B Immunity. Are booster immunisations needed for lifelong hepatitis B immunity? European Consensus Group on Hepatitis B Immunity. Lancet. 2000;355:561–5. [PubMed].
51. Łapiński TW, Stepaniuk J, Tomasiewicz K, Lebensztejn D, Kulikowski M, Flisiak R. Effect of hepatitis B virus (HBV) infection on the course of pregnancy and newborns' health status. Clin Exp Hepatol. 2015;3:112–6. https://doi.org/10.5114/ceh.2015.55568.
52. Han Y-T, Sun C, Liu C-X, Xie S-S, Xiao D, Liu L, Yu J-H, Li W-W, Li Q. Clinical features and outcome of acute hepatitis B in pregnancy. BMC Infectious Diseases. 2014;14:368. https://doi.org/10.1186/1471-2334-14-368.
53. 2016 UpToDate, Inc. Lee H, Lok ASF. Hepatitis B and pregnancy. http://www.uptodate.com/contents/hepatitis-b-and-pregnancy. Assessed 4 July, 2016.
54. Gower E, Estes C, Blach S, Razavi-Shearer K, Razavi H. Global epidemiology and genotype distribution of the hepatitis C virus infection. J Hepatol. 2014;61(1 Suppl):S45–57.
55. WHO. New recommendations in the updated WHO guidelines for the screening, care and treatment of persons with chronic hepatitis C infection. Policy Brief. 2016. WHO/HIV/2016.01. http://apps.who.int/iris/bitstream/10665/204452/1/WHO_HIV_2016.01_eng.pdf?ua=1. Assessed 5 July, 2016.
56. Arshad M, El-Kamary SS, Jhaveri R. Hepatitis C virus infection during pregnancy and the Newborn period. J Viral Hepat. 2011;18(4):229–36.
57. Frank C, Mohamed MK, Strickland GT, Lavanchy D, Arthur RR, et al. The role of parenteral antischistosomal therapy in the spread of hepatitis C virus in Egypt. Lancet. 2000;355:887–91.
58. Lauer GM, Walker BD. Hepatitis C virus infection. NEJM. 2001;345(1):41–52.
59. Arshad M, El-Kamary SS, Jhaveri R. Hepatitis C virus infection during pregnancy and the Newborn period. J Viral Hepat. 2011;18(4):229–36.
60. Onakewhor JUE, Okonofua FE. The prevalence of dual hepatitis C virus and human immunodeficiency virus infection in pregnancy in Benin City Nigeria. Afr J Reprod Health. 2009;13(2):97–108.
61. CDC Recommendations for Prevention and Control of Hepatitis C Virus (HCV) Infection and HCV-Related Chronic Disease MMWR October 16, 1998/47(RR19);1–39.

62. Foster GR, Goldin RD, Thomas HC. Chronic hepatitis C virus infection causes a significant reduction in quality of life in the absence of cirrhosis. Hepatology. 1998;27:209–12.
63. Canadian Paediatric Society. Hepatitis C in pregnancy. Paediatr Child Health. 2008;13(6):535. PMCID: PMC2532914.
64. Erhabor O, Ejele OA, Nwauche CA. The risk of transfusion-acquired hepatitis C infection among blood donors in Port Harcourt: the question of blood safety in Nigeria. Niger J Clin Pract. 2006;9(1):18–21.
65. Alfredo A, Clumeck N, Collins S, Gerlich W, Lundgren J, et al. The ECC Jury short statement of the first European consensus conference on the treatment of chronic hepatitis b and c in HIV co-infected patients. J Hepatol. 2005;42(5):615–24.
66. Wyld R, Robertson JR, Brettle RP, Mellor J, Prescott L, Simmonds P. Absence of hepatitis C virus transmission but frequent transmission of HIV-1 from sexual contact with doubly-infected individuals. J Infect. 1997;35:163–6.
67. Thomas DL, Villano SA, Riester KA, Hershow R, Mofenson LM, et al. Perinatal transmission of hepatitis C virus from human immunodeficiency virus type 1-infected mothers. Women and Infants Transmission Study. J Infect Dis. 1998. June;177(6):1480–8.
68. Annarosa floreani hepatitis C and pregnancy. World J Gastroenterol. 2013;19(40):6714–20. https://doi.org/10.3748/wjg.v19.i40.6714. PMCID: PMC3812470.
69. Ozaslan E, Yilmaz R, Simsek H, Tatar G. Interferon therapy for acute hepatitis C during pregnancy. Ann Pharmacother. 2002;36(11):1715–8.
70. Perinatology.com. Hepatitis C Infection. http://www.perinatology.com/exposures/Infection/HepatitisC.htm. Assessed 4 July, 2016.
71. WHO. New recommendations in the updated who guidelines for the screening, care and treatment of persons with chronic hepatitis C infection. Policy Brief. 2016. WHO/HIV/2016.01. http://apps.who.int/iris/bitstream/10665/204452/1/WHO_HIV_2016.01_eng.pdf?ua=1. Assessed 5 July, 2016.
72. WHO. Consolidated Guidelines on the use of antiretroviral drugs for treating and preventing HIV infection: recommendations for a public health approach. 2nd ed; 2016. p. 209.
73. Locatelli A, Roncaglia N, Arreghini A, Bellini P, Vergani P, Ghidini A. Hepatitis C virus infection is associated with a higher incidence of cholestasis of pregnancy. Br J Obstet Gynaecol. 1999;106(5):498–500.
74. Gordon Stirrat Hepatitis C Virus. Aids to obstetrics and gynaecology. New York: Churchill Livingstone; 1997. p. 110.
75. WHO. Rubella. Fact sheet. Reviewed March 2016. http://www.who.int/mediacentre/factsheets/fs367/en.
76. Onakewhor JU, Chiwuzie J. Seroprevalence survey of rubella infection in pregnancy at the University of Benin Teaching Hospital, Benin City, Nigeria. Niger J Clin Pract. 2011;14(2):140–5.
77. Rahman MM, Khan AM, Hafiz MM, Ronny FM, Ara S, Chowdhury SK, et al. Congenital hearing impairment associated with rubella: lessons from Bangladesh. Southeast Asian J Trop Med Public Health. 2002;33:811–7.
78. Banerji A, Ford-Jones EL, Kelly E, Robinson JL. Congenital rubella syndrome despite maternal antibodies. CMAJ. 2005;172(13):1678–9.
79. Edlich RF, Winters KL, Long WB 3rd, Gubler KD. Rubella and congenital rubella (German measles). J Long-Term Eff Med Implants. 2005;15(3):319–28.
80. Centers for Disease Control and Prevention. Progress toward elimination of rubella and congenital rubella syndrome – the Americas, 2003–2008. MMWR Morb Mortal Wkly Rep. 2008;57:1176–9.
81. Morice A, Carvajal X, León M, Machado M, Badilla X, Reef S, et al. Accelerated rubella control and congenital rubella syndrome prevention strengthen measles eradication: the Costa Rican experience. J Infect Dis. 2003;187:158–63.
82. Kelly H, Worth L, Karapanagiotidis T, Riddell M. Interruption of rubella virus transmission in Australia may require vaccination of adults males: evidence from a Victorian sero-survey. Commun Dis Intell Q Rep. 2004;28:69–73.
83. Castillo-Solorzano C, Carrasco P, Tambini G, Reef S, Brana M, de Quadros CA. New horizons in the control of rubella and prevention of congenital rubella syndrome in the Americas. J Infect Dis. 2003;187:S146–52.
84. Patient. Rubella and Pregnancy. http://patient.info/doctor/rubella-and-pregnancy. Assessed July, 2016.
85. National Antenatal Infections Screening Monitoring. Data tables: England 2005-2013; Public Health England, 2014.
86. Onyenekwe CC, Kehinde-Agbeyangi TA, Ofor US, Arinola OG. Prevalence of rubella-IgG antibody in women of childbearing age in Lagos, Nigeria. West Afr J Med. 2000;19:23–6.
87. Pennap G, Amauche G, Ajoge H, Gabadi S, Agwale S, Forbi J. Serologic survey of specific rubella virus IgM in the sera of pregnant women in Makurdi, Benue state, Nigeria. Afr J Reprod Health. 2009;13:69–73.
88. Bukbuk DN, el Nafaty AU, Obed JY. Prevalence of rubella-specific IgG antibody in non-immunized pregnant women in Maiduguri, north eastern Nigeria. Cent Eur J Public Health. 2002;10:21–3.
89. Bamgboye AE, Afolabi KA, Esumeh FI, Enweani IB. Prevalence of rubella antibody in pregnant women in Ibadan, Nigeria. West Afr J Med. 2004;23:245–8.
90. GOV.UK, viral rash in pregnancy; Public Health England, January 2011. https://www.gov.uk/government/publications/viral-rash-in-pregnancy. Assessed 4 July, 2016.
91. Centers for Disease Control and Prevention. Control and Prevention of Rubella: Evaluation and Management of Suspected Outbreaks, Rubella in Pregnant Women, and Surveillance for Congenital Rubella Syndrome. https://www.cdc.gov/mmwr/preview/mmwrhtml/rr5012a1.htm. Assessed 4 July,2016.
92. Centers for Disease Control and Prevention. Control and Prevention of Rubella: Evaluation and Management of Suspected Outbreaks, Rubella in Pregnant Women, and Surveillance for Congenital Rubella Syndrome. https://www.cdc.gov/mmwr/preview/mmwrhtml/rr5012a1.htm. Assessed 4 July, 2016.
93. Orenstein WA, Bart KJ, Hinman AR, Preblud SR, Greaves WL, Doster SW, et al. The opportunity and obligation to eliminate rubella from the United States. JAMA. 1984;251:1988–94.
94. Government of Canada. Prevention of rubella. 2015. http://www.healthycanadians.gc.ca/diseases-conditions-maladies-affections/disease-maladie/rubella-rubeole/prevention-eng.php. Assessed 6 July, 2016.
95. Nasiri R, Yoseffi J, Khajedaloe M, Sarafraz YM, Delgoshaei F. Congenital rubella syndrome after rubella vaccination in 1–4 weeks periconceptional period. Indian J Pediatr. 2009;76:279–82. dhepatitisalliance.org/en/news/feb-2016/world-hepatitis-day-2016-theme-announced. Assessed 5 July, 2016.

Neoplastic Diseases in Pregnancy

37

Michael Chudi Ezeanochie

Learning Objectives

At the end of this chapter, the reader should be able to:

- Understand the meaning of pregnancy-associated cancer
- Identify the cancers that are commonly associated with pregnancy
- Understand the overall principle for managing pregnancy-associated cancer
- Discuss the management of breast cancer in pregnancy
- Discuss the management of cervical cancer in pregnancy
- Discuss the management of ovarian cancer in pregnancy
- Understand the challenges associated with the management of pregnancy-associated cancers

37.1 Introduction

Neoplasms are abnormal tissue growths which arise from the proliferation of new cells. It is considered benign if it lacks the ability to invade neighbouring tissues or metastasize to distant sites. By contrast, malignant neoplasms or cancers invade surrounding tissues and can metastasize to distant sites usually uncontrollably.

This chapter will focus on the simultaneous occurrence of pregnancy and malignancies of the breast and the female reproductive tract. Pregnancy-associated cancer refers to instances in which the initial diagnosis of cancer is made during pregnancy or within 12 months of delivery [1–3]. Although rare, the incidence of malignant neoplasms occurring during pregnancy appears to be on the increase worldwide [4]. The overall estimated prevalence is between 1 in 1000 to 5000 pregnancies [5, 6]. Cancers of reproductive health importance that may occur in association with pregnancy includes breast cancer, cervical cancer, ovarian cancer and malignant trophoblastic disease.

Malignant neoplastic diseases in pregnancy present a diagnostic, therapeutic and ethical dilemma. This may arise if the cancer is diagnosed at a stage in pregnancy when the foetus is not viable for extrauterine survival or the standard recommended treatment modality is not very safe for use in pregnancy. Also, due to limited published literature on the subject, there is comparatively insufficient good quality evidence to guide decision making.

However, the overall principle of management should aim to provide the best available treatment for the woman while minimising harm to the developing foetus as much as possible. It should be within a multidisciplinary team setting and consider the risks, benefits and alternatives of the treatment choices and modalities. Also, the sociocultural, ethical, moral and spiritual dimensions of the treatment for the patient need to be considered.

37.2 Breast Cancer

37.2.1 Epidemiology

Breast cancer is one of the commonly diagnosed malignancies in pregnancy with a reported incidence of 1 in 3000 pregnancies [7]. Among women less than 50 years of age, 0.2–3.8% of breast cancers are pregnancy-associated [8]. The incidence is projected to rise in the future as more women delay the onset of pregnancy and childbirth for other life pursuits.

M. C. Ezeanochie (✉)
University of Benin Teaching Hospital, Benin City, Nigeria

Department of Obstetrics & Gynaecology, University of Benin, Benin City, Nigeria

F. Okonofua et al. (eds.), *Contemporary Obstetrics and Gynecology for Developing Countries*,
https://doi.org/10.1007/978-3-030-75385-6_37

37.2.2 Clinical Presentation

As observed in non-pregnant women, the most common presenting clinical feature is a painless lump in the breast. Occasionally, refusal by a nursing infant to feed from a lactating breast (milk rejection sign) may signify an occult carcinoma [9]. The physiological changes associated with pregnancy and lactation in the breast may make it a bit difficult for the patient and clinician to promptly identify masses on palpation and inadvertently lead to diagnostic delays. The differential diagnosis of a breast mass during pregnancy or lactation includes lactating adenoma, fibroadenoma, cystic disease, lobular hyperplasia, milk retention cyst (galactocoele), abscess, lipoma, lymphoma, sarcoma and tuberculosis.

37.2.3 Diagnosis

Breast imaging using ultrasound, mammogram or magnetic resonance imaging (MRI) is indicated when breast cancer is suspected during pregnancy or lactation from clinical history and examination. Ultrasound is usually preferred in pregnancy due to its safety for the foetus (avoids ionising radiation), availability and affordability. Mammography during pregnancy with abdominal and pelvic shielding, usually delivering negligible radiation dose of only 0.4 mrad to the foetus, is considered safe since its radiation exposure to the foetus is well below the acceptable upper limit of 5 rads (50mGray). Contrast-enhanced MRI is contraindicated as the Gadolinium contrast medium crosses the placenta and is teratogenic in rats.

Tissue confirmation in pregnant women with suspected breast cancer is the diagnostic gold standard for diagnosis [10]. Core needle biopsy, fine needle aspiration (FNA) and excisional biopsy are all acceptable modalities for tissue diagnosis. In lactating women, suspension of breastfeeding before the biopsy can reduce the incidence of milk fistula.

37.2.4 Treatment

The treatment of breast cancer in pregnancy follows the guidelines recommended for non-pregnant women and should be within a multidisciplinary team setting involving the obstetrician, oncologist, breast surgeon and geneticist. The aim of treatment is to control loco-regional disease and manage any systemic involvement while minimising foetal complications from therapy. Important factors considered in developing a treatment plan include the gestational age of the pregnancy, the stage of the disease and the preference of the patient. Therapeutic abortion is not indicated but may be considered if the patient desires it especially for cases diagnosed early in the first trimester.

Surgery, modified radical mastectomy with axillary dissection (MRM), is considered the standard of care for breast cancer that is considered operable in pregnancy as it may obviate the need for adjuvant radiation therapy with its associated foetal risks [10, 11]. Breast conserving treatment (BCT) such as lumpectomy with axillary dissection is feasible in pregnancy as a treatment option for women diagnosed in the second trimester or early third trimester [10]. In such cases, adjuvant radiation therapy is administered to the entire ipsilateral breast after delivery.

If the cancer is considered inoperable (advanced disease) in the first trimester, neo-adjuvant chemotherapy after the first trimester followed by surgery is acceptable when the patient desires to keep the pregnancy. Otherwise, termination of the pregnancy and further management as obtained in non-pregnant woman becomes the standard approach.

Breast cancer diagnosed in the second or third trimester of pregnancy can be managed with surgery followed by adjuvant chemotherapy if the disease is operable. It is important that chemotherapy isn't given within 3 weeks of planned delivery since it causes pancytopenia which increases the risk of infectious complications and haemorrhage [12]. If the cancer is inoperable (advanced disease), neo-adjuvant chemotherapy followed by surgery with or without radiotherapy is offered.

In terms of systemic therapy with drugs, chemotherapeutic drugs commonly used in the management of breast cancer in pregnancy include varying combinations of 5-fluorouracil, doxorubicin, epirubicin, cyclophosphamide and vinca alkaloids. Although they are considered teratogenic agents in pregnancy, limited published evidence considers them relatively safe for use in the second and third trimesters of pregnancy [11]. The use of newer drugs like monoclonal antibodies such as trastuzumab is still being evaluated for use in pregnancy. Tamoxifen use should be avoided in pregnancy because of its association with birth defects, such as Goldenhar syndrome (oculoauriculovertebral dysplasia), ambiguous genitalia and Pierre Robin sequence (triad of small mandible, cleft palate and glossoptosis) [11]. Other ancillary agents like ondasetron, metoclopramide, promethazine, erythropoietin and granulocyte colony stimulating factor are considered safe for use in pregnancy.

The prognosis for women managed for breast cancer in pregnancy is compares favourably with that for breast cancer outside of pregnancy with overall 5 year survival rate of 82% [13, 14]. Follow-up protocols are the same as for non-pregnant women. Since recurrent disease typically occurs within 3 years of treatment, further pregnancy should be delayed for at least 3 years. The impact of subsequent pregnancy on the overall prognosis is at yet uncertain.

37.3 Cervical Cancer

37.3.1 Epidemiology

This is the commonest malignancy of the reproductive tract worldwide with an estimated frequency of 5 cases per 1000 pregnancies [15]. It has been reported that a pregnant women is more likely to be diagnosed with cervical cancer in its early stages compared to non-pregnant controls [15, 16]. The increased surveillance and routine clinical evaluation of pregnant women during antenatal care may explain this observation.

37.3.2 Clinical Presentation

The physiological and hormonal changes that occur in pregnancy may result in structural changes on the cervix that can be confused with neoplasia. The cervix may be double or triple its pre-pregnant size at the end of pregnancy and under the influence of oestrogen, the transformation zone becomes more exuberant with eversion of the squamocolumnar junction onto the ectocervix.

The manifestation of cervical cancer in pregnancy is similar to disease in non-pregnant women. The commonest presenting symptom during pregnancy is abnormal vaginal bleeding which is often post-coital. Therefore, it is important that care providers should always recall that not all cases of vaginal bleeding in pregnancy are due to obstetric causes. Other symptoms may include abnormal fetid vaginal discharge, low abdominal or waist pains and haematuria.

37.3.3 Diagnosis

The diagnosis of cervical cancer in pregnancy is made after a suggestive history, finding of a cervical lesion on examination and histological confirmation from biopsy of the lesion. Cervical biopsy in pregnancy is considered safe with no undue increase in complications or pregnancy loss [16]. Ultrasound is helpful in the evaluation of the pregnancy and assessing the ureters and kidneys. A chest X-ray (with proper abdominal and pelvic shielding), cystoscopy and sigmoidoscopy can be used in the diagnostic workup and treatment planning of the patient when indicated. However, intravenous contrast-enhanced computed tomography (CT scan) or positron emission tomography (PET scan) is better avoided due to the foetal considerations from exposure to ionising radiation in pregnancy. Magnetic resonance imaging (MRI) has been shown to be safe in pregnancy and can be used to assess extracervical disease.

37.3.4 Treatment

The treatment of cervical cancer in pregnancy should be in a multidisciplinary team setting. Factors to be considered include the gestational age of the pregnancy, the clinical stage of the disease and the patient's fertility desires. Thorough documentation of the discussion and the decision taken is imperative. Although evidence suggests that moderate delay (range 3–32 weeks) in commencing definitive therapy for cervical cancer during pregnancy is associated with similar oncologic outcomes among women treated promptly [17], immediate patient treatment is advised if the diagnosis is made before the 16th week of pregnancy. This will inevitably imply a termination of the pregnancy.

Therefore, women diagnosed with early cervical cancer before 16 weeks are offered immediate treatment with an option of terminating the pregnancy while women diagnosed beyond 16 weeks of pregnancy are offered the option of delaying therapy until delivery later in pregnancy after foetal viability. For the occasional women who presents with advanced cervical pregnancy in pregnancy, the management has some considerations. In early pregnancy, delay of definitive treatment may worsen the prognosis and early treatment is therefore advised for maternal survival with unavoidable pregnancy loss. In later pregnancy, unduly delaying treatment for foetal viability may make a caesarean delivery more difficult with a cervical tumour in the lower segment.

The available treatment includes surgery (radical hysterectomy with lymphadenectomy) for early stage disease which usually follows a caesarean section in late pregnancy after foetal viability. It may be performed with the foetus in situ in early pregnancy. Transposition of the ovaries out of the pelvis in young women is advised during this surgery to preserve ovarian function especially if radiation therapy is subsequently required. Despite the changes associated with pregnancy, the evidence suggests that the outcome of radical hysterectomy performed during pregnancy is comparable to the outcome outside of pregnancy [15]. Advanced cervical cancer in pregnancy is best managed by prompt definitive treatment with chemoradiation irrespective of the gestational age.

Due to the bulky and friable nature of the cervix and the risk of significant haemorrhage, abdominal delivery is preferred to vaginal delivery in all cases of invasive cervical cancer [18]. Also, recurrence of cervical cancer at the site of episiotomy after vaginal delivery has been documented [19].

37.4 Ovarian Cancer

37.4.1 Epidemiology

Ovarian cancer is the next prevalent genital tract cancer diagnosed in pregnancy after cervical cancer and about 5% of ovarian tumours diagnosed in pregnancy are malignant [20]. The incidence of ovarian carcinoma complicating pregnancy has been reported as 0.11 and 0.073 per 1000 pregnancies [21, 22]. Most ovarian malignancies found in pregnancy are germ cell tumours and dysgerminoma is the commonest variant encountered. However, the incidence of epithelial ovarian malignancies diagnosed in pregnancy appears to be increasing as women defer childbearing later into their reproductive years.

37.4.2 Clinical Presentation

The course of the disease is asymptomatic in most cases and the initial diagnosis is typically made during a routine ultrasound examination in pregnancy. Occasionally, tumours greater than 8 centimetres may present with abdominal pain as a complications of ovarian torsion. Most cases are diagnosed in early stages of the disease [22].

37.4.3 Management

Due to its relative rarity, the management of ovarian cancer during pregnancy presents a considerable challenge due to the absence of clear standards of treatment. The options for treatment will consider the histologic type of the tumour, the extent of the disease, the gestational age of the pregnancy and the desires of the patient. Therefore, the management for ovarian cancer during pregnancy should be individualised and formulated within multidisciplinary team setting. Surgery and platinum-based chemotherapy still remains the mainstay of treatment as obtained in the non-pregnant population.

The treatment option presented here has been suggested [23]. For ovarian cancer diagnosed in early pregnancy, induced abortion followed by standard management of ovarian cancer as in non-pregnant women is acceptable. When pregnancy is desired, pregnancy-preserving surgery preferably done in mid-pregnancy (removal of diseased ovaries, omentectomy and excisional biopsy of visible lesions while sparing the uterus) followed by adjuvant chemotherapy. A planned caesarean delivery after foetal viability with a 'second look' at the surgery for optimal staging and debulking is performed.

Neo-adjuvant chemotherapy in pregnancy, planned delivery followed by debulking surgery during the postpartum period is also feasible especially for diagnosis made in the second half of pregnancy. There is abundant literature suggesting that chemotherapy after the first trimester of pregnancy appears not to be associated with untoward effects for the foetus [24]. It is however advisable to avoid the use of chemotherapy within 3 weeks of planned delivery or after 35 weeks of pregnancy.

37.5 Conclusion

Although the occurrence of neoplasms coexisting with pregnancy is relatively rare, pregnancy presents a unique opportunity for early diagnosis of some neoplastic conditions. This is because of the regular surveillance and clinical evaluation received in the course of antenatal care during pregnancy. The presence of the developing foetus along with a neoplasm in a woman presents diagnostic, therapeutic and ethical challenges for the managing team. In addition, the physical and hormonal changes associated with pregnancy presents additional dimensions different from the non-pregnant woman.

The gestational age of the pregnancy, the stage of the cancer at diagnosis and the fertility desires of the patient are important factors to be considered in deciding on a treatment plan. Surgery, radiation therapy and chemotherapy can be administered as treatment options with varying implications for maternal and foetal health. The primary treatment goal should be the physical and psychological health of the woman while making necessary modifications to therapy for better foetal outcome where possible.

37.6 Summary

The incidence of malignant neoplasms occurring during pregnancy appears to be on the increase worldwide. Cancers of reproductive health importance that may occur in association with pregnancy includes breast cancer, cervical cancer, ovarian cancer and malignant trophoblastic disease. They often present a diagnostic, therapeutic and ethical dilemma for Physicians especially when the cancer is diagnosed at a stage in pregnancy when the foetus is not viable for extra-uterine survival or the standard recommended treatment modality is not very safe for use in pregnancy. The goal of management should be to provide the best available treatment for the woman while minimising harm to the developing foetus as much as possible. Treatment should be provided within a multidisciplinary team setting should consider the risks, benefits and alternatives of the treatment modalities. Also, the sociocultural, ethical, moral and spiritual dimensions of the treatment for the patient are important factors that should be considered.

References

1. Hoellen F, Reibke R, Hornemann K, Thill M, Luedders DW, Kelling K, et al. Cancer in pregnancy. Part I: basic diagnostic and therapeutic principles and treatment of gynaecological malignancies. Arch Gynecol Obstet. 2011;285(1):195–205.
2. Van Calsteren K, Heyns L, De Smet F, Van Eycken L, Gziri MM, Van Gemert W, et al. Cancer during pregnancy: an analysis of 215

patients emphasising the obstetrical and the neonatal outcomes. J Clin Oncol. 2010;28:683–9.
3. Andersson TM, Johansson AL, Hsieh CC, Cnattingius S, Lambe M. Increasing incidence of pregnancy-associated breast cancer in Sweden. Obstet Gynecol. 2009;114:568–72.
4. Lee YY, Roberts CL, Dobbins T, Stavrou E, Black K, Morris J, et al. Incidence and outcomes of pregnancy-associated cancer in Australia, 1994–2008: a population-based linkage study. BJOG. 2012;119(13):1572–82.
5. Siegel R, Ward E, Brawley O, Jemal A. Cancer statistics, 2011: the impact of eliminating socioeconomic and racial disparities on premature cancer deaths. CA Cancer J Clin. 2011;61(4):212–36.
6. Antonelli NM, Dotters DJ, Katz VL, Kuller JA. Cancer in pregnancy: a review of the literature. Part I. Obstet Gynecol Surv. 1996;51:125–34.
7. Loibl S, von Minckwitz G, Gwyn K, et al. Breast carcinoma during pregnancy. International recommendations from an expert meeting. Cancer. 2006;106(2):237–46.
8. Merkel D. Pregnancy and breast cancer. Semin Surg Oncol. 1996;12:370–5.
9. Saber A, Dardik H, Ibrahim IM, Wolodiger F. The milk rejection sign: a natural tumour marker. Am Surg. 1996;62(12):998–9.
10. Navrozoglou I, Vrekoussis T, Kontostolis E, et al. Breast cancer during pregnancy: a mini-review. Eur J Surg Oncol. 2008;34(8):837–43.
11. Amant F, Deckers S, Van Calsteren K, Loibl S, Halaska M, Brepoels L, et al. Breast cancer in pregnancy: recommendations of an international consensus meeting. Eur J Cancer. 2010;46(180):3158–68.
12. Cardonick E, Iacobucci A. Use of chemotherapy during pregnancy. Lancet Oncol. 2004;5:283–91.
13. Murphy GC, Mallam D, Stein S, et al. Current and recent pregnancy is associated with adverse pathologic features but not impaired survival in early breast cancer. Cancer. 2012;118:3254–9.
14. Petrek JA, Dukoff R, Rogatko A. Prognosis of pregnancy-associated breast cancer. Cancer. 1991;67(4):869–72.
15. Traen K, Svane D, Kryger-Baggesen N, Bertelsen K, Mogensen O. Stage Ib cervical cancer during pregnancy: planned delay in treatment--case report. Eur J Gynaecol Oncol. 2006;27(6):615–7.
16. Gonçalves CV, Duarte G, Costa JS, Marcolin AC, Bianchi MS, Dias D, et al. Diagnosis and treatment of cervical cancer during pregnancy. Sao Paulo Med J. 2009;127(6):359–65.
17. Sood AK, Sorosky JI, Krogman S, Anderson B, Benda J, Buller RE. Surgical management of cervical cancer complicating pregnancy: a case-control study. Gynecol Oncol. 1996;63(3):294–8.
18. Van Calsteren K, Vergote I, Amant F. Cervical neoplasia during pregnancy: diagnosis, management and prognosis. Best Pract Res Clin Obstet Gynaecol. 2005;19(4):611–30.
19. Goldman NA, Goldberg GL. Late recurrence of squamous cell cervical cancer in an episiotomy site after vaginal delivery. Obstet Gynecol. 2003;101(5 Pt 2):1127–9.
20. Wróbel A, Rechberger E, Magnowska M, Banach P, Filipczak A, Nowak-Markwitz E, et al. Ovarian cancer during pregnancy--presentation of three cases and current diagnostic and treatment algorithms. Ginekol Pol. 2015;86(11):872–8.
21. Zhao XY, Huang HF, Lian LJ, Lang JH. Ovarian cancer in pregnancy: a clinicopathologic analysis of 22 cases and review of the literature. Int J Gynecol Cancer. 2006;16(1):8–15.
22. Machado F, Vegas C, Leon J, Perez A, Sanchez R, Parrilla JJ, et al. Ovarian cancer during pregnancy: analysis of 15 cases. Gynecol Oncol. 2007;105(2):446–50.
23. Mukhopadhyay A, Shinde A, Naik R. Ovarian cysts and cancer in pregnancy. Best Pract Res Clin Obstet Gynaecol. 2016;33:58–72.
24. Behtash N, Karimi Zarchi M, Modares Gilani M, Ghaemmaghami F, Mousavi A, Ghotbizadeh F. Ovarian carcinoma associated with pregnancy: a clinicopathologic analysis of 23 cases and review of the literature. BMC Pregnancy Childbirth. 2008;8:3.

Oral Health in Pregnancy

38

Foluso J. Owotade

Learning Objectives
At the conclusion of this chapter, the reader will be able to:

- Define oral health
- Articulate the importance of oral health in pregnancy
- Identify oral diseases peculiar to or aggravated in pregnancy
- Recognise the benefits of standardised oral care to the pregnant mother and the unborn baby
- Formulate a treatment plan to address oral health care in pregnancy

38.1 Definition of Oral Health

Oral health is a fundamental component of health, which includes physical and mental well-being, and it reflects the physiological, social and psychological attributes that are essential to the quality of life. Oral health is influenced by the person's changing experiences, perceptions, expectations and ability to adapt to circumstances.

The World Dental Federation (FDI) described oral health as being 'multifaceted and includes the ability to speak, smile, smell, taste, touch, chew, swallow, and convey a range of emotions through facial expressions with confidence and without pain, discomfort, and disease of the craniofacial complex' (FDI World Dental Federation 2016).

F. J. Owotade (✉)
Department of Oral & Maxillofacial Surgery and Oral Pathology, Faculty of Dentistry, Obafemi Awolowo University, Ile-Ife, Nigeria

38.1.1 Importance of Oral Health

The U.S. Surgeon General 2000 report titled 'Oral Health in America' emphasised that oral health is integral to general health and should not be seen as separate entities. The report changed the perception regarding oral health. Safe and effective measures exist to prevent the most common diseases, however, ignoring oral health problems can lead to needless pain and suffering. Individuals with poor oral health tend to have worse general health than those with good oral health. In addition, the negative impact of poor oral health on general health tends to worsen with age and poor oral health has been identified as a risk indicator of all-cause mortality. Furthermore, losses of teeth and poor oral care were significant predictors of poor general health, indicating that oral health and oral care are integral parts of general health.

In addition, the impact of oral health on quality of life is in relation to sociodemographic factors, age group and social class background, all of which influence education and access to health care. In some cases, poor oral health is due to a general lack of understanding of the importance of oral health care and restricted access to proper nutrition and medication.

38.1.2 Oral Health Status in Pregnancy

The physiologic changes and adaptation in pregnancy significantly affect the oral tissues. Increased production of hormones such as progesterone, estrogen and relaxin exert changes on the oral tissues with possible unfavourable local and systemic outcomes. These changes increase susceptibility to infection and reduce immunity leading to pathology of the hard and soft oral tissues. All the primary dentition and some permanent teeth form while the woman is pregnant and such teeth are also susceptible to damage due to complica-

F. Okonofua et al. (eds.), *Contemporary Obstetrics and Gynecology for Developing Countries*,
https://doi.org/10.1007/978-3-030-75385-6_38

tions or medications in pregnancy. In spite of the possibility of unfavourable changes, pregnancy offers an opportunity for oral health evaluation and intervention if the caregivers fully incorporated oral health evaluation into obstetric care. Pregnant women who attend antenatal care are exposed to sustained care and examination and have the opportunity of correcting practices inimical to their health and that of their unborn babies. Unfortunately, there is a high level of ignorance of oral health conditions in pregnant women and the antenatal visits do not always adequately address oral health education. Several oral conditions reported in pregnant women include gingivitis, periodontitis, pregnancy oral tumour and candidiasis and dental erosion. A recent systematic review summarised the prevalence of oral mucosal diseases as follows: The overall prevalence of oral mucosal disorders was 11.8%, gingival hyperplasia (17.1%), morsicatio buccarum (10%), oral candidiasis (4.4%), pyogenic granuloma (3%) and benign migratory glossitis (2.8%).

Furthermore, some existing oral diseases or concurrent oral conditions may also be aggravated or their management complicated by pregnancy.

(a) Gingivitis
This is inflammation of the gingival tissues and the most common oral finding in pregnancy. It is usually characterised by bleeding from the gums and usually aggravated in pregnancy even if it was pre-existing before pregnancy. The prevalence of gingivitis in pregnancy is variable and ranges from 30% to 100%. Pregnant women are more prone to gingivitis due to the presence of plaque which initiates the inflammatory process. In addition, the elevated levels of estrogen and progesterone in pregnancy coupled with the expression of estrogen receptor and progesterone receptor on the periodontium support the role of these hormones on inflammation of the supporting structures of the teeth. It is also believed that host response to alterations in the subgingival microbiome further damages the gingival and periodontal tissues. Although the results are not universally consistent, several bacterial organisms have been implicated in gingival inflammation in pregnancy. These include *Campylobacter rectus* and *Fusobacterium nucleatum*. There is also an observed impairment in neutrophil functions throughout pregnancy thereby increasing the susceptibility to inflammation.

(b) Periodontitis
This is inflammation of the supporting structures of the teeth leading to destruction and ultimately tooth mobility and tooth loss if unchecked. Pathogenic bacteria release toxins which stimulate chronic inflammatory response which leads to a breakdown of the periodontal tissues.

(c) Dental Caries
The prevalence to dental caries tends to increase during pregnancy as the teeth are more prone to caries due to reduced pH in the oral cavity. Furthermore, dietary changes and taste alterations lead to increased craving and consumption of cariogenic carbohydrates in pregnant women. There is also a loss of the cleansing and buffering action of saliva due to reduced saliva production. Pregnant women are also intolerant to the taste and smell of toothpaste and oral cleansing products due to olfactory and taste changes thereby making them more prone to dental caries.

(d) Pregnancy oral tumour
This is a benign swelling of the oral tissues seen exclusively in pregnant women, usually in the second trimester. A recent study in South Africa reported 8.5% prevalence in 443 women attending an antenatal facility. The presence of calculus acting as an irritant with the milieu created by oral bacteria and increased progesterone are causative factors. The gingival tissues are predominantly affected although it can occur on the tongue, the cheek and the palate. The swelling tends to disappear after pregnancy and may not require excision except if bleeding occurs and there is interference with mastication. Pregnancy tumour can be prevented by meticulous attention to oral hygiene and removal of plaque and calculus prior to or in early pregnancy.

Pyogenic granulomas may occur during pregnancy as an inflammatory reaction to dental plaque. It is a condition seen in the second or third trimester. It is a painless lesion that develops in response to irritation from plaque. It requires treatment by excision after giving birth.

(e) Oral candidiasis: Approximately, 50% of pregnant women are colonised with oral *Candida* and about 4% will have clinical infection (candidiasis). Increased sugar consumption as a result of dietary cravings increases the risk for *Candida* colonisation. Similarly, increased estrogen levels during pregnancy favours bacteria colonisation by enhancing the glycogen content of epithelia cells thereby providing a nutritional source for *Candida*.

(f) Ptyalism and perimylolysis
Ptyalism refers to excessive saliva production during early pregnancy in women who experience nausea, seems to subside when the nausea improves—at approximately 12–14 weeks' gestation. Nausea and vomiting are very common in pregnancy and affect between 50% and 85% of pregnancies. Vomiting of the gastric contents may lead to decreased pH in the oral cavity. Perimylolysis (acid erosion of tooth enamel), which occurs in patients who have bulimia nervosa, theoretically may occur during pregnancy if the gastric contents or the frequency and duration of vomiting are excessive. A case was reported in the literature of a patient with a gastrinoma that caused intractable vomiting, which resulted in severe dental enamel erosion.

(g) Dental erosion
Early pregnancy may be associated with morning sickness and attendant vomiting. Constant vomiting may predispose the teeth to dental erosion. Furthermore, in the latter stages

of pregnancy, acid reflux may be worsened due to the uterus pushing on a lax oesophageal sphincter. The palatal surfaces of the upper incisors are most severely affected in pregnancy-induced vomiting. Pregnant women with constant hyperemesis should be counselled to rinse the mouth immediately after vomiting with a fluoride mouth rinse or baking soda dissolved in plain water. Brushing with a hard brush and brushing immediately after vomiting should be avoided to prevent further loss of tooth tissue.

(h) Gestational diabetes
A well-known complication of pregnancy that is likely to affect the long-term periodontal health of the mother is gestational diabetes, which is currently estimated to occur in up to 4% of pregnant women. Women with gestational diabetes are more than nine times more likely to have periodontal diseases.

38.1.3 Impact of Mother's Health on the Unborn Baby

Poor oral health in pregnancy has implications for the unborn baby well beyond childbirth. Some of the unfavourable outcomes of poor maternal oral health on the unborn child include preterm birth, low birthweight and a higher propensity for early childhood caries. The initiation of optimal oral health for the unborn child starts with appropriate and purposeful care for the mother. The emphasis is on prevention of transmitting harmful oral microorganisms to the child via oral health education, oral prophylaxis and treatment of caries, gum disease and other pathologic oral health conditions in the mother.

(a) Preterm birth and low birthweight

Studies have suggested that periodontal infection may contribute to the birth of preterm/low birthweight babies. Periodontal disease is caused by Gram-negative anaerobic bacteria. The bacteria responsible for periodontal disease are capable of producing a variety of chemical inflammatory mediators such as prostaglandins, interleukins and tumour necrosis factor that can directly affect the pregnant woman. The individual host response, partially mediated by specific genotype, also plays an important role as a determinant of disease expression.

Adverse pregnancy outcomes included not only preterm/low birthweight but also miscarriage and pre-eclampsia. Studies have established an association between periodontal disease and increased risk of adverse pregnancy outcomes.

(b) Childhood caries

High *Streptococcus mutans* count in mothers can lead to higher caries susceptibility in their children. *S. mutans* is a major aetiologic factor in caries and count tends to correlate with caries experience. The first event is the acquisition of infection with *Streptococcus mutans*. The second event is the accumulation of *Streptococcus mutans* to pathogenic levels secondary to frequent and prolonged exposure to caries-promoting carbohydrates, particularly common sugar. The third event is rapid demineralisation of enamel, which if unchecked leads to cavitation.

Cariogenic bacteria are typically transmitted from mother or caregiver to child by behaviours that directly pass saliva, such as sharing a spoon when tasting baby food, cleaning a dropped pacifier by mouth or wiping the baby's mouth with saliva or premasticating food for the baby. For this reason, mothers who themselves have experienced extensive past or current caries need counselling on how to avoid early transmission of cariogenic bacteria to their offspring.

38.1.4 Recommendations for Oral Health Care in Pregnancy

Several guidelines have been published; however, there are no universally accepted and adopted guidelines on the appropriate oral and dental interventions in pregnancy. In the United States of America, regional and national organisations have published guidelines on the oral health care of pregnant women. Such organisations include the American College of Obstetricians and Gynaecologists with a policy guideline titled 'Oral Health Care During Pregnancy and Through the Lifespan: Committee Opinion'. Similar documents were published by the American Academy of Pediatric Dentistry titled 'Guideline on Oral Health Care for the Pregnant Adolescent (2015/2016)' and 'Guideline on Perinatal Oral Health Care (2015/2016)'.

The following interventions are highly recommended:

38.1.5 Prenatal Counselling

Infant oral health begins at the prenatal stage. It is important that prenatal oral health counselling for parents is commenced at this early stage. The main goal is to create awareness among the expectant mothers about the importance of prevention of dental disease by means of oral prophylaxis and restoring carious teeth. These procedures will decrease the microbial load in the oral cavity of the mother thereby reducing transmission to the child. Prenatal assessment begins with the oral health status of the expectant mother. If the expectant mothers are at risk, the dentist should provide preventive treatment such as oral prophylaxis, fluoride varnish application and educate them on good plaque control, followed by restorations if required and discuss the vertical transmissibility of *Streptococcus mutans*. Regular recall visits are planned to ensure effective oral hygiene measures and compliance with dietary habits. Thus, improving the expectant mothers' oral hygiene, modifying dietary habits and the use of mouthwashes can certainly have a significant impact on the child's oral health status, especially caries rate in the future.

38.1.6 Preventive Methods

Although a number of non-invasive preventive interventions are available, traditional health education is considered as the gold standard for imparting knowledge and encouraging parents on preventive interventions. 'Traditional health education' is a means of conducting counselling sessions by health care providers and/or the dissemination of information by means of pamphlets, posters and media campaigns. One crucial information to disseminate is the use of preventive agents in the oral cavity of pregnant women.

Xylitol and chlorhexidine reduce maternal oral bacterial load and reduce the vertical transmission of bacteria to infants when used late in pregnancy and/or in the postpartum period. Both topical agents are safe in pregnancy and during breastfeeding. Xylitol chewing gums of high dose had beneficial effects by reducing the plaque pH and on long-term use of xylitol chewing gums; it was found that there was significant reduction in the plaque pH and *Streptococcus mutans* saliva concentration.

38.1.7 Anticipatory Guidance

Anticipatory guidance is the process of providing practical, developmentally appropriate information about children's health to prepare parents for the significant physical, emotional and psychological milestones. General anticipatory guidance for the mother includes the following (Nowak and Casamassimo, 1995):

(a) Education concerning development and prevention of dental disease and also demonstration of oral hygiene procedures.
(b) Counselling to instill preventive attitudes and motivation.
(c) Educating the pregnant women about pregnancy gingivitis.
(d) Regular visit to a dentist for check-up, to reduce the gingivitis (pregnancy induced) and restoring all carious teeth as early as possible.
(e) Eating healthy foods containing proteins and vitamins, such as fresh fruits and vegetables, grains and dairy products such as milk and cheese. From the dental perspective, the expectant mother should take adequate nutrition during the third trimester because the enamel (primary or milk teeth) maturation of the child occurs in that phase.
(f) Limiting the amount of sugar consumption, if at all taken, it should be taken along with the meals. The frequency of snacking (food rich in sugar increases the risk of tooth decay) in between meals is to be avoided.
(g) Brushing the teeth thoroughly thrice a day with fluoridated toothpaste and flossing daily.
(h) Rinsing the oral cavity with an alcohol-free mouthwash before going to bed (preferably a fluoridated mouth rinse).
(i) Not smoking cigarettes or chewing tobacco.

38.1.8 Screening and Prevention

Oral examination should include both the soft tissue and hard tissue. Patients should be counselled to perform regular brushing with soft bristles and flossing the inter-dental areas, avoid frequent snacking with sugary snacks and carbonated drinks and to have frequent dental check-up. The oral health status, treatment plan and follow-ups should be documented to evaluate the oral health maintenance. Many healthcare providers including the dentists are often reluctant to treat the expectant mothers. This situation can be overcome by multi-specialty discussions, through which a clear communication and a better understanding can be obtained. Dentists can explain various dental materials, procedures and safety of dental treatment to the gynaecologists and the physicians so that they can explain them to the pregnant mothers and provide referral recommendations.

38.1.9 Diagnosis

Dental radiography (periapical, bite wing and occlusal) can be performed during pregnancy for emergency purposes. As much as is possible, radiographs should be delayed till the second trimester. Radiographs taken for regular check-ups should be postponed until delivery. Use of lead aprons and thyroid shields, collimators and E-speed films and avoidance of retakes will further reduce the risk of radiation exposure. The teratogenic risk of radiation exposure from intra-oral films is 1000 times less than the natural risk of spontaneous abortion or malformation.

38.1.10 Medications Used During Dental Procedures

Local anaesthetic solutions such as lidocaine (Xylocaine) and prilocaine (Citanest) mixed with epinephrine are safe for procedures when dosed appropriately. Sedatives such as benzodiazepines (e.g. midazolam), lorazepam (Ativan) and triazolam (Halcion) should be avoided. Use of nitrous oxide during pregnancy is still not rated, but its use is controversial.

38.1.11 Periodontal Therapy

There was a significant reduction of preterm birth or low birthweight rate in children in a randomised controlled trial consisting of 870 pregnant women for whom dental treatment was done. Such treatment included plaque control, daily rinsing using 0.12% chlorhexidine and manually performed supragingival removal of plaque every 2–3 weeks until delivery.

38.1.12 Restorative Dentistry

Amalgam is the most commonly used restorative material in dentistry. It has advantages over other restorative materials since it is not technique sensitive; however, there are concerns about release of mercury as vapour that can possibly be ingested or inhaled. There is no published evidence that amalgam exposure during pregnancy have deleterious effect such as spontaneous abortions or birth defects. In a longitudinal evaluation of filling materials on caries-active expectant mothers, it was concluded that highly viscous glass ionomer cement can be a material of choice in minimally invasive cavity preparations and composite restorations can be used for anterior teeth.

38.1.13 Dental Extraction

Dental pain has become a common complaint during pregnancy. Due to the hormonal changes during pregnancy, the gingiva is sensitive to irritation. The gingiva gets inflamed, turns red, bleeds and becomes painful. Brushing is difficult which gives way for plaque accumulation around the teeth.

This commonly occurs in the gingiva around the impacted third molar teeth. This could be an indication for extraction during pregnancy. Most dentists would wish to postpone dental extractions during pregnancy. There is a continuous stress when the expectant mother is in constant pain and this can jeopardise the health of the developing child.

38.1.14 Management of Acute Dental Conditions

In conditions such as mild cellulitis, first-line antibiotics such as penicillin, amoxicillin and cephalexin are the drugs of choice. In patients allergic to penicillin, erythromycin base (not erythromycin estolate, which is associated with cholestatic hepatitis in pregnancy) or clindamycin (Cleocin) can be used. In patients with severe cellulitis, the pregnant mother should be treated as an inpatient with intravenous infusion of cephalosporins or clindamycin. Acetaminophen is the drug of choice to relieve dental pain; ibuprofen and limited use of oxycodone are appropriate.

Various types of dental procedures that can be undertaken during each trimester are summarised as follows:

- First trimester: It is the most crucial period for growth of the foetus. Only emergency dental treatment should be undertaken in consultation with the patient's gynaecologist/physician when organogenesis is incomplete. If the expectant mother complains of dental pain, the dentist can do an emergency access opening, extirpate the inflamed pulp (or) drain the pus and relieve pain. Intra-canal medicaments such as chlorhexidine/metronidazole, calcium hydroxide can be used. Plaque and diet control programmes are initiated for the mother throughout pregnancy.
- Second trimester: This phase is considered the safest to treat patients among the three trimesters. Emergency as well as elective dental treatment can be provided in the second trimester. Treatment such as emergency dental extractions, periodontal surgeries and completion of root canal can be performed.
- Third trimester: If patient develops dental pain, an emergency treatment can be performed and definitive treatment can be postponed until after birth, if possible. There is a positional discomfort in the third trimester and the risk of compression of the vena cava. This can be overcome by repositioning them frequently and propping on their left side and most importantly, reducing the timings of appointments can minimise complications. Postponing dental treatment until delivery can be problematic because mothers are more focused on the care of their newborn child than their own health.

Further Reading

1. Africa CWJ, Turton M. Oral health status and treatment needs of pregnant women attending antenatal clinics in KwaZulu-Natal, South Africa. Int J Dent. 2019;2019:5475973.
2. Al-Rusan RM, Darwazeh AM, Lataifeh IM. The relationship of Candida colonisation of the oral and vaginal mucosae of mothers and oral mucosae of their newborns at birth. Oral Surg Oral Med Oral Pathol Oral Radiol. 2017;123(4):459–63.
3. Bartlett D. Intrinsic causes of erosion. Monogr Oral Sci. 2006;20:119–39.
4. Bett JVS, Batistella EA, Melo G, Munhoz EA, Silva CAB, Guerra E, et al. Prevalence of oral mucosal disorders during pregnancy: a systematic review and meta-analysis. J Oral Pathol Med. 2019;48(4):270–7.

5. Briggs GG, Wan SR. Drug therapy during labor and delivery, part 1. Am J Health Syst Pharm. 2006;63(11):1038–47.
6. Dabelea D, Snell-Bergeon JK, Hartsfield CL, Bischoff KJ, Hamman RF, McDuffie RS, et al. Increasing prevalence of gestational diabetes mellitus (GDM) over time and by birth cohort: Kaiser Permanente of Colorado GDM Screening Program. Diabetes Care. 2005;28(3):579–84.
7. Davis M. Nausea and vomiting of pregnancy: an evidence-based review. J Perinat Neonatal Nurs. 2004;18(4):312–28.
8. Evans RD, Briggs PF. Tooth-surface loss related to pregnancy-induced vomiting. Prim Dent Care. 1994;1(1):24–6.
9. Glick M, Williams DM, Kleinman DV, Vujicic M, Watt RG, Weyant RJ. A new definition for oral health developed by the FDI World Dental Federation opens the door to a universal definition of oral health. Int Dent J. 2016;66(6):322–4.
10. Iida H. Oral health interventions during pregnancy. Dent Clin N Am. 2017;61(3):467–81.
11. Kandan PM, Menaga V, Kumar RR. Oral health in pregnancy (guidelines to gynaecologists, general physicians & oral health care providers). J Pak Med Assoc. 2011;61(10):1009–14.
12. Lopez NJ, Da Silva I, Ipinza J, Gutierrez J. Periodontal therapy reduces the rate of preterm low birth weight in women with pregnancy-associated gingivitis. J Periodontol. 2005;76 Suppl 11S:2144–53.
13. Melkonian R, Baker D. Risks of industrial mercury exposure in pregnancy. Obstet Gynecol Surv. 1988;43(11):637–41.
14. Nowak AJ, Casamassimo PS. Using anticipatory guidance to provide early dental intervention. J Am Dent Assoc. 1995;126(8):1156–63.
15. Offenbacher S, Katz V, Fertik G, Collins J, Boyd D, Maynor G, et al. Periodontal infection as a possible risk factor for preterm low birth weight. J Periodontol. 1996;67(10):1103–13.
16. Owotade FJ, Ogundipe OK, Ugboko VI, Okoje VN, Olasoji HO, Makinde ON, et al. Awareness, knowledge and attitude on cleft lip and palate among antenatal clinic attendees of tertiary hospitals in Nigeria. Niger J Clin Pract. 2014;17(1):6–9.
17. Reyes L, Phillips P, Wolfe B, Golos TG, Walkenhorst M, Progulske-Fox A, et al. Porphyromonas gingivalis and adverse pregnancy outcome. J Oral Microbiol. 2018;10(1):1374153.
18. Silk H, Douglass AB, Douglass JM, Silk L. Oral health during pregnancy. Am Fam Physician. 2008;77(8):1139–44.
19. Smith RE, Badner VM, Morse DE, Freeman K. Maternal risk indicators for childhood caries in an inner city population. Community Dent Oral Epidemiol. 2002;30(3):176–81.
20. Sobel JD. Vulvovaginal candidosis. Lancet. 2007;369(9577):1961–71.
21. Soderling E, Isokangas P, Pienihakkinen K, Tenovuo J, Alanen P. Influence of maternal xylitol consumption on mother-child transmission of mutans streptococci: 6-year follow-up. Caries Res. 2001;35(3):173–7.
22. Sonbul H, Ashi H, Aljahdali E, Campus G, Lingstrom P. The influence of pregnancy on sweet taste perception and plaque acidogenicity. Matern Child Health J. 2017;21(5):1037–46.
23. Tettamanti L, Lauritano D, Nardone M, Gargari M, Silvestre-Rangil J, Gavoglio P, et al. Pregnancy and periodontal disease: does exist a two-way relationship? Oral Implantol (Rome). 2017;10(2):112–8.
24. Vamos CA, Thompson EL, Avendano M, Daley EM, Quinonez RB, Boggess K. Oral health promotion interventions during pregnancy: a systematic review. Community Dent Oral Epidemiol. 2015;43(5):385–96.
25. Wu M, Chen SW, Jiang SY. Relationship between gingival inflammation and pregnancy. Mediators Inflamm. 2015;2015:623427.
26. Xiong X, Buekens P, Fraser WD, Beck J, Offenbacher S. Periodontal disease and adverse pregnancy outcomes: a systematic review. BJOG. 2006;113(2):135–43.
27. Zanata RL, Navarro MF, Pereira JC, Franco EB, Lauris JR, Barbosa SH. Effect of caries preventive measures directed to expectant mothers on caries experience in their children. Braz Dent J. 2003;14(2):75–81.

Part IV

General Gynaecology

Ectopic Pregnancy

39

Friday Okonofua

Learning Objectives
After reading this chapter, the reader will be able to:

- Describe the different types of ectopic pregnancy (EP) and its epidemiology
- Articulate the causes and pathophysiology of the disease
- Discuss its clinical features including symptoms, signs and methods of diagnosis
- Describe the use of new technology and methods for the early diagnosis of unruptured EP
- Discern the various approaches that can be used for its prevention
- Discuss the clinical management and follow-up of women experiencing EP
- Contextualize research gaps in EP, with a particular focus on research needs in sub-Saharan African countries

39.1 Introduction

Ectopic pregnancy (EP) is the implantation of pregnancy outside the uterine cavity. Long known for generations, it is surprising that no permanent solution has been found to its occurrence. By contrast, it continues to increase in prevalence and incidence in both developed and developing countries. Because of the many diverse ways of clinical presentation and even sites of implantation that may confuse both the greenhorn and the expert alike, it has been referred to as the 'black beast' or 'big masquerader' in gynaecological practice [1].

Till date, ectopic pregnancy is a significant cause of maternal death and is a contributor to maternal mortality statistics in both developed and developing countries. The early diagnosis and management of EP require imaginative clinical knowledge and a high index of suspicion, along with available facilities to manage gynaecological emergencies. The fact that ectopic pregnancy still results in death and disability in all countries suggests the need for more concentrated efforts and innovations to deal with the problem. It requires more creative use of existing clinical infrastructure as well as new scientific discoveries to potentiate its early diagnosis and management.

This chapter will review the epidemiology, clinical features and management of ectopic pregnancy and suggest new lines of research and clinical practice to better manage the disease, especially within the context of developing countries.

39.1.1 Sites and Pathophysiology of Ectopic Pregnancy

Worldwide, EP constitutes 1.2–1.4% of all reported pregnancies [2], with the fallopian tube being the most common site of implantation. Tubal site implantation accounts for 95.5% of all ectopic pregnancies. Of all tubal EPs, the ampullary part of the fallopian tube is the most common site (75–80%), followed by the isthmus (10–15%) and then the fimbrial part (5%). Both fallopian tubes have equal chances of been involved in ectopic pregnancy. Bilateral tubal ectopic is rare and occurs in 1 in 200,000 pregnancies [3], while variants such as combined intra-uterine and extra-uterine gestation [4], hysteroscopic ectopic pregnancy with ruptured ectopic [5] and ectopic pregnancy with twin gestational sacs [6] have been described in various settings.

Other sites for EP include the ovary (3.2%) [7], interstitial pregnancy [8], abdominal pregnancy (1.3%) [9], the cervix (0.15%) [10] and caesarean scar pregnancy (1:1800 pregnancies). Of these, only some abdominal pregnancies have been reported to result in a live birth [11]. Unless otherwise indicated, most references to an ectopic pregnancy in this review

F. Okonofua (✉)
Centre of Excellence in Reproductive Health Innovation, Department of Obstetrics and Gynaecology, University of Benin, Benin City, Nigeria

Women's Health and Action Research Centre, Benin City, Nigeria

University of Medical Sciences, Ondo City, Ondo State, Nigeria

F. Okonofua et al. (eds.), *Contemporary Obstetrics and Gynecology for Developing Countries*,
https://doi.org/10.1007/978-3-030-75385-6_39

relate to ectopic tubal pregnancy rather than to other forms of ectopic pregnancy.

The underlying pathophysiology of ectopic pregnancies involves the deposition or entrapment of a fertilized egg or blastocyst at an extra-uterine site, followed by an attempt at decidua formation and progression of the pregnancy at the site. The extent to which the pregnancy develops is dependent on the available space. The fallopian tube with its small lumen and minimal musculature is quickly overwhelmed by the size of the growing embryo. Within 6–8 weeks, it has reached its maximum level of development, and with the associated increased vascularization, it tends to rupture when not detected earlier, with the risk of internal bleeding of various degrees. The bleeding is internal and ranges from mild to severe, depending on the level of vascularization and the site of implantation of the pregnancy. Thus, ectopic pregnancy may be classified as acute, when the bleeding is severe and profound and associated with hypotension and shock. It is subacute or chronic when the site of ectopic pregnancy is slow-leaking and is associated with progressive chronic anaemia and possibly infection over a more extended period.

39.1.2 Epidemiology of Ectopic Pregnancy

Ectopic pregnancy is linked to high rates of maternal morbidity and mortality worldwide. EP accounts for 4–10% of maternal deaths in developed countries [12], and possibly much more in developing countries. The case fatality associated with EP ranges between 1% and 3% in developing countries, which is ten times higher than in developed countries [13]. Strategies designed to reduce the incidence and death rates from EPs will contribute to global efforts to reduce maternal mortality rates and achieve the sustainable development goals.

Approximately 10,000 ectopic pregnancies are reported annually in the UK, with an annual incidence rate of 11.1 per 1000 pregnancies [14]. This prevalence rate is similar to the incidence rate of EP in most western countries. By contrast, the yearly incidence of the disease is not known with accuracy in many African countries due to the scarcity of data and missing cases as a result of the inaccurate diagnosis. But there has been a strong suggestion that the incidence of EP may be higher in African countries due to the higher frequency of the factors that predispose to the disease [13]. A population-based study in Yaoundé, the Republic of Cameroon [15] reported an annual incidence of 320 EPs per 40,100 live births – a prevalence of 0.79% (CI: 0.72–0.88). This lower incidence data as compared to those reported from Western countries may be due to under-reporting, as is suspected to be the case in many developing countries.

In both developed and developing countries, the incidence of EP has increased over the past 30 years [2], and the surges are mainly due to the increasing prevalence of predisposing factors as well as the emergence of the new reproductive technologies. For example, in Conakry, Guinea, the incidence of EP for all pregnancies increased from 0.41% to 1.5% [16].

Risk Factors Most cases of tubal EP arise as a result of previous damage to the fallopian tube from infection or tubal surgery. As such, the risk factors for tubal EP include the following:

- *Maternal Age:* The older the woman, the higher the chances of an ectopic pregnancy due to the greater likelihood that older women are more likely to have been exposed to tubal damage that leads to EP. Ectopic pregnancy is rare in women less than 20 years of age. Reports indicate a rising incidence of EP from 1.4% of all pregnancies at age 21 to 6.9% in those aged 46 years or more [16].
- *Behavioural Risk Factors*: Smoking has been shown to reduce ciliary motility and to predispose to EP in both animal and human models [17]. Smoking may promote embryo retention within the tube as a result of impaired smooth muscle contractility and alterations in the microenvironment of the tube. Alcohol intake has so far not been associated with increased risks of ectopic gestation. Previous ectopic pregnancy increases the risk for another EP because of the tendency to existing bilateral tubal damage, while the use of some contraceptives, notably intrauterine contraceptives devices, may increase the risk of EP, although this has not been confirmed in most settings [18].
- *Previous Pelvic Inflammatory Disease:* Women with past episodes of pelvic inflammatory disease are more likely to experience EP – 13% after the first episode of infection, 35% after a second episode and 75% after a third episode [2, 19]. These infections are mostly due to *Neisseria Gonorrhoea* and *Chlamydia trachomatis*. Due to the asymptomatic nature of infections with Chlamydia, it has been challenging to develop a public health approach for dealing with the problem. The difficulty is one factor that accounts for the rising incidence of EP, especially in developing countries.
- *Unsafe Abortion*: Unsafe abortion is a significant risk factor for ectopic pregnancy in societies where abortion is dangerous and restrictive. A large percentage of women in several sub-Saharan African countries are at risk of pelvic infection from poorly performed illicit abortions [20, 21], which has been shown to increase the risk of ectopic pregnancy compared to women who have never had abortion [22, 23]. Abortion safety and access are now recognised to be an essential strategy for reducing the prevalence of EP in many African countries.
- *Other Tubal Infections:* Infections with tuberculosis and schistosomiasis have been reported to lead to tubal dam-

age and increase the risk of EP [24]. Puerperal infections from women using unclean delivery places (such as homes of traditional birth attendants) can damage the fallopian tubes and predispose to EP in later pregnancies [23].

- *Previous Tubal Surgery:* Past tubal surgery from tubal ligation (either with surgery or laparoscopy), reversal surgery for tubal ligation, tubal repair surgeries (tubal adhesiolysis, salpingostomy, fimbrioplasty, etc.) all increase the risks of subsequent ectopic pregnancy [25].
- *Assisted Reproductive Technology:* The advent of the assisted reproductive technologies is now known to be associated with increased risk of EP [26]. The rate of tubal EP following in vitro fertilization has been reported to be twice as high as rate following spontaneous pregnancy [27]. This prevalence rate has been attributed to the technique of embryo transfer, and possibly the increased number of embryos transferred during in vitro fertilization (IVF).

39.1.3 Clinical Presentation of Ectopic Pregnancy

Lower abdominal pain after a period of secondary amenorrhea is the most common method of presentation of EP. However, amenorrhea does not always occur; it may follow an altered or normal menstrual flow, but abdominal pain is much more pathognomonic of EP. Abdominal pain should never happen in association with a healthy pregnancy at least in the first trimester of pregnancy. A 'normal' abdominal pain due to stretching of the round ligament or to 'Braxton Hicks' contraction may occur in the late second or third trimester. By contrast, any lower abdominal pain arising in the first trimester of pregnancy (when there is a missed period or positive pregnancy test) must be treated with suspicion until proven otherwise.

Therefore, the classic symptom of EP is lower abdominal pain followed by mild-to-moderate vaginal bleeding. The differential diagnosis with spontaneous abortion can be made because vaginal bleeding in EP is less severe than in spontaneous abortion. Also, vaginal bleeding precedes abdominal pain in spontaneous abortion, whereas lower abdominal pain is first experienced before vaginal bleeding in cases of ectopic pregnancy. This is because the significant bleeding in EP is intra-abdominal, while the significant bleeding in spontaneous abortion is external through a dilated cervix and the vagina.

The most severe type of EP – acute ectopic pregnancy – is characterised by tubal rupture and intra-abdominal bleeding and is often associated with severe abdominal pain, hypotension and shock. The degree of hypotension and shock depends on the extent of intra-abdominal bleeding. The more severe bleeding related to shock is an acute gynaecological emergency, which may occur suddenly and must be attended to by emergency surgical care if the woman is to survive.

By contrast, 'slowly leaking' ectopic pregnancies with slower intra-abdominal blood losses may be more confusing to clinicians as sudden hypotension and shock do not occur, while anaemia may take a longer time to develop. In some of these cases, blood or blood clots may collect either in the pouch of Douglas, in the pelvis, or the general abdominal cavity. This manifestation may lead to other complications such as chronic infection and the formation of adhesions, cysts and omental crusts.

The most daunting cases of EP is when the tubal has not yet ruptured, frequently referred to as an unruptured ectopic pregnancy. The symptoms and clinical presentations may be much more nebulous. Apart from amenorrhea and mild abdominal pain, nothing else may be evident. The diagnosis of EP then depends on a high level of suspicion, great clinical insight and experience and the use of modern technology. If the diagnosis of unruptured EP is not made and the patient is wrongly discharged home, it could lead to sudden rupture later on and pose a real danger to the woman. So, it is imperative that a diagnosis of ectopic pregnancy is excluded by all means before a woman with associated symptoms is discharged home.

39.1.3.1 Diagnosis of Unruptured Ectopic Pregnancy

In clinical practice, when the diagnosis of EP is suspected, the first step is to carry out a urine or serum pregnancy test. If any of these tests are positive, it suggests the need to pursue the diagnosis further. However, a negative pregnancy test may not always be sufficient to exclude an existing EP; if available, a beta-subunit human chorionic gonadotropin (hCG) assay should be done to confirm the presence or absence of a slowly growing pregnancy. Before now, many resorted to laparoscopy to establish the presence or absence of a suspected extra-uterine pregnancy. However, the advent of trans-vaginal ultrasound scan has upturned the practice, as the technique is now the gold standard in the diagnosis of unruptured ectopic pregnancy [28]. In experienced hands, the sensitivity of trans-vaginal ultrasound in the diagnosis of unruptured EP has been reported to be as high as 99% [2]. The range of ultrasonic findings in EP is broad. The most diagnostic is the presence of a gestational sac outside the uterine cavity containing a yolk sac, with or without embryonic echoes.

The use of computerised tomography and MRI have been suggested [2], but these are generally not used in pregnancy because of radiation effects on the growing foetus. However, in acute abdominal emergencies, computerised tomography is highly accurate in pinpointing the exact cause and site of bleeding. In the case of suspected EP, this should be used sparingly because of the possibility that a wanted intrauterine pregnancy exists.

Serum levels of enzyme markers such as vascular endothelial growth factor [29], creatine kinase [30] and a disintegrin and metalloprotease-2 (Adam-12) [31] have been reported to be significantly higher in EP as compared to controls. In routine clinical practice, they may not be used, but they are especially useful in groups of EPs with low levels of beta sub-unit hCG. They will be helpful in future research for identifying creative ways to make a rapid diagnosis of EP.

39.1.4 Management of Ectopic Pregnancy

Acute Ectopic Pregnancy The treatment of EP is a surgical emergency if it presents acutely with severe haemorrhage, hypotension and shock. Time should not be wasted. An intravenous line should immediately be started, and the woman transfused with normal saline or any available intravenous fluids pending the availability of whole blood. In acute blood loss, whole blood (which includes plasma) should be transfused rather than packed cells or partially packed cells. However, if blood is not immediately available, time should not be wasted looking for blood. Immediate steps should be put in place to take the patient to the theatre and to carry out laparotomy, while the patient is receiving massive intravenous fluids to prevent her from sliding into irreversible shock. Our experience indicates that when prompt action is taken to open the abdomen, identify the site of ruptured EP and stop haemorrhage, the approach will be more useful in saving the life of the woman than fruitless efforts concentrated at trying to obtain blood for transfusion before surgery. This is one example in clinical surgical practice where the assertion of waiting to get blood before surgery is started, can be overlooked with overwhelming evidence that this is the better approach.

Indeed, in many developing countries blood may not always be available to transfuse women experiencing an acute ectopic pregnancy. The lack of blood for transfusion accounts for the presently high case-fatality rates associated with EP in many African countries. However, the lack of blood should not be an excuse for inaction, as various methods have been reported in the literature that clinicians working in difficult situations have used to overcome this. The principal method is an intra-operative autologous blood transfusion, which has been reported as life-saving in many sub-Saharan African settings [32–34]. In this method, blood obtained from the abdominal cavity in women undergoing surgery for EP is cleared of clots and contaminants and then used to auto-transfuse the women during the surgery. Tremendous beneficial surgical outcomes and safety for affected women have been reported for this procedure, without any significant reported adverse side effects [35]. It is recommended for the management of acute EPs, especially in countries with limited access to blood for emergency transfusion.

During laparotomy for ectopic pregnancy, the immediate concern should be to identify the bleeding site and secure hemostasis and to ensure adequate intravascular volume. Thereafter, the surgeon can take the proper time to perform the definitive surgery and to clean up the abdomen. Partial or total salpingectomy is recommended, while the contra-lateral tube should always be inspected to determine its functionality and to exclude another EP.

The surgeon should avoid the temptation of trying to carry out a conservative surgery on the involved tube as our experience shows that this is counter-productive. It is time-wasting and reduces the time to the hemodynamic recovery of the patient and exposes her to the risk of a repeat ectopic in the same site.

39.1.4.1 Sub-acute (Slow-Leaking) Ectopic Pregnancy

Slow-leaking EP is often complicated by chronic anaemia and infection. The patient is more chronically ill, and therefore time must be taken to resuscitate her before definitive surgical treatment. Rather than whole blood, anaemia should be treated with packed cells or partially packed cells, to prevent relapse into cardiac failure as a result of an overload of the circulation. If packed cells are not available, intravenous frusemide or ethacrynic acid should be given with the transfusion, which should be done slowly over some time.

Broad-spectrum antibiotics should also be given – a good choice being one of the third of fourth-generation cephalosporin, combined with gentamycin and metronidazole. These would cover all possible infections and provide a foundation for manipulation of the ectopic pregnancy site and prevent dissemination of infection.

Surgery for the repair of a slow-leaking EP is best done with a lower midline incision to provide adequate surgical space, should adjacent organs be involved. Since the ectopic pregnancy may involve the omentum, the small and large intestine, it is best that the operation is undertaken jointly with a general surgeon who will deal with associated surgical complications. After surgery, the abdomen and pelvis should be cleaned with adequate saline lavage, and if considered necessary, a drain should be inserted to deal with the following collection of fluid or infected products. Additionally, closure of the wound should be with anticipation of possible infection, with the use of interrupted non-absorbable sutures (e.g. 2/0 nylon) for the closing of the abdominal fascia.

39.1.5 Treatment of Unruptured Ectopic Pregnancy

Three types of options are available for the management of unruptured EP. These include (1) expectant management, (2) medical management and (3) surgical management.

Expectant Management It is based on the notion that the trophoblast could regress in growth if not in a favourable environment [36]. This type of management is recommended in settings where there are adequate methods of laboratory investigations, high-quality ultrasound examination and proper protocol for follow-up that is adhered to by patients and clinicians alike. The American College of Obstetricians and Gynaecologists [37] recommends this method when the beta sub-unit hCG is less than 200 mIU/ml and has been demonstrated to be in the declining phase. There is evidence that all EPs spontaneously resolve when the beta sub-unit hCG reaches a level of 15 mIU/ml or less. This method is not recommended for use in resource-poor countries where there may not be adequate facilities and trained personnel to undertake the high-level investigations and monitoring needed.

Medical Management Various medications have been reported to be useful for the treatment of unruptured EP [38, 39]. These include systemic and local methotrexate, local potassium chloride, hyperosmolar glucose, prostaglandins, danazol, etoposide and mifepristone. The local administration of these drugs has been reported following laparoscopy and the instillation of the drugs at the site of the EPs.

However, most reviews of medical treatment have focused more on methotrexate treatment. A single dose of methotrexate 0.4–1.0 mg/kg body weight or 50 mg/m^2 is recommended without the use of folinic acid rescue. However, multiple combinations of cytotoxic drugs may also be used, but this is associated with higher rates of side effects without substantial additional benefits. The follow-up measurement of the beta-subunit hCG every week is recommended when this regimen is used. If the hCG has not declined by 25% during the first 1 week of follow-up, then the second dose of methotrexate should be given. Follow-up monitoring should include weekly trans-vaginal ultrasound to ensure progressive vanishing of the pregnancy site. Side effects associated with the use of methotrexate include nausea, vomiting, diarrhoea, abnormal liver function tests and neutropenia. Barnhart et al. [40] in a meta-analysis of published studies has reported success rates of 88–93% following the correct use of methotrexate for the medical treatment of EP.

Surgical Treatment In many developing countries where there may not be facilities for endoscopic surgery, most practitioners resort to laparotomy or mini-laparotomy for the treatment of unruptured EP. The method of choice of treatment at laparotomy is conservative salpingostomy, whereby an incision is made on the fallopian tube over the swelling. The pregnancy is then removed with forceps and continuous saline irrigation. After that, the incision is closed with fine interrupted non-absorbable sutures, or it may be left to heal by secondary intention.

However, where facilities are available, the preferred method of treatment of unruptured EP is diagnostic laparoscopy with salgingostomy [2, 41]. This will enable the tube to be preserved more precisely without the additional risk of pelvic adhesions that may occur with laparotomy.

39.1.6 Prevention of Ectopic Pregnancy

The prevention of ectopic pregnancy is best considered under three categories – primary, secondary and tertiary prevention.

Primary prevention is to prevent ectopic pregnancy from occurring in the first place. Interventions designed to reduce the incidence and prevalence of EP will be more impactful in the long run in reducing the health burdens posed by the disease. Primary prevention includes the prevention of sexually transmitted infections, unsafe abortion, unclean deliveries and various infections (schistosomiasis, tuberculosis, etc.) that lead to tubal damage and subsequent ectopic pregnancy. A system-wide approach to preventing these infections within existing health care systems should be adopted as a better and more sustainable method that will yield measurable results. Risks can also be reduced from other causes of EP such as the assisted reproductive technology if available protocols are adhered to, and clinicians are adequately trained to use the procedures.

Secondary prevention is the prompt emergency treatment of women when they experience complications of ectopic pregnancy. This includes both demand and supply components. On the demand side, women need to be taught to identify possible symptoms of ectopic pregnancy and to report in health facilities as soon as they experience such symptoms. On the demand side, referral facilities must be business-ready to receive women who experience symptoms of gynaecological emergencies and to treat them promptly and efficiently. These include preparations made for emergency gynaecological care on a 24-hour basis with available staff, including preparations for blood transfusion, intensive care and emergency surgery. Such facilities may not always exist in resource-poor countries, but first referral centres with pooled resources could be considered in such settings.

Tertiary prevention is the rehabilitation of a woman after she has experienced complications of EP. These include forecasting and the counselling of at-risk women to prevent a repeat ectopic pregnancy. Women who have completed their family sizes should be counselled to undergo permanent contraception such as with bilateral or unilateral tubal ligation as the case may be. Women not willing to endure permanent contraception should be advised to receive effective contraceptives depending on their preference on a regular basis.

Women with pre-existing infertility or sub-fertility should be guided to achieve a future pregnancy using conventional treatment approaches, or with assisted reproductive techniques. Efforts should be made to prevent a repeat EP in such cases and to manage the resultant pregnancies until delivery effectively.

39.1.7 Needed Research in Ectopic Pregnancy

Although ectopic pregnancy is common in developing countries, there has been limited research and relevant data globally. The limited research on EP from developing countries has been from single hospitals and retrospectively designed studies. As such, the findings have been less useful for targeting interventions. Some suggestions for future research relating to EP in developing countries include the following:

- Multi-centre prospective cohort studies that utilised optimum sample sizes to assess the prevalence, incidence, and outcomes of management of EP.
- Clinical trials that evaluate different modes of treatment of EP – such as comparison of medical versus surgical treatment of unruptured EPs, etc.
- Assessment of the health services used for the management of gynaecological emergencies, including EPs. The investigations should include quality of care assessment and the evaluation of the knowledge and preparedness of providers to deal with EP. It is essential to determine the training needs for the improved system management and prevention of EP.
- Assessing the knowledge and cultural barriers to health seeking for EP and other early complications of pregnancy would be highly relevant. Are their cultural hindrances to health seeking, and what other factors constrain the use of emergency services for EP in resource-challenged environments? These are critical questions that would enable the design of programmes and policies for educating the general public about EP and its consequences.
- Intervention and translational investigations that identify ways to prevent and manage EP, with evidence demonstrated of effective translation of the results of such research for policy development and implementation.

39.2 Conclusion

Ectopic pregnancy is a significant complication of pregnancy in both developed and developing countries. Its rising incidence in all countries is evidence of the increasing prevalence of factors – sexually transmitted infections assisted reproductive technologies, etc. – that predispose to the disease. Although EP is prevalent in both developed and developing countries, it is in developing countries that the condition makes its most profound negative consequences on the health and social well-being of women. Early diagnosis and the prompt, efficient and effective method of medical and surgical treatments is the best approach to prevent and manage the disease in all countries. This chapter is a call to action to health practitioners, especially obstetricians and gynaecologists in developing countries to learn the application of various new methods and skills that are relevant for the prevention and management of the condition to save the lives of women.

References

1. Medicine EB. Complications of pregnancy, Part 1: early pregnancy. Accessed from https://www.ebmedicine.net/topics.php?paction=showTopicsSeg&topic_id=130&seg_id=2554 on December 29, 2018.
2. Poonama R, Imaran K, Pajbala S, et al. Ectopic pregnancy: a review. Arch Gynecol Obstet. 2013;288:747–57. https://doi.org/10.1007/s00404-013-2929-3.
3. Brady J, Wilson M. Spontaneous bilateral tubal ectopic pregnancy. J R Soc Med. 2005;98(3):120–1. https://doi.org/10.1258/jrsm.98.3.120.
4. Franke C, Rohrborn A, Thiele H, Glatz J. Combined intrauterine and extra-uterine gestation. A rare cause of acute abdominal pain. Arch Gynecol Obstet. 2001;265(1):51–2.
5. Varras M, Akrivis C, Hadjopoulos G, Antonious N. Heterotopic pregnancy in a natural conception cycle presenting with tubal rupture: a case report. Eur J Obstet Gynecol Reprod Biol. 2003;106(1):79–89.
6. Okonofua FE, Nganwuchu A, Onwudiegwu U. Dizygotic twin ectopic gestation in a Nigerian woman. J Obstet Gynaecol. 1990:52;527–9.
7. Odejinmi F, Rizzuto M, MacRae R, Olowu O, Hussain M. Diagnosis and laparoscopic management of 12 consecutive cases of ovarian pregnancy and review of the literature. J Minim Invasive Gynaecol. 2009;16:354–9.
8. Katz DL, Barrett JP, Sanfilippo JS, Badway DM. Combined hysteroscopy and laparoscopy in the treatment of interstitial pregnancy. Am J Obstet Gynecol. 2003;188:1113–4.
9. Yildizham R, Kurdoglu M, Kolusari A, Erten R. Primary omental pregnancy. Saudi Med J. 2008;29:606–9.
10. Webb EM, Green GE, Scoutt LM. Adnexal mass with pelvic pain. Radiol Clin North Am. 2004;42:329–48.
11. Isah AY, Amed Y, Nwobodo EI, Ekele BA. Abdominal pregnancy with a full-term live foetus: a case report. Ann Afr Med. 2008;7(4):198–9.

12. Marion LL, Meeks GR. Ectopic pregnancy: history, incidence, epidemiology and risk factors. Clin Obstet Gynaecol. 2012;55:376–86.
13. Goyan N, Leke R, Keita N, Thonneau P. Ectopic pregnancy in African countries. Acta Obstet Gynaecol Scan. 2003;82(4):304–12.
14. Boufous Quartararo M, Molisin M. Trends in the incidence of ectopic pregnancy in New South Wales between 1990–1998. Aust N Z Obstet Gynaecol. 2001;41:436–8.
15. Leke RJ, Goyaux N, Matsuda T, Thonneau PF. Ectopic pregnancy in Africa: a population-based study. Obstet Gynecol. 2004;103(4):692–7.
16. Thonneau P, Jijazi Y, Goyaux N, Calvez T, Keita N. Ectopic pregnancy in Conakry, Guinea. Bull World Health Organ. 2002;80(5):365–70.
17. Bouyer J, Coste J, Shojaci T. Risk factors for ectopic pregnancy: a comprehensive analysis based on a large case-control, population-based study in France. Am J Epidemiol. 2003;157:185–94.
18. Furlong LA. Ectopic pregnancy risk when contraception fails: a review. J Reprod Med. 2002;47:881–5.
19. Bakken IJ. Chlamydia trachomatis and ectopic pregnancy: recent epidemiological findings. Curr Opin Infect Dis. 2008;21:77–82.
20. Okonofua FE. Abortion and maternal mortality in the developing world. J Obstet Gynaecol Can. 2006;28(11):974–9.
21. Grimes DA, Benson J, Singh S, Romero M, Ganatra B, Okonofua FE, Shah I. Unsafe abortion: the preventable pandemic. The lancet special issue on women's reproductive health series, edited by Glasier, and Gulmezolu; Oct 2006. p. 65–76.
22. Okonofua FE. Induced abortion: a risk factor for infertility in Nigerian women. J Obstet Gynaecol. 1994;12:272–6.
23. Okonofua FE. Causes and management of infertility in sub-Saharan Africa. Medical Forum International. Gynaecol Forum. 1999;4(4):10–4.
24. Okonofua FE, Ojo OS, Odunsi OA, Odesanmi WO. Ectopic pregnancy associated with tubal schistosomiasis in a Nigerian woman. Int J Gynaecol Obstet. 1990;32:281–4.
25. Madhuri P. Ectopic pregnancy after infertility treatment. J Human Reprod Sci. 2012;5:154–65.
26. Clayton HB, Schieve LA, Peterson AB, Jamieson DR, Reynolds MA, Wright VC. Ectopic pregnancy risk with assisted reproductive technology procedures. Obstet Gynecol. 2006;107:595–604.
27. Strandell A, Thorburn J, Hamberger L. Risk factors for ectopic pregnancy in assisted reproduction. Fertil Steril. 1999;71:282–6.
28. Condous G. Ectopic pregnancy – risk factor and diagnosis. Aust Fam Physician. 2006;35:854–7.
29. Daponte A, Pournaras S, et al. The value of a single combined measurement of VEGF, glycodelin, progesterone, PAPP-A, HPL and LIF for differentiating between ectopic and abnormal intra-uterine pregnancies. Hum Reprod. 2005;20:3163–6.
30. Katsikis J, Rousso D, et al. Creatine phosphokinase in ectopic pregnancy revisited: significant value of its MB and MM isoenzyme fractions. Am J Obstet Gynecol. 2006;194:86–91.
31. Yagami HT, Sato T, et al. A metalloprotease – disintegrin participating in myoblast fusion. Nature. 1995;377:652–6.
32. Adama O, Rodrigues SS, Pegwande A, et al. Place of autologous intra-operative blood transfusion in the treatment of broken ectopic pregnancy at the Chiphra Hospital in Ouagadougou, Burkina Faso. Open J Obstet Gynaecol. 2017;7(10):1035–43. https://doi.org/10.4236/0jog.ojog.2017/710104.
33. Selo-Ojeme DO, Onwudiegwu U, Durosinmi M, Owolabi AT. Emergency autologous blood transfusion in the management of ruptured ectopic pregnancy. J Obstet Gynaecol. 1997;17:353–5.
34. Jongen VH. Autotransfusion and ectopic pregnancy: an experience from Tanzania Ndala Hospital. Tanzan Med Doct J. 2007;27:78–9.
35. Silva PD, Beguin EA Jr. Intra-operative rapid autologous blood transfusion. Am J Obstet Gynaecol. 2009;160:1226–7.
36. Rajesh V, Lawrence M. Evidence-based management of ectopic pregnancy. Current Obstet Gynecol. 2002;12:191–9.
37. American College of Obstetricians and Gynaecologists. Medical management of tubal pregnancy. ACOG Practice Bulletin no 3. Obstet Gynecol. 1998;92:1–7.
38. Raughley MJ, Frishman GN. Local treatment of ectopic pregnancy. Semin Reprod Med. 2007;25(2):99–115.
39. van Mello MN, Mol F, Mol BW, Hajenius PJ. Conservative management of tubal ectopic pregnancy. Best Pract Res. 2009;23:509–18.
40. Barnhart KT, Gosman G, Ashby R, Sammel M. The medical management of ectopic pregnancy: a meta-analysis comparing "single dose and "multidose" regimens. Obstet Gynecol. 2003;101:778–84.
41. Rodrigues SP, de Buriet KJ, Hiemstra E, Twijinstra AR, van Zwet W, et al. Ectopic pregnancy: when is expectant management safe? Gynaecol Surg. 2012;9:421–6.

Prevention and Management of Recurrent Miscarriage

40

Chioma Uchenna Chilaka, Nasreen M. N. Soliman, and Victor N. Chilaka

Learning Objectives

By the end of the chapter, the reader should be able to:

- Define recurrent pregnancy loss (RPL) and appreciate the importance of the topic and the significance to affected patients
- Should be able to appreciate the signs and symptoms of RPL and be able to make the diagnosis and be able to investigate the condition even in poorly resourced health services Should understand the diagnostic criteria for antiphospholipid syndrome
- Should be able initiate simple management and counselling for the affected patient
- Critically evaluate the different options available for the management of these patients and be able to refer appropriately for further management
- Have a good idea of management of the woman if she gets pregnant understanding the advantages and limitations of medications as progesterone, aspirin, low-molecular-weight heparins and folic acid

40.1 Introduction

Miscarriage can be a challenging and traumatic experience for any woman. Multiple miscarriages can be heart-breaking for a couple, especially in the developing world with limited resources for investigation, lower standards of education and diverse cultural practices. It can lead to enormous pressures on the couple, and this might push them to seek remedies that might be harmful to their health.

Miscarriage is defined as the spontaneous loss of pregnancy before the foetus reaches viability (i.e. before 24 weeks of completed gestation). Recurrent miscarriage, defined as the loss of three or more *consecutive* pregnancies affects about 1% of couples who are trying to conceive [1]. The overall risk of spontaneous miscarriage in pregnancy is about 15–20% [2]. Late miscarriage occurs between 12 and 24 weeks gestation. This is less common and affects about 1% of pregnancies [2].

There is limited information regarding the management of recurrent miscarriages in the developing world and so needs constant reviews and research.

40.1.1 Clinical Presentation

Patients with recurrent miscarriage in the developed world, usually present to a gynaecology outpatient setup. In developing countries, they are more likely to present in the acute setting, at the time of miscarriage. It is therefore essential to capture the history and initiate management at this time. The patient will commonly present with vaginal bleeding and, or abdominal pain. There may be an associated sub-optimal rise or even drop of beta-human chorionic gonadotropin (B-HCG) levels. It is essential to rule out ectopic pregnancy in these women.

In the gynaecology outpatient setup, patients will usually present at a general gynaecology clinic or a fertility clinic. The recommendation of the Royal College of Obstetricians and Gynaecologists (RCOG) is to have a dedicated clinic for recurrent miscarriages [1]. This may not be feasible in developing countries, but they can be merged with closely associated clinics like infertility clinics. These specialist clinics help in the patient's experience and provide psychological and emotional support to them. Often in these clinics, investigations are reviewed and the patients

C. U. Chilaka
Specialty Registrar, East Midlands, UK

N. M. N. Soliman
Shrewsbury & Telford Hospitals NHS Trust, Shrewsbury, UK

V. N. Chilaka (✉)
Women's Wellness and Research Centre, Hamad Medical Corporation, Doha, Qatar

F. Okonofua et al. (eds.), *Contemporary Obstetrics and Gynecology for Developing Countries*,
https://doi.org/10.1007/978-3-030-75385-6_40

Table 40.1 Age-dependent risk of miscarriages

Age (Years)	Risk of miscarriage (Percentage)
12–19	13.3%
20–24	11.1%
25–29	11.9%
30–34	15.0%
35–39	24.6%
40–44	51.0%
45 or more	93.4%.

Table 40.2 Causes of recurrent miscarriage

	Factor	Percentage
1	Genetic	2–5
2	Anatomic	10–15
3	Autoimmune	20
4	Infections	0.5–5
5	Endocrine	17–20
6	Unexplained	40–50

are counselled. The development of written protocols to run the clinics is very helpful.

40.1.2 Risk Factors for Recurrent Pregnancy Loss

The aetiology of recurrent miscarriage is multifactorial and ranges from genetic factors to implantation difficulties and pregnancy factors. Some of these factors can be mitigated to reduce the risk of further miscarriages, but up to 50% of miscarriages will have no clear cause [3].

40.1.2.1 Epidemiological Factors

(a) *Age-Related:*

Increased maternal age is an independent risk factor for miscarriage. There is a decrease in the amount and quality of oocytes with increasing maternal age. Foetal loss is much higher in women in their 30s and older (Table 40.1).

(b) *Obesity*

Obesity is a risk factor for sporadic and recurrent miscarriages [3, 4]. There is a general increase in miscarriage rates in women with a body mass index (BMI) greater than 25 kg/m^2 when compared with women of normal weight, regardless of the method of conception [4]. It is therefore recommended to advise women to lose weight if they are overweight or obese to help reduce the chance of recurrent miscarriage [1]. Obesity is also associated with increased pregnancy complications [4].

(c) *Previous Reproductive History*

A previous miscarriage is a risk factor for further miscarriages. This risk increases with each further pregnancy loss and by the time a woman has three consecutive miscarriages, her risk of further miscarriage is about 40% [5].

(d) *Environmental Risk Factors*

There have been some studies trying to identify the links, if any, between recurrent miscarriage and environmental factors. It is obviously difficult to establish singular causes and risk factors because of the confounding nature of the various suspected risk factors. Some studies have looked at these associations and found out that there may be a dose-dependent link between recurrent miscarriages and maternal cigarette smoking as well as heavy alcohol consumption.

There is also some emerging evidence that there may be a link between heavy metals in the developing world with miscarriages and stillbirths [5]. There is a suggestion that the accumulation of environmental heavy metals such as lead and mercury in the system could be embryotoxic. The effect of anaesthetic gases on theatre workers is inconclusive [6].

(e) *Antiphospholipid Syndrome (APS)*

Antiphospholipid syndrome (APS) is one of the most important treatable causes of recurrent miscarriage. Antiphospholipid syndrome refers to the association between antiphospholipid antibodies, lupus anticoagulant (LA), anticardiolipin (aCL) antibodies and anti-B2 glycoprotein-1 antibodies and adverse pregnancy outcome or vascular thrombosis [7]. It is typically characterised by the presence of antiphospholipid antibodies. Adverse pregnancy outcomes include three or more consecutive miscarriages before ten weeks of gestation, one or more morphologically normal foetal losses after the 10th week of gestation and one or more preterm births before the 34th week of gestation due to placental disease.

There is a great variation in the prevalence of APS in women with recurrent miscarriages. It occurs in about 15% of women with recurrent pregnancy loss (RPL) compared with 2% in normal women without RPL [8]. Diagnosis is by the presence of one clinical criterion (as above) associated with one laboratory criterion.

The mechanisms by which antiphospholipid antibodies cause problems in pregnancy include inhibition of trophoblastic function and differentiation, activation of complement pathways at the maternal-foetal interface resulting in a local inflammatory response and in later pregnancy thrombosis of the uteroplacental vasculature [1]. It is also linked to increased obstetric complications such as pre-eclampsia and late foetal demise. There are limited data on the efficacy of the prevention of obstetric complications of APS with low-dose aspirin and low-molecular-weight (LMW) heparin. However, many clinicians still use these medications in the absence of other effective alternatives (Table 40.2).

40.1.2.2 Genetic Factors

Parental Chromosomal Rearrangements

The prevalence of a balanced structural chromosomal anomaly in one of the couples affected with RPL is about 2–5% and the most common is a balanced reciprocal or Robertsonian translocation [9]. These carriers of a balanced translocation are usually phenotypically normal, but their pregnancies are at increased risk of miscarriage and may result in a live birth with multiple congenital malformations.

Abnormal Embryonic (Foetal) Karyotypes

Chromosomal abnormalities are the most important causes of miscarriages before 10 weeks [10]. The vast majority of early pregnancy losses are due to chromosomal abnormalities. Up to 90% of chromosomally abnormal embryos are spontaneously aborted [8]. Embryonic aneuploidy is the most common cause of early pregnancy loss. The risk of embryonic aneuploidy increases with maternal age. In couples with recurrent miscarriage, chromosomal abnormalities of the embryo account for 30–57% of further miscarriages [10] (Table 40.3).

Table 40.3 Diagnostic criteria for antiphospholipid syndrome

(one clinical criterion and one laboratory criterion)	
Clinical criteria	Laboratory criteria
Vascular thrombosis 1. One or more clinical episodes of an arterial, venous or small vessel thrombosis, in any tissue or organ 2. Confirmed by imaging or Doppler studies or histopathology except for superficial venous thrombosis 3. Histology: thrombosis without significant evidence of inflammation in the vessel wall	1. Anticardiolipin antibody (IgG and/or IgM isotype) in serum or plasma, present in medium or high titre (i.e. >40 GPL or MPL, or >99th percentile, or > mean þ 3SD of 40 healthy controls), on two or more occasions, at least 12 weeks apart 2. Lupus anticoagulant present in plasma, on two or more occasions at least 12 weeks apart
Pregnancy morbidity 1. One or more unexplained deaths of a morphologically normal foetus at or beyond the 10th week of gestation, with normal foetal morphology documented by ultrasound or by direct examination of the foetus or 2. One or more premature births of a morphologically normal neonate before the 34th week of gestation because of eclampsia/severe pre-eclampsia or recognised features of placental insufficiency or 3. Three or more unexplained consecutive spontaneous miscarriages before the 10th week of gestation, without maternal anatomic or hormonal abnormalities and paternal and maternal chromosomal anomalies	3. Anti-β2 glycoprotein-I antibody (IgG and/or IgM isotype) in serum or plasma, present on two or more occasions, at least 12 weeks apart, measured by a standardised enzyme-linked immunosorbent assay

40.1.2.3 Anatomical Factors

Congenital Uterine Malformations

Uterine abnormalities can be congenital or acquired. They are thought to affect the pregnancy by affecting the blood supply and the placentation. The reported prevalence of uterine anomalies in recurrent miscarriage populations ranges between 1.8% and 37.6%, but the prevalence in the normal population is unknown [11]. The prevalence of uterine malformations appears to be higher in women with second-trimester miscarriages compared with women who have first trimester miscarriages. This may be related to the cervical weakness that is frequently associated with uterine malformation. The timing of miscarriage may be affected by the type of uterine malformation: with uterine septae occurring in the first trimester and arcuate uteri occurring in the second trimester.

Acquired abnormalities include uterine adhesions, myomas and polyps.

Cervical Incompetence

Cervical incompetence usually results in mid-trimester loss and preterm labour, and the true incidence is unknown. There is currently no satisfactory objective test that can identify women with cervical weakness in the non-pregnant state. The diagnostic features are as follows:

- Clinical history: It is usually seen with patients who have painless dilatation and recurrent mid-trimester loss.
- Ultrasound scan (USS) findings: Transvaginal cervical length measurements that show cervical length of less than 25 mm before 24 weeks gestation.
- Clinical presentation on examination: Silent dilation and effacement of the cervix with or without prolapsing membranes before 27 weeks gestation.

Risk factors will include damage to the cervix like surgical evacuation of the uterus and cervical treatment in cervical cancer.

Endocrine Disorders

Hypothyroidism, luteal phase defect, polycystic ovarian syndrome (PCOS), diabetes mellitus, thyroid disease, hyperprolactinemia have all been associated with recurrent miscarriage [12].

Hypothyroidism has an association with poor obstetric outcome, including recurrent miscarriages and subfertility. There is limited evidence on the link between subclinical hypothyroidism and recurrent pregnancies [13].

Hyperprolactinemia is associated with infertility and miscarriage by altering the hypothalamic–pituitary–ovarian axis, thus leading to impaired folliculogenesis and anovulation. There is suggestion that treating hyperprolactinemia with dopamine agonist may help in the reduction of recurrent miscarriages [14]; however, the data are very limited.

Polycystic ovary syndrome (PCOS) is an endocrine disorder involving many different mechanisms. The increased risk of miscarriage in women with PCOS has been recently attributed to insulin resistance, hyperinsulinaemia and hyperandrogenaemia. The prevalence of insulin resistance is increased in women with recurrent miscarriage compared with matched fertile controls [15]. Metformin has been shown to improve insulin sensitivity, and aid in weight loss and can also improve fertility in patients with PCOS. There are conflicting data to conclude that metformin treatment really reduced the incidence of recurrent miscarriages. Some studies have shown that there is some benefit [16]. Metformin is known to be safe in pregnancy and not teratogenic.

Luteal phase deficiency remains a highly controversial area in reproductive medicine. It is thought that the reduced progesterone affects the implantation process, thus leading to miscarriage. Conditions that affect the hypothalamic–pituitary–ovarian axis and gonadotropin secretion are thought to lead to the deficiency of progesterone. Treatment options include treatment of the underlying causative factors for the hormonal imbalance. The most routinely used treatment all over the world is supplementary vaginal progesterone. There is, however, little evidence to suggest that this improves birth rates in women with recurrent miscarriages [8].

Infection

The role of infection in recurrent miscarriage is unclear as such infections will have to be able to persist undetected for so long and will not systemically upset the woman [1]. Chronic endometritis is a chronic inflammation of the endometrium, and there are suggestions that it may affect implantation by stromal infiltration of plasma cells. This can alter gene expression and affect implantation and lead to recurrent pregnancy losses as well as failed in vitro fertilisation (IVF). The gold standard for diagnosing this is immunohistochemistry stains that identify plasma cells in the endometrial stroma. Toxoplasmosis, rubella, cytomegalovirus and herpes (TORCH), and listeria infections do not fulfil these criteria and routine TORCH screening should be abandoned [17]. There is some evidence that bacterial vaginosis (*Mycoplasma hominis, Ureaplasma urealyticum*), brucellosis, syphilis, cytomegalovirus, dengue fever, human immunodeficiency virus, rubella and malaria are more frequently found in women with spontaneous miscarriages [8]. There is suggestion that treatment with doxycycline may help, but more data are needed before this can be an established management plan [18].

Inherited Thrombophilias

Inherent thrombophilias include: Factor V Leiden mutation, prothrombin gene mutation (PT 20210A) and deficiencies of natural anticoagulants protein C, protein S and antithrombin III, hyperhomocysteinaemia. They are associated with increased miscarriages [12]. Thrombophilias are thought to affect placental function due to systemic thrombosis. There are limited data to clearly demonstrate the evidence for the association between recurrent pregnancy loss and thrombophilia, nor is there adequate evidence to show that anticoagulation reduced the rate of recurrent miscarriages [19–24].

Immunology

Immunological abnormalities and dysregulation have been proposed as a theory to recurrent miscarriages. Maternal immune tolerance allows for normal placentation. Any dysregulation of the following could lead to implantation failure and pregnancy loss: normal CD4 T-helper cell (Th), uterine natural killer (NK) activity and a Th imbalance in the endometrium. There are suggestions that immunoregulation may help increase the live birth rate in women with recurrent pregnancy loss [25]. However, there needs to be a lot more research and large randomised control trials (RCTs) in this area to give definitive answers. It is important however to note that there is no clear evidence to support the hypothesis of human leukocyte antigen (HLA) incompatibility between couples, the absence of maternal leucocytotoxic antibodies or the absence of maternal blocking antibodies. There is, therefore, no need to offer couples these tests routinely in the investigation of recurrent miscarriage [1].

Unexplained Miscarriages

About 50% of miscarriages are unexplained with no obvious cause. Unexplained recurrent pregnancy losses are associated with significant adverse psychological consequences for the couple. Apart from the grief of each miscarriage, there is a lot of anxiety and insecurity associated with each positive pregnancy test.

40.1.2.4 Clinical Assessment

In the developing world, it can be very difficult to work up patients for a non-life-threatening condition when there may be other pressing conditions affecting patients and their families. The social stigma and pressures faced by women without children should not be underestimated. It is important to encourage them and signpost patients to get answers and scientific explanations to their conditions. These can also help to liberate, exonerate and provide solutions to them as there may also be male factors contributing to the condition. More so, investigations with or without positive answers can help to reassure the woman that there is nothing fundamentally wrong with her and to just keep trying.

History
A full obstetric history including presumed gestations, relevant scans and outcome should be taken. A gynaecological history, smear history (including treatment depth), sexual history and family history should be taken. A detailed discussion about potential environmental factors is essential.

Investigations
Investigations should be initiated after three miscarriages. There is evolving evidence that this should take place after two miscarriages depending on patient-specific circumstances. Considerations should be given on individual bases to each patient depending on history, age and other risk factors. Investigations can be sooner rather than later in some situations especially in women over the age of 35. Partners of women with recurrent pregnancy losses may have to be investigated to rule out chromosomal abnormalities that may be contributing to the condition.

40.1.2.5 Blood Tests

- Full blood count
- Thrombophilia screen
- Lupus anticoagulant (LA)
- Anticardiolipin antibody (aCL)
- Anti-β II glycoprotein I antibodies
- Thyroid function test in the content of symptoms – thyroid-stimulating hormone (TSH)
- Endocrine disorders – prolactin, HbA1C/fasting glucose
- Inherited thrombophilias – if there is a personally history or string family history of thrombosis

Imaging
Imaging is helpful in investigating anatomical abnormalities. Ideally, a 3D ultrasound scan (USS) would give and assessment of the uterine cavity and is not invasive. This may not always be an available option in the developing world. Depending on availably facilities, a hysterosalpingogram, USS and hysteroscopy can help in the diagnosis of uterine abnormalities.

Cervical length screening should also be done with ultrasonography.

40.1.2.6 Genetic Factors

Parental Karyotyping
Chromosomal analysis of the miscarried pregnancy may help. Chromosomal aneuploidy is the most common form accounting for 50% of miscarriages [26].

Infection
There is some association between an increased rate of miscarriage and preterm delivery. Bacterial vaginosis is a risk factor for preterm delivery and late miscarriage.

There is an established association between miscarriage and systemic infections such as malaria, brucellosis, cytomegalovirus and human immunodeficiency virus, dengue fever, influenza virus and of vaginal infection with bacterial vaginosis [17]. However, there still needs to be more research in this area to establish a proper cause-effect relationship.

Management
Ideally women who have undergone recurrent miscarriages should be managed by a specialist preferably in a dedicated clinic. This is more likely to provide additional psychological support that the patients may need.

When counselling women, it is important to remember that 50% of recurrent miscarriages are unexplained and they need support and encouragement to keep trying. Couples with recurrent pregnancy loss should be informed that the chances for a future successful pregnancy could be as high as 50–70% and depend mostly on maternal age and the number of previous losses [8].

General Advice
Patients should be advised on weight reduction and nutrition. They should ideally aim for a BMI below 25 (but at the very least a BMI of 30 or below). They should also be advised to take 400 micrograms of folic acid for neuroprotection of their babies should pregnancy occur. Those with increased risk factors such as diabetes mellitus, on antiepileptic medication, or have a family history of neural tube defects should have higher doses of folic acid, 5 mg. Folate/Folic acid can also be found in green vegetables, citrus fruits, beans, avocado, okra, seeds and nuts and fortified breads.

Thrombophilias
Low-dose aspirin and prophylactic low-molecular-weight heparin can be used for patients with antiphospholipid syndrome. This should be started as soon as there is a positive pregnancy test and is usually carried on throughout pregnancy and 6 weeks post-natal as there is an increased risk of thrombotic events in pregnancy and puerperium.

Cervical Weakness
Medical or surgical management can be considered. Vaginal progesterone can be given or a cervical cerclage inserted between 16 and 24 weeks. A rescue cerclage can be considered when there is painless dilatation of the cervix and exposed foetal membranes. It is usually performed between 16 and 27 + 6 in the absence of signs of infection, active vaginal bleeding or uterine contractions.

Chromosomal Abnormalities
Genetic counselling and support with genetic conditions should be part and parcel of management of recurrent pregnancy losses. IVF may be considered with pre-implantation

genetic testing. The alternative is to consider donor gametes if culturally acceptable to the couple.

Pre-implantation genetic screening (PGS) may reduce miscarriage rate in patients with balanced translocations [8].

Endocrine Abnormalities

In women with PCOS, metformin should be considered. This will help with their weight loss and improve sensitisation of insulin and reduced androgen production.

In women with thyroid diseases, the aim would be for euthyroid TSH levels. Those who are clinically suspected to have diabetes mellitus should be investigated fully. Oral glucose tolerance test may be the best test to clinch the diagnosis [26]. To help reduce the rate of foetal abnormalities, conception should be advised when HbA1c levels are in the normal range. These patients should be on a high dose of folic acid (5 mg once a day prior to conception and stay on it through the first trimester).

Medications (Table 40.4)

Infection

Treatment for infection is only recommended if there are clinical or bacteriological signs of infection. Triple swabs should be taken and infections should be treated accordingly.

Progesterone Dysfunction

There is no evidence that first-trimester progesterone therapy improves outcomes in women with a history of unexplained recurrent miscarriages. Adjuvant treatments in unexplained recurrent miscarriage have no significant benefit on future live birth rates.

Intra-uterine Foetal Demise

Worldwide the rate of still birth has been falling and stands at around 15 deaths/1000 live births [27] (GBD 2015). The still births rates are much higher in developing countries and often occur around the time of delivery. When an intra-uterine foetal demise occurs, there should be a comprehensive work up of the mother to investigate causes. The placenta should also be sent for histologic assessment to see if there are any other causes that can be treated to prevent recurrence. Closer surveillance should be performed for subsequent pregnancies (Table 40.5).

Treatment in Low-Resource Countries

There are real challenges in the availability of resources, expertise in investigations and management of recurrent miscarriage. It is unlikely that governments and health-providers will effectively resource this area with their scarce funds. However, the psychological impact of recurrent miscarriage to a patient and their partners should not be underestimated [28]. In the absence of resources, good advice and prescribing folic acid and low-dose aspirin might encourage the patients enough not to seek futile and potentially harmful solutions to this complex problem.

40.2 Conclusion

Recurrent miscarriage constitutes an important reproductive health issue more so in the developing countries with paucity of resources personnel. A lot of progress has been made over the years in identifying and treating the causes of RPL. A full workup can be initiated following two or three consecutive pregnancy losses to identify treatable causes that include uterine abnormalities, APS, endocrine diseases and balanced translocations.

Table 40.5 Risk factors of intra-uterine foetal demise

Maternal	Foetal	Pregnancy
Diabetes mellitus	Arrhythmias	Abruption
Obesity	Genetic abnormalities	Ascending infection
Previous still birth	Multiple pregnancy	Foetal-maternal haemorrhage
Smoking and illicit drug use		Hypertensive disorders
Uterine abnormalities		Placental abnormalities
Unknown		

Table 40.4 Medications and their benefits in pregnancy

Medication	Condition to try	Benefit	Dosage
Aspirin	Antiphospholipid syndrome	Anticoagulant limited benefit	75 mg once a day throughout pregnancy
Progesterone	Luteal phase deficiency	Little or no benefits	Oral or vaginal
Adjuvant treatment	Unexplained RPL	Little or no benefits	N/a
Low molecular weight heparin	Autoimmune conditions, thrombophilias	Limited	Weight-dependent prophylactic dose Once daily in pregnancy and 6 weeks postnatal
Folic acid	Risk of neural tube defects raised BMI	Protection against neural tube defects	400 μg or 4 mg once a day

Life style modifications in the form of weight loss, diet and nutrition should also be implemented to improve reproductive prognosis. Despite all these, almost half of the cases remain unexplained, and research and developments will probably throw more light on these areas. Regardless of the cause, a thorough clinical work-up and adequate follow-up with psychological support can help many couples achieve a successful live birth.

References

1. Royal College Obstetricians and Gynaecologists (RCOG). The investigation and treatment of couples with recurrent first-trimester and second-trimester miscarriage. R Coll Obstet Gynaecol. 2011. https://doi.org/10.4103/2230-8210.107834.
2. Sagali H, Divers M. Modern management of miscarriage - review. Obstet Gynecol. 2007;9(2):102–8.
3. Lashen H, Fear K, Sturdee DW. Obesity is associated with increased risk of first trimester and recurrent miscarriage: matched case-control study. Hum Reprod. 2004. https://doi.org/10.1093/humrep/deh277.
4. Moussa HN, Alrais MA, Leon MG, Abbas EL, Sibai BM. Obesity epidemic: impact from preconception to postpartum. Futur Sci OA. 2016. https://doi.org/10.4155/fsoa-2016-0035.
5. Amadi CN, Igweze ZN, Orisakwe OE. Heavy metals in miscarriages and stillbirths in developing nations. Middle East Fertil Soc J. 2017. https://doi.org/10.1016/j.mefs.2017.03.003.
6. McGregor DG. Occupational exposure to trace concentrations of waste anaesthetic gases. Mayo Clin Proc. 2000. https://doi.org/10.4065/75.3.273.
7. Miyakis S, Lockshin MD, Atsumi T, et al. International consensus statement on an update of the classification criteria for definite antiphospholipid syndrome (APS). J Thromb Haemost. 2006. https://doi.org/10.1111/j.1538-7836.2006.01753.x.
8. El Hachem H, Crepaux V, May-Panloup P, Descamps P, Legendre G, Bouet PE. Recurrent pregnancy loss: current perspectives. Int J Womens Health. 2017. https://doi.org/10.2147/IJWH.S100817.
9. Stephenson MD, Sierra S. Reproductive outcomes in recurrent pregnancy loss associated with a parental carrier of a structural chromosome rearrangement. Hum Reprod. 2006. https://doi.org/10.1093/humrep/dei417.
10. Sugiura-Ogasawara M, Ozaki Y, Suzumori N. Management of recurrent miscarriage. J Obstet Gynaecol Res. 2014. https://doi.org/10.1111/jog.12388.
11. Salim R, Regan L, Woelfer B, Backos M, Jurkovic D. A comparative study of the morphology of congenital uterine anomalies in women with and without a history of recurrent first trimester miscarriage. Hum Reprod. 2003. https://doi.org/10.1093/humrep/deg030.
12. Ford HB, Schust DJ. Recurrent pregnancy loss: etiology, diagnosis, and therapy. Rev Obstet Gynecol. 2009;2:76–83.
13. Rushworth FH, Backos M, Rai R, Chilcott IT, Baxter N, Regan L. Prospective pregnancy outcome in untreated recurrent miscarriers with thyroid autoantibodies. Hum Reprod. 2000. https://doi.org/10.1093/humrep/15.7.1637.
14. Chen H, Lina H. Dopamine agonists for preventing future miscarriage in women with idiopathic hyperprolactinemia and recurrent miscarriage history. Cochrane Database Syst Rev. 2010;(7). https://doi.org/10.1002/14651858.CD008883.pub2.
15. Craig LTB, Ke RW, Kutteh WH. Increased prevalence of insulin resistance in women with a history of recurrent pregnancy loss. Fertil Steril. 2002. https://doi.org/10.1016/S0015-0282(02)03247-8.
16. Glueck CJ, Phillips H, Cameron D, Sieve-Smith L, Wang P. Continuing metformin throughout pregnancy in women with polycystic ovary syndrome appears to safely reduce first-trimester spontaneous abortion: a pilot study. Fertil Steril 2001. https://doi.org/10.1016/S0015-0282(00)01666-6.
17. Giakoumelou S, Wheelhouse N, Cuschieri K, Entrican G, Howie SEM, Horne AW. The role of infection in miscarriage. Hum Reprod Update. 2016. https://doi.org/10.1093/humupd/dmv041.
18. McQueen DB, Perfetto CO, Hazard FK, Lathi RB. Pregnancy outcomes in women with chronic endometritis and recurrent pregnancy loss. Fertil Steril. 2015. https://doi.org/10.1016/j.fertnstert.2015.06.044.
19. Rey E, Kahn SR, David M, Shrier I. Thrombophilic disorders and fetal loss: a meta-analysis. Lancet. 2003. https://doi.org/10.1016/S0140-6736(03)12771-7.
20. Nelen WLDM, Blom HJ, Steegers EAP, Den Heijer M, Eskes TKAB. Hyperhomocysteinemia and recurrent early pregnancy loss: a meta-analysis. Fertil Steril. 2000. https://doi.org/10.1016/S0015-0282(00)01595-8.
21. Lissalde-Lavigne G, Fabbro-Peray P, Cochery-Nouvellon E, et al. Factor V Leiden and prothrombin G20210A polymorphisms as risk factors for miscarriage during a first intended pregnancy: the matched case-control "NOHA first" study. J Thromb Haemost. 2005. https://doi.org/10.1111/j.1538-7836.2005.01581.x.
22. Dizon-Townson D, Miller C, Sibai B, et al. The relationship of the factor V Leiden mutation and pregnancy outcomes for mother and foetus. Obstet Gynecol. 2005. https://doi.org/10.1097/01.AOG.0000173986.32528.ca.
23. Silver RM, Zhao Y, Spong CY, et al. Prothrombin gene G20210A mutation and obstetric complications. Obstet Gynecol. 2010. https://doi.org/10.1097/AOG.0b013e3181c88918.
24. Kaandorp SP, Goddijn M, Van Der Post JAM, et al. Aspirin plus heparin or aspirin alone in women with recurrent miscarriage. Obstet Gynecol Surv. 2010. https://doi.org/10.1097/OGX.0b013e3182021f71.
25. Mekinian A, Cohen J, Alijotas-Reig J, et al. Unexplained recurrent miscarriage and recurrent implantation failure: is there a place for immunomodulation? Am J Reprod Immunol. 2016. https://doi.org/10.1111/aji.12493.
26. Jeve Y, Davies W. Evidence-based management of recurrent miscarriages. J Hum Reprod Sci. 2014. https://doi.org/10.4103/0974-1208.142475.
27. Global, regional, national, and selected subnational levels of stillbirths, neonatal, infant, and under-5 mortality, 1980–2015: a systematic analysis for the Global Burden of Disease Study 2015. Lancet (London, England). 2016. https://doi.org/10.1016/S0140-6736(16)31575-6
28. Farren J, Jalmbrant M, Ameye L, et al. Post-traumatic stress anxiety and depression following miscarriage or ectopic pregnancy: a prospective cohort study. BMJ Open. 2016. https://doi.org/10.1136/bmjopen-2016-011864.

41 Control of Sexually Transmitted Infections Through Integrated Reproductive Health Services

Lindsay Edouard and Olufemi A. Olatunbosun

Learning Objectives

At the end of this chapter, the reader will be able to:

- Identify challenges for an evidence-based approach to the control of sexually transmitted infections in developing countries
- Describe linkages with other components of sexual and reproductive health
- Discuss the relative value of alternative strategies
- Adapt available protocols and tools for preventive care, risk assessment, diagnosis and treatment to local circumstances
- Appreciate the need for integrating community-based interventions with clinical treatment

41.1 Introduction

With the increasing provision of comprehensive reproductive health services, it is compelling to integrate the control of sexually transmitted infections (STIs). Efforts at achieving effective and sustainable integration have had variable success. The move towards integration requires a considerable paradigm shift in the role of healthcare providers. Moreover, there is a critical need for clarity about the precise model of integration of programmes besides evidence from operational research on the feasibility and cost-effectiveness of integration. In this chapter, we examine approaches, challenges and strategies for prevention and control of STIs through integrated reproductive health services.

Globally, more than one million sexually transmitted infections are acquired every day with one of the following four STIs: chlamydia, gonorrhoea, syphilis and trichomoniasis. STIs can have profound consequences beyond the immediate impact of the infection including: (a) enhanced risk of HIV acquisition, (b) mother-to-child transmission resulting in congenital malformation, prematurity, low birthweight and neonatal death, (c) pelvic inflammatory disease leading to chronic pelvic pain and infertility and (d) cervical cancer related to human papilloma virus (HPV) infection. Current STI control efforts are hampered by several behavioural and implementation challenges including a large proportion of asymptomatic infections, lack of readily available diagnostic tests, repeat infections, drug resistance and barriers regarding access to care [1].

41.1.1 Integrated Reproductive Health Services

The word 'integrate' means to coordinate or blend into a functioning or unified whole; to unite one thing with another; to incorporate something into a larger unit; or to end the segregation of something. All of these are descriptive of what it means to talk about sexual and reproductive health (SRH) services being integrated in national health services. In order to have a lasting impact, activities cannot be isolated events but must be integrated into a larger framework. The rationale behind integration is simple. Individuals with known or suspected STI would feel more at ease seeking care at facilities that they are already familiar with instead of seeking care at an STI clinic. Incorporating STI diagnosis, treatment and prevention into reproductive health services may enhance contraceptive uptake and maternal and perinatal outcomes because STIs impact both maternal and foetal health. Integrated reproductive health services may be seen as a network of pathways aimed at linking the various systems to strengthen reproductive health policy, training and services. Utilising existing infrastructure for the control of STIs represents a potential cost-saving model of 'one-stop shopping' that is particularly relevant to low-resource countries. As

L. Edouard (✉) · O. A. Olatunbosun
Department of Obstetrics and Gynaecology, College of Medicine, University of Saskatchewan, Saskatoon, SK, Canada

F. Okonofua et al. (eds.), *Contemporary Obstetrics and Gynecology for Developing Countries*,
https://doi.org/10.1007/978-3-030-75385-6_41

noted earlier, there is an urgent need for clarity about the precise model and operational methodology of integration STI control into reproductive health services. An emerging concept is the use of risk assessment tools.

41.1.2 STI Risk Assessment

STI risk assessment is a practical tool that uses responses of clients regarding symptoms and demographic characteristics besides behavioural and clinical information, other than laboratory test results, to assess the likelihood that persons are currently infected with an STI or are at high risk of future infection. Risk assessment can be done in various ways and used for various purposes. It can be used as part of prevention counselling, as a way to determine who should be tested or treated for STIs, or as an adjunct to syndromic management algorithms [2]. These factors can be either incorporated into guidelines for clinical management of specific patients or aggregated into graduated scales predicting STI risk. The results can then be used as tools for effective STI management and appropriate family planning counselling. For example, individual clients determined to be at increased risk of current or future STIs would be poor candidates for intrauterine devices (IUDs) but may be good candidates for barrier methods. By helping family planning providers assist women in choosing the most appropriate contraceptive method, STI risk assessment provides a unified pathway for integrated reproductive health services. Having been a traditional part of disease control programmes for decades, STI risk assessment can help make the most cost-effective use of increasingly limited resources. Since the risk of infection is an important consideration in choosing a contraceptive method, family planning providers can use STI risk assessment not only for disease control but also for counselling clients about behavioural and contraceptive choices that will help them achieve their future childbearing goals.

41.1.3 Programme Linkage

The control of STIs, provision of contraceptive services and maternal health care are intimately linked through sexual intercourse and constitute central elements of SRH. The prevention of STIs, including HIV, has lost importance to interest in the treatment of infection with the human immunodeficiency virus (HIV) and acquired immunodeficiency syndrome (AIDS). Unfortunately, the relationship of STIs with other components of reproductive health has been largely neglected over the years in most countries albeit for commonalities pertaining to HIV/AIDS: sexual transmission being the most common mode of infection besides blood products and vertical transmission from mother to child.

HIV infections are overwhelmingly associated with SRH, whether through sexual transmission, pregnancy, delivery or breastfeeding [3]. Interest for an integrated approach for the control of HIV has led to unexpected opportunities for the management of STIs, both for prevention and treatment through integrated reproductive health services [4, 5]. The treatment of STIs has been shown to be one of the most effective interventions to reduce the transmission of HIV in resource-scarce settings [6].

It is difficult to determine the actual prevalence of STIs because (a) those infections are often asymptomatic, (b) individuals with symptoms might not seek health services and (c) the epidemiological reporting system is often deficient. However, the extent of the problem can often be estimated from the incidence of STIs among well-defined populations such as pregnant women receiving antenatal care and individuals attending family planning clinics.

With an annual incidence of around 500 million cases, curable STIs consist largely of syphilis, gonorrhoea, chlamydia and trichomoniasis. Among women of reproductive age in Africa, the prevalence of syphilis is around 3.5% as opposed to 2.3% for gonorrhoea, 2.6% for chlamydia and 20% for trichomoniasis [7]. Among the viral STIs, the most important ones for SRH are hepatitis B, human papillomavirus and herpes simplex virus type 2 (HSV-2). As hepatitis B is transmitted through blood and affects the liver, its importance for reproductive health is often overlooked despite the importance of direct transmission from mother to child and through the exchange of body fluids during sexual intercourse.

41.1.4 International Agreements

Current efforts for international development focus on attaining the Sustainable Development Goals where reproductive health features prominently in the third goal with its consolidation of health issues [8]. It is noteworthy that the issue of universal access to reproductive health, as agreed upon at the International Conference on Population and Development, has now been given increased importance by being included not only within the health goal 3 but also in the gender goal 5 of the Sustainable Development Goals [9].

Targets of the health goal include the reduction of maternal, neonatal and child mortality besides ending the epidemics of AIDS and communicable diseases by 2030 and ensuring universal health coverage including access to reproductive health services. Major challenges will consist of addressing inequity in the provision of services and producing reliable health statistics to monitor progress in meeting those targets [10, 11].

41.1.5 Strategy

The strategy for controlling STIs consists of three prongs: (a) decreasing the infectivity of sexual partners, (b) decreasing the risk of transmission from sexual partners and (c) reducing the number of sexual partners. The overlap between those three components can be appreciated from the fact that a decrease in the infectivity of sexual partners can be achieved by the prompt treatment of infections, contact tracing to decrease the pool of infections and in some cases, long-term therapy and vaccines.

Moreover, related activities could be perceived along a different set of axes to consist of healthy sexual practices of individuals and accessible health care at the community level. Special attention should be paid to disadvantaged populations, such as poor people and adolescents, with their decreased access to health care.

41.1.6 Prevention

A clear distinction between individual and community perspective must be made so that the value of interventions can be appreciated. Whereas the individual is concerned with personal outcomes, the community should have the wider perspective on the effective use of scarce resources. As far as possible, prevention should go hand in hand with treatment. Numerous preventive interventions are described much later on under the rubric of integrated reproductive health services, but the following three topics deserve a separate consideration immediately below.

41.1.6.1 Screening

Effectiveness should by no means be the only criterion for the implementation of a screening programme as other considerations such as cost-benefit, nature of test, age and sex groups are critically important. Screening for chlamydia can be effective [12], but the modality of how it should be used has yet to be decided. As the case has not yet been made for its use for mass screening, it should be used largely for opportunistic screening. A prime example is in the United Kingdom where proposals for mass screening subsequently faced major problems when implementation issues were considered.

Opportunistic screening should ensure that it occurs in situations such as contraceptive services, antenatal care, youth clinics including street children and high-risk groups such as commercial sex workers, prisoners, men having sex with men, refugees and during clinical consultations after gender-based violence.

41.1.6.2 Risk for HIV

The presence of an STI lesion, whether of an ulcerative or untreated inflammatory nature, increases the risk at an individual level for HIV transmission. With genital ulcer disease being responsible for a substantial proportion of heterosexual transmission of HIV in sub-Saharan Africa, the control of STI is a central pillar in the strategy to fight HIV [13]. However, it should be appreciated that STIs of a non-ulcerative nature are as important in the aetiology of HIV when a population perspective is considered: despite a lower magnitude in the level of the relative risk, the population attributable risk may be as great with their much increased prevalence in the community. For programmatic purposes, it is imperative to go beyond the philosophy of comparisons of attribution to aetiology so as to appreciate the concept of the impact of interventions. It is reassuring to know that a randomised trial at the primary care level in Mwanza demonstrated that case management of STIs decreased the incidence of HIV by about 40% in a rural population [14].

41.1.6.3 Vaccines

The sexual transmission of hepatitis B is well documented [15], and for more than a decade, it has been recommended that vaccination should occur at puberty, and this has not caused any controversy. However, the introduction of a vaccine against HPV has already led to controversy because the preventable outcome relates to an STI as compared to a liver condition without an obvious direct sexual association [16, 17].

With HPV being present on both male and female external genitalia, barrier methods have a limited role in preventing its transmission, and primary prevention will depend largely on prophylactic HPV vaccines. Operationalisation issues for the introduction of HPV vaccine will need to draw upon a sexual health approach as opposed to an infectious disease one. Special attention needs to be paid to gender issues besides sexual and reproductive health services as entry points for reaching adolescents [18, 19].

41.1.7 Clinical Presentations

In women health settings, STIs usually present as vaginal discharge, genital lesion or lower abdominal pain. Special consideration should be given to STIs in pregnancy as pertaining to congenital syphilis and neonatal ophthalmia.

Although the emphasis in this chapter is on the health care of women for the sake of brevity, it is appreciated that services for men are important. Nevertheless, the implications regarding numerous issues have commonalities whether for men having sex with men or women having sex with women [20].

41.1.7.1 Vaginal Discharge

Vaginal discharge represents a most common presentation in clinical consultations in reproductive settings. Lactobacilli in the vaginal flora protect from infection by promoting an acidic environment in the vagina with a pH around 4.0. Personal perceptions are primordial in the self-reporting that leads to the consideration of an abnormality in vaginal discharge, and it is likely that psychosocial factors play a substantial role [21]. Whereas the aetiology of a presenting symptom of vaginal discharge is usually physiological, it is important to exclude pathological causes that include both infective and non-infective ones such as neoplasms, fistulae and foreign bodies. Neoplasms consist commonly of cervical ectopy and polyps that typically lead to copious clear discharge, but genital cancer is also a cause. When left in the vagina for a prolonged period of time, condoms and tampons usually lead to a foul-smelling discharge. With those numerous causes, vaginal discharge is not a reliable indicator of an STI, but its presence often leads to worry and decision to obtain screening. Special consideration should be given to the clinical management of vaginal discharge as related to either pregnancy, children or the menopause.

Among the causes of vaginal discharge, *Trichomonas vaginalis*, *Chlamydia trachomatis and Neisseria gonorrhoeae* are STIs, whereas bacterial vaginosis and candidiasis are infections that are not sexually transmitted.

41.1.7.2 Bacterial Vaginosis

Usually presenting as a mild non-itchy white discharge with a fishy smell, bacterial vaginosis is the usual cause of vaginal discharge of infectious aetiology when lactobacilli are overtaken by other organisms such as *Gardnerella vaginalis*. It occurs when there is disruption of the vaginal flora, as can happen with vaginal douching [22], and the possibility of sexual transmission is gaining more credibility.

41.1.7.3 Candida albicans

Under certain circumstances, *Candida albicans*, which is a commensal organism in the vagina of about a fifth of asymptomatic individuals, can become so prominent as to lead to a vaginal discharge from vulvovaginal candidiasis, another cause being *Candida glabrata*. Presenting typically as a thick white cheesy vaginal discharge with vulval pruritus, vulvovaginal candidiasis is commonly caused by oestrogen and antibiotic therapy.

41.1.7.4 Trichomoniasis

Presenting typically with a frothy yellow offensive discharge and sometimes accompanied by a strawberry cervix, trichomoniasis is associated with poverty [23].

41.1.7.5 Gonorrhoea

The symptom of vaginal discharge occurs in only half of women with gonorrhoea which causes cervicitis. Whereas diagnosis is feasible through culture of a high vaginal swab on chocolate agar, it is better to use an endocervical swab.

41.1.7.6 Chlamydia Trachomatis

The presence of *Chlamydia trachomatis* is asymptomatic in about 80% of cases. When they occur, symptoms include intermenstrual or postcoital bleeding, dyspareunia and lower abdominal pain. Cervicitis causes vaginal discharge.

41.1.8 Genital Lesion

The aetiology of genital ulcers varies tremendously according to the regional variations in the prevalence of infections: herpes, syphilis, chancroid, lymphogranuloma venereum and granuloma inguinale. Whatever the cause, genital ulcers are important as the presence of an open skin surface increases the risk of transmission of HIV.

Genital herpes is caused by the herpes simplex virus type 2 (HSV2) that is the commonest cause of genital ulcerative disease. Whereas there is no cure for herpes, the prompt administration of systemic acyclovir decreases the severity of symptoms. Recurrent episodes are common, and repeat treatment from the outset of a new episode is beneficial. Neonatal herpes is a risk in cases where the primary infection occurred just prior to delivery: consideration should be given to delivery by caesarean section in those cases [24].

Primary syphilis usually consists of an ulcer at the site where the infection was transmitted, whereas secondary syphilis manifests itself as extensive lymphadenopathy and skin rash.

Genital warts and cervical cancer are caused by the human papillomavirus. There is no known treatment for HPV itself. Whilst only 30 of the more than 100 types of HPV cause genital infections, the latter are largely asymptomatic. However, they infect transiently about two-thirds of women who are sexually active. Whereas some HPV types, such as 6 and 11, are non-oncogenic but lead to genital warts, types 16 and 18 are high risk for the development of cervical cancer, accounting for two-thirds of cases. As HPV is present in around 99% of squamous cell carcinoma of the cervix, preventive vaccines against HPV have recently been introduced into health services. However, protection would be effective only if vaccination occurs before sexual debut.

41.1.9 Lower Abdominal Pain

The diagnosis of pelvic inflammatory disease should be considered when lower abdominal pain is associated with abnormal vaginal discharge, dyspareunia and tenderness upon cervical motion and in the vaginal adnexae. Pelvic inflammatory disease is important sequelae of infections with *Chlamydia trachomatis and Neisseria gonorrhoeae* with the risk of infertility and ectopic pregnancy from damage to the fallopian tubes [25].

41.1.10 Pregnancy

A distinction should be made between congenital syphilis which is an antenatal infection and those, such as herpes, gonorrhoea and chlamydia, which occur around the time of birth. Congenital syphilis is fully preventable through screening at the first antenatal visit and in high-risk areas, with repeat testing around 28 weeks of pregnancy and at delivery. Around a million cases of congenital syphilis continue to occur annually due to the lack of awareness of the problem, political will and commitment to strengthen available services for the appropriate tasks: early antenatal attendance, decentralised blood testing and presumptive treatment of partners [26].

Ophthalmia neonatorum can be due to *Neisseria gonorrhoeae* and *Chlamydia trachomatis*. Delay in treatment can cause blindness. The mainstay in the management of ophthalmia neonatorum consists of prophylaxis for all infants immediately after delivery: careful cleaning of the eyes prior to the application of 1% tetracycline ointment as compared to the original prophylaxis with an aqueous solution of silver nitrate which is not that effective against chlamydia besides sometimes causing chemical conjunctivitis [27]. When the mother is known to have either a gonococcal or chlamydial infection, the neonate should be treated accordingly with supplementary therapy.

41.1.11 Diagnostic Challenges

In the ideal situation, laboratories provide services for both the identification of organisms and their sensitivities to antimicrobials. In developing countries, the operational level of laboratories can vary enormously as exemplified by a national reference laboratory, this role being often assumed by a university laboratory as opposed to a peripheral one attached to a dispensary. Although an infection may be suspected because of disease in a partner or the presence of another STI, the infection may be diagnosed only by a specific laboratory test. This approach, with laboratory confirmation of clinical diagnoses, often cannot be used in resource-scarce settings: besides being expensive, there is delay in initiating treatment in situations where the individual is unlikely to return for a follow-up visit.

Around 2000, WHO had focussed on syndromic case management as a pragmatic tool to enable treatment for individuals with clinical features, whether symptoms or signs, in low-resource settings without any recourse to laboratory tests: its algorithms had to be adapted to local epidemiological characteristics of STIs and the approach could not be used for screening. Modelling of flowcharts should incorporate factors such as the prevalence of organisms besides their clinical relevance, pattern of resistance to antimicrobials and their cost [28, 29]. Furthermore, periodic aetiological assessments are necessary to validate treatment recommendations [30].

Syndromic case management alone is inadequate because infections with important pathogens such as *Chlamydia trachomatis* and *Neisseria gonorrhoea* may be present without any symptoms or findings. Besides, syndromic approach can either overdiagnose STIs, thereby exposing individuals to unnecessary treatment, or fail to diagnose an existing infection or even cause relationship problems when partners are given a false result. With those severe limitations of syndromic case management, WHO now promotes a move towards an aetiological approach. With the identification of the causative organism becoming very important, the WHO monograph on laboratory services has become a very valuable resource [31].

The diagnosis of vaginal discharge is aided by a high vaginal swab for microscopy, gram stain and culture for bacterial vaginosis, *Trichomonas vaginalis* and *Candida*. Resources should be sought to enable on-site microscopy [32].

Candida albicans can be diagnosed at the bedside by direct wet mount microscopy. A high vaginal swab is put in saline before placing a drop on to a slide and adding a drop of potassium hydroxide solution. Light microscopy shows the presence of yeast or mycelia. It is also possible do a Gram stain from the swab. When this is not satisfactory for the identification of yeast cells, the diagnosis of *Candida albicans* can be confirmed through culture using Sabouraud's agar.

The diagnosis of *Trichomonas vaginalis* is made easily by microscopy: a vaginal swab from the posterior fornix is placed in a saline solution and a wet mount leads to the bedside diagnosis through the visualisation of motile flagellate protozoa.

The diagnosis of bacterial vaginosis is made from a high vaginal swab with microscopy and Gram stain to satisfy Amsel's criteria which consist of the presence of at least three of the following four items: (1) sticky greyish white discharge on vaginal wall, (2) positive whiff amine test consisting of a fishy smell upon adding a drop of 10% solution of potassium hydroxide, (3) vaginal pH greater than 4.5 and (4) clue cells consisting of bacteria around epithelial cells of the vagina.

The identification of *Neisseria gonorrhoeae* by microscopy of a Gram stain of a urethral specimen, with the visualisation of gram-negative diplococci, is easy in men but not in women as there are other similar-looking organisms in the endocervix. Whereas Gram staining, as currently used in most developing countries, is simple and inexpensive, it is relatively insensitive. The identification of *Neisseria gonorrhoeae* and *Chlamydia trachomatis* remains problematic. Although highly sensitive for chlamydia and gonorrhoea, the nucleic acid amplification tests are expensive and complex thereby limiting their utility in low-income countries. Being simple and able to provide rapid results for clinical decisions and follow-up, rapid point-of-care tests [33] have demonstrated promising value for chlamydia and gonorrhoea: whereas some tests have reported specificity (98%) in field trials, their sensitivity in symptomatic women (50–70%) is considered to be low for widespread use and their utility in asymptomatic women has not been fully investigated. It seems prudent to utilise a combination of syndromic management, effective laboratory testing and emerging point-of-care tests for the diagnosis of many STIs in low-resource situations.

Rapid laboratory testing for HIV and syphilis currently exists in many low-resource countries. The tests are simple, accurate and provide results within 15–20 minutes. Testing for these infections is especially important for preconception and antenatal care of women to reduce the burden of mother-to-child transmission of infection. *Treponema pallidum* can only be identified directly by using a specimen from a lesion, and as laboratory culture is not possible, dark-field microscopy is used to demonstrate the typical coil-like morphology. Non-treponemal tests, such as the rapid plasma reagin (RPR), are valuable for screening for syphilis: they are sensitive besides being simple and cheap to carry out provided that facilities enable the refrigeration of reagents and have electrical power. Excellent for detecting early syphilis, they suffer from a relatively high false positive rate which constitutes around 25% of positive results for tests carried out during pregnancy. A treponemal test, such as *Treponema pallidum* haemagglutination assay or fluorescent treponemal antibody absorption test, must be performed subsequently to confirm positive cases. Serologic tests for syphilis are simple to perform, and both the test and treatment are inexpensive. Experience in developing countries has shown that clinic staff with little or no laboratory experience can be trained to perform syphilis blood tests with a high level of accuracy.

Human papillomavirus and herpes simplex, the two common viral infections of the genital tract, are often subclinical. Laboratory detection techniques for the diagnosis of HPV are still largely limited to research settings. The laboratory diagnosis of genital herpes simplex consists of cell culture from a swab.

41.1.12 Drug Treatment

Access to appropriate antimicrobial therapy is crucial for the control of STIs, whether the diagnosis was made on the laboratory identification of organism with antimicrobial sensitivity or syndromic approach with locally determined algorithms. The selection of antimicrobials for the control of STIs is facilitated by use of the WHO model list of essential medicines which allows countries to make the final selection of essential drugs by taking into account local circumstances such as cost [34]. It should be appreciated that commodities such as intrauterine devices and condoms might not be, strictly speaking, considered as being drugs. However, in the control of STIs, it is imperative that this wider perspective be acknowledged. Whenever the term condoms is mentioned, both female and male condoms should be considered whilst appreciating that much more evidence is available for male as compared to female condoms. For both contraception and the control of STI including HIV, the cost of drugs and consolidated procurement procedures must be considered.

Antimicrobial resistance is increasingly leading to worries in global health [35], and the emergence of resistant strains of *N. gonorrhoeae* is so serious that the risk of untreatable gonorrhoea is being discussed seriously [30]. Resistance of organisms to antimicrobials is usually due to inappropriate selection of drugs, inadequate dose or too short duration of therapy. With the success of directly observed therapy in the management of tuberculosis, there is interest in single-dose therapy for STIs. This approach is especially appealing with the anticipated decrease in cost due to the expiration of patents on certain antimicrobials. The global surveillance system that has been set up by WHO to monitor antimicrobial resistance will be useful for routine reports regarding appropriate treatment for gonorrhoea.

As gonococci are now largely resistant to antibiotics such as penicillin and tetracycline, treatment of uncomplicated gonorrhoea in gynaecological practice normally consists of a single dose whether orally, with ciprofloxacin or cefixime, or intramuscularly, with ceftriaxone or spectinomycin. Besides being contraindicated in pregnancy, ciproflaxin should be avoided in the treatment of adolescents. Antimicrobial resistance to gonorrhoea shows such marked geographical differences that ideally each jurisdiction should decide on recommended treatment regimens by drawing upon the best available information. Azithromycin should not usually be used for treating gonorrhoea in view of increasing resistance but is still appropriate for treating chlamydial infections. With the strong association between infections with gonorrhoea and chlamydia, it is advisable for treatment to be provided for both unless there is laboratory evidence for the absence of chlamydia.

The treatment of uncomplicated chlamydia consists of oral therapy usually with either a single dose of azithromycin or a 7-day course of doxycycline, but it is also possible to prescribe a 7-day course of amoxycillin, tetracycline, erythromycin or ofloxacin. There is a contraindication for use of doxycycline and other tetracyclines during pregnancy and breastfeeding as opposed to erythromycin estolate during pregnancy only.

Candidiasis is treated with a 3-day course of intravaginal clotrimazole or miconazole or a single dose of intravaginal clotrimazole or oral fluconazole. Trichomoniasis is treated with oral metronidazole or tinidazole, either as a single dose or a 7-day course. Bacterial vaginosis is usually treated with a 7-day course of oral metronidazole and otherwise as a single dose besides the intravaginal application of metronidazole gel for 4 days or clindamycin cream for 7 days. During pregnancy, a 7-day course of oral metronidazole is given from the second trimester but as a single dose if treatment is needed earlier.

Symptomatic treatment of genital herpes consists of oral acyclovir or valaciclovir for 7 days for the first episode but 5 days for recurrent infections.

External genital warts can be treated with the local application of podophyllin, trichloroacetic acid, podophyllotoxin or imiquimod: the latter two have the advantage of self-application and should be tried first, but it might be necessary to use cryotherapy with liquid nitrogen or surgery. Treatment of vaginal warts consists of cryotherapy using liquid nitrogen, podophyllin or trichloroacetic acid.

Early syphilis is treated by the intramuscular administration of a single dose of benzathine benzylpenicillin or alternatively with a 10-day course of intramuscular procaine benzylpenicillin. Those individuals who are allergic to penicillin should receive a 14-day oral course of either doxycycline or tetracycline with erythromycin being used for treatment during pregnancy. Congenital syphilis is treated with intravenous aqueous benzylpenicillin for the newborn during the first 17 days of the neonatal period.

41.1.13 Coverage

In common with the control of other infections, success with STIs depends largely on coverage to decrease the presence of the incriminated organism in the population. Therefore, all opportunities should be used whether within the health sector or other sectors such as education, work and youth.

Within the health sector, STIs are related to most components of reproductive health services, prime examples being family planning, adolescent health and gender violence besides maternal, newborn and child health. Those relationships should be formally acknowledged at the local level through integrated reproductive health services by strengthening linkages for mutual benefits, especially increased coverage.

It is imperative to ensure the collaboration of the private sector in view of their extensive implication in the provision of services for the treatment of STIs. Even poor individuals would rather pay for private services that are perceived as being of better quality, than receive free public services.

41.1.14 Adapting Protocols

In view of the specificities of each country, it is important that protocols be adapted as necessary to meet the local situation even if it necessitates certain changes to reflect the unique situation in each country. Those specifications include social and cultural norms with their implications for behavioural aspects of health-seeking behaviour, economic conditions with their effect on the availability of resources for health service provision.

The control of STIs has faced major issues associated with stigma, whereby symptomatic individuals either fail to seek care altogether or attend too late, leading to further spread of the STI in the intervening period. Stigma is often the reason for seeking private health care, whether from medical practitioners, nurses or pharmacists besides over-the-counter purchases and encounters with traditional healers simply for easier access to care which is unfortunately related to human rights issues such as privacy and confidentiality. The situation is made even more complex because affected individuals are often asymptomatic when infected or, as in the case of men with trichomonas, even infested. Therapy can become complicated when the issue of treatment of partners is raised.

The identification of individuals with asymptomatic infections consists of either mass screening or case finding. Whereas mass screening aims at comprehensive coverage of a community without any emphasis on clinic attendance, case finding focusses on a specific group such as attendees at clinics providing reproductive health services such as contraception or antenatal care. Screening poses major logistical problems, and the well-entrenched procedures for the testing of blood donations for infections, such as HIV, syphilis and hepatitis B, reflect the importance that is attached to the perceived risk for recipients of blood products. The prime example of case finding in antenatal care refers to the detection of congenital syphilis.

41.1.15 Service Standards

As was the case with family planning services more than a decade ago, bold actions are needed to ensure that services for the control of STIs are effective through the elimination of medical barriers and the promotion of appropriate healthcare-seeking approaches.

Women often seek STI services from health facilities that do not have dedicated STI clinics, prime examples being primary health care and specialist obstetric and gynaecological clinics. Beyond prevention, STI control emphasises case management with its four-pronged approach: diagnosis, antimicrobial therapy, behaviour change communication including condoms and finally, treatment of sexual partners. High-risk groups deserve targeted services but not to the detriment of coverage of the rest of the population even at low risk as a reflection of the epidemiological concept of population attributable risk.

41.1.16 Contact Tracing

Contact tracing with partner notification leads to treatment which serves as primary prevention to prevent infection of others besides persistent or recurrent infection of the index case [36]. This aspect of the management of STIs is sensitive for various reasons.

The selection of drugs for treatment, also called epidemiological treatment, simply follows the same regimen that was adopted for the index case. A careful approach, respecting privacy and confidentiality in accordance with the accepted principles of human rights, should be used for partner notification whilst respecting the sociocultural context and avoiding any coercion.

41.1.17 Surveillance

With sparse and scarce data in most jurisdictions, an excellent case can be made for ensuring that STIs are notifiable like many infectious diseases. However, the limited resources that are available in resource-poor settings raise the issue of a balance between resources for services as opposed to data. Besides the usual aspects of monitoring and evaluation that are in common with other reproductive health services, epidemiological surveillance of STIs is important for detecting antimicrobial resistance which should not be limited to the central referral hospital but sentinel posts should also cover the entire community specially to ensure that rural areas are monitored.

STI surveillance should be complemented by ad hoc studies to investigate issues as they arise, prime examples being the investigation of outbreaks. It is desirable for data from surveillance to be linked to other healthcare utilisation data in order to facilitate community-wide epidemiological investigations.

41.1.18 Implementing Integrated Reproductive Health Services

A life-cycle approach should be used to address reproductive health with special attention to women empowerment and male responsibility [37] besides the consideration of social capital regarding gender and sexuality. The integration of reproductive health services was recommended for the last two decades but major issues have been encountered during attempts at its implementation especially in the configuration of linkages for service delivery. The integration of services for STI and family planning tends to occur de facto at the peripheral level with the employment of multipurpose staff, but at the more central level, there seems to be missed opportunities from the dispersed units of the management structure. Further epidemiological studies on the cost-benefit of integration are needed [38].

41.1.18.1 Contraception

The basic principle in the provision of contraceptive services is to enable individuals to have access to a range of safe and effective methods so that they can exert their choice in the selection of the best method to suit their need. The intrinsic linkages of sexuality with the implications of sexual intercourse for STIs must emphasise the close association of the management, both prevention and treatment, of STIs to the provision of contraceptive services by promoting dual method use. However, the close interface between contraception and STI leads to important considerations to ensure that the selection of contraceptive method is appropriate. With the risk of both a pregnancy and an STI from sexual intercourse, it is not all surprising that there has been much interest in a relation between contraception and the acquisition of STIs.

Whatever the nature of any association, the relatively low use of barrier methods is worrying. When used correctly and consistently, male condoms are effective for preventing the transmission of HIV, syphilis, gonorrhoea, chlamydia, genital HSV-2 and trichomonas [39]. In view of their contraceptive effect, male condoms are therefore extremely valuable for dual protection against pregnancy and STIs, including HIV. As the prevention of STIs is often ignored when condom users change method to more effective hormonal contraceptives, consistent use of condoms is more common when used for contraception as opposed to hormonal methods. Whilst recognising the value of condoms for dual protection, it should be acknowledged that dual-method use is preferable for those who prefer to combine the excellent contraception from hormonal methods with condoms for preventing STIs. The production, marketing and distribution of female condoms will need to complement other activities to promote their utilisation, like male condoms, for dual protection [40]. Furthermore, there is much interest in a revival of the diaphragm as a female-controlled method [41].

An increase in the risk of infections from sex hormones could be due to cervical ectopy, higher vaginal pH from a decrease in lactobacilli, increased infectivity of certain microbes, suppression of the immune system with local humoral dysfunction of the cervix and for HIV, increased shedding in vaginal and cervical secretion. With the impossibility of carrying out a randomised trial, an observational approach is needed.

There is concern that those women who harbour STIs might be at increased risk from pelvic inflammatory disease from use of the intrauterine contraceptive device through an ascending infection with transfer of organisms, during the insertion procedure, from the lower genital tract through cervical canal and uterine cavity to the upper genital tract. Whereas users with an STI have a higher risk with insertion, the lack of comparable data for non-users makes it impossible to determine whether there is any increased risk with the insertion of an intrauterine contraceptive device. Medical eligibility criteria of the World Health Organization for the utilisation of contraceptive methods are useful as service guidelines to guide clinical practice [42, 43]. Nonoxynol-9, a spermicide considered to have microbicidal properties, was impregnated into male condoms, but this well-intentioned approach was squashed with the finding of an increased risk of HIV acquisition when nonoxynol-9 was used often by high-risk women [44].

41.1.18.2 Fertility

STIs can have adverse effects on fertility such as increased incidence of ectopic pregnancy and foetal mortality. The role of STIs in the aetiology of male infertility can be substantial [45], and affected individuals have a pattern of inappropriate health-seeking behaviour regarding STIs [46].

41.1.18.3 HIV Programmes

The intertwining of STIs and HIV with numerous components of reproductive health is well recognised. Moreover, the coexistence of STIs and HIV should be fully appreciated as treatment of STIs has the potential to decrease HIV transmission [47]. With shared causal determinants for undesired outcomes in those diverse areas, relevant interventions would be complementary and intensified linkages should be sought to improve impact, a win-win situation for the major investments in reproductive health services.

Service providers should be fully aware of their potential role in the control of HIV and STIs through integrated reproductive health. The interface of STI and HIV control programmes includes areas such as advocacy for increased resources both for donors and national authorities to improve joint services. Sexual behaviour change, communication to decrease risk including the availability, accessibility and utilisation of both female and male condoms are important. Counselling regarding both screening for STIs and voluntary testing for HIV and implementation of policies for the inclusion of the comprehensive range of reproductive health commodities, especially antimicrobials for the treatment of STIs and condoms, both female and male, in national lists of essential medicines are essential components of integrated reproductive health services. The primacy of joint services is of such importance that there have been international declarations in this area. Whereas much is being done to ensure common activities, it would be valuable for substantial resources to be allocated only for joint activities with the conditionality that those funds would be released only upon full agreement of policy makers and managers of STI and HIV programmes.

41.1.18.4 Maternal, Newborn and Child Health

The effect of STIs on maternal, foetal and neonatal morbidity and mortality is exemplified by conditions such as congenital syphilis, low birthweight and ophthalmia neonatorum. The high incidence of asymptomatic STIs in pregnant women is well recognised [48], and much can be achieved during antenatal care.

With increasing evidence in 2016 of its sexual transmission, the Zika virus became an emerging STI with concerns for complications such as microcephaly and Guillain-Barré syndrome. WHO issued recommendations for safer sexual practices during pregnancy in affected areas besides for 8 weeks afterwards by visitors who should also avoid pregnancy for 6 months [49].

41.1.18.5 Adolescent Health

Services for the control of STIs provide a most valuable entry point for HIV prevention through the treatment of STI, counselling with voluntary testing, promotion of healthy sexual behaviour and provision of barrier methods of contraception. Sexual health education of adolescents does not increase their sexual activity [50], and it is crucial that they understand their sexuality for protection from STIs through the provision of sex education, including negotiation skills before puberty [51].

Adolescents often seek services from the informal sector for treatment of STIs, the likely reason being confidentiality of services but the quality of care is usually poor. Gender-specific messages should be directed at adolescents. Also, counselling of adolescents tends to be poor in both the formal and informal parts of the health sector [52, 53]. Much needs to be done to draw upon the value of the private sector both for public-private partnerships and the involvement of a wide range of private non-medical health workers for the management of STIs [54].

Youth-friendly services should be accessible and appropriate to local circumstances to be welcoming to address their disadvantage regarding lack of information and access to services. There is a need to safeguard the privacy and confidentiality of adolescents to services with special attention to the special vulnerability of adolescent girls due to their social circumstances and biological factors. Efforts should include the provision of services through multiple outlets such as youth centres and school clinics to take advantage of circumstances.

The aetiologies of cervical and liver cancer have commonalities through infections with HPV and hepatitis B, respectively, that are both preventable through vaccination in adolescence. It would be most unfortunate when the introduction of HPV vaccine faces opposition due to a misconception as being a sex vaccine with moralistic implications [1].

41.1.19 Barriers to Integration and Opportunities for Change

Despite recent positive signs that governments in many developing countries are in favour of integrated reproductive health services, service provision is full of barriers that are unnecessary and often discouraging to both providers and potential users. Such barriers include lack of adequate training and resources, socio-cultural barriers, lack of strong and active government commitment and resistance to integration by health professionals who believe that reproductive services should be provided only in a medical setting using unnecessary and time-consuming medical and laboratory examinations [55, 56]. Significant reduction in outside funding also affects integration of STI prevention into reproductive health services because of urgent priorities including the HIV/AIDS epidemic. When resources for social sector activities are reduced, those who suffer the most are disadvantaged populations, such as those in rural areas, because that share of the resources is usually cut first. Besides, most health activities in urban centres have higher associated costs that are not readily discernable in the form of staff salary and other recurrent costs.

Recently, there has been heightened awareness of the importance of STI prevention to HIV/AIDS control with a new appreciation of the pivotal role of the impact of untreated STIs to reproductive health. Renewed attempts at integration of reproductive health services are investing in operational research to develop sound methodology for integration [57]. Concerted efforts are needed to strengthen the infrastructure, trainers and curricula in pre-service training of service providers to provide family planning and STI services for immediate on-the-job application upon graduation. Besides technical capacity building for STI control, efforts are being directed towards changing the provider attitudes to deal with these infections. Operational research evidence is needed to identify the best approach to integration of STI control into family planning and services for mothers and adolescents in different settings and identify other potential options where full integration is not feasible.

41.1.20 Sector-Wide Approach

Scaling-up implies increased coverage of the population with quality services and long-term sustainability, a situation that is likely to necessitate resource mobilisation through the availability of funds from a sector-wide approach mechanism in line with national priorities for reproductive health. Therefore, the ultimate control of STIs will rely upon political commitment for resource mobilisation besides the complementary short-term objective of exploiting the current opportunity whereby increasingly available funds for HIV activities could be used for common resources that will benefit tasks pertaining also to STIs.

Experience should draw upon the lessons learned from the failures of primary health care to ensure that the delivery of reproductive health services would achieve the goals that were feasible for the available level of resources. A sector-wide approach should promote health sector reform to emphasise coordinated activities as opposed to vertical programmes besides a holistic perspective to include issues such as male involvement which is crucial to address gender inequalities in the context of masculinity as pertaining to social norms for behaviour change communication [58] including solutions to overcome problems that were faced by the approach focussing on information, education and communication for population education. Nevertheless, health professionals will continue to devote much precious resources, especially in the form of their time, to address rumours from the public and misinformation from professionals that merely constitute a distraction from priority tasks that would advance the control of STIs.

Capacity building constitutes a major task. Training in STIs should be incorporated in the curricula of health professional schools [59] besides being incorporated in on-the-job training especially in conjunction with supervisory visits.

41.1.21 Programme Effectiveness

The evaluation of the effectiveness of STI control programmes is a complex process yielding mixed findings in both developed and developing countries. Overall, the prevalence of STIs has shown a decline over the past three decades. Several countries in Asia have reported sharp decline in the incidence of common STIs, such as gonorrhoea and chlamydia, following the introduction of integrated STI control programmes, public sexual health education, condom utilisation and improved access by commercial sex workers to STI services. On the contrary, some industrialised countries in Europe and North America have observed a rise in the occurrence of some STIs. However, it is unclear whether those observed increases are due to an actual surge in STIs or merely more accurate diagnostic and reporting procedures. Nevertheless, STIs remain a public health concern for most developing countries particularly in Africa where resources are lacking for STI control efforts besides inadequate surveillance that prevent the assessment of time trends. As STI control is a relatively dynamic process that is vulnerable to political, social and economic change, a coordinated and integrated effort is needed for a sustainable outcome.

41.1.22 Conclusions and Recommendations

With the close interactions of STIs with contraception, maternal health, adolescent health and sexuality besides other components of sexual and reproductive health, opportunities should be used to form strategic partnerships specially to produce the evidence base, bridge the gap in service provision, promote synergies for reproductive health and scale-up activities [60, 61].

Much can be done for the prevention, diagnosis and treatment of STIs by exploiting the potential of services, particularly for women and adolescents, that have been recognised globally [62]. Procedures, especially for diagnosis, will depend largely on the availability of resources, especially human and laboratory. A contraceptive service should serve as an entry point for the control of STIs, whether prevention or treatment, and encourage healthy behaviour including the utilisation of condoms whether for dual protection or dual method use. Integrated reproductive health services should be promoted so that various interventions can be implemented.

References

1. Gottlieb SL, Low N, Newman LM, Bolan G, Kamb M, Broutet N. Toward global prevention of sexually transmitted infections (STIs): the need for STI vaccines. Vaccine. 2014;32:1527–35.
2. Bourgeois A, Henzel D, Dibanga G, et al. Prospective evaluation of a flow chart using a risk assessment for the diagnosis of STDs in primary healthcare centres in Libreville, Gabon. Sex Transm Infect. 1998;74 Suppl 1:S128–32.
3. UNAIDS. The gap report. Geneva: Joint United Nations Programme on HIV/AIDS; 2014.
4. World Health Organization. Progress report of the implementation of the global strategy for prevention and control of sexually transmitted infections: 2006–2015. Geneva: World Health Organization; 2015.
5. United Nations. Transforming our world: the 2030 agenda for sustainable development. Resolution adopted by the General Assembly on 25 September 2015. Document A/RES/70/1. New York: United Nations; 2015.
6. Hogan DR, Baltussen R, Hayashi C, Lauer JA, Salomon JA. Cost effectiveness analysis of strategies to combat HIV/AIDS in developing countries. BMJ. 2005;331:1431–7.
7. World Health Organization. Global incidence and prevalence of selected curable sexually transmitted infections, 2008. Geneva: World Health Organization; 2012. p. 4–5.
8. World Health Organization. Health in the 2030 agenda for sustainable development. Sixty-ninth World Health Assembly. Document A69/15. Geneva: World Health Organization; 2016.
9. Magar V. Gender, health and the sustainable development goals. Bull World Health Organ. 2015;93:743.
10. Kuruvilla S, Bustreo F, Kuo T, et al. The global strategy for women's, children's and adolescents' health (2016–2030): a roadmap based on evidence and country experiences. Bull World Health Organ. 2016;94:398–400.
11. Edouard L, Bernstein S. Challenges for measuring progress towards the Sustainable Development Goals. Afr J Reprod Health. 2016;20:45–54.
12. Scholes D, Stergachis A, Heidrich FE, Andrilla H, Holmes KK, Stamm WE. Prevention of pelvic inflammatory disease by screening for cervical Chlamydia infection. N Engl J Med. 1996;334:1362–6.
13. World Health Organization. Global health sector strategy on sexually transmitted infections, 2016–2021. Geneva: World Health Organization; 2015.
14. Hayes RJ, Schulz KF, Plummer FA. The cofactor effect of genital ulcers on the per-exposure risk of HIV transmission in Sub-Saharan Africa. J Trop Med Hyg. 1995;98:1–8.
15. Ogunkunle MO, Oni AA, Odaibo GN, Olaleye OD. Hepatitis B surface antigen (HbsAg) in blood and genital secretions of patients with sexually transmitted diseases in Ibadan, Nigeria. West Afr J Med. 2005;24:206–8.
16. Edouard L. Sex and the cervix: hormones, infections and cancers. J Fam Plann Reprod Health Care. 2005;31:338–9.
17. Pollack AE, Balkin M, Edouard L, Cutts F, Broutet N. Ensuring access to HPV vaccines through integrated services: a reproductive health perspective. Bull World Health Organ. 2007;85:57–63.
18. Daley EM, Vamos CA, Zimet GD, Rosberger Z, Thompson EL, Merrell L. The feminization of HPV: reversing gender biases in US human papillomavirus policy. Am J Public Health. 2016;106:983–4.
19. Izugbara CO. Tasting the forbidden fruit: the social context of debut sexual encounters among young persons in a rural Nigerian community. Afr J Reprod Health. 2001;5:22–9.
20. Hughes C, Evans A. Health needs of women who have sex with women. BMJ. 2003;327:939–40.
21. Patel V, Pednekar S, Weiss H, et al. Why do women complain of vaginal discharge? Int J Epidemiol. 2005;34:853–62.
22. Mitchell H. Vaginal discharge – causes, diagnosis, and treatment. BMJ. 2004;328:1306–8.
23. Hotez PJ. Neglected infections of poverty in the United States of America. PLoS Negl Trop Dis. 2008;2:e256.
24. James SH, Kimberlin DW. Neonatal herpes simplex virus infection: epidemiology and treatment. Clin Perinatol. 2015;42:47–59.
25. Brunham RC, Gottlieb SL, Paavonen J. Pelvic inflammatory disease. N Engl J Med. 2015;372:2039–48.
26. World Health Organization. Elimination of mother-to-child transmission (EMTCT) of HIV and syphilis - global guidance on criteria

and processes for validation. Geneva: World Health Organization; 2014.
27. Schaller UC, Klauss V. Is Crede's prophylaxis for ophthalmia neonatorum still valid? Bull WHO. 2001;79:262–3.
28. World Health Organization. Guidelines for the management of sexually transmitted infections. Geneva: World Health Organization; 2003.
29. World Health Organization. Sexually transmitted and other reproductive tract infections – a guide to essential practice. Geneva: World Health Organization; 2005.
30. World Health Organization. Draft global health sector strategies – sexually transmitted infections, 2016–2021. Paragraphs 14–15, 52–54, 127, 130. Document A69/33. Geneva: World Health Organization; 2016.
31. Unemo M, editor. Laboratory diagnosis of sexually transmitted infections, including human immunodeficiency virus. Geneva: World Health Organization; 2013.
32. Melville C, Nandwani R, Bigrigg A, McMahon AD. A comparative study of clinical management strategies for vaginal discharge in family planning and genitourinary medicine settings. J Fam Plann Reprod Health Care. 2005;31:26–30.
33. Jain A, Ison CA. Chlamydia point-of-care testing: where are we now? Sex Transm Infect. 2013;89:88–9.
34. World Health Organization. The selection and use of essential medicines: twentieth report of the WHO Expert Committee 2015 including the 19th WHO Model List of Essential Medicines and 5th WHO Model List of Essential Medicines for Children. WHO Technical Report Series number 994. Geneva: World Health Organization; 2015.
35. World Health Organization. Global action plan on antimicrobial resistance. Sixty-ninth World Health Assembly. Document A69/24. Geneva: World Health Organization; 2016.
36. Golden MR, Whittington WL, Handsfield HH, et al. Effect of expedited treatment of sex partners on recurrent or persistent gonorrhoea or chlamydial infection. N Engl J Med. 2005;352: 676–85.
37. Ezumah NN. Gender issues in the prevention and control of STIs and HIV/AIDS: lessons from Awka and Agulu, Anambra State, Nigeria. Afr J Reprod Health. 2003;7:89–99.
38. Dehne K, Snow R. Integrating STI management into family planning services: what are the benefits? Document WHO/RHR/99.10. Geneva: World Health Organization, 1; 1999.
39. Holmes KK, Levine R, Weaver M. Effectiveness of condoms in preventing sexually transmitted infections. Bull World Health Organ. 2004;82:454–61.
40. Francis-Chizororo M, Natshalaga NR. The female condom: acceptability and perception among rural women in Zimbabwe. Afr J Reprod Health. 2003;7:101–16.
41. van der Straten A, Kang MS, Posner SF, Kamba M, Chipato T, Padian NS. Predictors of diaphragm use as a potential sexually transmitted disease/HIV prevention method in Zimbabwe. Sex Transm Dis. 2005;32:64–71.
42. World Health Organization. Medical eligibility criteria for contraceptive use. 5th ed. Geneva: World Health Organization; 2015.
43. World Health Organization. Selected practice recommendations for contraceptive use. 2nd ed. Geneva: World Health Organization; 2004.
44. World Health Organization/CONRAD. WHO/CONRAD technical consultation on nonoxynol-9: summary report. Document WHO/RHR/03.08. Geneva: World Health Organization; 2003.
45. Nwabuisi C, Onile BA. Male infertility among sexually transmitted diseases clinic attendees in Ilorin, Nigeria. Niger J Med. 2001;10:68–71.
46. Okonofua F, Menakaya U, Onemu SO, Omo-Aghoja LO, Bergstrom S. A case-control study of risk factors for male infertility in Nigeria. Asian J Androl. 2005;7:351–61.
47. Kehinde AO, Lawoyin TO. STI/HIV co-infections in UCH, Ibadan, Nigeria. Afr J Reprod Health. 2005;9:42–8.
48. Akerele J, Abhulimen P, Okonofua F. Prevalence of asymptomatic genital infection among pregnant women in Benin City, Nigeria. Afr J Reprod Health. 2002;6:93–7.
49. World Health Organization. Prevention of sexual transmission of Zika virus: interim guidance update, 30 May 2016. Document WHO/ZIKV/MOC/16.1 Rev.1. Geneva: World Health Organization; 2016.
50. UNAIDS. Impact of HIV and sexual health education on the sexual behaviour of young people. Document UNAIDS/97.4. Geneva: Joint United Nations Programme on HIV/AIDS; 1997. p. 5.
51. Richter L, Mabaso M, Ramjith J, Norris SA. Early sexual debut: voluntary or coerced? Evidence from longitudinal data in South Africa – the Birth to Twenty Plus study. S Afr Med J. 2015;105:304–7.
52. Okonofua FE, Ogonor JI, Omorodion FI, et al. Assessment of health services for treatment of sexually transmitted infections among Nigerian adolescents. Sex Transm Dis. 1999;26:184–90.
53. Muntean N, Kereta W, Mitchell KR. Addressing the sexual and reproductive health needs of young people in Ethiopia: an analysis of the current situation. Afr J Reprod Health. 2015;19:87–99.
54. Imogie AO, Agwubike EO, Aluko K. Assessing the role of traditional birth attendants (TBAs) in health care delivery in Edo State, Nigeria. Afr J Reprod Health. 2002;6:94–100.
55. Edouard L. Sexually transmitted infections – breaking the cycle of transmission. New York: United Nations Population Fund; 2004.
56. World Health Organization. Breaking the chain of transmission - global strategy for the prevention and control of sexually transmitted infections. Document WHO/RHR/05.16. Geneva: World Health Organization; 2006.
57. Haire BG, Folayan MO, Brown B. Standards and guidelines for HIV prevention research: considerations for local context in the interpretation of global ethical standards. Afr J Reprod Health. 2014;18:55–65.
58. UNAIDS. Men and AIDS: a gendered approach. Geneva: Joint United Nations Programme on HIV/AIDS; 2000.
59. Haslegrave M, Olatunbosun OA. Incorporating sexual and reproductive health care in the medical curriculum in developing countries. Reprod Health Matters. 2003;11:49–58.
60. Chukwujekwu O, Chabikuli NO, Merrigan M, Awi D, Hamelmann C. Integrating reproductive health and HIV indicators into the Nigerian health system – building an evidence base for action. Afr J Reprod Health. 2010;14:109–16.
61. Broutet N, Edouard L. Sexually transmitted infections: key issues for clinical practice. Int J Gynaecol Obstet. 2007;97:229–31.
62. World Health Organization. Resolutions of the sixty-ninth World Health Assembly, 28 May 2016. Geneva: World Health Organization; 2016.

Uterine Fibroid and Hysterectomy

42

Friday Okonofua

Learning Objectives
After reading this chapter, the reader will be able to:

- Describe the epidemiology and risk factors for uterine fibroid
- Discuss the clinical features and modes of presentation of the disease
- Articulate the methods of diagnosis and indications for treatment
- Discuss the medical and surgical treatment of the disease
- Discern the indications for medical and surgical treatment
- Describe the skills and methods for the surgical procedure with myomectomy and hysterectomy
- Identify the research gaps relating to uterine fibroids, with a particular focus on research needs in sub-Saharan African countries

42.1 Introduction

Uterine fibroid, also called leiomyoma, is the most common benign growth of the female reproductive tract. It occurs in both developed and developing countries, but it has an unusually high prevalence and adverse health consequences in sub-Saharan African countries. While it may appear as a single growth within the uterine musculature, it tends to occur more frequently as multiple benign growths with a low proclivity to transform into a malignancy.

A uterine fibroid is one of the most common reasons for gynecological consultation in many African countries [1, 2], and unquestionably accounts for the most frequent indication for hysterectomy in women. It has been posited that "the fear of uterine fibroid is the beginning of wisdom for women" for women in developing countries. This age-long cautionary tale is still true till this day, due to the high prevalence of fibroid, as well as the numerous complications that women experience when they seek health care for fibroid in resource-challenged settings. In countries where women are under pressure to achieve high fertility, the diagnosis of fibroid is considered a major catastrophe as it is perceived to be associated with infertility that attracts important health, psychological, and social consequences for women.

This chapter reviews the epidemiology and clinical features of uterine fibroid and summarizes the most relevant aspects of its current medical and surgical management. Given its high prevalence in developing countries, it is crucial that clinicians in developing countries develop and implement an impeccable protocol for its management to reduce associated myths and bring assistance to women.

42.1.1 Pathophysiology of Uterine Fibroids

The exact cause of uterine fibroid is not understood with certainty, but several linkages with hormones, epigenetic factors, diet, and behavioral factors have been suggested and will be discussed further in the next section. Regardless of its mode of initiation, the primary pathology is the development of a large amount of extracellular matrix in the smooth muscle cells of the myometrium. The tumors are well circumscribed and separated from the normal uterine muscle by a pseudo-capsule that is made up of thin muscle fibers. Uterine fibroids tend to be parasitic as they often borrow vascularization from surrounding structures. They disrupt the delicate network associated with the vascularization of the normal myomectum leading to altered multiple patterns of neovascularization.

F. Okonofua (✉)
Centre of Excellence in Reproductive Health Innovation, Department of Obstetrics and Gynaecology, University of Benin, Benin City, Nigeria

Women's Health and Action Research Centre, Benin City, Nigeria

University of Medical Sciences, Ondo City, Ondo State, Nigeria

F. Okonofua et al. (eds.), *Contemporary Obstetrics and Gynecology for Developing Countries*,
https://doi.org/10.1007/978-3-030-75385-6_42

Fibroids are often classified according to their location within the uterus as follows:

- Subserous—when the fibroids are located underneath the subserous layer of the uterus.
- Intramural—when the fibroids are buried mostly within the uterine musculature with the muscle having to be cut before they can be removed.
- Submucous—the fibroid lies underneath the surface of the lining (endometrium) of the uterus. This type of fibroid often expands the endometrium and increases the amount of bleeding during menstruation.

Both subserous and submucous fibroids may be pedunculated, with nodules of fibroids left connected to the uterus both externally and internally with long layers of fibrous tissue and muscle. The subserous fibroids, in particular, can attach to adjacent organs and stimulate tissue reaction and, with possible additional infection, cause the formation of various degrees of adhesions. Adhesion formation is responsible for other manifestations of fibroids, including the destruction of the fallopian tubes and ovaries, and multiple distortions of the pelvic cavity.

Both in clinical practice and research, several factors have been known to influence the growth or regression of uterine fibroids [3]. These include:

- Estrogen—stimulates the growth of fibroids both in animals and in humans. There is evidence that fibroids grow considerably in situations of high estrogen output especially in pregnancy, in the presence of estrogen-producing tumors and when exogenic estrogens or its derivatives are used for therapeutic purposes.
- Progesterone—inhibits the growth of the uterus as has been shown in various animal models. The progesterone receptors within the tumors are inhibitory, and this informs the use of GnRH analogs and progesterone derivatives for the treatment of fibroids. Although pregnancy also produces a large amount of progesterone, the aggregate effect is to stimulate the growth of existing fibroids due to the higher levels of various types of estrogen also provided by the placenta in pregnancy.

Cytokines and growth factors (e.g., epidermal growth factor, transforming growth factor-alpha, insulin-like growth factor, vascular endothelial growth factor, basic fibroblast growth factor, etc.) have been reported [4] to play roles in the growth of fibroid, especially in synergistic action with estrogen and progesterone. This is particularly relevant in pregnancy when both estrogen and progesterone are produced.

42.1.2 Epidemiology

The reported prevalence rates of fibroids vary considerably depending on the population of women studied and the diagnostic techniques used. Prevalence rates range from 5.4% to 77% [5], with evidence indicating that the incidence is lower in Europe as compared to the United States.

There are no existing population-based data on the prevalence of fibroids in sub-Saharan African countries. However, it has been well documented that the incidence and prevalence of fibroids are higher in women of African descent in the United States [6], and possibly in black women elsewhere. The intensity and clinical manifestations of fibroid are also more severe in African women, while several reports are indicating that many obstetricians and gynecologists in African countries spend a lot of their time attending to women with fibroid and its complications [1, 2]. Hospital data show a prevalence of 6.8% among women attending routine ultrasound scan in Ekiti, South-west Nigeria [7]. A retrospective review at the Irrua Teaching Hospital also reported an overall incidence of 19.8% [8]. Although these figures are low when compared to data from developed countries, its possibility suggests under-reporting, knowing that these are prevalence data obtained from hospitals often self-selected by women for care, while data collection from retrospective reviews may have been suboptimal. There is a need for population-based research that investigates the incidence and prevalence of uterine fibroids in African countries, to enable the development of appropriate policies and programs to tackle the problem.

42.1.3 Risk Factors

Several risk factors have been associated with the risk of development of uterine fibroids as follows:

Age Fibroids occur in the reproductive age group, while up to 40% are diagnosed after the age of 40 years and decrease considerably in the postmenopausal years reflecting declining estrogen levels [9]. They are rare in the pubertal age and tend to occur more frequently in women who had experienced earlier ages of menarche.

Race and genetics Uterine fibroids are more common in black women and rarest in women of the Asian race [5]. This pattern has stimulated considerable research into the role of epigenetics in the causation of fibroids. Some scientific evidence that suggests a role for genetics in uterine fibroids includes the observation that fibroids sometimes occur in families [10], the higher frequency of fibroids in monozygotic twins compared to di-zygotic twins [11], and cytogenetic studies which show tumor-specific chromosomal abnormalities in approximately 40% of tumor samples [12]. Research to determine the role of genetics is still in progress, but the aberrant expression of micro-RNA (a class of non-coding RNAs that regulate cell proliferation, differentiation, and death) is one mechanism that has been proposed and is currently being investigated [5].

Reproductive risk factors The association of late pregnancy with increased risk of uterine fibroid is well known [12] while increasing number of pregnancies decrease the risk of the fibroid. Fibroids have increased prevalence in women with polycystic ovary syndrome due to the persistently elevated levels of luteinizing hormone [12]. Also, increased exogenous use and endogenous production of estrogens raise the risk of fibroid in reproductive age women [5].

Lifestyle factors Various lifestyle factors such as diet, smoking, physical activities, and stress have been reported to potentiate the likelihood of uterine fibroids [13]. Diet with high glycemic index and those rich in red meat have been reported to increase the risk of fibroids [14]. By contrast, the diet rich in fruit, vegetables, fish, vitamin A and D, carotenoids, and bioflavonoids reduce the risk of fibroids. However, these results need to be validated in various populations through a large sample of case-control studies that investigate the dietary habits of women with fibroids compared with age-matched controls.

Few studies have been conducted to determine the effect of physical exercise on the risk of developing fibroids. However, a reduced risk has been established in women who regularly exercise and have a healthy body weight in all racial groups studied [14]. While alcohol intake has been shown to increase the risk of the fibroid, no such effect has been demonstrated for coffee, tea, and caffeine consumption, at least in African women [15]. Similarly, the impact of smoking and stress on fibroid risk has not shown any significant untoward effects [5, 16].

Infection and uterine injury A practice-based case-control study demonstrated a significant increase in fibroids in women with previously diagnosed episodes of pelvic inflammatory disease [17]. This study stimulated discussion as to whether pelvic inflammatory disease may increase the risk of fibroids, at least in women of African descent. However, the study has never been replicated, and as such the possible role of pelvic inflammatory disease and its mechanism of action in fibroid causation remains a matter of conjecture. In particular, it needs to be established whether the infection is a cause rather than a consequence of fibroid through appropriately designed follow-up cohort studies.

Other risk factors Several studies in Western countries have demonstrated an increase in the prevalence of fibroid in women with diabetes mellitus and arterial hypertension [13]. Such studies need to be replicated in African countries where the incidence of diabetes and hypertension may differ from those of women in Western countries.

42.1.4 Clinical Features

Despite the high prevalence of uterine fibroids, a large proportion is clinically asymptomatic and may only be routinely diagnosed on routine gynecological examination or at pelvic ultrasound scan. However, when fibroids present in clinical facilities, the standard modes of presentation are: the presence of a substantial abdominal mass possibly associated with pressure effects, menstrual irregularities/abnormal uterine bleeding, chronic abdominal pain, pregnancy complications, and in association with the management of infertility.

Abdominal Mass with or Without Pressure Symptoms Some uterine fibroids present when women felt a hard mass in the abdomen, with or without specific symptoms. They may report that their abdomen has grown in size, that their clothes no longer fit them, or that their friends or relatives have complained of the increase in the dimensions of their abdomen. All of these symptoms suggest the presence of a growing uterine fibroid that has risen above the pelvic cavity.

Huge fibroid masses in the abdomen may give rise to pressure symptoms. Common pressure symptoms include frequency of micturition, cystitis, urinary tract infection, and even difficulty in emptying the bladder. We have reported the case of a 43-year-old Nigerian woman with huge multiple uterine fibroids with evidence of obstruction of both ureters (hydro-ureters) and hydronephrosis, resulting in elevated serum urea and creatinine [18]. These abnormalities returned to normal as soon as the woman underwent a total abdominal hysterectomy.

Huge fibroids may sometimes also compress the colon and the rectum and lead to difficulty in passing stools and constipation, while prolonged compression of the small intestines may lead to the malabsorption syndrome and chronic malnutrition of women. A rare symptom in women with substantial uterine fibroid is the occasional passage of a massive quantity of clear fluid through the vagina. This tends to occur irregularly and unexpectedly and may occur in embarrassing situations with the women unprepared for it. Hydrorrhea frequently happens when huge submucous fibroids are present either in the lower segment of the uterus or in the cervix.

Menstrual Irregularities This is the most dramatic clinical presentation associated with uterine fibroid. Menorrhagia occurs in the presence of submucous fibroids and is due to endometrial hyperplasia and expanded endometrial bleeding surface. Women frequently report this as both an elongation in the number of days of bleeding, the passage of clots, and increased severity of bleeding. Careful menstrual history by the attending clinician will help to determine the duration of the heavy menstrual bleeding, which will enable an assessment of anemia that may be associated with this complication.

Moderate to severe dysmenorrhea is also frequently associated with uterine fibroid. It often presents as secondary dysmenorrhea, implying that the woman previously had pain-free menstrual cycles before the onset of painful periods. The pain precedes the onset of bleeding by a few days, while the intensity of pain reduces after the beginning of the menstrual bleeding. Dysmenorrhea is due to vascular congestion of the pelvis, as well as irregular contractions of the uterine muscle at the time of menstruation. Other menstrual irregularities, especially oligomenorrhea and intermenstrual bleeding, are often not caused by fibroids, although they may occur in association with uterine fibroids.

Chronic Abdominal Pain Uterine fibroid may cause severe chronic pelvic and lower abdominal pain that is unrelated to the menstrual period. The pain is due to pelvic congestion, especially when the fibroid fills the entire pelvis and compresses the pelvic nerves. Such fibroids may also cause painful sexual intercourse (deep dyspareunia) and lower backache.

Pregnancy Complications Fibroids frequently coexist with healthy pregnancies. In such cases, they may be discovered incidentally at cesarean sections. However, fibroids may cause irregular contractions and abdominal pain during pregnancy. Abdominal pain in association with fibroids in pregnancy is sometimes due to red degeneration [19], a process whereby the coexisting fibroid undergoes substantial growth with bleeding within its internal architecture. Red degeneration is not an indication for operative intervention during pregnancy, but merely a call for more observation, painful relief, and careful monitoring of the pregnancy. Abdominal pain also is due to torsion of a pedunculated subserous fibroid, which is more common in the pregnant than in the nonpregnant state.

As a result of irregular contractions, their number and positions in the uterus, fibroids may cause several complications in pregnancy [20]. These include second-trimester spontaneous abortion, premature onset of labor and prematurity, and fetal malpresentation. Uterine fibroid also increases the incidence of placenta previa and abruptio placenta. Such complications may warrant the increased use of cesarean section for delivery in women with fibroids, but we must caution that no attempt should be made to remove fibroids at any time when they coexist with pregnancy. Although there are reports of successful myomectomy at cesarean sections [21, 22], there are also reports of instances when such operations went sour and were associated with massive intraoperative bleeding that led to the death of patients [23]. Overall, efforts to remove the fibroid during pregnancy should be discouraged especially in countries with a limited resource as it may be associated with heavy bleeding and may compromise the life of the woman and the baby.

Uterine fibroids may prevent uterine contractility in the third stage of labor and predispose women to primary postpartum bleeding, retained placenta or retained placenta products, puerperal infection, and postpartum subinvolution of the uterus.

Association with Infertility Fibroid is not necessarily a cause of infertility, as many women with fibroids often become pregnant and carry such pregnancies to term, with normal vaginal delivery. However, fertility may be delayed if there are multiple uterine fibroids, if the fibroids are in the submucous position where they can distort the endometrium and prevent normal implantation, or if the fibroids are in the cornual or interstitial parts of the tube where they block the entry of the fallopian tubes into the uterus.

Infertility may also be due to peritubal adhesions that are elicited by uterine fibroids, and also to anovulation caused by the involvement of the ovaries in the pelvic adhesions.

A wise counsel is that despite the presence of fibroids, it should not always be assumed that they are the causes of infertility in individual cases. Efforts should still be made to exclude other causes of infertility such as oligo/azoospermia, anovulation, and hormonal factors, cervical factors, etc. before a decision is reached about the possible role of fibroids as a causal factor. Our experience indicates that fibroid always coexists with other elements in cases of infertility where they manifest. Clinicians must resist the temptation often suggested by infertile couples that any existing fibroid is the sole cause of the infertility.

42.1.5 Diagnosis of Fibroids

If the fibroid is moderately sized or large, diagnosis can easily be made with an abdominal or vaginal examination. Abdominal palpation will show an irregularly firm and nontender mass, which has a delineable upper limit, but difficult to determine its lower limit. This is because of the pelvic origin of the mass, which can be confirmed with a bimanual vaginal examination. In experienced hands, the vaginal examination is useful for the diagnosis of moderate-sized uterine fibroids. The primary differential diagnosis that should be considered includes adenomyosis, adnexal masses, and ovarian tumors. A careful vaginal examination will show that the masses arise from the uterus and are continuous with the body of the uterus as demonstrated by the manipulation of the cervix and that they are firm and irregular as distinct from the firm and regular consistency of adenomyosis.

When still in doubt, an abdominal or transvaginal scan will resolve the diagnosis. The most common ultrasonic feature of uterine fibroid is a hypoechoic well-circumscribed area of the uterus, in comparison with the surrounding normal myometrium. Sometimes, the area could be isoechoic or even hyper-echoic. When the fibroid has undergone calcification, it will be seen as echogenic foci associated with shadowing.

Other investigations required to assess the effects of the fibroid fully include hematocrit estimation and full blood count, urine analysis and urine culture, and estimation of serum electrolytes, urea, and creatinine. When the fibroids are multiple and huge, an intravenous urography would be necessary to exclude pressure effects on the pelvic ureter, especially if the serum electrolytes, urea, and creatinine are abnormal.

In women with fibroid and infertility, a full assessment of infertility should be undertaken. These include evaluation of ovulation with day 21 serum progesterone, and day 2/3 serum follicle stimulating hormone and luteinizing hormone, as well as a full semen analysis. In all such women, hysterosalpingography should always be undertaken to assess the patency of the fallopian tubes, and if available a hysteroscopy should be done to determine the status of the endometrium and determine the presence of submucous fibroid and their location.

42.1.6 Management of Uterine Fibroids

Depending on the mode of presentation, the management of uterine fibroid can be with surgery or with medical treatment. Medical treatment alone is seldom used and will be described either as an adjunct to the surgical procedure or as primary treatment in women not desiring surgery. The surgical treatments for uterine fibroid are myomectomy and hysterectomy—the frequency of each method depends on country-specific contexts and the preference of the woman.

Myomectomy has traditionally been the preferred method of surgical treatment in young women (<40 years old) who may have been infertile or subfertile and desire more children. However, with the advent of the new reproductive technologies, myomectomy can still be done in older women who prefer to retain their uterus for the sake of an assisted pregnancy with the use of donor eggs. This procedure is particularly useful in women who may be ending their reproductive lives without having been pregnant. Myomectomy is the surgical removal of fibroid nodules while preserving the uterus, achieved through laparotomy or laparoscopy. Intraoperative bleeding is the life-threatening complication associated with myomectomy, especially when the fibroids are huge and multiple. Consequently, the need to reduce blood loss is one of the most important considerations during myomectomy.

Various methods have described the control of blood loss at myomectomy. These include intra-myometrial vasopressin, peri-cervical tourniquets, misoprostol, bupivacaine plus epinephrine, intravenous and topical tranexamic acid, methylergonovine, and the preoperative administration of GnRH analog and sublingual or rectal misoprostol [24–26].

The use of a temporary tourniquet tied around the lower part of the uterus during myomectomy operation deserves a special mention as we have used this method in 224 myomectomies over 20 years without a single case of severe bleeding and any of the women being transfused postoperatively [18]. The technique is performed with Foley's urethral catheter applied as low as possible at the base of the uterus before enucleating the fibroid masses. This method is cheap and safe and effectively reduces blood loss during myomectomy. It also significantly reduces transfusion rate while not adding to the complications due to the operation [27].

The use of an absorbable tourniquet that is left in situ around the uterine arteries to reduce perioperative bleeding and subsequent pelvic adhesions [27] is a novel idea, but its effectiveness still needs to be examined in an appropriately powered study.

Temporary clipping of the uterine arteries before laparoscopic myomectomy is a safe procedure for controlling excessive blood loss without jeopardizing the uterine blood supply [28, 29]. Temporary occlusion of the uterine arteries may be an alternative approach to minimize intraoperative blood loss during laparoscopic myomectomy and should be considered in patients with challenging myomas at higher risk of bleeding.

After securing control of blood loss, the fibroid nodules are removed with enucleation or through the use of a myomectomy screw. Attempts should be made to remove all fibroids because any little nodules left behind may regrow after surgery. The sites from which the fibroids are removed are then closed carefully with multiple layers of absorbable sutures. The external layer of the uterus should be closed with a delayed absorbable suture such as vicryl to reduce the chances of development of postoperative adhesions.

As much as possible, every attempt should be made to avoid incisions to the posterior wall of the uterus, as these could lead to the formation of adhesions with the small or large bowel and cause intestinal obstruction postoperatively. Similarly, entry into the endometrium should be avoided as much as possible to prevent the development of intrauterine adhesions and reduced menstrual flow later. If the endometrium is breached at myometrium, the insertion of a postoperative urethral catheter to the uterine cavity for a few days will reduce the incidence of post-myomectomy uterine adhesions.

42.1.7 Hysterectomy

Hysterectomy is the total removal of the uterus and the cervix either through abdominal laparotomy or by laparoscopy. In many developing countries, a total hysterectomy is mostly done through laparotomy because of the lack of skills for operative laparoscopy, and also because laparotomy provides an opportunity for the surgeon to deal with other abdominal or pelvic pathologies. Recent advances have led to the development and use of minimally invasive robotic procedures for performing hysterectomy [30]. In this method, the surgeon uses a high-definition 3-D, robotic technology and miniature instruments to view, manipulate, and remove the uterus. The procedure is associated with minimal pain and postoperative complications, and the patient is often discharged home the same day.

Subtotal hysterectomy that was sometimes done in the past primarily to provide an opportunity for young women to continue to experience some modicum of menstruation is no longer recommended [31]. It increases the incidence of postoperative morbidity and exposes the women to the risk of future cervical cancer. The prophylactic removal of both ovaries at hysterectomy, when not involved in any significant pathology, has been a subject of debate for decades. The consensus is that such ovaries should not be routinely removed in women aged 45 years or less but could be removed in older women to reduce the risk of future development of ovarian cancer [32].

A uterine fibroid is the most common indication for hysterectomy in most developing countries. Other indications for hysterectomy include severe pelvic inflammatory disease from botched unsafe abortion; chronic pelvic inflammatory disease that is unresponsive to treatment; endometriosis, as part of treatment for malignancies of the ovary and the fallopian tubes; endometrial hyperplasia/malignancy; cervical intraepithelial neoplasia (CIN); uterine malignancy (e.g., leiomyosarcoma); and adenomyosis [33–35].

In many sub-Saharan African countries, hysterectomy is not to be taken lightly but should only be undertaken after deep considerations. This is because of women's reluctance to accept the removal of their uteruses either because of cultural reasons or because of the desire to retain fertility and continuing menstruation [36, 37]. The removal of the uterus in a woman without the partner's approval could attract considerable family tension and disapproval. As a result, time must be taken to fully explain the procedure to the woman (and possibly her close relatives), and to ensure that she accepts the procedure on her terms before it is carried out.

Thus, the procedure should be undertaken after extensive counselling—if possible, a social worker should be involved in the counselling process. The woman should then be assessed for her hematological status; blood should be cross-matched and made ready for possible use during the surgery; screening for coinfection (HIV, hepatitis B and C, and syphilis) should be carried out; and full investigation for her medical status with blood pressure assessment, exclusion of diabetes mellitus and assessment of her renal state, must be undertaken.

Abdominal hysterectomy is best undertaken with balanced general anesthesia. But in resource-poor countries, spinal or epidural anesthesia can be safely used. Depending on the size of the fibroid, a midline, paramedian, or Pfannenstiel incisions should be used for entering the abdomen. The experience of the surgeon dramatically influences the choice of incision. There should never be pressure to use a fanciful or cosmetic incision when the size of the uterus and its associated pathologies calls for the use of an incision that will enable the surgeon to gain adequate access to the abdomen. It is for this reason that a midline or paramedian incision is often preferred, as it gives the option to extend the incision above the umbilicus when necessary.

Several techniques for abdominal hysterectomy have been well described in various publications and textbooks [38]. It is not within the scope of this book to explain this in detail. It is recommended that the reader should read any of these texts, assist an experienced surgeon in performing up to ten hysterectomies, and be assisted in doing at least five cases before embarking on a solo effort at hysterectomy. The intra-fascial technique of hysterectomy is the method this author has used for more than 25 years, with minimal risks of intraoperative and postoperative complications. This method is recommended and is well described in Techniques of Operative Gynaecology [38]; readers are advised to consult the book for further details.

42.1.8 Conservative Surgical Treatment

These can either be by surgery or by conservative medical treatment. Conservative surgical procedure can either be with uterine artery embolization or with MRI-guided focused ultrasound. Uterine artery embolization has been approved for the treatment of uterine fibroids by the Royal College of Obstetricians and Gynaecologists [39]. It is performed under radiological screening when the uterine arteries are catheterized via the femoral arteries. Particles are then injected, most commonly polyvinyl alcohol, to embolize the uterine vascular bed. It is carried out under local anesthesia with limited complications, the most common being postoperative pain. Fibroid shrinkage is progressive reaching a mean of about 60% at 6 months post surgery [40].

MRI-guided focused ultrasound involves the use of high-frequency, high-energy ultrasound beam to destroy fibroid tissues by coagulative necrosis [41]. The technique is new and currently being developed, while its assessment is still small scale and undergoing refinement. It, however, holds promise for the future improvement in the outpatient management of uterine fibroids resulting in uterine preservation.

42.1.9 Conservative Medical Treatment

There is currently substantive evidence for the use of medical treatment for uterine fibroids. Some of these include nonhormonal treatment, combined oral contraceptives, levonorgestrel-releasing intrauterine systems, progestogens and androgens, antiprogesterone/selective progesterone receptor modulators (mifepristone), and gonadotropin-releasing hormone (GnRH) analogs. These are briefly reviewed below.

Nonhormonal Treatment Nonsteroidal anti-inflammatory drugs are useful in the management of the pain associated with uterine fibroids, although they are not effective in the control of blood loss. As such, they could be used on a short-term basis in patients experiencing severe pain from fibroids pending definitive treatment. As for the medical treatment of menorrhagia, there has been a report from a nonrandomized trial that antifibrinolytic, such as tranexamic acid, may reduce blood loss by up to 50% in women experiencing massive blood loss from fibroids [42]. These could also be tried as well, albeit on a short-term basis.

Combined Oral Contraceptives Uterine fibroid is not a contraindication to the use of the combined oral contraceptive (OC) pills. Indeed, there is evidence that the long-term use of OC may protect women from developing uterine fibroids [43]. A small randomized controlled study has shown a 13% reduction in measured blood loss with a regimen containing the standard dose of OC used for contraception as compared to women who did not take the contraceptives [44]. More such studies are required—an example being case-control studies that investigate the self-reported use of OC in women with fibroids as compared to age-matched women without fibroids. Also, more extensive clinical trials on the effect of OC on ultrasonically determined fibroid sizes in women on the pill as compared to those not taking the OC would also be relevant.

Levonorgestrel-Releasing Intrauterine Systems There is evidence that levonorgestrel-releasing intrauterine devices (LNG-IUD) may reduce the quantity of menstrual blood loss and improve hematological parameters in women with fibroids, without significantly reducing the size of the fibroids [45]. However, although women with distorted uterine cavities and those with uterine fibroids greater than 12 weeks size were excluded, LNG-IUD use in women with fibroids was still associated with high rates of spontaneous expulsion of the device and more cases of breakthrough bleeding. Thus, LNG-IUD use for treatment of fibroid-associated heavy menstrual bleeding is restricted to women with fibroids less than 12 weeks in size without distortion of the uterine cavity.

Progestogens and Androgens Progestogens even in high doses do not reduce the size of uterine fibroids. They should therefore not be used routinely for the treatment of fibroids. The long-term use of depot medroxyprogesterone acetate (Depo-Provera) may protect against the development of fibroids but is not useful in the treatment of fibroid-related symptoms [46].

However, the androgen danazol and the androgenic anti-progesterone gastronome have been shown to be effective in reducing the sizes of fibroids and menstrual blood loss. Gastronome is preferred because of its fewer side effects as compared to danazol and could be used in the short-term control of fibroid-related menstrual blood loss.

Anti-progesterone/Selective Progesterone Receptor Modulators Mifepristone is a known anti-progesterone agent that is active as a progesterone receptor modulator. At a dose of 5–10 mg daily for up to 6 months, mifepristone has been shown to reduce menstrual blood loss when compared to a placebo, without an effect on the uterine size or volume [47]. Similar results were obtained with the anti-progesterone, ulipristal [48], which does better than mifepristone by reducing uterine volume as well as blood loss. Further evidence for the use of anti-progesterone in the treatment of fibroids is still being awaited.

Gonadotropin-Releasing Hormone Analogs Treatment with the GnRH buserelin and leuprolide acetate has been shown to reduce the size of fibroids [49]. The mechanism of action is through suppression of ovarian function, which in itself reduces fertility and predisposes women to the risk of increased bone loss. However, its use is mainly recommended for shrinking the sizes of fibroids before hysteroscopic, laparoscopic, or conventional surgery. When used in combination with iron therapy, it can significantly improve hematological parameters and reduce intraoperative blood loss.

Gonadotropin-releasing hormone analogs may also be useful in women who decline surgery and in whom other medical treatments have failed. It is recommended that the analogs should be given for at least 3 months before the addition of low-dose hormone replacement therapy to overcome the consequences of low estrogen levels. Backup treatment with tibolone will maintain the fibroid shrinkage while reducing the associated vasomotor symptoms.

42.1.10 Prevention

The prevention of uterine fibroid is divided into three major categories: (1) primary prevention—the prevention of fibroids from occurring in the first place; (2) secondary prevention—the practical and prompt management of fibroids when they occur; and (3) tertiary prevention—the rehabilitation of women after they have had fibroid treatment.

Primary Prevention Because the exact cause of fibroid is not yet known, it is difficult to recommend specific methods that women can use for the primary prevention of fibroids. However, attention needs to be paid to diet and appropriate lifestyles, while the use of combined oral contraceptives has been shown to reduce fibroid risk in the long term.

Also, since fibroid tends to develop in older infertile women, it may be worthwhile counselling women to complete their family sizes in earlier ages to reduce the risk and consequences of fibroids.

Secondary Prevention This depends mostly on the early recognition and prompt treatment of fibroids. A major constraint in many developing countries is that women often delay in seeking treatment for fibroids and its complications. Clinical experiences indicate that women often find treatment after having had fibroids for several years, and in the face of irreversible damage and severe complications. This may be due to cultural or religious considerations, the excessive fear of surgery, or to reasons of costs. Consequently, efforts should be put in place to educate women on fibroids and its prevention and treatment, with the hope that this will increase early health-care seeking for fibroids.

Physicians in developing countries also need to be trained on the use of various modalities for early fibroid management, especially those that involve the use of small surgery and conservative medical and surgical treatments. The procedures will increase the likelihood that women will accept initial treatment for fibroids.

Tertiary Prevention In women undergoing hysterectomy, postsurgical management and counselling will enable women to cope with the psychological and sexual effects of the removal of the uterus. This is particularly the case in relatively younger women whose ovaries had been removed. Hormone replacement therapy may assist such women in coping with the related changes.

For younger women who have had myomectomy or other conservative treatments, the primary consideration is future fertility. There is evidence that women can become pregnant within months of myomectomy. Therefore, they should be advised to try for pregnancy as soon as healing has taken place. Indeed, our experience indicates that pregnancy in such instances reduces the tendency for the women to develop recurrent fibroids.

For women that had myomectomy in the presence of severe tubal disease or other severe cases of infertility, treatment with assisted reproductive technology should be recommended. When or else fails, women and couples should be counseled to accept their infertility or to adopt a child.

42.1.11 Research Gaps

Some suggested research gaps, particularly in African countries, include the following:

- Epidemiological studies, especially those that provide population-based data on the incidence and prevalence, as well as the risk factors for fibroids.
- Clinical case-control studies that determine the association of various risk factors for the likelihood of developing countries. Such factors include smoking, use of alcohol, specific dietary practices, contraceptive practices, and previous sexually transmitted infections
- The investigation into local treatments for the prevention and treatment of fibroids, including local herbs that have been reported in local folklores as useful in the treatment of fibroids.
- Clinical trials that compared different modalities and approaches for the treatment of fibroids.
- Qualitative studies to determine women's perceptions and beliefs (and other stakeholders) toward fibroids and its management.
- Intervention studies that compare the effectiveness of teaching and training programs in building the knowledge and skills of communities and health providers on fibroid treatment and prevention.

42.1.12 Summary

Uterine fibroid is one of the most frequent gynecological disorders in developing countries. It has severe consequences for the reproductive health and social well-being of women.

As such, its management and prevention deserve priority attention among obstetricians and gynecologists practicing in these countries. Hopefully, this chapter has provided sufficient information to enable practitioners to understand the various ways that fibroids present clinically, at least within the context of developing countries, and to manage them effectively and efficiently. Continuous in-service training will build local capacity for the management of fibroid and its complications.

References

1. Okogbo FO, Ezechi OC, Loto OM, Ezeobi PM. Uterine leiomyomata in Southwest Nigeria: a clinical study of presentation and management outcomes. Afr Health Sci. 2011;11(2):271–8.
2. Okezie O, Ezegwi HU. Management of uterine fibroids in Enugu, Nigeria. J Obstet Gynecol. 2006;26(4):363–5.
3. Fleischer R, Weston GC, Vollenhoven BJ, Rogers A. Pathophysiology of fibroid disease angiogenesis and regulation of smooth muscle proliferation. Best Pract Res Clin Obstet Gynaecol. 2008;22(4):603–14.
4. Ciarmela P, Islam Md S, Reis F, Gray PC, et al. Growth factors and myometrium: biological effects in uterine fibroid and possible implications. Hum Reprod Update. 2011;17(6):772–90. https://doi.org/10.1093/humupd/dmr031.
5. Sparic R, Mirkovic L, Malvais A, Tinelli A. Epidemiology of uterine myomas: a review. Int J Fert Steril. 2016;9(4):424–35.
6. Jacoby VL, Fujimoto VJ, Gocidice LC, Kupperman M, Washington AE. Racial and ethnic disparities in benign gynaecologic conditions and associated surgeries. Am J Obstet Gynecol. 2010;202(2):514–21.
7. Ukwenya V, Maduemezia N, Afolayan O, Alese O, Thomas W. Prevalence of uterine fibroid in South-Western Nigerian population: a sonographic study. J Exi Clin Anat (serial Online). 2015;14:24–9.
8. Elugwaraoru O, Okojie AI, Oyadoghan GP. The incidence of uterine fibroid among reproductive age women: a five year review of cases at ISTH, Irrua, Edo State, Nigeria. Int J Basic Appl Innov Res. 2013;2(3):55–60.
9. Othman EE, Al-Hendy A. Molecular genetics and racial disparities of uterine leiomyomas. Best Pract Clin Obstet Gynecol. 2008;22(4):589–601.
10. Uimari O, Suomalainen-Konig S, et al. Natural history of familial myomas. Eur J Obstet Gynecol Reprod Biol. 2006;125(2):255–8.
11. Luoto R, Kaprio J, Tutanen EM, Taipale P, Perola M, Koskenvuo M. Heritability and risk factors for uterine fibroids – the Finnish twin cohort study. Maturitas. 2000;37(1):15–26.
12. Wise LA, Laughlin-Tommaso SK. Uterine leiomyomata. In: Goldman MB, Troisi R, Rexrode KM, editors. Women and health. San Diego: Academic Press; 2013. p. 285–306.
13. He Y, Zeng Q, Dong S, et al. Associations between uterine fibroids and lifestyles including diet, physical activity and stress: a case control study in China. Asia Pac Clin Nutr. 2013;22(1):109–17.
14. Parker WH. Etiology, symptomatology and diagnosis of uterine myomas. Fertil Steril. 2007;87(4):725–36.
15. Wise LA, Palmer JR, Harlow BL, et al. Risk of uterine leiomyomata in relation to tobacco, alcohol and caffeine consumption in the Black Women's Health Study. Hum Reprod. 2004;19(8):1746–54.
16. Vines AI, Ta M, Esserman DA. The association between self-reported major lifestyle events and the presence of uterine fibroids. Womens Health Issues. 2010;20(4):294–8.
17. Faerstein E, Szkio M, Rosenshein NB. Risk factors for uterine leiomyoma: a practice based case-control study. II Atherogenic risk factors and potential sources of uterine irritation. Am J Epidemiol. 2001;153(1):11–9.
18. Okonofua FE, et al. Reducing blood loss at open myomectomy: a review of 224 cases over 20 years. Afr J Reprod Health. In Press.
19. Lee HJ, Norwitz ER, Shaw J. Contemporary management of fibroids in pregnancy. Rev Obstet Gynecol. 2010;3(1):20–7.
20. Klatsky PC, Tran ND, Caughey AB, Fujimoro VY. Fibroids and reproductive outcomes: a systematic literature review from conception to delivery. Am J Obstet Gynecol. 2008;198:357–66.
21. Gucemmeghami F, Karmi-Zarchi M, Gharebaghian M, Kernani J. Successful myomectomy during caesarean section: a case report and literature review. Int J Biomed Sci. 2017;13(2):119–21.
22. Song D, Zhang W, Chames MC, Guo J. Myomectomy during caesarean delivery. Int J Gynecol Obstet. 2013;121(3):208–13.
23. Kwon DH, Song JE, Yoon KR, Lee KY. The safety of caesarean myomectomy in women with large fibroids. Obstet Gynecol Sci. 2014;57(5):367–72.
24. Ragab D, El-Sayed El-Shamy, Ayman S. Methylerogonovine infusion may decrease blood loss during abdominal myomectomy: a 3-year observational study. J Gynecol Women's Health. 2018;10(5):555796. https://doi.org/10.19080/JGWH.2018.10.555796.
25. Vahdat M, Kashanian M, Asadollah S, Yazdkhasti P, Nikravan N. The effect of misoprostol on intraoperative blood loss after myomectomy. Int J Reprod Contracept Obstet Gynecol. 2015;4:776–9.
26. Berna Aslan Çetin, Begüm Aydoğan Mathyk, Nadiye Köroğlu, Ali Soydar, Gökhan Demirayak and Tayfur Çift, Oxytocin infusion reduces bleeding during abdominal myomectomies: a randomised controlled trial, Arch Gynaecol Obstet, 2019; 299:151–157. https://doi.org/10.1007/s00404-018-4944-9
27. Taylor A, Sharma M, Tsirkas P, Di Spiezio Sardo SA, Setchel M. Reducing blood loss at open myomectomy using triple tourniquets: a randomised controlled trial. BJOG. 2005;112(3):340–5.
28. Voss M, Koehler C, Elger F, et al. Temporary clipping of the uterine artery during laparoscopic myomectomy: a new technique and the results of the first cased. Gynecol Surg. 2007;4:101. Available at https://doi.org/10.1007/s10397-007-0280-y. Accessed on 2 Jan 2019.
29. dos Santos Martin RL, Zomer MT, Hayashi R, Ribeiro R, Kondo W. How do I perform temporary occlusion of the uterine arteries during laparoscopic myomectomy? Gynecol Obstet (Sunnyvale). 2015;5:278. https://doi.org/10.4172/2161-0932.1000278.
30. Stanford Health Care. Our approach to hysterectomy. Available at
31. https://standfordhealthcare.org/medical-treatment/h/hysterectomy/technigues.html.
32. Accessed on January 2, 2019.
33. Studd J. Hysterectomy for benign disease – total versus sub-total. In: Progress in obstetrics and gynaecology; J Studd;14:238–40; Churchill Livingstone, Edinburgh, Scotland; 2000.
34. Evans EC, Matteson KA, Orejuela FJ, et al. Salpingo-oophorectomy at the time of benign hysterectomy: a systematic review. Obstet Gynecol. 2016;128(3):476–85. https://doi.org/10.1097/AOG/0000000000001592.
35. Arowojolu AO. Hysterectomy. In: Okonofua F, Odunsi K, editors. Contemporary obstetrics and gynaecology for developing countries. Women's Health and Action Research Centre (WHARC). Nigeria: Benin City; 2003. p. 227–42.
36. Bukar M, Audu B, Yahaya U. Hysterectomy for benign gynaecological conditions at Gombe, North Eastern Nigeria. Niger Med J. 2010;51:35–8.
37. Ahmed ZD, Taiwo N. Indications and outcome of gynaecological hysterectomy at the Aminu Kano Teaching Hospital, Kano: a 5-year review. Open J Obstet Gynecol. 2015;5(5):298–304. https://doi.org/10.4236/ojog.2015.075043.
38. Adegbesan-Omilabu MA, Okunade KS, Gbadegesin A. Knowledge of, perception of, and attitude towards uterine fibroids among women with fibroids in Lagos, Nigeria. Scientifica. 2014; article

ID 809536. Available at https://doi.org/10.1155/2014/809536. Accessed on 2 Jan 2019.
39. Onyeabochukwu DA, Duke-Onyeabo C, et al. A six year review of hysterectomy for benign gynaecological conditions at the Federal Medical Centre, Owerri. Int J Reprod Contracep Obstet Gynaecol. 2014;3(2):352–6.
40. Jones HW, Rock JA. Telinde's operative gynaecology. 2015, July. ISBN/ISSN: 9781451177367.
41. RCOG. Clinical recommendations on the use of uterine artery embolization (UAE) in the management of uterine fibroids. 3rd ed. London: RCOG and RCR; 2013.
42. Khaund A, Moss HG, McMillan N, Lumsden MA. Evaluation of the effect of uterine artery embolization on menstrual blood loss and uterine volume. BHOG. 2004;111:700–5.
43. Hesley GK, Gorny KR, Woodrum DA. MR-guided focused ultrasound for the treatment of uterine fibroids. Cardiovasc Intervent Radiol. 2013;36:5–13.
44. Nilsson L, Rybo G. Treatment of menorrhagia. Am J Obstet Gynecol. 1971;10:713–20.
45. Qin J, Yang T, Kong F, Zhou Q. Oral contraceptives use and uterine leiomyoma risk: a meta-analysis based on cohort and case-control studies. Arch Gynecol Obstet. 2013;288:139–48.
46. Sayed GH, Zakherah MS, El-Hashar SA, Shaaban MM. A randomised clinical trial of a levonorgestrel intra-uterine contraceptive system and a low-dose combined oral contraceptive for fibroid-related menorrhagia. Int J Gynecol Obstet. 2011;112:126–30.
47. Zapata LB, Whiteman MK, Tepper NK, Jamieson DJ, Marchbanks PA, Curtis KM. Intrauterine device use among women with uterine fibroids: a systematic review. Contraception. 2010;82:41–55.
48. Lumbiganon P, Rugpao S, Phandhu-fund S, et al. Protective effect of depo-medroxyprogesterone acetate on surgically treated uterine leiomyomas: a multi-centre case-control study. BJOG. 1995;103:909–14.
49. Tristan M, Ozozco LI, Steed A, et al. Mifepristone for uterine fibroids. Cochrane Database Syst Rev. 2012;(8). Art. No: CD007687. https://doi.org/10.1002/14651858. CD 007687. Pub2.

Endometriosis

43

Uche A. Menakaya

Learning Objectives

After studying this chapter, the reader should be able to:

- Improve their understanding of endometriosis, including the health and socio-economic impact of the disease
- Arrange appropriate investigations for women presenting with a clinical suspicion of endometriosis
- Triage women with endometriosis to the most appropriate form of treatment
- Understand the limitations of managing endometriosis in resource-restricted countries

43.1 Introduction

Endometriosis is a gynaecological disorder characterised by the growth of endometrial tissue outside the uterine cavity [1]. It is a heterogeneous disease with various morphologic phenotypes that include typical and atypical peritoneal implants, ovarian endometriomas and/or deep infiltrating endometriotic (DIE) nodules [2, 3]. It may also be associated with various degrees of pelvic adhesions including ovarian/tubal adhesions and/or adhesion in the pouch of Douglas [2, 3].

Endometriosis is a hereditary disease and is thought to arise through retrograde endometrial tissue loss during menstruation [4–6]. Other theories for endometriosis include coelomic metaplasia [7], endometriotic disease theory [8] and lymphatic spread in immunologically and genetically susceptible individuals [9]. It is an oestrogen-dependent, benign, inflammatory disease that affects predominantly reproductive age women. However, it has been reported in premenarcheal girls and in 2–5% of postmenopausal women [10, 11].

43.1.1 Incidence and Prevalence

The prevalence rates for endometriosis in the general population are unknown, because some women are asymptomatic and a definitive diagnosis is established only at laparoscopy. However, based on community prevalence estimates of symptoms [12–14], endometriosis probably affects 10% of all women and 30–50% of symptomatic premenopausal women [15] representing about 176 million women worldwide [16]. In Australia, it is estimated that up to 800,000 women have endometriosis.

In Africa and other developing countries, studies on prevalence of endometriosis are scarce compared to those from developed countries owing to the inadequate laparoscopic facilities and specific training of African gynaecologists to diagnose and treat endometriosis [17]. However, in a recent cross-sectional study among women aged 18–45 years from Nigeria scheduled for their first diagnostic laparoscopy for gynaecologic indications, endometriosis lesions were visualised in 48.1% of the study population [18].

43.1.2 Clinical Presentation

The clinical presentation for endometriosis is variable. It may be asymptomatic in some women with the diagnosis made incidentally during surgery or during imaging procedures for other indications. It can also present as chronic pelvic pain or infertility.

In symptomatic women, endometriosis may present as chronic abdominopelvic pain, ovulation pain, dyschezia, dysuria and/or dysmenorrhoea. Dysmenorrhea associated

U. A. Menakaya (✉)
JUNIC Specialist Imaging and Women's Centre, Coombs, ACT, Australia

Calvary Public Hospital, Bruce, ACT, Australia

Calvary Private Hospital, Bruce, ACT, Australia
e-mail: info@junicimaging.com.au

F. Okonofua et al. (eds.), *Contemporary Obstetrics and Gynecology for Developing Countries*,
https://doi.org/10.1007/978-3-030-75385-6_43

with endometriosis is characterised as dull or crampy pelvic pain that typically begins 1–2 days before menses, persists throughout menses and can continue for several days afterwards. Chronic abdominopelvic pain can be described as dull, throbbing, sharp and/or burning [19, 20].

Adnexal masses (e.g. endometrioma) related to endometriosis may present with pelvic pain or pressure symptoms [21]. Additional endometriosis symptoms may include bowel and bladder dysfunction, abnormal uterine bleeding, low back pain or chronic fatigue [22–25].

These symptoms can occur alone or in combination. An increased number of symptoms have been associated with increased likelihood of endometriosis [26, 27]. A cohort study including over 600 women with endometriosis identified a visceral syndrome of seven symptoms associated with endometriosis that included abdominal pain with no relation to menstruation, pain during urination, pain during defecation, constipation or diarrhoea, irregular bleeding, nausea or vomiting and feeling tired or lacking energy [27]. Women with endometriosis were more likely to report five to seven symptoms compared with unaffected women (20% versus 2%) [27].

The European Society of Human Reproduction and Embryology (ESHRE) recommends a diagnosis of endometriosis in the presence of gynaecological symptoms such as dysmenorrhoea, non-cyclical pelvic pain, deep dyspareunia, infertility and non-gynaecological cyclical symptoms like dyschezia, dysuria, haematuria and rectal bleeding, shoulder tip pain and fatigue in women of reproductive age [25].

Women with endometriosis can also present with reduced fertility. An increased prevalence of endometriosis has been reported in women with subfertility (up to 50%) compared to women with proven fertility (5–10%), and a reduced monthly fecundity rate is noted in women with endometriosis (2–10%) compared with fertile couples (15–20%) [12, 28, 29].

Endometriosis impairs fertility by causing a local inflammatory state, inducing progesterone resistance, impairing oocyte release and reducing sperm and embryo transport [30]. In addition to the local inflammatory state, endometriosis can result in decreased endometrial receptivity, cause mechanical obstruction and alter sexual function [30].

There are reports of a strong association between severity of endometriosis and impact on fertility, probably due to impaired tubo-ovarian function, the presence of ovarian endometrioma, subclinical pelvic inflammation, possibly reduced oocyte quality and reduced endometrial receptivity to implantation [31]. Both endometriosis and adenomyosis (lesions occurring in the uterine intramural muscular layer) reduce the chance of success of assisted reproductive treatment. [32, 33] Others have not demonstrated any correlation between the stage/extent of disease and the reproductive outcome or recurrence risk [34].

43.2 Investigation

43.2.1 Physical Examination

A physical examination is recommended in all women with clinically suspected endometriosis. In cases where a vaginal examination may be inappropriate for adolescents and/or women without previous coital experience, a rectal examination should be considered.

Findings from a physical examination may include tenderness on vaginal examination, immobility or displacement of pelvic structures, painful induration and/or nodules of the rectovaginal septum or visible vaginal nodules in the posterior vaginal fornix [35, 36]. Ovarian endometriomas should also be considered in women with adnexal masses detected during physical examination [36–38].

A diagnosis of endometriosis should still be considered in women with clinically suspected endometriosis whose physical examination is normal as routine clinical examination may not be sufficient to diagnose and locate deeply infiltrating endometriosis [39].

43.2.2 Laboratory Tests

There are no pathognomic laboratory tests for endometriosis at present. Although CA 125 may be elevated in women with endometriosis, its role in the primary diagnosis of endometriosis is undefined [22]. A number of other serum biomarkers like leptin, monocyte chemotactic protein-1 (MCP-1), regulated on activation normal T cell expressed and secreted (RANTES) and macrophage migration inhibitory factor (MIF) have been the focus of more recent research; however, they have not been useful diagnostic predictors owing to poor sensitivity or specificity, small sample size or inadequate validation of their accuracy [40]. Other research interests have focused on endometrial immunohistochemistry for nerve fibre density [41, 42] and on urinary markers (cytokeratin 19, urinary peptide 1.8 kDa), [40] but these require future formal and robust evaluation of their accuracy [9].

It is good practice to offer screening for sexually transmitted disease to sexually active women presenting with chronic pelvic pain [43].

43.2.3 Imaging

A number of imaging modalities are now available for the preoperative diagnosis of endometriosis. [44, 47–50]. These imaging modalities can be useful for diagnosing deep infiltrating endometriosis lesions and the presence of pelvic adhesions prior to surgical treatment.

These imaging modalities provide a cost-effective approach to pre-operative diagnosis of endometriosis by reducing the need for expensive diagnostic laparoscopic surgery and limiting surgery to only those women who need it [51]. This is consistent with the current paradigm for a cost-effective approach to the management of women with endometriosis [9]. Furthermore, these imaging tests provide laparoscopic surgeons with the information they need to plan and improve their surgical approach when these tests accurately predict the location of endometriotic lesions [44].

The imaging modalities for endometriosis include transvaginal ultrasound, magnetic resonance imaging and computed tomographic colonography.

43.3 Transvaginal Ultrasound

Transvaginal ultrasound (TVS) is now considered the first-line imaging modality in the diagnosis of pelvic endometriosis including deep infiltrating endometriosis [52, 53]. A significant body of research have demonstrated evidence for the diagnostic performance of TVS in the diagnosis of ovarian and extra-ovarian endometriosis and their markers of local invasiveness when compared to gold standard laparoscopy. [45, 46, 50, 54–56]

The low cost of TVS, absence of harmful radiation, its ubiquitous availability and acceptability as well as its real-time dynamic ability that provides opportunities for pre-operative assessment of status of POD and interactive pain mapping are significant added advantages [49, 51, 53].

The diagnostic performance of transvaginal ultrasound for different non-ovarian phenotypes of endometriosis was reported in a meta-analysis [57, 58] (see Tables 43.1 and 43.2).

Table 43.1 Diagnostic accuracy of transvaginal ultrasound for diagnosis of deep endometriosis regarding locations other than recto-sigmoid: systematic review and meta-analysis

Location of lesion	Sensitivity % (CI)	Specificity % (CI)	Pre-test probability %	Post-test probability %
Uterosacral	53 (35–70)	93 (83–97)	42	85
Vaginal	58 (40–74)	96 (87–99)	18	77
Bladder	62 (40–80)	100 (97–100)	6	93
Recto-vaginal septum	49 (36–62)	98 (95–99)	26	90

Table 43.2 Diagnostic accuracy of transvaginal ultrasound for diagnosis of deep endometriosis in the recto-sigmoid: a meta-analysis

Location of lesion	Sensitivity % (CI)	Specificity % (CI)	LR+	LR-
Recto-sigmoid *8–12%*	91 (85–94)	98 (96–99)	38.4 (20.2–73.1)	0.09 (0.06–0.16)
POD obliteration	83–96	92–97	10.7–29.2	0.12–0.17

43.3.1 Performing an Endometriosis Scan

Studies have shown that TVS is an accurate and highly reproducible method for non-invasive diagnosis of deep endometriosis when performed by well-trained professionals [59]. The sonographic techniques for eliciting these phenotypes of endometriosis have been described [49, 60], providing opportunities for a 'protocolised' approach to capacity building programmes for endometriosis imaging in resource-restricted countries [51, 61, 62] (see Table 43.3).

43.3.2 Ultrasound-Based Staging System for Endometriosis

The diagnostic performance of TVS for different phenotypes of endometriosis has resulted in a proposed pre-operative ultrasound-based staging system that classifies endometriosis in a way that focuses on the anticipated complexity of laparoscopic surgery for endometriosis [63]. The proposed ultrasound-based endometriosis staging system (UBESS) demonstrated acceptable accuracy (84.9%) and high correlation (*weighted Cohen's kappa (K)*: 0.82) with predicting the level of surgical complexity expected at laparoscopy (*see* Table 43.3) [63].

UBESS has the potential to streamline referral pathways for women with symptomatic severe endometriosis at their primary clinical interface [63]. It has been suggested that integrating and mainstreaming this approach in clinical practice could improve the quality and value of care provided to women with severe endometriosis especially in resource-restricted countries [61, 64] (Table 43.4).

43.4 Computed Tomography Colonoscopy

The conventional virtual colonoscopy (VC) scan, also known as CT colonography (CTC), is a non-invasive multi-detector computed tomographic (MDCT) scan of the abdomen and pelvis performed while the colon is insufflated with air or carbon dioxide via a rectal catheter, usually after a bowel cleansing laxative preparation. Evidence suggest that it provides accurate data on the length and height of colorectal involvement by deep endometriosis and any associated ste-

Table 43.3 Five domain-based TVS approach for the evaluation of the pelvis in women with suspected endometriosis, correlating sonomorphologic features with predicted phenotypes of endometriosis

Domains		Objective	Sonologic sign (s)	Phenotypes of endometriosis
I		Routine assessment of the uterus and adnexa	Myometrial cysts, streaky echogenic lines, thickened posterior myometrium, loss of endometrial/myometrial interface on 3D Thick-walled ovarian cysts with homogenous low-level internal echoes 'Ground glass appearance'	Adenomyosis Endometriomata
II		Tenderness-guided assessment	Site-specific tenderness	Possible peritoneal endometriosis
III		Assessment of Organ mobility		
	IIIa	Ovarian mobility	Ovarian immobility	Ovarian adhesions
	IIIb	Status of the pouch of Douglas (POD)	Real-time dynamic 'sliding sign'	POD obliteration/adhesions
IV		Assessing for Non-Bowel deep infiltrating endometriosis (DIE) Anterior, lateral and posterior pelvic compartment	Nodules – Solid hypoechoic Rounded shape lesions Linear thickenings – Hypo echoic linear thickening Plaques – Hypo echoic lesions With irregular shape	Extra-ovarian non-bowel deep infiltrating endometriosis (DIE)
V		Assessment for bowel deep infiltrating endometriosis	Non-compressible hypoechoic lesion on muscularis propria (may infiltrate the mucosa layer)	Extra-ovarian bowel DIE

Table 43.4 The ultrasound-based endometriosis staging system (UBESS) with sonographic features assessed with TVS (+/− enhanced TVS techniques) and the correlation with RCOG levels of surgical complexity

UBESS stages	Features assessed on transvaginal ultrasound (+/−enhanced TVS techniques)	Level of surgical complexity
Stage I	Normal mobile ovaries, absent non-bowel or bowel DIE, normal POD +/− SST	Level 1 (Negative laparoscopy or Mild stage disease)
Stage II	Endometrioma +/− immobile ovaries, +/− non-bowel DIE, absent bowel DIE +/− normal POD	Level 2 Moderate stage disease
Stage III	Bowel DIE +/− immobile endometrioma +/− abnormal POD	Level 3 Higher stage disease

Legend: *DIE* deep infiltrating endometriosis, *POD* pouch of Douglas, *SST* site-specific tenderness. Levels 1–3 based on RCOG laparoscopic levels of surgical complexity [65]

Reproduced with permission from Menakaya et al. [63]

nosis of the digestive lumen. Such information on the extent of bowel involvement in endometriosis, as well as the existence of bowel stenosis enables informed decision making regarding the feasibility of conservative bowel surgery versus a more radical bowel resection [48, 66].

43.5 Magnetic Resonance Imaging

MRI can be helpful in diagnosing endometriosis of the ureters, bladder and recto-sigmoid. However, it is inadequate for detecting pelvic adhesions or superficial peritoneal implants.

43.6 Diagnosis

Delays in the diagnosis of endometriosis is a significant challenge in the management of endometriosis worldwide. In Europe, an overall diagnostic delay of 10 years in Germany and Austria, 8 years in the UK and Spain, 7 years in Norway, 7–10 years in Italy and 4–5 years in Ireland and Belgium have been reported [67–69]. In Nigeria, diagnostic delays of 5–7 years have been reported [68].

Overall, these delays mainly occur at the primary level of care with women reporting an average of seven visits before specialist referral [68]. The 'discrediting' nature of menstrual irregularities and associated risk of stigmatisation may also delay women from seeking help [67, 70]. These delays contribute to unnecessary patient sufferings, reduced quality of life and significant personal and societal costs associated with endometriosis [68, 71]. Indeed, the annual costs (per employed woman) of endometriosis-associated work productivity loss varies from US$208 in Nigeria to US$23,712 in Italy [68].

Proposed strategies to reduce the substantial delays associated with diagnosis of endometriosis have included a number of symptom-based models for early evaluating and identifying women with endometriosis [72]. One large retrospective analysis described symptoms that are predictive of the diagnosis of endometriosis. These include severe dysmenorrhoea, abdominopelvic pain, heavy menstrual bleeding, infertility, dyspareunia, postcoital bleeding and/or previous diagnosis of ovarian cyst, irritable bowel syndrome or pelvic inflammatory disease [18, 26] and early age at menarche (<12 years old) [73].

Other symptom-based models have demonstrated good accuracy with predicting moderate to severe endometriosis [72]. Predictive tools based on these symptom-based models could help prioritise women for surgical investigation in clinical practice and thus contribute to reducing time to diagnosis [72]. This is especially important in resource-restricted countries with limited access to expensive laparoscopic services.

43.7 Reducing Diagnostic Delays in Resource-Restricted Countries

Globally, there is strong consensus that diagnosis and management of endometriosis should be incorporated into the primary health care of women worldwide [9]. In low-resource settings, strategies to reduce diagnostic delays must therefore include a formal integration of endometriosis education and community awareness with other women's healthcare strategies, appropriate training of healthcare providers, a systematic evaluation of historical variables related to endometriosis using symptom-based models and the utilisation of transvaginal ultrasound to identify and triage those women with clinically suspected endometriosis who would benefit from medical or surgical management [9, 18, 61, 72].

43.8 Management

Treatment for endometriosis should aim to improve quality of life, reduce symptoms and prevent recurrence and the development of more severe disease [9]. In addition, treatment should also reduce the likelihood of compromised future fertility [9]. In developing a management plan in symptomatic women with endometriosis, it is important to note that the stage of a woman's life is an important determinant of her requirement for treatment options [9].

Standardised questionnaires like the Endometriosis Health Profile (EPH 30) questionnaire can also provide an unbiased tool for assessing improvements in symptoms after any given interventions in women diagnosed with endometriosis [74].

43.9 Medical Treatment

In women with a high clinical suspicion of endometriosis, an empirical treatment with analgesics and hormonal medication as first-line option is recommended [25]. This is due to the invasive nature and costs associated with laparoscopic diagnosis especially in resource-restricted countries and the relative ease of prescribing hormonal contraceptives. This empirical approach also considers endometriosis and pelvic pain as a continuum of disease and can potentially avoid excluding women who lack laparoscopic confirmation of a diagnosis of endometriosis from treatment [9].

Well-tolerated, low-cost, easily accessible options such as non-steroidal anti-inflammatory drugs (NSAIDs), other analgesics, combined OCP and progestins should be considered for use as first-line empirical medical treatment [9]. Other second-line medical treatment with LNG-IUS may be considered for use as empirical medical treatment for women who are not optimally treated with first-line empirical therapy prior to surgical diagnosis and treatment [9]. Prior to starting empirical treatment for endometriosis, it is important to exclude other potential causes of pelvic pain like pelvic inflammatory disease.

A role for endometriosis support groups as a valuable forum for women with endometriosis have been recommended [9, 25]. These support groups have the potential to assist women with endometriosis to improve their quality of life by teaching coping mechanisms and sharing experiences. Furthermore, involvement of experienced and skilled medical practitioners, accredited educators and other stakeholders brings strength to these support groups [9].

43.10 Surgical Treatment

Endometriosis lesions are commonly found on the ovaries, uterus, fallopian tubes, uterosacral ligaments, broad ligaments, round ligaments, cul-de-sac or ovarian fossa, as well as on the appendix, large bowel, ureters, bladder or recto-vaginal septum. Other rarer locations of the disease may include the upper abdomen, diaphragm, abdominal wall or abdominal scar tissue and lungs.

A number of staging systems have been proposed for intraoperative classification of pelvic endometriosis. The revised American Society for Reproductive Medicine (rASRM) classification is the most commonly used staging system [75].

Surgical treatment of endometriosis is effective in reducing endometriosis-associated pain and improving fertility in women with minimal to mild endometriosis [76, 77]. However, in women with moderate to severe endometriosis, studies are yet to evaluate if fertility improves with surgery [9]. In these groups of women, the functional appearance of the fallopian tubes and ovaries at the end of the surgical procedure appears to predict the chance of natural conception post-operatively [78]. Among women with endometriomas experiencing infertility, it is important to consider their ovarian reserve prior to surgical treatment as current evidence demonstrates that surgical removal of endometriomas can reduce ovarian reserve [79].

Laparotomy and laparoscopy are equally effective in the treatment of endometriosis-associated pain, but laparoscopic surgery is usually associated with less pain, intraoperative magnification, shorter hospital stay and quicker recovery as well as better cosmetic outcome; hence, it is usually preferred to open surgery [9, 25]. Irrespective of mode of surgery, appropriate surgical training to recognise and treat endometriosis is key to achieving the best outcomes for the patients with endometriosis.

References

1. Kennedy S, Bergqvist A, Chapron C, d'Hooghe T, Dunselman G, Greb R, et al. ESHRE guideline for the diagnosis and treatment of endometriosis. Hum Reprod. 2005;20:2698–704.
2. Giudice LC. Clinical practice. Endometriosis. N Engl J Med. 2010;362:2389–98.
3. American Society for Reproductive Medicine. Endometriosis and infertility: a committee opinion. Fertil Steril. 2012;98(3):591–8.
4. Kennedy S, Mardon H, Barlow D. Familial endometriosis. J Assist Reprod Genet. 1995;12(1):3234.
5. Kennedy S, Hadfield R, Mardon H, Barlow D. Age of onset of pain symptoms in non-twin sisters concordant for endometriosis. Hum Reprod. 1996;11(2):403–5.
6. Sampson JA. The development of the implantation theory for the origin of peritoneal endometriosis. Am J Obstet Gynaecol. 1940;40:549–57.
7. Gruenwald P. Origin of endometriosis from the mesenchyme of the coelomic walls. Am J Obstet Gynaecol. 1942;44(3):470–4.
8. Koninckx PR, Kennedy SH, Barlow DH. Endometriotic disease the role of peritoneal fluid. Human Reprod Update. 1998;4(5):741–51.
9. Johnson NP, Hummelshoj L, World Endometriosis Society Montpellier Consortium. Consensus on current management of endometriosis. Hum Reprod. 2013;28:1552–68.
10. Laufer MR. Premenarcheal endometriosis without an associated obstructive anomaly: presentation, diagnosis, and treatment. Fertil Steril. 2000;74:S15.
11. Nezhat F, Datta MS, Hanson V, Pejovic T, Nezhat C. The relationship of endometriosis and ovarian malignancy: a review. Fertil Steril. 2008;90(5):1559.
12. Eskenazi B, Warner ML. Epidemiology of endometriosis. Obstet Gynecol Clin North Am. 1997;13:235–58.
13. Zondervan KT, Yudkin PL, Vessey MP, Jenkinson CP, Dawes MG, Barlow DH, et al. The community prevalence of chronic pelvic pain in women and associated illness behaviour. Br J Gen Pract. 2001;51(468):541–7.
14. Zondervan KT, Cardon LR, Kennedy SH. What makes a good case-control study? Design issues for complex traits such as endometriosis. Hum Reprod. 2002;17:1415–23.
15. Rogers PAW, d'Hooghe TM, Fazleabas A, Gargett CE, Giudice LC, Montgomery GW, et al. Priorities for endometriosis research: recommendations from an international consensus workshop. Reprod Sci Reprod Sci. 2009;16:335–46.
16. Adamson GD, Kennedy SH, Hummelshoj L. Creating solutions in endometriosis: global collaboration through the World Endometriosis Research Foundation. J Endometriosis. 2010;2:3–6.
17. Kyama CM, Mwenda JM, Machoki J, Mihalyi A, Simsa P, Chai DC, D'Hooghe TM. Endometriosis in African women. A review. Women's Health. 2007;3(5):629–35.
18. Fawole AO, Bello FA, Ogunbode O, Odukogbe AT, Nkwocha GC, Nnoaham KE, Zondervan KT, Akintan A, Abdus-Salam RA, Okunlola MA. Endometriosis and associated symptoms among Nigerian women. Int J Gynaecol Obstet. 2015;130(2):190–4.
19. Brawn J, Morotti M, Zondervan KT, et al. Central changes associated with chronic pelvic pain and endometriosis. Hum Reprod Update. 2014;20:737.
20. Bajaj P, Bajaj P, Madsen H, Arendt-Nielsen L. Endometriosis is associated with central sensitization: a psychophysical controlled study. J Pain. 2003;4:372.
21. Givens V, Mitchell GE, Harraway-Smith C, et al. Diagnosis and management of adnexal masses. Am Fam Physician. 2009;80:815.
22. Vercellini P, Viganò P, Somigliana E, Fedele L. Endometriosis: pathogenesis and treatment. Nat Rev Endocrinol. 2014;10:261.
23. Sinaii N, Plumb K, Cotton L, et al. Differences in characteristics among 1,000 women with endometriosis based on extent of disease. Fertil Steril. 2008;89:538.
24. Engemise S, Gordon C, Konje JC. Endometriosis. BMJ. 2010;340:c2168.
25. Dunselman GA, Vermeulen N, Becker C, et al. ESHRE guideline: management of women with endometriosis. Hum Reprod. 2014;29:400.
26. Ballard KD, Seaman HE, de Vries CS, Wright JT. Can symptomatology help in the diagnosis of endometriosis? Findings from a national case-control study—part 1. BJOG. 2008;115:1382.
27. Hansen KE, Kesmodel US, Baldursson EB, et al. Visceral syndrome in endometriosis patients. Eur J Obstet Gynecol Reprod Biol. 2014;179:198.
28. The Practice Committee of the American Society for Reproductive Medicine. Endometriosis and infertility. Fertil Steril. 2004;81:1441–6.
29. D'Hooghe T, Debrock S, Hill J, Meuleman C. Endometriosis and subfertility: is the relationship resolved? Semin Reprod Med. 2003;21:243–54.
30. Koch J, Rowan K, Rombauts L, Yazdani A, Chapman M, Johnson N. Endometriosis and Infertility – A Consensus Statement From ACCEPT (Australasian CREI Consensus Expert Panel On Trial Evidence). ANZJOG. 2012;52:513–22.
31. Lessey DA. Assessment of endometrial receptivity. Fertil Steril. 2011;96:522–9.
32. Barnhart K, Dunsmoor-Su R, Coutifaris C. Effect of endometriosis on in vitro fertilization. Fertil Steril. 2002;77:1148–55.
33. Maubon A, Faury A, Kapella M, Pouquet M, Piver P. Uterine junctional zone at magnetic resonance imaging: a predictor of in vitro fertilization implantation failure. J Obstet Gynaecol Res. 2010;36:611–8.
34. Adamson GD. Endometriosis classification: an update. Curr Opin Obstet Gynecol. 2011;23:213–20.
35. Hickey M, Ballard K, Farquhar C. Endometriosis. BMJ. 2014;348:1752.
36. Bazot M, Lafont C, Rouzier R, Roseau G, Thomassin-Naggara I, Darai E. Diagnostic accuracy of physical examination, transvaginal sonography, rectal endoscopic sonography, and magnetic resonance imaging to diagnose deep infiltrating endometriosis. Fertil Steril. 2009;92:1825–33.
37. Eskenazi B, Warner M, Bonsignore L, Olive D, Samuels S, Vercellini P. Validation study of nonsurgical diagnosis of endometriosis. Fertil Steril. 2001;76:929–35.
38. Condous G, Van Calster B, Van Huffel S, Lam A. What is the value of preoperative bimanual pelvic examination in women undergoing laparoscopic total hysterectomy? J Minim Invasive Gynecol. 2007;14:334–8.
39. Chapron C, Dubuisson JB, Pansini V, Vieira M, Fauconnier A, Barakat H, Dousset B. Routine clinical examination is not sufficient for diagnosing and locating deeply infiltrating endometriosis. J Am Assoc Gynecol Laparosc. 2002;9:115–9.

40. May KE, Conduit-Hulbert SA, Villar J, Kirtley S, Kennedy SH, Becker CM. Peripheral biomarkers of endometriosis: a systematic review. Hum Reprod Update. 2010;16:651–74.
41. Al-Jefout M, Dezarnaulds G, Cooper M, Tokushige N, Luscombe GM, Markham R, Fraser IS. Diagnosis of endometriosis by detection of nerve fibres in an endometrial biopsy: a double blind study. Hum Reprod. 2009;24:3019–24.
42. Bokor A, Kyama CM, Vercruysse L, Fassbender A, Gevaert O, Vodolazkaia A, De Moor B, Fulop V, D'Hooghe T. Density of small diameter sensory nerve fibres in endometrium: a semi–invasive diagnostic test for minimal to mild endometriosis. Hum Reprod. 2009;24:3025–32.
43. Royal College of Obstetricians and Gynaecologists. *Management of acute pelvic inflammatory disease*. In: Green-top Guideline No. 32. London: RCOG; 2008. www.rcog.org.uk/womens-health/clinical-guidance/management-acute-pelvicinflammatory-disease-32.
44. Nisenblat V, Bossuyt PMM, Farquhar C, Johnson N, Hull ML. Imaging modalities for the non-invasive diagnosis of endometriosis. Cochrane Database Syst Rev. 2016;2(2):CD009591.
45. Hudelist G, English J, Thomas AE, Tinelli A, Singer CF, Keckstein J. Diagnostic accuracy of transvaginal ultrasound for non-invasive diagnosis of bowel endometriosis: systematic review and meta-analysis. Ultrasound Obstet Gynecol. 2011;37:257–63.
46. Holland TK, Yazbek J, Cutner A, Saridogan E, Hoo LW, Jurkovic D. Value of transvaginal ultrasound in assessing severity of pelvic endometriosis. Ultrasound Obstet Gynecol. 2010;36:241–8.
47. Hsu AL, Khachikyan I, Stratton P. Invasive and non-invasive methods for the diagnosis of endometriosis. Clin Obstet Gynecol. 2010;53(2):413–9.
48. Van Der Wat J, Kaplan MD. Modified virtual colonoscopy in the diagnosis and quantification of bowel and disseminated endometriosis. Surg Technol Int. 2015;26:19–24.
49. Menakaya UA, Reid S, Infante F, Condous G. The systematic evaluation of women with suspected endometriosis using a five domain ultrasound based approach. J Ultrasound Med. 2015;34:937–47.
50. Dessole S, Farina M, Rubattu G, Cosmi E, Ambrosini G, Nardelli GB. Sonovaginography is a new technique for assessing rectovaginal endometriosis. Fertil Steril. 2003;79(4):1023–7.
51. Menakaya UA, Rombauts L, Johnson NP. Diagnostic laparoscopy in pre-surgical planning for higher stage endometriosis: Is it still relevant? Aust N Z J Obstet Gynaecol. 2016;56(5):518–22.
52. Benacerraf BR, Groszmann Y. Sonography should be the first imaging examination done to evaluate patients with suspected endometriosis. J Ultrasound Med. 2012;31:651–3.
53. Savelli L. Transvaginal sonography for the assessment of ovarian and pelvic endometriosis: how deep is our understanding? Ultrasound Obstet Gynecol. 2009;33:497–501.
54. Reid S, Lu C, Hardy N, Casikar I, Reid G, Cario G, Chou D, Almashat D, Condous G. Office gel sonovaginography for the prediction of posterior deep infiltrating endometriosis: a multicentre prospective observational study. Ultrasound Obstet Gynecol. 2014;44:710–8.
55. Bazot M, Thomassin I, Hourani R, Cortez A, Darai E. Diagnostic accuracy of transvaginal sonography for deep pelvic endometriosis. Ultrasound Obstet Gynecol. 2004;24:180–5.
56. Menakaya UA, Reid S, Infante F, Condous G. The "sliding sign" in conjunction with Sonovaginography: Is this the optimal approach for the Diagnosis of Pouch of Douglas Obliteration and Posterior Compartment deep infiltrating endometriosis? AJUM. 2013;16(3):118–23.
57. Guerriero S, Ajossa S, Angel Minguez J, Jurado M, Mais V, Melis GB, Alcazar JL. Diagnostic accuracy of transvaginal ultrasound for diagnosis of deep endometriosis regarding locations other than recto-sigmoid: systematic review and meta-analysis. Ultrasound Obstet Gynecol. 2015. https://doi.org/10.1002/uog.15667. Epub ahead of print.
58. Guerriero S, Ajossa S, Orozco R, Perniciano M, Jurado M, Melis GB and Alcazar JL. Diagnostic accuracy of transvaginal ultrasound for diagnosis of deep endometriosis in the recto-sigmoid: a meta-analysis. Ultrasound Obstet Gynecol. 2015. https://doi.org/10.1002/uog.15662. Epub ahead of print.
59. Tammaa A, Fritzer N, Lozano P, Krell A, Salzer H, Aslama M, et al. Interobserver agreement and accuaracy of non invasive diagnosis of endometirosis by TVS. Ultrasound Obstet Gynecol. 2015;46(6):737–40.
60. Guerriero S, Condous G, van den Bosch T, Valentin L, Menakaya U, et al. Systematic approach to sonographic evaluation of the pelvis in women with suspected endometriosis, including terms, definitions and measurements: a consensus opinion from the International Deep Endometriosis Analysis (IDEA) group. Ultrasound Obstet Gynecol. 2016;48(3):318–32.
61. Menakaya UA. Managing endometriosis in sub-Saharan Africa: emerging concepts and new techniques. Afr J Reprod Health. 2015;19(2):13–6.
62. Menakaya UA. Capacity building in endometriosis ultrasound: are we there yet? Aust J Ultrasound Med. 2015;18(4):129–31.
63. Menakaya U, Reid S, Lu C, Bassem G, Infante F, Condous G. Performance of an ultrasound based endometriosis staging system (UBESS) for predicting the level of complexity of laparoscopic surgery for endometriosis. Ultrasound Obstet Gynecol. 2016;48(6):786–95.
64. Menakaya UA, Adno A, Lanzarone V, Johnson NP, Condous G. Integrating the concept of advanced gynaecological imaging for endometriosis. ANZJOG. 2015;55:409–12.
65. Royal College of Obstetricians and Gynaecologists (RCOG). Classification of laparoscopic procedures per level of difficulty. Report of the RCOG working party on training in gynaecological endoscopic surgery. 2001.
66. Roman H, Carilho J, Da Costa C, De Vecchi C, et al. Computed tomography-based virtual colonoscopy in the assessment of bowel endometriosis: the surgeon' point of view. Gynecol Obstet Fertil. 2016;44(1):3–10.
67. Ballard K, Lowton K, Wright J. What's the delay? A qualitative study of women's experiences of reaching a diagnosis of endometriosis. Fertil Steril. 2006;86:1296–301.
68. Nnoaham KE, Hummelshoj L, Webster P, d'Hooghe T, de Cicco NF, de Cicco NC, Jenkinson C, Kennedy SH, Zondervan KT, World Endometriosis Research Foundation Global Study of Women's Health Consortium. Impact of endometriosis on quality of life and work productivity: a multicentre study across ten countries. Fertil Steril. 2011;96:366–73. e368
69. Hudelist G, Fritzer N, Thomas A, Niehues C, Oppelt P, Haas D, Tammaa A, Salzer H. Diagnostic delay for endometriosis in Austria and Germany: causes and possible consequences. Hum Reprod. 2012;27:3412–6.
70. Seear K. The etiquette of endometriosis: stigmatisation, menstrual concealment and the diagnostic delay. Soc Sci Med. 2009;69:1220–7.
71. Harvey J, Warwick I. Endometriosis. BMJ. 2010;340:c2661.
72. Nnoaham KE, Hummelshoj L, Kennedy SH, Jenkinson C, Zondervan KT, World Endometriosis Research Foundation Women's Health Symptom Survey Consortium. Developing symptom-based predictive models of endometriosis as a clinical screening tool: results from a multi Centre study. Fertil Steril. 2012;98:692–701.
73. Nnoaham KE, Webster P, Kumbang J, Kennedy SH, Zondervan KT. Is early age at menarche a risk factor for endometriosis? A systematic review and meta-analysis of case-control studies. Fertil Steril. 2012;98:702–12.

74. Jones G, Kennedy S, Barnard A, Wong J, Jenkinson C. Development of an endometriosis quality of life instrument: the endometrioisis health profile- 30. Obstet Gynecol. 2001;98(2):258–64.
75. Revised American Society for Reproductive Medicine. Classification of endometriosis. Fertil Steril. 1997;67(5):817–21.
76. Jacobson TZ, Duffy JM, Barlow D, Koninckx PR, Garry R. Laparoscopic surgery for pelvic pain associated with endometriosis. Cochrane Database Syst Rev. 2009;4:CD001300.
77. Jacobson TZ, Duffy JM, Barlow D, Farquhar C, Koninckx PR, Olive D. Laparoscopic surgery for subfertility associated with endometriosis. Cochrane Database Syst Rev. 2010;20:CD001398.
78. Adamson GD, Pasta DJ. Endometriosis fertility index: the new, validated endometriosis staging system. Fertil Steril. 2010;94:1609–15.
79. Pellicano M, Bramante S, Guida M, Bifulco G, Di Spiezio SA, Cirillo D, Nappi C. Ovarian endometrioma: postoperative adhesions following bipolar coagulation and suture. Fertil Steril. 2008;89:796–9.

Chronic Pelvic Pain

44

Tarek Elshamy, Olukunle Ajayi, and Victor N. Chilaka

Learning Objectives

By the end of the chapter, the reader should be able to:

- Highlight the impact of chronic pelvic pain on the quality of life and the magnitude of the problem
- Discuss the differential diagnosis and common associations of chronic pelvic pain
- Highlight the importance of careful history taking and clinical examination in the evaluation of women with CPP
- Stress on the importance of multidisciplinary approach in the management of CPP

44.1 Introduction

Chronic pelvic pain is a common problem affecting up to 24% of women worldwide. In the UK, it is estimated that 38 per 1000 women present to the primary care with chronic pelvic pain each year. This rate is as frequent as those of bronchial asthma (37 per 1000) and back pain (41 per 1000) [1].

Chronic pelvic pain represents a challenge to the gynaecologist. It is important to remember that it is a symptom rather than a diagnosis. Patients usually present with other associated problems including bowel, bladder or sexual dysfunction. In addition, anxiety, depression and sleep deprivation are common sequelae. Furthermore, it may not be possible to identify the cause of the pain, and a significant number of women presenting with chronic pelvic pain do not receive a definitive diagnosis despite years of investigations and interventions.

According to the International Association for the study of Pain (IASP), pain is defined as "unpleasant sensory and emotional experience associated with actual or potential tissue damage, or described in terms of such damage" [2].

In acute pain situations, pain is sudden in onset and lasts for short duration of time. It usually disappears after the affected tissue has healed. On the other hand, chronic pain persists.

There are many definitions for chronic pelvic pain (CCP) in the literature. The widely acceptable definition is "intermittent or constant pain in the lower abdomen or pelvis of a woman of at least 6 months in duration, not occurring exclusively with menstruation or intercourse and not associated with pregnancy" [3].

44.2 Differential Diagnosis of Chronic Pelvic Pain and Common Associations

These can be grouped into gynaecological and non-gynaecological causes.

The gynaecological causes include:

- Endometriosis
- Adenomyosis
- Pelvic inflammatory disease (PID)
- Pelvic adhesions
- Residual ovary syndrome
- Ovarian remnant syndrome
- Pelvic congestion syndrome
- Vulvodynia

T. Elshamy
West Middlesex University Hospital, London, UK

O. Ajayi
York Teaching Hospital NHS, East Riding Hospital, and Scarborough Hospital, York, UK

V. N. Chilaka (✉)
Women's Wellness and Research Centre, Hamad Medical Corporation, Doha, Qatar

F. Okonofua et al. (eds.), *Contemporary Obstetrics and Gynecology for Developing Countries*,
https://doi.org/10.1007/978-3-030-75385-6_44

The non-gynaecological causes include:

- Irritable bowel syndrome (IBS)
- Inflammatory bowel disease
- Interstitial cystitis (IC)
- Urethral syndrome
- Nerve entrapment
- Neuropathic and referred pain
- Pelvic congestion syndrome
- Psychosocial factors
- Physical and sexual abuse

44.3 Clinical Assessment

44.3.1 History Taking

Adequate time should be allocated for the initial consultation. The gynaecologist should encourage the patient to tell her story. This will help to build rapport with the patient and improve her experience.

A detailed history taking is essential using both open-ended and closed-ended questions. In addition to routine obstetric and gynaecological history, analysis of the pain is essential including site, onset, character, severity, radiation, time course, exacerbating and relieving factors of pain. The relationship of pain to the menstrual cycle is important. Presence or absence of dysmenorrhea or dyspareunia and association with other problems should be identified, for example, bladder and bowel symptoms, psychological problems, as well as the effect of movement and posture on the pain [4].

The gynaecologist should identify 'red flag' symptoms, and refer or treat appropriately. These symptoms include:

- Rectal bleeding
- New onset IBS like symptoms (>50 years old)
- Irregular vaginal bleeding (>40 years old)
- Haematuria
- Post-coital bleeding
- Pelvic mass
- Excessive weight loss
- New onset pain after menopause
- Suicidal ideation

Screening for irritable bowel syndrome (IBS) can be achieved by using one of the common symptom-based tools, for example, the Rome II criteria, which include:

- At least 12 weeks continuous or recurrent abdominal pain or discomfort associated with ≥2 of the following
- A change in the frequency of stool
- Abnormal appearance or form of stool
- Pain relieved by defecation [5]

The use of simple screening questionnaires, such as the two-question Patient Health Questionnaire, may help in identifying depression which is a common association with CPP [3].

History of physical or sexual abuse may be associated with chronic pelvic pain. Sensitive questioning is essential.

After the initial visit, the patient should be encouraged to complete a pain diary for two or three menstrual cycles. This will aid the gynaecologist in identifying provoking factors, activities or temporal associations [4].

44.3.2 Physical Examination

Thorough abdominal and pelvic examination is an essential component of the initial assessment of women presenting with chronic pelvic pain.

44.3.3 General Examination

This should include assessment of posture and gait (when musculoskeletal cause is suspected).

44.3.4 Abdominal Examination

The examination is done in supine position. Inspection of the abdomen may reveal scars of previous surgery or pelvi-abdominal masses or generalised distention.

Abdominal palpation should be done in a systematic approach covering the whole abdomen and starting from pain-free region. Any tender areas, obvious masses or loaded bowel should be noted.

44.3.5 Pelvic Examination

The aim is to identify trigger points in the pelvis. This part of the examination is conducted in lithotomy position and should include the following:

- Inspection of the vulva and the perineum
- Evaluation for trigger points using a cotton-tipped swab
- Speculum examination of the vagina and cervix
- Bimanual pelvic examination (to identify any cervical motion tenderness, size and position of the uterus, any adnexal masses or tenderness)
- Assessment of pelvic floor muscle tone
- Recto-vaginal examination to identify deeply infiltrating endometriosis (in the rectovaginal septum)

44.4 Investigations

44.4.1 *Urinalysis*

Looking for signs of urinary tract infection. Midstream urine sample (MSU) should be sent for culture and antibiotic sensitivity when appropriate.

44.4.2 Screening for Infection

Genital swabs for chlamydia trachomatis and gonorrhoea should be taken when pelvic inflammatory disease (PID) is suspected in sexually active women; antibiotics should be started while awaiting results.

44.4.3 Diagnostic Imaging

Ultrasonography is becoming more readily available in low resource setting.

Transvaginal ultrasonography (TVUS) is an essential tool to identify and characterise many pathological conditions including ovarian endometrioma, adenomyosis and uterine fibroids. In addition, the use of ultrasonography can provide some reassurance to the patient and help in her counselling [4].

Other imaging modalities including magnetic resonance imaging (MRI) can detect deeply infiltrating endometriosis, adenomyosis and ovarian endometriomas. In selected cases, MRI can replace diagnostic laparoscopy [6].

44.4.4 Diagnostic Laparoscopy

Diagnostic laparoscopy is considered the 'gold standard' test for chronic pelvic pain. At present, it is the main investigation to diagnose pelvic adhesions and peritoneal endometriosis. However, it is estimated that 50% of diagnostic laparoscopies are negative. In addition, it cannot diagnose adenomyosis, painful bladder syndrome or IBS [7].

44.4.5 Empirical Treatment

The Royal College of Obstetricians and Gynaecologists guideline on the management of CPP recommends that women with cyclical pain should have a therapeutic trial using hormonal treatment for 3–6 months before being offered laparoscopy. Similarly, women with IBS should be encouraged to amend their diet and be offered a trial of antispasmodics [3].

44.4.6 Cystoscopy

To rule out urological causes, for example, interstitial cystitis and urinary bladder stones.

44.4.7 Proctoscopy and Colonoscopy and Barium Enema

These tests are reserved for cases when bowel-related problem is suspected.

44.5 Management

Management of chronic pelvic pain is complex and good doctor-patient relationship is crucial. Care should be provided by a multidisciplinary team in a pain clinic where available. The team includes gynaecologist, urologist, gastroenterologist, psychotherapist, physiotherapist and specialist nurse working together to formulate a management plan. It is important to treat each patient as an individual and the management plan should be tailored according to patient needs and fertility wishes. The objectives of the treatment should be restoration of function and improving the overall quality of life. Regular follow-up appointments should be arranged after the initial visit [8].

44.5.1 Medical Treatment

This includes hormonal or non-hormonal options.

1. Non-hormonal treatment

   This involves simple analgesics, for example, paracetamol, aspirin and non-steroidal anti-inflammatory drugs (NSAID), for example, ibuprofen and diclofenac. If simple analgesia is not successful in controlling the pain, opioids (e.g. codeine) and anticonvulsants (e.g. gabapentin) could be considered especially in cases of neuropathic pain. Some patients may benefit from tricyclic antidepressants (TCA). Amitriptyline is the most frequently used TCA in these situations. Selective serotonin uptake inhibitors (SSRIs) such as fluoxetine and sertraline can also be used in selected cases.
2. Hormonal treatment

   This entails the manipulation of the hypothalamo-pituitary-ovarian axis by means of hormonal treatment can be effective in cases of cyclical chronic pelvic pain, for example, endometriosis and adenomyosis-related pain.

Options include combination of oestrogen and progestin, for example (combined oral contraceptive pill), progestin alone, danazol and gonadotropin-releasing hormone (GnRH) analogue.

44.5.2 Combined Oral Contraceptive Pill

These are inexpensive and well tolerated by women. They can be given cyclically or continuously.

44.5.3 Progestogens

These are cheaper than GnRH analogues and can be administered by different routes including orally, for example, medroxyprogesterone acetate (MPA), intramuscular injection, implant or intrauterine system (e.g. levonorgestrel IUS).

The main side effects of progestin therapy are bloating, water retention, weight gain and irregular bleeding. Prolonged use of depot medroxyprogesterone acetate (MPA) can result in loss of bone mass.

44.5.4 GnRH Analogues

GnRha can be given either by intramuscular, subcutaneous injection or by nasal spray. Examples include triptorelin, naferelin and goserelin. They are usually given in combination with add-back therapy (e.g. tibolone). The recommended duration of GnRH analogues intake is 6 months. The main side effects include menopausal symptoms and osteoporosis.

44.5.5 Surgical Treatment

Many women with chronic pelvic pain undergo several laparoscopic procedures for adhesiolysis or ablation of endometriosis and may eventually undergo hysterectomy with or without oophorectomy in an attempt to improve their symptoms. However, and despite multiple surgical procedures, CPP often persists. Therefore, preoperative counselling by an experienced gynaecologist regarding the risk of persistence of pain is essential.

1. Adhesiolysis

   The procedure is usually undertaken through the laparoscopic route. There is no evidence to support routine adhesiolysis in the treatment of CPP. Therefore, more selective approach may be more appropriate such as releasing adhesions surrounding the fallopian tube and resulting in hydrsalpinx which is consistent with patient's symptoms.
2. Hysterectomy

Hysterectomy can be performed though open or laparoscopic approach with or without oophorectomy. Nevertheless, it is estimated that 30% of women continue to report persistent pelvic pain following hysterectomy. Therefore, hysterectomy should not be considered as a definitive treatment for CPP [9].

It is also worth mentioning that there is no evidence to support surgical procedures such as laparoscopic uterine nerve ablation (LUNA) in the management of women with CPP [3].

44.5.6 Adjunctive Therapies

These include physical therapy and psychoeducational interventions such as cognitive behavioural therapy, psychotherapy and patient education. A meta-analysis by Allegrante suggested that a combination of interventions can have a significant impact on improving the functional status and reducing pain especially of musculoskeletal origin [10].

44.6 Summary

Chronic pelvic pain is common among the general population. However, in many women, the cause of chronic pelvic pain cannot be identified despite years of investigations. Moreover, the cause of CPP is often multifactorial and not related to one pathology.

There are several treatment options for chronic pelvic pain including medical, surgical, and adjunctive therapies. However, it is important to remember that proper counselling, multidisciplinary team approach, and individualised care are essential in order to improve the woman's satisfaction with the quality of care.

References

1. Latthe P, Latthe M, Say L, Gulmezoglu M, Khan KS. WHO systematic review of prevalence of chronic pelvic pain: a neglected reproductive health morbidity. BMC Public Health. 2006;6:177.
2. IASP Task Force on Taxonomy. Classification of chronic pain. 2nd ed. Seattle: IASP Press; 1994.
3. RCOG Guidelines and Audit Committee. The initial management of chronic pelvic pain. London: Royal College of Obstetricians and Gynaecologists; 2005. Report No.: Greentop guideline 41.
4. Arulkumaran S, Regan L, Papageorghiou A, Monga A, Farquharson D. Oxford desk reference: obstetrics and gynaecology. Oxford: Oxford University Press; 2011.

5. Drossman DA. The functional gastrointestinal disorders and the Rome III process. Gastroenterology. 2006;130(5):1377–90. https://doi.org/10.1053/j.gastro.2006.03.008. PMID: 16678553.
6. Cody J, Ascher SM. Diagnostic value of radiological tests in chronic pelvic pain. Baillieres Best Pract Res Clin Obstet Gynaecol. 2000;14:433–66.
7. Howard FM. The role of laparoscopy as a diagnostic tool in chronic pelvic pain. Best Pract Res Clin Obstet Gynaecol. 2000; 14:467–94.
8. American College of Obstetricians and Gynaecologists (ACOG). Chronic pelvic pain. Washington, DC: American College of Obstetricians and Gynaecologists (ACOG); 2004. p. 17. (ACOG practice bulletin; no. 51).
9. Brandsborg B, Nikolajsen L, Kehlet H, Jensen TS. Chronic pain after hysterectomy. Acta Anaesthesiol Scand. 2008;52(3):327–31.
10. Allegrante JP. The role of adjunctive therapy in the management of chronic nonmalignant pain. Am J Med. 1996;101:S33–9.

Infertility

45

Friday Okonofua

Learning Objectives

At the conclusion of this chapter, the reader will be able to:

- Understand the definition, causes and epidemiology of infertility
- Come to terms with the clinical presentation and the methods of clinical investigation
- Be knowledgeable about the current management of infertility including the use of assisted reproductive technology (ART)
- Appreciate the importance and approaches for preventing infertility, especially within the context of developing countries
- Recognise unmet areas for research and programming for addressing infertility as a major reproductive health concern in developing countries

45.1 Introduction

Different definitions of infertility have been used within sociological, demographic and clinical literature. In the context of this chapter, we will use the restricted definition of infertility recommended by the World Health Organization [1] as "the failure to achieve a clinical pregnancy after 12 months or more of regular unprotected intercourse." Although there has been suggestion to include the context of marriage in this definition, this is yet to attain worldwide acceptance. As such, we will limit the definition of infertility to this widely accepted norm, and also not argue about the duration of the absence of pregnancy as a component. The use of this accepted WHO definition allows cross-national and regional comparisons and also standardises the methods and procedures for research and clinical interventions across countries.

Infertility is one of the most daunting challenges in sexual and reproductive health in many developing countries. While it is correct to say that developing countries in sub-Saharan Africa have the highest fertility rates in the world, it is paradoxical that the region also has the highest rates of infertility. While high fertility bestows cultural and sociological acceptance and recognition to women, the converse of infertility is one of the most serious social opprobrium that women face within the context of marriage in sub-Saharan African countries. Although infertility affects both men and women, it is now evident that women are mostly affected by the adverse consequences of infertility.

In this chapter, we will review the epidemiology and clinical management and the prevention of infertility. While the management of infertility has improved in recent times with the uptake of the new reproductive techniques of management, we posit that a focus on the preventative approach will best suit the peculiar circumstances of couples in developing countries.

45.2 Epidemiology of Infertility

Worldwide, it has been estimated that nearly 70 million couples experience infertility, the majority of which are in developing countries. Sub-Saharan African countries have the highest rates of infertility in the world averaging 10.1% [2], with a high of 30% in some African countries [3]. There is an infertility belt in Central Africa that stretches from Tanzania in the East to Gabon in the West [4, 5], with couples in this zone experiencing some of the highest prevalence rates of infertility in the world.

F. Okonofua (✉)
Centre of Excellence in Reproductive Health Innovation, Department of Obstetrics and Gynaecology, University of Benin, Benin City, Nigeria

Women's Health and Action Research Centre, Benin City, Nigeria

University of Medical Sciences, Ondo City, Ondo State, Nigeria

F. Okonofua et al. (eds.), *Contemporary Obstetrics and Gynecology for Developing Countries*,
https://doi.org/10.1007/978-3-030-75385-6_45

Infertility is described as primary infertility, if the couples have never been pregnant, while it is secondary if they have had at least a pregnancy including a spontaneous or induced abortion. Several studies indicate that sub-Saharan African countries have higher rates of secondary infertility, mainly due to the fact that most infertility cases in sub-Saharan Africa are due to secondary causes. By contrast, there have been more cases of primary infertility reported in Western countries.

There is increasing evidence that the incidence of infertility is rising in both developed and developing countries [6]. In sub-Saharan Africa, this increase is likely due to the increase in rates of sexually transmitted infections and other forms of infections that lead to infertility in both men and women. Additionally, the increasing availability of new methods for diagnosing and managing infertility with couples more inclined to present for investigation and management may also account for the documented increase. This may be more relevant in developed countries.

45.3 Causes of Infertility

Infertility is a disorder of couples, and cannot be said to exist unless there is regular sexual intercourse between consenting men and women. Thus, infertility may be due to defects in the man or the woman in a relationship. The proportion of infertility attributable to factors in either partner varies from country to country, and even between regions within the same country. However, global estimates suggest that in about 35% of cases of infertility, a male factor is involved, while the female factor is involved in 50% [7]. Increasingly, reports from many sub-Saharan African countries [8–11] indicate that both male and female factors are jointly involved in 10%, while in the remaining 5%, no cause may be identifiable.

In sub-Saharan Africa, primary infertility is uncommon, and may be due to age-related factors when couples delay pregnancies until later ages as the effects of secondary factors or diseases then set in. In a worldwide survey of the causes of infertility, the World Health Organization reported that most cases of male and female infertility in sub-Saharan Africa are due to infections of the genital tract [12]. By contrast, most causes in Western countries tend to be structural, epigenetic/congenital or due to hormonal anomalies.

Beginning with infertility in the female, within the context of sub-Saharan African countries, most causes tend to be tubal or uterine factors, while a few may be due to failure of ovulation and endometriosis. Male infertility, on the other hand, is often due to primary testicular disease or to secondary factors. The case of the normally infertile couple or unexplained infertility will be discussed separately.

45.3.1 Tubal Infertility

Estimates indicate that up to 40% of cases of female infertility are due to damage to the fallopian tubes [2]. The WHO study reported that bilateral tubal occlusion is three times more common in sub-Saharan Africa as compared to developed countries (49% vs. 11%) [12].

The fallopian tube plays active role in conception as it actively mobilises the sperm to unite with the oocyte, and is the point at which ovulation occurs. As such any damage to the tube will hinder this process. While damage to only one tube could still enable the woman to become pregnant through the second tube, it is often that the infection that damaged one tube often damages, albeit partially the other tube. Thus, although bilateral tubal occlusion is the diagnosis that jeopardises fertility, even the damage to only one tube could still place the woman in a difficult position, especially if there are existing peri-tubal pelvic adhesions that compromise the integrity and functionality of the contralateral tube.

Pelvic inflammatory disease (PID) due to sexually transmitted infections is the most common cause of tubal damage that leads to tubal infertility. As a result of their "silent" nature and due to the lack of awareness about their reproductive health effects, *Chlamydia trachomatis* and *Mycoplasma genitalium* are now regarded to be the most common causes of PID in sub-Saharan Africa [13]. Acute PID due to *Neisseria gonorrhoea* is now less common, but is still seen frequently in rural and impoverished communities. Additional causes of tubal damage include pelvic infections (PI) arising from exogenous and possibly endogenous infections affecting the pelvic cavity and the tubes. The most common of these infections in sub-Saharan Africa include post-abortal infections from complications of induced or spontaneous abortion and infectious complications after full-term deliveries. These infections are usually by a combination of gram positive and gram negative bacteria, and could be very severe leading to extensive tubal damage if the woman recovers. The other causes of severe pelvic infections, tubal damage and infertility include infections from complicated appendicitis, tuberculosis, schistosomiasis, viral infections and abdominal inflammatory disorders such as Crohn's disease. Tubal damage may also occur directly from tubal ligation, and pelvic endometriosis, or indirectly as a consequence of pelvic or abdominal surgery.

45.3.2 Uterine Infertility

Defects in the uterus are potential causes of infertility. Congenital uterine malformations such as absent uteri (as in testicular feminisation syndrome), uterine didelphys, and septate uteri are known causes of infertility in the female. However, most uterine causes of infertility are acquired, the most common of which is uterine leiomyomata (uterine fibroids), especially in sub-Saharan African countries. The association between uterine fibroids and female infertility has been well documented [14], but not all fibroids result in infertility. Fibroids cause infertility when they are multiple and huge eliciting multiple pelvic adhesions; when they underlie the uterine cavity (submucous fibroids) thereby distorting the cavity; and when they are located in the cornual ends of the uterus, thereby blocking the point of entry of the fallopian tubes into the uterus.

Other uterine causes of infertility include the presence of intra-uterine adhesions (synechae) also called *Asherman's syndrome* due to damage to the stratum basalis of the endometrium. Such damage is frequently due to botched and unsafe abortions done in settings where induced abortion is legally restricted. Asherman syndrome may also be due to uterine curettage done in the presence of an existing endometritis, from caesarean section, uteroplasty or myomectomy. Uterine infections from tuberculous endometritis may also lead to infertility.

45.3.3 Endometriosis

Moderate-to-severe endometriosis can occlude the fallopian tubes through the formation of adhesions by endometriotic deposits. Pelvic endometriosis was initially thought to be rare in African women, but it is now increasingly diagnosed because of the increasing use of diagnostic laparoscopy and newer technologies [15]. Adenomyosis, which is the presence of endometrial tissues within the uterine myometrium, is much more common in the African continent. It causes moderate-to-severe enlargement of the uterus and severe pelvic pain [16], while the associated infertility may be severe and irreversible.

45.3.4 Anovulatory Infertility

Anovulation (failure of ovulation) is increasingly identified as a cause of female infertility in sub-Saharan African countries, although much less common than in developed countries. Four main causes of anovulation have been described: ovarian dysfunction with normal levels of gonadotrophins (such as polycystic ovarian syndrome [PCOS]), hypergonadotrophic hypogonadism (so-called premature ovarian failure), hyperprolactinaemia and hypogonadotrophic hypogonadism. In our experience in Nigeria, polycystic ovarian disease and hyperprolactinaemia are the most common, while premature ovarian failure is now more frequently diagnosed. By contrast, hypogonadotrophic hypogonadism (low levels of pituitary hormone) is relatively uncommon.

Polycystic ovarian syndrome (PCOS) is one of the most common endocrine disorders in women of reproductive age. It consists of multiple symptoms and signs including oligomenorrhoea/amenorrhoea, hyper-androgenism, obesity and infertility. It has been linked with a metabolic disorder, the most important component being insulin resistance and elevated levels of insulin. The ovaries often show multiple centric cysts on ultrasound. The diagnosis of PCOS is therefore often made with trans-vaginal ultrasound scan and/or hormone assay. The early cases of PCOS may not show the classical ultrasound or hormonal features, and are better classified as milder cases and managed as ovarian dysfunction.

Although elevated levels of prolactin (hyperprolactinaemia) may be found in women undergoing infertility investigations, with some women demonstrating expressible galactorrhoea, the exact contribution of hyperprolactinaemia as a cause of female anovulatory infertility has not been quantified [17]. Theoretically, because both prolactin and gonadotrophins are produced from the same part of the pituitary gland, it would be expected that high levels prolactin will result in lower levels of gonadotrophins. Although this pattern has been well demonstrated, it is not clear whether this causes infertility, and the actual mechanisms associated with hyperprolactinaemia as a possible cause of infertility. Clearly, more research is needed.

There is evidence of increasing incidence of premature ovarian failure that manifests as high levels of follicle stimulating hormone in women less than 40 years of age (also called hypergonadotrophic hypergonadism). The pathogenesis of premature ovarian failure remains unknown. However, it has been attributed to possible genetic abnormalities, metabolic disorders, autoimmunity, environmental pollution and nutritional factors [18]. The increasing incidence of infertility in women who delay pregnancies to older ages, often associated with ovarian insufficiency, is an important concern in most infertility clinics in Africa.

In our experience, the least common of the major causes of anovulatory infertility at least within the context of sub-Saharan Africa, is hypogonodotropic hypogonadism, which is the failure of the pituitary glands to produce adequate levels of gonadotropins that stimulate the ovaries. Some disorders of the pituitary glands that lead to decreased production of follicle stimulating hormone (FSH) include the destruction of the anterior pituitary gland as a result of tumours such as craniopharyngiomas, by infections such as tuberculosis or by a post-haemorrhagic event such as Sheehan's syndrome. Also, rare congenital malformations of the pituitary gland may occur, for example, the Laurence-Moon-Bell syndrome, Kallmann's or the Prader-Willi syndromes. However, in our experience, these are rare in sub-Saharan African women.

45.3.5 Male Infertility

Male infertility is often epitomised as reduced quality and quantity of spermatozoa in the seminal fluid (oligozoosperma/asthenozoospermia) or the complete absence of spermatozoa (azoospermia). There is evidence that the quality and quantity of spermatozoa has been declining gradually worldwide over the past decades [19]. This decline has also occurred in developing countries [20] and may account for the increasing proportion of infertility attributable to the male factor. The causes of the declining numbers and quality of spermatozoa are not known with accuracy but it may be due to the prevailing climate change with increasing scrotal temperatures or to other environmental factors.

The production of spermatozoa takes place in the testes under the influence of gonadotropin releasing hormones (FSH and luteinizing hormone [LH]) from the pituitary gland. The spermatozoa then undergo further maturation and are transported through the rete testis, the epididymis, and vas deferens to the penile urethra where they are ejaculated.

The causes of male infertility can therefore be categorised into primary testicular disease, obstructive male infertility, hormonal anomalies, autoimmune disorders, environmental factors, varicocoele, drugs and ejaculatory factors.

Primary testicular disease is arguably the most common cause of male factor infertility, the cause of which is largely unknown. Some cases of azoospermia and oligospermia have been linked to the deletion of genes on the Y-chromosome, Klinfester syndrome, testicular maldescent, mumps orchitis, testicular trauma and as a complication following drug use (e.g. anti-cancer drugs) [21]. Increasingly, research is ongoing in many parts of the world to uncover the primary causes of male infertility.

Obstruction at the levels of the rete testis, vas deferens, and the epididymis may also cause male factor infertility. Such obstructions have been attributed to congenital, iatrogenic and infectious causes. Male infertility may be due to the congenital absence of the vas deferens, to previous vasectomy or to sexually transmitted infections caused by *Chlamydia trachomatis* or *Neisseria gonorrhoea*. In our recent study [22], we showed that previous self-reporting of a sexually transmitted infection was a significant risk factor for male infertility in Nigerian men. Therefore the role of infections, especially within the context of developing countries is paramount.

Endocrinological causes of male infertility, although much rarer have also been reported. These include hypogonadotrophic hypogonadism, hyperprolactinaemia, diabetes mellitus, thyroid and adrenal endocrine malfunctions. These conditions should also be considered as treatment when identified is straightforward. Other causes of male infertility include auto-immune disorders (the formation of anti-sperm antibodies), which occur in up to 10% of men with infertility; the use of drugs such as anabolic steroids, cigarettes, opiates and marijuana, anti-depressants, anti-hypertensives; and environmental factors such as exposure of the scrotal sacs to excessive heat and chemicals (such as pesticides, paints and organic solvents).

For years, varicocoeles have been implicated as causes of male infertility, and as such varicocoelectomy has been pushed forward as possible treatment. However, there has been no substantive evidence to indicate that varicocoeles cause male infertility and that their treatment through surgical repair increases the chances of infertility [23]. With the current discovery of new methods of treating male factor infertility, it is doubtful if the treatment of varicocele yields any superior results.

By contrast, erectile and ejaculatory disorders are distinct disorders that account for the male factor as a cause of infertility. These include retrograde ejaculation, all of which can follow from neurological disorders, diabetes mellitus or prostrate surgery. It may also be due to psychological difficulties which in our experience often occur when couples are trying to get pregnant the first time.

45.4 Investigation of Infertility

As infertility is a disorder of couples, it is important that the male and female partner be investigated and treated simultaneously, and that the first visit to the practitioner is by both couples. In our experience in Nigeria, this is often not the case, with up to 80% of infertile women often visiting the clinics alone without their partners. Indeed, many male partners often fail to visit the clinic insisting either that they have no problems or that the woman should start the treatment before they join. Our more detailed investigation of this scenario indicates that men are often afraid to receive negative report of their infertility or reduced fertility status. While practitioners in more developed countries may be reluctant to continue infertility investigation as a result of the non-cooperation of the male partner, our practice is to continue with the investigation of the female partner with the hope that the male partner will agree to be investigated at a later date, especially when the results of the female partner are known. Additionally, there are now novel methods such as the post-coital test (PCT) to indirectly examine the role of the male partner as a cause of infertility.

The investigation of infertility begins with detailed history taking. This consists of personal history from both partners – age, occupational history, exposure to possible risk factors such as excessive heat by the male partner, intake of alcohol and cigarettes and use of recreational drugs. The menstrual history of the female partner is crucial. This should include the age of menarche, date of the last menstrual period, frequency and length of the menstrual cycle, the regularity of the menstrual cycle and the existence of dysmenorrhoea (primary or secondary). The previous use of contraceptives should be explored especially oral contraceptives, long-acting progestogens and the intra-uterine contraceptive device.

Also, questions should be asked about previous pregnancies and their outcomes in the current and previous relationships for both the man and the woman. For men in polygamous relationships, questions should be asked about pregnancies and the outcomes in other women in the relationships as well as pregnancies men may have had in non-marital relationships. In African countries where extra-marital and polygamous relationships are common amongst men, it is important to investigate the extant fertility experiences of the men, as this may provide substantive insights into the possible contribution of the male factor to the infertility.

The other information that needs to be elicited during history taking is the past or current presence of medical or surgical conditions in both the man and the woman, and the nature of any treatment presently or previously taken. The possible impact of any prescription or non-prescription drugs or even traditional medications should also be obtained.

Also, and most importantly the couple's frequency of sexual intercourse and associated problems such as dyspareunia or ejaculatory problems should be solicited. Inquiries should include request on information about personal and family history of diabetes, hypertension, endometriosis and polycystic ovarian disease as well as information about recent or previous tests for HIV, hepatitis B and C, rubella vaccination and the use of folic acid.

45.5 Clinical Examination of the Infertile Couple

The clinical examination of the couple often begins with the woman – the male partner will only need to be examined after the results of the semen analysis show subnormal semen parameters. Indeed, even for the female partner, unless there is evidence that clinical examination will throw up additional information, there seems to be nothing to be gained from routine clinical examination. However, in my experience some woman gain confidence and trust in the clinician when they are examined even when nothing is found. The indications from the history that would prompt a detailed clinical examination of the woman include secondary dysmenorrhoea, menorrhagia, dyspareunia or history of vaginal discharge.

Physical examination should include the elicitation of vital signs, body mass index and the examination for features of hormonal abnormalities such as hirsutism, male-type baldness and galactorrhoea. Abdominal examination should be done to exclude a huge abdominal mass such as from uterine fibroid or ovarian mass, while a pelvic examination would be necessary to investigate the nature of a vaginal discharge. Vaginal examination should begin with a careful bivalve speculum examination which is necessary to take high vaginal or cervical swabs for culture and sensitivity tests. Bimanual examination will then follow to examine the size and position of the uterus as well as the presence or absence of an adnexal mass or tenderness.

45.6 Laboratory Investigations, Imaging and Endoscopy

Table 45.1 shows some of the basic tests that need to be done to establish the cause of infertility and to determine the nature of treatment. It is important that all of these tests are done before treatment is initiated as the infertility may be due to multiple causes in the male or/and the female.

The most basic tests consist of (1) tests of ovulation and ovarian reserve; (2) tubal patency and uterine assessment tests; (3) the post-coital test; and (4) semen analysis and male function test.

45.6.1 Tests of Ovulation and Ovarian Reserve

Assessment of ovulation has historically consisted of the use of the basal body temperature tracing. Biphasic tracing is the norm due to the effect of progesterone in elevating the basal temperature in the second half of the cycle. Other tests that have been used include endometrial biopsy and histology, and examination of the cervical mucus. However, these days, the estimation of the level of serum progesterone on Day 21 of the menstrual cycle (mid-luteal phase) is the gold standard

Table 45.1 Schema for investigating female and male infertility

Test	Results	Interpretation
Progesterone assay on day 21 of the menstrual cycle	<20 nmol/l	Anovulation
Serum FSH on day 2 or 3 of the menstrual cycle	>10 IU/l	Reduced ovarian reserve, possibly premature ovarian failure
Serum LH on day 2 or 3 of the menstrual cycle	>10 IU/l	Suggests polycystic ovarian disease, to be confirmed with pelvic ultrasound scan
Increased LH/FSH ratio	>2	Suggests polycystic ovarian disease, to be confirmed with pelvic ultrasound case
Testosterone	>2.5 nmol/l	May be polycystic ovarian disease. To confirm with ultrasound scan
Prolactin	>1000 IU/L	May be pituitary adenoma. Repeat the test and exclude hypothyroidism
Hysterosalpingography (HSG)	Abnormal results	May be tubal disease
Laparoscopy	Blocked tubes Endometriosis Pelvic adhesions	Tubal factor infertility
Semen analysis	Reduced sperm count or sperm quality	Follow up with hormone assay and anti-sperm antibodies

for assessing ovulation, especially because accurate and simpler methods for measuring serum progesterone are now widely available.

The history of regular menstrual periods normally suggests ovulation. But in our practice, the measurement of serum progesterone is done for all women who present with complaints of infertility, whether or not they report a normal menstrual cycle. This is because we have seen several cases where women with "self-reported normal cycles" were found to be anovulatory. Accuracy of reporting of menstrual cycles has not been investigated, but we believe this may vary with different cultures, and may account for the inconsistency between the self-reporting of menstrual patterns and the results of serum progesterone.

When the results of the progesterone are found to be low, ovarian reserve tests are done to determine the quality of follicular reserve in the ovaries. This is particularly necessary in women with advanced age (>30 years) and those with prior ovarian surgery. The testing includes a day 2 or 3 assessment of serum follicular stimulating hormone (FSH), luteinizing hormone (LH), oestradiol and possibly trans-vaginal scan to determine ovarian antral follicle count.

45.6.2 Tubal Patency and Uterine Assessment Tests

Three methods are now routinely used for assessing the patency of the fallopian tubes. These include ultrasound scan with hydrotubation, also called hysterosalpingo-contrast sonography (HyCoSy), hysterosalpingography (HSG) and laparoscopy and dye test.

HSG is a radiological procedure that consists of the injection of a radio-opaque contrast medium into the uterus through the cervix, with X-rays taken at timed intervals during and after the injection. The images consist of the uterine outline, the outline of the fallopian tubes and the free spillage of the dye into the pelvic peritoneum. HSG should be carried out during the first 10 days of the menstrual cycle in order to prevent the disruption of a growing embryo when done in the peri-ovulatory period.

The complications of HSG include mild-to-moderate pain, severe pain which could lead to vaso-vagal attack in some cases and flare up of existing in up to 3% of cases. When done correctly, HSG has been reported to have a sensitivity of 65% and specificity of 85% [24] in the prediction of tubal disease.

The HyCoSy is a more recent non-invasive device for investigating tubal patency using trans-vaginal ultrasound scan [25]. It consists of the slow injection of a contrast medium into the uterine cavity under ultrasound visualisation, with imaging of the uterus and the fallopian tubes. It is then relatively easy to see the contours of the uterine cavity and then the evidence of tubal patency and spillage of the contrast into the peritoneal cavity. The method is easy and safe as it does not expose the woman to X-rays. There is now some evidence that the HyCoSy method [26] compares reasonably well with the HSG in the investigation of tubal infertility, especially when the procedure is carried out by an expert.

Laparoscopy and dye test appears to be the most reliable and accurate method for investigating tubal infertility. This is because it is able to diagnose the intra-luminal integrity of the fallopian tubes as well as extra-tubal peritoneal factors that may hinder the performance of the tube in carrying out its fertility functions. However, it is more expensive and potentially carries more complications. It is also possible to carry out some treatment procedures through laparoscopy, including electrocoagulation of endometriotic spots, peritubal adhesiolysis and even myomectomy.

The history and standard method of laparoscopy has been very described in many textbooks. It is not the intention of this chapter to repeat such descriptions. Interested readers are advised to consult such textbooks as well as a recent systematic review of laparoscopic surgery [27] which elegantly summarised the procedure and its complications. In brief, laparoscopy is often carried out under general anaesthetic, and requires the instillation of gas into the peritoneal cavity to enable the insertion of the laparoscope and inspection of the pelvic organs. The instillation of a dye through the cervix will enable the determination of the patency of both fallopian tubes. Apart from laparoscopy being a necessary procedure in women with intractable infertility, it normally should be considered in women with suspected endometriosis, previous pelvic inflammatory disease and those with previous pelvic surgery. In good hands, laparoscopy is safe, but the procedure carries the risks of visceral injury and intra-abdominal haemorrhage.

In our setting, we have compared the effectiveness of laparoscopy with HSG in the diagnosis of tubal infertility [28] and have found identical results. However, laparoscopy is more accurate in diagnosing peri-tubal pathologies, especially when the procedure is carried out by skilled specialists.

Another useful procedure is hysteroscopy, which is the visualisation of the uterine cavity through the hysteroscope. This is usually done at the time of laparoscopy and allows the concomitant inspection of the uterine cavity to exclude disorders such as Asherman syndrome and endometrial polyps.

45.6.3 The Post-coital Test

The post-coital test (PCT) is intended to provide information on the quality of the spermatozoa, adequacy of sexual intercourse and the ability of the spermatozoa to survive in the cervical mucus. It consists of the microscopic examination of cervical mucus samples taken soon after sexual intercourse. The mucus is examined for the presence of active, live and progressively mobile spermatozoa, which if present suggests a positive PCT. However, the absence of spermatozoa or of dead or immobile spermatozoa is referred to as negative PCT and suggests either the presence of anti-sperm antibodies, inadequate sexual intercourse or low sperm count. In the context of developing countries when men tend not to attend for infertility investigations, the PCT is an indirect method of assessing male fertility. However, the method has been criticised for being associated with high rates of false-positive results [29] and also for not being predictive of pregnancy rates [30].

45.6.4 Semen Analysis and Male Function Tests

The schema for investigating male infertility includes an initial semen analysis for all male partners of women presenting with infertility. If the results of the semen analysis reveal poor results, the male partner would be examined, following which more investigations would be undertaken. This is in contradistinction to the female partner who would be first clinically examined before the investigations are undertaken. In our experience, there is nothing to be gained by examining all men, before an assessment of a semen sample is carried out.

Semen analysis is often requested from men after at least 3 days of abstinence and with the use of masturbation. The semen samples are immediately forwarded to the laboratory and analysed through microscopic and, in more recent times, automated methods. Routine semen analyses are best performed using the criteria recently updated by the WHO (see Table 45.2). This includes the volume of the ejaculate, concentration, motility and percentage of normal forms. The criteria have been revised based on the lowest probability for achieving pregnancies, and are based on international standards, with little variation between countries.

When the results are abnormal, history taking and examination of the man should be undertaken. These include histories of previous illnesses and surgeries, including sexually transmitted infection, diabetes, hypertension and drug use. The physical examination should encompass general examination to identify any stigmata of chromosomal anomalies to detect the level of masculinisation and to exclude inguinal hernia, prostate enlargement, gynaecomastia and evidence of systemic illnesses. Genital examination should include the examination of the testes, epididymis, vas deferens and the presence of scrotal swelling or varicocele.

Table 45.2 Reference values for semen analysis based on the updated World Health Organization Guidelines, 2010

Volume	Lower reference limit
Semen volume (ml)	1.5 (1.4–1.7)
Total Sperm Number (10^6 per ejaculate)	39 (33–40)
Sperm Concentration (10^6 per ml)	15 (12–16)
Progressive motility (PR, %)	32 (31–34)
Sperm morphology (normal forms, %)	4 (3.0–4.0)
Vitality (live sperms, %)	58 (55–63)
pH	≥7.2

With unexplained abnormal semen analysis results, further tests are warranted. The measurement of serum FSH if normal, suggests obstruction as the cause of the abnormal spermatozoa (especially azoospermia) as it indicates that the testis is functioning properly. However, if the FSH is elevated, it suggests disorders of spermatogenesis and primary testicular failure as being the cause. Other important tests that can complement the investigation include serum LH, sex hormone binding globulin and serum testosterone. Serum inhibin assay is also a marker for spermatogenesis and can also be performed to provide more insights. Other useful investigations include testicular ultrasound scan (with or without Doppler), testicular biopsy (especially when in vitro fertilisation [IVF is an option) and karyotyping. Male function tests also include the objective assessment of motility (such as with an automatic machine), hypo-osmotic swelling test, tests for sperm nuclear maturation, measure of acrosome status, acrosome reaction and acrosin activity, hamster zona-free oocyte penetration test and human sperm zona binding and penetration.

45.7 Management of Infertility

In our practice, we recommend an approach based on prevention as a foundational principle in managing infertility in developing countries. This is because of the high costs of managing infertility and the relative low cost-effectiveness of the presently available methods. Since infertility is largely preventable within the context of developing countries because of its association with infections in men and women, it makes sense to emphasise prevention as a central point in the discussion of its management. It also enables the consistent education of couples as many seek treatment late after initial consultations of inappropriate channels such as traditional and religious outlets. It is important that the education of couples be made a central focus of infertility management in developing countries.

The management of infertility can therefore be categorised into primary prevention, secondary prevention and tertiary prevention. Primary prevention of infertility is the prevention of infertility from occurring in the first place, while secondary infertility is the early treatment of infertility after it has occurred. By contrast, the tertiary prevention component of infertility is to counsel women and men with irreversible infertility to accept other options if they desire to nurture children.

45.7.1 Primary Prevention of Infertility

The primary prevention of infertility involves the prevention of sexually transmitted infections, pelvic infections and post-abortion infections that lead to irreparable tubal damage. Preventable measures should include the provision of sexuality education for the youth as many of these infections originate during the adolescent years. It includes keeping girls in school not only to reduce their age of first sexual debut, but also to provide an opportunity for them to acquire livelihood and life skills education and information necessary to orientate them for future development. Abstinence at an early age is also an option for both boys and girls. However, when they become sexually active, they should have appropriate information and skills to negotiate safe sex, to enable them avoid multiple sexual relationships, and to avoid the use of unguarded sex. Education on family planning and the use of contraceptives should be available to men and women of all ages for the prevention of unwanted pregnancies. Barrier contraception (male and female condoms) will help reduce the risk of sexually transmitted infections, including those due to *Neisseria gonorrhoea* and *Chlamydial trachomatis*.

For women with unwanted and mis-timed pregnancies who desire termination of such pregnancies, there is now world-wide consensus that for human right, social justice and gender equality reasons, it is best to allow such women to have easy access to safe abortion care. The high prevalence of unsafe abortion is the dominant reason for the high prevalence of pelvic infections due to abortion, and the subsequent high prevalence of tubal infertility in many African countries where abortion is legally restricted.

45.7.2 Secondary Prevention of Infertility

Secondary prevention of infertility is the treatment of infertility after it has been diagnosed. The emphasis should be on early diagnosis and treatment of infertility as this would increase the chances for successful treatment outcome. Our experience is that couples with infertility often delay in seeking orthodox treatment, with many first consulting traditional and religious methods of treatment. It is only when initial treatments with traditional practitioners fail that they seek orthodox treatment, at which point the causes of the infertility may have intensified or further damage may have been done with attempts at traditional and religious methods of treatment. Consequently, public health education needs to be provided as part of the approach to effective treatment of infertility on the need for early treatment and the avoidance of ineffective and potentially dangerous methods of treatment.

The medical treatment of infertility when it has occurred is broadly divided into two broad categories: (1) conventional treatment and (2) treatment with the assisted reproductive technologies. Conventional infertility involves the identification of the causes of infertility followed by treatment/rectification of the specific causes, with the hope that natural pregnancy would occur. By contrast, assisted reproductive technology is a term used collectively for all non-coital methods that have been developed for the treatment of infertility.

45.8 Conventional Methods of Infertility Treatment

The conventional methods of treatment of infertility that would be described in this chapter include ovulation induction, tubal surgery, male infertility treatment and treatment of unexplained infertility.

45.8.1 Tubal Surgery

Tubal surgery is indicated when there is evidence of tubal occlusion, including when there are demonstrable peritubal adhesions. Tubal surgery was a major undertaking in the early days of infertility treatment and was carried out by trained specialist surgeons who used either macrosurgical methods or treatment with the operating microscope (microscopic surgery) or with laparoscopy. Some of the surgical methods are well described in standard textbooks, and they include tubal re-anastomosis, fimbrioplasty, salpingostomy, salpingolysis and cornual implantation. Unfortunately, the results of tubal repair in terms of attainment of pregnancy were not always satisfactory. Indeed, except in minor cases of tubal damage for which minimal tubal repair techniques are required, the results with severe tubal damage are consistently poor. With the advent of in vitro fertilisation and embryo transfer (IVF-ET), major degrees of tuboplasty are no longer done because of better results obtained for pregnancy attainment with IVF-ET. Both procedures are equally expensive but the cost-effectiveness analysis increasingly favours IVF-ET, especially in countries that have equal expertise to perform the two procedures.

Another relatively non-invasive procedure for treating tubal infertility is selective salpingography and tubal cannulation. The procedure is often done under image intensification or at hysteroscopy for women with proximal tubal obstruction. It consists of selective salpingography and tubal catheterisation, while at hysteroscopy, tubal cannulation is also possible. All procedures increase the chances of pregnancy.

45.8.2 Treatment of Anovulation

Failure of ovulation (anovulation) is treated with ovulation induction. Failure of ovulation may be due to recent life changes such as anxiety, depression and obesity. The normalisation of body weight can help return normal ovulatory cycles. Anxiety occasionally sets in when women are attempting to get pregnant the first time. Such anxiety can actually reduce the chances of a pregnancy because it may trigger anovulation. It is therefore important that women are counselled to avoid anxiety in order to lower their risk of anovulation.

The most common cause of anovulation in our practice is PCOS. Ovulation induction can easily be achieved in such cases with the anti-oestrogens clomiphene citrate and tamoxifen or with gonadotropins with high rates of success. Treatment with the anti-oestrogens is normally continued for 1 year, before alternative methods are sought. Women receiving clomiphene citrate or tamoxifen should be followed up with trans-vaginal follicular monitoring at least during the first cycle of treatment to ensure appropriate dosage and reduce the likelihood of multiple pregnancies.

Other treatments which have been reported for the PCOS, especially in those that fail to respond to clomiphene citrate include surgical drilling or wedge biopsy of the ovaries. However, wedge biopsy, although resulted in some pregnancies, has fell into disrepute as a result of associated high rates of complications including tubal damage and adhesion formation. By contrast, ovarian drilling involves focal destruction of the ovarian stroma with laser or diathermy, often applied through laparoscopy. Indeed, ovarian drilling is superior to wedge resection and achieves equivalent pregnancy rates as clomiphene citrate. It has less risk of multiple gestation and other complications such as the ovarian hyperstimulation syndrome (OHSS) that is a complication of medical ovulation.

When anovulation is proven to be due to hyperprolactinoma, treatment with bromo-ergocriptine would help restore ovulation. However, in our experience this is a rare cause of anovulation, rarer still is anovulation due to hypogonadotrophic hypogonadism. If present, ovulation can be induced with the pulsatile administration of gonadotrophin releasing hormone (GnRH) or by the daily injection of gonadotrophins.

45.8.3 Treatment of Infertility Due to Uterine Abnormalities

Infertility due to congenital defects of the uterus, leiomyoma, endometrial polyps and intra-uterine adhesions can easily be treated. The methods of treatment include myomectomy carried out laparoscopically or by laparotomy as previously described. Sub-mucous fibroids are most likely to cause infertility. It is therefore important that efforts be made to remove such fibroids during open myomectomy. Submucous fibroids and any intra-uterine adhesions are best removed through hysteroscopy, when this technique is available. Hysteroscopy is now increasingly done in many hospitals in Nigeria. Complications such as haemorrhage, tubal damage, uterine perforation and endometrial scarring may occur. It is therefore important that operators gain proficiency before they embark on the procedure.

45.8.4 Conventional Treatment of Male Infertility

In our experience, male infertility is difficult to treat conventionally, possibly because most cases are due to testicular failure. The rate of pregnancy is notoriously poor with conventional treatment when a diagnosis of moderate-to-severe male infertility is diagnosed. Some conventional treatments that have been tried include varicocelectomy in men found to have varicoceles. However, to date varicocelectomy have not been found to be uniformly effective in the treatment of male infertility. For men with anti-sperm antibodies, the use of condoms, corticosteroids and the intrauterine insemination of washed semen at the time of ovulation are sometimes effective.

Hormonal treatment of male infertility is also not regularly successful because only a few men have so-called Kallman's syndrome that can be successfully treated with pulsatile GnRH. By contrast, men with idiopathic semen anomalies should not be given androgens, anti-oestrogens, bromo-ergocryptine or any such drugs as they have not been shown anywhere to be effective.

45.8.5 Treatment of Unexplained Infertility

Unexplained infertility is when there is no obvious cause for infertility after all investigations have been carried out in the man and the woman. Pregnancy may sometimes occur spontaneously in this group, especially after the physiology of ovulation and mechanisms of pregnancy are explained to the couple. Spontaneous pregnancy has also been found after the woman undergoes HSG or trans-ultrasound flushing of the fallopian tubes. Most often, unexplained infertility is treated with ovulation induction, follicular monitoring and timing of the intercourse. This requires cooperation with the couple, which sometimes may be difficult. Some men may find it difficult to ejaculate and may even experience sexual difficulties should they be advised on timing of intercourse. In such cases, the use of artificial insemination using the husband's full or washed semen has proven to be effective.

The use of controlled ovarian stimulation (COS) with gonadotrophins followed by intra-uterine insemination (IUI) has proven to be most successful in the treatment of unexplained infertility. If the COS-IUI regime fails to achieve pregnancy after two to three cycles, it is advised to proceed to either gamete intra-fallopian transfer (GIFT) or IVF-ET.

45.9 Assisted Reproductive Techniques

Assisted reproductive technology (ART) [31] came into being when the first baby conceived with the technique was delivered in the UK in 1978. Since then, several babies have been delivered with ART throughout the world. The most common technique which is the focus of this chapter is in vitro fertilisation and embryo transfer (IVF-ET). The technique has also spread to many developing countries including Nigeria with high rate of successful reproducibility. There are now several IVF centres in Nigeria offering quality services that are comparable to those in other parts of the world. Up to ten fully functional and effective clinics are private clinics while five public teaching hospitals in the country have also opened IVF centres.

At the onset of IVF, doubts were raised about the possibility of carrying out the procedure in developing countries [32], especially because of cost- and effectiveness-related issues. We also wondered at that point in time whether developing countries should adopt the highly expensive IVF procedures that would benefit a few rather than preventive measures that will benefit the majority. In these days of activism for universal health coverage, the question remains unanswered.

To date, IVF has proven to be very effective within the context of developing countries. The Bridge Fertility Centre, Lagos, one of Nigeria's leading IVF clinics was opened in 1999. Twenty years after (in 2019), the clinic has recorded more than 2000 babies born with various IVF techniques including intra-cytoplasmic sperm transfer (ICSI). Other Clinics including the Nordica Fertility in Lagos and the Nisa Fertility Centre in Abuja, have recorded similar successes. Thus, it's now evident that the full scientific armamentariums for the treatment of infertility are now available in developing countries. But issues relating to equity and social justice and the question as to who is served by these clinics still need to be addressed.

Several assisted reproductive techniques (ART) have been described and are currently in use. These include IVF (using standard techniques), IVF with ICSI (with the micro-injection of sperm into the oocyte, gamete intra-fallopian transfer (GIFT), frozen embryo transfer (FET), IVF using sperm donation, IVF using oocyte donation, IVF using embryo donation, IVF using surrogacy and many more.

Within the context of developing countries and for reasons of costs and ethics, the management of infertility in developing countries should always begin with conventional treatment. It is when conventional treatment fails, and there are guidelines to determine failure, that recourse should be made to the ART. The indication for ART can therefore be categorised into irreversible bilateral tubal occlusion, low ovarian reserve (premature ovarian failure or the resistant ovary syndrome), age-related infertility, severe oligospermia or azoospermia, ejaculatory dysfunction and medical indications.

The techniques of the various ART procedures are described in standard textbooks. Interested readers are advised to consult such texts and also to endeavour to attend the many workshops now held around the world for training and capacity building on the ARTs. To summarise, a typical IVF cycle involves pituitary suppression, induction of multiple ovulation with gonadotropins, the monitoring of follicular maturation, the retrieval of oocytes through trans-vaginal ultrasound scan, sperm insemination and fertilisation and fertilisation (in the case of men with low sperm count, ICSI would be performed at this stage), embryo development followed by trans-vaginal transfer, luteal phase support, and followed by confirmation of treatment. The team is normally interdisciplinary specialists and consists of obstetricians and gynaecologists, nurses/midwives, embryologists and administrators. Both couples should be mandatorily screened for HIV, and hepatitis B and C before the onset of the procedure.

45.10 Tertiary Prevention of Infertility

The tertiary prevention of infertility is any measure taken to rehabilitate the couple when they have irreversible infertility and when all measures at secondary prevention have failed. Our experience has shown that women in sub-Saharan African countries rather than men [33] suffer inordinate social, psychological and economic adverse consequences as a result of infertility. They are often blamed for the problem even when the infertility is due to the male factor. As such, it is important and critical that the joint counselling of the couple be made part of the management of infertility from the very onset. Providing regular counselling to the couple during the infertility management will help them come to terms with the situation and will enable them to finally accept the reality of infertility should treatment fail.

Specific support and counselling should be given to the woman. One of the best ways to do this is to conduct individual sessions with the woman to understand how the infertility is affecting her in the marital and social relationships. Such individual sessions will enable the clinician to play the role of an adviser, and supporter to the woman and also provide specific counselling relating to the woman's specific needs. When all else fails, the couple should be advised on adoption and fostering. Fostering occurs naturally in African societies but adoption is less easily accepted. However, in modernising African communities, it is noteworthy that there has been increasing uptake of adoption as a method for resolving infertility.

45.11 Conclusion

Infertility is a common diagnosis in women seeking gynaecological care in many developing countries. It is paradoxical that many developing countries, especially sub-Saharan African countries have high rates of infertility as well as fertility. It is important that equal attention is paid to the management of infertility in order to stimulate community support for the management of fertility.

Infertility management in sub-Saharan African countries is difficult, costly and not always successful. As such it is important and critical to use a preventative mindset for managing all cases of infertility. Preventive approaches help reduce the costs of management and will be more successful at scale for reducing the burden of infertility. Infertility is one of the most challenging issues for women in the developing world, and one that elicits gender, human rights and social justice sentiments. It is therefore important that clinicians are able to do more to prevent and treat all cases of infertility.

References

1. Gurunath S, Pandimu Z, et al. Defining infertility – a systematic review of prevalence studies. Hum Reprod Update. 2011;5:575–88. https://doi.org/10.1093/humudp/dmr015.
2. Cerais AS, Rushwan H. Infertility in Africa. Pop Sci. 1992;12:25–46.
3. Adetoro OO, Ebomoyi A. The prevalence of infertility in a rural Nigerian community. Afr J Med Med Sci 1991;20(1):23–7.
4. Bongaarts J, Frank O, et al. The proximate determinants of fertility in sub-Saharan Africa. Popul Dev Rev. 1984;10:511–37.
5. Larsen U. Infertility in Central Africa. Tropical Med Int Health. 2003;8:354–67.
6. Maya NM, Seth RF, Ties Boerma, et al. National, regional and global trends in infertility prevalence since 1990: A systematic analysis of 277 health surveys. Plos Med. 2012. https://doi.org/10.1371/journal.pmed.1001350.
7. El-Toukhy TA, Khalaf Y. Treatment of unexplained infertility. BMJ. 2008;337. https://doi.org/10.1136/bmj.a772.
8. Panti AA, Sununu YT. The profile of infertility in a teaching hospital in North-west Nigeria. Sahel Med J. 2014;17(1):7–11.
9. Ulla L. Trends in infertility in Cameroon and Nigeria. International Family Planning Perspectives. 1995;21:138–142 & 166.
10. Okonofua F. Female and male infertility in Nigeria. PhD Thesis Dissertation. Department of Public Health Sciences Division of International Health (IHCAR). Stockholm, Sweden: Karolinska Institutet, 2005.
11. Olatunji AO, Sule-Odu AO. The pattern of infertility cases at a University Hospital. West Afr J Med. 2003;3:205–7.
12. World Health Organization. Infections, pregnancies and infertility: perspectives on prevention. Fertil Steril. 1987;47:964–8.
13. Nkwabong E, Dingom MAN. Acute pelvic inflammatory disease in Cameroon: A cross-sectional descriptive study. African Journal of Reproductive Health. 2015;19(4):87–91.
14. Van Heertum K, Barmat L. Uterine fibroids associated with infertility. Women's Health (London). 2014;10(6):645–53. https://doi.org/10.2217/whe.14.27.
15. Menakaya UA. Managing endometriosis in sub-Saharan Africa: emerging concepts and new technologies. Afr J Reprod Health. 2015;19(2):13–6.
16. Taran FA, Stewart EA, Brucker S. Adenomyosis: epidemiology, risk factors, clinical phenotype and surgical interventional alternatives to hysterectomy. Geburtshilfe Frauenheikd. 2013;73(9):924–31. https://doi.org/10.1055/s-0033-1350840.
17. Hamoda H, Khalak Y, Caroll P. Hyperprolactinaemia and female reproductive function: what does the evidence say? Obstet Gynaecol. 2012;14:81–6.
18. Rudnicke E, Kruszewska J, et al. Premature ovarian failure: aetiology, epidemiology and diagnostic evaluation. Menopause Review. Prz Meopauzalmy. 2018;17(3):105–8. https://doi.org/10.5114/pm.2018.78550.
19. Sengupta P, Dutta S. The disappearing sperms: Analysis of reports published between 1980 and 2015. Am J Men's Health. 2017;11(4):1279–304. EPUB 2016, April 19.
20. Sengupta P, Nwagha U, Dutta S, et al. Evidence for decreasing sperm count in African population from 1965 to 2015. Afr Health Sci. 2017;17(2):418–27. https://doi.org/10.4314/ahs.v17i2.16).
21. Abarikwu SO. Causes and risk factors for male factor infertility in Nigeria: a review. Afr J Reprod Health. 2013;17(4):150–66.
22. Okonofua FE, Menakaya U, Bergstrom S. A case control study of risk factors for male infertility in Nigeria. Asian J Androl. 2005;7(4):351–61. https://doi.org/10.1111/j.1745-7262.2015.00046.x.
23. Miyaoka R, Esteves S. A critical appraisal on the role of varicocele in male infertility. Adv Androl. 2012:597495. 9 pages, 2012. https://doi.org/10.1155/2012/597495.
24. Letterie GS, Haggerty MF, Fellows DW. Sensitivity of Hysterosalpingography after tubal surgery. Arch Gynecol Obstet. 1992;251(4):175–80.
25. Oguntoyinbo AE, Amole AOD, Komolafe OF. Sonographic assessment of fallopian tube patency in the investigation of female infertility in Ilorin. Nigeria Afr J Reprod Health. 2001;5(1):100–5.
26. Dasan A, Basawaraj NG. A comparative study of the saline infused sonohysterography and conventional hysterosalpingography in the evaluation of female infertility. West Afr J Radiol. 2016;23:124–9.
27. Bura A, Stockhausen F, Hanisch E. Laparoscopic surgery: a qualified systematic review. World J Methodol. 2015;5(4):238–54. https://doi.org/10.5662/wjm.v5.i4.238.

28. Okonofua FE, Esen UI, Nimalaraj T. Hysterosalpingography versus laparoscopy in tubal infertility: comparison based on findings at laparoscopy. Int J Gynaecol Obstet. 1989;28:143–8.
29. Oei SG, Helmerhorst FM, et al. Effectiveness of the postcoital test: a randomised controlled trial. Br Med J. 1998. https://doi.org/10.1136/bmj.317.7157.502.
30. Leushuis E, van der Steeg JW, et al. Prognostic value of the postcoital test for spontaneous pregnancy. Fertil Steril. 2011; https://doi.org/10.1016/j.fertnstert.2011.02.038.
31. Steptoe PC, Edwards RG. Re-implantation of a human embryo with subsequent tubal pregnancy. Lancet. 1976;I:880–2.
32. Okonofua FE. The case against the development of reproductive technology in developing countries. Br J Obstet Gynaecol. 1996;103:957–62.
33. Okonofua FE, Harris D, Zerai A, Odebiyi A, Snow RC. The social meaning of infertility in Southwest Nigeria. Health Transit Rev. 1997;7:205–20.

Laparoscopy

46

Dan O. Selo-Ojeme

Learning Objectives

At the conclusion of this chapter, the reader will be able to:

- Determine the correct patient selection for operative laparoscopy
- Adequately prepare the patient for operative laparoscopy
- Demonstrate an understanding of proper theatre set up for operative laparoscopy
- Understand the entry and exit safe zones in laparoscopy
- Recognise and manage complications associated with laparoscopy

46.1 Introduction

There have been significant improvements in laparoscopic surgery over the last couple of decades and this has transformed the surgical management of several gynaecological conditions to the extent that laparoscopy now plays a primary role in general and specialist gynaecological practice. Initially, the practice of laparoscopy was mainly used in gynaecology for occlusion of the fallopian tubes in female sterilisation and for the diagnosis of pelvic pain and infertility. It is now commonly employed in the surgical management of benign gynaecological conditions, in pelvic reconstructive surgery, geriatric gynaecology, urogynaecology, and gynaecological oncology.

Before embarking on operative laparoscopic gynaecology, it is essential that the surgeon is conversant with the rudiments of safe intraperitoneal insufflation, safe entry and insertion of various ports and instruments, and have a good knowledge of the complications that can occur during laparoscopy and how to avoid them. The aim of this chapter is to expose the reader to a framework upon which the safe utilisation of gynaecological laparoscopy can be built. It is not a treatise on operative gynaecological laparoscopy. Table 46.1 lists some of the conditions amenable to gynaecologic laparoscopy. It is important that no laparoscopic surgeon attempt any procedure that is beyond his level of competence.

46.2 Relevant Anatomy

A good working knowledge of surgical anatomy of the pelvis is fundamental to the practice of gynaecological laparoscopy. This ensures that the displacement and or alteration of organs by disease conditions are recognised so that the risk of complications during surgery is reduced. The disposition of visceral organs such as the bowel and extraperitoneal organs must be ascertained.

46.3 Patient Selection and Preoperative Assessment

As with any surgical practice, good outcome is dependent on appropriate case selection and adequate preoperative preparation. Consideration must be given to patient-related factors, including relevant comorbidities. Some of these can be improved prior to surgery while others dictate caution.

The use of intraoperative prophylactic antibiotics should be discussed and any allergies noted. It may be prudent to reduce the size of large fibroids with a 3-month course of a long-acting GnRH agonist before attempting a myomectomy or Laparoscopi Assisted vaginal Hysterectomy (LAVH).

D. O. Selo-Ojeme (✉)
Urogynaecological Services, Barnet and Chase Farm Hospital, The Royal Free London NHS Foundation Trust, London, UK
e-mail: Dan.Selo-Ojeme@nhs.net

F. Okonofua et al. (eds.), *Contemporary Obstetrics and Gynecology for Developing Countries*,
https://doi.org/10.1007/978-3-030-75385-6_46

Table 46.1 Use of laparoscopy in gynaecology

Organ/Condition	Laparoscopic Procedure
Uterus	Myomectomy, metroplasty, hysterectomy for benign disease
Tubes	Salpingectomy, salpingostomy (ectopic pregnancy)
Ovaries	Cystectomy, oophorectomy
Urogynaecology	Colposuspension, Sacral colpopexy, hysteropexy, fascioplasties
Gynaecological oncology	Radical hysterectomy, lymphadenectomy
Infertility	Tubal occlusion, salpingectomy (hydrosalpinx)
Chronic pelvic pain	Ablation/excision of endometriosis, adhesiolysis

Table 46.2 Risk assessment for thromboprophylaxis

Low risk	Age less than 40 years No additional risk factors Surgery is less than 30 minutes
Medium risk	Age > 40 years Obesity Immobility > 4 days Past history of Deep Vein Thrombosis (DVT) Major concurrent illness Gross varicose veins Surgery of any duration
High risk	Three or more moderate risk factors Major surgery for malignancy Major surgery in patient with previous history of DVT/PE or thrombophilia

The use of thromboprophylaxis should also be discussed in detail. While thromboprophylaxis may not be necessary in low-risk patients, pneumatic compression/compression stocking and low-molecular-weight heparin should be used in patients at moderate and high risk. The risk classification is as shown in Table 46.2.

The usual precautions regarding preoperative fasting should apply to avoid the risk of aspiration. There should be nothing by mouth after midnight for morning surgery and clear liquids up until 2 hours prior to surgery for cases that are scheduled for later in the day. Such practice makes the patient more comfortable and decreases the degree of preoperative dehydration.

The absolute and relative contraindications to laparoscopy are listed in Table 46.3.

46.4 Consenting

A detailed explanation of the intended procedure along with the associated risks must be discussed with the patient [1]. Every patient scheduled for a laparoscopic procedure must be informed of the risk of laparotomy either to complete the procedure or to deal with any complication that may arise from the procedure.

Table 46.3 Contraindications to laparoscopic surgery

Absolute	Large abdominopelvic mass (>14 weeks) Paralytic ileus Generalised peritonitis Cardiac or respiratory failure Clinical Shock
Relative	Multiple abdominal incisions Extreme body weight Previous peritonitis Multiple abdominal incisions Hiatus hernia Coagulopathies

46.5 Theatre and Patient Setup

General anaesthesia with endotracheal intubation is the preferred mode of anaesthesia for laparoscopy. This is because of the increased risk of aspiration and discomfort associated with high intra-abdominal pressures and Trendelenburg position.

It is essential that the surgeon has a good knowledge of the laparoscopy stack, the laparoscopy instruments (scissors, graspers and dissectors) and the operating room set up. There are myriads of both reusable and disposable instruments for laparoscopic surgery. The choice of instruments is really dependent on the condition of the available reusable equipment and the cost of the disposable equipment.

It is also essential that other members of the operating room team (scrub nurses, runners, operating theatre assistant) are adequately trained and understand their respective roles. This includes being able to solve all technical problems which could occur during the procedure. Nothing is more frustrating for a laparoscopic surgeon than to have a laparoscopy-virgin scrub nurse. As a rule, one assistant and one surgical nurse is enough but certain indications may require an additional assistant.

The operating room should be large enough to accommodate all the necessary equipment.

Before starting the surgery, it is prudent to check the instruments, particularly the insufflation device, the electrodiathermy system, as well as the irrigation system to ensure that they are in good working condition. The stack (Fig. 46.1), consisting of a screen, data storage unit, light source, insufflator, carbon dioxide cylinder and printer, should be checked to ensure that the components are working properly. The scope should be connected to the camera and light source and a 'white balance' confirmed. The insufflation lead should also be connected and tested. The stack should be positioned close to the right foot of the patient with the screen facing the surgeon standing on the left side of the patient. All the equipment monitors must be visible to the surgeon and the screen positioned at the eye level of the surgeon. The operating table is positioned at or below the level of the surgeon's waist. These ergonomic positions prevent undue fatigue and cramps to the neck and shoulders.

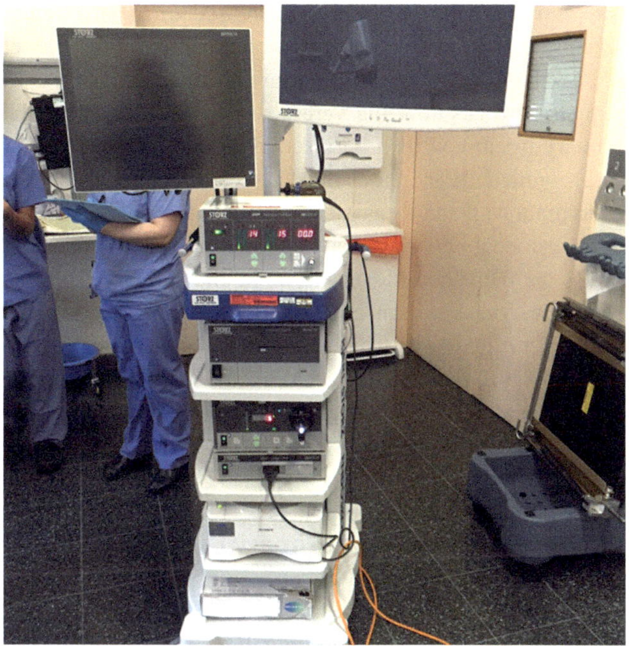

Fig. 46.1 Typical laparoscopy stack

46.5.1 Patient Positioning and Preparation

Appropriate patient positioning is a critical component of gynaecologic laparoscopy that is often overlooked. The patient should be in a low dorsal lithotomy position to allow vaginal access for uterine manipulation. The thighs are flexed such that the trunk-to-thigh angle is approximately 170 degrees. Lesser degrees of flexion might increase the strain on the obturator nerve [2]. The thighs should not be placed below the plane of the table (trunk-to-thigh angle >180 degrees) as this unnatural position places significant strain on the lumbar spine. Lithotomy stirrups such as the Allen Yellofins® Elite Stirrups with Lift-Assist™ are the best support for the lower extremities during gynaecologic laparoscopy.

The Trendelenburg position should be used only after the primary trocar has been inserted. This is because in that position, the sacral promontory with the overlying vessels, are brought into the axis of insertion of the primary trocar.

Routine surgical cleaning of the abdomen, perineum and vagina is performed to achieve a sterile operating field. Traditionally, complete emptying of the urinary bladder with an in-and-out catheter is performed to minimise the risk of bladder injury. Although some surgeons believe that the patient can void immediately prior to entering the operating room, this should be discouraged as there may be a significant amount of bladder distention either because of incomplete emptying or rapid bladder filling or unexpected prolonged surgery. In-and-out catheterisation is associated with minimal risk of iatrogenic urinary tract infection. An indwelling catheter is placed when a long procedure is anticipated.

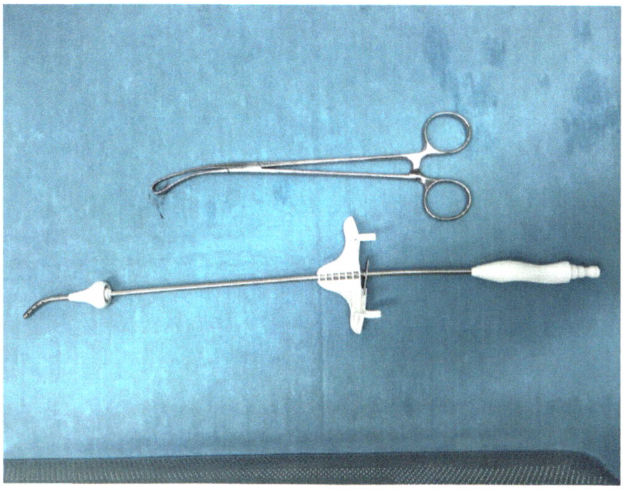

Fig. 46.2 Disposable Spackman's Cannula

The placement of a uterine manipulator is essential for good exposure at laparoscopy. By anteverting or retroverting the uterus, the anterior wall, the vesicouterine fold, the posterior wall and uterosacral ligaments are easily visualised. Lateral movements enable the exposure of the infundibulopelvic ligaments, the utero-ovarian ligaments, and the anterior and posterior leaves of the broad ligament. The elevation movement is important when investigating or treating rectovaginal pathology such as endometriosis. Over a dozen disposable uterine manipulators are currently available on the market but the spackman cannula is usually adequate (Fig. 46.2).

46.5.2 Creation of Pneumoperitoneum

Pneumoperitoneum is essential for laparoscopic surgery. The space it creates enables good visualisation of intraperitoneal anatomy and facilitates dissection and haemostasis. The gas can be introduced via a Veress needle, by direct insertion of a trocar, or through an open laparoscopy.

The introduction of the Veress needle must be done with utmost care as it is responsible for about 90% of vascular and visceral injuries [3]. The Veress needle should be sharp, with a good spring action. A disposable Veress needle is recommended (Fig. 46.3).

The umbilicus is the preferred area for placing the Veress needle solely because there is less subcutaneous and preperitoneal tissue in this area making the distance between the skin and peritoneum shorter than anywhere else on the anterior abdominal wall. The correct technique for inserting the Veress needle is to make an intraumbilical incision, lift up the anterior abdominal wall to increase the distance to the large vessels and then insert the needle. The angle at which the needle is inserted varies from a slant at 45 degrees in non-obese women to perpendicular at 90 degrees in very obese women [4]. One should feel the needle piercing first the aponeurosis and next

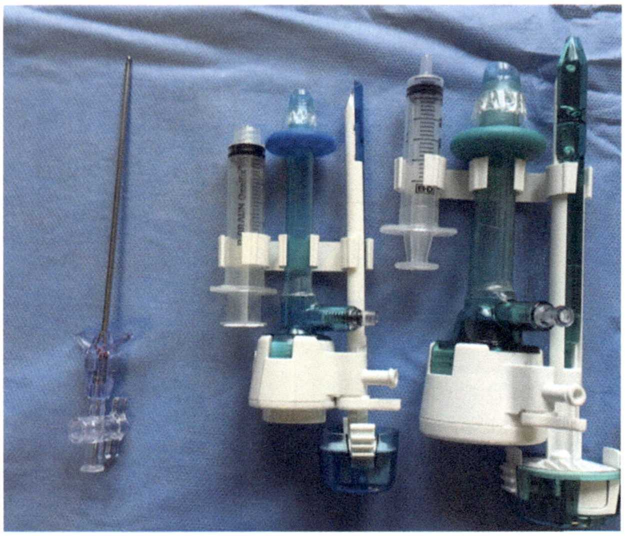

Fig. 46.3 Disposable Veress needle, balloon self-retaining 5 mm and 10 mm trocars

the peritoneum. It is necessary to feel or hear these two clicks in other to avoid needle placement between the aponeurosis and peritoneum with the resultant formation of preperitioneal surgical emphysema. During insertion, the tap should be open and gas unconnected so that once the negative pressure inside the peritoneal cavity is encountered room air enters and bowel and omentum fall away from the needle tip.

There are different ways to confirm appropriate intraperitoneal placement. The syringe test is the most widely used. A 10 ml syringe is filled with saline and attached to the inserted Veress needle. Correct needle placement is verified in three simple steps. The first is aspiration. The syringe plunger is withdrawn and this must not produce blood or matter indicating vascular or bowel perforation. In the second step, about 5 ml of saline is injected which should be free flowing. The third step is an attempt to re-aspirate the injected liquid which will not be possible as it would have dispersed into the peritoneal cavity. There should be a rapid free flow of the fluid in the Veress needle into the peritoneal cavity when the syringe is detached. Connection of the Veress needle to the insufflator machine should then indicate a negative or very low intraperitoneal pressure (<8 mmHg). Studies have shown that an initial intraperitoneal insufflation pressure of 10 mm Hg or less indicates correct Veress needle placement [5, 6]. Where the initial pressure is high or there is return of fluid, the needle should be removed and repositioned. The limit of the intraperitoneal insufflation pressure should be set at 20–25 mmHg with the patient lying flat on the operating table. This provides the necessary safe tension in the anterior abdominal wall for the safe introduction of the umbilical primary trocar. The greater the gas bubble and abdominal wall tension the lesser the risk of bowel injury.

The gas flow is commenced at a low rate of 1 L/min when confirming the initial low intra-abdominal pressure (<8 mmHg). The flow rate is increased to the maximum when safe pressure is confirmed with the cut off pressure set at 20–25 mmHg. Once this pressure is achieved with a consequent zero gas flow, the Veress needle is removed and the primary trocar can then be inserted as this maximum pressure significantly increases the distance between the anterior abdominal wall and the great vessels. It is imperative that the intraperitoneal pressure is reduced and maintained at 12–15 mmHg once the insertion of the primary trocar is complete. The Veress needle should be removed and reinserted if it is uncertain whether the insufflation is intraperitoneal. This is to prevent the development of too much surgical emphysema making subsequent attempts more difficult. The longer 15 cm Veress needle should be used for obese patients.

46.5.3 Insertion of the Primary Umbilical Trocar

There are different ways of inserting the primary umbilical trocar. By far, the commonest is the Veress needle technique where trocar insertion follows immediately after the creation of a pneumoperitoneum. Other methods include the direct trocar insertion, open laparoscopy and left upper quadrant insertion. The surgeon's experience and familiarity with the method has a significant impact on the safety of each technique.

The Veress Needle Technique Following the creation of pneumoperitoneum with the Veress needle, the primary trocar is introduced at an angle of 90 degrees to the skin, through the umbilical incision used for inserting the Veress needle. The incision may be extended to suit the trocar size which should be appropriate for the scope. Pressure exerted on the upper abdomen with the left palm in the area between the umbilicus and xiphisternum forces gas into the lower abdomen and increases the pressure in the peritoneal gas bubble thus increasing the distance to the great vessels. It is not necessary to lift the anterior abdominal wall as this will only cause unpleasant bruising. It is helpful to use a pointed trocar which is introduced using a rotating screw-like motion. One should have the tactile sensation of passing through the fascia and penetrating the abdominal cavity as a sudden 'give'. The common errors associated with this technique are inadequate stabilisation or tenting of the anterior abdominal wall during Veress needle insertion, inadequate pneumoperitoneum prior to insertion of the trocar, application of excessive or poorly controlled force with the trocar, and excessive resistance to trocar insertion due to inadequately sized incision.

In the technique of direct trocar insertion, there is no prior creation of pneumoperitoneum [7–8]. The primary trocar is inserted directly into the abdominal cavity in a manner similar to the introduction of the Veress needle. The sleeve from the trocar is then used to insufflate the abdomen with carbon dioxide gas. This method is thought to be as safe as the Veress needle technique with a 0.06% and 0.09% risk of bowel injury [8].

The open laparoscopy technique, commonly exemplified by the Hasson technique [9–10], involves lifting up the edges of the umbilicus with a pair of Littlewoods and making an infraumbilical incision followed by dissection and incision of the anterior rectus fascia. The peritoneum is then entered bluntly with a pair of artery forceps. A blunt-tipped trocar with sleeve is placed into the peritoneal cavity and anchored with sutures. The pneumoperitoneum is then created. The open laparoscopy technique significantly reduces the risk of injury to the bowel and retroperitoneal vessels.

The left upper quadrant insertion technique is used when there are large pelvic masses or high risk of midline adhesions or for patients in the second trimester of pregnancy. This method is contraindicated in the presence of ascites, hepatomegaly, or splenomegaly. The stomach must be emptied with a gastric tube before this procedure. An incision is made 2–4 cm below the costal margin in the left midclavicular line. A 5-mm trocar is introduced into the peritoneal cavity by gentle motion in the direction of the pelvis on the tented abdominal wall at an angle of 45° from the horizontal plane. A pneumoperitoneum is then created.

A review of the various methods did not show any evidence of an advantage in using any single technique in terms of preventing major vascular or visceral complications [11]. No evidence of difference in the rates of vascular or visceral injuries was also shown with regards to the use of different types of trocars [12].

46.5.4 Initial Inspection

Prior to insertion of a secondary trocar, efforts must be made to study the anatomy of the pelvis following insertion of the laparoscope. This step is crucial to safe operative laparoscopy and must never be omitted as each individual pelvis looks different. The omentum, bowel and bifurcation of the major vessels must be carefully inspected for any injury that may have occurred during the introduction of the Veress needle or primary trocar.

The patient is then placed in a steep Trendelenburg position for a systematic and detailed inspection of the pelvis to identify any pathology such as endometriosis or adhesions. The scope is held close to the peritoneal surface to reveal any subtle or atypical appearance of the tissue. The pelvic side wall is inspected to determine the course of the ureters which is normally 1–2 cm lateral to the uterosacral ligaments. The ovarian fossa, posterior surface of the ovary and broad ligament, pouch of Douglas and the uterovesical peritoneum are all carefully inspected.

Attention is then turned to the upper abdomen to look for other evidence of disease such as perihepatic adhesions (Fitz-Hugh-Curtis syndrome).

46.5.5 Insertion of the Secondary Trocars

The patient should be in a steep Trendelenburg position for secondary trocar placement. This position forces back the bowel and gives good exposure to the pelvis. The location and number of secondary ports are determined by the nature of the procedure and preference of the surgeon. Some surgeons prefer unilateral secondary ports while others use bilateral secondary ports. These can be located in the lower abdominal quadrant or upper abdominal quadrant. It is necessary to take into account the variations in age and body mass index, and insert the secondary trocars in that area located in the outer third of the distance from the midline to the sagittal plane through the anterior superior iliac spine [13–15]. This is regarded as the 'safe zone' (Fig. 46.4).

This is achieved by identifying the epigastric vessels by trans-illumination and placing the trocars laterally in the safe zone. This usually corresponds to 2 cm medial to the anterior superior iliac spine for low quadrant ports or 8 cm from the midline and 8 cm above the pubic symphysis for high quadrant ports. Midline trocars are placed 3 cm above the pubic symphysis.

As a rule, all secondary trocars must be inserted under direct vision to avoid the risk of injury to the bowel (Fig. 46.5). Secondary trocars are usually 5 mm trocars with the 10 mm trocars used for the midline suprapubic ports (Fig. 46.6).

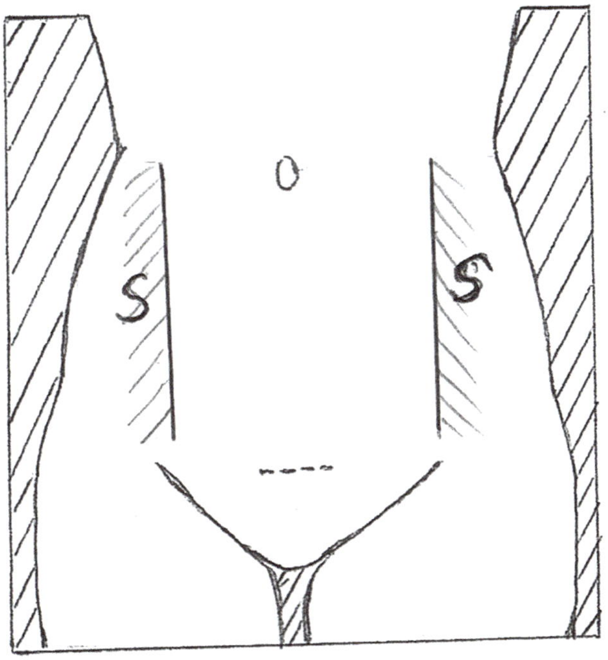

Fig. 46.4 Safe zone [S] for secondary trocar placement

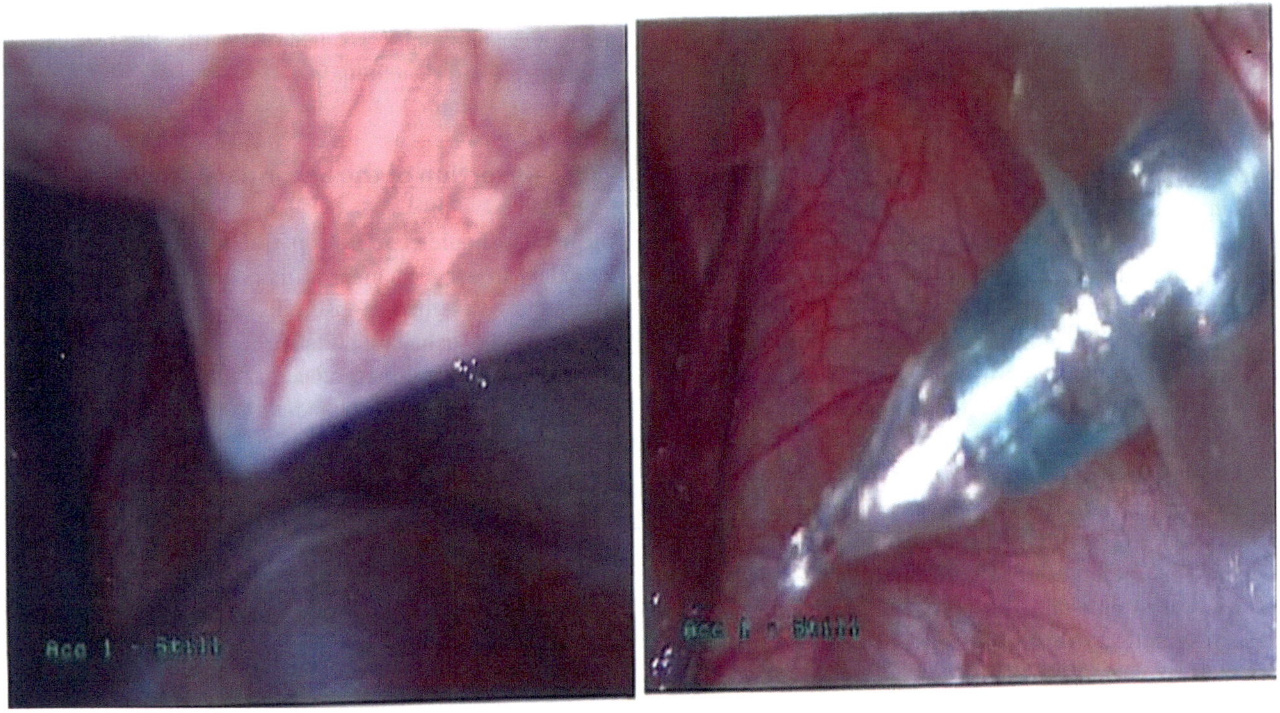

Fig. 46.5 Secondary trocar inserted under direct vision

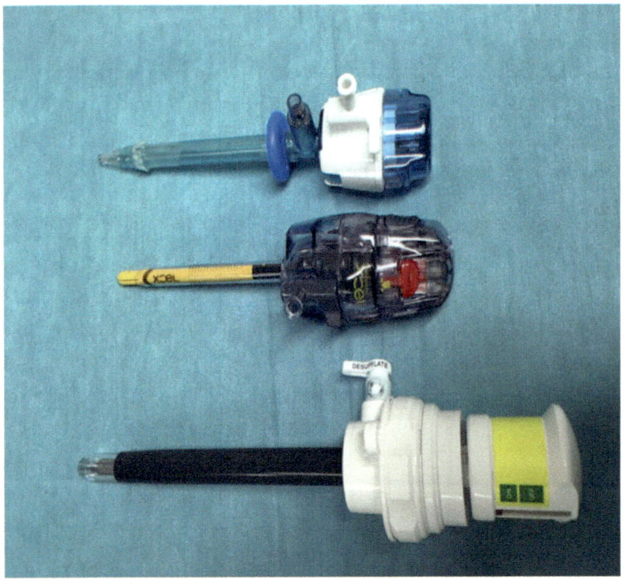

Fig. 46.6 Different 10 mm and 5 mm disposable trocars

46.5.6 Exit Techniques and Closure

All laparoscopy instruments and ports should be removed under direct vision. This is to identify any bleeding or injury to omentum and bowel. These injuries may be partial or complete and if left unidentified, they could lead to serious morbidity or indeed mortality.

Residual pneumoperitoneum can result in uncomfortable post-operative chest and shoulder pain. This is from gas irritation of the diaphragm when the patient sits upright. This situation is best avoided by maintaining the Trendelenburg position when the trumpet valve of the umbilical trocar sleeve is opened to release gas from the abdominal cavity. Only after the sleeve is removed should the Trendelenburg position be discontinued.

It is necessary to close the fascia to avoid the risk of bowel herniation following the use and removal of large trocars (>7 mm). Infiltration of the incision site with a local anaesthetic agent reduces the incidence of post-operative port site pain.

46.6 Energy Sources and Power

The use of energy is indispensable in operative laparoscopy and the surgeon must be familiar with the workings of the energy source being used. Simply put, it is either monopolar electrosurgery where the patient is part of the electrical circuit or bipolar electrosurgery, where the electrical circuit is between the tips of the electrosurgical instrument. The latter has the advantage of reducing the risk of injury to neighbouring tissues because of the limited thermal spread.

Recent advances have seen the introduction of other energy sources that are more precise as a result of much reduced lateral thermal spread. These include the impedance-controlled bipolar devises and the harmonic scalpel (Ethicon Endo-Surgery, Inc., Cincinnati, Ohio). Unlike electrosurgery, the harmonic scalpel uses ultrasonic vibrations instead of electric current to cut and cauterise tissue. The scalpel surface itself cuts through tissue by vibrating in the range of 55,500 Hz. The high frequency vibration of tissue molecules generates stress and friction in tissue. This produces heat and resultant protein denaturation. This technique causes minimal energy transfer to surrounding tissue, potentially limiting collateral damage. It is available as a 5-mm rounded scalpel with a blunt or hooked edge or as a 5-to-10-mm shear or Harmonic ACE that can also be used to grasp tissue.

The impedance-controlled bipolar devices include the Enseal (Ethicon), The ENSEAL® Round Tip for bipolar coagulation and mechanical transection of tissue allows simultaneous seal and transection of vessels and large tissue bundles up to 7 mm with minimal thermal damage.

Other devices such as the LigaSure® (LigaSure®, Valley Lab, Inc., Boulder, Colorado) use radiofrequency energy. This energy output is conveyed through a complex, computer-controlled algorithm that constantly processes resistance and alters the energy output to produce a measured current that denatures protein and elastin in vessel walls with resultant vessel sealing. The LigaSure® technology seals vessels of at least 7 mm in diameter and the sealed vessels can withstand more than three times the systolic blood pressure of the patient.

46.7 Intracorporal Instrument Handling

Once introduced into the peritoneal cavity, laparoscopic instruments should be handled in such a way that optimises performance. Half to two-thirds of the instrument should be inside the abdomen and an angle of 60 degrees should be maintained between two instrument tips. The distance between the optic trocar and the working trocar should be as maximum as possible. The level of the operating table should be such that the surgeon's elbow and hands are not raised up in the American Bikers' position. It should be about waist level and allow comfortable hand movements.

46.8 Post-Operative Care

Although laparoscopic incisions are small, some patients may have had a lot of surgery performed inside them. Therefore, some measure of soreness or discomfort should be expected in the week following the procedure. Nevertheless, recovery following laparoscopic surgery should take no more than 3–7 days. It may take longer with major procedures. An elevated temperature is unusual beyond the first day and the patient should be informed to report any other rise in temperature. They should also be warned to expect some vaginal bleeding from the use of the intrauterine manipulator.

In general, there should be improvement with each passing hour following laparoscopic surgery. The patients should be counselled to report back to the ward for clinical assessment should they experience increasing pain or malaise. It is important that there is no delay in diagnosing peritonitis from unrecognised bowel injury. The occurrence of worsening abdominal pain associated with distension should raise alarm bells and be treated with extreme urgency. It is essential to recognise that occult injury of bowel may take days to develop. Thus, there should be a low threshold for admission and clinical assessment to avoid serious morbidity.

46.9 Complications of Gynaecologic Laparoscopy

The complication rate for gynaecologic laparoscopy ranges from 0.2% to 10.3% [16]. Early recognition and intervention reduces the risk of morbidity and mortality. The majority of complications associated with laparoscopy occur during the introduction of instruments for pneumoperitoneum and use of energy sources. A brief account of some common complications is as follows:

46.9.1 Complications Involving the Bowel

The incidence of bowel injury is reported to be 0% to 0.5% [16]. The presence of bowel adhesion to the anterior abdominal wall is the biggest cause for this. Bowel adhesions may occur as a result of previous abdominal surgeries and intra-abdominal infections. The introduction of disposable trocars with a safety shield designed to extend over the blade once in the peritoneal cavity reduces the risk of bowel lacerations. Thermal injury to the bowel can result from the use of monopolar electrocautery when an arc of electricity involves the bowel. The use of bipolar electrodes reduces the chance of stray current injury.

Bowel injuries lead to life-threatening peritonitis if unrecognised. It is for this reason that this complication is thought to be the most common cause of laparoscopy-related mortality [17]. In general, minor injuries caused by the Veress needle may be managed expectantly as these are mostly small punctures. Trocar injuries, on the other hand, are larger and warrant open repair. Thermal injuries require resection of the damaged segment of bowel and this can be accomplished laparoscopically by a well-trained surgeon [18].

Some unrecognised injuries often manifest 24–48 hours after surgery. Hence patient counselling is of utmost importance. They should be made aware of symptoms requiring attention such as abdominal pain, fever, nausea and vomiting.

46.9.2 Complications Involving the Ureters

The locations where ureteric injuries mostly occur are at the pelvic brim (where the ureters lie beneath the insertions of the infundibulopelvic ligaments), at the ovarian fossa and at the ureteral canal [19]. Risk of ureteric injury occurs in any procedure involving instrumentation near the ureters. Thermal injuries may not be apparent for days after the surgery. The surgeon must be acutely aware of the position of the ureter when power instrument are used. Cautery in close proximity to the ureter should be avoided as much as possible. Inadvertent ligation of the ureter results in presentation with flank pain from hydro nephrosis. Transection leads to the development of urinoma or ascites and the patient presents 1–5 days after surgery with abdominal pain and fever. About 20% of ureteric injuries occur during laparoscopic-assisted vaginal hysterectomy, 11% during oophorectomy, 10% during laparoscopic pelvic lymphadenectomy, 7% during laparoscopic sterilisation, 7% during excision of endometriosis and 6% during endometriosis ablation [20].

46.9.3 Complications Involving Abdominal Wall Vessels

The incidence of abdominal wall bleeding from vessel injury is 0.3–0.5% [16]. The main vessels at risk are the epigastric vessels (inferior and superficial) and the superficial circumflex iliac vessel. The inferior epigastric vessel arises from the external iliac vessel, and the superficial vessel originates from the femoral vessel. These injuries usually occur in during insertion of secondary ports. A good knowledge of the anatomy of these vessels is fundamental to avoiding injury. The superficial vessels can be identified by trans-illuminating the anterior abdominal wall with the laparoscope. Because of their location, the inferior epigastric artery cannot be trans-illuminated but can be seen laparoscopically beneath the peritoneum between the insertion of the round ligament at the inguinal canal and the obliterated umbilical artery. If these vessels cannot be visualised, the operator can improve the chance of successfully avoiding the vessels by placing the trocars in the safe zone described earlier.

Immediate steps must be taken to control bleeding when any of these vessels are injured. Coagulation with electrocautery is an initial option. In the event that no other ancillary port is available to use electrocautery, a Foley catheter can be placed through the trocar and the balloon inflated with saline. Traction on the catheter, maintained with a clamp on the abdominal side, tamponades the bleeding thus providing the opportunity to institute more definitive measures. Electrocautery can be used once a second port is established. If this is unsuccessful, the vessel should be ligated following enlargement of the incision.

46.9.4 Complications Involving Retroperitoneal Major Vessels

The incidence of major vessel injury range from 0.04% to 0.5% [21, 22] with a reported mortality rate of 6–11% [23, 24]. These injuries often occur during the insertion of the Veress needle and the primary or secondary trocar. It often does not depend on the complexity of case [25–26]. Because most surgeons are right-handed and stand on the left side of the table during insertion, the distal aorta and the right common iliac artery are the vessels commonly susceptible to injury [27]. The bifurcation of the aorta (and branching of the right common iliac artery) is only 3–4 cm directly below the umbilicus in the anaesthetised abdomen. This distance is increased to 8–14 cm with pneumoperitoneum.

Inserting the Veress needle or primary trocar through the umbilicus directed towards the hollow of the pelvis would avoid trauma to the aorta and inferior vena cava. It must be noted that in some cases, the bifurcation is above or below L4. Thin patients are particularly at risk as the distance from the umbilicus to the retroperitoneal vessels may be as short as 2–3 cm. In obese patients, the umbilicus may not lie over L4. In this case, a good guide to the position of the bifurcation is palpation of the iliac crest which is in the same plane lateral to L4. Open laparoscopy remains a safe alternative for avoiding retroperitoneal injury.

When placing the Veress needle, the patient must be in the horizontal position (not Trendelenburg). Inadequate intraperitoneal pressure prior to trocar insertion, excessive force and or poor control of force on trocar and Veress needle, lack of counter traction (usually achieved by lifting the anterior abdominal wall), instrument tips pointing downwards rather than towards the pelvis in the horizontal patient, and inserting the Veress needle and primary trocar with the patient in the Trendelenburg position all increase the risk of major vessel injury.

It is prudent to have good inspection of the peritoneal cavity immediately after entry as any active bleeding may be immediately obvious. Blood may also be noticed to be flowing from the open Veress needle. Unexpected and unexplained changes in the patient's vital signs should prompt suspicion of major vessel injury and warrant urgent action as the peritoneal cavity may not show signs of bleeding in a retroperitoneal haemorrhage. Timely identification is vital to patient survival. The anaesthetist must be alerted once a major vessel injury is suspected so that consideration may be given to the placement of a central line and ordering of blood products.

The Veress needle or trocars should not be removed when vessel injury is identified as this can result in profuse bleeding with resultant difficulty in identifying the site of bleeding. The vascular injury must be repaired immediately via a laparotomy by a competent vascular surgeon.

46.9.5 Complications Involving Nerves

Nerve injuries during laparoscopic surgery are uncommon. However, to reduce the risk of positional nerve injuries it is important for the surgeon to have a good knowledge of the nerves at risk of injury during laparoscopy and ensure that each patient is positioned appropriately. Long periods in the lithotomy position can cause injuries to the femoral, lateral femoral cutaneous, obturator, sciatic and common peroneal nerves. Sensory deficit are reported to be in the region of 1.5% of case done in the lithotomy position. Motor deficits are reported to be 0.03% [28]. The use of lithotomy stirrups appears to decrease the risk of nerve injuries.

46.10 Troubleshooting

- *Hazy Pictures/shadows on screen*: This can occur if the camera is out of focus. Adjusting the focus usually resolves this. If the picture is still hazy and there appears to be shadows then the scope should be detached and the lenses cleaned with spirit. The camera head should also be cleaned.
- *Fogging:* Fogging occurs as a result of the differential temperature between the scope and peritoneal cavity. Various commercial anti-fog solutions are available. Inserting the scope in a warm saline solution or a commercial warmer tube brings the scope temperature up to that of the body and prevents fogging. Other techniques include cleaning the scope end with spirit solution and touching a swab or bowel wall.
- *High Insufflation Pressures:* In the first instance, ensure correct intraperitoneal placement of the Veress needle. Then flush the needle as the tip may be blocked by tissue. Grasp and lift up the abdominal wall to seperate viscera from the needle tip.
- *Distorted Pelvic Anatomy*: Ensure that the camera is held in the correct alignment such that the organs are seen in the correct anatomical position. This is often a problem if the assistant is a novice.

46.11 Robotic Surgery

Currently, the only commercially available robotic system is the da Vinci® Surgery System (Intuitive Surgical Inc. Sunnyvale, California, USA). The system is made up of three parts: a 3D high-definition vision system, a surgeon's console and a robotic platform with three or four robotic arm that holds the Endowrist® Instruments and camera.

Robotic surgery offers all the advantages of laparoscopic surgery in addition to the following; robotic movements are reduced by up to 10 times, assured precision with microsurgical dissection and a very stable camera with 3D vision. The hand movements are intuitive when using the robot as the instruments move in the same direction as the surgeon's hands. This is in contrast to straight stick laparoscopy where the hand and instrument movements are counterintuitive.

Robotic surgery attracts a prohibitive capital cost in the range of $1–2.5 million [29]. When this is added to the cost of maintenance and instruments cost, it is exceedingly more expensive that conventional laparoscopy.

An excellent up-to-date review of the role of robotic surgery in gynaecology is provided by Nair et al. [30].

46.12 Summary

Advances in minimal access surgery are ever evolving and has largely replaced open surgery in the management of both benign and malignant gynaecological conditions. It is necessary for the modern-day gynaecologist to be well equipped with the knowledge and skills of basic and or advanced laparoscopy so as to offer patients the optimum routes for gynaecological surgery.

References

1. RCOG Consent Advice No2. http://bsge.org.uk/wp-content/uploads/2016/03/ca2-15072010.pdf.
2. Warner MA, Warner DO, Harper CM, Schroeder DR, Maxson PM. Lower extremity neuropathies associated with lithotomy positions. Anesthesiology. 2000;93(4):938–42.
3. Azevedo JL, Azevedo OC, Miyahira SA, Miguel GP, Becker OM Jr, Hypólito OH, Machado AC, Cardia W, Yamaguchi GA, Godinho L, Freire D, Almeida CE, Moreira CH, Freire DF. Injuries caused by Veress needle insertion for creation of pneumoperitoneum: A systematic literature review. Surg Endosc. 2009;23(7):1428–32.
4. Hurd WW, Bude RD, De Lancey JOL, Gavin JM, Aisen AM. Abdominal wall characterisation with magnetic resonance imaging and computed tomography: the effect of obesity in the laparoscopic approach. J Reprod Med. 1991;26:473–6.
5. Teoh B, Sen R, Abbott J. An evaluation of four tests used to ascertain Veress needle placement at closed laparoscopy. J Minim Invasive Gynecol. 2005;12:153–8.
6. Vilos AG, Vilos GA, Abu-Rafea B, Hollet-Caines J, Al-Omran M. Effect of body habitus and parity on the initial Veres intraperitoneal (VIP) C02 insufflation pressure during laparoscopic access in women. J Minim Invasive Gynecol. 2006;13(2):108–13.
7. Theodoropoulou K, Lethaby DR, Bradpiece HA, Lo TL, Parihar A. Direct trocar insertion technique: an alternative for creation of pneumoperitoneum. JSLS. 2008;12(2):156–8.
8. Agresta F, Mazzarolo G, Bedin N. Direct trocar insertion for laparoscopy. JSLS. 2012;16(2):255–9.
9. Lal P, Singh L, Agarwal PN, Kant R. Open port placement of the first laparoscopic port: a safe technique. JSLS. 2004;8(4):364–6.
10. Hasson HM. Open laparoscopy. Biom Bull. 1984;5(1):1–6.
11. Ahmad G, Gent D, Henderson D, O'Flynn H, Phillips K, Watson A. Laparoscopic entry techniques. Cochrane Database Syst Rev. 2015;8:CD006583. https://doi.org/10.1002/14651858.CD006583.pub4.

12. la Chapelle CF, Swank HA, Wessels ME, Mol BW, Rubinstein SM, Jansen FW. Trocar types in laparoscopy. Cochrane Database Syst Rev. 2015;12:CD009814. https://doi.org/10.1002/14651858.CD009814.pub2.
13. Epstein J, Arora A, Ellis H. Surface anatomy of the inferior epigastric artery in relation to laparoscopic injury. Clin Anat. 2004;17:400–8.
14. Bhatti AF, Iqbal S, Lee TC. Variation in surface marking of superior epigastric vessels. A guide to safe laparoscopic port insertion. Surgeon. 2008;6:50–2.
15. Vázquez-Frias JA, Huete-Echandi F, Cueto-Garcia J, Padilla-Paz LA. Prevention and treatment of abdominal wall bleeding complications at trocar sites: review of the literature. Surg Laparosc Endosc Percutan Tech. 2009;19:195–7.
16. Magrina JF. Complications of laparoscopic surgery. Clin Obstet Gynecol. 2002;45:469–80.
17. Peterson HB, DeStefano F, Rubin GL, et al. Deaths attributable to tubal sterilization in the United States, 1977 to 1981. Am J Obstet Gynecol. 1983;146:131–6.
18. Reich H, McGlynn F, Budin R. Laparoscopic repair of full-thickness bowel injury. J Laparoendosc Surg. 1991;1:119–22.
19. Gordon AG, Lewis BV. Complications of laparoscopy. In: Gordon AG, Lewis BV, DeCherney AH, editors. Atlas of gynaecologic endoscopy. New York: Mosby-Wolfe; 1995. p. 136–42.
20. Ostrzenski A, Radolinski B, Ostrzenska KM. A review of laparoscopic ureteral injury in pelvic surgery. Obstet Gynecol Surv. 2003;58:794–9.
21. Munro MG. Laparoscopic access: complications, technologies, and techniques. Curr Opin Obstet Gynecol. 2002;14:365–74.
22. Aksu T, Coskun F. Complications of gynaecological laparoscopy—a retrospective analysis of 3572 cases from a single institute. J Obstet Gynaecol. 2004;24:813–6.
23. Chandler JG, Corson SL, Way LW. Three spectra of laparoscopic entry access injuries. J Am Coll Surg. 2001;192:478–91.
24. Bhoyrul S, Vierra MA, Nezhat CR, Krummel TM, Way LW. Trocar injuries in laparoscopic surgery. J Am Coll Surg. 2001;192:677–83.
25. Nordestgaard AG, Bodily KC, Osborne RW, Buttorff JD. Major vascular injuries during laparoscopic procedures. Am J Surg. 1995;169:543–5.
26. Vilos GA, Ternamian A, Dempster J, Laberge PY. Laparoscopic entry: a review of techniques, technologies, and complications. The society of obstetricians and gynaecologists of Canada. J Obstet Gynaecol Can. 2007;29:433–65.
27. Philips PA, Amaral JF. Abdominal access complications in laparoscopic surgery. J Am Coll Surg. 2001;192:525–36.
28. Warner MA, Martin JT, Schroeder DR, Offord KP, Chute CG Lower-extremity motor neuropathy associated with surgery performed on patients in a lithotomy position. Anesthesiology. 1994;81(1):6–12.
29. Barbash GI, Glied SA. New technology and health care costs—the case of robot-assisted surgery. N Eng J Med. 2010;363:701–4.
30. Nair R, Killicaot K, Ind TEJ. Robotic surgery in gynaecology. Obstet Gynaecol. 2016;18:221–2.

Pelvic Organ Prolapse

47

Olukunle Ajayi and Victor N. Chilaka

Learning Objectives

By the end of the chapter, the reader should be able to:

- Define pelvic organ prolapse (POP) and appreciate its prevalence and significance in contemporary practice
- Understand the significant aetiological factors in POP and be able to take a good history from the patients with this condition and initiate necessary investigations
- Examine POP showing understanding of the various compartments involved and understand the principles of grading POP using the POP-Q system
- Understand the principles of management of the different forms and combinations of pelvic organ prolapse:
  - (a) The preventive measures and pelvic floor health
  - (b) Strengths and limitations of pelvic floor physiotherapy
  - (c) The pros and cons of using vaginal pessaries
  - (d) The principles of surgical correction of POPs and surgical complications
  - (e) The advantages of the use of surgical mesh and its limitations

47.1 Introduction

Pelvic organ prolapse is defined as the descent or herniation of pelvic organ from their normal anatomical position. Pelvic floor dysfunction covers a broader range of conditions, including pelvic organ prolapse (POP), urinary incontinence (UI) and faecal incontinence (FI) [1]. As life expectancy increases in the developed countries, the prevalence of POP will continue to rise, and it is a matter of time before the same trend is observed in developing countries. It is expected that the United States will experience a 46% increase in pelvic organ prolapse between 2010 and 2050 [2]. The demand for treatment of non-communicable disease and age-related medical conditions such as pelvic organ prolapse is set to continue to increase as the health of the population improves.

47.2 Prevalence

Surgery for prolapse accounts for approximately 20% of elective major gynaecological surgery and up to 59% of operations in older women.

The lifetime risk of having surgery for prolapse is 11%, and a third of these are for recurrent prolapses. As many as 50% of parous women have some form of prolapse, but only about 20% will be symptomatic.

The prevalence of POP in post-menopausal women is as follows: anterior prolapse – 51%, posterior prolapse – 27%, and uterine/vault prolapse – 20% [3]. Vault prolapse is also seen in 1.8% of women who have had a hysterectomy for benign conditions, but in 11.6% in those who had a hysterectomy because of prolapse [4, 5].

Classification

Traditionally, POP is classified as follows:

(i) Anterior compartment prolapse (cystourethrocele) when the bladder and/or urethra herniated through the anterior vagina wall
(ii) Posterior compartment prolapse (rectocoele) occurs when the rectum herniates through the posterior vaginal wall

O. Ajayi
York Teaching Hospital NHS, East Riding Hospital, and Scarborough Hospital, York, UK

V. N. Chilaka (✉)
Women's Wellness and Research Centre, Hamad Medical Corporation, Doha, Qatar

F. Okonofua et al. (eds.), *Contemporary Obstetrics and Gynecology for Developing Countries*,
https://doi.org/10.1007/978-3-030-75385-6_47

(iii) Apical compartment prolapse (utero-vagina prolapse/ vault prolapse) occurs when the cervix and uterus or the bowel herniating through the vagina vault in patients who had a hysterectomy

Grading Systems

(a) General System of Grading Prolapses:

First Degree:

Lowest part of prolapse descends halfway down the vaginal axis to the introitus.

Second Degree:

Lowest part of the prolapse extends to the level of the introitus and through the introitus on straining.

Third Degree:

Lowest part of the prolapse extends through the introitus and lies outside the vagina. Procidentia describes a third-degree uterine prolapse.

(b) *Baden and Walker Classification (1972)*:

Grade I	Descent of any organ to the vaginal mid-plane
Grade II	Descent to the hymenal ring
Grade III	Descent halfway through the introitus
Grade IV	Complete eversion

These systems lacked scientific accuracy.

(c) *The Pelvic Organ Prolapse Quantification (POP-Q) and Scoring System*

ICS committee on standardisation [6]. This ICS accredited staging is similar to Baden and Walker system but involves well-defined anatomic relations. Measurements are taken in the left lateral position at rest and maximal Valsalva, thus providing an accurate and reproducible method of quantification.

Grade O: No descent in pelvic organs during straining

Grade I: Leading surface of prolapse does not descend below 1 cm above the hymenal ring

Grade II: Leading edge of prolapse extends from 1 cm above to 1 cm below the hymenal ring

Grade III: From 1 cm below the hymenal ring but without complete vaginal eversion

Grade IV: Complete vaginal eversion

Anatomic Relations for the POP-Q Systems

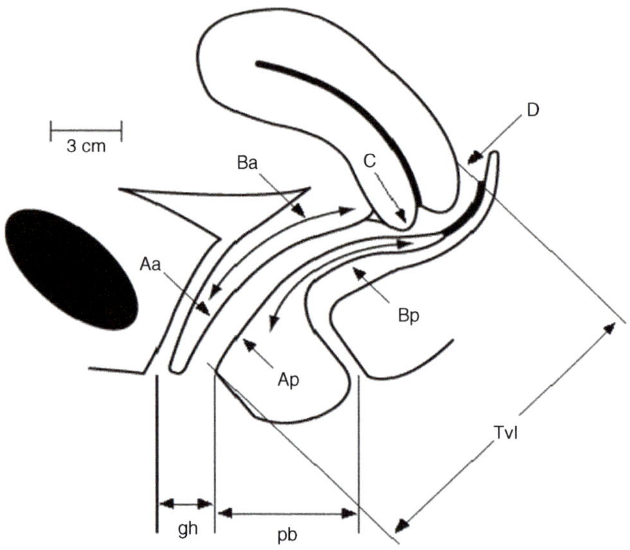

gh	Genital hiatus
pb	Perineal body
tvl	Total vaginal length
Aa	Midline point of the anterior vaginal wall 3 cm proximal to the ext. meatus
Ba	Most distal/dependent position of the anterior vaginal wall from the vaginal vault or anterior fornix to Aa
C	Most distal/dependent edge of cervix or vault
D	Location of the posterior fornix
Bp	Most distal/dependent position on posterior vaginal wall from the vaginal vault or posterior fornix to Ap
Ap	Point on midline posterior vaginal wall 3 cm proximal to the hymen

Examples

Normal Anatomy

−3 Aa	−3 Ba	−8 C
2 gh	3 pb	10 tvl
−3 Ap	−3 Bp	10 D

Complete Vaginal Vault Eversion

+3 Aa	+8 Ba	+8 C
4.5 gh	1.5 pb	8 tvl
+3 Ap	+8 Bp	– D

47.3 Aetiological Factors

The triad of age, childbirth injury and increased intra-abdominal pressure are the main contributing factors to pelvic organ prolapse. The striated muscles of the pelvic floor in common with other striated muscles undergo gradual denervation with age that results in weakening of the muscles. Also, denervation injury occurs commonly at childbirth. These, coupled with a marked reduction of oestrogen in the menopausal women and increased intra-abdominal pressure in patients with obesity, chronic cough and constipation, are common aetiological factors in the development of POP.

Other factors include some exercises as weight lifting, high-impact aerobics and long-distance running increase.

Surgical operations as Burch colposuspension, needle suspension (Pereyra & Stamey), Manchester and even hysterectomies can predispose women to POP.

Genetics may also be an essential factor in the aetiology of POP as it has been observed that it may be commoner in whites when compared with black populations.

47.4 Epidemiology

Few epidemiological studies concerned with the prevalence of pelvic floor dysfunction have been carried out in developing countries. As the vast majority of developing countries resources are directed at life-threatening conditions such as post-partum haemorrhage, unsafe abortion, cervical cancer, violence against women and gender inequality, research into pelvic organ prolapse has taken backstage. Moreover, significant cultural barriers in reaching women in certain parts of Africa, the sensitive nature of the questions and examinations concerned with the evaluation of pelvic floor dysfunction have contributed to less research in this area. A review of the demographics of pelvic floor disorders indicates that a fifth of parous women have a pelvic organ prolapse. It is generally accepted that 50% of women will develop pelvic organ prolapse (POP), but only 10–20% of those seek evaluation for their condition. The peak incidence of symptoms attributed to POP is between the ages of 70 and 79, while POP symptoms are still relatively common in younger women [7]. A North American Actuarial analysis revealed that a woman up to the age of 80 years has 11% risk of needing surgery for pelvic floor weakness and if she has an operation, she has a 29% risk of requiring further surgery [8].

POP seems commoner in Whites, although good epidemiological data are still lacking. Van Dongen [9] concluded that genital prolapse was 80 times commoner in Whites than Blacks in South Africa. He proposed five factors to explain this observation:

1. The smaller circumference of the pelvis in Blacks requires shorter suspensory ligaments from the pelvic sidewalls to the cervix and vagina, and shorter ligaments are less likely to stretch than longer ones.
2. The deeper pelvis in black women allows for a thicker cardinal and uterosacral ligaments, which because of their vast bulk are less likely to stretch or tear.
3. The longer supra-vaginal cervix in black women allows larger and stronger attachments for the cardinal and uterosacral ligaments.
4. Blacks inherently have tougher connective tissue than their white counterparts based on preliminary histological studies, showing a higher collagen content in their ligaments.
5. The more significant lumber lordosis in Blacks results in the diversion of abdominal forces towards the pubic bone and anterior abdominal wall rather than towards the pelvic diaphragm.

More work is required to identify the reasons for the observed racial differences.

Clinical Presentation Clinical presentation depends on the compartment mainly affected and could be a combination of the compartments involved as well as sexual. Careful history taking is essential in evaluating pelvic dysfunction. It is crucial to ascertain the patient's symptoms, the severity of the symptoms, the patient's perception of the problems and what the patient wishes or their specific goals for consultation.

47.4.1 General Symptoms

These may vary in magnitude and depends on the site of prolapse. Feeling of discomfort or heaviness in the pelvis with 'lump or something coming down' is quite common. This sensation tends to worsen with prolonged standing and towards the end of the day. They may also experience difficulty in inserting tampons or tampons could be spontaneously extruded. A good number will complain of chronic low backache. In advanced prolapse, there could also be decubitus ulcerations and lichenification, with vaginal discharge or bleeding.

Sexual symptoms are not uncommon, and they may experience dyspareunia with slackness at coitus, lack of sensations, sexual satisfaction and orgasms. In severe cases, there could be apareunia, urinary incontinence during sexual intercourse, embarrassment or fear of leaking urine to the avoidance of intercourse altogether. There is, therefore, an essential need to ask about sexual functions as many women in the developing countries may not volunteer this information, but it could be a significant part of their distress.

47.4.2 Anterior Compartment

Apart from complaining of something coming down, protrusion or mass par vaginam, LUTS (hesitancy urgency frequency and sensation of incomplete emptying) are very common complaints of anterior compartment prolapse. There could also be digitation or positional change to help voiding. They also tend to present with recurrent UTIs, terminal urinary dribbling, and at times difficulty in initiating urination (hesitancy).

47.4.3 Posterior Compartment

They may have difficulty in opening the bowels, tenesmus, faecal urgency, with anal or vaginal digitation to defecate. There could also be incomplete bowel emptying, incontinence of flatus or stool, and faecal urgency. In cases of rectal prolapse, there may be a painful lump at the anal margins.

47.4.4 Others

Symptoms of other underlying condition that could precipitate or worsen pelvic floor dysfunction should be determined for instance: chronic cough/chronic obstructive pumonary disease, ascites, abdominopelvic mass such as big uterine fibroids, chronic constipation. The quality of life (QoL) assessment reveals the severity of symptoms and quantifies the impact on the quality of life. It is always good practice to recheck QoL after interventions to determine their impact. It is essential to ascertain if the woman wishes to resume sexual activity (if stopped prior to consultation). This has an implication on the choice of conservative management like the vaginal pessary, or surgical approach to the treatment of POP.

47.4.5 Examination

It is essential to offer an explanation of the steps involved in the examination to the patient, and ensure verbal consent and a chaperone. General examination including Body Mass Index (BMI) assessment, relevant systems, such as chest for features of COPD, abdomen for masses and the neurological system should be examined in detail.

47.4.6 Pelvic Examination

This should start with an inspection of the vulva. Procidentia is immediately visible. Ulcerations may be present posteriorly. A speculum examination should be done in the dorsal position to inspect vaginal wall and cervix, followed by a digital examination to assess the uterine size, and adnexa. The pelvic floor muscle tone and the patient's ability to perform a pelvic floor contraction should also be assessed. The patient is then examined in the left lateral position with the aid of a Sim's speculum. Pelvic organ prolapse quantification (POP-Q) method or the more widely used Baden-Walker halfway system is used to grade the stage of prolapse.

At times, it may be necessary to have the patient to stand up and strain in other to demonstrate the prolapse adequately.

Rarely, a rectal examination may be indicated to check for anal sphincteric tone, pelvic floor tone and stool consistency.

47.4.7 Investigation

Clinical assessment is sufficient in most cases of POP. However, if urinary symptoms are present, a midstream urine should be dipped and if suspicious of infection be sent for microscopy, culture and sensitivity.)

Urodynamic studies are indicated if there are concomitant lower urinary tract symptoms as stress incontinence urgency and urge incontinence or suspected voiding disorders. It is noteworthy that USI may be unmasked by anterior colporrhaphy. It is always good practice to check for urinary incontinence during examination for POP, and if USI is confirmed, a continence procedure may be done at the same time as the repair.

Other investigations that are rarely required include renal tract ultrasound, which should be considered in chronic urinary residual and recurrent UTIs. Severe may be associated with obstructive uropathy, and intravenous urogram may be useful. Procidentia is often associated with some degree of ureteric obstruction.

Pelvic fluoroscopy or MRIs may be used in detecting enterocoeles, and Isotope defaecography can be used in detecting rectocoeles.

Cystourethroscopy can be used to investigate severe irritative symptoms, to exclude chronic follicular or interstitial cystitis.

47.5 Management of POP

The current approach to the management of POP involves:

(i) Preventive measures (obstetric and non-obstetric measures)
(ii) Conservative management using a combination of lifestyle interventions, behavioural strategies, physical or physiotherapy
(iii) Surgical management

47.5.1 Preventive Measures

47.5.1.1 Eradicate Harmful Obstetric Practices: Fundal Pressure

The use of fundal pressure to accelerate labour or aid the bearing down urge during childbirth has no place in modern obstetric practice but still employed by some birth attendants in developing countries.

Limit Prolonged Second Stage

Avoidance of prolonged second stage of labour through careful monitoring employment of partograph as well as assisted vaginal delivery reduces the impact of excessive denervation injury that almost invariably accompanies childbirth.

Eradicate Prolonged Obstructed Labour

It is essential to sustain the efforts over the past decades of ensuring trained birth attendant in labour. Partograph use in labour is essential for early diagnosis and intervention to limit pelvic floor damage. It is also essential to address the causes of delay in the transfer of women in labour and accessing emergency obstetric services.

Non-obstetric Factors

It is necessary to avoid and also treat any factor that leads to chronic increases in intra-abdominal pressure (constipation, obesity, chronic chest conditions and obstructive airways disease and asthma).

Hormone Replacement Therapy (HRT) with estrogens may also decrease the incidence of prolapse, but randomised controlled trials (RCTs) are needed to support this view. HRT is rarely used in developing countries but does reduce the lower genital tract symptoms.

There is also a need to emphasise smaller family size and improvements in antenatal and intrapartum to maintain a healthier pelvic floor. Caesarean section seems protective of urogenital prolapse. Antenatal and postnatal pelvic floor exercises have not been shown conclusively to reduce the incidence of prolapse, but may be protective.

Pelvic floor exercises (PFE) have not been shown to prevent prolapses, but may slow its progression and prevent urinary stress incontinence and should be encouraged. PFE may have a role in cases of mild prolapse in younger women who are yet to complete their family.

Lifestyle Interventions

This may include dietary advice, weight loss, laxative use, avoidance of high-impact exercise.

Pelvic Floor Re-education or Pelvic Floor Muscle Training: (PFMT) Graded muscle training alone, or in combination with physical adjuncts such as vaginal cones, electrical stimulation and biofeedback are used to re-educate the pelvic floor muscles. In stress incontinence, PFMT works by increasing the tone and strength of the pelvic muscles. PFMT has also been shown to reduce the rate of progression of pelvic organ prolapse. PFMT success depends on the patient's ability to perform the exercise correctly [10].

47.6 Pelvic Floor Exercise

The pelvic muscle is graded using the Oxford scale from 0 to 5. (Table 47.1). A 2014 multicentre randomised controlled trial (RCT) comparing individualised pelvic floor muscle training with no intervention found a statistically significant improvement in subjective assessment of prolapse symptoms in the intervention group. No significant improvement in objective assessment of anatomy, as assessed by the pelvic organ prolapse quantification system (POP-Q), was reported [11].

47.6.1 Vaginal Pessaries

Vagina pessaries have been available in some form for over 4000 years. The first pessaries described were pomegranate skins [12]. The commonest pessary in use is the ring type. Made of polypropylene, easy to insert and remove. It could be inserted and removed by well-motivated patients (at bedtime or before coitus as the patient deems fit. It does not preclude sex. The optimal size is usually determined by trial and error. It is essential that the pessary is shown to the patients to allay fear and ensure compliance. The optimal time interval for change of pessary has not been determined. Most clinicians change pessaries between 4 and 6 months in order to rule out pressure ulceration or impaction. Slight blood loss during pessary use may indicate ulceration, but care is needed in the post-menopausal women to rule our cervical or endometrial cancer by proper clinical evaluation. If there is ulceration, do not replace pessary, use oestrogen cream vaginally to encourage healing and pessary is replaced after heal-

Table 47.1 Modified Oxford grading of pelvic floor muscle

Grade	Characteristics
0	No discernible contraction
1	Flickering contraction, not visible on inspection of the perineum
2	Weak squeeze, distinctly palpable contraction. No lift
3	Moderate squeeze, palpable upward and forward movement. Definite lift
4	Good muscle strength, elevation possible against slight resistance. Good squeeze with lift
5	Very strong muscle strength, contraction possible against vigorous resistance. Strong squeeze with lift

ing. Pessary offers several advantages: It is effective, no risk of anaesthesia, affordable, reusable and it is authors' opinion that pessary use should be widely advocated in combination with supervised pelvic floor exercise in a resource-poor setting. Space occupying pessaries like the shelf pessary precludes sexual intercourse and are therefore unsuitable for sexually active women. The shelf pessary may be quite challenging to change and be embedded in the vaginal wall. Some pessaries are designed for stress incontinence while others have dual action for stress incontinence as well as control of pelvic organ prolapse symptoms.

Complications of the pessary include pain, urinary incontinence and retention, vaginal discharge and ulcerations, which can lead to fistula formation if neglected. Before using these in the tropics, it is essential to ensure that the patient must be able to keep follow-up appointments A simple guideline for pessary selection is provided in Table 47.2.

47.7 Surgical Management of Pelvic Organ Prolapse

Surgery aims to restore the anatomy of the vagina and pelvic floor, as well as sexual functions, and the correction of urinary and faecal incontinence. It is also essential to have it in mind to reduce and prevent recurrent and de novo prolapses, urinary and faecal incontinence.

Table 47.2 Pessary selection guide

Pessary	1st/2nd degree Prolapse	3rd degree Prolapse	SUI	Cystocoele	Rectocoele
Ring	√			√	
Ring with support	√		√		
Gellhorn standard		√		√	√
Gellhorn short		√		√	√
Shaatz	√			√	
Ring with knob	√	√	√	√	
Cube		√		√	√
Donut		√		√	√
Dish	√	√	√	√	
Dish with support	√		√	√	
Hodge	√			√	
Gehrung		√		√	√
Gehrung with knob		√	√	√	√
Inflatoball		√			
Shelf		√			

47.7.1 Anterior Repair

White described the paravaginal repair of cystocoele in 1909. Four years later, Kelly described the anterior vaginal repair with a central plication of pubo-cervical fascia using interrupted and absorbable sutures. Cautious trimming of excess vaginal skin is done by many but offers no advantage to a good plication. The vaginal is then closed with interrupted or continuous locking sutures. Conventional anterior repair is the most commonly performed operation for cystocoele and now looked upon as traditional repair. Permanent or absorbable meshes may be used for recurrent prolapses. De novo stress incontinence (5%) and de novo detrusor overactivity (5%) are known urinary complications of anterior repair [12].

47.7.2 Posterior Repair

This is the traditional way for the correction of rectocoele and deficient perineum. It is the meeting point of colorectal surgeons (trans-anal correction), and the gynaecologists (transvaginal or posterior repair). It involves levator plication, but recent reports of only fascial repair yielded about 80% success rate with fewer complications.

The procedure involves excision of any perineal scarring and the posterior vaginal wall opened. The rectocoele is mobilised from the vaginal epithelium by blunt and sharp dissection. The para-rectal and rectovaginal fasciae from each side are approximated using interrupted polyglycolic (Vicryl, Ethicon) sutures. The posterior wall is closed with continuous locked polyglycolic (Vicryl, Ethicon) sutures. Perineoplasty is done by placing deeper absorbable sutures into the perineal muscles and fascia.

47.8 Vaginal Hysterectomy

The conventional approach is vaginal hysterectomy with the additional repair of the vaginal walls. The first successful vaginal hysterectomy was credited to Langenback in 1813. The Moschowitz procedure (closure of the peritoneum of the cul-de-sac); McCall culdoplasty (approximating the utero-sacral ligaments to obliterate the peritoneum of the posterior cul-de-sac as high as possible) and suturing the cardinal and uterosacral ligaments to the vaginal cuff may also reduce subsequent enterocoele and vault prolapse [13, 14].

Manchester repair is no longer as popular as it used to be. Described in 1888 Archibald Donald. It is an alternative to vaginal hysterectomy for patients with uterine prolapse, although this may have been a more useful technique for patients with an elongated cervix rather than real uterine descent.

In 1966, Williams [15] described a technique for transvaginal uterosacral-cervical ligament plication. He reported on the outcomes of 20 women undergoing this procedure, with three 'failures' encountered within a 6-month follow-up period. His method involved a posterior colpotomy with the division of the uterosacral ligaments from the cervix. The ligaments are then plicated across the midline and reinsertion into the cervix. The cardinal ligaments are then plicated anteriorly across the midline.

Richardson [16] first described the concept of sacrospinous hysteropexy in 1989. The cervix or uterosacral ligament is transfixed to the sacrospinous ligament using either permanent or delayed absorbable sutures. In 2001, Maher [17] reported a small comparison study between sacrospinous hysteropexy and vaginal hysterectomy with sacrospinous vault fixation, with no differences in objective or subjective outcomes at follow-up. The technique of posterior vaginal slingplasty was first described in 2001 [18], using a mesh kit to create 'neo-uterosacral ligaments'. One prospective comparison study quoted a 91.4% patient satisfaction rate post-surgery, Conservation of the prolapsed uterus is a valid option: medium-term results of a prospective comparative study with cumulative data suggest a high incidence of mesh complications with up to a 21% mesh erosion rate [19].

47.9 Vaginal Vault Prolapse Surgeries

Sacrospinous fixation either unilateral (commonly on the right) or bilaterally (rarely performed) is the commonest surgery for treatment of vaginal vault prolapse. It involves the fixation of the vaginal vault to the sacrospinous ligament. It has a very high success rate, but surgery is done under limited visibility with the risk of injury to the pudendal nerves and vessels. The procedure was modified by Miya using a unique hook (Miya Hook) to attach stitch to the sacrospinous ligament. The stitch is then passed through the vaginal vault to attach it to the sacrospinous ligament. Recent advancement in surgical instrumentation has led to a new generation of stitching devices as Capio (Boston Scientific) Fixt (Bard) and I-Stitch (AMI). These have a significant advantage over the Miya hook, which requires more extensive dissection [1]. Success rates of 98% have been reported, but there is a small risk of cystocoele formation, urinary stress incontinence and post-operative dyspareunia.

Alternative fixation to the ileo-coccygeal ligament (ICF) is equally successful but has a lower satisfaction rate because of the higher incidence of cystocoeles.

Re-attachment of the vault to the pubo-cervical fascia, rectovaginal fascia, and uterosacral ligaments have also been described, but these operations are complicated and carry a high risk of injuries to ureters.

47.10 Abdominal Approach to POP Surgery

Several methods for open abdominal hysteropexy have been described, including transfixing the uterus to the anterior abdominal wall and ventral fixation to the pectineal ligaments. Most techniques use the sacral promontory as the fixation point, giving rise to the term 'abdominal sacrohysteropexy'. Abdominal suture sacrohysteropexy was described as early as 1957 [20], with the uterine fundus being fixed to the sacral promontory with silk sutures.

More recent techniques have utilised a variety of synthetic meshes to aid fixation. In 1993, Addison [21] first described a technique for resuspending the uterus to the sacrum using MersileneTM (Ethicon US, LLC USA) polyester fibre mesh. Leron and Stanton [22] followed-up 13 women undergoing abdominal sacrohysteropexy and found it to be a safe and effective surgery for the management of uterine prolapse. Farkas et al. [23] described a technique for uterine suspension using a 'wrap-around' insert of Gore-Tex (W.L. Gore & Associates, Inc., Newark, USA) for women with prolapse secondary to bladder exstrophy.

47.11 Laparoscopic Approach

The advantages of laparoscopic surgery are well documented. Several laparoscopic uterine suspension procedures have been described using different methods. Laparoscopic ventrosuspension involves suturing the round ligaments to the rectus sheath. It has been shown to have poor outcomes, with one case series of nine women reporting recurrent prolapse in all but one patient within 6 months [24]. Chen et al. [25] used mesh to suspend the uterus by attachment to the anterior abdominal wall. While they reported good outcomes, all patients experienced significant pain or dragging sensations over the mesh attachment site. Laparoscopic uterosacral ligament plication was first described by Wu et al. [26] in 1997, with excellent results in a small case series. Maher et al. [27] modified this technique to include re-attachment of the uterosacral ligaments to the cervix and closure of the pouch of Douglas, with an objective success rate of 79% in 43 women at 12 months. Recent techniques have focused on the use of the sacral promontory as a point of fixation. Krause et al. [28] carried out laparoscopic sacral suture hysteropexy, placing sutures through the posterior aspect of the cervix and transfixing to the sacral promontory via the right uterosacral ligament. Objective correction of prolapse was seen in 94% of patients at a mean of 20.3 months follow-up. Cutner et al. [29] developed the technique of laparoscopic uterine sling suspension. The peritoneum is opened over the sacral promontory, and the rectum is reflected laterally. A tunnel is created by blunt dissection underneath the peritoneum from the sacral promontory to the insertion of the uterosacral ligament complex into the cervix on either side. Mersilene tape on a needle is placed through the cervix, through the uterosacral ligaments and through the peritoneal tunnels on each side, before being bilaterally tacked to the sacral promontory to suspend the uterus. This technique aims for the sling to resemble newly created uterosacral ligaments. The laparoscopic polypropylene cervical en-cerclage hysteropexy was recently modified in Oxford. A method of complete cervical en-cerclage was developed using a bifurcated polypropylene mesh [30]. The technique involves using a 5 cm wide strip of polypropylene under the peritoneum and attached to the sacral promontory [31].

47.12 Controversies in Surgical Management of Pelvic Organ Prolapse

While vaginal hysterectomy has served patients and gynaecologists well for many years, its continued routine use has been subject to debate.

Many gynaecologists argue that the uterus itself is healthy and the underlying pathophysiology is a connective tissue deficiency [32], whether congenital or acquired through childbirth or ageing, and that uterine prolapse is merely a symptom, not the disease. Vaginal hysterectomy fails to address this underlying deficiency in connective tissue, with relatively high recurrence rates of 10–40% described in the literature [3, 33]. When there is a loss of apical support, a traditional vaginal hysterectomy will not correct the defect. This is most readily apparent when women present with procidentia. Furthermore, hysterectomy removes a healthy organ that may play a role in a woman's individual and sexual identity. Finally, the satisfaction rate of vaginal hysterectomy for prolapse are not significantly different from uterine preservation [34].

47.13 Use of Mesh in Surgical Repair of POP

Use of synthetic mesh is becoming increasingly common in urogynaecological practice. It does offer additional support to endopelvic fascia and vaginal epithelium. The ideal mesh (Type 1) should be durable and flexible, allowing ease of use, and should have an adequate pore size (>75 microns). This allows access to leucocytes and fibroblasts to control infection around it and also reduces the risk of rejection. Dyspareunia is often seen with synthetic meshes and may be associated with erosion into the vagina, lower urinary tract and rectum. The use of mesh should therefore be reserved for those with recurrent defects in specialist pelvic floor reconstructive surgery units.

The use of Type 1 mesh is well established and has common usage in sacrocolpopexy and mid-urethral slings. However, the medical community has become aware of some of the complications that have attracted high media attention. because of potential litigations. The use of mesh for prolapse and incontinence in gynaecology is now under intense scrutiny. This has been secondary to a realisation that vaginal mesh extrusion rates are higher than previously thought. Indeed, the use of transvaginal mesh for vaginal prolapse appears to have a relatively high complication rate, with mesh erosion reported in up to 10% of cases [35]. This is secondary to mesh lying adjacent to the vaginal wall that has been weakened by a surgical incision and subsequent scarring. With an abdominal approach, the mesh extrusion rate is considerably less, as the vaginal incision is avoided.

47.14 Conclusions

POP continues to afflict millions of women in sub-Saharan Africa, and as life expectancy increases, there is bound to be an increase in demand for treatment. POP, in many cases, arise as a consequence of carrying out biological functions. Managing POP is mainly by instituting relatively inexpensive measures – simple lifestyle modifications, pelvic floor exercise, use of vagina pessaries and surgical management. Although misconceptions and beliefs of women arise in developing countries about the aetiology of POP, ignorance and the poor help-seeking behaviour of women suffering from POP are well documented. The problem is compounded by a dearth of professionals, lack of resources and political will to fund health education and research in this area. With renewed interest in women's health in the sustainable development goal, continued local and national efforts to partner with patient, healthcare planners and providers, pelvic organ prolapse on women in the sub-Saharan Africa will receive the attention it deserves.

References

1. Ajayi OA, Chilaka VN. Preventing pelvic floor dysfunction. In: Okonofua F, editor. Confronting the challenge of reproductive health in Africa: a textbook for students and development practitioners. Boca Raton: BrownWalker; 2014. p. 423–38.
2. Wu JM, Hundley AF, Fulton RG, Myers ER. Forecasting the prevalence of pelvic floor disorders in U.S. Women: 2010 to 2050. Obstet Gynecol. 2009;114(6):1278.
3. Versi E, Harvey MA, Cardozo L, Brincat M, Studd JW. Urogenital prolapse and atrophy at menopause: a prevalence study. Int Urogynecol J Pelvic Floor Dysfunct. 2001;12(2):107–10. https://doi.org/10.1007/s001920170074.
4. Marchionni M, Bracco GL, Checcucci V, Carabaneanu A, Coccia EM, Mecacci F, Scarselli G. True incidence of vaginal vault prolapse. Thirteen years of experience. J Reprod Med. 1999;44(8):679–84. PMID: 10483537.

5. Marchionni M, Bracco GL, Checcucci V, Carabaneanu A, Coccia EM, Mecacci F, et al. True incidence of vaginal vault prolapse. Thirteen years' experience. J Reprod Med. 1999;44:679–84.
6. Bump RC, Mattiasson A, Bo K, et al. The standardisation of terminology of female pelvic organ prolapse and pelvic floor dysfunction. Am J Obstetr Gynaecol. 1996;175:10–7. https://doi.org/10.1016/s0002-9378(96)70243-0.
7. Luber KM, Boero S, Choe JY. The demographics of pelvic floor disorders: current observations and future projections. Am J Obstet Gynecol. 2001;184(7):1496–501.
8. Olsen AL, Smith VJ, Bergstrom JO, Colling JC, Clark AL. Epidemiology of surgically managed pelvic organ prolapse and urinary incontinence. Obstet Gynecol. 1997;89(4):501–6.
9. Dongen V. The anatomy of genital prolapse. S Afr Med J. 1981;60(9):357–9.
10. Abrams P, Artibani W, Cardozo L, Khoury S, Wein A, editors. Clinical manual of incontinence in women. Health Publications Ltd; Paris. 2005.
11. Hagen S, Stark D, Glazener C, Dickson S, Barry S, Elders A, et al. Individualised pelvic floor muscle training in women with pelvic organ prolapse (POPPY): a multicentre randomised controlled trial. Lancet. 2014;383:796–806.
12. Smith A. Pelvic floor dysfunction I: Uterovaginal prolapse. Urinary incontinence. Chapter 49. In: Edmonds K, editor. Dewhurst's textbook of obstetrics and gynaecology. 7th ed. Blackwell Publishing; Oxford United Kingdom. 2007.
13. Cruikshank SH, Kovac SR. Randomised comparison of three surgical methods used at the time of vaginal hysterectomy to prevent posterior enterocele. Am J Obstet Gynecol. 1999;180:859–65.
14. Cruikshank SH. Preventing post-hysterectomy vaginal vault prolapse and enterocele during vaginal hysterectomy. Am J Obstet Gynecol. 1987;155:1433–40.
15. Williams BFP. Surgical treatment for uterine prolapse in young women. AmJ Obstet Gynaecol. 1966;95:967–71.
16. Richardson DA, Scotti RJ, Ostergard DR. Surgical management of uterine prolapse in young women. J Reprod Med. 1989;34:388–92.
17. Maher CF, Cary MP, Slack CJ, Murray CJ, Milligan M, Schluter P. Uterine preservation or hysterectomy at sacrospinous colpopexy for uterovaginal prolapse? Int Urogynecol J. 2001;12:381–4.
18. Petros PE. Vault prolapse II: restoration of dynamic vaginal supports by infracoccygeal sacropexy, an axial day-case vaginal procedure. Int Urogynecol J Pelvic Floor Dysfunct. 2001;12:296–303.
19. Dietz V, Schraffordt Koops SE, van der Vaart CH. Vaginal surgery for uterine descent; which options do we have? A review of the literature. Int Urogynecol J Pelvic Floor Dysfunct. 2009;20:349–56.
20. Arthure HG, Savage D. Uterine prolapse and prolapse of the vaginal vault treated by sacral hysteropexy. J Obstet Gynaecol Br Emp. 1957;64:355–60.
21. Addison WA, Timmons MC. Abdominal approach to vaginal eversion. Clin Obstet Gynecol. 1993;36:995–1004.
22. Leron E, Stanton SL. Sacrohysteropexy with synthetic mesh for the management of uterovaginal prolapse. BJOG. 2011;108:629–33.
23. Farkas AG, Shepherd JH, Woodhouse CRJ. Hysterosacropexy for uterine prolapse with associated urinary tract abnormalities. J Obstet Gynaecol. 1993;13:358–60.
24. O'Brien PM, Ibrahim J. Failure of laparoscopic uterine suspension to provide a lasting cure for uterovaginal prolapse. Br J Obstet Gynaecol. 1994;101:707–8.
25. Chen G, Wu D, Zhao W. Modified laparoscopic extraperitoneal uterine suspension to the anterior abdominal wall: the easier way to treat uterine prolapse. Int Urogynecol J. 2012;23:887–91.
26. Wu MP. Laparoscopic uterine suspension for the treatment of uterovaginal prolapse. Int J Gynaecol Obstet. 1997;59:259–60.
27. Maher CF, Carey MP, Murray CJ. Laparoscopic suture hysteropexy for uterine prolapse. Obstet Gynecol. 2001;97:1010–4.
28. Krause HG, Goh JT, Sloane K, Higgs P, Carey MP. Laparoscopic sacral suture hysteropexy for uterine prolapse. Int Urogynecol J Pelvic Floor Dysfunct. 2006;17:378–81.
29. Cutner A, Kearney R, Vashisht A. Laparoscopic uterine sling suspension: a new technique of uterine suspension in women desiring surgical management of uterine prolapse with uterine conservation. BJOG. 2007;114:1159–62.
30. Price N, Slack A, Jackson SR. Laparoscopic hysteropexy: the initial results of a uterine suspension procedure for uterovaginal prolapse. BJOG. 2010;117:62–8.
31. Jefferis H, Jackson SR, Price N. Management of uterine prolapse: is hysterectomy necessary? Obstetr Gynaecol. 2016;18:17–23. https://doi.org/10.1111/tog.12220.
32. Jackson SR, Avery NC, Tarlton JF, Eckford SD, Abrams P, Bailey AJ. Changes in metabolism of collagen in genitourinary prolapse. Lancet. 1996;347:1658–61.
33. Symmonds R, Williams T, Lee R, Webb M. Post hysterectomy enterocele and vaginal vault prolapse. Am J Obstet Gynecol. 1981;140:852.
34. Roovers JP, van der Vaart CH, van der Bom JG, van Leeuwen JH, Scholten PC, Heintz AP. A randomised controlled trial comparing abdominal and vaginal prolapse surgery: effects on urogenital function. BJOG. 2004;111:50–6.
35. Maher CM, Feiner B, Baessler K, Glazener CM. Surgical management of pelvic organ prolapse in women: the updated summary version Cochrane review. Int Urogynecol J. 2011;22:1445–57.

Urogynaecology

48

Victor N. Chilaka, Olukunle Ajayi, and Tarek Elshamy

Learning Objectives

By the end of the chapter, the reader should be able to:

- Define urinary incontinence and appreciate the prevalence and importance of the condition and the impact on affected patients
- Obtain a basic understanding of the neurological connections that are essential for the control of micturition
- Appreciate the signs and symptoms of urinary incontinence and be able to make the clinically assess patients with the condition and investigate them appropriately
- Obtain a basic idea of multichannel urodynamics and be able to read and understand a urodynamics chat
- Understand the principles of diagnosis for the commonest causes of urinary incontinence (USI) and DO and be able recommend initial management in these conditions
- Have a choice of drugs in the management of incontinence
- Understand the limitations of pelvic floor exercises and surgery for incontinence
- Understand the surgical steps in the management of and appreciate the major limitations of these procedures and be able to counsel patients on surgical complications
- Understand his limits and know when to refer patients with challenging conditions

48.1 Urinary Incontinence

Urinary incontinence is defined as involuntary loss of urine [1]. It is a prevalent condition in women of all ages, and the prevalence tends to increase with age. It occurs in approximately 25% in young women (aged 14–21 years) [2], 44–57% in middle-aged and post-menopausal women (aged 40–60 years) [3], and 75% in elderly women (aged ≥75 years) [4] At least, a third of females over the age of 35 years do experience urinary incontinence twice or more in a month [5]. In psychogeriatric hospital wards, the incidence may be as high as 91% [6]. The Market Opinion Research Institute (MORI) poll in 1991 indicated that in the United Kingdom, 3.5 million women suffer from incontinence [7]. About 50–75% of sufferers do not seek advice for various reasons. Such reasons include not recognising the condition as abnormal or considering it a minor inconvenience, while others feel either too embarrassed to talk about urinary incontinence or feel that nothing can be done about it [8, 9]. If this poor reporting is taken into consideration, the number of sufferers in the United Kingdom could be closer to ten million.

The enormity of the problem reflects the estimated national cost of urinary incontinence in the US in 2007 at $65.9 billion, with projected costs of $76.2 billion in 2015 and $82.6 billion in 2020 [10]. The prevalence of urinary incontinence is probably about the same all over the world and depends on such characteristics as age, beliefs, culture, tradition, and educational background of the population (Table 48.1).

Clinical experience suggests racial differences in the prevalence of incontinence, but very little epidemiological data are available to support the observation, as data from the tropics are scanty [18]. In a recent study, of a mixed American population, Bump [19] noted that Urodynamic Stress Incontinence (USI) was 2.3 times commoner in Whites than in Blacks while Detrusor Overactivity (DO) was twice as common in Blacks than in Whites. Similarly, Peacock et al. [20] reported a higher prevalence of DO in Blacks compared

V. N. Chilaka (✉)
Women's Wellness and Research Centre, Hamad Medical Corporation, Doha, Qatar

O. Ajayi
York Teaching Hospital NHS, East Riding Hospital, and Scarborough Hospital, York, UK

T. Elshamy
West Middlesex University Hospital, London, UK
e-mail: tarek.elshamy@nhs.net

F. Okonofua et al. (eds.), *Contemporary Obstetrics and Gynecology for Developing Countries*,
https://doi.org/10.1007/978-3-030-75385-6_48

Table 48.1 Prevalence of urinary incontinence

Source and country	Number(n)	Incontinence (%)	Patient population
MORI (1991), UK [7]	2980	14	Population survey 30–70+ years
Harrison and Memel (1994) UK [11]	314	53.2	Epidemiological survey 20–80 years
Samuelsson et al. (1997) Sweden [12]	491	27.7	Population survey 20–59 years
Turan et al. (1996) Turkey [13]	1250	24.5	Epidemiological survey 18–44 years
Nygard & Lemke (1996) USA [14]	2025	55.1	Cohort study 65+ years
Thomas et al. (1980) UK [5]	20,000 (Approx.)	8.5 11.6	Epidemiological survey 15–64 years 65+ years
Diokono et al. (1986, MESA Study) [15]	1145	37.6	Population survey 60+ years
Nemir & Middleton (1954) USA [16]	1327	52	Epidemiological survey Nulliparous American students
Brocklehurst et al. (1972) UK [17]	454	57	General practice survey 45–64 years

with the white population studies, which showed a higher prevalence of USI.

The reasons for these racial differences are not clear. In trying to find an explanation for them, Knobel [21] compared various measures of lower urinary tract functions in Indians and Blacks in South Africa. He concluded that Blacks had bladder necks that were higher in the pelvis and closer to the inferior border of the symphysis pubis, urethras that were longer with higher resting pressures, and pelvic floor muscles that were more contractile than those of the Indians. More work is required to identify the reasons for the observed racial differences.

Urogynaecology is a rapidly developing subspecialty. This development has followed detailed basic science research into the structure and functions of the urothelium and bladder wall. Control of detrusor muscle and bladder neck has been studied at molecular level [22]. Advanced imaging techniques (X-rays, MRI) in combination with video-recording has led to a more and in-depth understanding of the complex and dynamic structure and functions of the lower urinary tract [23, 24]. Results of long-term follow-up of different surgical techniques are becoming available [25], [26]. New techniques and new drugs are being tried, and minimally invasive surgical techniques are being used more than ever before in this area [26].

It is common knowledge to gynaecologists in many developing countries that urogynaecology is under-practised, except in the area of obstetric vesicovaginal fistula. This does not imply that other causes of incontinence do not exist, but they have probably given a much lower priority. Emphasis is still on more acute and life-threatening conditions like infections and infestations, vesicovaginal fistulas, prevention of maternal deaths, improving foetal and child survival and other acute conditions. However, with improving standards of living, and education, there is no doubt that the demands on urogynaecological services will begin to expand.

48.1.1 Functional Physiology of the Lower Urinary Tract

The bladder functions as a low-pressure reservoir for the temporary storage of urine until socially convenient voiding is achieved. Urine continuously enters the bladder at the rate of between 2.5 and 5 ml/min, and the first sensation of bladder filling and a strong desire to void usually felt at about half and three-quarters of cystometric capacity, respectively. During physiological filling, the intravesical pressure changes minimally and usually does not exceed 15 cm of water at full capacity.

As the bladder fills, the stretch receptors in its wall pass impulses through the pelvic plexus to the S2–4 segment of the spinal cord through the visceral afferent fibres in the pelvic splanchnic nerves. These impulses ascend the cord through the lateral spinothalamic tracts and are mediated by both excitatory and inhibitory centres higher up in the central nervous system (Fig. 48.1). During this phase, the sympathetic control of the striated urethral sphincter as well as the pudendal motor neurons is activated by the vesical afferent input, whereas during micturition, motor neurons are reciprocally inhibited [27]. The basal ganglia subconsciously inhibit the reflex arc in the early phase, but as filling continues, the sensation is brought to the consciousness of the cerebral cortex and the first sensation to void is appreciated. Further bladder filling reinforces these afferent impulses, and cortical inhibition of micturition is maintained until a convenient voiding is achieved. Micturition is mediated by the activation of the sacral parasympathetic efferent pathway to the bladder, and reciprocal inhibition of the somatic pathway to the urethral sphincter. The result is a fall of the urethral pressure, which occurs prior to an increase in the bladder pressure. Once micturition is initiated, the intravesical pressure remains constant for the rest of the act. At the end of voiding, the pelvic floor and the intrinsic striated muscles of the urethra contract and any urine which is left in the proximal urethra is milked back into the bladder. After this, the subconscious inhibition of micturition is re-established.

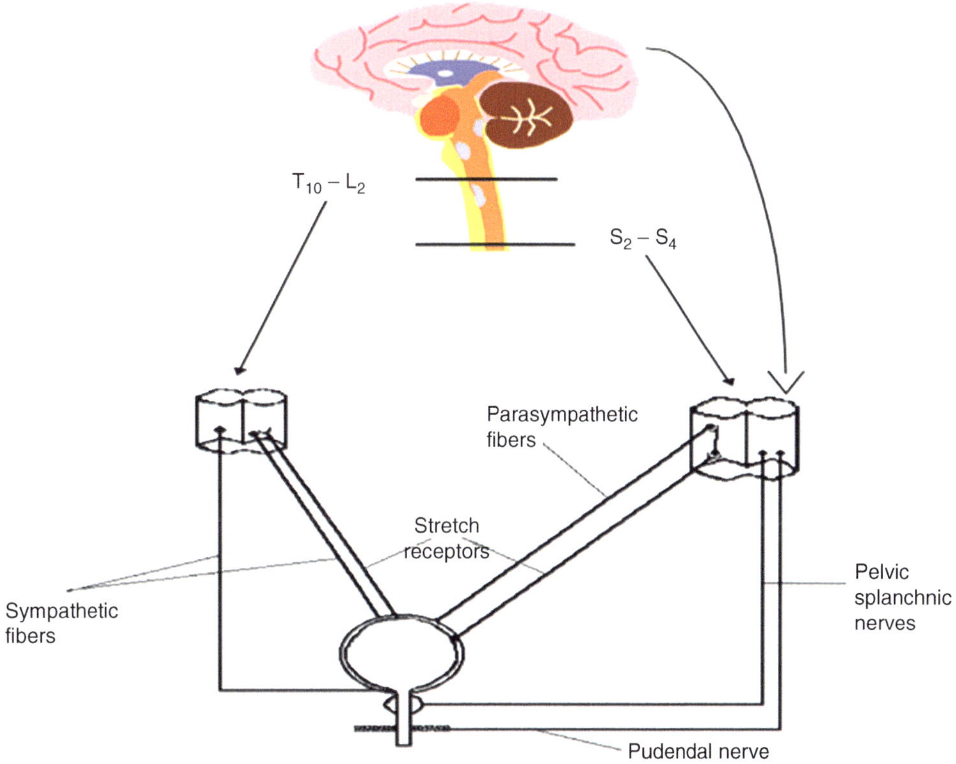

Fig. 48.1 Control and innervation of the lower urinary tract

48.1.2 Pathophysiology of Urinary Incontinence

For the maintenance of urinary continence, the urethral pressure (Pura) must always exceed the intravesical pressure (Pves) [28]. The source of Pura seems to result from a group of interrelated but separate mechanisms involving the hermetic seal of the proximal urethra achieved by the innate softness of its walls, inner urethral compression and outer urethral wall tension [29]. If the balance is lost, incontinence results and this could be due to:

(i). Weakened urethral sphincter mechanism (urodynamic stress incontinence – USI)
(ii). Excessive detrusor pressure (detrusor overactivity – DO)
(iii). Combination of (i) and (ii)

Various factors have been associated with the incompetence of the urethral sphincter mechanism. The weakening of the pubourethral ligament and damage to the pelvic floor musculature (levator ani) may lead to bladder neck displacement. The proximal urethra is intra-abdominal, supported above the pelvic floor by the pubourethral ligament. Increases in intra-abdominal pressures are transmitted to the proximal urethra, and this reinforces the positive urethral closure pressure (Fig. 48.2). This anatomical advantage is lost when there has been a descent of the bladder neck through the pelvic floor. In USI, pressure transmission to the proximal urethra tends to fall or collapse after a series of coughs [30].

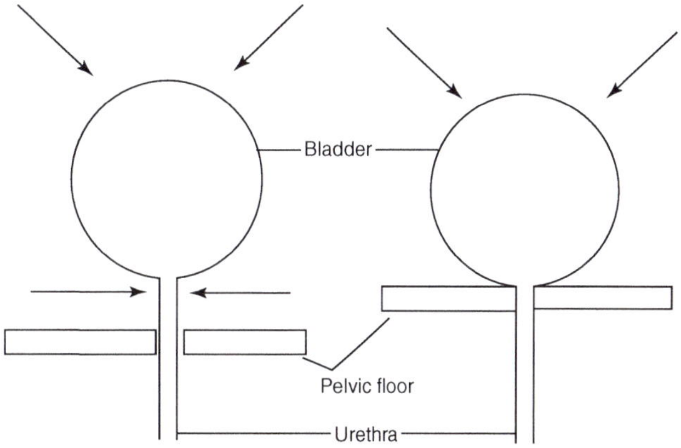

Fig. 48.2 Effect of bladder neck displacement on the continence mechanism

Parturition causes denervation and weakening of the pelvic floor, with the most damage inflicted by long active second stage [31]. Other factors include oestrogen deficiency (menopause, ovarian ablation), urethral scarring (surgery, recurrent urethritis, radiotherapy amongst others) and chronic elevation of intra-abdominal pressure (obesity, ascites, chronic cough and abdominal masses).

A weak sphincter at rest might be able to maintain a positive urethral closure pressure but becomes overwhelmed during increases in intra-abdominal pressure.

In detrusor overactivity, abnormal detrusor contractions occur spontaneously at rest or during the filling phase to overwhelm a normal maximum urethral pressure and cause leakage of urine. A poorly compliant bladder generates high detrusor pressures during bladder filling (Table 48.2).

48.2 Clinical Presentation

In developing countries with limited resources for investigations, a detailed history and examination are essential. Unfortunately, the bladder is an unreliable witness with a weak correlation between clinical presentation and urodynamic diagnosis [32]. The precise nature of the patients' symptoms should be characterised and quantified as accurately as possible. It is a common feature that most patients presenting for assessment will have a mixture of symptoms [33]. When this is the case, the patients' assessment of the relative severity of each symptom should be carefully noted.

The usual presenting symptoms of lower urinary tract dysfunction include:

(a) Incontinence
(b) Sensory-motor complaints (urgency, frequency, dysuria, hesitancy, enuresis, etc.)
(c) Voiding difficulties (hesitancy, weak or intermittent urinary stream)

Stress incontinence is, however, the most common symptom presented by patients [11–13]. It is essential to identify the factors associated with it, for example, sneezing, coughing, running, walking bending, rising, aerobics, etc. It is also important to note whether a few drops are lost at a time or uncontrollable voiding occurs. Urge incontinence is described as incontinence resulting from overwhelming urgency and is more associated with detrusor overactivity. Incontinence may also be associated with exposure to the cold, the sound of running water, etc. Evidence of existing or childhood nocturnal enuresis should also be sought.

Table 48.2 Aetiologic classification of urinary incontinence

Urodynamic stress incontinence (USI)
Detrusor overactivity (DO)
Overflow incontinence
Neurological, obstructive
Urethral diverticulum
Abnormal urinary openings
Congenital
Acquired, for example
Vesicovagina fistula, malignancies, radiotherapy, surgical trauma
Neuropathic incontinence
Spina bifida, cord injury, multiple sclerosis
Diabetic neuropathy
Miscellaneous
Functional incontinence, for example, mental ill health, age
Temporary, for example, urinary tract infections, faecal impaction, loss of mobility

Urinary frequency can be reactive or irritative. Incontinent patients soon learn that keeping their bladders empty temporarily relieves the symptom. The desire to keep the bladder empty, fluid intake and the emotional state of the patient affect the daytime frequency so much that nocturia is a better measure of irritation primarily when there is associated dysuria, haematuria or low abdominal pain. Difficulty in initiating voiding (hesitancy), reduced or intermittent urinary stream, recurrent attacks of urinary tract infection, or a history of urinary retention could point to voiding difficulties. Post-micturition dribbling is commonly seen with urethral diverticulum.

Urine loss may be subjectively quantified by assessing the amount of sanitary protection (pads or devices) used per day, and how frequently these are changed. As with menstrual loss, there is a wide margin of error with patients' self-quantification of urine loss, and objective assessment is important [33]. It is however essential to assess how their social life has been affected by incontinence. Drinking habits should also be noted, taking into account the high insensible water loss in the tropics.

A full obstetrics, gynaecological and medical history is essential as many of these women do not get frequent opportunities for medical consultation. Multiparity, which is common in the tropics, has a well-recognised association with stress incontinence [34]. Also, uterine fibroids, which are much commoner in Blacks [35], can compress the bladder and cause urinary frequency and urgency [36]. The symptoms of genital prolapse (pressure, protrusion and pain) should be asked.

Particular emphasis should be laid on the bowel and neurological functions. Urinary incontinence may be the first manifestation of a neurological problem, for example, multiple sclerosis, or polyneuropathies [37] Tropical myeloneuropathies, which include tropical ataxic neuropathy and tropical spastic paraparesis, are common and doctors should be conscious of their local prevalence. These disorders occur in geographic isolates in several developing countries and are associated with malnutrition, cyanide intoxication from cassava consumption, tropical malabsorption, vegetarian diets and lathyrism [38]. Drugs such as diuretics may increase urine output and cause frequency and urgency. Other drugs as β-blockers, antidepressants, and major tranquilisers can also affect detrusor functions (Table 48.3).

Clinical examination should consist of a full assessment of all the systems again with particular emphasis on the mental state, neurological and urinary systems. The demeanour, gait and mobility should be observed as the patient enters the room. The chest should be examined for signs of chronic chest conditions, and the abdomen for a distended bladder, organomegalies and hernias. On pelvic examination, atrophic changes may point to oestrogen deficiency, while excoriation

Table 48.3 Medications that can worsen urinary incontinence

Medication	Potential and/or actual effect
α-Adrenoceptor antagonists	Reduce smooth muscle tone in the urethra and can cause stress incontinence in women
Angiotensin-converting enzyme inhibitors	Cause cough that can worsen stress incontinence
Agents with antimuscarinic properties	Reduce bladder and bowel tone and cause ineffective voiding and constipation. Some do cause cognitive impairment and reduce effective toileting ability (high dose, if cognitively at risk)
Calcium channel blockers	May cause constipation (verapamil) that can contribute to incontinence. Can cause dependent oedema (amlodipine, nifedipine), and contribute to nocturnal polyuria
Cholinesterase inhibitors	Can cause urge incontinence through cholinergic action
Diuretics	Diuresis urinary urgency and incontinence
Lithium	Can cause polyuria due to a diabetes insipidus-like state
Opioid analgesics	Can cause constipation, confusion, and immobility e all of which can contribute to incontinence
Psychotropic drugs	Can cause confusion, impaired mobility and incontinence
Sedatives, hypnotics, antipsychotics Histamine-1 receptor antagonists	Most have anticholinergic effects
Selective serotonin reuptake inhibitors (sertraline identified)	Increase cholinergic transmission and can lead to urgency UI
Gabapentin Non-steroidal anti-inflammatory agents	Can cause oedema, lead to polyuria while supine and worsen nocturnal polyuria and night-time incontinence
Glitazones	Can lead to an osmotic diuresis and predispose to incontinence and perhaps urinary tract infection

may indicate long-standing incontinence. Objective demonstration of incontinence will confirm the patient's story but is not diagnostic of any condition. Pelvic organ prolapses should be looked for, and the uterus and adnexae examined carefully. If a neurological lesion is suspected, the cranial nerves and sacral nerve roots S2–4 should be examined. The sacral dermatomes are evaluated by assessing the anal sphincter tone and control, peri-anal sensations, and the bulbocavernosus reflex [39] . It is important to note that this reflex is not detected in up to 30% of otherwise healthy women [40].

48.3 Investigations

The importance of investigations cannot be overemphasised as it has been demonstrated that there is always a margin of error when the final urodynamic diagnosis is compared with clinical evaluation no matter how accurate the latter is. In a meta-analysis involving 19 articles from 29 studies and 6042 patients (USI – 3092, DO – 2950), Jensen et al. [43], 52 studies found a weak correlation between clinical history and eventual urodynamic diagnosis (Table 48.4). Using a standard Gaudenz-Incontinence-Questionnaire on 1938 patients, Haeusler et al. [41] revealed that the sensitivity and specificity of clinical evaluation in diagnosing USI were 0.559 and 0.447, respectively, and 0.615 and 0.563 for DO. In another small series, Ng et al. [42], as part of an audit, carried out urodynamic studies on patients who were ready for treatment after a full clinical evaluation and changed the intended management in 21% of cases.

Table 48.4 History and diagnosis of stress incontinence

History consistent with ↓	Sensitivity	Specificity	Positive Pr. value	Negative Pr. value
USI	0.906	0.511	0.749	0.711
DO	0.735	0.552	0.561	0.728

Adapted from Jensen et al. [43]

Table 48.5 Investigation of female urinary incontinence

General investigations:	Midstream urine (for culture and sensitivity)
	Frequency volume chart
	Pad weighing
Basic urodynamics	Uroflowmetry
	Cystometry
	(Video) Cystourethrography
Specialised tests	
	Urethral pressure profilometry (resting/stress)
	Vaginal ultrasonography
	Intravenous urography
	Micturition cystography
	Electromyography
	Sacral nerve studies
	Urethral electrical conductance
	Cystourethroscopy

A large number of tests (Table 48.5) are available for a full evaluation of incontinent patients. Even in developed countries, the full range of tests is available only in specialised urogynaecology centres. A sensible choice of tests depending on the circumstances of the patient is, therefore, desirable.

A midstream specimen of urine should always be sent for culture and sensitivity, and any urinary tract infection (UTI) is treated before considering any other form of investigations. Apart from contributing to the irritative symptoms, instrumentation in the presence of UTI can affect the outcome of the assessments and precipitate generalised sepsis. The frequency volume chart provides beneficial information but requires some level of literacy, and its use should be encouraged in selected cases. The pad-weighing test after a series of standard exercises [44, 45] is also beneficial but should be interpreted with caution considering the faster rates of evaporation and perspiration in the tropical environment. A supervised 1e-hour test will probably be more reliable than the 24- and 48-hour tests.

Urodynamic studies refer to a series of tests employed to determine the functions of the lower urinary tract as it performs its dynamic functions of urine collection, storage and voiding. Observed urine loss during multichannel urodynamics is the best diagnostic test for incontinence [46].

In a standard subtracted cystometrogram (Fig. 48.3), a filling line and pressure transducer are inserted into the bladder, and another pressure transducer is inserted into the rectum (or vagina) to record the intra-abdominal pressure. The transducer in the bladder measures the total bladder pressure (P_1), which is the sum of the detrusor, and intra-abdominal pressures, while the rectal/vaginal transducer measures only the intra-abdominal pressure (P_2). The detrusor pressure (P_{det}) is calculated by subtracting P_2 from P_1 [47]. The bladder is usually filled with physiological saline at body temperature. When the patient is filled to capacity, the filling line is removed, and she is asked to cough in the supine sitting and standing positions, and at times heel-bounce while observing for incontinence. The patient then sits and waits for a short time, while water is run to her hearing. Her hands may be immersed in cold water while observing for detrusor contractions. At the end of the test, she is asked to empty her bladder with pressure transducers in situ. After achieving a steady stream, she may be asked to interrupt her urinary stream, and the resulting rise in detrusor pressure (isometric detrusor contraction) is noted. A normal urodynamics tracing is shown in Fig. 48.4.

During cystometry, the following pieces of information should be available:

1. Free flow voiding rate (peak flow rate of up to and above 15 ml/s)
2. Post voiding residual volume (usually less than 50 ml)
3. The sensation of first desire to void (50% cystometric capacity)
4. The sensation of a strong desire to void (75% cystometric capacity)
5. Cystometric capacity (400–600 ml)
6. A rise in detrusor pressure with or without leakage:
   - Gradual rise of more than 15 cm of water (non-compliant)
   - Systolic detrusor contractions (instability)
7. Opening detrusor pressure (pressure at the onset of urine flow)
8. Voiding pressure (usually less than 60 cm of water)
9. Peak or isometric detrusor contraction pressure
10. After-contractions (of doubtful significance)

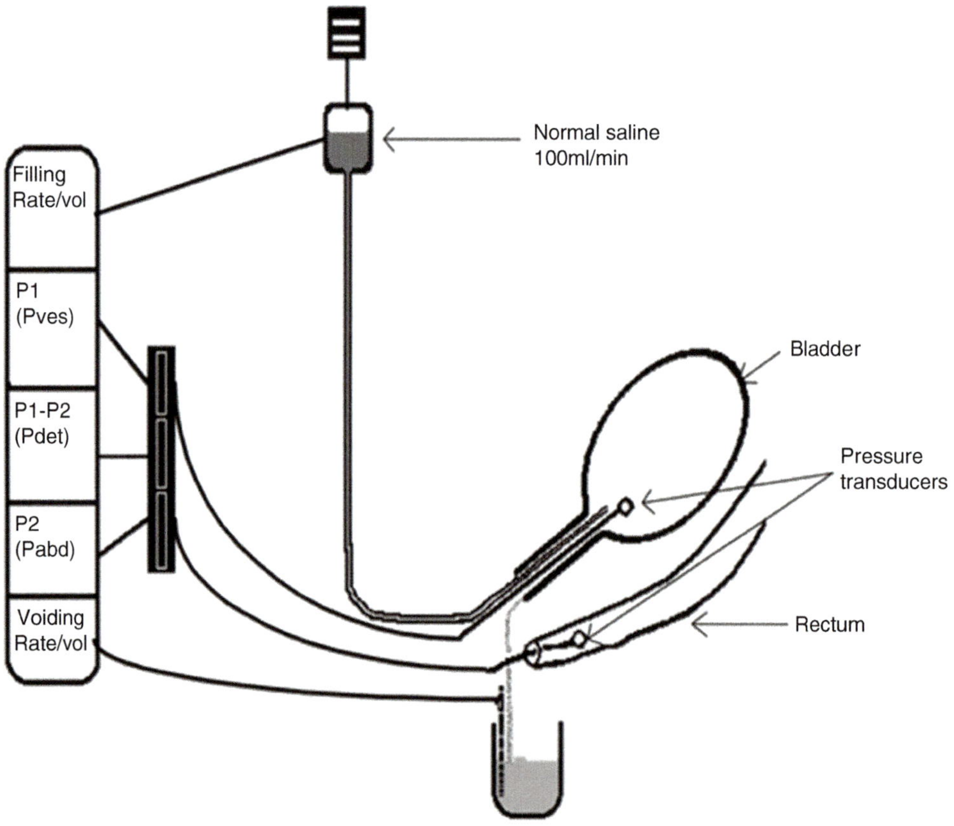

Fig. 48.3 Set up of dual channel cystometry

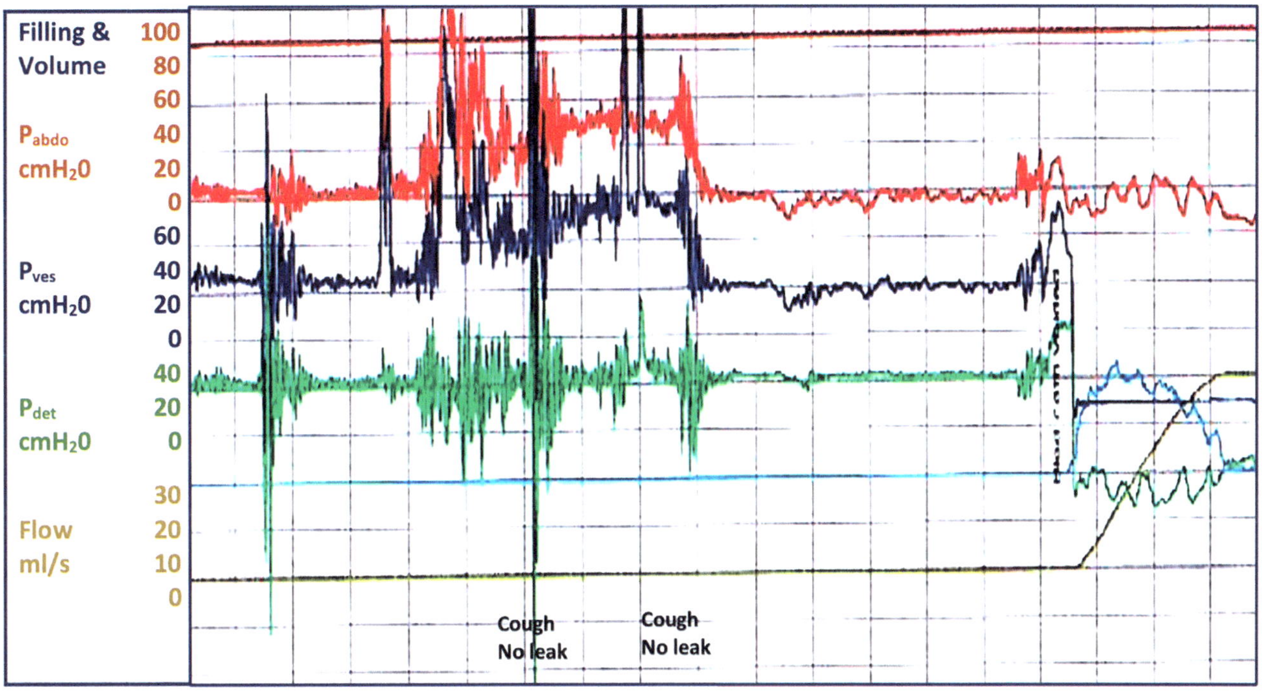

Fig. 48.4 Normal urodynamics trace

Uroflowmetry is the measurement of urine flow, and when done in conjunction with detrusor pressure recording, it is very informative. The urine peak flow rate should be at least 15 ml/s if a volume of up to 150 ml is voided. A low flow rate with high detrusor pressure may imply obstruction while with low or normal pressure becomes more difficult to interpret. It may be secondary to detrusor hypotonia, poor motor coordination, etc. Patients with a preoperative poor flow rate seem more likely to develop post-operative voiding difficulties.

Videocystourethrography (VCU) combines cystometry, uroflowmetry and radiological real-time observation of the bladder and urethra [48]. It is the most informative urodynamic investigation but expensive and time-consuming [49]. It will objectively demonstrate the extent of bladder neck descent, and leakage of contrast into the urethra during stress. It will also reveal bony abnormalities, abnormal bladder morphology, vesicoureteric reflux, trabeculation, vesicovaginal fistulas, and bladder or urethral diverticulae. All the information can be recorded on video for reference. VCU is particularly useful in patients in whom previous incontinence procedures have failed, and when there are mixed, unusual, or neurological problems [50].

Other specialised investigations include urethral pressure profilometry (UPP). Important information that can be derived from this includes the maximal urethral closure pressure, functional urethral length, pressure transmission ratio (the increment in urethral pressure on stress as a percentage of the simultaneously recorded increment in intravesical pressure), urethral instability and relaxation [28]. UPP is not essential in making the diagnosis of USI [51], but helpful in failed incontinence surgery and voiding disorders [50].

Micturition cystography has been replaced mainly by VCU. It can still be used to diagnose anatomical problems as fistulas, tumours, foreign bodies, bladder and urethral diverticulae. Intravenous urography (IVU) is essential in cases of recurrent urinary tract infections, haematuria, voiding difficulties and vesicourethral reflux. It will also help with the diagnosis of ureteric fistula, renal tumours and calculi.

Ultrasonography has become very useful in investigating the lower and upper urinary tracts. In the lower urinary tract, it can be used to measure the bladder capacity and to estimate residual volumes. Vaginal probes have been used to visualise detrusor contractions [52] while rectal and perineal probes have been used to examine the mobility and anatomy of the bladder neck and urethra [53, 54]. Ultrasound is, however, no match to urodynamic investigations which examine the dynamic functions rather than the morphology of the lower urinary tract. Magnetic resonance imaging (MRI) has also contributed a lot to the understanding of the anatomy and morphology of the lower urinary tract [55], but its place if any in routine investigations is still not decided.

Electromyography, which is employed to assess the integrity of nerve supply to a muscle, is not of much use in the routine evaluation of patients with uncomplicated incontinence. It may, however, be useful in cases with suspected neurological anomalies, voiding problems and urinary retention. Recently, sacral nerve assessment and stimulation has become an essential pre-assessment procedure in patients who are being considered for sacral nerve implantation for the treatment of intractable detrusor overactivity [56]. Urethral electrical conductance measures the passage of urine along the urethra by registering the change in conductivity as different conductivity patterns are associated with different urodynamic diagnoses, although equivocal results have been observed [57, 58].

Urodynamic studies are done in unfamiliar surroundings, in the presence of unfamiliar people and with unfamiliar objects in the urinary tract. The tests are not strictly physiological and at times, can be invasive. In order to approach physiological standards, ambulatory urodynamics has been introduced [59] but has not yet become part of routine assessment of the incontinent patient.

Cystourethroscopy is essential when there is haematuria, recurrent urinary tract infections, or when there are persistent sensory symptoms with normal urodynamic findings. Abnormalities such as tumours, papillomas, ulcers and inflammatory changes of infections or interstitial cystitis may be seen. Biopsies can then be taken to ascertain the diagnosis.

48.3.1 Management of Urinary Incontinence

In the tropics and developing countries, it is absolutely essential that the limited resources for investigations and treatment be carefully used to achieve the best possible results. The principle should be a detailed history and right choice of essential investigations, starting with the most affordable ones. Every patient should have midstream urine analysed. A simple dipstick should be done on all women with lower urinary tract symptoms (LUTS), and if there is a suspicion of infection a sample should be sent for microscopy, culture and sensitivity, and infections treated. Cystometry and uroflowmetry should then be considered if the facilities are available, and if not, the weight of the symptoms will have to be taken into consideration to initiate reasonable treatment. Unfortunately, most patients will present with mixed symptoms. USI and DO are the most prevalent causes of urinary incontinence, and 56% of black incontinent patients may have a mixed picture [17, 60]. However, those with overwhelmingly stress symptoms can be started on available forms of pelvic floor physiotherapy, while others with primarily sensory symptoms of frequency, urgency and urge incontinence can be started on bladder re-training and behaviour modification techniques. It may be worthwhile to start conservative management for both conditions in patients with mixed symptoms if urodynamics is not available. Bladder re-training or short therapeutic trial with anticholinergic drugs (e.g. oxybutynin tolterodine solifenacin, etc.) might be an essential diagnostic step in those with mainly sensory symptoms. If any form of surgical management is being considered, simple cystometry with uroflowmetry should be considered [61].

48.3.2 General Measures

A good standard of living with proper health education can prevent or limit the effects of urinary incontinence. Information dissemination on incontinence is very poor in most developing countries. Discussing urinary incontinence can be embarrassing to the women. Health education issues on the subject and the concept of pelvic floor exercises should be introduced as early in life as possible and intensified during the childbearing years. Very good care of the second stage of labour is also critical to avoid over-stretching hence damage and denervation of the pelvic floor.

Women with chronic constipation and chest infections (chronic bronchitis, tuberculosis and other causes of raised Intra-abdominal pressure) should be treated adequately. Stress incontinence is very troublesome with chronic cough, and surgery can be dangerous with a poor outcome. Overweight patients should be encouraged to lose weight, and smoking discouraged. The place of oestrogen replacement therapy remains equivocal [62, 63] and very few women in the developing countries receive it. There is as yet no clear indication to use it to prevent or cure incontinence.

It is essential to appreciate that all cases of incontinence cannot be cured. A sympathetic, advisory and humane approach to the patients may be all that can be offered. The patients should be advised on suitable incontinence pads and pants. Women with long-standing incontinence may develop excoriation (ammoniacal dermatitis), and protective creams as (Vaseline or Zinc emulsion in castor oil) can be applied. In some cases, where the patient is very frail or terminally ill, an in-dwelling catheter may be considered.

48.3.3 Temporary Causes

Urinary tract infections, when diagnosed, should be treated with suitable antibiotics. The benefits of medications such as diuretics that may exaggerate or contribute to symptoms should be evaluated, and treatment is stopped or changed if appropriate. Modifying and/or changing the timing of medications may be necessary to achieve reasonable periods of rest. Those with limited mobility can be helped with rehabilitation, and if necessary, to relocate toilets to make them easily assessable.

Functional incontinence where no organic cause can be found is often associated with old age, anxiety, depression and other mental conditions. Such conditions should be recognised and treated appropriately. Support with personal hygiene may be required in the elderly.

Faecal impaction, uterine fibroids, and other abdomino-pelvic tumours that can compress or obstruct the bladder may require surgical intervention.

48.3.4 Urodynamic Stress Incontinence (USI)

This is defined as involuntary loss of urine when intravesical pressure exceeds maximum urethral closure pressure in the absence of detrusor activity [1]. It is the most frequent cause of incontinence, although the incidence seems to be higher in the Caucasian population [21].

The typical presentation of USI is stress incontinence without sensory symptoms of frequency urgency or urge incontinence. When this is the case, and stress incontinence is demonstrated during coughing, the chance of diagnosing USI on urodynamic testing is about 95%. However, only 2% of patients will present like this, and the majority will have mixed symptoms [64].

48.4 Conservative Treatment

This should be the first choice of treatment. It is also indicated when patients do not want surgery or are unfit for it or when there is a desire to have more children. Unfortunately, the success rate in terms of complete cure is poor [77, 78], but the improvement of symptoms has been recorded in about 60–70% of patients [65]. Conservative methods of managing USI are shown in Table 48.6.

Mechanical devices are being used more than ever before. These can be intravaginal, intraurethral or meatal. The intravaginal devices are designed to support the bladder neck while the others are used to either plug the urethra or the urethral meatus. It is essential to choose a simple device that patients can apply easily. Intraurethral devices are associated with high incidences of urinary tract infections and can get displaced into the bladder [79].

Oestrogen therapy alone has not been shown to be helpful, but in combination with other measures has been shown to reduce incontinence objectively and subjectively [80, 81].

48.4.1 Surgery

This is the most effective treatment for USI with success rates of between 85% and 95% [67, 82]. The general aim of the surgery is to elevate the bladder neck and proximal urethra into an intra-abdominal position or to support the mid-urethra and increase its resistance to the leakage of urine [67].

Table 48.6 Treatment of USI

Conservative
Pelvic floor physiotherapy (30–70%) [65, 66]
Pelvic floor exercises (Kegel)
Vaginal cones
Faradism
Perineometry
Interferential therapy
Maximum electrical stimulation
Mechanical devices:
Vaginal tampons
Intraurethral/meatal plugging devices
Drugs:
α-Adrenergic agonists and oestrogens[b]
Surgery:
Sub-urethral tapes (TVT/TOT) (85–95%)[a] [67]
Colposuspension (80–95%) [68, 69]
Marshal-Marchetti-Krantz (70–92%) [70].
Bladder neck suspension (Raz, Stamey, slings) (67–100%) [42, 71, 72]
Collagen injections (25–70%) [73, 74]
Anterior repair (35–69%) [75, 76].
Artificial sphincter
Urinary diversion

[a]Numbers in parenthesis represent approximate cure rates, [b]See text

Many gynaecologists favoured the Burch colposuspension as first choice surgery for the correction of female USI [69, 76] when there is no vaginal scarring or narrowing. The cure rate varies from 80% to 95% depending on outcome measures and duration of follow-up [70, 76]. It involves the approximation of the para-vaginal fascia with long-lasting or non-absorbable sutures to the ipsi-lateral ileo-pectineal ligament. A suction drain is usually inserted in the retropubic space and the bladder drained with a supra-pubic or urethral catheter until voiding function resumes. The surgery can also be done laparoscopically with equivalent outcome results [26], although there is some evidence that the open technique may have a slightly better outcome in long-term follow-up, but this remains unsubstantiated [83].

Complications of colposuspension include voiding disorders (5–12%), detrusor overactivity (10–27%, genital prolapse (8–20%) and dyspareunia (4%) [84]. Others are inadvertent bladder and ureteric injuries [85] retropubic and wound haematomas. Also, urinary tract infections are common in the immediate post-operative period [86] and can become recurrent with time [87]. It is necessary to administer prophylactic antibiotics. Single intraoperative antibiotics may be adequate in patients requiring short periods of catheterisation, but those who remain on a catheter for much longer will require a course of prophylactic antibiotics [86]. This may well be the preferred surgical technique in the tropics and poor resource-setting since it does not require tapes and insertion devices which may not be affordable.

The sub-urethral or tension-free vaginal tape (TVT) procedure has become the first choice operative treatment of USI in many centres. It is performed under spinal or local anaesthetic with sedation often on outpatient or day-case basis. It involves the placement of tape for urethral support without elevating the bladder neck or fixing the proximal ends of the tape. The technique followed from experimental work by Ulmsten [88], and subsequent clinical trials demonstrated its safety and efficacy [82, 89], even on long-term follow-up [25].

It is simple, with minimum peri-operative morbidity, and short hospital stay [67, 88]. The cure rate (75–95%) is comparable with the best invasive surgical techniques [69]. Complications of the TVT procedure include bladder perforation (0–25%) [82, 84], bleeding, and pelvic haematomas, urinary retention (10%) [84], urge incontinence (8–10%) [82, 84], healing problems with a very low incidence of graft rejection and erosion [82].

In the Marshal-Marchetti-Krantz procedure, the paraurethral tissue at the level of the bladder neck is secured to the periosteum of the posterior aspect of the pubic symphysis. A cure rate of 70–85% is expected [68, 70], but it does not correct cystoceles and is associated with osteitis pubis in 5–10% of cases [90].

Sling procedures also have excellent success rates. The rectus sheath is commonly used, but inorganic materials (e.g. Mersilene, silastic, etc.) can also be used with similar results. Post-operative voiding difficulties are commoner with sling procedures [91]. Endoscopic bladder neck suspensions [92, 93] are simple, quick and easy to perform and can be done under regional analgesia with quick discharge from hospital. They, however, rely on two sutures only which can break or pull through. Voiding problems are frequent, and long-term results are poorer [91, 92].

Bulking agents composed of synthetic materials, bovine collagen, or autologous substances increase urethral resistance to urinary flow. Cure rates as high as 70% have been recorded in some series [73, 94] after repeated injections. The durability of the injected material often determines their long-term outcome. A lot of research is still going on to develop safer and more durable bulking agents. It, however, has the advantage of being done as day surgery, and under regional or local anaesthesia. It is particularly suitable for women who have undergone several previous operations with fixed and fibrosed urethras, and in those at increased risk of general anaesthesia. It could also be considered for use in women who have embarrassing USI but have not completed their families. More recently, investigations of stem cell injections have shown promise for use not only as a bulking agent but also as the potential to regenerate damaged or weakened rhabdosphincter [95].

Anterior colporrhaphy produces a poor cure rate of only 35–69% [75]. It is the operation of choice for cystourethroceles, but when these co-exist with urodynamic stress incontinence, priority should be given to the latter, since it is more difficult to cure. It also makes further surgery for incontinence more complicated and probably less successful.

The best chance of cure is with the first operation. The efficacy of each operation has to be balanced with its complications, and if in doubt, the experience of a urogynaecologist should be sought. Unfortunately, conventional surgery might fail after many trials in some patients. In these, an artificial sphincter or urinary diversion may be considered.

48.4.2 Detrusor Overactivity (DO)

This is defined as a condition in which the detrusor is objectively shown to contract either spontaneously, or on provocation, during bladder filling while the subject is trying to inhibit micturition [1] (Fig. 48.5). Over the years, various terms have been used to describe the phenomenon, for example, hypertonic bladder, unstable bladder, detrusor hyperreflexia, urge syndrome, etc. It is the second commonest cause of incontinence (30–40%), and the incidence increases with age [50].

The cause of DO is unknown. It is often associated with inadequate bladder training in childhood, emotional or psychosomatic factors. In some cases, it may occur in association with upper motor neuron lesions (e.g. multiple sclerosis) when it is referred to as detrusor hyperreflexia. In men, it commonly results from outflow obstruction, and this may explain its high incidence in women following incontinence surgery. The autonomic imbalance between parasympathetic and sympathetic systems has been suspected, and in some cases, non-adrenergic, non-cholinergic (NANC) mechanisms may act as modulators [105].

The common presenting symptoms of DO include urgency and urge incontinence, frequency and nocturia, coital and giggling incontinence, and at times stress incontinence. The diagnosis is based on urodynamic findings.

48.4.3 Conservative Treatment

The large number of treatment modalities for DO (Table 48.7) implies that none is universally satisfactory. Behaviour modification is aimed at regaining control of micturition by re-establishing cortical control over the hyper-excitable micturition reflex. Subjective and objective improvement is achieved in about 80% and 50% of patients respectively, but nearly half of the cases relapse with time [105, 106]. Bladder re-training, which was pioneered by Frewen [106] involves regulating the amount of fluid intake and the frequency of voiding. Advice on fluid restriction should take into account

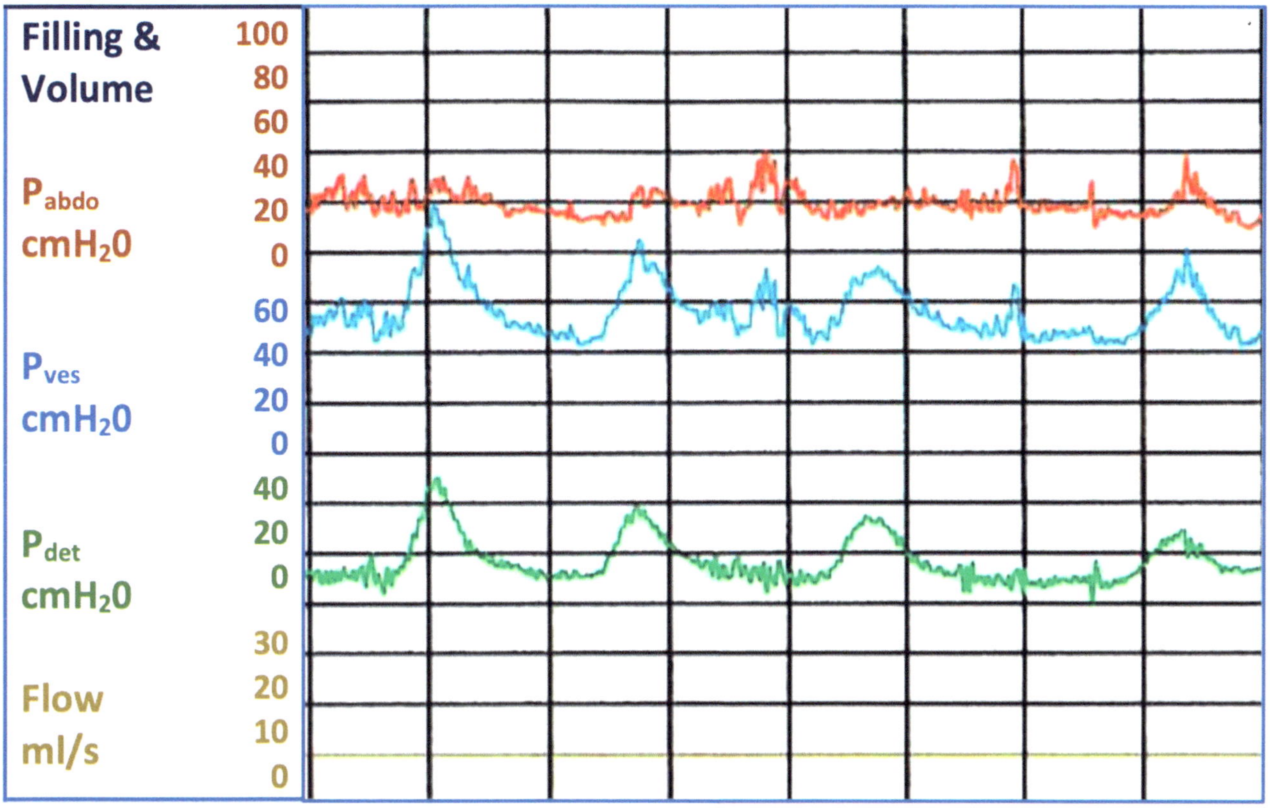

Fig. 48.5 Urodynamics trace of detrusor overactivity (DO)

Table 48.7 Treatment of DO

Conservative	
	Behaviour modification
	Bladder drills (27% dry, 87% improve)[a] [96]
	Bio-feedback techniques (40% dry) [97]
	Hypnotherapy (58% improve, 50% relapse) [98]
	Acupuncture (69% improve) [99]
Drugs[b]:	
	Anticholinergics, β3 agonist, tricyclic antidepressants
	Anti-prostaglandins, calcium channel blockers
	ADH analogues, etc.
Surgical	
	Cystoscopy + Cystodistension (23%) [100]
	Botox injection to the bladder [101, 102]
	Trans-vesical phenol injections [103]
	Bladder transection [104]
	Sacral nerve stimulation [56]
	Vaginal denervation
	Sacral neurectomy
	Augmentation cystoplasty

[a]Numbers in parenthesis represent approximate cure rates, [b]See text

the high rate of insensitive water loss in the tropics, to avoid dehydration. Improvements often seen in some women who move from the temperate to the tropical regions are associated with this higher rate of perspiration. Group psychotherapy, hypnotherapy [98] and acupuncture [99] have also been shown to benefit some patients.

Anticholinergic agents (oxybutynin, tolterodine solifenacin, etc.) are the most common drugs in use for controlling DO. Other useful drugs are calcium channel blockers (nifedipine, flumazine, etc.). Dry mouth, which is one of the common side effects of anticholinergic therapy, is uncomfortable to these patients in whom fluid restriction is also often advised.

Recently, the β3 agonist Mirabegron has been introduced as an effective treatment of DO. Mirabegron activates β3 adrenergic receptors in the detrusor muscle in the bladder, which leads to muscle relaxation and an increase in bladder capacity. It carries the potential to eliminate the side effects of anticholinergic medications as dry mouth, constipation, etc. [107]. It will be particularly useful in symptomatic patients who suffer from closed-angle glaucoma in whom anti-cholinergic drugs are contraindicated. There is also the enormous potential of using it in combination with other anticholinergic medications in resistant DO [108].

The vasopressin analogue – DDAVP used in controlling nocturnal enuresis significantly reduces nocturia and provides for more extended periods of night rest. Tricyclic antidepressants (imipramine, etc.) have central and peripheral anticholinergic, central sedative, and β-adrenergic agonist effects. It has been shown to produce 60% continence in patients with DO [109] and can also be used in conjunction with other anticholinergics to improve efficacy.

48.4.4 Surgical Treatment

Surgical treatment of DO is far from satisfactory. Bladder distention causes degeneration of unmyelinated nerve fibres of the bladder, thus reducing sensory and motor functions [100]. Subjective rates of improvement are high, but the cure rate is under 10% [100, 110].

Botulinum toxin A (BTX-A), a potent neurotoxin produced by the bacterium *Clostridium botulinum*, has been introduced for the treatment of idiopathic detrusor overactivity, especially in patients who did not respond to oral treatment. It prevents the release of acetylcholine at the neuromuscular junction. This effect, in turn, inhibits depolarisation of the detrusor muscle, resulting in chemical denervation of the bladder. Botox is administered directly into the detrusor muscle via cystoscopic technique and is generally safe and well tolerated. In clinical trials, the effects last typically for 3–6 months. In patients with over active bladder symptoms (OAB), Botox injection resulted in increased bladder capacity, increased bladder compliance, and improved quality of life [102, 111].

Augmentation 'Clam' enterocystoplasty with a cure rate of 80–90% is the most successful operation for detrusor overactivity [112, 113]. The bladder is sub-totally transected in the coronal or sagittal plane, and a strip of detubularised bowel is interposed into the defect. Complications include voiding problems, electrolyte imbalance (hyperchloremic metabolic acidosis), mucus production and more recently, suspected risks of malignancy [114].

Sacral nerve stimulation techniques are based on experimental and clinical evidence that electrical stimulation activates the urethral musculature and inhibits the detrusor muscle [56]. Consistent good results have been reported [115], and the technique is becoming more popular.

Bladder denervation surgery can be performed trans-abdominally, trans-vaginally, or by injecting an aqueous solution of phenol into the bladder base [103]. The complications of these operations are high, and the success rate is no more than 50% [103, 116].

Reports that bladder transections yield 74% success rate [104] has not been consistently reproduced by other observers [117] and the procedure is gradually falling into disrepute.

Occasional patients may not benefit from any of these modalities of treatment, and urinary diversion may be the only option to achieve any reasonable quality of life.

48.4.5 Mixed Incontinence

In many patients, USI and DO co-exist. In these, medical treatment should be tried in conjunction with pelvic floor physiotherapy. If stress incontinence remains the dominant feature, surgical correction can be considered, as improvements in DO are not uncommon after correction of USI [118].

48.4.6 Overflow Incontinence

Overflow incontinence can be defined as involuntary loss of urine associated with over-distention of the bladder. Overflow occurs in association with neurological disorders, obstruction of the urethra (stenosis/stricture, pelvic masses, etc.), drugs (anticholinergic agents, tricyclic antidepressants, epidural analgesia) inflammatory conditions (urethritis, vulvitis or vaginitis, etc.) and atonic detrusor secondary to over-distention. It is also seen in some medical conditions as diabetic neuropathy, hypothyroidism, psychosis, anxiety, etc.

The presenting symptoms vary from dribbling, frequency, and stress incontinence to recurrent urinary infections. Clinical examination will reveal a large bladder, and on catheterisation, a residual volume greater than 50% of bladder capacity will be recovered. The voiding peak flow might be reduced.

The most crucial step in the management is to ascertain the cause of the overflow and address it.

If it is secondary to obstruction, urethral dilation or urethrotomy may be required. In cases of hypotonic detrusor, cholinergic agents (e.g. Bethanechol) can be tried. In some cases, where no cause is found, clean intermittent self-catheterisation (CISC) may be tried [119], although its acceptance in the developing countries remains to be tested.

Overflow incontinence can be prevented in many cases by simple measures. It is always essential to avoid sustained over-distension of the bladder. The human bladder, once over-distended, may never contract normally again [120]. In radical pelvic surgery and incontinent procedures, where postoperative urine retention is likely, adequate bladder drainage is essential. Also following difficult vaginal deliveries, caesarean sections or when spinal or epidural analgesia is used for surgical procedures, etc., an indwelling catheter should be left in situ for 12–24 hours to avoid over-distending the bladder.

48.4.7 Urethral Diverticulum

The condition was first described by Hey in 1805. It was thought to be rare but is currently estimated to occur in 1–6% of adult females [121]. It generally occurs between the ages of 20 and 60 years (with an average of 40 years) and has a predilection for Blacks [122]. Some cases have been described in young infants, but the majority seem to be acquired secondary to urethral infections, birth trauma, high intravesical pressures, instrumentation, urethral calculi, or urethral/anterior vaginal wall surgery.

It classically presents with post-micturition dribbling or stress incontinence immediately after voiding, but can also present with pain (especially after voiding) or dyspareunia. The diagnosis can be made by micturating cystourethrogram, videocystourethrogram or urethroscopy. Treatment should be conservative if the patient is asymptomatic. Intermittent courses of antibiotics can be used to control mild symptoms, and surgery considered if symptoms are severe. The standard operation done to correct the condition is sub-total diverticulectomy with urethral reconstruction. However, a simple marsupialisation can also be employed for diverticulae in the distal third of the urethra away from the intrinsic and external sphincter mechanisms [121].

48.4.8 Other Lower Urinary Tract Problems

48.4.8.1 Urethral Prolapse

This condition is defined as the complete eversion of the urethral mucosa through the external urethral meatus [123]. It commonly affects young girls, usually between the ages of 5 and 10 years and often affects post-menopausal women. There is a higher prevalence in black pre-menarchal girls [124], but it is not uncommon in Whites [125]. The aetiology is not clear but seems to be related to an inherent anatomic defect in association with episodic increases in intra-abdominal pressure and oestrogen deficiency [126].

It commonly presents with pre-menarchal vaginal bleeding and a peri-urethral mass, which is reddish and encompasses the whole circumference of the external urethral meatus [126]. If uncomplicated, it is usually painless [127] but may be associated with dysuria and urethral discharge [124]. Over the years, the preferred treatment has been by excision or cautery [126]. Conservative management with treatment for the cause of raised intra-abdominal pressure (cough constipation and other causes of raised intra-abdominal pressure), and the use of topical oestrogens with local hygiene have yielded consistently good result [125, 128]. This should be the first line of treatment, and surgery offered only if conservative methods fail.

48.4.8.2 Urethral Caruncle

This is a benign polypoid mass of the urethral meatus of uncertain aetiology, usually found on the posterior aspect of the external urethral meatus [129]. It is covered with transitional epithelium and may cause pain, dysuria and bleeding. It occurs commonly in post-menopausal women and is treated by excision followed by local or systemic oestrogens. It can mimic a malignancy or tuberculosis and requires histopathological examination after excision [129].

48.4.8.3 Urethral Stricture

This is uncommon in women and may result from chronic urethritis, or trauma from either repeated urethral dilatation or urethral surgery. It commonly becomes manifest after the menopause and presents as voiding difficulties or recurrent urinary tract infections. Diagnosis can be made by cystometry with uroflowmetry or videocystourethrography. The lesion can be localised with the aid of urethral pressure profilometry or cystourethroscopy. The treatment is urethrotomy (Otis or open) and oestrogen replacement therapy in post-menopausal women.

48.4.8.4 Carcinoma of the Urethra

This is a rare condition that usually involves the proximal urethra. Primary urethral tumours are usually transitional, but secondary tumours can affect the urethra from adjacent structures (endometrium, bladder, vagina or vulva). It commonly presents with haematuria, vaginal bleeding or discharge, recurrent urinary tract infections or voiding difficulties. The diagnosis is based on histology of biopsy specimens taken during cystourethroscopy. Treatment of proximal or entire urethral tumours is by radical surgery (cystourethrectomy with urinary diversion) followed by radiotherapy while either surgery or radiotherapy can treat early distal tumours without exenterative procedures [130]. Advanced tumours will require a multidisciplinary approach involving surgery, radiotherapy, and chemotherapy.

References

1. Haylen BT, de Ridder D, Freeman RM, et al. An International Urogynaecological Association (IUGA)/International Continence Society (ICS) joint report on the terminology for female pelvic floor dysfunction. Neurourol Urodyn. 2010;29(1):4–20. https://doi.org/10.1002/nau.20798.
2. Carls C. The prevalence of stress urinary incontinence in high school and college-age female athletes in the Midwest: implications for education and prevention. Urol Nurs. 2007;27(1):21–24,39. http://www.ncbi.nlm.nih.gov/pubmed/17390923
3. Kinchen KS, Lee J, Fireman B, Hunkeler E, Nehemiah JL, Curtice TG. The prevalence, burden, and treatment of urinary incontinence among women in a managed care plan. J Womens Health. 2007;16(3):415–22. https://doi.org/10.1089/jwh.2006.0122.
4. Sampselle CM, Harlow SD, Skurnick J, Brubaker L, Bondarenko I. Urinary incontinence predictors and life impact in ethnically diverse perimenopausal women. Obstet Gynecol. 2002;100(6):1230–8. http://www.ncbi.nlm.nih.gov/pubmed/12468167
5. Thomas TM, Plymat KR, Blannin J, Meade TW. Prevalence of urinary incontinence. Br Med J. 1980;281(6250):1243–5. http://www.ncbi.nlm.nih.gov/pubmed/7427654
6. McLaren SM, McPherson FM, Sinclair F, Ballinger BR. Prevalence and severity of incontinence among hospitalised, female psychogeriatric patients. Health Bull. 1981;39(3):157–61. http://www.ncbi.nlm.nih.gov/pubmed/7251350
7. MORI. Survey of prevalence and attitudes to incontinence. 1991.
8. Yarnell JW, Voyle GJ, Richards CJ, Stephenson TP. The prevalence and severity of urinary incontinence in women. J Epidemiol

Community Heal. 1981;35(1):71–4. http://www.ncbi.nlm.nih.gov/pubmed/7264536
9. Cox L, Rovner ES. Lower urinary tract symptoms in women: epidemiology, diagnosis, and management. Curr Opin Urol. 2016; https://doi.org/10.1097/MOU.0000000000000283.
10. Coyne KS, Wein A, Nicholson S, Kvasz M, Chen CI, Milsom I. Economic burden of urgency urinary incontinence in the United States: a systematic review. J Manag Care Pharm. 2014;20(2):130–40. https://doi.org/10.18553/jmcp.2014.20.2.130.
11. Harrison GL, Memel DS. Urinary incontinence in women: its prevalence and its management in a health promotion clinic. Br J Gen Pr. 1994;44(381):149–52. http://www.ncbi.nlm.nih.gov/pubmed/8185987
12. Samuelsson E, Victor A, Tibblin G. A population study of urinary incontinence and nocturia among women aged 20-59 years. Prevalence, well-being and wish for treatment. Acta Obs Gynecol Scand. 1997;76(1):74–80. http://www.ncbi.nlm.nih.gov/pubmed/9033249
13. Turan C, Zorlu CG, Ekin M, Hancerlioğullari N, Saraçoğlu F. Urinary incontinence in women of reproductive age. Gynecol Obs Invest. 1996;41(2):132–4. http://www.ncbi.nlm.nih.gov/pubmed/8838975
14. Nygaard IE, Lemke JH. Urinary incontinence in rural older women: prevalence, incidence and remission. J Am Geriatr Soc. 1996;44(9):1049–54. http://www.ncbi.nlm.nih.gov/pubmed/8790229
15. Diokno AC. Epidemiology of urinary incontinence. J Gerontol A Biol Sci Med Sci. 2001;56(1):M3–4. http://www.ncbi.nlm.nih.gov/pubmed/11193229
16. NEMIR A, MIDDLETON RP. Stress incontinence in young nulliparous women; a statistical study. Am J Obs Gynecol. 1954;68(4):1166–8. http://www.ncbi.nlm.nih.gov/pubmed/13197481
17. Brocklehurst JC. Treatment of urinary incontinence in the elderly. Postgr Med. 1972;51(4):184–7. http://www.ncbi.nlm.nih.gov/pubmed/5027882
18. Coyne KS, Sexton CC, Bell JA, et al. The prevalence of lower urinary tract symptoms (LUTS) and overactive bladder (OAB) by racial/ethnic group and age: results from OAB-POLL. Neurourol Urodyn. 2013;32(3):230–7. https://doi.org/10.1002/nau.22295.
19. Bump RC. Racial comparisons and contrasts in urinary incontinence and pelvic organ prolapse. Obstet Gynecol. 1993;81(3):421–5. http://www.ncbi.nlm.nih.gov/pubmed/8437798
20. Peacock LM, Wiskind AK, Wall LL. Clinical features of urinary incontinence and urogenital prolapse in a black inner-city population. Am J Obs Gynecol. 1994;171(6):1464–71. http://www.ncbi.nlm.nih.gov/pubmed/7802055
21. Knobel J. Stress incontinence in the Black female. S Afr Med J. 1975;49(12):430–2. http://www.ncbi.nlm.nih.gov/pubmed/1171526
22. Blakeman P, Hilton P. Cellular and molecular biology in urogynaecology. Curr Opin Obs Gynecol. 1996;8(5):357–60. http://www.ncbi.nlm.nih.gov/pubmed/8941434
23. Swami SK, Abrams P. Urge incontinence. Urol Clin North Am. 1996;23(3):417–25. http://www.ncbi.nlm.nih.gov/pubmed/8701556
24. Veenboer PW, Bosch JL, Rosier PF, et al. Cross-sectional study of determinants of upper and lower urinary tract outcomes in adults with spinal dysraphism–new recommendations for urodynamic followup guidelines? J Urol. 2014;192(2):477–82. https://doi.org/10.1016/j.juro.2014.02.2566.
25. Nilsson CG, Palva K, Aarnio R, Morcos E, Falconer C. Seventeen years' follow-up of the tension-free vaginal tape procedure for female stress urinary incontinence. Int Urogynecol J. 2013;24(8):1265–9. https://doi.org/10.1007/s00192-013-2090-2.
26. Hong JH, Choo MS, Lee KS. Long-term results of laparoscopic Burch colposuspension for stress urinary incontinence in women. J Korean Med Sci. 2009;24(6):1182–6. https://doi.org/10.3346/jkms.2009.24.6.1182.
27. Clemens JQ. Basic bladder neurophysiology. Urol Clin North Am. 2010;37(4):487–94. https://doi.org/10.1016/j.ucl.2010.06.006.
28. Enhorning G. Simultaneous recording of intravesical and intraurethral pressure. A study on urethral closure in normal and stress incontinent women. Acta Chir Scand Suppl. 1961;Suppl 276:1–68. http://www.ncbi.nlm.nih.gov/pubmed/13696922.
29. Delancey JO, Ashton-Miller JA. Pathophysiology of adult urinary incontinence. Gastroenterology. 2004;126(1 Suppl 1):S23–32. http://www.ncbi.nlm.nih.gov/pubmed/14978635
30. Hilton P, Stanton SL. Urethral pressure measurement by microtransducer: the results in symptom-free women and in those with genuine stress incontinence. Br J Obs Gynaecol. 1983;90(10):919–33. http://www.ncbi.nlm.nih.gov/pubmed/6684949
31. Alperin M, Cook M, Tuttle LJ, Esparza MC, Lieber RL. Impact of vaginal parity and aging on the architectural design of pelvic floor muscles. Am J Obs Gynecol. 2016; https://doi.org/10.1016/j.ajog.2016.02.033.
32. Jarvis GJ, Hall S, Stamp S, Millar DR, Johnson A. An assessment of urodynamic examination in incontinent women. Br J Obs Gynaecol. 1980;87(10):893–6. http://www.ncbi.nlm.nih.gov/pubmed/7426486
33. Frazer MI, Haylen BT, Sutherst JR. The severity of urinary incontinence in women. Comparison of subjective and objective tests. Br J Urol. 1989;63(1):14–5. http://www.ncbi.nlm.nih.gov/pubmed/2920255
34. Rogers RG, Leeman LM, Borders N, et al. Contribution of the second stage of labour to pelvic floor dysfunction: a prospective cohort comparison of nulliparous women. BJOG. 2014;121(9):1145–53; discussion 1154. https://doi.org/10.1111/1471-0528.12571.
35. Wise LA, Ruiz-Narvaez EA, Palmer JR, et al. African ancestry and genetic risk for uterine leiomyomata. Am J Epidemiol. 2012;176(12):1159–68. https://doi.org/10.1093/aje/kws276.
36. Langer R, Golan A, Neuman M, Schneider D, Bukovsky I, Caspi E. The effect of large uterine fibroids on urinary bladder function and symptoms. Am J Obs Gynecol. 1990;163(4 Pt 1):1139–41. http://www.ncbi.nlm.nih.gov/pubmed/2145766
37. Varma JS, Fidas A, McInnes A, Smith AN, Chisholm GD. Neurophysiological abnormalities in genuine female stress urinary incontinence. Br J Obs Gynaecol. 1988;95(7):705–10. http://www.ncbi.nlm.nih.gov/pubmed/3415936
38. Román GC. Tropical myelopathies. Handb Clin Neurol. 2014;121:1521–48. https://doi.org/10.1016/B978-0-7020-4088-7.00102-4.
39. Vodušek DB. The role of clinical neurophysiology in urogynaecology. Int Urogynecol J. 2011;22(12):1473–7. https://doi.org/10.1007/s00192-011-1485-1.
40. Blaivas JG, Zayed AA, Labib KB. The bulbocavernosus reflex in urology: a prospective study of 299 patients. J Urol. 1981;126(2):197–9. http://www.ncbi.nlm.nih.gov/pubmed/7265365
41. Haeusler G, Hanzal E, Joura E, Sam C, Koelbl H. Differential diagnosis of detrusor instability and stress-incontinence by patient history: the Gaudenz-incontinence-questionnaire revisited. Acta Obs Gynecol Scand. 1995;74(8):635–7. http://www.ncbi.nlm.nih.gov/pubmed/7660771
42. Ng RK, Murray A. Can we afford to take short cuts in the management of stress urinary incontinence? Singap Med J. 1993;34(2):121–4. http://www.ncbi.nlm.nih.gov/pubmed/8266149
43. Jensen JK, Nielsen FR, Ostergard DR. The role of patient history in the diagnosis of urinary incontinence. Obstet Gynecol. 1994;83(5 Pt 2):904–10. http://www.ncbi.nlm.nih.gov/pubmed/8159393
44. Ferreira CH, Bø K. The pad test for urinary incontinence in women. J Physiother. 2015;61(2):98. https://doi.org/10.1016/j.jphys.2014.12.001.

45. Versi E, Orrego G, Hardy E, Seddon G, Smith P, Anand D. Evaluation of the home pad test in the investigation of female urinary incontinence. Br J Obs Gynaecol. 1996;103(2):162–7. http://www.ncbi.nlm.nih.gov/pubmed/8616134
46. Swift SE, Ostergard DR. Evaluation of current urodynamic testing methods in the diagnosis of genuine stress incontinence. Obstet Gynecol. 1995;86(1):85–91. https://doi.org/10.1016/0029-7844(95)00106-2.
47. Abrams P, Cardozo L, Wein A. 3rd international consultation on incontinence--research society 2011. Neurourol Urodyn. 2012;31(3):291–2. https://doi.org/10.1002/nau.22221.
48. McGuire EJ, Cespedes RD, Cross CA, O'Connell HE. Videourodynamic studies. Urol Clin North Am. 1996;23(2):309–21. http://www.ncbi.nlm.nih.gov/pubmed/8659029
49. Bates CP, Corney CE. Synchronous cine-pressure-flow cystography: a method of routine urodynamic investigation. Br J Radiol. 1971;44(517):44–50. https://doi.org/10.1259/0007-1285-44-517-44.
50. Robinson D, and Cardozo L, Urinary incontinence. Chapter 49: In Edmonds DK, Editor. Dewhurst's Textbook of Obstetrics & Gynaecology. P504 – 559. 7th Edition, 2007. Blackwell Publishing, Oxford, UK. ISBN: 978-1-4051-5667-7.
51. Versi E, Cardozo L, Cooper DJ. Urethral pressures: analysis of transmission pressure ratios. Br J Urol. 1991;68(3):266–70. http://www.ncbi.nlm.nih.gov/pubmed/1913067
52. Quinn MJ, Beynon J, Mortensen NJ, Smith PJ. Transvaginal endosonography: a new method to study the anatomy of the lower urinary tract in urinary stress incontinence. Br J Urol. 1988;62(5):414–8. http://www.ncbi.nlm.nih.gov/pubmed/3061556
53. Bergman A, McKenzie CJ, Richmond J, Ballard CA, Platt LD. Transrectal ultrasound versus cystography in the evaluation of anatomical stress urinary incontinence. Br J Urol. 1988;62(3):228–34. http://www.ncbi.nlm.nih.gov/pubmed/3056562
54. Gordon D, Pearce M, Norton P, Stanton SL. Comparison of ultrasound and lateral chain urethrocystography in the determination of bladder neck descent. Am J Obs Gynecol. 1989;160(1):182–5. http://www.ncbi.nlm.nih.gov/pubmed/2643321
55. Strohbehn K, Quint LE, Prince MR, Wojno KJ, Delancey JO. Magnetic resonance imaging anatomy of the female urethra: a direct histologic comparison. Obstet Gynecol. 1996;88(5):750–6. https://doi.org/10.1016/0029-7844(96)00323-7.
56. Ruud Bosch JL, Groen J. Treatment of refractory urge urinary incontinence with sacral spinal nerve stimulation in multiple sclerosis patients. Lancet. 1996;348(9029):717–9. http://www.ncbi.nlm.nih.gov/pubmed/8806291
57. Creighton SM, Plevnik S, Stanton SL. Distal urethral electrical conductance (DUEC)--a preliminary assessment of its role as a quick screening test for incontinent women. Br J Obs Gynaecol. 1991;98(1):69–72. http://www.ncbi.nlm.nih.gov/pubmed/1998636
58. Adekanmi OA, Freeman RM, Reed H, Bombieri L. Improving the diagnosis of genuine stress incontinence in symptomatic women with negative cough stress test: the Distal Urethral Electrical Conductance test (DUEC) revisited. Int Urogynecol J Pelvic Floor Dysfunct. 2003;14(1):9–12; discussion 12. https://doi.org/10.1007/s00192-002-0998-z.
59. Gorton E, Stanton S. Ambulatory urodynamics: do they help clinical management? BJOG. 2000;107(3):316–9.
60. Burgio KL, Locher JL, Zyczynski H, Hardin JM, Singh K. Urinary incontinence during pregnancy in a racially mixed sample: characteristics and predisposing factors. Int Urogynecol J Pelvic Floor Dysfunct. 1996;7(2):69–73. http://www.ncbi.nlm.nih.gov/pubmed/8798089
61. Agur W, Housami F, Drake M, Abrams P. Could the National Institute for Health and Clinical Excellence guidelines on urodynamics in urinary incontinence put some women at risk of a bad outcome from stress incontinence surgery? BJU Int. 2009;103(5):635–9. https://doi.org/10.1111/j.1464-410X.2008.08121.x.
62. Lachowsky M, Nappi RE. The effects of estrogen on urogenital health. Maturitas. 2009;63(2):149–51. https://doi.org/10.1016/j.maturitas.2009.03.012.
63. Cardozo LD, Kelleher CJ. Sex hormones, the menopause and urinary problems. Gynecol Endocrinol. 1995;9(1):75–84. http://www.ncbi.nlm.nih.gov/pubmed/7793304
64. Sultan AH, Monga AK, Stanton SL. The pelvic floor sequelae of childbirth. Br J Hosp Med. 1996;55(9):575–9. http://www.ncbi.nlm.nih.gov/pubmed/8735035
65. Cammu H, Van Nylen M, Amy JJ. A 10-year follow-up after Kegel pelvic floor muscle exercises for genuine stress incontinence. BJU Int. 2000;85(6):655–8. http://www.ncbi.nlm.nih.gov/pubmed/10759660
66. Wilson PD, Al Samarrai T, Deakin M, Kolbe E, Brown AD. An objective assessment of physiotherapy for female genuine stress incontinence. Br J Obs Gynaecol. 1987;94(6):575–82. http://www.ncbi.nlm.nih.gov/pubmed/3497667
67. Ross S, Tang S, Eliasziw M, et al. Transobturator tape versus retropubic tension-free vaginal tape for stress urinary incontinence: 5-year safety and effectiveness outcomes following a randomised trial. Int Urogynecol J. 2015; https://doi.org/10.1007/s00192-015-2902-7.
68. Colombo M, Scalambrino S, Maggioni A, Milani R. Burch colposuspension versus modified Marshall-Marchetti-Krantz urethropexy for primary genuine stress urinary incontinence: a prospective, randomised clinical trial. Am J Obs Gynecol. 1994;171(6):1573–9. http://www.ncbi.nlm.nih.gov/pubmed/7802070
69. Eriksen BC, Hagen B, Eik-Nes SH, Molne K, Mjølnerød OK, Romslo I. Long-term effectiveness of the Burch colposuspension in female urinary stress incontinence. Acta Obs Gynecol Scand. 1990;69(1):45–50. http://www.ncbi.nlm.nih.gov/pubmed/2346079
70. Demirci F, Yildirim U, Demirci E, Ayas S, Arioglu P, Kuyumcuoglu U. Ten-year results of Marshall Marchetti Krantz and anterior colporrhaphy procedures. Aust N Z J Obs Gynaecol. 2002;42(5):513–4. http://www.ncbi.nlm.nih.gov/pubmed/12495097
71. Stanton SL, Reynolds SF, Creighton SM. The modified Pereyra (Raz) procedure for genuine stress incontinence-A useful option in the elderly or frail patient? Int Urogynecol J Pelvic Floor Dysfunct. 1995;6(1):22–5. https://doi.org/10.1007/BF01961844.
72. Conrad S, Heinzer H, Fernandez de la Maza S, Schwaibold H, Huland H. Long-term results of Stamey bladder neck suspension. Effect of data analysis technique on surgical result. Urologe A. 1997;36(5):432–9.
73. Cross CA, English SF, Cespedes RD, McGuire EJ. A followup on transurethral collagen injection therapy for urinary incontinence. J Urol. 1998;159(1):106–8. http://www.ncbi.nlm.nih.gov/pubmed/9400447
74. Kang D, Han J, Neuberger MM, et al. Transurethral radiofrequency collagen denaturation for the treatment of women with urinary incontinence. Cochrane Database Syst Rev. 2015;3:CD010217. https://doi.org/10.1002/14651858.CD010217.pub2.
75. Glazener CM, Cooper K. Anterior vaginal repair for urinary incontinence in women. Cochrane Database Syst Rev. 2000;2:CD001755. https://doi.org/10.1002/14651858.CD001755.
76. Chinegwundoh FI, Nayeem N. Outcome of Burch colposuspension in a district general hospital. Br J Clin Pr. 1995;49(1):41–2. http://www.ncbi.nlm.nih.gov/pubmed/7742186
77. Roda OP, López MA, Paniagua JV, González MS, Bellido PD, Gómez JJ. Adherence to pelvic floor muscle training with or without vaginal spheres in women with urinary incontinence: a secondary analysis from a randomised trial. Int Urogynecol J. 2016; https://doi.org/10.1007/s00192-015-2941-0.

78. Jurczak I, Chrzęszczyk M. The impact assessment of pelvic floor exercises to reduce symptoms and quality of life of women with stress urinary incontinence. Pol Merkur Lek. 2016;40(237):168–72. http://www.ncbi.nlm.nih.gov/pubmed/27088198
79. Nielsen KK, Walter S, Maegaard E, Kromann-Andersen B. The urethral plug II: an alternative treatment in women with genuine urinary stress incontinence. Br J Urol. 1993;72(4):428–32. http://www.ncbi.nlm.nih.gov/pubmed/8261298
80. Hilton P, Stanton SL. The use of intravaginal estrogen cream in genuine stress incontinence. Br J Obs Gynaecol. 1983;90(10):940–4. http://www.ncbi.nlm.nih.gov/pubmed/6313035
81. Cody JD, Jacobs ML, Richardson K, Moehrer B, Hextall A. Oestrogen therapy for urinary incontinence in post-menopausal women. Cochrane Database Syst Rev. 2012;10:CD001405. https://doi.org/10.1002/14651858.CD001405.pub3.
82. Tincello DG, Botha T, Grier D, et al. The TVT worldwide observational registry for long-term data: safety and efficacy of suburethral sling insertion approaches for stress urinary incontinence in women. J Urol. 2011;186(6):2310–5. https://doi.org/10.1016/j.juro.2011.07.078.
83. Carey MP, Goh JT, Rosamilia A, et al. Laparoscopic versus open Burch colposuspension: a randomised controlled trial. BJOG An Int J Obstet Gynaecol. 2006;113(9):999–1006. https://doi.org/10.1111/j.1471-0528.2006.01037.x.
84. Ward K, Hilton P. Prospective multicentre randomised trial of tension-free vaginal tape and colposuspension as primary treatment for stress incontinence. BMJ. 2002;325(7355):67. https://doi.org/10.1136/bmj.325.7355.67.
85. Rosen D, Korda AR, Waugh RC. Ureteric injury at Burch Colposuspension 4 case reports and literature review. Aust New Zeal J Obstet Gynaecol. 1996;36(3):354–8.
86. Chilaka VN, Mayne CJ. Postoperative urinary tract infections (UTIs) following single-dose intraoperative antibiotic prophylaxis in colposuspension patients. Int Urogynecol J Pelvic Floor Dysfunct. 1998;9(3):132–5. https://doi.org/10.1007/BF02001080.
87. Alcalay M, Monga A, Stanton SL. Burch colposuspension: a 10-20 year follow up. Br J Obstet Gynaecol. 1995;102(9):740–5. https://doi.org/10.1111/j.1471-0528.1995.tb11434.x.
88. Ulmsten U. An introduction to tension-free vaginal tape (TVT)–a new surgical procedure for treatment of female urinary incontinence. Int Urogynecol J Pelvic Floor Dysfunct. 2001;12(Suppl 2):S3–4. http://www.ncbi.nlm.nih.gov/pubmed/11450978
89. Agur W, Riad M, Secco S, et al. Surgical treatment of recurrent stress urinary incontinence in women: a systematic review and meta-analysis of randomised controlled trials. Eur Urol. 2013;64(2):323–36. https://doi.org/10.1016/j.eururo.2013.04.034.
90. Garcia-Porrua C, Picallo JA, Gonzalez-Gay MA. Osteitis pubis after Marshall-Marchetti-Krantz urethropexy. Jt Bone Spine. 2003;70(1):61–3. https://doi.org/10.1016/S1297-319X(02)00013-1.
91. Wang AC. Burch colposuspension vs. Stamey bladder neck suspension. A comparison of complications with special emphasis on detrusor instability and voiding dysfunction. J Reprod Med. 1996;41(7):529–33.
92. Ashken MH, Abrams PH, Lawrence WT. Stamey endoscopic bladder neck suspension for stress incontinence. Br J Urol. 1984;56(6):629–34. http://www.ncbi.nlm.nih.gov/pubmed/6534480
93. Stamey TA. Endoscopic suspension of the vesical neck for urinary incontinence in females. Report on 203 consecutive patients. Ann Surg. 1980;192(4):465–71. http://www.pubmedcentral.nih.gov/articlerender.fcgi?artid=1346989&tool=pmcentrez&rendertype=abstract.
94. Davis NF, Kheradmand F, Creagh T. Injectable biomaterials for the treatment of stress urinary incontinence: their potential and pitfalls as urethral bulking agents. Int Urogynecol J Pelvic Floor Dysfunct. 2013;24(6):913–9. https://doi.org/10.1007/s00192-012-2011-9.
95. Zhou S, Zhang K, Atala A, et al. Stem cell therapy for treatment of stress urinary incontinence: the current status and challenges. Stem Cells Int. 2016;2016:7060975. https://doi.org/10.1155/2016/7060975.
96. Burgio KL, Locher JL, Zyczynski H, et al. Bladder training–3 years on. Br J Urol. 1981;55(1):660–4. http://www.ncbi.nlm.nih.gov/pubmed/7456206
97. Cardozo LD, Abrams PD, Stanton SL, Feneley RC. Idiopathic bladder instability treated by biofeedback. Br J Urol. 1978;50(7):521–3. http://www.ncbi.nlm.nih.gov/pubmed/753504
98. Freeman RM, Baxby K. Hypnotherapy for incontinence caused by the unstable detrusor. Br Med J (Clin Res Ed). 1982;284(6332):1831–4. http://www.pubmedcentral.nih.gov/articlerender.fcgi?artid=1498778&tool=pmcentrez&rendertype=abstract.
99. Philp T, Shah PJ, Worth PH. Acupuncture in the treatment of bladder instability. Br J Urol. 1988;61(6):490–3. http://www.ncbi.nlm.nih.gov/entrez/query.fcgi?cmd=Retrieve&db=PubMed&dopt=Citation&list_uids=3401657.
100. Pengelly AW, Stephenson TP, Milroy EJ, Whiteside CG, Turner-Warwick R. Results of prolonged bladder distension as treatment for detrusor instability. Br J Urol. 1978;50(4):243–5. http://www.ncbi.nlm.nih.gov/entrez/query.fcgi?cmd=Retrieve&db=PubMed&dopt=Citation&list_uids=753469.
101. Mohee A, Khan A, Harris N, Eardley I. Long-term outcome of the use of intravesical botulinum toxin for the treatment of overactive bladder (OAB). BJU Int. 2013;111(1):106–13. https://doi.org/10.1111/j.1464-410X.2012.11282.x.
102. Dmochowski R, Chapple C, Nitti VW, et al. Efficacy and safety of onabotulinumtoxinA for idiopathic overactive bladder: a double-blind, placebo controlled, randomised, dose ranging trial. J Urol. 2010;184(6):2416–22. https://doi.org/10.1016/j.juro.2010.08.021.
103. Chapple CR, Hampson SJ, Turner-Warwick RT, Worth PH. Subtrigonal phenol injection. How safe and effective is it? Br J Urol. 1991;68(5):483–6. http://www.ncbi.nlm.nih.gov/pubmed/1747722
104. Parsons KF, O'Boyle PJ, Gibbon NO. A further assessment of bladder transection in the management of adult enuresis and allied conditions. Br J Urol. 1977;49(6):509–14. http://www.ncbi.nlm.nih.gov/entrez/query.fcgi?cmd=Retrieve&db=PubMed&dopt=Citation&list_uids=588955.
105. Berghmans LCM, Hendriks HJM, de Bie RA, et al. Conservative treatment of urge urinary incontinence in women: a systematic review of randomised clinical trials. BJU Int. 2000;85(3):254–63. https://doi.org/10.1046/j.1464-410x.2000.00434.x.
106. Frewen W. Role of bladder training in the treatment of the unstable bladder in the female. Urol Clin North Am. 1979;6(1):273–7. http://www.ncbi.nlm.nih.gov/pubmed/432996. . Accessed April 24, 2016
107. Matsukawa Y, Takai S, Funahashi Y, Yamamoto T, Gotoh M. Urodynamic evaluation of the efficacy of mirabegron on storage and voiding functions in women with overactive bladder. Urology. 2015;85(4):786–90. https://doi.org/10.1016/j.urology.2015.01.002.
108. Wada N, Okazaki S, Kobayashi S, et al. Efficacy of combination therapy with mirabegron for anticholinergic-resistant neurogenic bladder: videourodynamic evaluation. Hinyokika Kiyo. 2015;61(1):7–11. http://www.ncbi.nlm.nih.gov/pubmed/25656013
109. Castleden CM, George CF, Renwick AG, Asher MJ. Imipramine–a possible alternative to current therapy for urinary incontinence in the elderly. J Urol. 1981;125(3):318–20. http://www.ncbi.nlm.nih.gov/pubmed/7009892. Accessed April 24, 2016
110. Sehn JT. Anatomic effect of distention therapy in unstable bladder: new approach. Urology. 1978;11(6):581–7. https://doi.org/10.1016/0090-4295(78)90007-9.

111. Anger JT, Weinberg A, Suttorp MJ, Litwin MS, Shekelle PG. Outcomes of intravesical botulinum toxin for idiopathic overactive bladder symptoms: a systematic review of the literature. J Urol. 2010;183(6):2258–64. https://doi.org/10.1016/j.juro.2010.02.009.
112. Mundy AR, Stephenson TP. "Clam" ileocystoplasty for the treatment of refractory urge incontinence. Br J Urol. 1985;57(6):641–6. http://www.ncbi.nlm.nih.gov/pubmed/4084722
113. Snow BW, Cartwright PC. Bladder autoaugmentation. Urol Clin North Am. 1996;23(2):323–31. https://doi.org/10.1016/S0094-0143(05)70314-1.
114. Biardeau X, Chartier-Kastler E, Rouprêt M, Phé V. Risk of malignancy after augmentation cystoplasty: A systematic review. Neurourol Urodyn. April 2015. https://doi.org/10.1002/nau.22775.
115. Schreiner L, Dos Santos TG, De Souza ABA, Nygaard CC, Da Silva Filho IG. Electrical stimulation for urinary incontinence in women: a systematic review. Int Braz J Urol. 2013;39(4):454–64. https://doi.org/10.1590/S1677-5538.IBJU.2013.04.02.
116. Ramsay IN, Clancy S, Hilton P. Subtrigonal phenol injections in the treatment of idiopathic detrusor instability in the female–a long-term urodynamic follow-up. Br J Urol. 1992;69(4):363–5. https://doi.org/10.1111/j.1464-410X.1992.tb15558.x.
117. Mundy AR. Long-term results of bladder transection for urge incontinence. Br J Urol. 1983;55(6):642–4. http://www.ncbi.nlm.nih.gov/pubmed/6652432
118. Zyczynski HM, Albo ME, Goldman HB, et al. Change in overactive bladder symptoms after surgery for stress urinary incontinence in women. Obstet Gynecol. 2015;126(2):423–30. https://doi.org/10.1097/AOG.0000000000000929.
119. Elbiss HM, Moran PA, Hammad FT. Teaching patients clean intermittent self-catheterisation prior to anti-incontinence or prolapse surgery: is it necessary in women with obstructive voiding dysfunction? Int Urol Nephrol. 2012;44(3):739–43. https://doi.org/10.1007/s11255-011-0072-1.
120. Shah PJ. Pathophysiology of voiding disorders. In: Drife JO, Hilton P, Stanton SL, editors. Micturition. London: Springer; 1990.
121. Young GP, Whale GR, Raz S. Female urethral diverticulum. In: Raz S, editor. Raz female urology. 2nd ed. Philadelphia: WB Saunders; 1996.
122. Benjamin J, Elliott L, Cooper JF, Bjornson L. Urethral diverticulum in adult female. Clinical aspects, operative procedure, and pathology. Urology. 1974;3(1):1–7. https://doi.org/10.1016/S0090-4295(74)80048-8.
123. Antosh DD, Gutman RE. Diagnosis and management of female urethral diverticulum. Female Pelvic Med Reconstr Surg. 2011;17(6):264–71. https://doi.org/10.1097/SPV.0b013e318234a242.
124. John COO, Alegbeleye JO, Enyinda CE. Childhood urethral mucosa prolapse in Port Harcourt, Nigeria: an 11-year experience. Niger Heal J. 2016;15(2):79.
125. Rudin JE, Geldt VG, Alecseev EB. Prolapse of urethral mucosa in white female children: experience with 58 cases. J Paediatr Surg. 1997;32:423–5. https://doi.org/10.1016/S0022-3468(97)90596-0.
126. Lowe FC, Hill GS, Jeffs RD, Brendler CB. Urethral prolapse in children: insights into etiology and management. J Urol. 1986;135(1):100–3. http://www.ncbi.nlm.nih.gov/pubmed/3941438. . Accessed April 24, 2016
127. Sanda G, Soumana A, Oumarou H. The urethral mucosal prolapse in young girls: a series of 22 cases and a literature review. African J Urol. 2012;18(2):93–6. https://doi.org/10.4314/aju.v18i2.
128. Wright M. Urethral prolapse in children--alternative management. S Afr Med J. 1987;72(8):551–2. http://www.ncbi.nlm.nih.gov/pubmed/3672273. Accessed April 24, 2016
129. Conces MR, Williamson SR, Montironi R, Lopez-Beltran A, Scarpelli M, Cheng L. Urethral caruncle: clinicopathologic features of 41 cases. Hum Pathol. 2012;43(9):1400–4. https://doi.org/10.1016/j.humpath.2011.10.015.
130. Thyavihally YB, Wuntkal R, Bakshi G, Uppin S, Tongaonkar HB. Primary carcinoma of the female urethra: single centre experience of 18 cases. Jpn J Clin Oncol. 2005;35(2):84–7. https://doi.org/10.1093/jjco/hyi024.

49 Amenorrhea and Abnormal Uterine Bleeding

Stephen C. Collins, J. Ryan Martin, and Lubna Pal

Learning Objectives

After studying this chapter, the reader should be able to:

- Distinguish between primary and secondary amenorrhea
- Delineate the common hormonal and structural causes of amenorrhea
- Recall the evaluation of amenorrhea
- Explain the goals and approaches to treating amenorrhea, when necessary
- Describe the PALM-COEIN system for characterising the causes of abnormal uterine bleeding
- Evaluate patients with abnormal uterine bleeding
- Know the approaches to management of abnormal uterine bleeding

The normal menstrual cycle is the manifestation of the interplay between the hypothalamus, pituitary, ovaries and uterus as they enable the establishment of pregnancy or end in menses (Fig. 49.1).

Dysfunction in this synchrony between multiple players can lead to abnormalities in the menstrual cycle, ranging from an absence of menstrual flow (amenorrhea) to cycles of abnormal duration, frequency or pattern (abnormal uterine bleeding, AUB). In this chapter, we will review the common causes and approach to the evaluation and management of patients presenting with such disorders of the menstrual cycle.

49.1 Amenorrhea

49.1.1 Background

Amenorrhea is, quite simply, the absence of menses. Primary amenorrhea is diagnosed in girls who have not had menarche by age 15, despite normal secondary sexual development. (Girls lacking secondary sexual development by age 13 should be evaluated for abnormal pubertal development, which can be a similar evaluation to primary amenorrhea; please refer to Chap. 61 of this textbook for further details on delayed puberty.) Secondary amenorrhea is generally considered to be 3 months without menstrual bleeding in women with previously normal cycles [1]. Although some have proposed that secondary amenorrhea should require 6 months without menses in women with irregular menstrual cycles at baseline [2], this semantic distinction is not clinically useful, as infrequent menses alone merit a similar clinical evaluation to the workup for secondary amenorrhea.

The prevalence of primary amenorrhea varies substantially throughout the world. In the United States, for instance, 2% of women experience primary amenorrhea [3]. However, in Kenya, the median age at menarche is 15, so by this definition, 50% of Kenyan women meet criteria for primary amenorrhea [4]. Median age at menarche correlates with a variety of factors, including nutritional status and physical activity level; energy balance among children in developing countries seems to favour later age at menarche [5]. Likely for some of the same reasons, secondary amenorrhea is also more common in the developing world, ranging from 5% to 9% prevalence [6] (as compared to 3–4% prevalence in the United States [1]).

While the absence of menses is not inherently detrimental to health, amenorrhea is linked with women's wellbeing in several important ways. Women may experience amenorrhea as a

S. C. Collins (✉)
Yale University School of Medicine, New Haven, CT, USA
e-mail: Stephen.c.collins@yale.edu

J. R. Martin
Shady Grove Fertility, Warrington, PA, USA
e-mail: Ryan.Martin@sgfertility.com

L. Pal
Division of Reproductive Endocrinology & Infertility, Department of Obstetrics, Gynaecology and Reproductive Sciences, Yale School of Medicine, New Haven, CT, USA
e-mail: lubna.pal@yale.edu

F. Okonofua et al. (eds.), *Contemporary Obstetrics and Gynecology for Developing Countries*,
https://doi.org/10.1007/978-3-030-75385-6_49

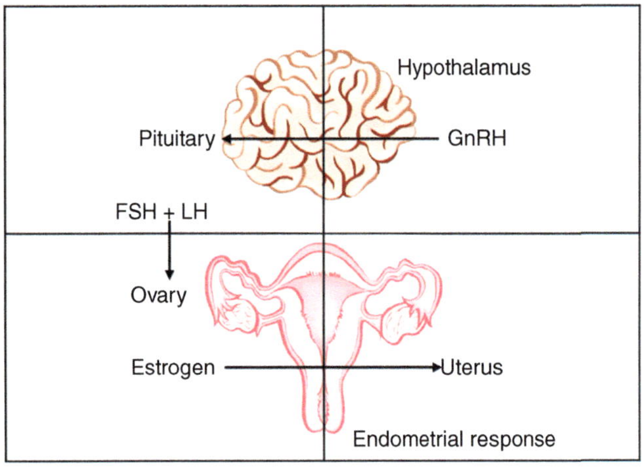

Fig. 49.1 HPO axis

Table 49.1 Causes of amenorrhea

Endocrine causes	
Hypothalamic:	Functional hypothalamic amenorrhea (e.g. emotional stress, nutritional deficiency, excess exercise, systemic disease)
	Congenital GnRH deficiency
	Hypothalamic tumours or infections (e.g. TB, encephalitis)
	Iatrogenic (e.g. chronic opioid use)
Pituitary:	Hyperprolactinaemia
	Pituitary disease (e.g. sellar masses, Sheehan syndrome, radiation)
Ovarian:	Gonadal dysgenesis (e.g. Turner syndrome, Swyer syndrome)
	Primary ovarian insufficiency (genetic, autoimmune, chemo, radiation)
Mixed:	Polycystic ovary syndrome
Other:	Thyroid disease
Structural causes	
Inborn:	Transverse vaginal septum
	Imperforate hymen
	Müllerian agenesis (Mayer-Rokitansky-Küster-Hauser syndrome)
	46,XY with AIS, 5α-reductase deficiency, etc.
Acquired:	Asherman's syndrome
	Cervical stenosis

consequence of an underlying disease in need of attention, such as acquired immune deficiency syndrome (AIDS) or tuberculosis [6]. Amenorrhea commonly associates with infertility, and these two intertwined processes must often be addressed as one in order to enable reproduction. If hypoestrogenism is present as part of the amenorrhea process, bone health may suffer, particularly when compounded with an underlying nutritional deficiency. Finally, although women's sentiments vary across the world, women in some cultures place a value upon the normalcy of monthly menses. For example, 81% of women in Nigeria like to have periods, feeling it allows them "to get rid of bad blood." Thus, the loss of menses in secondary amenorrhea can be a source of distress [7].

49.1.2 Causes

The World Health Organization (WHO) has classified amenorrhea into three categories based upon its cause. In WHO group I, amenorrhea occurs in the setting of low/normal gonadotropin levels and low oestrogen levels, but omits patients with abnormal prolactin levels or structural lesions in the brain. WHO group II includes patients with normal FSH and normal oestrogen levels, but no menses. Patients with gonadal failure, notable for low oestrogen and high FSH levels, fall into WHO group III [1]. However, because this WHO classification scheme does not have a place for all amenorrheic patients (e.g. women with hyperprolactinaemia or pituitary tumours), it is helpful to consider the differential diagnosis for amenorrhea with respect to the possible involved organs within the hypothalamic-pituitary-ovarian-uterine axis (Table 49.1).

The most common cause of hypothalamic amenorrhea is *functional* hypothalamic amenorrhea. In this process, disruption of the pulsatile release of GnRH by the hypothalamus, and consequently a disordered release of pituitary gonadotropins (specifically FSH), prevents normal ovarian follicular development; a lack of endometrial proliferation secondary to hypoestrogenism and anovulation are consequences of disordered or arrested ovarian follicular development, resulting in amenorrhea. Functional hypothalamic amenorrhea is most commonly caused by disruptions to the energy balance; nutritional deficiency (whether as a result of limited access to food, malabsorptive gastrointestinal diseases such as celiac sprue or eating disorders such as anorexia or bulimia) and excess energy expenditure (either occupationally or through exercise, an example commonly encountered in competitive female athletes) are the chief instigators. Excess psychological stress and severe systemic illness have also been implicated [8].

Functional hypothalamic amenorrhea is a diagnosis of exclusion, so consideration must also be given to other causes for impaired hypothalamic function. Congenital GnRH deficiency is a rare clinical entity where a variety of genetic mutations cause the patient to not produce GnRH, leading to low levels of gonadotropins and oestrogen and thus to primary amenorrhea. Constitutional delay of puberty can present in a similar fashion; clues in favour of congenital GnRH deficiency, however, include a positive family history of the same condition, the presence of anosmia (as seen in the Kallmann syndrome) and a lack of delay in pubic hair development (as adrenal androgens still drive pubic hair development when there is an isolated GnRH deficiency) [9, 10]. Hypothalamic tumours can also cause dysfunctional GnRH release and should be considered in the patient with hypogonadotropic hypogonadism and concomitant headaches or visual disturbance [1]. Certain infections are able to cause hypothalamic amenorrhea. Tuberculosis, for instance, is known to frequently lead to amenorrhea even in women with no evidence of genital disease; this has been attributed to its impact on hypothalamic function [11]. Finally, amenorrhea associated with use of certain medications such as methadone [12] as well as with use of hormonal contraceptives (e.g. continuous combined hormonal contraception or injectable depot progestins [7]) has hypothalamic origins.

At the level of the pituitary, the most common cause of amenorrhea is secondary to prolactin excess, which underlies 13% of all cases of secondary amenorrhea [13]. Elevated prolactin levels cause suppression of GnRH release, leading to low levels of pituitary gonadotropins, with consequent hypoestrogenism and amenorrhea [14]. The greater the elevation in prolactin level, the more severe the menstrual phenotype; thus, while women with mild hyperprolactinaemia may have menstrual irregularities, amenorrhea is more commonly seen in women with substantially elevated prolactin (e.g. >100 ng/ml). Women with hyperprolactinaemia may also present with galactorrhea, headache, or visual disturbance, but these symptoms are found only in a minority of patients [15]. Prolactinoma, a benign overgrowth of the lactotroph cell population within the anterior pituitary, is a common cause of hyperprolactinaemia; additional causes of prolactin excess include primary hypothyroidism (a compensatory increase in the hypothalamic TRH is deemed a mechanism for disrupting the dopamine mediated suppression of pituitary lactotrophs) or due to exposure to medications that disrupt normal dopaminergic signalling to the pituitary (Table 49.2) [14].

Generalised hypopituitarism can also result in amenorrhea. This can be caused by a variety of processes, including cranial radiation exposure, prior pituitary surgery and infection by pathogens such as tuberculosis [16]. One cause of particular note in the developing world is Sheehan's syndrome, an infarction of the pituitary that follows a profound ischemic insult, such as caused by a massive postpartum haemorrhage. Although access to advanced obstetric care has made this an uncommon entity in the developed world, Sheehan's syndrome remains the most common cause of hypopituitarism in the developing world [17].

Table 49.2 Drugs implicated in hyperprolactinaemia[75]

Drug class	Specific drugs
Typical antipsychotics	Haloperidol, fluphenazine, chlorpromazine
Atypical antipsychotics	Paliperidone, risperidone, molindone
Tricyclic antidepressants	Clomipramine
Monoamine oxidase inhibitors (MAO-I)	Pargyline, clorgyline
Antiemetics/prokinetics	Metoclopramide, domperidone
Antihypertensives	Methyldopa, verapamil
Opioids	Methadone, morphine

Primary ovarian mechanisms are the most common cause of primary amenorrhea and an important contributor to both primary and secondary amenorrhea. Gonadal dysgenesis, which underlies greater than 40% of all cases of primary amenorrhea [18], is characterised by an abnormal developmental process in which the follicles and oocytes are prematurely depleted, often in utero. Turner syndrome (45,X) or Turner mosaicism (e.g. 45,X/46XX, among others) and Swyer syndrome (46,XY) are classic examples of amenorrhea (primary or secondary) with genetic underpinnings; rarely, gonadal dysgenesis can be seen with a normal 46,XX karyotype. Primary ovarian insufficiency (POI) is described in women who have premature depletion of follicles and oocytes later in life but before age 40. The underlying causes of POI include prior chemotherapy or radiation exposure, genetic mutations (including the fragile X premutation and galactosemia, among others) and autoimmunity [19]. Women with autoimmune POI are more likely to have other concomitant autoimmune disorders; the most common is thyroiditis, but insulin-dependent diabetes, myasthenia gravis, parathyroid disease and adrenal insufficiency are also associated with POI. Thus, when an amenorrheic patient is diagnosed with POI, it is important to consider the possibility of these concurrent disease processes which hold serious health implications [20–22].

Polycystic ovary syndrome (PCOS) is a common condition with menstrual dysfunction often being the initial presenting symptom. PCOS is a chronic disorder of hyperandrogenism (clinical and/or biochemical) and anovulation that is often associated with insulin resistance. PCOS is diagnosed by clinical criteria; the most commonly used diagnostic criteria are from the Rotterdam ESHRE/ASRM-sponsored PCOS Consensus Workshop Group. This scheme requires two out of three criteria to be met: (1) hyperandrogenism (as defined by biochemical evidence of elevated serum androgens or symptoms such as acne or hirsutism), (2) oligomenorrhea or amenorrhea and (3) polycystic-appearing ovaries on transvaginal pelvic ultrasound (as defined by the presence of 12 or more follicles measuring 2–9 mm per ovary and/or ovarian volume greater than 10 cm^3). PCOS is a diagnosis of exclusion, so other causes for the clinical presentation must be considered before assigning the diagnosis [23]. For further description of other hyperandrogenic disorders, please refer to Chap. 64 of this textbook. Because the anovulatory cycles seen in PCOS are more likely to lead to infrequent menses than to amenorrhea [1], discussion of the management of the menstrual pattern of PCOS will be reserved for the section on AUB.

Menstrual dysfunction is common in the setting of untreated thyroid dysfunction (both hypothyroidism and hyperthyroidism) and can present as amenorrhea. Although the role of thyroid disease in disorders of the menstrual cycle is not as significant as was once thought [24, 25], there appears to be a small (albeit nonsignificant) increase in secondary amenorrhea among women with hyperthyroidism and with severe hypothyroidism [25].

Anatomical underpinnings to amenorrhea are of particular relevance for patients with primary amenorrhea, as well as in those developing secondary amenorrhea in appropriate clinical settings. Anatomical causes can be identified in approximately 20% of cases of primary amenorrhea [18]. Mayer-Rokitansky-Küster-Hauser syndrome (MRKHS) refers to a lack of development of the Müllerian structures (uterus, cervix, vagina or a combination) with the patient presenting with primary amenorrhea in the setting of normal external sexual development. The phenotype of MRKHS shares similarities with a less common entity of complete androgen insensitivity syndrome (CAIS); absent pubic and axillary hair in CAIS and chromosomal distinction differentiate the two (46,XX karyotype of MRKHS contrasts with the 46,XY karyotype of CAIS). Disrupted Müllerian duct developments of lesser magnitude than MRKHS or defects of distal vaginal canalisation that can result in outflow tract obstruction, such as an imperforate hymen or, less frequently, a transverse vaginal septum, must be considered in the differential diagnosis of primary amenorrhea. These anomalies will often present with progressively worsening cyclic pelvic pain and bladder or bowel symptoms in addition to primary amenorrhea, due to the cyclic build-up of endometrium and menses without a means of egress [1].

Secondary amenorrhea can result from acquired anatomical abnormalities involving the outflow tract. *Cervical stenosis* most often develops after procedures involving the cervix, radiation to the cervix or the development of a gynaecologic malignancy (e.g. cervical cancer). Disruption of the regenerative endometrial epithelial zona basalis is a recognised mechanism for secondary amenorrhea, commonly referred to as Asherman's syndrome. Predisposing conditions for the development of Asherman's syndrome include post-abortal and postpartum endometrial curettage undertaken for removal of products of conception, the use of uterine compressive sutures for a postpartum haemorrhage, surgeries on the uterus including myomectomy and endometrial ablation and intrauterine infections [26]. In the developing world, two infections of particular note are genital tuberculosis and schistosomiasis, which have both been implicated in causation of Asherman's syndrome [27]. Both cervical stenosis and Asherman's syndrome can present with cyclic pelvic pain in addition to amenorrhea, as the outflow obstruction can cause functional endometrium to yield monthly hematometra [26].

49.1.3 Evaluation

The first step of evaluation of the amenorrheic patient is to obtain a thorough history. Because amenorrhea is a presenting symptom in pregnancy, lactation and age-appropriate menopause, these physiologic processes must be excluded before pursuing additional evaluation. Consideration should be given to whether the patient's amenorrhea is primary or secondary as the list of differential diagnoses varies between these two entities; although there is substantial overlap in their differential diagnoses, some causes will only apply to one or the other. If, on the one hand, the patient has primary amenorrhea, an assessment of her overall growth and physical development, including height, weight and development of secondary sexual characteristics (including breasts, axillary/pubic hair and appearance of external genitalia), is crucial. If, on the other hand, the patient is experiencing secondary amenorrhea, a full menstrual history should be obtained. The age at menarche, typical intermenstrual interval, recent intermenstrual interval and time since her last menses and temporal relationship with lifestyle, psychological and iatrogenic events should be assessed. A recent pattern of infrequent menses before the onset of amenorrhea with accompanying symptoms of vasomotor instability and vaginal dryness may suggest ovarian insufficiency; in contrast, secondary amenorrhea in the setting of progressive weight gain may reflect a hypothyroidism-related anovulatory process as the mechanism for secondary amenorrhea. The presence of cyclic symptoms during the period of amenorrhea, such as pelvic pain or moliminal symptoms (e.g. breast tenderness, fatigue or mood changes) should raise concerns for an underlying structural defect of the menstrual outflow tract as a mechanism for amenorrhea.

Medical history should be reviewed, with particular attention paid to systemic diseases which may cause amenorrhea (such as malabsorptive disorders, AIDS, tuberculosis, autoimmune disease or cancers treated with pelvic or cranial radiation or systemic chemotherapy). Relevant surgical history would include prior intracranial or uterine procedures, including myomectomy and endometrial curettage. Obstetric history may hold a clue; history of postpartum haemorrhage increases suspicion for Sheehan's syndrome, while a history of post-abortal or postpartum curettage should raise concerns for Asherman's syndrome. Medication use should be assessed, including use of methadone and hormonal contraceptives (which can cause hypothalamic amenorrhea), as well as antipsychotics and metoclopramide (which can cause hyperprolactinaemia). Social history should focus on dietary patterns, physical activity and life stressors, as these can inform the risk assessment for functional hypothalamic amenorrhea. The family history should focus on female relatives' age at menarche and menopause, as well as insulin resistance or autoimmune disorders in other family members (which may increase suspicion of PCOS or autoimmune POI, respectively). A focused review of systems should assess for symptoms of hypoestrogenism (including vaginal dryness, sleep disturbance, hot flushes and mood liability), hyperandrogenism (such as acne, excessive facial and/or bodily hair growth and scalp hair loss), galactorrhea and headache or visual changes (which may indicate a prolactinoma or another intracranial mass lesion impacting the hypothalamus or the pituitary).

Physical examination can provide meaningful information about the underlying mechanisms for amenorrhea. The patient's height and weight can give suggestion of constitutional delay or Turner syndrome (shorter girls with primary amenorrhea), functional hypothalamic amenorrhea (often with low body mass index-BMI) or PCOS (often with elevated BMI). General examination may reveal stigmata of Turner syndrome (including shield-shaped chest, widely spaced nipples and webbed neck) or evidence of hyperandrogenism (acne, hirsutism or thinning of scalp hair) or insulin resistance (acanthosis nigricans). Breast exam will provide evidence of pubertal development of the patient with primary amenorrhea and can reveal galactorrhea in patients with hyperprolactinaemia. For patients with primary amenorrhea, the pelvic examination may allow the identification of Müllerian anomalies, such as the absence of vagina or uterus, and for other structural abnormalities, including an imperforate hymen or transverse vaginal septum. A complete absence of pubic hair at a chronologically appropriate age (13 or older) should raise concerns for CAIS (in a patient with no uterus) or constitutionally delayed puberty (in a patient who has a uterus). Evidence of genital atrophy, and thereby hypoestrogenism, should raise concerns for POI in a woman with primary or secondary amenorrhea.

Figure 49.2 presents an algorithm that outlines a systematic approach to the evaluation of amenorrhea, facilitating identification of mechanism/s underlying the clinical picture while maintaining due regard to the cost of testing and interventions; these latter considerations can be particularly meaningful in low-resource settings as are commonly encountered in the developing world.

The first test to perform is the pregnancy test; urinary HCG point of care testing has the benefit of lower cost and no need for a centralized lab, but the serum bHCG is a more sensitive test and preferred when available. If the patient is not pregnant, the next step is to perform the progestin challenge test. In the progestin challenge test, an amenorrheic patient is given an oral progestin (e.g. medroxyprogesterone acetate 10 mg PO daily for 10 days); if a withdrawal bleed happens, it both proves that estradiol levels are adequate to allow endometrial proliferation and rules out an outflow tract obstruction. This scenario most often is seen in patients with anovulation from PCOS. Follow-up testing for such patients should include serum androgens (including testosterone, free testosterone, DHEA-S and 17-OH progesterone); as per Chap. 64 of this textbook, these tests are useful both in order to establish a diagnosis of PCOS and to exclude other causes of hyperandrogenism. Serum prolactin should also be tested; although marked elevations in prolactin typically cause hypoestrogenaemia, lower level elevations can still have menstrual implications. Finally, thyroid-stimulating hormone (TSH) levels are needed to rule out underlying thyroid dysfunction. However, in resource-limited settings, one can consider omitting this test unless clinical suspicion is high, as only overt hypo- and hyperthyroidism seem to associate with amenorrhea [25].

If no withdrawal bleed occurs with the progestin challenge test, a follow-up test can be performed with administration of either a combined oral contraceptive or an oestrogen (e.g. conjugated equine oestrogen 1.25 mg PO daily for 21 days) followed by a progestin (e.g. medroxyprogesterone acetate 10 mg PO daily for 10 days) [28]. Hypoestrogenic patients will have a withdrawal bleed with this test, as exogenous oestrogen will allow endometrial proliferation, but women with a structural anomaly or outflow tract obstruction will not [29]. In the patient with primary amenorrhea, pelvic ultrasound, an economical and accessible imaging approach for many providers throughout the world [30], can complement the physical exam to identify structural anomalies. Haematocolpos can be seen in patients with an imperforate hymen or transverse vaginal septum. Ultrasound may confirm or reveal the absence of a uterus in a patient with CAIS or MRKHS. If a uterus is not present, serum androgens are useful in distinguishing between patients with Müllerian agenesis and CAIS, as the androgens will be markedly elevated in a CAIS patient. Karyotype is another way to diagnose CAIS, as the patient will be 46,XY.

For patients with secondary amenorrhea who fail the oestrogen-progestin challenge test, the presence of hematometra on ultrasound can suggest an acquired outflow tract obstruction (Fig. 49.3a). When available, pelvic ultrasound supplemented with saline infusion can allow visualisation of the constricted uterine cavity of Asherman's syndrome (Fig. 49.3b). Fluoroscopic hysterosalpingography is equally effective for detecting Asherman's syndrome [31] and is a reasonable alternative in settings where this is the more accessible imaging modality [32]. Hysteroscopy is the gold standard for diagnosis of Asherman's syndrome and offers the added benefit of concomitant diagnosis and treatment [26]. Finally, when there is concern of Asherman's syndrome, testing for tuberculosis and schistosomiasis should be considered for patients in endemic areas or with known exposures [27].

Patients who have a bleed to the oestrogen-progestin challenge test are the group with the broadest differential diagnosis to work through. The next step in evaluation of such patients is to test their serum follicle-stimulating hormone

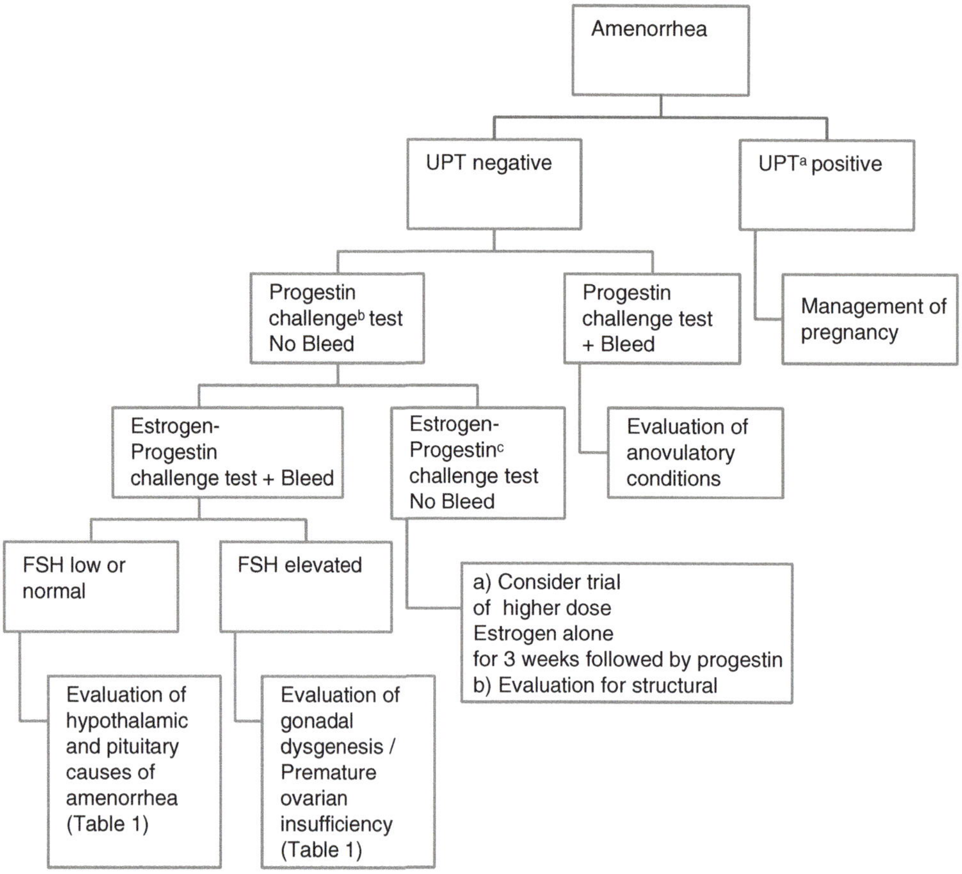

Fig. 49.2 Algorithm for the evaluation of amenorrhea. (**a**) UPT – urine pregnancy test. (**b**) A 7- to 10-day course of a locally available progestin (e.g. 10 mg daily of medroxyprogesterone acetate or 5 mg daily of norethindrone acetate). (**c**) Three-week course of a locally available hormonal contraceptive (combined oestrogen plus progestin) formulation is usually effective; in the absence of any contraindications, preferentially consider formulations containing moderate doses of oestrogen (e.g. 25–30 microgram ethinylestradiol) over lesser oestrogen dose contraceptives for this trial

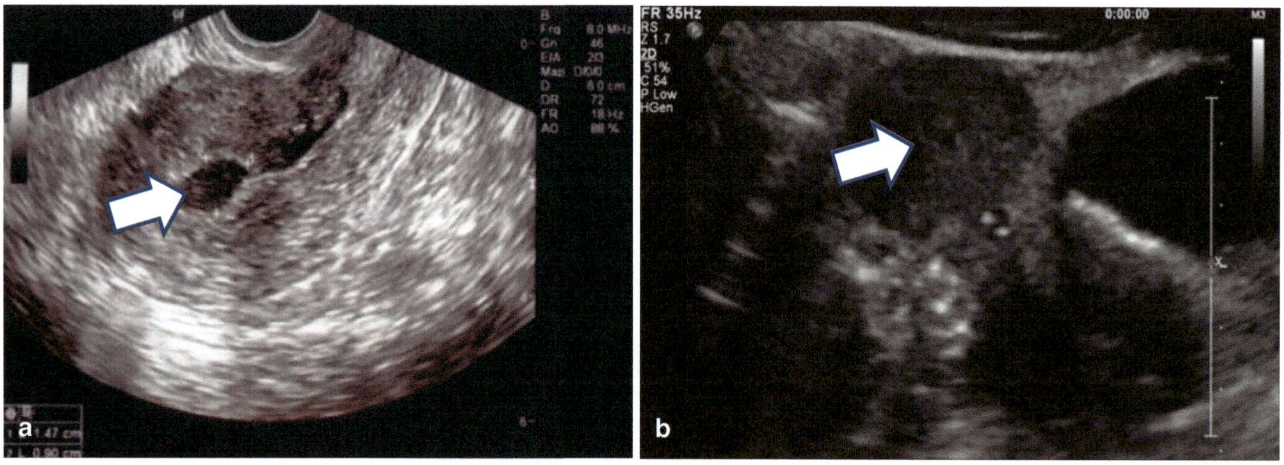

Fig. 49.3 Medical imaging in amenorrhea. (**a**) Transvaginal ultrasound showing hematometra (white arrow) from cervical stenosis. (**b**) Transabdominal ultrasound during saline infusion showing minimal cavity distension (white arrow), secondary to Asherman's syndrome

(FSH), as it distinguishes patients with hypogonadotropic hypogonadism (i.e. WHO class I) from those with hypergonadotropic hypogonadism (i.e. WHO class III). For patients with a low or normal FSH (hypogonadotropic hypogonadism), prolactin is also an essential test, as hyperprolactinaemia must be excluded when considering this class of patients. As discussed for the patients who failed the progestin challenge test, TSH can also be obtained in patients with hypogonadotropic hypogonadism in order to rule out thyroid dysfunction, particularly if clinical suspicion of thyroid disease is high. MRI of the brain is recommended in amenorrheic women who have lab evidence of hyperprolactinaemia (after two elevated values, due to the high false positive rate of the test), manifest symptoms of an intracranial process (e.g. headache or visual disturbance) or who do not have any clear explanation for hypogonadotropic hypogonadism, as these patients may have an underlying intracranial mass manifesting as amenorrhea.

Patients with evidence of hypergonadotropic hypogonadism should be evaluated for the various causes of gonadal dysgenesis and POI. A karyotype should be obtained to diagnose Turner syndrome, Turner mosaicism or Swyer syndrome. It is important to identify such patients, as 45% of women with Turner syndrome have some form of congenital heart disease [33] and 25% of women with a Y chromosome will develop gonadal tumours [34]. Genetic testing for mutations implicated in POI, such as the fragile X premutation, is prudent when available for women with hypergonadotropic hypogonadism. Antiadrenal antibodies should be assessed in women with unexplained POI, due to the high rate of autoimmunity in this population and the ramifications of undiagnosed adrenal insufficiency.

49.1.4 Treatment

Treatment strategies for amenorrhea can be grouped into two categories: targeted treatments for symptomatic underlying causes and goal-directed therapies. Symptomatic underlying causes which can be managed primarily include endocrinopathies, outflow tract obstructions, infections, systemic disease and malnutrition. Goal-directed therapies are those which do not correct the amenorrhea primarily, but rather address the associated problems of hypoestrogenism, endometrial hyperplasia risk and infertility.

Among the symptomatic underlying causes, the endocrinopathies of hyperprolactinaemia and thyroid dysfunction are among the most common. Hyperprolactinaemia is primarily managed medically with dopamine agonists such as bromocriptine or cabergoline. While both are effective, cabergoline has a superior side effect profile, but bromocriptine has more safety data for use in pregnancy. If the patient has MRI evidence of a pituitary macroadenoma (i.e. a prolactinoma larger than 1 cm in size) which is not responding to medical therapy, or if symptoms worsen despite multiple attempts at medical treatment, the patient should be referred for neurosurgical consultation [14]. Patients with hypothyroidism should be initiated on thyroxine supplementation. Hyperthyroidism merits further evaluation to determine the underlying process (e.g. Grave's disease versus toxic nodule), and the patient should be referred to an endocrinologist for a thorough discussion of the risks and benefits of medical, radioactive and surgical approaches to management.

Women with amenorrhea due to outflow tract obstructions benefit primarily from surgical correction, although menstrual suppression through continuous use of a combined hormonal contraceptive or ovarian suppression through hypothalamo-pituitary suppression using a GnRH analogue can be temporary considerations in providing symptomatic relief in the setting of pain resulting from cryptomenorrhea. Primary amenorrhea resulting from a vaginal septum or imperforate hymen will often need surgery for relief of haematocolpos and associated discomfort and to minimise risk for endometriosis resulting from exaggerated retrograde menstrual spill. In contrast to those with distal outlet obstruction (such as cervical stenosis, transverse vaginal septum or imperforate hymen), women with Asherman's syndrome may or may not experience cyclic discomfort, depending on the degree of residual functional endometrium proximal to the area of uterine cavity scarring and whether their endometrium is capable of proliferating and yielding concealed menses. Thus, the need for surgical correction for patients with Asherman's is driven more by a patient's desire for future fertility rather than symptom bother. If surgery is desired for the correction of Asherman's syndrome, it is carried out hysteroscopically, and preferably under ultrasound guidance; the historical use of blind dilation and curettage has high rates of uterine perforation and is considered obsolete [26]. Following hysteroscopic correction of the uterine cavity, data show a benefit to the post-operative use of exogenous oestrogen to promote endometrial regrowth and return of menses [35]. Additionally, many providers will place an intrauterine balloon, uterine Foley catheter or IUD at the time of surgery to minimise re-approximation of the opposing uterine walls during the process of healing to prevent re-formation of adhesions [26].

Amenorrhea associated with infections, systemic disease and malnutrition may resolve with adequate medical treatment of the underlying problem. For instance, roughly three-quarters of women with pulmonary tuberculosis resume normal menses after completion of standard TB treatment [36].

Many patients with amenorrhea, including those with gonadal dysgenesis, POI and hypothalamic amenorrhea, live in a sustained hypoestrogenic state. This can impair normal pubertal development and be deleterious to cardiovascular and bone health. Details about management of delayed puberty can be found in Chap. 61 of this textbook, so such discussion will be deferred here. Observational data suggest that early menopause can be associated with increases in total morbidity and mortality due to ischemic heart disease and possibly stroke [37–39]. However, current data do not suggest a benefit to oestrogen supplementation for preventing these outcomes. On the other hand, bone health does benefit from oestrogen supplementation. Women who develop POI prior to peak bone mass attainment are at particular risk for osteoporotic fractures [40, 41]. For this reason, women with POI should be offered oestrogen replacement in the form of oral birth control pills or oestrogen/progestin hormone replacement. In the case of hypoestrogenism caused by hypothalamic amenorrhea, treatment with oral contraceptives has been shown to help bone density. However, weight gain shows a greater effect on bone mineral density, and therefore, behavioural modification should be recommended as the first-line strategy for optimising bone health in this patient population [42, 43].

For patients who have amenorrhea secondary to anovulatory conditions such as PCOS, an essential part of treatment is the reduction of endometrial hyperplasia risk conferred by the prolonged unopposed oestrogen state. Because PCOS more often causes infrequent menses and abnormal uterine bleeding, further discussion on this aspect of management will be deferred to the subsequent section on AUB.

Amenorrheic patients may be infertile for a variety of reasons, and a desire for fertility may be what directs their management. Anovulatory PCOS patients, on the one hand, may be able to conceive with the use of an oral ovulation induction medication, such as clomiphene citrate or letrozole. Patients with hypothalamic amenorrhea, on the other hand, may require injectable exogenous gonadotropins for folliculogenesis and ovulation for in vitro fertilization (IVF). Patients with gonadal dysgenesis or POI may not be capable of reproducing with their own oocytes, and thus would only have the option of donor oocyte IVF if they wish to pursue child-bearing. Patients with infertility due to Asherman's syndrome, as described above, would require surgical correction in order to carry a pregnancy. Women who fail Asherman's syndrome corrective surgery or have Müllerian agenesis would need to use a gestational carrier or undergo uterine transplantation [44] in order to have children. For further details on these fertility treatments, please refer to Chap. 65.

49.1.5 Amenorrhea and Public Health in the Developing World

While amenorrhea itself does not pose a public health risk, the associated conditions of hypoestrogenism and infertility create a burden for society. The most significant and preventable contributors to amenorrhea in the developing world are consequent to interventions that are undertaken during the course of management of obstetric haemorrhage (endometrial curettage to control PPH) or pregnancy termination, with resulting endometrial scarring, or infection and malnutrition. Efforts to improve eradication of causal diseases, such as tuberculosis and schistosomiasis, may result in decreased rates of amenorrhea. Improved nutrition would also be expected to reduce the prevalence of amenorrhea throughout the developing world.

49.2 Abnormal Uterine Bleeding

49.2.1 Background

Abnormal uterine bleeding (AUB) is a general term encompassing a large variety of disordered bleeding patterns and is the manifestation of a diverse array of disease processes. Throughout the developed [45] and developing world [6], AUB is one of the most common gynaecologic concerns that brings women to seek healthcare. In the United States, the annual prevalence of AUB has been estimated at 5.3% [46], with prevalence estimates as high as 15% across the developing world [6].

Abnormal uterine bleeding impacts women's lives in several key ways. It is a sign of underlying disease, commonly serving as the first indication of a serious disease process. For instance, adolescent women with an inherited coagulopathy will commonly be diagnosed after menarche due to their heavy menstrual bleeding, and women with endometrial hyperplasia or cancer will frequently present with AUB as their first symptom. AUB can also be a direct cause of morbidity by contributing to anaemia through blood loss. This is of particular consequence in the developing countries of Africa, where nutritional deficiencies contribute to the highest rates of anaemia in the world [47]. Beyond its influence on direct measures of health, AUB also has significant impact on women's quality of life and access to opportunities within society, due to missed days of work or school and social isolation from embarrassment, fatigue and discomfort [48].

As an umbrella term, abnormal uterine bleeding includes menses of abnormal quantity, duration and schedule (Table 49.3).

Heavy menstrual bleeding (HMB), formerly termed menorrhagia, is defined for research purposes as menses with greater than 80 mL of blood loss. Clinically, it is more meaningful to define this symptom from the patient's subjective perception of her bleeding [45], as the practicality and accuracy of measuring menstrual flow is limited. Furthermore, the quality-of-life impact of HMB cannot easily be measured objectively, so the benefit of treatment can be best determined by a patient's subjective perception of need. (Of

Table 49.3 Normal and abnormal uterine bleeding [45, 46]

Volume of monthly blood loss	Normal: ≤80 mL
	Heavy menstrual bleeding (HMB): >80 mL
Duration of menses	Normal: 3–6 days
	Prolonged: ≥7 days
Frequency of menses	Normal: 21–35 days
	Frequent: <21 days
	Infrequent: >35 days
Intermenstrual bleeding	Bleeding between menses

course, objective evidence of hemodynamic compromise from HMB, such as significant blood loss anaemia or vital sign abnormalities, merits immediate clinical attention irrespective of a patient's subjective perceptions.) Prolonged menses (i.e. those lasting 7 days or longer) can also lead to excessive blood loss and should be evaluated. A disordered menstrual schedule can indicate underlying pathology and be a nuisance to the patient. Frequent menses (formerly termed polymenorrhea [49]) occur more often than every 21 days, and infrequent menses (formerly termed oligomenorrhea [49]) occur less often than every 35 days [45]. While intermenstrual bleeding can be a normal periovulatory event in 1–2% of women, the possibility of a more serious cause makes this symptom worthy of assessment as well [49].

Abnormal uterine bleeding can be further categorised into acute AUB and chronic AUB. Acute AUB is defined by the International Federation of Gynaecology and Obstetrics (FIGO) as "an episode of bleeding in a woman of reproductive age, who is not pregnant, that is of sufficient quantity to require immediate intervention to prevent further blood loss." [49] Thus, acute AUB, on the one hand, is typically the result of HMB or prolonged menses, although it can emerge in the context of a disordered menstrual schedule. Chronic AUB, on the other hand, is defined as AUB that has been present for the majority of the prior 6 months [49].

49.2.2 Causes

Since AUB can result from a wide array of underlying causes, FIGO has developed a classification system to further delineate subtypes of AUB. This system, known by the acronym PALM-COEIN, was developed with the input of clinicians from six continents to maximise its utility across different healthcare settings throughout the developed and developing world. The PALM-COEIN system distinguishes AUB caused by nine distinct aetiologies (Table 49.4) and forms the basis of a differential diagnosis for AUB. The structural causes of AUB are represented by the PALM categories, while the non-structural causes (e.g. haematologic, endocrinologic, etc.) are encompassed in the COEIN categories [50].

Table 49.4 FIGO classification system (PALM-COEIN) for causes of abnormal uterine bleeding [50]

Polyp		**C**oagulopathy
Adenomyosis		**O**vulatory dysfunction
Leiomyomata	**SM** – submucosal	**E**ndometrial
	O – other	**I**atrogenic
Malignancy/hyperplasia		**N**ot yet classified

AUB-P is abnormal bleeding caused by endometrial polyps, which are intrauterine growths of vascularized endometrial glands and stroma. Polyps can be sessile or pedunculated, and single or in multiples; they range in size from millimetres to centimetres and can originate from anywhere within the uterine cavity. Ageing, obesity and tamoxifen use are risk factors for the development of polyps. Two-thirds of women with endometrial polyps will experience AUB, with intermenstrual bleeding and HMB as the most common patterns [51]. In premenopausal women, endometrial polyps have only a 1.7% chance of malignancy, but the risk is increased if the patient has AUB. Thus, for patients with AUB-P, polyp removal is recommended to both address the presenting symptom and assess for malignancy [52].

AUB-A is abnormal bleeding associated with adenomyosis, a disorder defined by the presence of endometrial glands and stroma within the myometrium. Women with adenomyosis may experience HMB (50%), dysmenorrhea (30%) and intermenstrual bleeding (20%). Adenomyosis has historically been diagnosed only by histologic evaluation after hysterectomy, so while the lifetime prevalence is estimated to be approximately 20%, the true prevalence is unknown [53]. According to FIGO, AUB-A can be diagnosed if imaging criteria consistent with adenomyosis are met [50]. Although MRI has greater sensitivity and specificity for identifying adenomyosis in certain clinical contexts (e.g. when a patient also has leiomyomata) [53], FIGO recognises ultrasonographic evidence as adequate for diagnosis of AUB-A, given restricted access to MRI in settings with limited resources such as the developing world [50].

A third category of structural AUB is abnormal uterine bleeding from leiomyomata (AUB-L). Leiomyomata, also known as fibroids, are benign growths of myometrial smooth muscle. The pattern of AUB they most frequently cause is HMB, which is mediated by alteration to the usual haemostatic mechanisms of the uterus through changes in vascular compression and the release of vasoactive growth factors [54]. AUB-L is the only FIGO category currently with subcategories; AUB-L_{SM} and AUB-L_{O} (submucosal leiomyoma vs. other leiomyoma) distinguish between the leiomyoma locations with greater and lesser impact on AUB, respectively [50].

AUB-M includes bleeding associated with uterine malignancy and hyperplasia. The bleeding pattern of AUB-M may be intermenstrual bleeding, frequent menses, HMB or prolonged bleeding. AUB is often the first clinical evidence of hyperplasia or neoplasia, so this must be considered in patients with risk factors such as increased age, exposure to unopposed oestrogen, obesity and Lynch syndrome [55]. All patients with AUB who are older than age 45 should have endometrial sampling to evaluate for these processes, as should all women with AUB younger than age 45 but with history of unopposed oestrogen exposure (e.g. anovulation, obesity, tamoxifen use), failed medical management of AUB or high-risk family/genetic histories [45].

Impaired haemostasis underlies the abnormal bleeding of AUB-C (coagulopathy). The coagulopathy can be innate, such as von Willebrand disease or inherited platelet dysfunction, or acquired, such as in patients with uraemia from renal disease or on anticoagulant medications [50]. The most common cause of AUB-C is von Willebrand disease. In a systematic review of North American and European studies, the prevalence of vWD among women with AUB was 13%, although some of these women had other reasons for AUB as well. The prevalence of vWD among women with AUB may be lower in an African population, if the lower prevalence seen in North American women of African ancestry is genetic in origin [56]. One cause of AUB-C which is more common in the developing world is dengue haemorrhagic fever, where HMB can ensue among other haemorrhagic complications [6].

AUB-O is abnormal bleeding caused by ovulatory dysfunction. Anovulation leads to a lack of cyclic progesterone and continued endometrial proliferation. With no cyclic progesterone exposure and withdrawal, the endometrium has partial shedding in an unpredictable fashion, which manifests as menses with unpredictable timing and sometimes HMB. Anovulation and oligo-ovulation can result from a variety of endocrinologic disturbances to the hypothalamic-pituitary-ovarian (HPO) axis, including thyroid disease (hyper- and hypothyroidism), hyperprolactinaemia, polycystic ovary syndrome and hypothalamic dysfunction (e.g. nutritional deficiency, systemic illness and stress). Additionally, the HPO axis is commonly dysfunctional at the extremes of reproductive age, with post-menarchal and perimenopausal women frequently experiencing AUB-O [57].

AUB-E results from defects in the mechanisms of endometrial haemostasis, such as deficiencies in vasoconstrictors like endothelin-1, and excesses of vasodilators, such as prostaglandin E_2 [50]. Alterations in these mechanisms may be the way in which pelvic infections lead to AUB. Although the association between chronic endometritis and AUB is debated [58], acute endometritis in the postpartum or postabortal period can cause HMB. AUB has also been described in patients with subclinical *Chlamydia trachomatis* infections [59], pelvic inflammatory disease [60], and endometrial tuberculosis [6].

Iatrogenic causes of disordered menstruation are included in AUB-I. This category predominantly includes the effects of contraceptive devices and medications. Copper intrauterine devices can cause HMB and intermenstrual bleeding [61], causing anaemic users to have worsening of their anaemia and iron stores [62]. The etonogestrel implant, on the one hand, causes AUB in up to 50% of its users, and the progesterone-only contraceptive pill causes an irregular bleeding pattern in 30–40% of women. The levonorgestrel intrauterine device, on the other hand, will only cause irregular cycles and HMB (in some users) for the first 3–6 months, after which the menses typically lighten substantially, with some women becoming amenorrheic. Similarly, injectable depot medroxyprogesterone acetate can cause menstrual disturbances for the first 3 months of use, but 70% of women are amenorrheic after 1 year of use [63]. Combined hormonal contraceptives, such as the pill, patch and ring, do not generally cause AUB after the first 3 months of use, unless doses are missed or delayed [50]. Other medications which can iatrogenically contribute to AUB include those which induce hyperprolactinaemia, such as first-generation antipsychotic medications and tricyclic antidepressants, by causing anovulation [64].

The final FIGO category for abnormal uterine bleeding is AUB-N (not yet classified). This category includes unvalidated and poorly defined clinical entities which may have an association with AUB, but further investigation is needed [50].

49.2.3 Evaluation

The evaluation of a patient presenting with abnormal uterine bleeding begins with a detailed history. Primary attention should be paid to the patient's menstrual history, including age at menarche; her cycle length and regularity, her menstrual flow amount and duration, the presence of intermenstrual bleeding or spotting and any recent changes to her menses. As noted above, the differential diagnosis of what underlies AUB can be narrowed based upon the observed menstrual pattern. For women with irregular or infrequent cycles, it may also be helpful to assess for the presence of moliminal symptoms prior to the menses, as these would not be seen in anovulatory cycles. Other important aspects of a patient's gynaecologic history include a sexual history (which may increase or decrease the likelihood of pregnancy or underlying infection), the use of contraception (which may lead to iatrogenic AUB), her cervical screening history (which may suggest a non-uterine cause of bleeding) and the presence of pelvic pain or dyspareunia (which may point to infection or adenomyosis). Recent genital or sexual trauma can indicate a lower genital tract source of bleeding (such as from the cervix, vagina or vulva), which is distinct from AUB [45].

When evaluating AUB, aspects of the patient's broader health history must be considered as well. Non-gynaecologic bleeding can masquerade as AUB, so the clinician should assess for whether haematuria or rectal bleeding is what the patient is truly experiencing. Relevant aspects of a woman's medical history include renal disease (which may lead to coagulopathy), evidence of endocrinopathy (such as thyroid disease or hyperprolactinaemia) or hyperandrogenism (commonly seen in polycystic ovary syndrome), obesity (which may predispose to endometrial hyperplasia/malignancy and ovulatory dysfunction) or nutritional deficiency (either due to limited food access, eating disorder or gastrointestinal dysfunction such as celiac disease). A history of prior gynaecologic surgery, such as myomectomy or polypectomy, can increase suspicion of recurrent pathology. Family history of coagulopathy and cancer syndromes (e.g. Lynch syndrome) increase suspicion of heritable causes of AUB. A review of the patient's medications can reveal iatrogenic causes of abnormal bleeding, as reviewed above [50].

Physical examination is the next step in evaluation of AUB. Vital signs should be assessed to identify any evidence of haemodynamic compromise or anaemia. The pelvic examination provides an essential source of information; in developing countries where access to medical imaging may be more limited, the pelvic exam has an even more vital role. A speculum examination can reveal lower genital tract sources of bleeding, such as lesions on the cervix or trauma to the vagina or vulva. It also can allow a quantification of active ongoing uterine bleeding, which is important in the patient with acute AUB. The bimanual examination can reveal evidence of structural causes of AUB, if the patient has palpable leiomyomata or a boggy and globular uterus suggestive of adenomyosis. Tenderness elicited on bimanual examination or with cervical motion may suggest adenomyosis or an infectious cause of AUB, such as endometritis, chlamydial infection or pelvic inflammatory disease. The possibility of a non-gynaecologic source of bleeding can be further assessed by inspecting the urethra and anus, with digital rectal examination if indicated. Finally, during general physical exam, attention should be paid for physical stigmata of anaemia (such as pallor, tachycardia), of iron deficiency (angular cheilosis, atrophic glossitis or koilonychia), of liver disease (including portal hypertension, caput medusa and hepatosplenomegaly) which may predispose to coagulopathy, of insulin resistance (e.g. acanthosis nigricans, central obesity) or hyperandrogenism (suggestive of polycystic ovary syndrome), and of thyroid abnormalities (irregularity, nodularity, enlargement or tenderness), and galactorrhea should be assessed (consistent with hyperprolactinaemia) [45].

Laboratory evaluation is required for true diagnosis and severity assessment in many cases of AUB. The first test to consider is pregnancy testing with serum or urinary human chorionic gonadotropin (hCG), as pregnancy must be ruled out to consider AUB. The other essential lab test to perform is an assessment of the patient's haemoglobin to identify evidence of anaemia [65]. Both of these tests are available as a point-of-care test, which may be of benefit in the developing world when access to full laboratories is limited [66]. Laboratory evaluation is also required for identifying underlying coagulopathies and endocrinopathies. Coagulopathy should be considered in patients with a history of lifelong HMB, excess bleeding with surgeries or dental work or postpartum haemorrhage; the appropriate lab tests to obtain depend on patient-specific factors and what tests are available in each particular low-resource setting. Endocrinopathies are common causes of AUB-O, and the patient's clinical presentation may suggest the presence of one or another. Thyroid function does not need to be measured in all patients with AUB, but rather for those women with an irregular menstrual pattern suggestive of anovulation or a family history of thyroid disease [65]. Androgen levels can help to differentiate between polycystic ovary syndrome and other disorders of androgen excess, such as androgen-secreting tumours. For further details on androgen excess, please refer to Chap. 64.

Medical imaging can help to identify various structural causes of AUB. In the developing world, this predominantly would be done with ultrasound where available. Decreasing costs, improving technology, portability and lack of need for dedicated services (e.g. film, technicians and radiologists) have made ultrasound a particularly appealing imaging modality through the developing world [30]. When available, transvaginal ultrasonography allows for an improved visualization of the pelvic organs in most women (as compared to transabdominal ultrasonography). If an intracavitary lesion is suspected, such as an endometrial polyp or submucosal myoma, the imaging may be enhanced with saline-infusion sonography or hysteroscopy, when available (Fig. 49.4) [45].

A final, but important, component of evaluation for selected women with AUB is endometrial sampling. While endometrial sampling may be used for the detection of chlamydial infections of the endometrium, its primary role is in screening for endometrial hyperplasia or malignancy [50]. Risk factors for hyperplasia or malignancy and indications for screening were reviewed above. Sampling can be obtained with an office biopsy, global dilation and curettage or hysteroscopically directed biopsies. Surgical approaches are more expensive and require more infrastructure without significant diagnostic benefit. Thus, office biopsy is the first-line approach to endometrial sampling [55], and this holds true in low-resource settings like the developing world.

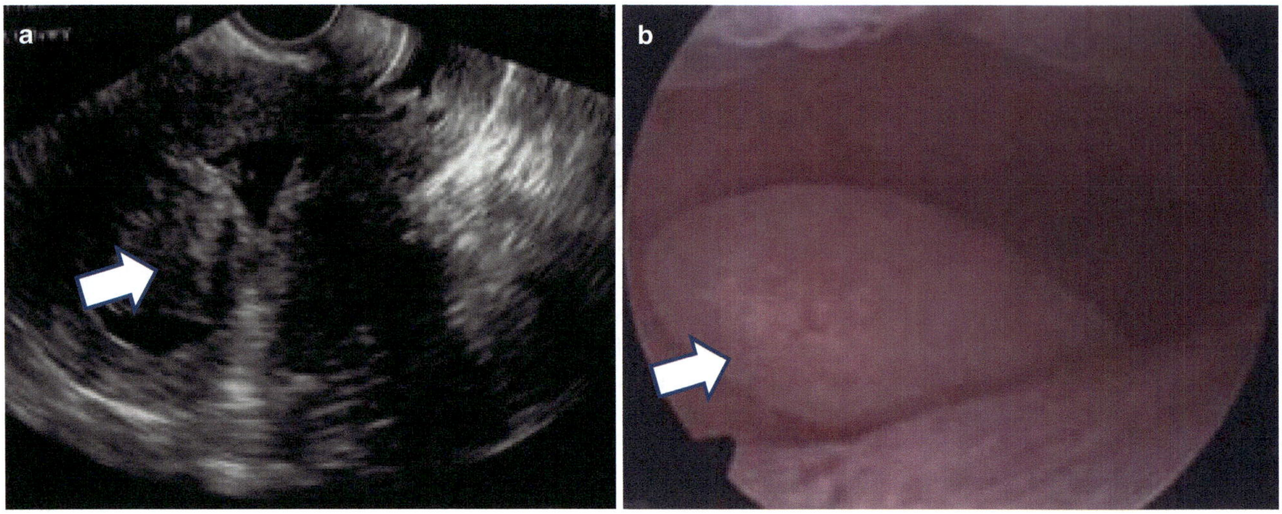

Fig. 49.4 Medical imaging in AUB. (**a**) Saline infusion sonography showing submucosal leiomyoma (white arrow). (**b**) Hysteroscopy showing endometrial polyp (white arrow)

49.2.4 Treatment

Patients presenting with acute episodes of AUB often require quick interventions with quick results, in order to keep a patient from becoming unstable or to stabilize a haemodynamically compromised patient. If a patient with acute AUB is unstable, the first step in management is establishment of reliable large-bore intravenous access for fluid resuscitation or blood transfusion, if indicated. As a temporizing measure, intrauterine tamponade can be attained using a Foley catheter (30 cc balloon) or gauze packing. Medical management options to consider include IV oestrogen (e.g. conjugated equine oestrogens 25 mg every 4–6 hours for 24 hours), high dose combined oral contraceptive pill regimens (e.g. combined oral contraceptive three times per day for 7 days) or oral progestins (e.g. medroxyprogesterone acetate 20 mg every 8 hours for 7 days). Moderate oestrogen dose formulations (e.g. those containing 30–35 microgram ethinylestradiol) should be preferentially considered for the high dose hormonal contraceptive regimens for control of HMB.

A non-hormonal medical option is tranexamic acid, an antifibrinolytic which can be given intravenously or orally. Of these medical options, IV oestrogen yields the quickest response, giving significant improvement to bleeding within the course of hours. Surgical management can be used if the patient will not be stable over the course of hours, or if these medicines are unavailable or contraindicated. Fertility-sparing surgery is limited to dilation and curettage, which can stabilize the bleeding but does not prevent recurrence; effective surgeries for patients not desiring future fertility include endometrial ablation and hysterectomy [67].

An expanded set of management options is available to control chronic AUB. The treatment is chosen with consideration to the underlying cause of the AUB and the patient's overall goals of care, particularly with reference to current and future fertility plans. If, for instance, a patient's AUB results from coagulopathy, hyperprolactinaemia or thyroid disease, the primary approach to management is to correct the underlying problem. Table 49.5 summarises the major treatment options for chronic AUB, which can be categorised into medical/hormonal, medical/nonhormonal and surgical.

There are several hormonal medications which can benefit the patient with AUB (Table 49.5a). The first option for many women is an oestrogen/progestin hormonal contraceptive, such as the pill, patch or vaginal ring. Oestrogen/progestin contraceptives are effective at regulating irregular menstrual cycles, decreasing the menstrual blood loss and reducing dysmenorrhea [68]. Cyclic regimens with a shorter number of med-free (i.e. placebo) days generally have less blood loss with each menses when compared to women with seven med-free days each month [69]. Oestrogen/progestin contraceptives can also be administered in extended or continuous courses, where med-free days only occur every several months or not at all; this can benefit women for whom menstrual bleeding poses a significant health risk or life disturbance. These medicines are not safe for all women, such as those who use tobacco or who have hypertension, migraine with aura or stroke. A full list of medical eligibility criteria is published by the World Health Organization in its Medical Eligibility Criteria for contraceptive use [70]. For further details on oestrogen/progestin contraceptives, please refer to Chap. 49 of this textbook.

Another first-line approach for many women with AUB is the levonorgestrel intrauterine system (LNG-IUS). LNG-IUS is effective for the treatment of HMB and endometrial protection while providing highly effective long-acting contraception. Many women become amenorrheic with the LNG-IUS in place, and the reduction in menstrual bleeding

Table 49.5 Treatment options for management of abnormal uterine bleeding (AUB). Note that causes of AUB are categorised per FIGO classification system (PALM-COEIN) terminology [50] (Table 49.4)

(a) *Hormonal treatment options for management of AUB*			
Medication	**Beneficiaries**	**Pros**	**Cons**
Oestrogen/progestin contraceptives	HMB AUB-O [a]AUB-A, L, C, I	Contraception Endometrial protection Extended/continuous option	Larger contraindication list
LNG-IUS	HMB AUB-A, M, C, O, I [a]AUB-L	High rate of amenorrhea Contraception Endometrial protection	Procedure/indwelling Cavity shape/size Cost
Oral progestin	HMB AUB-M, O [a]AUB-L, C, I	Endometrial protection Fewer contraindications	Not proven contraceptive Side effect profile
Injected progestin	HMB AUB-O [a]AUB-L, C, I	High rate of amenorrhea Contraception	Not approved for endometrial protection
Injected GnRH agonist	HMB AUB-A, L, C, I	Can reduce size of pathology	Side effect profile Cost
(b) *Non-hormonal treatment options for management of AUB*			
Medication	**Beneficiaries**	**Pros**	**Cons**
NSAIDs	HMB	Only needed during menses Can be used in months attempting conception Treats dysmenorrhea Low cost Low risk	Less effective
Tranexamic acid	HMB AUB-L, C	Only needed during menses Can be used in months attempting conception	Contraindicated if VTE risk
(c) *Surgical options for management of AUB*			
Surgery	**Beneficiaries**	**Pros**	**Cons**
Hysteroscopy polypectomy	AUB-P	Outpatient procedure Targeted treatment for polypfertility sparing	Polyp recurrence
Myomectomy	AUB-L	Fertility sparing Definitive treatment of fibroids	Fibroid recurrence Surgical morbidity Surgical recovery
Dilation and curettage	HMB AUB-P	Outpatient procedure Acute bleeding control	Short duration of benefit
Endometrial ablation	HMB AUB-L, C, I [a]AUB-O	High rate of amenorrhea Outpatient/office surgery	Needs concomitant contraception – Future pregnancy contraindicated Contraindicated in hyperplasia
Hysterectomy	All AUB	Definitive management for AUB	Loss of fertility Surgical morbidity Surgical recovery
Uterine artery embolization	AUB-L [a]AUB-A	Quicker recovery than hysterectomy	Future pregnancy contraindicated

HMB heavy menstrual bleeding.
[a]*Indicates inconclusive data or patient-specific aspects to benefit. Treatment method not first-line approach for these aetiologies of AUB*

is superior to oestrogen/progestin contraceptives [68]. The LNG-IUS has fewer contraindications than oestrogen/progestin contraceptives; these predominantly relate to the uterine shape (e.g. large submucosal fibroids and uterine anomalies) [70]. Another limitation to broad usage of the LNG-IUS in the developing world is its cost. Although providers and users throughout Africa have found the LNG-IUS to be an appealing medical device, access has remained limited [71]. A low-cost version of the device has been developed (marketed as Liletta in the United States and as Levosert in the rest of the world), which will hopefully improve access to the product throughout the developing world [72].

Second-line hormonal medical approaches can be considered in patients for whom first-line approaches are unavailable or contraindicated. These would include high-dose oral progestins, injectable progestins and GnRH agonists. High-dose oral progestin regimens, such as medroxyprogesterone 5 mg daily, are better than placebo, but not as effective as combined contraceptives, for improving AUB [65]. These oral progestins have not been validated as effective contraceptives, so additional contraception may be needed by the patient. Injectable progestins, such as depot medroxyprogesterone acetate, are effective for contraception and can successfully induce amenorrhea or decrease bleeding, and thus could be a reasonable approach for some patients. Injectable GnRH agonists, such as leuprolide, are effective at inducing amenorrhea. However, due to its cost and side effect profile (from resultant hypoestrogenism), this method is only typically used in settings where a specific benefit from this approach is sought, such as reducing the size of leiomyomata before surgery, rather than as a maintenance medication for AUB [65].

Nonhormonal medications are also successful strategies for the management of AUB (Table 49.5b). The most successful nonhormonal option is tranexamic acid, an antifibrinolytic medication which has been shown to cause a 26–54% reduction in uterine bleeding among women with AUB [68]. Tranexamic acid can be used during months where conception is being actively attempted if used around the time of the menses, giving it a unique advantage over hormonal approaches for the couple desiring imminent pregnancy [65]. NSAIDs, such as naproxen, are also somewhat effective at reducing menstrual bleeding in women with AUB [68]. Although their effect is more moderate, they are typically easier to access and have fewer contraindications than many of the hormonal approaches [65].

Surgical management for AUB can be done in a fertility-sparing or fertility-sacrificing manner (Table 49.5c). Fertility-sparing surgeries target a specific structural abnormality. For patients with AUB-P, the treatment of choice is hysteroscopic polypectomy, which has been shown to have greater sensitivity than blind polypectomy or dilatation and curettage (D&C) [73]. Patients with HMB due to uterine leiomyomata who desire to preserve their fertility can be treated with myomectomy; depending on fibroid size and location, this may be accomplishable hysteroscopically, laparoscopically (utilising traditional approach or with robotic assistance), abdominally or even vaginally. For further details on myomectomy, please refer to Chap. 51 of this textbook.

Surgical options available to women preferring surgical management of AUB who no longer desire fertility include endometrial ablation, hysterectomy or uterine artery embolisation. Endometrial ablation is a less invasive procedure that can be performed in an office setting, provided the necessary equipment is available. It is not recommended in patients with anovulation or with current hyperplasia, due to the risk of development of a concealed uterine malignancy [73]. After 1–2 years of the procedure, endometrial ablation does not offer any superior quality of life or reduction in blood loss when compared to the more accessible LNG-IUS [73], making commercially available ablation options an approach of limited utility in low-resource settings. There have been reports of low-cost ablation systems, using such approaches as a Foley catheter in the uterus for thermal ablation, which suggest that endometrial ablation may be accomplishable in the developing world, but long-term data are lacking [74]. Hysterectomy offers the most definitive management of AUB, albeit with the highest rates of major complications among the various AUB management strategies [73]. For further information on hysterectomy, please see Chap. 52 of this textbook. Uterine artery embolisation is an approach to AUB which requires specialised interventional radiology facilities. These facilities may not be available in low-resource settings and therefore are beyond the scope of this textbook.

49.2.5 AUB and Public Health in the Developing World

Abnormal uterine bleeding has several public health considerations of particular importance in the developing world. Of foremost concern are the issues that pertain to blood loss anaemia. Africa has the highest rates of anaemia in the world, largely driven by nutritional deficiencies. In women with AUB, blood loss compounds this anaemia, leading to increased morbidity [47]. Studies have shown that women in developing countries with AUB are often not aware of the need for (or do not have access to) iron supplementation to prevent worsening anaemia [6]. Improved education about the relationship between AUB, anaemia and wellness, along with increased access to iron supplementation and improved nutrition, would be of great benefit. Additionally, the lower cost of the copper IUD has made this the more accessible IUD in much of the developing world. However, the copper IUD can worsen AUB and, subsequently, anaemia. Thus, efforts to improve access to the LNG-IUS for contraception may reduce the burden of AUB-related anaemia in the developing world [71].

Cultural views of the menses can also impact the diagnosis and treatment of AUB in the developing world. For instance, in Gambia, menses are customarily only discussed between mother and daughter. This may reduce the likelihood of seeking clinical assessment for heavy bleeding. Additionally, South Asian women have been reported to value heavy menses, as this is believed to have a cleansing benefit. Similar cultural belief systems can normalise pathology, even if it leads to morbid sequelae like blood loss anaemia [6].

49.3 Conclusion

Disorders of the menstrual cycle are of far-ranging significance across the globe, serving as consequences of morbid systemic disease, reflections of nutritional status and indicators of reduced fertility. Prompt recognition and evaluation of such disorders are essential for the early detection and prevention of many long-term health issues, ranging from uterine cancer to anaemia to osteoporosis.

Treatment of amenorrhea is based upon the goals of care. For some amenorrheic women, unopposed oestrogen increases the risk of endometrial hyperplasia and malignancy, so endometrial protection becomes the priority in care. Other amenorrheic women are hypoestrogenic, whether due to POI or hypothalamic amenorrhea, and benefit from strategies to maximise bone and heart health. Managing infertility in the amenorrheic patient is an additional consideration in the lives of many affected women.

On the other hand, treatment of AUB is generally focused on reducing the burden of blood loss on the patient. AUB can compound with iron-deficiency anaemia of dietary origin to worsen the morbidity of the patient's anaemia. Prolonged menstrual flow can be disruptive to social, educational and employment opportunities. By recognising and treating AUB, these burdens can be lessened for women throughout the developing world.

References

1. Practice Committee of American Society for Reproductive Medicine. Current evaluation of amenorrhea. Fertil Steril. 2008;90(5 Suppl):S219–25.
2. Deligeoroglou E, Athanasopoulos N, Tsimaris P, Dimopoulos KD, Vrachnis N, Creatsas G. Evaluation and management of adolescent amenorrhea. Ann N Y Acad Sci. 2010;1205:23–32.
3. ACOG Committee Opinion No. 651: menstruation in girls and adolescents: using the menstrual cycle as a vital sign. Obstet Gynecol. 2015;126(6):e143–6.
4. Morabia A, Costanza MC. International variability in ages at menarche, first livebirth, and menopause. World Health Organization Collaborative Study of Neoplasia and Steroid Contraceptives. Am J Epidemiol. 1998;148(12):1195–205.
5. Thomas F, Renaud F, Benefice E, de Meeus T, Guegan JF. International variability of ages at menarche and menopause: patterns and main determinants. Hum Biol. 2001;73(2):271–90.
6. Harlow SD, Campbell OM. Epidemiology of menstrual disorders in developing countries: a systematic review. BJOG. 2004;111(1):6–16.
7. Glasier AF, Smith KB, van der Spuy ZM, Ho PC, Cheng L, Dada K, Wellings K, Baird DT. Amenorrhea associated with contraception-an international study on acceptability. Contraception. 2003;67(1):1–8.
8. Gordon CM. Clinical practice. Functional hypothalamic amenorrhea. N Engl J Med. 2010;363(4):365–71.
9. Sedlmeyer IL, Palmert MR. Delayed puberty: analysis of a large case series from an academic Centre. J Clin Endocrinol Metab. 2002;87(4):1613–20.
10. Palmert MR, Dunkel L. Clinical practice. Delayed puberty. N Engl J Med. 2012;366(5):443–53.
11. Fallahian M, Ilkhani M. Menstrual disorders in nongenital tuberculosis. Infect Dis Obstet Gynecol. 2006;2006:18452.
12. Santen FJ, Sofsky J, Bilic N, Lippert R. Mechanism of action of narcotics in the production of menstrual dysfunction in women. Fertil Steril. 1975;26(6):538–48.
13. Reindollar RH, Novak M, Tho SP, McDonough PG. Adult-onset amenorrhea: a study of 262 patients. Am J Obstet Gynecol. 1986;155(3):531–43.
14. Capozzi A, Scambia G, Pontecorvi A, Lello S. Hyperprolactinemia: pathophysiology and therapeutic approach. Gynecol Endocrinol. 2015;31(7):506–10.
15. Bayrak A, Saadat P, Mor E, Chong L, Paulson RJ, Sokol RZ. Pituitary imaging is indicated for the evaluation of hyperprolactinemia. Fertil Steril. 2005;84(1):181–5.
16. Lam KS, Sham MM, Tam SC, Ng MM, Ma HT. Hypopituitarism after tuberculous meningitis in childhood. Ann Intern Med. 1993;118(9):701–6.
17. Zargar AH, Singh B, Laway BA, Masoodi SR, Wani AI, Bashir MI. Epidemiologic aspects of postpartum pituitary hypofunction (Sheehan's syndrome). Fertil Steril. 2005;84(2):523–8.
18. Reindollar RH, Byrd JR, McDonough PG. Delayed sexual development: a study of 252 patients. Am J Obstet Gynecol. 1981;140(4):371–80.
19. Cox L, Liu JH. Primary ovarian insufficiency: an update. Int J Women's Health. 2014;6:235–43.
20. Bakalov VK, Anasti JN, Calis KA, Vanderhoof VH, Premkumar A, Chen S, Furmaniak J, Smith BR, Merino MJ, Nelson LM. Autoimmune oophoritis as a mechanism of follicular dysfunction in women with 46,XX spontaneous premature ovarian failure. Fertil Steril. 2005;84(4):958–65.
21. Bakalov VK, Vanderhoof VH, Bondy CA, Nelson LM. Adrenal antibodies detect asymptomatic auto-immune adrenal insufficiency in young women with spontaneous premature ovarian failure. Hum Reprod. 2002;17(8):2096–100.
22. Kim TJ, Anasti JN, Flack MR, Kimzey LM, Defensor RA, Nelson LM. Routine endocrine screening for patients with karyotypically normal spontaneous premature ovarian failure. Obstet Gynaecol. 1997;89(5):777–9.
23. Rotterdam ESHRE/ASRM-Sponsored PCOS Consensus Workshop Group. Revised 2003 consensus on diagnostic criteria and long-term health risks related to polycystic ovary syndrome. Fertil Steril. 2004;81(1):19–25.
24. Krassas GE, Pontikides N, Kaltsas T, Papadopoulou P, Paunkovic J, Paunkovic N, Duntas LH. Disturbances of menstruation in hypothyroidism. Clin Endocrinol. 1999;50(5):655–9.
25. Kakuno Y, Amino N, Kanoh M, Kawai M, Fujiwara M, Kimura M, Kamitani A, Saya K, Shakuta R, Nitta S, Hayashida Y, Kudo T, Kubota S, Miyauchi A. Menstrual disturbances in various thyroid diseases. Endocr J. 2010;57(12):1017–22.
26. Conforti A, Alviggi C, Mollo A, De Placido G, Magos A. The management of Asherman syndrome: a review of literature. Reprod Biol Endocrinol. 2013;11:118.
27. Krolikowski A, Janowski K, Larsen JV. Asherman syndrome caused by schistosomiasis. Obstet Gynecol. 1995;85(5 Pt 2):898–9.
28. Master-Hunter T, Heiman DL. Amenorrhea: evaluation and treatment. Am Fam Physician. 2006;73(8):1374–82.
29. Nakamura S, Douchi T, Oki T, Ijuin H, Yamamoto S, Nagata Y. Relationship between sonographic endometrial thickness and progestin-induced withdrawal bleeding. Obstet Gynecol. 1996;87(5 Pt 1):722–5.
30. Sippel S, Muruganandan K, Levine A, Shah S. Review article: use of ultrasound in the developing world. Int J Emerg Med. 2011;4:72.
31. Soares SR, Barbosa dos Reis MM, Camargos AF. Diagnostic accuracy of sonohysterography, transvaginal sonography, and hysterosalpingography in patients with uterine cavity diseases. Fertil Steril. 2000;73(2):406–11.
32. Ozumba B, Ezegwui H. Intrauterine adhesions in an African population. Int J Gynaecol Obstet. 2002;77(1):37–8.
33. Cramer JW, Bartz PJ, Simpson PM, Zangwill SD. The spectrum of congenital heart disease and outcomes after surgical repair among

children with Turner syndrome: a single-centre review. Pediatr Cardiol. 2014;35(2):253–60.
34. Manuel M, Katayama PK, Jones HW Jr. The age of occurrence of gonadal tumours in intersex patients with a Y chromosome. Am J Obstet Gynecol. 1976;124(3):293–300.
35. Johary J, Xue M, Zhu X, Xu D, Velu PP. Efficacy of estrogen therapy in patients with intrauterine adhesions: systematic review. J Minim Invasive Gynecol. 2014;21(1):44–54.
36. Hassan WA, Darwish AM. Impact of pulmonary tuberculosis on menstrual pattern and fertility. Clin Respir J. 2010;4(3):157–61.
37. de Kleijn MJJ, van der Schouw YT, Verbeek ALM, Peeters PHM, Banga JD, van der Graaf Y. Endogenous estrogen exposure and cardiovascular mortality risk in postmenopausal women. Am J Epidemiol. 2002;155(4):339–45.
38. Jacobsen BK, Knutsen SF, Fraser GE. Age at natural menopause and total mortality and mortality from ischemic heart disease: the Adventist health study. J Clin Epidem. 1999;52(4):303–7.
39. Rocca WA, Grossardt BR, Miller VM, Shuster LT, Brown RD. Premature menopause or early menopause and risk of ischemic stroke. Menopause. 2012;19(3):272–7.
40. Anasti JN, Kalantaridou SN, Kimzey LM, Defensor RA, Nelson LM. Bone loss in young women with karyotypically normal spontaneous premature ovarian failure. Obstet Gynecol. 1998; 91(1):12–5.
41. Gallagher JC. Effect of early menopause on bone mineral density and fractures. Menopause. 2007;14(3):567–71.
42. Rickenlund A, Carlstrom K, Ekblom B, Brismar TB, von Schoultz B, Hirschberg AL. Effects of oral contraceptives on body composition and physical performance in female athletes. J Clin Endocrinol Metab. 2004;89(9):4364–70.
43. Warren MP, Miller KK, Olson WH, Grinspoon SK, Friedman A. Effects of an oral contraceptive (norgestimate/ethinyl estradiol) on bone mineral density in women with hypothalamic amenorrhea and osteopenia: an open-label extension of a double-blind, placebo-controlled study. Contraception. 2005;72(3):206–11.
44. Brannstrom M, Johannesson L, Bokstrom H, Kvarnstrom N, Molne J, Dahm-Kahler P, Enskog A, Milenkovic M, Ekberg J, Diaz-Garcia C, Gabel M, Hanafy A, Hagberg H, Olausson M, Nilsson L. Livebirth after uterus transplantation. Lancet. 2015;385(9968):607–16.
45. ACOG Committee on Practice Bulletins-Gynaecology. Practice bulletin no. 128: diagnosis of abnormal uterine bleeding in reproductive-aged women. Obstet Gynecol. 2012;120(1):197–206. Kjerulff KH, Erickson BA, Langenberg PW. Chronic gynaecological conditions reported by US women: findings from the National Health Interview Survey, 1984 to 1992. Am J Public Health. 1996;86(2):195–9.
46. Haverkate M, Smits J, Meijerink H, van der Ven A. Socioeconomic determinants of haemoglobin levels of African women are less sin areas with more health facilities: a multilevel analysis. J Epidemiol Community Health. 2014;68(2):116–22.
47. Cote I, Jacobs P, Cumming DC. Use of health services associated with increased menstrual loss in the United States. Am J Obstet Gynecol. 2003;188(2):343–8.
48. Fraser IS, Critchley HO, Broder M, Munro MG. The FIGO recommendations on terminologies and definitions for normal and abnormal uterine bleeding. Semin Reprod Med. 2011;29(5):383–90.
49. Munro MG, Critchley HO, Broder MS, Fraser IS, Disorders FWGoM. FIGO classification system (PALM-COEIN) for causes of abnormal uterine bleeding in nongravid women of reproductive age. Int J Gynaecol Obstet. 2011;113(1):3–13.
50. Salim S, Won H, Nesbitt-Hawes E, Campbell N, Abbott J. Diagnosis and management of endometrial polyps: a critical review of the literature. J Minim Invasive Gynecol. 2011;18(5):569–81.
51. Lee SC, Kaunitz AM, Sanchez-Ramos L, Rhatigan RM. The oncogenic potential of endometrial polyps: a systematic review and meta-analysis. Obstet Gynecol. 2010;116(5):1197–205.
52. Garcia L, Isaacson K. Adenomyosis: review of the literature. J Minim Invasive Gynecol. 2011;18(4):428–37.
53. Doherty L, Mutlu L, Sinclair D, Taylor H. Uterine fibroids: clinical manifestations and contemporary management. Reprod Sci. 2014;21(9):1067–92.
54. ACOG Committee on Practice Bulletins—Gynaecology and the Society of Gynaecologic Oncology. Practice Bulletin No. 149: Endometrial cancer. Obstet Gynecol. 2015;125(4): 1006–26.
55. Shankar M, Lee CA, Sabin CA, Economides DL, Kadir RA. von Willebrand disease in women with menorrhagia: a systematic review. BJOG. 2004;111(7):734–40.
56. ACOG Committee on Practice Bulletins—Gynaecology. Practice bulletin no. 136: management of abnormal uterine bleeding associated with ovulatory dysfunction. Obstet Gynecol. 2013;122(1):176–85.
57. Heatley MK. The association between clinical and pathological features in histologically identified chronic endometritis. J Obstet Gynaecol. 2004;24(7):801–3.
58. Toth M, Patton DL, Esquenazi B, Shevchuk M, Thaler H, Divon M. Association between chlamydia trachomatis and abnormal uterine bleeding. Am J Reprod Immunol. 2007;57(5):361–6. Wiesenfeld HC, Sweet RL, Ness RB, Krohn MA, Amortegui AJ, Hillier SL. Comparison of acute and subclinical pelvic inflammatory disease. Sex Transm Dis. 2005;32(7):400–5.
59. Diedrich JT, Desai S, Zhao Q, Secura G, Madden T, Peipert JF. Association of short-term bleeding and cramping patterns with long-acting reversible contraceptive method satisfaction. Am J Obstet Gynecol. 2015;212(1):50.e1–8.
60. Lowe RF, Prata N. Haemoglobin and serum ferritin levels in women using copper-releasing or levonorgestrel-releasing intrauterine devices: a systematic review. Contraception. 2013;87(4): 486–96.
61. Faculty of Family Planning and Reproductive Health Care Clinical Effectiveness Unit. Management of Unscheduled Bleeding in Women Using Hormonal Contraception. 2009.
62. Torre DL, Falorni A. Pharmacological causes of hyperprolactinemia. Ther Clin Risk Manag. 2007;3(5):929–51.
63. Marret H, Fauconnier A, Chabbert-Buffet N, Cravello L, Golfier F, Gondry J, Agostini A, Bazot M, Brailly-Tabard S, Brun JL, De Raucourt E, Gervaise A, Gompel A, Graesslin O, Huchon C, Lucot JP, Plu-Bureau G, Roman H, Fernandez H, Francais CCNdGeO. Clinical practice guidelines on menorrhagia: management of abnormal uterine bleeding before menopause. Eur J Obstet Gynecol Reprod Biol. 2010;152(2):133–7.
64. St John A, Price CP. Existing and emerging technologies for point-of-care testing. Clin Biochem Rev. 2014;35(3):155–67.
65. ACOG Committee on Practice Bulletins—Gynaecology. ACOG committee opinion no. 557: management of acute abnormal uterine bleeding in nonpregnant reproductive-aged women. Obstet Gynecol. 2013;121(4):891–6.
66. Matteson KA, Rahn DD, Wheeler TL 2nd, Casiano E, Siddiqui NY, Harvie HS, Mamik MM, Balk EM, Sung VW, Society of Gynaecologic Surgeons Systematic Review G. Nonsurgical management of heavy menstrual bleeding: a systematic review. Obstet Gynecol. 2013;121(3):632–43.
67. Nakajima ST, Archer DF, Ellman H. Efficacy and safety of a new 24-day oral contraceptive regimen of norethindrone acetate 1 mg/ethinyl estradiol 20 micro g (Loestrin 24 Fe). Contraception. 2007;75(1):16–22.

68. World Health Organization. Medical eligibility criteria for contraceptive use. 5th ed. World Health Organization. Geneva; 2015.
69. Hubacher D. The Levonorgestrel intrauterine system: reasons to expand access to the public sector of Africa. Glob Health Sci Pract. 2015;3(4):532–7.
70. Jacobstein R, Shelton JD. The Levonorgestrel intrauterine system: a pragmatic view of an excellent contraceptive. Glob Health Sci Pract. 2015;3(4):538–43.
71. Brooks PG, Serden SP. Hysteroscopic findings after unsuccessful dilatation and curettage for abnormal uterine bleeding. Am J Obstet Gynecol. 1988;158(6 Pt 1):1354–7.
72. ACOG Committee on Practice Bulletins. Practice bulletin number 81: endometrial ablation. Obstet Gynecol. 2007;109(5):1233–48.
73. Marjoribanks J, Lethaby A, Farquhar C. Surgery versus medical therapy for heavy menstrual bleeding. Cochrane Database Syst Rev. 2016;1:CD003855.
74. Helal AS, Abdel-Hady el S, Mashaly Ael M, Shafaie ME, Sherif L. Modified thermal balloon endometrial ablation in low resource settings: a cost-effective method using Foley's catheter. Arch Gynecol Obstet. 2011;284(3):671–5.
75. Molitch ME. Drugs and prolactin. Pituitary. 2008;11(2):209–18.

Menopause

50

Victor N. Chilaka and Abdulmalik Bako

Learning Objectives

After studying this chapter, the reader should be able to:

- Define the menopause and the climacteric and understand the principles of "reproductive ageing"
- Understand that managing the menopause has become an essential part of gynaecology
- Recognise the signs and symptoms of the menopause and be able to diagnose the condition
- Recognise and differentiate the menopause from premature ovarian failure
- Show very good understanding of hormone replacement therapy (HRT) and be able to counsel patients on their benefits and side effects
- Understand the place of non-hormonal management of menopausal symptoms
- Recommend HRT regimen for menopausal women at different stages of the menopause
- Understand the limitations and potential side effects of HRT and be able to counsel patients on these appropriately
- Make adequate referral in complicated cases

50.1 Definition

Menopause is defined as occurring after 12 months of amenorrhea that results from the loss of ovarian follicular activity that cannot be attributed to another physiologic or pathologic cause [1]. The final menstrual period is always determined retrospectively. The menopause occurs averagely about the age of 51 years [1].

50.1.1 Reproductive Ageing

The reproductive age of a woman spans from puberty (menarche) to the menopause. Menarche describes the first menstruation in a woman's life. Once started, it establishes and regularises, and the woman soon reaches the peak of her reproductive life and after that begins to decline. Anovulation, associated with menstrual irregularities is quite common leading up to the menopause. The complete physiology behind this is still not very well understood and can be explained by ovarian ageing associated with a decline in oocyte and follicular pool. During early embryonic development, cells from the dorsal endoderm of the yolk sac begin to migrate along the hindgut to the gonadal ridge to join the forming ovary. These primordial germ cells that will eventually give rise to the oocytes multiply by mitosis and are referred to as oogonia within the gonadal ridge. Their number reaches a peak of 6–7 million at about 20 weeks of pregnancy, and after that, their number begins to reduce. At birth, there are about 1.5–2 million follicles. In humans, no new ones are formed after birth. Follicular atresia, however, continues throughout life, and at menarche, there are 300,000–400,000 follicles. The loss of ovarian follicles accelerates when the total number of follicles reaches about 25,000 and when the numbers are sufficiently depleted (<1000), menopause occurs. Generally, fertility begins to decline at about the age of 32 with a rapid decline starting approximately about the age of 37 [2] (Fig. 50.1).

V. N. Chilaka
Women's Wellness and Research Centre, Hamad Medical Corporation, Doha, Qatar

A. Bako (✉)
Women's Wellness and Research Centre, Hamad Medical Corporation, Doha, Qatar

Weill Cornell Medicine-Qatar, Doha, Qatar

F. Okonofua et al. (eds.), *Contemporary Obstetrics and Gynecology for Developing Countries*,
https://doi.org/10.1007/978-3-030-75385-6_50

50.1.2 Perimenopause

The term 'perimenopause' has been defined as commencing when the first clinical signs of approaching menopause begin (the most common being the onset of cycle irregularity) and finishing 1 year after the last menstruation [3]. Perimenopause follows a period of declining fertility and precedes menopause. It is characterised mainly by cycle irregularity (shortening then lengthening) and increasing symptoms of the menopause. The perimenopause could last from 2 to 8 years (average of 4 years) [3].

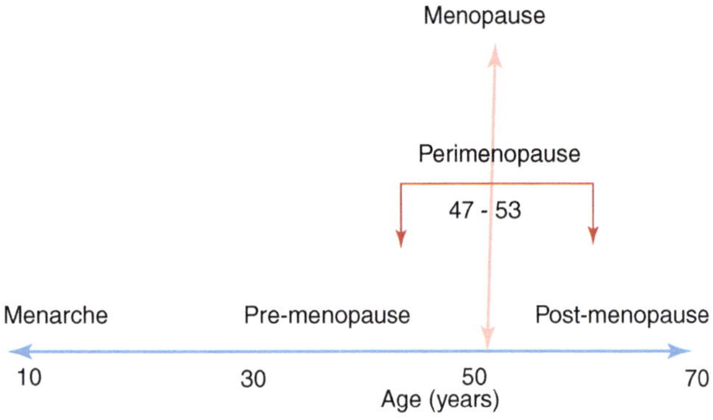

Fig. 50.1 Menstrual life of women

50.1.3 The Menopause

The menopause marks the end of reproductive life and is diagnosed after cessation of menses (final menstrual period) for 12 months. It should be a clinical diagnosis and not a laboratory diagnosis in women aged over the age of 45 years [1, 4]. Menopause can happen due to egg depletion and cessation of estrogen production by the ovary, which may happen naturally from ageing or surgically induced following removal or irradiation of the ovaries. In younger women who are less than 45 years of age with amenorrhoea and menopausal symptoms, the diagnosis can be confirmed by laboratory investigations. The management of the menopause has become even more critical than ever as life expectancy in the developed countries such as in Europe and the United States is averaging above 84 years implying that many women live around 50–55% of their adult life as menopausal females [5] (Fig. 50.2).

50.1.4 Symptoms of the Menopause

The manifestation of the symptoms of the menopause is variable in timing, severity and duration. The hormonal shifts

Final Menstrual Period

Stages	**-5**	**-4**	**-3**	**-2**	**-1**		**+1**	**+2**
Terminology	**Reproductive**			**Menopausal Transition**			**Post-menopause**	
	Early	Peak	Late	Early	Late		Early	Late
				Perimenopause				
Duration of satge	Variable			Variable		1yr	4 years	For rest of life
Menstrual cycle	Variable to regular	Regular		Variable cycle length	≥2 skipped cycles & an interval of amenorrhoea ≥2 60 days	Amenorrhea >12 months	None	
Endocrine	**Normal FSH**			**↑FSH**	**↑FSH**		**↑FSH**	

Fig. 50.2 Stages of reproductive ageing. (Adapted from Harlow et al. [6])

Table 50.1 Categories of menopausal symptoms

Acute symptoms	
	Vasomotor: hot flushes, night sweats, headaches
	Psychological: mood changes and irritability
	Memory and concentration loss
	Sexual dysfunction: vaginal dryness, altered libido
Long-term consequences	
	Cardiovascular disease
	Osteoporosis
	Urogenital atrophy
	Joint and muscle stiffness
	Dementia

associated with this period of life predispose women to a wide range of signs and symptoms which include hot flushes, night sweats, palpitations, irregular or absent menstrual periods and vaginal dryness which may cause dyspareunia. There may also be behavioural and other neurophysiological problems like mood swings, insomnia, anxiety and depression, forgetfulness and impaired concentration. Some may also experience altered libido, paraesthesia, nervousness, melancholia, vertigo, weakness, lower urinary tract problems (such as urge and stress incontinence), arthralgia/myalgia, headache and formication (Table 50.1).

50.1.4.1 Vasomotor Symptoms

Women generally describe hot flushes as a sensation of warmth that is frequently accompanied by skin flushing and perspiration. They vary in intensity, duration and frequency. They can occur occasionally or frequently and may last from seconds to an hour. In some women, it is perceived as a minor nuisance, while in others, it can disrupt rest, work, sleep and daily activities and can affect the quality of life adversely. Hot flush is the menopausal symptom that has the strongest association with depression and reduced quality of life. The consistent relationship between hot flushes and the menopause and perimenopause justifies its designation as a definite perimenopausal and postmenopausal symptom [7].

Hot flushes tend to start commonly during the perimenopause and are reported in 14–80% of women within 2 years of their final menstrual bleeding [7]. The proportion of women who report hot flushes may be as high as 80% in Western Europe and America [8] but may be as low as 10% in some East Asian countries [8]. The causes of these variations are not apparent. The frequency of hot flushes is also known to be unusually low in the African population. Hot flushes, however, diminish spontaneously or become more tolerable as the time from the menopause increases [7].

50.1.4.2 Depression

In some studies, women who present for evaluation and treatment at menopausal clinics have rates of clinical depression as high as 45% [9]. However, a good number of longitudinal population-based studies do not report any association between the menopausal transition and depression [10]. A Canadian cohort study has shown that 51% of menopausal women screened with the Centre for Epidemiologic Studies Depression Scale were positive for depressive symptoms at least once during the 3 years of observation within the study. It was however shown that high scores of depression were related to poor perception of health and not specifically to the menopause [11]. A few other studies, however, indicated that those who were at high risk of depression seemed to be those who have suffered from a depressive illness earlier in life [12]. These tend to support the vulnerability theory that women who had previously suffered from affective disorders may be at increased risk of mood disturbance during the menopausal transition [12].

50.1.4.3 Vaginal Atrophy

Symptoms of dyspareunia, vaginal dryness, itching and irritation are common presentations in the menopause. Vaginal atrophy may be a cause of postmenopausal bleeding. The finding of epithelial pallor, petechiae, friability and absence of rugae in the vagina may suggest a diagnosis of vulvovaginal atrophy. It is noteworthy to realise that these signs may be present in the absence of symptoms and may not be found in symptomatic women. Histological examination of the vaginal epithelium in the menopause does reveal a shift of the maturation index to the left (i.e., towards the less mature cell types). This shift to the left involves all the layers of the vaginal epithelium from the parabasal cells (least mature), to intermediate, and the superficial cells (most mature) [12]. The degree of cell change seems to correspond poorly to symptoms; hence, the diagnosis of atrophic vaginitis remains a clinical one and not a histological diagnosis [12].

50.1.4.4 Sexual Dysfunction

Some evidence suggests that sexual function declines over the menopausal transition [13]. It is not completely clear whether this decline is due to the menopause itself, natural ageing, psychological function or partner's factors such as availability and or other health issues. It is obvious that some of the menopause-related symptoms interfere with female sexuality. Estrogen withdrawal can lead to vaginal atrophy and dryness that can result in dyspareunia, and in some women, this can culminate to reduced sexual arousal.

50.1.4.5 Coronary Heart Disease

There exists an aetiological and biochemical relationship between menopause and increased risk of cardiovascular disease, and the reason for this may be in part be due to changes in cardiovascular risk factors such as lipid profiles that begin to alter during the perimenopause [14]. There is a higher age-adjusted rate of cardiovascular disease among women who have had bilateral oophorectomy compared to those who have their ovaries conserved [14]. Postmenopausal women have a twofold higher risk of developing coronary cardiovascular disease than premenopausal women, after adjustment for age [14]. In the Postmenopausal Estrogen/Progestins Intervention (PEPI) Trial, conjugated equine estrogens produced the most significant increase in high-density lipoproteins [15]. Combination treatment with conjugated equine estrogens and cyclical micronised progesterone resulted in slightly less increase in HDL, compared with conjugated equine estrogen alone [15].

50.1.4.6 Osteoporosis

The menopause is associated with loss of bone mineral density and is causally related to higher rates of osteoporotic fractures in postmenopausal women when compared with premenopausal women [16]. Hormone replacement therapy after the menopause results in the preservation of bone mineral density. There is also clear evidence (mainly from cohort studies) that postmenopausal HRT users have fewer fractures than non-users [14]. The varying rates of bone loss after menopause in different women, however, raises the question of whether there is a group of women who become demineralised more rapidly than others, and whether this subset of women can be identified. If it is possible to identify them, they might be targeted for screening and counselling about osteoporosis prevention and they may also require unique therapeutic interventions [17].

50.1.4.7 Urinary Incontinence

There is no established relationship between urinary incontinence and the menopause. The reports on the prevalence of urinary incontinence are not consistent. Some studies report a higher prevalence, but when adjusted for age, the difference seems to disappear. Some of the changes that occur in the urinary tract during menopause include atrophy of the bladder trigone and urethral mucosa; decreased sensitivity of alpha-adrenergic receptors of the bladder neck and urethral sphincter [14]. These changes may account for overactive bladder and voiding symptoms (frequency and urgency) as well as some of the observed increase in urinary incontinence [14]. Pelvic floor damage with ageing and childbirth seems to be more associated with stress urinary incontinence.

50.1.4.8 Urinary Tract Infection (UTI)

There is no definite causal relationship between urinary tract infection and the menopause. Physiological changes that occur after the menopause may, however, lead to increased susceptibility to such UTI. These changes include an alteration in the vaginal flora to predominantly Gram-negative organisms because of increasing vaginal pH, which is the main factor predisposing the lower genito-urinary tract to infections.

50.1.4.9 Other Morbidities

A good number of epidemiological studies tend to show associations between menopause, HRT and the occurrence of some chronic conditions. Since most of these diseases tend to also occur with ageing, it is difficult to establish a causal relationship. Some conditions associated with the menopause include Alzheimer's disease, cognitive decline, ovarian cancer, skin atrophy arthritis, cataracts, colonic cancer and dental and periodontal diseases [14, 16].

50.1.5 Premature Ovarian Insufficiency (POI)

Premature ovarian insufficiency (POI) occurs when there is a cessation of ovarian function before the age of 40 years [18]. It is characterised by elevated gonadotrophins that are associated with hypoestrogenism and loss of residual follicles. These, therefore, result in menstrual abnormalities, pregnancy failures and often decreased health-related quality of life that is associated with menopausal symptoms [18]. POI can occur at any age, but the overall prevalence is estimated at 1% in women under 40 years old, 0.1% in those under 30% and 0.01% in those under the age of 20 years [19]. The aetiology of premature ovarian insufficiency in the majority of cases is not well understood and is therefore termed spontaneous or idiopathic. Some known associations are shown in Table 50.2 [4].

Table 50.2 Conditions associated with premature ovarian failure

Genetic abnormalities (10%)	Turner syndrome and its variants (X-monosomy) Conditions manifesting as gonadal dysgenesis that is associated with the presence of the Y chromosome
Autoimmunity (30%)	Close relation with other autoimmune diseases as Sjögren's syndrome, rheumatoid arthritis, Hashimoto's thyroiditis, type 1 diabetes mellitus, multiple sclerosis, myasthenia gravis systemic lupus erythematosus, inflammatory bowel diseases and alopecia
Impaired metabolism	Close association with 17-OH deficiency and classic galactosaemia
Iatrogenic causes	Radiation, chemotherapeutic agents and surgery
Infections	Epidemic parotitis virus which is responsible for mumps oophoritis, HIV infection and antiretroviral therapy may impair ovarian function
Environmental factors	Environmental pollutants and toxins. Suspected agents include bisphenol A (a component of plastic used for food packing), polychlorinated biphenyls, genistein, dioxins, pesticides, polycyclic aromatic hydrocarbons and cigarette smoke

50.1.6 Diagnosis

The diagnosis of POI is made when oligomenorrhoea/amenorrhoea of more than 4 months' duration occurs in association with elevated gonadotropins (FSH >40 IU/l) measured at least on two occasions, 4–6 weeks apart in ladies under the age of 40 [19]. The quantification of serum FSH level is the gold standard test for the diagnosis of POI [19]. Other helpful biochemical markers include reduced oestradiol, inhibin and anti-Müllerian hormone (AMH). AMH should be interpreted together with the FSH and estrogen levels. Pelvic ultrasound and total follicular count may be useful. Bone density (DEXA) scan may be done to exclude osteoporosis. Karyotyping may be necessary for establishing the aetiology of POI [4].

50.1.7 Management of the Menopause

50.1.7.1 Diagnosis

The diagnosis of the menopause and perimenopause should be based on signs and symptoms in otherwise healthy women aged over 45 years with symptoms of the menopausal. The perimenopause should be based on vasomotor symptoms and irregular periods while menopause is diagnosed in women after at least 12 months of amenorrhoea when they are not on hormonal treatment [4] or other drugs that cause amenorrhea. There is no need to run hormone assays or imaging in this group of women [4, 20]. However, in younger women, FSH assays are quite useful to establish the diagnosis of premature menopause or POI. Surgical menopause is diagnosed in the immediate post-oophorectomy period.

50.1.7.2 Information and Advice

Poor understanding of the physiology of the menopause and poor perception of health are strongly associated with depression and reduced quality of life [4]. NICE (2015) recommends that the provision of appropriate information to menopausal women as well as to their families and carers is an essential part of their treatment [4]. Information given should include a clear explanation of typical menopausal symptoms and signs, the method of diagnosis and stages of menopause. Information should also be given on the options of treatment including personalised lifestyle changes and interventions that could help to improve general health and wellbeing of the woman. There is also a need to inform them of the risks and benefits of treatments, as well as long-term health issues that the menopause can pose. Information should be comprehensive and should include the merits and demerits of hormonal therapy (HRT), non-hormonal treatment (e.g., clonidine) and non-pharmacological therapy (e.g., cognitive behavioural therapy (CBT). Contraceptive information should be given to women who are in the perimenopausal period who may be at risk of pregnancy. It is recommended that information about menopause and fertility should be given before treatment is commenced. If the primary or secondary health-care physician is uncomfortable with managing the patient, she should be referred to a health-care professional with the expertise in the management of the menopause [4].

50.1.7.3 Psychotherapy

Cognitive behavioural therapy (CBT) has been shown to be a helpful tool in managing vasomotor symptoms during the menopause [21]. CBT on its own has not been shown to improve the intensity or frequency of vasomotor symptoms, but it is associated with a significant reduction of hot flush frequency when combined with HRT. CBT also significantly reduces anxiety and personal ratings of hot flushes, and the changes were sustained for a reasonable length of time [21, 22].

50.1.7.4 Non-hormonal Drug Treatment

There is some evidence that drugs such as clonidine, gabapentin, paroxetine, venlafaxine and black cohosh may benefit some women with vasomotor symptoms [22]. Vasomotor symptoms may be treated with clonidine hydrochloride in women who have contraindications to estrogen [23]. Clonidine stimulates the norepinephrine receptors that are implicated in the initiation of flushes and is generally used as an antihypertensive medication [23]. Following a multicentre double-placebo trial, it has been shown that clonidine has relatively mild side effects. Also, the absence of potentially harmful estrogenic effects of clonidine in the dose range of 25–75 μg twice daily makes it a useful addition or an alternative therapy for menopausal who are suffering from vasomotor symptoms [23]. Side effects of clonidine include postural hypotension, salivary gland pain, sexual dysfunction and sleep disturbance, and these may be unpleasant to the patient.

Gabapentin is an anticonvulsant useful in treating neuropathic pain and has been shown to reduce hot flushes through an unknown mechanism. Selective serotonin or serotonin-norepinephrine reuptake inhibitors are mainly used as antidepressants as they increase the levels of serotonin and norepinephrine. Both of these neurotransmitters are implicated in the generation of hot flushes in menopausal women. Clonidine, SSRIs and SNRIs and gabapentin, when combined with relaxation therapy, showed a mild to moderate effect in relieving hot flushes in women who have suffered from breast cancer [22].

There is no evidence yet to support the use of fluoxetine, red clover, phytoestrogens, Ginseng, evening primrose, dong quai and vitamin E in the management of the menopause. The side effects of these therapies should be considered and seem to outweigh any benefits that might be achieved by their use [24].

Bisphosphonates are very useful in women with accelerated bone loss, osteopenia or osteoporosis. It is important to note that bisphosphonate can be incorporated in the matrix of bones over a long period of time [19]. There is limited evidence assessing long-term reproductive implications associated with the use of biphosphinates, and caution should, therefore, be exercised with their use in women with POI and those in the reproductive age group who may wish to achieve a pregnancy [19].

50.1.7.5 Hormone Replacement Treatment (HRT)

All manifestations of the menopause are related to estrogen deficiency; hence, estrogen replacement therapy can reverse or prevent all these manifestations. Knowledge of HRT in the menopause and the climacteric is an essential part of the current care of women, and the principles of therapy should be clearly understood.

HRT aims to be physiological where possible to maintain estrogen-dependent tissues and prevent hypoestrogenic-related atrophy in tissues and organs that are dependent on estrogen. The goals of treatment may differ in different women and can vary from short-term control of vasomotor symptoms, vaginal dryness to long-term treatment or chronic indications such as osteoporosis prevention.

50.1.7.6 Estrogens

Estrogens can be given by mouth, injection or via transdermal (by patch, skin cream), intradermal (pellet) or vaginal route. With the non-oral administration of estrogen, the first-pass through the liver is avoided, and this can be particularly useful in women with compromised liver functions with or without high triglycerides. In warmer climates, skin patches may be troublesome because of sweating and irritation, and gels might be a better option. Oestradiol implants are crystalline 17-beta-oestradiol pellets which can be inserted into the buttocks or anterior abdominal wall. However, when there are side effects, the pellets may be difficult to extract. Most vaginal preparations seem to exert their effect locally and are very useful in treating vaginal symptoms of the menopause. However, there is significant systemic absorption to preserve bone density with Estring pessary [4]. Systemically administered estrogen in the perimenopause and after menopause diminishes postmenopausal osteoporosis.

50.1.7.7 Progestogens

Progestogens are used to treat or prevent endometrial hyperplasia in women with an in situ uterus. There is, therefore, no need to give progestogen to a woman who has had a hysterectomy. There are three subgroups of progestogens used for hormone replacement therapy:

(a) C-21 derivatives of progesterone (medroxyprogesterone acetate, dydrogesterone)
(b) C-19 derivatives of nortestosterone (norethisterone)
(c) Natural progesterone

Medroxyprogesterone acetate has very minimal androgenic effect, but it does counteract the rise in HDL produced by unopposed estrogen therapy [15]. Dydrogesterone has no androgenic and estrogenic effect and also does not antagonise the beneficial effects of estrogen on lipids [13]. However, no practical advantages have been demonstrated based on these mild biochemical differences [12].

The route of administration of progestogens can be either oral or incorporated with intra-uterine contraceptive devices (IUCDs). With IUCDs, virtually all endometrial hyperplasia caused by any of the estrogens is suppressed, but it is worth noting that their effect is not only local as they can induce changes in lipid profile that is comparable to that of 1 mg norethisterone daily [25].

50.1.7.8 Combination of Estrogens and Progestogens

Combined estrogens and progestogens can be offered to women with a uterus. Adding a progestogen to estrogen in women with a uterus has the potential to prevent hyperplasia of the endometrial lining, and therefore, suppress possible transformation to endometrial malignancy. Combined HRT may be given continuously after 12 months of the final menstruation, or cyclically in the peri-menopausal period and within 12 months of the menopause. Women on continuous HRT may have irregular bleeding in the early stages of treatment, and if persistent, endometrial pathology should be excluded, and it may be worthwhile considering a change to cyclical HRT.

Combined HRT can be given to ladies with early natural or surgically induced menopause (before age 45 years) as they may be at high risk of osteoporosis. In this group, HRT can be given up until the approximate age of natural menopause. If osteoporosis is, however, the main concern, alternatives to HRT may be considered.

50.1.7.9 Tibolone

Tibolone is a synthetic steroid which has estrogenic, progestogenic and weak androgenic activity. It can, therefore, be given continuously without the need for progestogens. It is unsuitable for use in the peri-menopause and within 12 months of the final menstruation. If commencing tibolone after cyclical HRT, it is recommended to start at the end of the cyclical HRT regimen and at any time if transferring from continuous-combined HRT. Tibolone is also licensed for prophylaxis of osteoporosis in women at high risk of fractures especially when other medications as estrogens are contraindicated [4].

50.1.8 Selective Estrogen Receptor Modulators (*SERMs*)

These drugs have the potential to act as partial estrogen receptor agonists or antagonist depending on their interaction with the estrogen receptors in the target tissues. Examples include tamoxifen, raloxifen and bazedoxifen. Tamoxifen is an estrogen receptor agonist and can lead to endometrial hyperplasia and polyp production, while raloxifene is an estrogen receptor antagonist on the uterus. Bazedoxifene has similar effects to that of raloxifene. The combination of bazedoxifene and conjugated estrogen is available in the United States for the management of menopausal hot flushes and for preventing osteoporosis [26]. This combination prevents estrogen-induced endometrial hyperplasia rendering the co-administration of a progestin unnecessary [27]. This combination is indicated in women with bothersome hot flushes and who have breast tenderness with standard HRT. It is also beneficial in women who cannot tolerate any progestin therapy because of side effects. However, the risk of VTE is increased with bazedoxifene [27, 28].

50.1.9 Testosterone

Postmenopausal women with reduced libido may benefit from adding some testosterone to their HRT [23]. This combined therapy may, however, be associated with testosterone-specific side effects such as unpleasant hair growth, acne and a reduction in HDL cholesterol. The prevalence of these side effects may be affected by the different doses and routes of administration. There is however a paucity of evidence to determine the effects of the long-term use of testosterone in menopausal women [29].

50.1.10 Regimens of HRT

Several factors influence the choice of HRT. It is essential to balance the benefits (relief of the bothersome symptoms) and the risks and side effects of HRT. Women with a uterus in the perimenopause or within 12 months of their last menstruation should be offered estrogen with an additional cyclical progestogen in the last 12–14 days of the menstrual cycle or preparations that contain both estrogen and progesterone as a single preparation in a cyclical pattern. For those who are over 12 months of their last menstrual period, they can be offered continuous combined preparations or tibolone. A woman without a uterus can be offered continuous estrogen or tibolone. However, the addition of progestogen should be considered in women with a history of endometriosis as endometrial foci may remain indifferent area despite hysterectomy and oophorectomy. In administering HRT, the minimum effective dose should be prescribed and for the shortest duration and response to therapy should be assessed every 6–12 months [4].

50.1.11 Risks of HRT

50.1.11.1 Venous Thromboembolism (VTE)

It is essential to review the need for combined or estrogen-only HRT in women with predisposing factors to VTE because of increased risk in these women. The predisposing factors include personal or family history of deep vein thrombosis or pulmonary embolism, smoking, obesity, prolonged bed rest, severe varicose veins and travel that involve prolonged immobility. The risk of VTE is unusually high in the first year of use [4] and may be lower with the transdermal route [30]. Available data do not suggest a higher risk of VTE with tibolone compared with other forms of combined HRT or in women not taking HRT at all.

50.1.11.2 Risk of Endometrial Cancer

The use of estrogen-only HRT is associated with an increase in the risk of endometrial cancer. This increased risk depends on the dose and length of use of estrogen-only HRT. The increased risk seems to be eliminated if a progestogen is given continuously; however, the addition of a cyclical progestogen (for at least 10 days per 28-day cycle) reduces the risk.[31] The risk of endometrial cancer in women using combined HRT should, however, be weighed against the potential increased risk of breast cancer.

50.1.11.3 Risk of Breast Cancer

The risk of breast cancer is increased over the background population risk in women using combined HRT and becomes apparent after about 5 years of therapy [31]. The duration of use of HRT influences the risk, and the risk diminishes within 5 years of stopping HRT. Estrogen-only HRT is not associated with an increased risk of breast cancer [31]. Progesterone therapy is associated with a higher risk of breast cancer but seems to reduce the risk of bowel cancer [30]. Tibolone seems to increase the risk of breast cancer but to a lesser extent when compared with combined HRT. It is also associated with increases in the risk of recurrence in women who have had breast cancer in the past.

50.1.11.4 Risk of Cerebrovascular Accidents (Stroke)

The risk of cerebrovascular accidents (CVA) in women using combined HRT is increased slightly. The risk becomes apparent after about 5 years of use. Tibolone may slightly increase the risk of CVA in women over age 60 [32].

50.1.11.5 Risk of Ovarian Cancer

There is a small increase in the prevalence of ovarian cancer in women on long-term use of HRT. A large but detailed meta-analysis of 52 epidemiological studies involving 21,488 postmenopausal women with ovarian cancer suggests that there is a small excess risk of ovarian cancer in menopausal women taking HRT [33]. The excess risk, however, tends to disappear within a few years of stopping treatment.

50.1.11.6 Risk of Coronary Heart Disease

An increase in the risk of coronary heart disease has been noted in women who start combined HRT more than 10 years into the menopause. Coronary heart risk becomes apparent after about 5 years of use and becomes more significant after 10 years of use. Studies suggest a lower risk in younger women who commence HRT close to their menopause compared to older women. Starting HRT late in the menopause does not prevent coronary heart disease and should therefore not be offered for this purpose [27].

50.2 Summary

Menopause is a physiological phenomenon that can be associated with a variety of symptoms. Some of the symptoms of menopause can significantly reduce the quality of life in women. Management of symptoms of the menopause requires careful individualisation based on each woman's symptoms, impact on quality of life, personal circumstances of the woman, risk factors as well as anticipated and real side effects. The minimum effective dosage of HRT should be prescribed and for the shortest duration of treatment. The response to treatment and assessment of progress and side effects should be reviewed at least annually (Table 50.3).`

Table 50.3 Tips on HRT and the menopause

Counselling for HRT		
Risks	Benefits	Caution:
Breast cancer Related to the duration of treatment and no increased risk with estrogen only *Thrombosis* Risk 2–3/10,000 per year (less with patch/gel: non-oral) *Stroke* Risk for older group/hypertensive and dose related *CV disease* Risk in older patients commencing HRT	Menopausal symptoms relieved Quality of life improvements Osteoporosis/fractures reduced Bowel cancer, reduced risk	Hormone-dependent cancers Previous or high risk of thrombosis (non-oral) High-risk CV disease Abnormal bleeding
Starting HRT If still menstruating: sequential or cyclical HRT If stopped menstruating >12 months: continuous combined HRT Titrate dose (offer the lowest effective dose) Caution if starting older women on HRT (>10 years postmenopausal) Older women need a lower dose	*If she has had a hysterectomy + oophorectomy* Treat with estrogen-only HRT Titrate dose against symptoms Benefits outweigh risks generally No increased risk of breast cancer No decreased risk of bowel cancer Consider combined HRT if hysterectomy + oophorectomy was for endometriosis	*Early menopause (<45)* Benefits > risks in younger women Younger women may need higher doses Treat until 51 years of age, and then consider whether to continue COC or HRT in younger women – both effective
Mirena and HRT Provides adequate progestogen for estrogen HRT Licensed for 4 years duration Most likely to give bleed-free HRT at any age Titrate dose of estrogen to symptom relief	*Local (vaginal) HRT* Vaginal dryness/soreness Recurrent UTIs Sensory urinary symptoms (frequency, urgency, UTIs) At recommended doses, (treatment twice weekly), 2 years treatment is fine At low doses, more extended treatment should be fine	*Stopping HRT* No arbitrary time limit on HRT Aim for lowest effective dose Stop HRT slowly by gradually reducing the dose Don't be worried about restarting if bothersome symptoms return

References

1. Research on the menopause in the 1990s. World Heal Organ Tech Rep Ser:1996. https://doi.org/10.1016/0378-5122(95)00967-1.
2. Faddy MJ, Gosden RG, Gougeon A, Richardson SJ, Nelson JF. Accelerated disappearance of ovarian follicles in mid-life: implications for forecasting menopause. Hum Reprod. 1992; https://doi.org/10.1093/oxfordjournals.humrep.a137570.
3. Hay AG, Bancroft J, Johnstone EC. Affective symptoms in women attending a menopause clinic. Br J Psychiatry. 1994; https://doi.org/10.1192/bjp.164.4.513.
4. National Institute for Health and Care Excellence. Menopause: Diagnosis and Management. Nice. 2015. https://doi.org/10.3109/13697137.2010.522875.
5. Beshay VE, Carr BR. Hypothalamic-pituitary-ovarian axis and control of the menstrual cycle. In: Clinical reproductive medicine and surgery; 2013. https://doi.org/10.1007/978-1-4614-6837-0_2.
6. Harlow SD, Gass M, Hall JE, Lobo R, Maki P, Rebar RW, Sherman S, Sluss PM, de Villiers TJ, et al. Executive summary of the stages of reproductive aging workshop + 10: addressing the unfinished agenda of staging reproductive aging. J Clin Endocrinol Metab. 2012; https://doi.org/10.1210/jc.2011-3362
7. Thompson B, Hart SA, Durno D. Menopausal age and symptomatology in a general practice. J Biosoc Sci. 1973; https://doi.org/10.1017/S0021932000008956.
8. Krailo MD, Pike MC. Estimation of the distribution of age at natural menopause from prevalence data. Am J Epidemiol. 1983; https://doi.org/10.1093/oxfordjournals.aje.a113548.
9. Beyene Y. Cultural significance and physiological manifestations of menopause a biocultural analysis. Cult Med Psychiatry. 1986; https://doi.org/10.1007/BF00053262.
10. Pearlstein T, Rosen K, Stone AB. Mood disorders and menopause. Endocrinol Metab Clin N Am. 1997; https://doi.org/10.1016/S0889-8529(05)70247-4.
11. Vivian-Taylor J, Hickey M. Menopause and depression: is there a link? Maturitas. 2014; https://doi.org/10.1016/j.maturitas.2014.05.014.
12. Avis NE, Brambilla D, McKinlay SM, Vass K. A longitudinal analysis of the association between menopause and depression results from the Massachusetts women's health study. Ann Epidemiol. 1994; https://doi.org/10.1016/1047-2797(94)90099-X.
13. Avis NE, Colvin A, Karlamangla AS, et al. Change in sexual functioning over the menopausal transition: results from the study of Women's Health Across the Nation. Menopause. 2017; https://doi.org/10.1097/GME.0000000000000770.
14. Greendale GA, Judd HL. The menopause: health implications and clinical management. J Am Geriatr Soc. 1993; https://doi.org/10.1111/j.1532-5415.1993.tb06953.x.
15. Mebane Sims IL. Effects of estrogen or estrogen/ progestin regimens on heart disease risk factors in postmenopausal women: the postmenopausal estrogen/progestin interventions (PEPI) trial. J Am Med Assoc. 1995; https://doi.org/10.1001/jama.273.3.199.
16. Dugan SA, Powell LH, Kravitz HM, Everson Rose SA, Karavolos K, Luborsky J. Musculoskeletal pain and menopausal status. Clin J Pain. 2006; https://doi.org/10.1097/01.ajp.0000208249.07949.d5.
17. Hansen MA, Overgaard K, Riis BJ, Christiansen C. Role of peak bone mass and bone loss in postmenopausal osteoporosis: 12 year study. BMJ. 1991; https://doi.org/10.1136/bmj.303.6808.961.
18. Davies M, Webber L, Anderson R, et al. ESHRE guideline: management of women with premature ovarian insufficiency. Hum Reprod. 2014;
19. Hamoda H. The British Menopause Society and Women's Health Concern recommendations on the management of women with premature ovarian insufficiency. Post Reprod Heal. 2017; https://doi.org/10.1177/2053369117699358.
20. Webber L, Davies M, Anderson R, et al. ESHRE guideline: management of women with premature ovarian insufficiency. Hum Reprod. 2016; https://doi.org/10.1093/humrep/dew027.
21. Hunter MS, Liao KLM. Evaluation of a four-session cognitive - behavioural intervention for menopausal hot flushes. Br J Health Psychol. 1996; https://doi.org/10.1111/j.2044-8287.1996.tb00496.x.
22. Cheema D, Coomarasamy A, El-Toukhy T. Non-hormonal therapy of post-menopausal vasomotor symptoms: a structured evidence-based review. Arch Gynecol Obstet. 2007; https://doi.org/10.1007/s00404-007-0390-9.
23. Clayden JR, Bell JW, Pollard P, CN-C-00009937. Menopausal flushing: double-blind trial of a non-hormonal medication. Br Med J. 1974;1(5905):409–12.
24. Medicines and Healthcare products Regulatory Agency. Hormone-replacement therapy: updated advice – GOV.UK. GOV.UK. https://www.gov.uk/drug-safety-update/hormone-replacement-therapy-updated-advice. Published 2014. Accessed December 16, 2018.
25. Raudaskoski TH, Lahti EI, Kauppila AJ, Apaja-Sarkkinen MA, Laatikainen TJ. Transdermal estrogen with a levonorgestrel-releasing intrauterine device for climacteric complaints: clinical and endometrial responses. Am J Obstet Gynecol. 1995; https://doi.org/10.1016/0002-9378(95)90095-0.
26. Lobo RA, Pinkerton JAV, Gass MLS, et al. Evaluation of bazedoxifene/conjugated estrogens for the treatment of menopausal symptoms and effects on metabolic parameters and overall safety profile. Fertil Steril. 2009; https://doi.org/10.1016/j.fertnstert.2009.03.113.
27. Kagan R, Goldstein SR, Pickar JH, Komm BS. Patient considerations in the management of menopausal symptoms: role of conjugated estrogens with bazedoxifene. Ther Clin Risk Manag. 2016; https://doi.org/10.2147/TCRM.S63833.
28. Solomon ZJ, Mirabal JR, Mazur DJ, Kohn TP, Lipshultz LI, Pastuszak AW. Selective androgen receptor modulators: current knowledge and clinical applications. Sex Med Rev. 2018; https://doi.org/10.1016/j.sxmr.2018.09.006.
29. Sherwin BB. Estrogen and/or androgen replacement therapy and cognitive functioning in surgically menopausal women. Psychoneuroendocrinology. 1988;13(4):345–57. https://doi.org/10.1016/0306-4530(88)90060-1.
30. Lobo RA. Hormone-replacement therapy: current thinking. Nat Rev Endocrinol. 2017; https://doi.org/10.1038/nrendo.2016.164.
31. Writing Group for the Women's Health Initiative Investigators. Risks and benefits of estrogen plus progestin in healthy postmenopausal women: principal results from the Women's Health Initiative Randomised Controlled Trial. J Am Med Assoc. 2002; https://doi.org/10.1001/jama.288.3.321.
32. Formoso G, Perrone E, Maltoni S, et al. Short-term and long-term effects of tibolone in postmenopausal women. Cochrane Database Syst Rev. 2016; https://doi.org/10.1002/14651858.CD008536.pub3.
33. Menopausal hormone use and ovarian cancer risk: individual participant meta-analysis of 52 epidemiological studies. Lancet. 2015; https://doi.org/10.1016/S0140-6736(14)61687-1.

Physiotherapy in Obstetrics and Gynaecology

51

Joseph A. Balogun

Learning Objectives

After reading this chapter, the reader will be able to:

- Describe the composition and functions of the members of the obstetrics and gynaecology healthcare team
- List the primary obstetrics and gynaecological disorders that are amenable to physiotherapy
- Discuss the physiotherapy modalities used to treat obstetrics and gynaecological disorders and its associated sequelae
- Enunciate the obstetrics and gynaecological disorders in which Kegel's exercise is indicated
- Describe the essential conditions that must be addressed for Kegel's exercise training to be clinically effective
- Articulate the need for a comprehensive evaluation of patients with chronic pelvic and abdomen pain

51.1 Introduction

In the last ten decades, the breathtaking and exhilarating scientific and medical discoveries involved the cooperation of different professionals. Today, healthcare practice is a collaborative team effort, and each professional in the team brings a unique perspective and expertise in the management of the patient. Some team members diagnose disease, perform surgery and treat with medications; other professionals manage illness using physical agents or behaviour modification strategies. Unfortunately, many health professionals have no firm knowledge of the roles and responsibilities of the other disciplines outside their niche.

Although reproductive diseases and associated complications are a significant cause of mortality and morbidity in Africa [1], many obstetricians and gynaecologists (Ob-Gyns) are not familiar with the reproductive diseases and disabilities that are amenable to physiotherapy. Previous studies revealed that timely referral to specialists is associated with slowed disease progression, fewer hospital admissions, reduced treatment costs and improved quality of life and number of survivals [2–6]. Quite often, physicians find it difficult to make early referrals to other practitioners and specialists because they are not sure of the disease process and periods of remission. This is compounded by the fact that they lack appropriate communication skill and limited understanding of the interdisciplinary team concept of healthcare delivery [2, 3, 7].

Physiotherapists are often underutilised in the management of obstetrics and gynaecological conditions because most Ob-Gyns are not familiar with their clinical expertise, causing late referral for physiotherapy services. The delay accentuates the lingering debilitating symptoms of the disease and impedes the improvement of the impairments associated with reproductive disorders [7].

This chapter presents the role of physiotherapy in the management of obstetrics and gynaecological disorders and will particularly be useful to Ob-Gyns. The discussion of the physical modalities used to treat them will be of unique interest to physiotherapist readers of this chapter. The description of the hands-on techniques for administering the modalities identified is beyond the scope of this book.

51.2 Operational Definitions

The term physiotherapy has its origin in the United Kingdom in 1894, and the analogous name physical therapy was coined in the USA in 1914.[1] *Physiotherapists* are quintes-

[1] https://www.physiotherapy-treatment.com/history-of-physical-therapy.html

J. A. Balogun (✉)
Chicago State University, Chicago, IL, USA

University of Medical Sciences, Ondo City, Nigeria

Centre of Excellence in Reproductive Health Innovation, University of Benin, Benin City, Nigeria
e-mail: jbalogun@csu.edu; jbalogun@unimed.edu.ng

F. Okonofua et al. (eds.), *Contemporary Obstetrics and Gynecology for Developing Countries*,
https://doi.org/10.1007/978-3-030-75385-6_51

sentially non-invasive healthcare professionals trained to use physical modalities, health education and behavioural modification counselling measures to manage the sequelae associated with obstetrics and gynaecological conditions, by educating patients to stop smoking, adopt positive nutrition habits, manage weight, engage in monitored physical activity and reduce stress. Also, physiotherapists remediate impairments, restore function, optimise the quality of life and promote patients' health and well-being.

51.3 The Obstetrics and Gynaecology Healthcare Team

The management of reproductive diseases falls within the purview of obstetrics and gynaecology – the medical specialty that deals with pregnancy, child delivery and the postpartum period care of the female reproductive system (breast, vagina, uterus and ovaries), including the management of the disorders of the male prostate and the external structures such as the penis, scrotum and testicles [8]. The general public tends to associate obstetrics and gynaecology exclusively to the sub-specialty of women's health, forgetting that men also have significant medical disorders such as ejaculatory/orgasmic dysfunction, prostatitis, urinary stress incontinence and erectile dysfunction following prostatectomy. Around the world, many professional organisations contribute to this misinformation by creating 'Section on Women's Health' instead of the more inclusive and non-gender bias name: 'Section on Obstetrics and Gynaecology'.

The obstetrics and gynaecology healthcare team treat the diseases that impair the functioning of the reproductive systems during all phases of life, and the associated sequelae inform of disabilities from congenital malformation, neurological and developmental disorders, low birth weight, preterm birth, reduced fertility, impotence and menstrual disorders. In the USA, the typical obstetrics and gynaecology healthcare team consist of an Ob-Gyn, a nurse, genetic counsellor, mental health therapist, clinical psychologist, medical laboratory technologist and a physiotherapist (Fig. 51.1).

Of all the members of the obstetrics and gynaecology healthcare team, it is the physiotherapist whose role is least known and appreciated. This is because in most clinical settings, there is little interaction between the medical practitioners and the physiotherapists. This unfortunate situation often leads to unnecessary delay in referring patients with obstetrics and gynaecological diseases for physiotherapy.

In most developing countries, the profession of genetic counselling and mental health therapy is alien to the healthcare system, and their roles warrant exposition here. The genetic counsellor in an obstetrics and gynaecology healthcare team educates the patients to understand the medical, psychological and familial impact of gene disorder and helps to promote informed choices and assesses the chance of disease occurring or recurring. The mental health therapist provides women undergoing fertility treatments and experiencing ongoing loss of interest, low mood, strained relationships, high levels of anxiety, changes in sleep or appetite, excessive guilt/anger or social isolation with individual, couples and group therapy for those undergoing fertility treatments [8].

The roles and responsibilities of the other members of the healthcare team are well known. The Ob-Gyns perform surgical procedures ranging from in vitro processes, oocyte

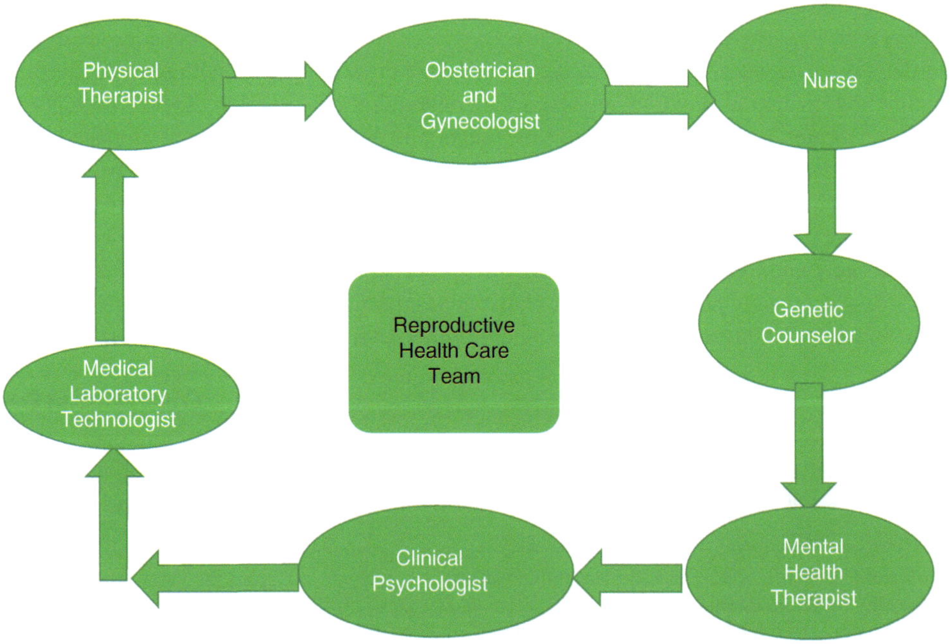

Fig. 51.1 The obstetrics and gynaecology healthcare team

identification to the preparation of embryos for transfer, semen processing, insemination, embryo assessment, cryopreservation, thawing, abortion and child delivery. The nurse assists the Ob-Gyns and anaesthesiologist with preoperative checklist and getting patients ready for surgery. They also provide care before and following surgery and provide orientation and injection training classes and as an excellent resource for answering routine questions during the hospitalisation period [8].

The clinical psychologist in an obstetrics and gynaecology healthcare team provides psychological assessments and support for patients contemplating abortion or after abortion, donors and patients experiencing third-party reproduction. The medical laboratory technologist performs phlebotomy, hormone and semen testing and any additional laboratory tests. Aside from the management of the impairments associated with physical disabilities, there are other obstetrics and gynaecological diseases that physiotherapists play a significant role in their treatment as discussed below.

51.4 Physiotherapy Modalities Used in Obstetrics and Gynaecology Practice

To treat their patients, physiotherapists utilise various physical agents such as: thermotherapy (infrared radiation, moist heat, paraffin wax bath, micro and shortwave diathermy), ultrasound, phonophoresis, cryotherapy, electrotherapeutics (interferential current, pre-modulated current, high volt galvanic stimulation, direct current, transcutaneous electrical nerve stimulation, microcurrent and functional electrical nerve stimulation, iontophoresis), light therapy (ultraviolet radiation and cold laser bio-stimulation therapy), vasopneumatic compression, therapeutic procedures and exercises, mechanical traction (computerised lumbar and cervical traction), manual therapeutics (massage, myofascial and connective tissue release techniques, mobilisation and manipulation), repositioning procedures, postural training, body mechanics/ergonomics, gait training, balance/coordination training and therapeutic exercise prescription [9, 10].

Before discussing the obstetrics and gynaecological disorders amenable to physiotherapy intervention, it is appropriate to provide an overview of the specific physical agents that are used to manage them. The core preventive physiotherapy intervention for managing obstetrics and gynaecological disorders include pelvic floor strengthening exercise and adjunctive therapies such as electrical stimulation (ES), electromyography (EMG) biofeedback, vaginal cones, shortwave diathermy (SWD) and transcutaneous electrical stimulation (TENS). *Kegel exercise* (*also known as pelvic floor-strengthening or pubococcygeus contraction exercise*) was named after Dr. Arnold Kegel who developed the protocol in the late 1940s to help women regain control of their bladders after childbirth. The pubococcygeus contraction exercise training (PCET) protocol is used to strengthen and stretch the weak pubococcygeus muscles in patients with urinary and faecal incontinence [11]. The exercise is indicated to restore bladder control after prostate surgery [11] and recommended for treating erectile dysfunction [12] and prevent premature ejaculation [13].

In young adults, the pubococcygeus muscles are typically taut and robust; they become weak and stretched with aging, during pregnancy or childbirth, after prostate cancer surgery or patients with bladder or bowel problems or other unknown factors. This situation negatively affects bladder control and sex life. Luckily, as with any muscle in the body, pubococcygeus muscles can be strengthened with targeted exercise workouts [11]. The PCET protocol is the same in both men and women. First, find the pubococcygeus muscles while urinating by stopping peeing mid-stream. The muscles used to hold back the urine or avoid passing gas are the pubococcygeus muscles. In males, the testicles will also rise when the pubococcygeus muscles contract. After locating the pubococcygeus muscles, proceed to practice flexing them by contracting and holding the pubococcygeus muscles for 5–20 seconds and then release them. Repeat this process 10–20 times in a row, 3–4 times a day and gradually increase the number of contractions completed and the holding time for each contraction. Practicing the above simple exercise can strengthen the pubococcygeus muscles and improve bladder control and sexual function [11].

Various adaptation of the PCET can be used by contracting and releasing the pubococcygeus muscles quickly, or slowly several times in succession. The activity can be performed in standing, sitting or supine. While doing PCET, breath normally and keep the rest of the body relaxed. Avoid tightening the abdominals, glutei or the quadriceps. The risks associated with doing PCET is minimal; it is easy to perform anywhere with no cost associated. Most patients tend to perform PCET at a low intensity or frequency based on their strength; over-exercising the pubococcygeus muscle tends to create muscle soreness and lead to a decrease in muscle performance, which means incontinence may worsen. Under-exercise is not going to be effective. Therefore, learning the correct and balanced protocol is critical in achieving the desired positive outcome [14]. In addition to PCET, other intervention includes educating the patients on the appropriate diet to avoid, and food and drinks that may irritate the bladder and how to change the behaviours that make the symptoms worse by decreasing urinary urge and frequency [9]. The PCET may be implemented in combination with ES, medication and biofeedback bladder training [11].

ES was first described more than 80 years ago as a conservative treatment option. Subsequently, its mechanism of action was investigated in animal models and found to inhibit the parasympathetic motor neurons causing the bladder to relax. ES also causes contractions of the pelvic floor and increase the number of muscle fibres with a rapid contraction property that is responsible for continence during stress [15].

TENS unit (Fig. 51.2) sends small electrical currents through the skin to specific body parts by modulating abnormally excited nerves and release endorphins [15]. The device is usually connected to the skin surface via two or more electrodes and applied at high frequency (>50 Hz) with an intensity below motor contraction (sensory intensity) or low frequency (<10 Hz) with an intensity that produces a motor contraction. TENS is commonly recommended to treat many conditions, but there is controversy over which disorders the device should be used to treat.

Surface EMG (sEMG) device (Fig. 51.3) is one of the conventional methods available to physiotherapists to evaluate stress urinary incontinence treatment outcome. The process allows the recording of the change in voltage over the muscle fibre membrane that initiates the muscle contraction via the impulses in the motor nerves. In skeletal muscles, there is a relationship between EMG activity and the force generated, which means the higher the EMG activity level, the stronger the power produced [15].

The Pathway MR-20 Surface EMG (Fig. 51.3) is a two-channel sEMG biofeedback system that enables the clinician to observe the behaviour of muscle and used to modulate hypertonic muscle, strengthen weak or atrophied muscle. It is recommended for pelvic muscle rehabilitation to treat muscle incoordination, pelvic pain and sexual dysfunction.

EMG biofeedback is used to treat obstetrics and gynaecological disorders by promoting correct control of muscle contraction and visualisation because many patients, both men and women, cannot voluntarily contract their pelvic floor muscles, and they, therefore, require some assistance to initiate and reinforce the movement. Biofeedback uses electrodes to transmit muscle potentials in the form of audible or visual signals. The process enables the patients to increase or decrease their muscle activity level volitionally [15, 16].

The Myo200 (Fig. 51.4) is a two-channel EMG feedback therapy and stimulation device with the adjustable audio signal upon attaining the target value and one channel pressure feedback in mmHg – used for treating urinary incontinence by way of perineal re-education. The vaginal and anal probes are non-implanted electrical devices applied to the pelvic floor musculature and surrounding structures for treatment of urinary incontinence. Transvaginal ES is the non-invasive application of electrical current to stimulate the pelvic floor muscles to contract and relax using electrodes placed within the vagina. The stimulation if repeated over some time will strengthen the muscles and ease stress urinary incontinence which may also help control urgency by stimulating the nerves and decreasing bladder irritability.

Short wave diathermy (SWD) is a deep-heating thermal agent available in the armamentarium of the physiotherapists to treat chronic pelvic diseases. It utilises electromagnetic radio waves to convert energy to deep heat and exert its therapeutic effects by both thermal and non-thermal mechanisms [16, 17]. In the USA, the use of SWD has been on the

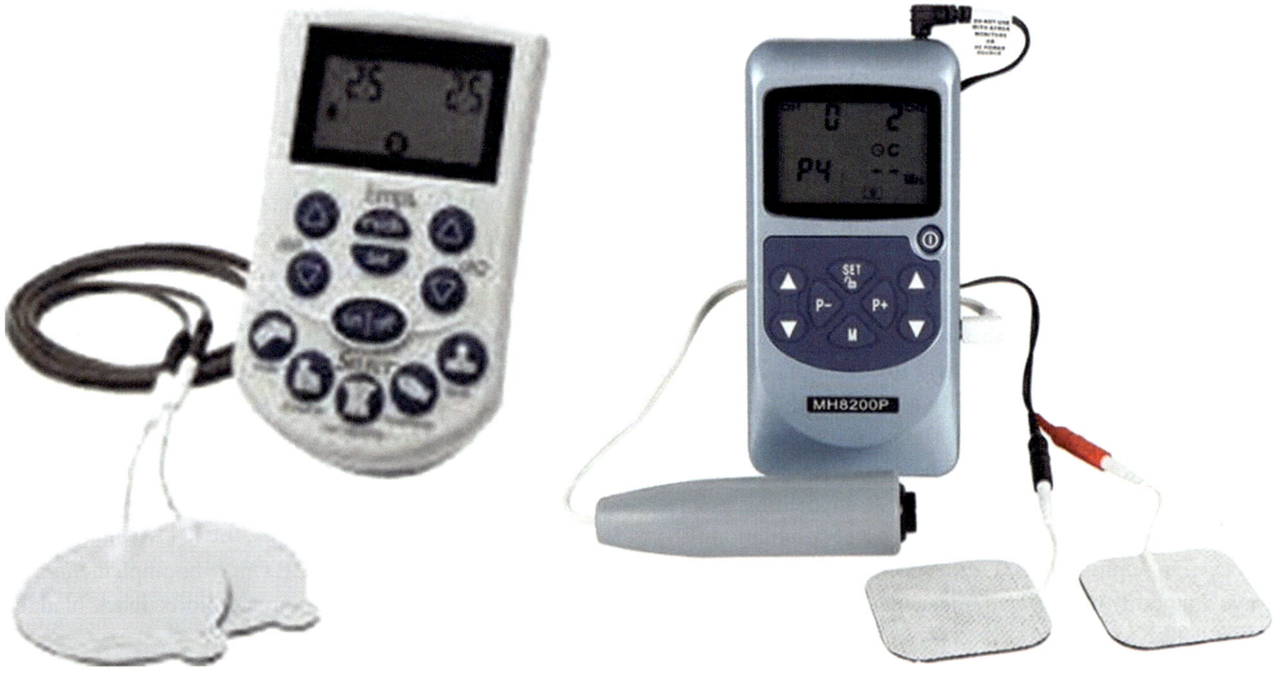

Fig. 51.2 TENS units†

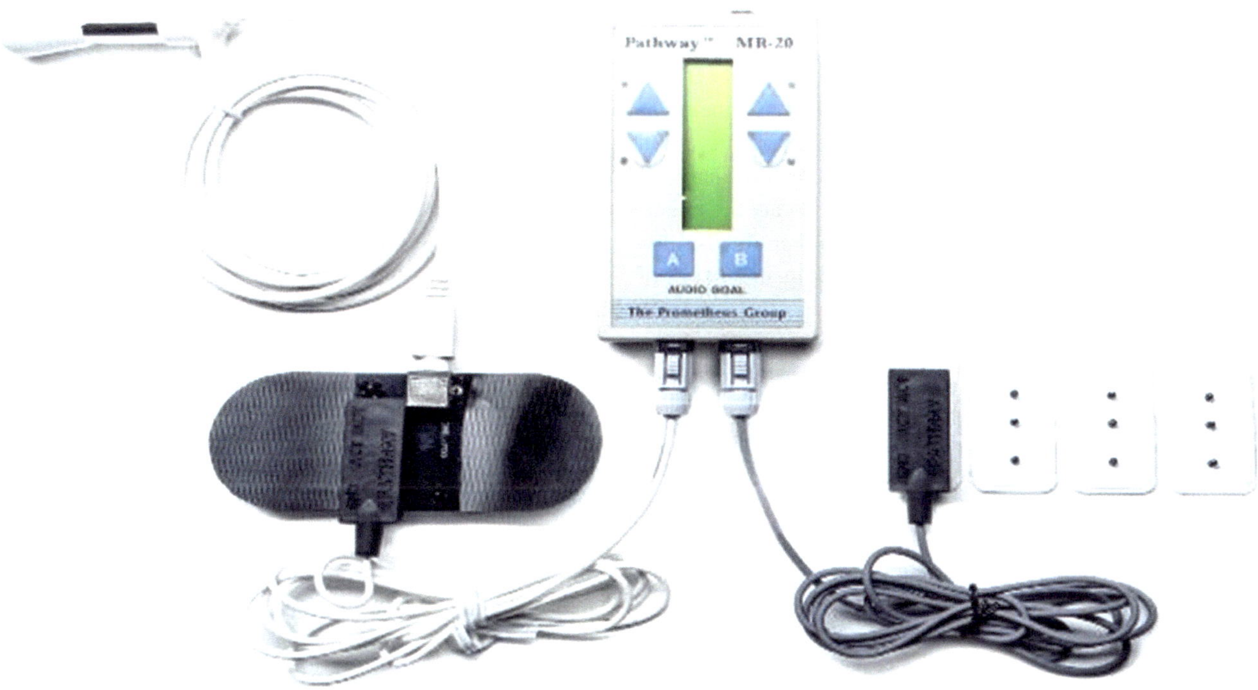

Fig. 51.3 The Pathway MR-20 Surface EMG‡

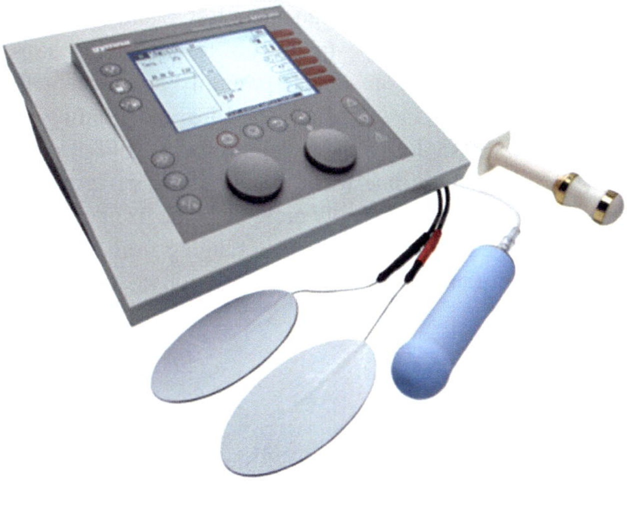

Fig. 51.4 EMG biofeedback Gymna Myo200*

decline for decades because of its large size and heavyweight (Fig. 51.5). Recent technology has produced a more compact and lightweight product that can be easily transported within the clinic and use in the home setting. An example of portable SWD device is the Mettler Auto-Therm 390 (Fig. 51.6).

The Mettler Auto-Therm 390 SWD machine (Fig. 51.6) is a pulsed, continuous wave unit with two (12 × 18 cm) soft-rubber plate capacitive applicators with flexible cables and six felt spacers. The device weighs only 7 kg and can be easily carried between treatment rooms and the patient's home.

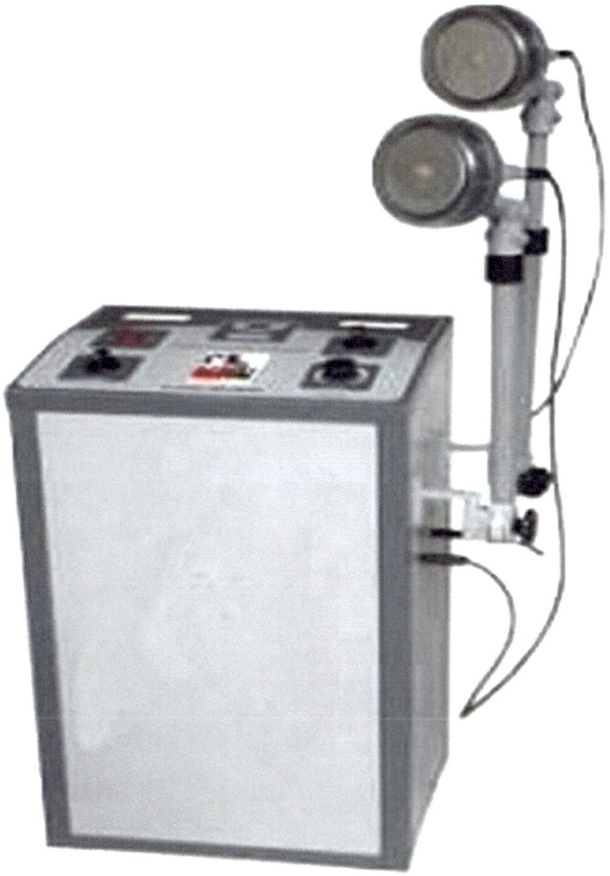

Fig. 51.5 The standard shortwave diathermy§

51.5 Reproductive Diseases and Associated Sequelae Amenable to Physiotherapy

An in-depth knowledge of the anatomy of the perineum as illustrated in Figs. 51.7 and 51.8 is critical in the successful management of male and female reproductive disorders.

Physiotherapy intervention aims to ameliorate the lingering debilitating symptoms associated with reproductive diseases and improve physical function and the quality of life of the patients. The common obstetrics and gynaecological diseases that are amenable to physiotherapy intervention are summarised in Fig. 51.9.

51.5.1 Urinary and Faecal Incontinence

Reliable population-based data on the prevalence of incontinence in developing countries, including Nigeria, are not available. In the USA, the prevalence of incontinence among women in the general population in 1995 is relatively low, particularly few cases in early life, but the incidence peak close to menopause and then rises steadily between the ages of 60 and 80 years with a prevalence of 10% among 15–19-year-olds and 18% in 20–24-year-olds [18]. More recent data in 2013 revealed that 10–30% of women in the USA aged 15–64 years have urinary incontinence. The incidence of incontinence in men is much lower than in women [16]. Overall, about 3–11% of men have urge incontinence, while stress incontinence accounts for less than 10% of cases and they are attributed primarily to prostate surgery, trauma, or neurological injury. The incidence of incontinence in men also increases with age, but severe cases in 70–80-year-old men are about half of that in women. In China, the overall incidence of stress urinary incontinence is about 20%, and it occurs mostly in women aged 45–59 years [19, 20].

Of this disorder, stress urinary incontinence is the most common type and is manifested by the involuntary loss of urine during physical exertion [18]. The predisposing risk factors for stress urinary incontinence include attenuation of the elasticity of the connective tissue, strenuous physical work, vaginal delivery, obesity and old age [16]. The outcome measures commonly used for stress urinary incontinence are both subjective (patient self-assessment, validated questionnaires, voiding diaries, patient satisfaction and quality of life) and objective (cough stress test, pad test and urodynamic evaluation). The treatments for managing stress urinary incontinence are aimed primarily at reducing the occurrence of the incontinence episodes and limiting the impact of the disorder on the patient's quality of life [16].

Urinary incontinence (*also known as stress, urge and mixed incontinence*) clinically presents in the form of loss of control of the bladder with severity ranging from occasionally leaking of urine when the individual cough, laugh, jump

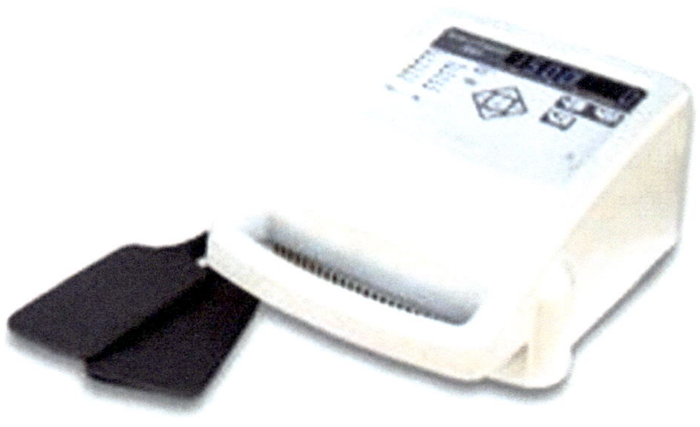

Fig. 51.6 The Mettler Auto-Therm 390®

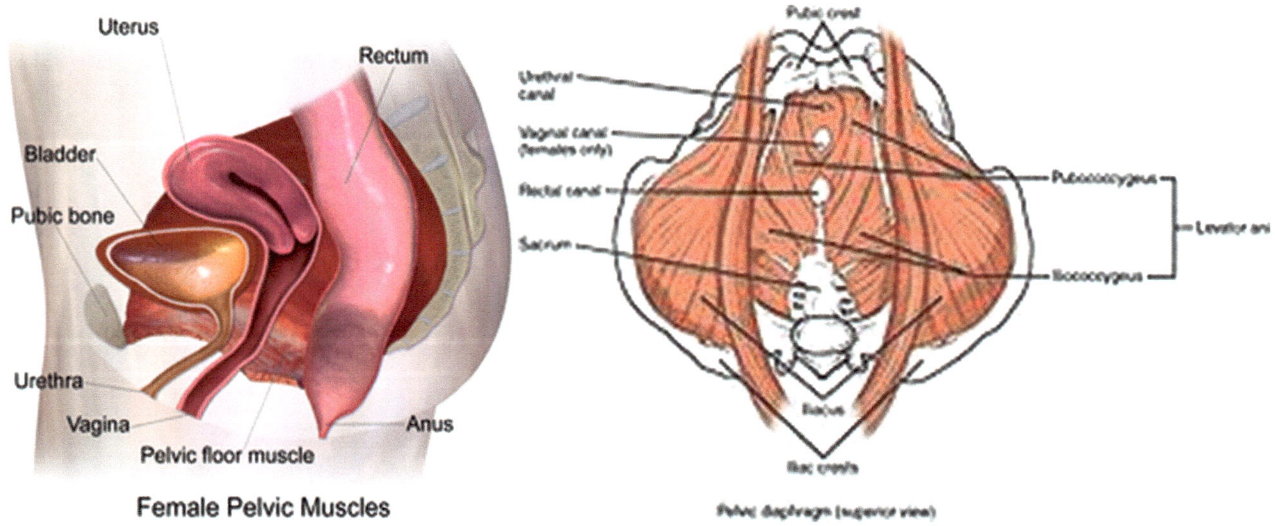

Fig. 51.7 The female perineum (pelvic floor: https://en.wikipedia.org/wiki/Pelvic_floor)

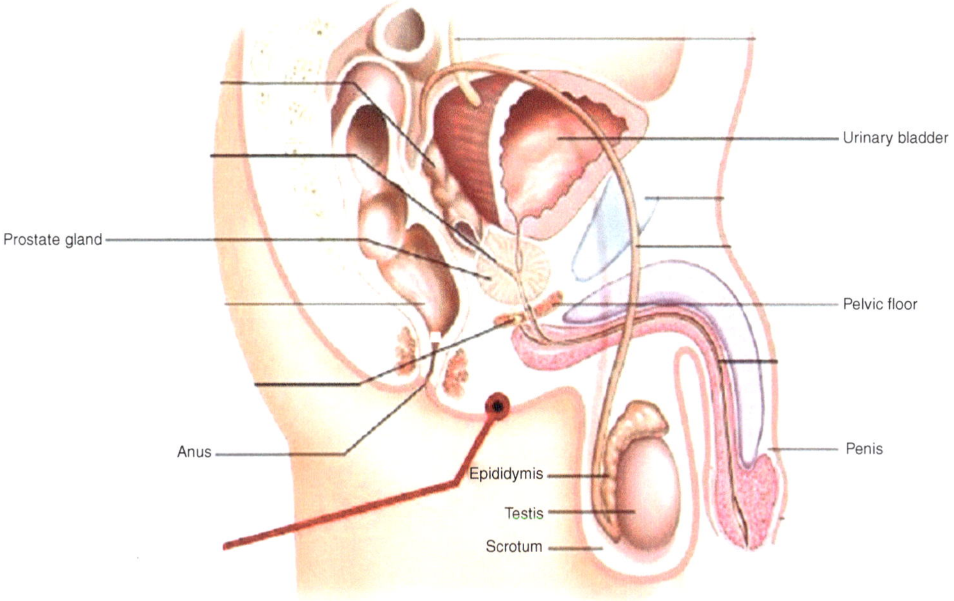

Fig. 51.8 The male perineum© (©https://images.search.yahoo.com/yhs/search?p=picture+of+the+male+perineum&fr=yhs-sz-002&hspart=sz&hsimp=yhs-002&imgurl=https%3A%2F%2Fi.ytimg.com%2Fvi%2FNiZ5W6kM57c%2Fmaxresdefault.jpg#id=0&iurl=https%3A%2F%2Fi.pinimg.com%2Foriginals%2F1a%2Fea%2F21%2F1aea21d70c4cae168f9dba95887f660c.jpg&action=click)

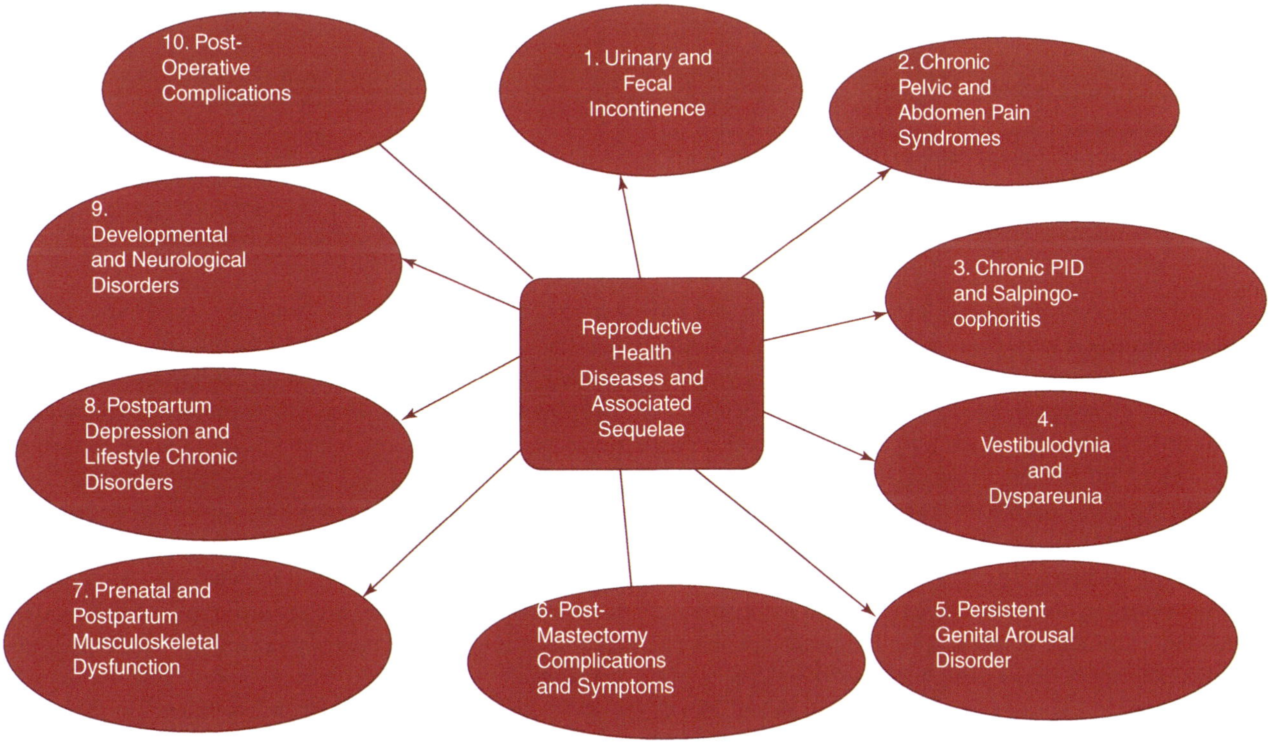

Fig. 51.9 Reproductive health diseases amenable to physical therapy intervention

or sneeze to having an urge to urinate that is so sudden and strong that he/she cannot get to a toilet in time (Fig. 51.10). Leakage of the urine occurs due to weak pelvic floor muscles and poor ligament. On the other hand, faecal incontinence is the loss of control of the bowel movements, causing an unexpected leak of stool (faeces) from the rectum – patients with

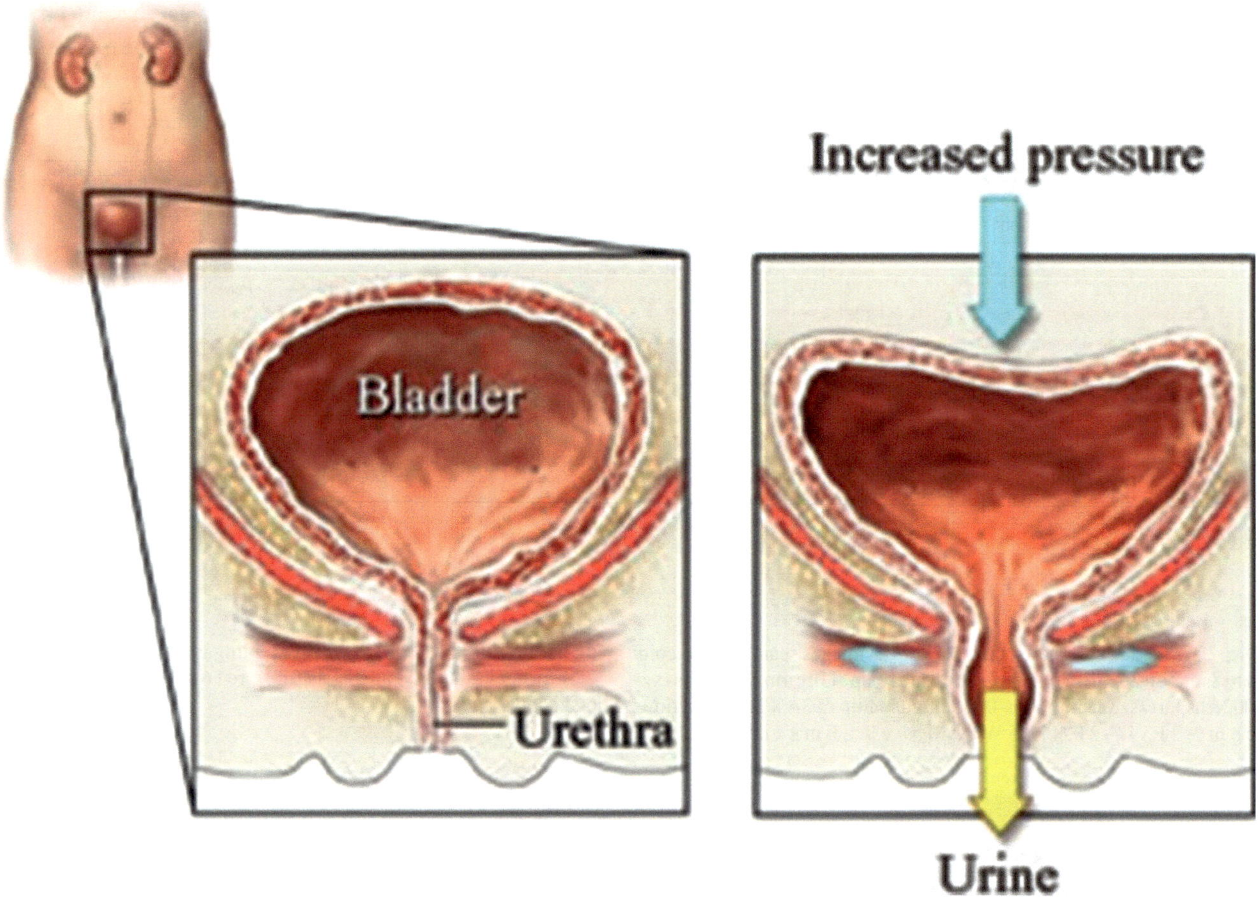

Fig. 51.10 Bladder and bowel control of urinary incontienece https://images.search.yahoo.com/yhs/search?p=picture+of+1.+Urinary+and+Fecal+Incontinence&fr=yhs-sz-002&hspart=sz&hsimp=yhs-002&imgurl=http%3A%2F%2Fwww.physiotherapyvictoria.ca%2Fwp-content%2Fuploads%2F2015%2F05%2FBladder-Control-Incontinence-Victoria-BC.png#id=17&iurl=https%3A%2F%2Fssl.adam.com%2Fgraphics%2Fimages%2Fen%2F9439.jpg&action=click)

chronic lower gastrointestinal tracts dysfunction present with uncoordinated or no relaxation of the associated muscles [18].

Faecal incontinence is usually a common complication of childbirth when using forceps and episiotomy deliveries, rectal surgery, inflammatory bowel disease or an abscess in the perirectal area following muscle damage. It may also occur as a result of nerve damage during childbirth, severe constipation, diabetes, spinal cord tumours and multiple sclerosis damaging the pudendal nerve, which innervates the rectal sphincter that controls bowel movements. Faecal incontinence can be caused by decreased elasticity of the perirectal muscle following surgery, radiation and childbirth leading to scarring of the rectum, causing it to stiffen and as a complication of the mechanical dysfunction of the anal sphincter – muscle and fascia strain that occurs following child delivery due to straining when voiding [18].

The physiotherapy management of urinary and faecal incontinence includes pubococcygeus exercise to strengthen and stretch the pubococcygeus muscles – Fig. 51.8 (normalise pelvic floor function at rest and upon contraction), ES to improve the awareness and strength of the muscles using vaginal and rectal internal or external electrodes and myofascial release techniques to increase or decrease muscle tension. It also includes the use of weights using rectal or vaginal air pressure devices (Figs. 51.11 and 51.12), EMG biofeedback that shows the patient how the muscles are working during exercise and home exercise program for the pelvic floor and core stabilisation muscles – including the strengthening of the back extensors and abdominal flexor muscles to augment spine support.

A study published in the American Journal of Obstetrics and Gynaecology in the early 1990s by Bump and associates and recently cited by Elite Pelvic Rehab evaluated the reproducibility of Kegels' exercise after a brief verbal instruction of women with urinary incontinence [14]. The women were taught the Kegels' protocol and re-tested again. Paradoxically, only 49% of the women performed the exercise correctly, and only 25% of them completed the task in a way that is

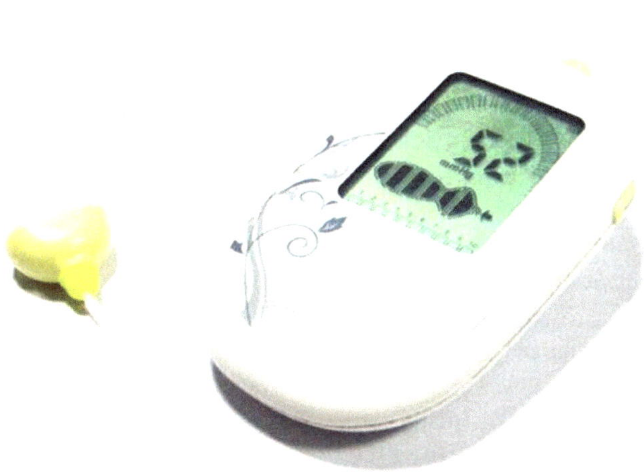

Fig. 51.11 SuperBid pelvic floor muscle Kegels' exerciser

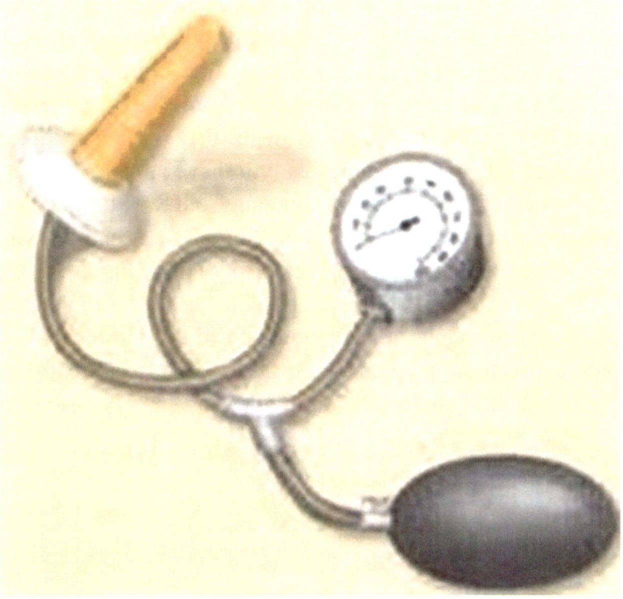

Fig. 51.12 The new Kegels' device

beneficial in the management of the incontinence. The findings led the authors to conclude that simple written or verbal instruction is inadequate when implementing a PCET program.

Over the years, many clinicians have postulated that PCET improves erectile function, ejaculation control and orgasm intensity in men with chronic prostatitis or chronic pelvic pain syndrome [11, 21, 22]. In 2014, Siegel posited that PCET is effective in the management of stress urinary incontinence complication after prostate surgery, postvoid dribbling, overactive bladder, erectile dysfunction, premature ejaculation and pelvic pain due to levator muscle spasm. This speculation has been buttressed by recent empirical studies that showed that PCET improve sexual function in women [23–25] and men [26, 27].

In 2012, Van Kampen reported that Glazener and colleagues found a significantly high rate of urinary incontinence in men following radical prostatectomy and transurethral resection of the prostate [26]. One year after the surgery, 76% of the men who had a radical prostatectomy and 65% of those who had transurethral resection of the prostate were still incontinent. Only 35% of the men in trial 1 and 27% in trial 2 still perform PCET daily. The efficacy of the intervention is rather low. Six weeks to 12 months after radical prostatectomy and PCET intervention, the reduction of incontinence ranged from 100% to 76% and from 100% to 65% after transurethral resection of the prostate. Based on the findings from the study, Glazener and colleagues concluded that four or fewer guided one-to-one conservative physiotherapy treatment for men with incontinence after prostate surgery is unlikely to be effective.

In 2016, García-Sánchez and associates analysed the content of several published studies that evaluated the efficacy of physical exercise and PCET training program in the management of urinary incontinence among women [28]. They searched seven electronic databases published in the last 10 years and identified three studies on urinary incontinence in women athletes and another six studies that investigated urinary incontinence in women. The nine studies reviewed showed improvement in their urinary incontinence status following intervention. Based on the findings from the available systematic reviews and meta-analyses, it is prudent to conclude that PCET has a beneficial effect in the management of urinary incontinence [23–27].

51.5.2 Chronic Pelvic and Abdomen Pain Syndromes

A referral from Ob-Gyns with a diagnosis of chronic pelvic or abdominal pain is of no clinical significance to the physiotherapist because such non-specific term does not clarify the genesis or cause of the pain. As such, the physiotherapist must meticulously evaluate the patient to arrive at a physical diagnosis that will exclude pain originating from internal organs or the spine and referred to the pelvis and abdomen. The physical assessment should include a detailed obstetrics and gynaecological history and screening for gastrointestinal, urologic, musculoskeletal and neurological disorders. Gynaecologic causes of chronic pelvic or abdominal pain include PID, endometriosis, adhesive disease, ovarian retention syndrome, pelvic congestion syndrome, ovarian remnant syndrome, adenomyosis and leiomyomas. Non-gynaecologic causes of pain referred from the pelvis and abdomen may be due to irritable bowel syndrome, painful bladder syndrome and interstitial cystitis. It may also be due to pelvic floor tension myalgia or abdominal myofascial pain syndrome [29]. Pain in the pelvic and abdomen may be different from chronic pelvic pain syndrome and pelvic and pudendal neuralgia.

Chronic pelvic pain syndrome which clinically present in the form of increased pelvic muscle tenderness and pelvic floor dysfunction is prevalent among males 35–45 years old. Women and girls with *pelvic pain* are also referred for physiotherapy. Aching or burning discomfort characterises the pelvic pain in the lower abdomen, pelvis or perineum. The condition is described as chronic when the pain and any other symptoms have been present for more than 6 months. Other symptoms of pelvic pain include pain in the hip, buttock, tailbone, joints of the pelvis and pain during sexual intercourse. Other symptoms include tender points in the abdominal muscles, decreased hip and lumbar spine range of motion, urinary frequency, urgency or incontinence, constipation and straining with bowel movements and painful bowel movements. The condition is caused by pelvic joint dysfunction, imbalance of the pelvic floor, trunk and/or pelvis muscles, incoordination of the muscles that control the bowel and bladder function, tender points and/or weakness of the pelvic floor muscles, pressure on the peripheral nerves in the pelvic area and scar tissue formation post abdominal or pelvic surgery. The aetiology of pelvic pain is at times unknown, and it may be associated with organic disease processes. Consequently, it is essential to have a correct diagnosis to confirm the cause of the pain before physiotherapy intervention [30].

Pelvic and pudendal neuralgia is common in men and characterised by chronic pelvic pain in the penis, scrotum, perineum or anorectal area which is aggravated by prolonged sitting. *Endometriosis* is another painful disorder which clinically presents in the form of pelvic pain, pain during intercourse, bowel movements/urination, and bowel disorders in the form of constipation, abdominal pain and small bowel obstruction.

Physiotherapists evaluate patients with chronic pelvic and abdomen pain to establish a physical diagnosis of the origin of the pain and develop a treatment plan to address the clinical problem. A lower-quarter screening that includes the use of provocative test of the vertebrae, mobility and neurological tests is conducted to identify dysfunction emanating from the lumbar, sacroiliac, hip, knee, ankle and foot joints and to rule out the pain of musculoskeletal origin [30]. The medical management of chronic pelvic or abdominal pain is focused on the treatment of the causes or general pain management or using both approaches [29].

Physiotherapy management of pelvic and pudendal neuralgia includes the use of TENS to decrease pain and increase the quality of life of the patients. Pelvic floor exercise is often recommended to alleviate the pain associated with endometriosis disorder. Bowel disorders are amenable to manual therapy, localised soft tissue massage, behaviour modification strategies and body mechanics retraining. Bladder control retraining is enhanced by regaining regular urinary cycles, lifestyle choices by selecting different food and drink options that are less irritable to the bladder.

51.5.3 Chronic Pelvic Inflammatory Disease and Salpingo-Oophoritis

Chronic pelvic inflammatory disease (PID) and *salpingo-oophoritis* (inflammation of the fallopian tube and ovary – Fig. 51.12) have lingering debilitating illness that is characterised by various symptoms such as persistent or recurrent lower abdominal pains, vaginal discharge, dyspareunia and menstrual disorders. Untreated sexually transmitted diseases can cause PID, a severe condition, in women. In the USA, one in eight women with chronic PID has difficulties getting pregnant [32]. Based on self-reported lifetime data, 2.5 million women of reproductive age (18–44 years) constitute a prevalence rate of 4.4% of the general population, and sexually active have PID. The prevalence is highest among women with previous sexually transmitted infections [31]. Data from a cohort of inpatients from Scandinavia indicated that women diagnosed with PID have six times increased rate and are more likely to have an ectopic pregnancy, tubal factor infertility (ranging from 8% after the first episode to as high as 40% after three events) and chronic pelvic pain (18% following one episode) [31] (Fig. 51.13).

The most serious clinical consequences of chronic PID and salpingo-oophoritis include infertility, chronic pelvic pain and ectopic pregnancy. Of these symptoms, treatment options such as analgesics, antibiotics and surgery have pro-

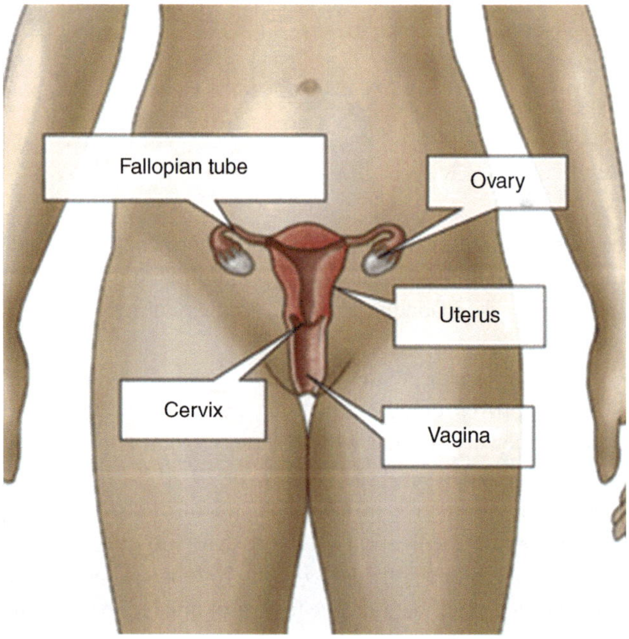

Fig. 51.13 The female reproductive system. (https://www.cdc.gov/std/pid/stdfact-pid.htm)

found side effects. The prolonged administration of anti-inflammatory analgesics is associated with maculopapular rash, agranulocytosis, aplastic anaemia, tinnitus and deafness, peptic ulceration and nephrotoxicity and development of resistant strains of organisms and predispose the patient to candidiasis. On the other hand, pelvic surgeries (including hysterectomy) have not been known to relieve symptoms in patients with chronic PID consistently. In some instances, the situation was made worse by the operative procedure. Luckily, the chronic pelvic pain associated with PID is effectively managed by SWD [30, 33–36].

51.5.4 Vestibulodynia and Dyspareunia

Vestibulodynia, also known as vulvar pain, clinically presents in the form of hypersensitivity reaction to a light touch of the vestibule, during sexual intercourse or on insertion of tampons. The severity of pain is variable among women. While some women with vestibulodynia can tolerate pain during sexual intercourse, other women experience pain on light tactile touch of the vestibule area or wearing tight pants and underwear. Deep pressure applied to the area produces soreness.

Vulvodynia affects about 8–12% of women during their lifetimes. Vulvar vestibulodynia which is the most common type of vulvodynia is characterised by pain when the vulvar vestibule is touched and causing entryway dyspareunia. The aetiology is multifactorial. Some experts posited that it is due to hormonal effects, muscle dysfunction, cognitive, personality and psychosocial factors, inflammatory mediators, pelvic floor muscle dysfunction and peripheral and central sensitisation to pain. Given its multiple aetiology, treatment is multimodal and consists of proper general vulvar hygiene and use of topical antinociceptive agents (lidocaine, capsaicin) and oral medications, anti-inflammatory agents (corticosteroids, interferon), neuromodulating medications (anticonvulsants and antidepressants), hormonal agents, and muscle relaxants (e.g., botulinum toxin) injectables, dietary changes with supplementations, acupuncture, hypnotherapy, surgery, cognitive behavioural therapy, surgery, and physiotherapy [37, 38]. Surgery (vestibulectomy) is indicated in cases that are not responsive to traditional treatment and the success rates are between 60% and 90%.

The physiotherapist must educate women with vestibulodynia or vulvar pain, how the pelvic-floor muscles tend to contract when pain is experienced. And women should be taught how to relax the pelvic-floor muscles during intercourse. The aforemnetioned exercise will decrease the sensation of pain considerably. Manual techniques used for proprioception, normalisation of muscle tone, pain modification and mobilisation technique applied on the surface of the perineum and internally by vaginal and sometimes anal palpation are indicated for treating vestibulodynia. These manual techniques include myofascial release, trigger-point pressures, massage, combined with EMG biofeedback monitored with surface and an intracavity vaginal probe displayed on a video monitor, bipolar, biphasic, low-frequency ES with a rectangular waveform used via the same intracavity probe as biofeedback and PCET. Home exercises for vestibulodynia include stretching exercise with a biofeedback unit and vaginal dilatation with dilators and dildos. Women are encouraged to involve their partner in the practice of these exercises and also perform manual stretching exercise techniques [38, 39].

Dyspareunia is characterised by painful sexual intercourse arising from medical or psychological aetiologies. The pain can be limited to the external surface of the genitalia, or more in-depth in the pelvis following deep pressure applied against the cervix. The pain can affect a small portion of the vulva or vagina or felt all over the area. Manual therapy and SWD are recommended for treating dyspareunia and vestibulodynia [39]; but there is presently no empirical evidence to support this recommendation. However, there is a strong evidence in the literature on the efficacy of a multidisciplinary treatment approach consisting of sex/psychotherapy, pelvic floor physiotherapy, transcutaneous ES, EMG biofeedback, fractional carbon dioxide laser therapy and medication to manage dyspareunia and sexual dysfunctions in women with provoked vestibulodynia and dyspareunia [40–43].

51.5.5 Persistent Genital Arousal Disorder

Persistent genital arousal disorder, a medical condition that is common mostly in women, clinically presents in the form of unrelenting, spontaneous, intrusive, uncontainable, unwanted physical arousal in the absence of conscious thoughts of sexual desire or sexual interest. The genital arousal often leads to ongoing physical pain, stress and psychological difficulties which may affect the regular performance of the activities of daily living tasks. In 2009, Korda, Pfaus, and Goldstein presented a case study of a 49-year-old woman with persistent genital arousal disorder treated with varenicline to control her smoking habit and within 2 weeks, she experienced a substantial reduction of her symptoms [44]. Each time varenicline was discontinued, the symptoms returned within 2 weeks. Today, varenicline is the first-line medication for treating persistent genital sexual arousal. The mechanism of action for the medication is mediated in part by the hypothalamic and limbic dopamine systems. Varenicline is a known partial agonist of the alpha2beta4 subtype of the nicotinic cholinergic receptor, and its unique pharmacological action stimulates the brain to release dopamine while blocking nicotine's ability to stimulate the further release of dopamine. In explaining their findings, the authors hypothesised that the central hyperactive dopamine release is a critical element of the pathophysiology of the disorder. They speculated that varenicline reduced the hyperstimulated central release of dopamine [44]. Follow-up randomised controlled studies are needed to demonstrate the safety and efficacy of varenicline in the treatment of persistent genital arousal disorder in women.

In addition to medication, physiotherapy is routinely recommended for persistent genital arousal disorder. The treatment is preceded by a comprehensive, individualised evaluation to establish a physical diagnosis and subsequently, the appropriate physical modalities selected to modulate pain, improve function and quality of life [15]. SWD and EMG biofeedback are recommended to modulate the symptoms of persistent genital arousal disorder by aiding genital muscle relaxation. The frequency of the treatment protocol is two to three times per week, lasting 6–8 weeks [39]. This recommendation should be taken with a dose of caution because they are not based on empirical evidence.

51.5.6 Post-Mastectomy Complications

Approximately 50% of survivors of breast cancer experience chronic sexual problems. Sadly, sexual dysfunction is generally underreported and undertreated in clinical practice. This schism is due to the limited evidence-based studies designed to improve women's sexual functioning [45].

Lymphedema and extremity pain are other complications associated with the resection of the axillary lymph node of women with breast cancer. Lymphedema is the dysfunction of the body's lymphatic system when it is not able to properly move the lymph fluid from the tissue spaces back to the bloodstream with a propensity to cause swelling in the extremities, trunk, genitalia, head or neck. Unlike normal oedema or swelling, lymphedema is made up of protein-rich fluid (lymph) that can only be drained by the lymphatic vessels. If the lymphatic system is not functioning correctly, the liquid and proteins will remain in the tissue spaces even when the part is elevated and may turn into a life-long chronic condition. Lymphedema is often caused by congenital anomaly, trauma, resection of the lymph node in the axillary (armpit) region during surgery for breast or other forms of cancers, infection and radiation treatment after the operation increases the risk for lymphedema. There is an increased risk for lymphedema if a patient has a history of one or more of the causes mentioned earlier [30].

The primary symptoms of lymphedema are swelling and 'pitting' of the tissues anywhere in the arm, hand, wrist or fingers after treatment for breast cancer. To diagnose lymphedema and before physiotherapy treatment, it is critical to rule out swelling due to dysfunction of the other organ systems such as the heart and kidneys. Early detection and treatment of lymphedema ensure faster and more successful outcomes. There is presently no known cure for lymphedema, but the condition can be managed with physiotherapy interventions designed to regain mobility and function of the body part. Breast cancer-related lymphedema impacts the activities of daily living skills of the women. They also often experience chronic and progressive swelling, recurrent skin infections and decreased self-image and quality of life [46].

Physiotherapists control and manage lymphedema using a complete decongestive therapy that includes manual lymphatic drainage, effleurage massage, followed by compression bandaging. It is sanguine to monitor the limb circumference before and after intervention to track treatment effectiveness. And once the limb girth returned to normal, the physiotherapist should provide home program exercise including the wearing of compression garments for maintenance [30].

51.5.7 Prenatal and Postpartum Musculoskeletal Dysfunctions

Prenatal and postpartum musculoskeletal dysfunction. The prenatal phase of pregnancy is associated with significant physical, emotional and hormonal changes. The alterations in the musculoskeletal system leads to muscle imbalances and changes in spinal mobility as the foetus develop. Postpartum, the hormone levels fluctuate, and this may cause hypermobility which in combination with the physical changes due to the delivery may contribute to excessive joint mobility, weakness of the core stabilisers and altered spinal mobility and function. The postural changes often cause some muscles to tighten, while other muscles are stretched and become weak causing muscle imbalance and potential for decreased stability. The spine adjusts to the changing posture when the foetus grows – it affects spinal mobility and can cause pain and dysfunction. The symptoms of musculoskeletal dysfunction during the prenatal and postpartum periods include pelvis or spinal pain, pain in the muscles of the hip joints, numbness in the lower extremities, and weakness of the abdominal muscles, causing pain during transitional movements or lifting. During the postpartum phase, urinary incontinence may manifest due to muscle weakness [9].

Physiotherapists provide patient-centred treatment for the musculoskeletal problems associated with pregnancy and during the different phases of life, from childbearing years to the postmenopausal period. Physiotherapists evaluate the patients and provide hands-on treatment for any observed spinal and pelvic joint dysfunction. The intervention typically includes mobilisation and manipulation to adjust faulty joint positioning, and muscle tightness. Other treatments include EMG biofeedback combined with pelvic floor muscle exercise to decrease pain or specific exercises to strengthen back extensors or the abdominal core muscles, postural and ergonomic training. Additionally, home program exercises are prescribed to address muscle weakness and imbalance and offer instruction on activities of daily living tasks that may be difficult during the prenatal and postpartum phases [9, 30].

51.5.8 Postpartum Depression and Lifestyle Chronic Disorders

Depression is a mental illness that affects over 340 million people globally [47], and is now one of the leading causes of disability and the second top contributor to the global burden of disease. People with mental disorders are more at risk of developing poor physical health. The promotion of physical development and mental well-being is one of the critical elements embedded in the WHO's definition for reproductive health [48, 49]. Non-communicable diseases such as heart disease, stroke, cancer, diabetes and lung disease are the primary cause of morbidity and mortality in industrialised countries, and it is becoming a contributing factor in many developing countries [50]. These diseases which are common in both men and women are strongly associated with risk behaviours, such as physical inactivity, unhealthy diet and tobacco use, and they are for the most part preventable [50]. The treatment of the lifestyle induced chronic conditions and the loss of time from work costs billions of dollars annually.

Physiotherapists play a significant role in promoting the physical and mental health of symptomatic and asymptomatic men and women. Several studies have demonstrated the positive effect of physical activity in the prevention and treatment of postpartum depression and the lifestyle of chronic diseases [51–56]. Today, physiotherapists routinely incorporate health and wellness into their practices to address the patients' behaviours relating to physical activity, nutrition and weight management, smoking cessation, sleep and stress management [57]. Following graded exercise testing, physiotherapists use the results to prescribe the type and dosage (intensity and frequency) of exercise and monitor the implementation of the intervention to ensure safety and effectiveness. Better outcomes occur when the exercise program designed for patients with postpartum depression and lifestyle chronic disorders is delivered by physiotherapists moving through advice and exercise programs [47, 50, 58].

51.5.9 Developmental and Neurological Disorders

Developmental disorders are present in early life and are more prevalent among males than females. In childhood, they fall into a category of mental health conditions that involve severe impairment in different areas of language learning, motor, autism spectrum disorders, attention deficit hyperactivity disorder, antisocial behaviour and schizophrenia [59]. Many different theories have been postulated as the cause of developmental disorders. Some scientists linked developmental disorders to environmental (chemicals and early childhood traumatisation as in extreme stress) hazards that disrupt normal development. Others implicated developmental abnormalities that are genetically pre-determined or spontaneous genetic mutations.

Neurological disorders affect both genders of all ages. The primary causes of the neurological disorders that often lead to disability in women and girls of reproductive age are trauma (e.g. skull fracture, spinal cord injury), Erb's palsy and cerebrovascular accident (e.g. stroke and cerebral palsy) as well as common complication of childbirth, neoplasia (e.g. glioma), infection (e.g. meningitis), metabolic disorders (e.g. diabetic neuropathy), genetic disorders (e.g. Down's syndrome), environmental factors (e.g., heavy metal encephalopathies) and immunological factors (e.g., multiple sclerosis) [60]. Globally, between 250,000 and 500,000 people sustain spinal cord injury annually from road traffic accidents, falls or violence, and they are 2–5 times more likely to die prematurely [1]. In many developing countries, no reliable population-based data are available on the number of spinal cord injury. For example, in Nigeria, hospital-based data revealed the gender, male-to-female ratio is about two to one, and the duration of hospital stay ranges from 2 to 60 (Mean = 12, SD = 8.6) weeks [61]. And as of 2017, the National Orthopedic Hospital in Kano admits about 480 cases of spinal cord injury annually [62].

The impairments associated with developmental and neurological disorders are managed by a team of medical rehabilitation specialists that include a physician, surgeon, physiotherapist, occupational therapist, speech therapist, behavioural therapist, counsellor, dietician and clinical psychologist.

51.5.10 Postoperative Complications

In general, there are two types of complications associated with major surgical procedures. One is specific to the operation performed. For example, transient incontinence is a plausible complication of bladder surgery, but not for heart surgery. The second is the potential risk for most major types of operation such as an adverse reaction to the anaesthesia, post-surgical infection risk, bleeding during surgery, poor wound healing and blood clots. Adverse reactions to general anaesthesia are rare but occur in the form of wheezing, dizziness, fever, low blood pressure, confusion, agitation, a rash and liver problems. Most adverse reactions are mild and temporary, but patients who are malnourished, and those in poor general health, or who have a circulatory disease such as diabetes are more prone to postoperative complications [63].

Another common complication of surgery is a respiratory problem that occurs in about 15% of people given general anaesthesia. Lung congestion and pneumonia are known risks associated with major surgery. Postoperative physiotherapy informs of deep breathing exercises and spirometry during recovery generally prevent this risk. Major surgeries that involve the removal of a vascularised organ carries a higher risk of bleeding because of a sudden rise in blood pressure or blood vessel damage caused by postoperative infection. Avoiding blood-thinning medications before the surgery will reduce this risk. If bacteria invade the surgical wound, infection and delayed wound healing can occur. The ulcer is treated with topical dressing and antibiotic therapy. The reduced blood circulation due to limited physical activity after surgery causes wounds to heal slowly even in the absence of infection. Postoperative physiotherapy in the form of low-level aerobic exercise will promote wound healing because exercise improves blood circulation [63].

Deep vein thrombosis and blood clot are common complications associated with major surgeries which potentially may have fatal consequences that is preventable if diagnosed early. One of the risk factors for blood clots is reduced mobility post-surgery, as this also reduces circulation. With regular gentle physical activity or isometric exercises, blood thinning medication (if there is no risk of bleeding), support stockings to improve flow and elevation of the extremities, this risk can be overcome.

A common dogma taught to physiotherapy students is that any major surgical procedure that warrants general anaesthesia will benefit from pre- and postoperative physiotherapy. Such operations include total and partial joint replacements, knee and hip surgeries, ligament or tendon reconstructions, low back and cervical surgeries (discectomy, aminotomy, laminectomy, spinal fusion), meniscectomy, mastectomy, open heart and brain surgeries. The goals of preoperative physiotherapy are to prepare the patient for the surgical procedure mentally, to maximise joint motion, maintain muscle strength and endurance, improve muscular control to aid faster recovery, to train the patients on the immediate exercises and precautions needed after the operation and to improve the patient's overall fitness and wellbeing. All these goals of preoperative physiotherapy contributes to better recovery after the operation [63].

Following surgery, physiotherapists perform detailed evaluation and work with the patient to set realistic functional goals prior to the physiotherapy interventions. Such treatment includes gait, posture, balance and coordination training, and exercise to increase strength, flexibility and range of motion; manual therapy complemented by physical modalities such as ice, heat and ES and home exercise program. During the postoperative evaluation, physiotherapists typically conduct a comprehensive assessment of patient pain, mobility, strength, lifestyle behaviours and physical limitations. Postoperative physiotherapy intervention focuses on promoting wound healing, reducing pain and swelling and restoring joint mobility, flexibility and strength [64, 65].

Although physiotherapy is recommended routinely as an essential component in the management of patients undergoing any major surgery, but empirical evidence for their efficacy is yet to be established. In 2007, a cross-sectional study by Reeve and associates investigated the practices of pre- and post-physiotherapy for patients undergoing thoracotomy and the factors that influenced the practice among different providers [66]. The overwhelming majority of the patients following the thoracotomy were referred for physiotherapy assessment and treatment immediately after surgery. However, only in one-third of the cases were preoperative physiotherapy provided, and relatively few had physiotherapy treatment follow-up after discharge from the hospital. A decade after Reeve and associates' study, the effectiveness of pre- and postoperative physiotherapy practice remains unknown. Therefore, randomised controlled studies are needed to guide clinicians in determining the efficacy of these practices for patients undergoing major surgeries.

51.6 Conclusion

Physiotherapists evaluate and treat obstetrics and gynaecological conditions such as urinary and faecal incontinence, chronic PID and chronic salpingo-oophoritis, chronic pelvic and abdomen pain syndromes, vestibulodynia and dyspareunia. Also, they manage persistent genital arousal disorder, post-mastectomy complications, pre- and postnatal musculoskeletal dysfunctions, postpartum depression and lifestyle chronic disorders, developmental and neurological disorders and postoperative complications. In combination with medication, radiation, surgery and behavioural modification techniques, physiotherapy is indicated for the conditions mentioned above.

Available literature revealed that men's reproductive disorders are understudied, and PCET used to treat urinary and faecal (anal) incontinence is the most investigated physical therapy modality, followed by aerobic exercise used for postpartum depression, obesity, gestational diabetes mellitus and mastectomy complication prevention [67].

This chapter presents the 10 most common obstetrics and gynaecological disorders that are amenable to physiotherapy intervention. Understanding of this information by Ob-Gyns will promote timely referral of patients for physiotherapy and blunt the impact and progression of the disease process which can ultimately reduce healthcare costs and duplicative use of services without compromising outcomes.

References

1. World Health Organization (WHO). Disabilities – Africa. 2017. Accessed May 5, 2018.
2. Devi PS. A timely referral to palliative care team improves quality of life. Indian J Palliat Care. 2011; 17(Suppl): S14–6. https://www.ncbi.nlm.nih.gov/pmc/articles/PMC3140091/. Accessed: May 5, 2019.
3. Auguste BL, Naimark DMJ. Timely referral to outpatient nephrology care slows progression and reduces treatment costs of chronic kidney diseases. Kidney Int Rep. 2017;2(4):77. https://www.sciencedirect.com/science/article/pii/S2468024917301201. Accessed: May 5, 2019.
4. Fritz JM, Childs JD, Wainner RS, Flynn TW. Primary care referral of patients with low back pain to physical therapy: impact on future healthcare utilisation and costs. Spine. 2012;37(25):2114–21.
5. Fuhrmans V. A novel plan helps hospital wean itself off pricey tests. Wall Street J. 2007. https://www.wsj.com/articles/SB116857143155174786. Accessed: July 7, 2021.
6. Fuhrmans V. Timing of physical therapy initiation for nonsurgical management of musculoskeletal disorders and effects on patient outcomes: a systematic review. J Orthop Sports Phys Therap. 2016;46(2):56–70. https://pubmed.ncbi.nlm.nih.gov/26755406/.
7. Stubblefield MD. The underutilisation of rehabilitation to treat physical impairments in breast cancer survivors. 2017; PMR. 9(9S2): S317–23.
8. Standford Medicine. (n.d). Fertility and reproductive healthcare team. https://www.stanfordchildrens.org/en/service/fertility-and-reproductive-health/careteam Accessed: May 5, 2019.
9. Manske RC, Lehecka BJ, Reiman MP, Loudon JK. Orthopedic joint mobilisation and manipulation. Human Kinetics. 2018.
10. OrthoBalance Physical Therapy. Treatment modalities and procedures. 2019. https://www.orthobalancept.com/treatment-modalities-procedures/. Accessed: May 5, 2019.
11. Rogers G, Story CM. Kegel exercises for men: do they work? 2016. https://www.healthline.com/health/kegel-exercises-for-men. Accessed: May 5, 2019.
12. Bubnis D, Case L, Goldman C. Exercises to eliminate erectile dysfunction. 2017. https://www.healthline.com/health/erectile-dysfunction/exercises. Accessed: May 5, 2019.
13. Pletcher P, Schaefer A. How to last longer in bed. 2015. https://www.healthline.com/health/mens-health/how-to-last-longer-in-bed. Accessed: May 5, 2019.
14. Elite Pelvic Rehab. Don't try Kegels until you read this. 2015. https://elitepelvicrehab.wordpress.com/tag/elite-pelvic-rehab/. Accessed: May 5, 2019.
15. Hecox B, Mehreteab TA, Weisberg J, Sanko J, editors. Physical agents: a comprehensive text for physical therapists. 2nd ed. Norwalk: Appleton and Lange.
16. Terlikowski R, Dobrzycka B, Kinalski M, Kuryliszyn-Moskal A, Terlikowski SJ. Transvaginal electrical stimulation with surface-EMG biofeedback in managing stress urinary incontinence in women of premenopausal age: a double-blind, placebo-controlled, randomised clinical trial. Int Urogynecol J. 2013; 24(10):1631–8. https://www.ncbi.nlm.nih.gov/pmc/articles/PMC3779318/. Accessed: May 5, 2019.
17. Waldman SD. The physiologic effects of therapeutic heat. Pain Review 2009. https://www.sciencedirect.com/topics/medicine-and-dentistry/short-wave-diathermy. Accessed: May 5, 2019.
18. Nitti VM. The prevalence of urinary incontinence. Rev Urol. 2001;3(Suppl 1):S2–6. https://www.ncbi.nlm.nih.gov/pmc/articles/PMC1476070/. Accessed: May 5, 2019
19. Liu L, Zhang Y, Gong J, Chen X, Wu H, Zhu W. Effects of different treatment methods on the clinical and urodynamic state of perimenopausal women with stress urinary incontinence. Iran J Public Health. 2018;47(8):1090–7.
20. Wu PL, Lee M, Huang TT. Effectiveness of physical activity on patients with depression and Parkinson's disease: a systematic review. https://journals.plos.org/plosone/article?id=10.1371/journal.pone.0181515. 2017. Accessed: May 5, 2019.
21. Siegelab AL. Pelvic floor muscle training in males: practical applications. Urology. 2014;84(1):1–7. https://www.sciencedirect.com/science/article/pii/S0090429514002738. Accessed: May 5, 2019.
22. LaFlamme M, Ellen Ellis M. Prevention of chronic prostatitis.2016. https://www.healthline.com/health/chronic-prostatitis. Accessed: May 5, 2019.
23. Bø K. Pelvic floor muscle training in the treatment of female stress urinary incontinence, pelvic organ prolapse and sexual dysfunction. World J Urol. 2012;30(4):437–43. https://link.springer.com/article/10.1007%2Fs00345-011-0779-8. Accessed: May 5, 2019.
24. Adams SR, Dessie SG, Dodge LE, Mckinney JL, Hacker MR, Elkadry EA. Pelvic floor physical therapy as primary treatment of pelvic floor disorders with urinary urgency and frequency-predominant symptoms. Female Pelvic Med Reconstr Surg. 2015;21(5):252–6.
25. Homsi C, Ferreira J, Dwyer PL, Davidson M, De Souza A, Alvarez J, Ugarte H, Frawley C. Does pelvic floor muscle training improve female sexual function? A systematic review. Int Urogynaecol J. 2015; 26(12):1735–50. https://link.springer.com/article/10.1007/s00192-015-2749-y. Accessed: May 5, 2019.
26. Van Kampen M. Pelvic floor muscle training after prostate surgery. Lancet J. 2012;379(9811):120. https://www.thelancet.com/journals/lancet/article/PIIS0140-6736(12)60058-0/fulltext. Accessed: May 5, 2019.
27. Cohen D, Gonzale J, Goldstein I. The role of pelvic floor muscles in male sexual dysfunction and pelvic pain sexual medicine. Reviews. 2016;4(1):53–62. https://www.sciencedirect.com/science/article/pii/S2050052115000025. Accessed: May 5, 2019.
28. García-Sánchez E, Rubio-Arias JA Ávila-Gandía V, Ramos-Campo DJ, López-Román J. The effectiveness of pelvic floor muscle training in treating urinary incontinence in women: a current review. Actas Urol Esp. 2016;40(5):271–8. https://www.ncbi.nlm.nih.gov/pubmed/26614435. Accessed: May 5, 2019.
29. Oh S-T. The management of chronic pelvic pain. J Korean Med Assoc. 2008;51(1):53 https://www.researchgate.net/publication/272425195_The_Management_of_Chronic_Pelvic_Pain. Accessed: May 5, 2019.
30. American Physical Therapy Association (APTA). Section on Women's Health. https://www.womenshealthapta.org/patients/2019. Accessed: May 5, 2019.
31. Balogun JA, Okonofua FE. Management of chronic pelvic inflammatory disease with shortwave diathermy. A case report. Phys Ther. 1988;68(10):1541–5. https://www.researchgate.net/publication/20695857_Management_of_Chronic_Pelvic_Inflammatory_Disease_with_Shortwave_Diathermy_A_Case_Report. Accessed: May 5, 2019.
32. U.S. Department of Health and Human Services, Centre for Disease Control and Prevention (USDHHS-CDC). Pelvic inflammatory disease. 2017. https://www.cdc.gov/std/pid/stdfact-pid.htm; https://www.cdc.gov/std/pid/stdfact-pid-detailed.htm; https://images.search.yahoo.com/yhs/search?p=picture+of+1.+Urinary+and+Fecal+Incontinence&fr=yhs-sz-002&hspart=sz&hsimp=yhs-002&imgurl=http%3A%2F%2Fwww.physiotherapyvictoria.ca%2Fwp-content%2Fuploads%2F2015%2F05%2FBladder-Control-Incontinence-Victoria-BC.png#id=17&iurl=https%3A%2F%2Fssl.adam.com%2Fgraphics%2Fimages%2Fen%2F9439.jpg&action=click. Accessed: May 5, 2019.
33. Lamina S Hanif S. Shortwave in the management of chronic pelvic inflammatory disease: case reports. J Nigeria Soci Physiother. 2008;16(1):31–8. http://www.jnsp.org/index.php/

jnsp/article/viewFile/27/28; https://www.thefreelibrary.com/Shortwave+diathermy+in+the+management+of+chronic+pelvic+inflammatory...-a0190793591. Accessed: May 5, 2019.
34. Lamina S, Hanif S, Gagarawa YS. Short wave diathermy in the symptomatic management of chronic pelvic inflammatory disease pain: a randomised controlled trial. 2008. http://capenergy.com/assets/files/estudios/52-short-wave-diathermy-in-the-symptomatic.pdf. Accessed: May 5, 2019.
35. Sonali J, Kaur A, Mitra M. Effect of short-wave diathermy in reducing pain and improving function in patients with pelvic inflammatory diseases. Indian J Physiother Occup Ther. 2015;9:20–3. http://www.indianjournals.com/ijor.aspx?target=ijor:ijpot&volume=9&issue=2&article=005. Accessed: May 5, 2019.
36. Saif DS, Fotoh DS, EL Kholy RM, Morsi DI, Farag HM. Combined (physical and medical treatment) therapy versus physical treatment alone and medical treatment alone in the management of chronic pelvic inflammatory disease. Egypt Rheumatol Rehab. 2019;46:132. http://www.err.eg.net/article.asp?issn=1110-161X;year=2019;volume=46;issue=2;spage=132;epage=139;aulast=Saif. Accessed: May 5, 2019.
37. Rosen NO, Dawson SJ, Brooks M, Kellogg-Spadt S. Treatment of vulvodynia: pharmacological and non-pharmacological approaches. Drugs. 2019;79(5):483–93. https://doi.org/10.1007/s40265-019-01085-1. https://www.ncbi.nlm.nih.gov/pubmed/30847806. Accessed: May 5, 2019.
38. Bergeron S, Brown C, Lord MJ, Oala M, Binik YM, Khalifé S. Physical therapy for vulvar vestibulitis syndrome: a retrospective study. J Sex Marital Ther. 2002;28(3):183–92. https://www.ncbi.nlm.nih.gov/pubmed/11995597.
39. Wilkinson EJ. The vulvodynia guideline. J Low Genit Tract Dis. 2005; 9(1):40–51. https://www.ncbi.nlm.nih.gov/pubmed/15870521. Accessed: May 5, 2019.
40. Women's Health Physical Therapy and Men's Pelvic Health (n.d.). https://www.obgyn-physicaltherapy.com/. Accessed: May 5, 2019.
41. Brotto LA, Yong P, Smith KB, Sadownik LA. Impact of a multidisciplinary vulvodynia program on sexual functioning and dyspareunia. J Sex Med. 2015;12(1):238–47. https://www.ncbi.nlm.nih.gov/pubmed/25354520. Accessed: May 5, 2019
42. Davis SN, Bergeron S, Binik YM, Lambert B. Women with provoked vestibulodynia experience clinically significant reductions in pain regardless of treatment: results from a 2-year follow-up study. J Sex Med. 2013;10(12):3080–7. https://www.ncbi.nlm.nih.gov/pubmed/24034424. Accessed: May 5, 2019.
43. Dionisi B, Anglana F, Inghirami P, Lippa P, Senatori R. Use of transcutaneous electrical stimulation and biofeedback for the treatment of vulvodynia (vulvar vestibular syndrome): result of 3 years of experience. Minerva Ginecol. 2008; 60(6):485–91. https://www.ncbi.nlm.nih.gov/pubmed/18981976. Accessed: May 5, 2019.
44. Dionisi B, Senatori R. Effect of transcutaneous electrical nerve stimulation on the postpartum dyspareunia treatment. J Obstet Gynaecol Res. 2011; 37(7):750–3. https://www.ncbi.nlm.nih.gov/pubmed/21395897 Accessed: May 5, 2019.
45. Korda JB, Pfaus JG, Goldstein. Persistent genital arousal disorder: a case report in a woman with lifelong PGAD where serendipitous administration of varenicline tartrate resulted in symptomatic improvement. J Sex Med. 2009; 6(5):1479–86. https://www.ncbi.nlm.nih.gov/pubmed/19228278. Accessed: May 5, 2019.
46. Juraskova I, Jarvis S, Mok K, Peate M, Meiser B, Cheah BC, Mireskandari S, Friedlander M. The acceptability, feasibility, and efficacy (phase I/ II study) of the OVERcome (olive oil, vaginal exercise, and MoisturizeR) intervention to improve dyspareunia and alleviate sexual problems in women with breast cancer. J Sex Med. 2013;10(10):2549–58. https://www.ncbi.nlm.nih.gov/pubmed/23635341. Accessed: May 5, 2019.
47. Panchik D, Masco S, Zinnikas P, Hillriegel B, Lauder T, Suttmann E, Chinchilli V, McBeth M, Hermann W. Effect of exercise on breast cancer-related lymphedema: what the lymphatic surgeon needs to know. J Reconstr Microsurg. 2019;35(1):37–45.
48. Dinas PC, Koutedakis Y, Flouris AD. Effects of exercise and physical activity on depression. Irish J Med Sci. 2011;180(2):319–25. https://link.springer.com/article/10.1007%2Fs11845-010-0633-9. Accessed: May 5, 2019.
49. World Health Organization. Sexual and reproductive health https://www.who.int/reproductivehealth/en/; https://www.who.int/westernpacific/health-topics/reproductive-health 2008. Accessed: May 5, 2019.
50. World Health Organization. https://www.afro.who.int/health-topics/sexual-and-reproductive-health 2017. Accessed: May 5, 2019.
51. Bezner JR. Promoting health and wellness: implications for physical therapist practice. Phys Ther. 2015; 95(10):1433–44. https://academic.oup.com/ptj/article/95/10/1433/2686492 Accessed: May 5, 2019.
52. Dennis CL. Treatment of postpartum depression. Part 2: a critical review of nonbiological interventions. J Clin Psychiatry. 2004;65(9):1252–65.
53. Josefsson T, Lindwall M, Archer T. Physical exercise intervention in depressive disorders: meta-analysis and systematic review. Scand J Med Sci Sports. 2014;24(2):259–72. https://onlinelibrary.wiley.com/doi/full/10.1111/sms.12050. Accessed: May 5, 2019.
54. Kvam S, Kleppe CL, Nordhus IH, Hovland A. Exercise as a treatment for depression: a meta-analysis. J Affect Disord. 2016; 15;202:67–86. https://www.sciencedirect.com/science/article/pii/S0165032715314221?via%3Dihub. Accessed: May 5, 2019.
55. Saligheh M, Hackett D, Boyce P, Cobley S. Can exercise or physical activity help improve postnatal depression and weight loss? A systematic review. Arch Womens Ment Health. 2017; 20(5):595–611. https://link.springer.com/article/10.1007%2Fs00737-017-0750-9. Accessed: May 5, 2019.
56. Wu PL, Lee M, Huang TT. Effectiveness of physical activity on patients with depression and Parkinson's disease: a systematic review. 2017. https://journals.plos.org/plosone/article?id=10.1371/journal.pone.0181515. Accessed: May 5, 2019.
57. Soucy I, Provencher M, Fortier M, McFadden T. Efficacy of guided self-help behavioural activation and physical activity for depression: a randomised controlled trial. Cognit Behav Ther. 2017;46(6):493–506. https://www.tandfonline.com/doi/abs/10.1080/16506073.2017.1337806?journalCode=sbeh20 Accessed: May 5, 2019.
58. World Confederation for Physical Therapy-WCPT. Physical therapy and mental health. https://www.wcpt.org/sites/wcpt.org/files/files/wptday/18/Booklet/WPTD2018_Booklet_Final.pdf. Accessed: May 5, 2019.
59. Verhagen E, Engbers L. The physical therapist's role in physical activity promotion. Br J Sports Med. 2009;43(2). https://bjsm.bmj.com/content/43/2/99 Accessed: May 5, 2019.
60. Developmental disorders (n.d): https://en.wikipedia.org/wiki/Developmental_disorderAccessed: May 5, 2019.
61. Lowrie MB (n.d.). Neurological disorders and their main causes. http://www.icsmsu.com/exec/wp-content/uploads/2011/12/ABS-Neuroscience.pdf Accessed: May 5, 2019.
62. Obalum DC, Giwa SO, Adekoya-Cole TO, Enweluzo GO. Profile of spinal injuries in Lagos, Nigeria Spinal Cord. 2009;(47):134–7. https://wwwnaturecom/articles/sc200893. Accessed: May 5, 2019.
63. Shuaibu I. Nigeria: Dala orthopaedic hospital handles 480 spinal cord injuries annually. This Day Newspaper 2017. https://allafrica.com/stories/201709070805.html. Accessed: May 5, 2019.
64. Lloyd E. What are the common complications of surgery? 2019. https://www.healthguideinfo.com/first-aid/p67213/. Accessed: May 5, 2019.

65. ProActive Physical Therapy (n.d). Pre-and-post-operative care. https://www.proactivecolorado.com/services/pre-post-operative-care/. Accessed: May 5, 2019.
66. Reeve J, Denehy L, Stiller K. The physiotherapy management of patients undergoing thoracic surgery: a survey of current practice in Australia and New Zealand. Physiother Res Int. 2007;12(2):59–71. https://onlinelibrary.wiley.com/doi/abs/10.1002/pri.354?sid=nlm%3Apubmed Accessed: May 5, 2019.
67. Balogun JA. Efficacy of physical therapy in the management of reproductive disorders. 2020. In: Physical Therapy Effectiveness. Intech Open Book. ISBN: 978-1-83880-076-5. http://mts.intechopen.com/articles/show/title/efficacy-of-physical-therapy-in-the-management-of-reproductive-disorders. Accessed: June 15, 2020.

Part V

Gynaecological Malignancies

Rising Burden of Gynaecological Cancers in Developing Countries

52

Olusegun Kayode Ajenifuja and Kunle Odunsi

Learning Objectives

After reading this chapter, the reader will be able to:

- Discuss the epidemiology of the common types of cancers amongst women
- Describe the prevalence rate for cervical cancer, ovarian cancer, gestational trophoblastic diseases and endometrial cancer
- Articulate the role of the vaccine in the prevention of human papillomavirus infection
- Describe the global burden of the common cancers amongst women in developing countries

52.1 Introduction

The global burden of cancer is rising, and according to the latest GLOBOCAN cancer statistics, it is estimated that globally there will be 17.0 million cancer cases and 9.5 million cancer deaths excluding skin cancer worldwide in 2018. A significant proportion of the new cases of cancers will be diagnosed in middle- and low-income countries [1]. For public health, the complexity of cancer control increased enormously following the shift of the disease burden from wealthy to less affluent countries. According to the latest WHO statistics, cancer causes around 7.9 million deaths worldwide each year. Of these deaths, around 70%, or 5.5 million, are now occurring in the developing world. A disease once associated with affluence now places its heaviest burden on poor and disadvantaged populations.

One striking feature of cancer incidence and mortality in developing countries is that its global share of cancer deaths exceed its shares of cancer incidence [2]. The reason for the higher case fatality is that majority of cancers in developing countries are diagnosed at advanced stages where treatment is no longer effective. These developing countries, especially in Africa, lack the capacity, manpower, and equipment, to manage advanced malignancies. A notable feature of cancer in developing countries is that there is an admixture of cancers caused by infectious agents and transitional cancers often attributed to the adoption of western lifestyles. The rapid rise in population and increasing life expectancy have also been implicated as a cause of the increasing incidence of cancer [2]. Over 80% of the world population live in developing countries, and ironically, these parts of the world have the least resources to combat cancer [3]. To reduce the burden of cancer globally, the World Health Organization recommends that attention should be focused on surveillance, primary prevention, secondary prevention and a fourth area that includes diagnoses, treatment and palliation [4].

One of the problems mitigating against reducing the burden of gynaecological malignancies in developing countries especially in Africa is the lack of reliable cancer statistics. The absence of population-based cancer registries has tended to underestimate the magnitude of the problems. Most of the figures quoted are hospital based, and since many women do not have access to modern health care which is often located in urban areas far from the rural areas where most of the population resides, the magnitude of the burden is often understated. Another problem mitigating the fight against cancer in developing countries is the issue of brain drain. Many highly trained medical practitioners in developing countries are migrating to western countries due to lack of

O. K. Ajenifuja
College of Health Sciences, Obafemi Awolowo University, Ile-Ife, Nigeria

Obafemi Awolowo University Teaching Hospitals, Ile-Ife, Nigeria

K. Odunsi (✉)
Roswell Park Comprehensive Cancer Centre (Roswell Park), Buffalo, NY, USA

Department of Gynaecologic Oncology, Centre for Immunotherapy, Roswell Park, Buffalo, NY, USA

University of Buffalo, Buffalo, NY, USA
e-mail: Kunle.odunsi@roswellpark.org

F. Okonofua et al. (eds.), *Contemporary Obstetrics and Gynecology for Developing Countries*,
https://doi.org/10.1007/978-3-030-75385-6_52

job satisfaction, low renumeration and in search of better education for their children [5].

Health financing is another important impediment towards control of gynaecological malignancies. Many developing countries are still battling with many infectious diseases such as HIV/AIDS, tuberculosis, malaria and childhood diseases [6]. With reduced budgetary allocations to health, the little funds allocated to health is thinly spread among the various competing needs with little left for cancer treatment and research. Payment for treatment is often out of pocket which means that treatment is on a cash-and-carry basis, that is, health is only accessed by those able to afford it. A study in India found out that half of the households affected by cancer have to sell the family assets to finance cancer treatment [7].

Cervical Cancer The leading gynaecological cancer in many developing countries is cervical cancer. It is also the fourth leading cause of cancer and cancer deaths globally. It is the second most common cancer in females and the leading gynaecological malignancy in developing countries [8]. Cervical cancer is a highly preventable cause of death and is best prevented by early screening and treatment of detected cases. It used to be the leading gynaecological cause of death in many developed countries decades ago, but with the advent of cytological screening and prompt treatment of detected cases, the incidence has dramatically reduced. Unlike the situation in developed countries, the burden of cervical cancer is on the increase in many developing countries. It is estimated that there will be 570,000 new cases and 311,000 deaths from cervical cancer in 2018 [9]. Majority of cases and deaths are from the developing countries. It is a major reproductive health problem as it affects pre- and postmenopausal women with resultant social and economic implications for the affected communities. The highest burden of the disease was reported in Asia, Latin America and African countries [10], with high prevalence in Haiti (93·85 per 100,000 women), Zimbabwe (54 per 100,000 women) and Guinea (46 per 100,000 [11, 12]). These figures are mainly hospital based and are believed underreported as most cases do not come to the hospitals and the near absence of population-based cancer registries. Apart from bearing the greater burden of cervical cancer globally, mortality is also higher in developing countries due to the late presentation of cases. The women present late due to lack of screening services in many parts of developing countries, and the few available services are located in urban areas. There is also a lack of capacity to treat advanced cases. It has been estimated that over half of cancer patients will require radiotherapy during the course of their illness [13]. Yet despite having more than three-quarters of the global burden of cervical cancer, developing countries have only about one-third of the amount of radiotherapy machines. Radiotherapy needed to manage advanced cases are often lacking in many developing countries. Even the few cases that do come to the hospital hardly complete their course of prescribed treatment due to poverty and lack of health insurance [14] .

Various epidemiological studies have proven that cervical cancer is associated with persistent oncogenic human papillomavirus (HPV) infection which is sexually transmitted. HPV prevalence is very high in many developing countries even among women with normal cytology [15, 16]. The introduction of HPV vaccines has been a landmark achievement in the prevention of cervical cancer, but the delivery of the vaccines in developing countries has been hampered by cost, maintaining the cold chain and by the fact that many developing countries do not have immunisation schedules targeted to the age group needing the vaccines. The vaccines are prophylactic and cannot eradicate existing HPV infections; hence, secondary prevention is needed for the millions of women already infected with the virus. The cytology-based screening which has succeeded in reducing the incidence and mortality from cervical cancer in developed countries has failed to make the desired impact in developing countries. The inability of many developing countries to replicate the success of the cytology-based screening program is due to the reduced capacity of many developing countries in terms of manpower, infrastructure and logistics. Cervical cancer screening by cytology has moderate sensitivity. The success achieved by it was due to repeated screenings. This is hardly possible in developing countries due to poor pathological services and the fact that the woman has to make several visits to the health facility before she can receive treatment [2, 17–19].

The World Health Organization (WHO) has proposed alternatives for developing countries. Among these is direct visualisation of the cervix using acetic acid and Lugol's iodine [20]. Methods of direct visualisation of the cervix have been tested in many developing countries and have been found to have a higher sensitivity than conventional cytology though less specific. The advantages of the visual inspection techniques have been that they are relatively cheap, materials needed for the performance are easily obtained locally and, more importantly, results of the techniques are obtained immediately meaning that treatment can be administered at the same clinic visit. However, the concerns about direct visualisation techniques are that it is a technique of pattern/colour recognition and is thus operator dependent and not reproducible [21]. Many results on VIA, the most commonly used direct visualisation method, have given varied and conflicting results [18, 22, 23].

To reduce the burden of cervical cancer in developing countries, a method of screening with enough sensitivity to detect cases and specificity to minimize overtreatment, is required. Such methods must have a high negative predictive value to permit a longer screening interval, with a reduced visit to the health facility.

Primary HPV screening seems likely the screening method of choice. Primary HPV screening has a better sensitivity than Pap smear, and the high negative predictive value gives a long-term reassurance [24]. In a landmark study in rural India, Sankaranarayanan and colleagues were able to demonstrate that a single round of HPV screening was more effective in preventing death from cervical cancer than either cytology or visual inspection technique [25].

Ovarian Cancer Though it constitutes less than 5% of total gynaecological malignancies, ovarian cancer is responsible for about 25% of mortality from gynaecological cancers. It is the eighth most common cancer in females, and in 2018 alone, there are 300,000 new cases and over half of the women will die of their disease. Incidence has been reportedly low in developing countries; however, several studies have shown that it is the second most common gynaecological malignancy in Nigeria and in many African countries. [26, 27, 28, 29]

Like cervical cancer, ovarian cancer could be considered a major public health problem in many developing countries. Unlike in western countries, ovarian cancer occurs more in young premenopausal women in African countries. The high case fatality ratio is due to advanced stages at the presentation of almost all ovarian cancer patients. While survival has significantly improved in developed countries, survival is still poor in many developing countries due to late presentation, lack of adequate surgical treatment and inability to complete the prescribed dose of chemotherapy due to cost issues and availability [28]. Many patients cannot afford the high cost of chemotherapy because payment is out of pocket which limits access to the poor women. With the younger age at presentation and many of the patients are said to be multiparous unlike in western countries, there is the paucity of data with regard to the proportions of the women who have hereditary forms of cancer.

Gestational Trophoblastic Diseases (GTD) GTD is common in developing countries especially the Far Eastern countries. It is one of the most common gynaecological malignancies. The incidence in African countries though higher than in western countries is still lower compared with the Asian countries. It is a curable form of cancer but requires long-term follow-up to detect recurrence. Follow-up of patients with gynaecological malignancies has been particularly difficult in many African countries due to widespread poverty, limited access to the treatment centres in terms of roads and cost of treatment. This is particularly difficult for cases like molar pregnancies when the patient had the initial remission; this gives them an illusion of cure and will default from follow-up.

Endometrial Cancer In developing countries, the incidence of endometrial cancer is low [30]. In a 3-year review of 249 women with gynaecological malignancies managed at a tertiary centre in northern Nigeria, endometrial cancer constituted 11.25% [31], while at the University College Hospital in southern-western Nigeria [32], it accounted for 3.1% of the gynaecological malignancies managed there. In Ghana, endometrial malignancy constituted 7.43% of gynaecological malignancies at Korle Bu [26]. The incidence of endometrial cancer is generally low in developing countries of Africa. Reasons for this may not be unconnected with relative high parity found in these regions. This may be attributed to reduced life expectancy and high parity found in many developing countries in Africa. Other gynaecological malignancies like vulvar and vagina have low incidences in developing countries.

In conclusion, the burden of gynaecological malignancies is rising in many developing countries, and mortality is also rising due to late presentation and lack of effective strategies for cancer prevention and management. A lot needs to be done in terms of capacity building. There is an urgent need by policymakers to create an enabling environment and enactment of policies that will avert an impending crisis. These policies should cover the spectrum of prevention, screening for early detection, treatment and survivorship.

References

1. Murray CJL, López AD, editors. The global burden of disease: a comprehensive assessment of mortality and disability from diseases, injuries and risk factors in 1990 and projected to 2020. Cambridge, MA: Harvard University Press; 1996.
2. Kanavos P. The rising burden of cancer in the developing world. Ann Oncol. 2006;17(Supplement 8):viii15–23.
3. Hanna and Kangolle described four approaches; cancer prevention, early detection, diagnosis/treatment and palliation to cancer.
4. Ngoma T. World Health Organization cancer priorities in developing countries. Ann Oncol. 2006;17(Suppl. 8):viii9–14.
5. Sako S. Brain drain and Africa's development: a reflection. African Issues. 2002;30(1):25. https://doi.org/10.2307/1167086.
6. Vuyst D, et al. The burden of human papillomavirus infections and related diseases in Sub-Saharan Africa. Vaccine. 2013;31(05):F32–46. https://doi.org/10.1016/j.vaccine.2012.07.092.
7. Rajpal S, Kumar A, Joe W. Economic burden of cancer in India: evidence from cross-sectional nationally representative household survey. PLoS One. 2018;13(2):e0193320. https://doi.org/10.1371/journal.pone.0193320.
8. Catarino R, et al. Screening for cervical cancer screening in developing countries. World J Clin Oncol. 2015;6(6):281–90.
9. Bray F, Soerjomataram I, et al. Global cancer statistics 2018: GLOBOCAN estimates of incidence and mortality worldwide for 36 cancers in 185 countries. CA Cancer J Clin. 2018;68:394–424.
10. Pisani P, Parkin DM, Bray F, Ferlay J. Estimates of the worldwide mortality from 25 cancers in 1990. Int J Cancer. 1999;83:18–9.
11. Chokunonga E, Levy LM, Basset MT, et al. Cancer incidence in the African population of Harare, Zimbabwe: second results from the Cancer: registry 1993–1995. Int J Cancer. 2000;85(1):54–5.
12. Koulibaby M, Kabba IS, Cisse A, et al. Cancer incidence in Conakry Guinea: first results from the Cancer registry 1992–1995. Int J Cancer. 1997;6(70):39–5.
13. Samiei Massoud. Challenges of making radiotherapy accessible in developing countries.
14. Sankaranarayanan R, Ferlay J. Worldwide burden of gynaecological cancer: the size of the problem. Best Pract Res Clin

Obstet Gynaecol. 2006;20(2):207–25. https://doi.org/10.1016/j.bpobgyn.2005.10.007.
15. Gage JC, et al. The age-specific prevalence of human papillomavirus and risk of cytologic abnormalities in rural Nigeria: implications for screen-and-treat strategies. Int J Cancer. 2012;130: 2111–7.
16. Allan B, et al. Cervical Human Papillomavirus (HPV) infection in South African women: implications for HPV screening and vaccine strategies. J Clin Microbiol. 2008;46(2):740–2.
17. Kitchener HC, Castle PE, Cox JT. Chapter 7: achievements and limitations of cervical cytology screening. Vaccine. 2006;24(Suppl 3):S3/63–70.
18. Mwanza T, Rambau PF. Pathology practice in a resource-poor setting. Arch Pathol Lab Med. 2011;135(2):191–3. https://doi.org/10.1043/1543-2165-135.2.191.
19. Adesina A, Rhumba D, Nelson AM, et al. Improvement of pathology in sub-Saharan Africa. Lancet Oncol. 2013;14(4):e152–7.
20. World Health Organization (WHO). Guidelines for Screening and Treatment of Precancerous Lesions for Cervical Cancer Prevention: WHO Guidelines. Geneva: WHO; 2013. http://www.who.int/reproductivehealth/publications/cancers/screening_and_treatment_of_precancerous_lesions/en/.
21. Ajenifuja KO, Gage JC, Adepiti AC, et al. A population-based study of visual inspection with acetic acid (VIA) for cervical screening in rural Nigeria. Int J Gynecol Cancer. 2013;23(3):507–12.
22. Jeronimo J, Bansil P, Lim J, START-UP Study Group, et al. A multicountry evaluation of careHPV testing, visual inspection with acetic acid, and papanicolaou testing for the detection of cervical cancer. Int J Gynecol Cancer. 2014;24(3):576–585. CrossRef. Medline.
23. Gravitt PE, et al. Effectiveness of VIA, Pap, and HPV DNA testing in a cervical cancer screening program in a peri-urban community in Andhra Pradesh, India. PLoS One. 2010;5(10):e13711. CrossRef. Medline.
24. Rijkaart DC, Berkhof J, Rozendaal L, et al. Human papillomavirus testing for the detection of high-grade cervical intraepithelial neoplasia and cancer: final results of the POBASCAM randomised controlled trial. Lancet Oncol. 2012;13(1):78–88.
25. Sankaranarayanan R, et al. HPV screening for cervical cancer in Rural India. N Engl J Med. 2009;360:1385.
26. Nkyekyer K. Pattern of gynaecological cancers in Ghana. East Afr Med J. 2000;77:534–8.
27. Zayyan A, et al. Epidemiology of ovarian cancers in Zaria, Northern Nigeria: a 10-year study. Int J Womens Health. 2017;9:855–60.
28. Iyoke CA, Ifeadike CO, Nnebue CC. A ten-year review of ovarian cancer in Enugu, South East Nigeria. Afrimedic J. 2011;2(1):8–12.
29. Fatiregun OA, Ketiku KK, Popoola AO, Sowunmi AC, Iyare O. Incidence and management of ovarian cancer cases in a Tertiary Hospital – a 10 year review. IOSR J Dental Med Sci (IOSR-JDMS) e-ISSN: 2279-0853, p-ISSN: 2279-0861. 2015;14(12) Ver. VI:106–14.
30. Okunowo AA, Alakaloko MA, Ohazurike EO, Okunade KS, Anorlu RI. Trend and Characteristics of Endometrial Cancer in Lagos, Nigeria. Gulf J Oncolog. 2019;1(31):52–9.
31. Yakasai IA, Ugwa EA, Otubu J. Gynaecological malignancies in Aminu Kano Teaching Hospital Kano: a 3 year review. Niger J Clin Pract. 2013;16(1):63–6.
32. Adekanbi AOA, Jimoh MA, Akanji AM, Olubukola FA. Endometrial cancer in ibadan: epidemiological and clinicopathological features –10 year review. NY Sci J. 2016;9(3):19–23.

53 Molecular Biology of Gynaecological Cancers

Tanja Pejovic and Kunle Odunsi

Learning Objectives

At the end of the chapter, readers will be able to learn the following:

- The molecular and epigenetic origins of ovarian, endometrial, and other types of gynaecologic cancers.
- The role of the human papilloma virus in cervical, vaginal, and vulvar cancers.
- The role of specific immune responses and immunotherapy in the aetiology and management of gynaecologic cancers.
- The use of immunotherapy and vaccines in the primary and secondary prevention of gynaecologic cancers.
- Research and programmatic gaps in the molecular biology, genetics, and immunology of gynaecologic cancers.

Gynaecologic cancer research programmes have focused on molecular defects in oncogenes, tumour-suppressor genes, and DNA repair mechanisms. These efforts have led to a broad understanding of the molecular abnormalities that underlie malignancies of the female genital tract (vulva, vagina, cervix, uterus, ovaries, and fallopian tubes). It is clear that an improvement in outcome of these cancers can only be achieved if [1] early diagnosis is achieved, [2] there is accurate prediction of progression and response, and [3] new treatment options reflecting the molecular pathogenesis and progression are developed. This requires detailed disease-specific understanding of the diverse molecular changes in gynaecologic malignancies that ultimately lead cells to develop the following hallmarks of cancer: abnormalities in self-sufficiency of growth signals, evasion of apoptosis, insensitivity to antigrowth signals, limitless replicative potential, sustained angiogenesis, and tissue invasion and metastases. Moreover, there is growing evidence for the concept of cancer immunosurveillance and immunoediting based on [1] protection against development of spontaneous and chemically induced tumours in animal systems and [2] identification of targets for immune recognition of human cancer [1]. This concept is supported by several studies in gynaecologic cancers and has opened new avenues for the development of novel biomarkers and therapeutic targets. It is the purpose of this chapter to highlight and summarise some of the recent basic findings in gynaecologic malignancies, with an emphasis on clinically applicable developments.

T. Pejovic
Oregon Health and Science University, Portland, OR, USA

K. Odunsi (✉)
Roswell Park Comprehensive Cancer Centre (Roswell Park), Buffalo, NY, USA

Department of Gynaecologic Oncology, Centre for Immunotherapy, Roswell Park, Buffalo, NY, USA

University of Buffalo, Buffalo, NY, USA
e-mail: Kunle.odunsi@roswellpark.org

53.1 Ovarian Cancer

53.1.1 Origins of Epithelial Ovarian Cancer

Until recently, epithelial ovarian cancer (EOC) was thought to arise primarily from the ovarian surface epithelium (OSE), with a subset likely originating in the adjacent fimbria [2, 3]. The OSE forms a monolayer surrounding the ovary, but it is composed of relatively few cuboidal cells per ovary, or 0.05% of the entire organ. Developmentally it derives from the celomic epithelium, which also gives rise to the peritoneal mesothelium and oviductal epithelium [4]. The OSE appears generally stable, uniform, and quiescent, though it can undergo proliferation in vivo [5]. Despite the small number of cells within the OSE and their apparent inactivity, the risk for EOC is nearly 2%, suggesting a high malignant potential. No physiological role for the primate OSE has been established [6].

F. Okonofua et al. (eds.), *Contemporary Obstetrics and Gynecology for Developing Countries*,
https://doi.org/10.1007/978-3-030-75385-6_53

While premalignant lesions in OSE have not been identified [7], recently, occult noninvasive and invasive carcinomas in the fallopian tubes, typically in the fimbria, have been discovered in women undergoing prophylactic salpingo-oophorectomies because of a family history or germline mutations of *BRCA1* and *BRCA2* [8]. This led to the hypothesis that these occult tubal carcinomas might shed malignant cells, which then implant and grow on the ovary, simulating primary ovarian cancer. Moreover, gene expression studies have demonstrated that the expression profiles of ovarian high-grade serous cancers (HGSCs) more closely resembled fallopian tube epithelium (FTE) than the OSE [9]. Because the tubal carcinomas were associated with serous and not endometrioid, clear cell or mucinous carcinomas, the noninvasive tubal carcinomas have been designated "serous tubal intraepithelial carcinoma" (STIC).

The new paradigm for the pathogenesis of ovarian serous cancer based on a dualistic model and the recognition that the majority of these tumours originate outside the ovary, that is, Fallopian tube epithelium, facilitates the development of novel approaches to prevention, screening, and treatment. The low-grade serous tumours (type I) are generally indolent, present in stage I (tumour confined to the ovary) and develop from well-established precursors, and are characterised by specific mutations, including *KRAS, BRAF*, and *ERBB2,* but rarely *TP53*. They are relatively genetically stable. In contrast, the HGSCs (type II) are aggressive, present in advanced stage, and develop from STICs. They have a very high frequency of *TP53* mutations but rarely harbour the mutations detected in the low-grade serous tumours. While low-grade serous and HGSCs develop along different molecular pathways, both types may develop from FTE and secondarily involve the ovary [10].

53.1.2 Molecular Pathways to Ovarian Cancer

53.1.2.1 Inherited Syndromes of Ovarian Cancers

A family history of the disease is the most significant known risk factor for epithelial ovarian cancer (EOC). There is a threefold increased risk of developing the disease for an individual with a first-degree relative affected with ovarian cancer [11]. Inherited EOC most often occurs as part of families with both ovarian and breast cancer cases or in families with only multiple ovarian cancer cases. Inherited ovarian cancer is also part of Lynch syndrome or hereditary non-polyposis colorectal cancer (HNPCC), found in families with multiple cases of colon cancer. It is estimated that 5–10% of EOC cases are due to these familial syndromes [12].

Linkage analysis of familial breast and ovarian cancers provided some of the first insights into the molecular basis of ovarian cancer ultimately leading to identification of two genes *BRCA1* and *BRCA2*, each associated with a significant increased incidence of ovarian cancer. The frequency of *BRCA1* and *BRCA2* mutations in the general population is estimated to be 1 in 800 and 1 in 500, respectively [11, 12].

The *BRCA1* gene was cloned in 1994 [13] and has 24 exons spanning 80 kb of genomic DNA, and had a 7.8 kb transcript coding for an 1863 amino acid protein [13]. The *BRCA2* gene mapped to chromosome 13q12–13, has 27 exons (26 coding), spanning 70 kb of genomic DNA, and has an 11.4 kb transcript and coded a 3418 amino acid protein [14]. Hundreds of mutations in *BRCA1* have now been identified, most commonly loss of function nonsense or frame shift mutations. Two specific mutations, 185delAG and 5382insC, are found in 1% and 0.1% of Ashkenazi Jewish women. Some missense changes have been found to be pathogenic, but the majorities are polymorphisms or are unclassified variants (UV), also known as variants of uncertain significance (VUS). A high frequency of large genomic rearrangements (LGR) have been identified in both *BRCA1* and the *BRCA2* gene [15].

The position of mutations within large *BRCA1* and *BRCA 2* genes determines the risk of ovarian cancer. The *BRCA1* gene mutation within nucleotides 2402–4190 carries the high risk of ovarian cancer (and lower risk of breast cancer). Both genes show autosomal-dominant transmission of highly penetrant germline mutations and behave as tumour suppressor genes. Both proteins function in the double-strand DNA break repair pathway but may have additional functions; *BRCA1* functions in both checkpoint activation and DNA repair, *BRCA2* is a mediator of homologous recombination.

Functionally, *BRCA1* regulates *p53*, an oncogene frequently implicated in ovarian cancer. Thus, loss of *BRCA1* allows DNA damage to accumulate via a loss of its activation of *p53*. However, mutations in *BRCA1* also likely contribute to ovarian cancer by mechanisms other than its interactions with *p53*. Any understanding of the role of *BRCA1* in ovarian cancer is further complicated by reports of women with high-risk mutations in *BRCA1* who fail to develop ovarian cancer. These observations speak clearly to the role of genetic modifiers in determining whether *BRCA1* or *BRCA2* mutations ultimately lead to malignancy.

High-penetrance *BRCA1* and *BRCA2* gene mutation accounts for about 40% of ovarian cancer risk [16]. The remaining risk is due to very rare high-risk genes, very few moderate-risk genes, and/or multiple low-risk genes. International collaborative, Ovarian Cancer Association Consortium (OCAC) was established in 2005 to investigate the risk of SNPs (singe nucleotide polymorphisms) in ovarian cancer. At least 6 additional loci associated with risk of ovarian cancer have been reported: 2q31, 3q25, 8q24, 9p22.2, 17q21, and 19p13.1 [11].

BRCA1 indirectly and BRCA2 protein directly are associated with maintaining the genome stability, for example, a cell's ability to tolerate DNA damage. Interestingly, tumours with inactivated BRCA2 are responsive to cisplatin.

However, due to their low accuracy of DNA repair, these cells accumulate secondary genetic modifications that can lead to reversal of BRCA2 mutation, allowing these cells to acquire resistance to crosslinking agents [17].

Recently, mutations have been identified in four genes *RAD51C*, *RAD51D*, *BRIP1*, and *PALB2* in the BRCA DNA repair pathway. Mutations in the *RAD51C* and *RAD51D* genes were found in approximately 1% of breast/ovarian cancer families. The relative risk (RR) of ovarian cancer in *RAD51D* carriers was 6.3 (95% CI: 2.9–13.9). Mutations in *PALB2* (*FANCN*) were found in 3.4% of breast cancer families, and 55% of these families had family members with ovarian cancer. An Icelandic mutation in *BRIP1* (FANCJ) with a frequency of 0.41% increased the risk ovarian cancer, OR 8.1 (95% CI: 4.7–14.0). A Spanish *BRIP1* mutation had a frequency of 1.3% in ovarian cancer cases, and the risk of ovarian cancer was OR 25 (95% CI: 1.8–340) [11].

In 2010, Walsh et al. screened 21 DNA repair/tumour suppressor genes in mutations in 360 unselected ovarian, fallopian tube, or peritoneal cancer cases and found mutations in 6 additional genes (*BARD1*, *CHEK2*, *MRE11A*, *NBN*, *RAD50*, and *TP53* [18] in serous as well as non-serous carcinomas and in younger as well as in patients older than 70 years of age. These findings suggest that careful and comprehensive mutational screen of all women may identify that inherited risk of ovarian cancer is higher than originally thought and that early identification of the risk may ultimately lead to prevention of 24% of ovarian cancer cases.

Role of Poly (ADP-Ribose) Polymerase (PARP) and PARP Inhibitors in Gynaecologic Cancers

Abnormalities in DNA repair have been identified in many human epithelial cancers, including serous ovarian cancer. DNA repair is a complex process designed to repair specific abnormalities within the DNA. Single-stranded DNA breaks are repaired by a protein complex containing Poly ADP-ribose polymerase (PARP). In contrast, double-stranded breaks that are lethal for the cell require a different complex, which contains the BRCA proteins [19].

Since PARP proteins are intimately involved in the repair of single-stranded DNA breaks, inhibition of PARP function impedes single-stranded DNA break repair leading to the formation of double-stranded breaks. Research performed in multiple laboratories suggested that inhibition of PARP would be a lethal event in cells that have inactivation of BRCA1 or 2. This concept called "synthetic lethality" (first proposed for cancer therapeutics in 1997) was tested early in the development of PARP inhibitors [20]. Pre-clinical data strongly supported this concept with BRCA mutated cell lines showing 100–1000 fold sensitivity to parp inhibitors compared with wild-type control cell lines. This laboratory proof of principle led to a rapid transition into the clinic.

The clinical development of PARP inhibitors began in earnest in the mid-2000 where they were tested in early phase trials. The first phase I trial focused on women with germ line BRCA mutation of and yielded encouraging results. The expansion cohort of this study treated woman with ovarian cancer and recorded a 46% response rate in platinum-sensitive patients and a 33% response rate in platinum-resistant patients. Of note, the drug was well tolerated and its oral delivery made it quite convenient. This landmark trial led to a follow-up study that examined dose 100 mg to 400 mg and involved ovarian cancer mutation carriers. The response rate was dose dependent (13% to 33%) and again demonstrated significant activity in platinum-resistant disease. Parp inhibitors have also been tested in the maintenance setting after effective treatment of platinum-sensitive recurrent disease. A dramatic improvement in progression-free survival was demonstrated with a HR of 0.15 for mutation carriers. At this time, at least 8 different PARP inhibitors are in development. Continued enthusiasm for these agents has led three companies to recently design phase III trials to establish their role in the treatment of ovarian cancer.

It is important to note that most of these trials have tested the effectiveness of PARP inhibitors in mutation carriers. Recent work from large genomic studies support that a much larger percentage of serous ovarian cancers, about 50%, have homologous recombination deficiencies, and it is likely that these patients with acquired deficiencies in HR would also benefit from PARP inhibitors [19].

There are important unanswered questions and challenges involving the effective use of PARP inhibitors. Should PARP inhibitors be used up front with chemotherapy or later in maintenance or relapse disease? At present, there is little long-term safety data on PARP inhibition and given their mechanisms of action, there is concern about secondary malignancies such as leukaemia. This may be dependent on the mode of administration with chronic use versus intermittent being more problematic. Further, the mechanism(s) of PARP inhibitor resistance remains essentially unknown. Recent work has demonstrated an in-frame mutation in BRCA gene that restored the protein function in a small number of resistant tumours. Finally, other potential clinical settings for PARP inhibitors such as radiation sensitisers, in combination with chemotherapy, for cervical or endometrial cancers will need to be evaluated.

53.1.3 Angiogenesis

Growth of both primary ovarian cancers and their metastases requires the formation of new blood vessels to support adequate perfusion. This process, known as *angiogenesis*, mechanistically involves both the branching of new capillaries and the remodelling of larger vessels. Other processes, such as vasculogenic mimicry, have also been implicated in tumour angiogenesis.

Angiogenesis is tightly regulated by a balance of pro- and antiangiogenic factors. These include growth factors, such as TGF-β, VEGF, and platelet-derived growth factor; prostaglandins, such as prostaglandin E2; cytokines, such as interleukin 8; and other factors, such as the angiopoietins (Ang-1, Ang-2), and hypoxia-inducible factor-1α (HIF-1α). Many of these angiogenic factors have been implicated in ovarian cancer. For example, VEGF is a family of secreted polypeptides with critical roles in both normal development and human disease. Many cancers, including ovarian carcinomas, release VEGF in response to the hypoxic or acidic conditions typical in solid tumours. Near universal, albeit variable, levels of VEGF expression have been reported in ovarian cancers, in which higher levels correlate with advanced disease and poor clinical prognosis [20]. Circulating levels of VEGF have also been reported to be higher in the serum of women with ovarian cancers when compared with those with benign tumours. Expression of HIF-1 correlates well with microvessel density in ovarian cancers and has been proposed to upregulate VEGF expression [21]. Culturing ovarian cancer cell lines under hypoxic conditions stimulates the expression of both HIF-1α and VEGF expression; the addition of prostaglandin E2 potentiates the ability of hypoxia to induce the expression of both proangiogenic factors [22].

So far, anti-angiogenic targeting treatment has been used in combination with conventional chemotherapy in ovarian cancer. Phase III clinical trials have investigated the potential of VEGFi Bevacizumab as addition to carboplatin/paclitaxel for improving PFS in ovarian cancer patients at high risk for progression by approximately 4 months [23] .

53.2 Role of Specific Immune Responses and Immunotherapy

The novel observation by William Coley in the 1890s that severe bacterial infections could induce an anti-tumour response in patients with partially resected tumours has evolved into an understanding that the immune system can recognise tumour-associated antigens and direct a targeted response. The concept of "cancer immunoediting" suggests that the immune system not only protects the host against the development of primary cancers but also dynamically sculpts tumour immunogenicity [24]. In epithelial ovarian cancer, support for the role of immune surveillance of tumours comes from observations that the presence of infiltrating T lymphocytes (TILS) in tumours is associated with improved survival of patients with the disease [24, 25]. A recent meta-analysis of ten studies with 1815 ovarian cancer patients confirmed the observation that a lack of intraepithelial lymphocytes (TILs) is significantly associated with a worse survival among ovarian cancer patients (pooled HR: 2.24, 95% CI; 1.71–2.91) [9]. This effect was evident regardless of tumour grade, stage, or histologic subtype. In addition, encouraging results from large-scale clinical trials of immune system-provoking therapies [10–13] have re-kindled the promise of harnessing the immune system to attack cancers. Finally, advanced-stage ovarian cancer patients can have detectable tumour-specific cytotoxic T cell and antibody immunity. This was illustrated in a study that indicated that immunity to p53 predicted improved overall survival in patients with advanced-stage disease [26]. All of these observations support clinical trials of immunotherapy for epithelial ovarian cancer in an effort to elicit effective anti-tumour responses.

The major criteria required for the immunological destruction of tumours include generation of sufficient numbers of effector T cells with high avidity recognition of tumour antigens in vivo, trafficking and infiltration into the tumour, overcoming inhibitory networks in the tumour microenvironment, and persistence of the anti-tumour T cells. In the past decade, significant progress has been made in the development of interventions that mediate anti-tumour effects by initiating a *de novo* or boosting an existing immune response against cancer cells, and some have gained regulatory approval in other solid tumours. These interventions include cancer vaccines, cell-based therapy, immune checkpoint blockade, and oncolytic virus-based therapy. Major obstacles include the identification approaches to overcome tumour evasion of immune attack.

53.2.1 Ovarian Cancer-Specific Antigens

Human tumour antigens defined to date can be classified into one or more of the following categories: (1) differentiation antigens, such as tyrosinase, Melan-A/MART-1, and gp 100; (2) mutational antigens, such as CDK4, β-catenin, caspase-8, and P53; (3) amplification antigens, such as Her2/neu and p53; (4) splice variant antigens, such as NY-CO-37/PDZ-45, and ING1; (5) viral antigens, such as human papillomavirus (HPV) and Epstein-Barr virus; and (6) cancer-testis antigens, such as MAGE, NY-ESO-1, and LAGE-1. In considering an antigenic target for ovarian cancer immunotherapy, an ideal candidate antigen should not only demonstrate high-frequency expression in the tumour tissues and restricted expression in normal tissues, but also provide evidence for inherent immunogenicity. In this regard, the cancer-testis antigens are a distinct and unique class of differentiation antigens with high levels of expression in adult male germ cells, but generally not in other normal adult tissues, and aberrant expression in a variable proportion of a wide range of different cancer types. Among cancer-testis antigens, NY-ESO-1, initially defined by serologic analysis of recombinant cDNA expression (SEREX) libraries in oesophageal cancer, is particularly immunogenic, eliciting both cellular and humoral immune responses in a high proportion of patients with advanced NY-ESO-1 expressing ovarian cancer [27].

The reasons for the aberrant expression of cancer-testis antigens in cancer are currently unknown. Nevertheless, the fact that the expression of these antigens is restricted to cancers, gametes, and trophoblast suggests a link between cancer and gametogenesis. Although possible mechanisms include global demethylation and histone deacetylation, the induction of a "gametogenic" program in cancer has also been proposed [28]. Although several lines of evidence have shown that spontaneous or vaccine-induced tumour-antigen–specific T cells can recognise ovarian cancer targets, prolongation of survival in patients treated with immunisation has only rarely been observed. This is probably a reflection of several in vivo immunosuppressive mechanisms in tumour-bearing hosts. A recently described mechanism in ovarian cancer is the expression of inhibitory molecules such as programmed death-1 (PD-1) and lymphocyte activation gene-3 (LAG-3) [29]. Together, these molecules render ovarian tumour infiltrating CD8+ T cells "hyporesponsive," wherein effector function is most impaired in antigen-specific LAG-3 + PD-1 + CD8+ TILs.

Immunotherapy of Ovarian Cancer

Clinical progress in the field of cancer immunotherapy has been slow for many years, but within the last 5 years, breakthrough successes have brought immunotherapy to the forefront in cancer therapy. Promising results have been observed in a variety of cancers including solid tumours and haematological malignancies. These interventions include cancer vaccines, cell-based therapy, immune checkpoint blockade, and oncolytic virus-based therapy. Several groups have launched clinical trials testing various vaccination strategies of generating anti-tumour immune responses, either against specific tumour antigens [30, 31] or against autologous tumour lysate [32, 33]. Studies on vaccination combined with immune checkpoint blockade and studies of adoptive T-cell therapy utilising engineered T cells are ongoing at several institutions.

Several forms of dendritic cell (DC)-based vaccine approaches have been developed, most of which involve the isolation of patient-derived circulating monocytes and their differentiation ex vivo, in the presence of agents that promote DC maturation, such as granulocyte macrophage colony-stimulating factor (GM-CSF). These autologous DCs are injected into cancer patients upon exposure to a tumour antigen (protein, peptide, mRNAs, recombinant viral vectors encoding tumour antigen, tumour cell lysates). The antigen-pulsed DCs are able to prime tumour-targeting immune responses in vivo upon administration to patients. An additional strategy is to fuse tumour to mAbs that selectively bind to endocytosis receptors (e.g. mannose receptor or DEC-205) on the surface of DCs [34].

Advances in next-generation sequencing and epitope prediction now permit the rapid identification of mutant tumour neoantigens. This has led to efforts in utilising these mutant tumour neoantigens for personalising cancer immunotherapies. Deep-sequencing technologies permit easy identification of the mutations present within the protein-encoding part of the genome (the exome) of an individual tumour allowing for prediction of potential neoantigens. Several pre-clinical and clinical studies have now confirmed the possibility of identifying neoantigens on the basis of cancer exome data [35]. Although there are limitations of probing the mutational profile of a tumour in a single biopsy, it is evident that the vast majority of neoantigens occur within exonic sequence and do not lead to the formation of neoantigens that are recognised by autologous T cells. Consequently, a robust pipeline for filtering the cancer exome data is essential. Epitope presentation of neoantigens by MHC class I molecules may be predicted using previously established algorithms that analyse critical features such as the likelihood of proteasomal processing, transport into the endoplasmic reticulum, and affinity for the relevant MHC class I alleles. In order to predict epitope abundance, gene and/or protein expression levels can also be integrated into the analysis. Based on these considerations, it becomes of interest to stimulate neoantigen-specific T-cell responses in cancer patients using two possible approaches. The first is to synthesise long peptide vaccines that encode a set of predicted neoantigens. The second approach is to identify and expand pre-existing neoantigen-specific T-cell populations to create either bulk neoantigen-specific T-cell products or TCR-engineered T cells for adoptive therapy. These strategies are currently being tested in ovarian cancer patients in a few institutions in the United States. Adoptive T-cell therapy using natural host tumour infiltrating lymphocytes (TILs), host cells that have been genetically engineered with anti-tumour T-cell receptors (TCRs) or chimeric antigen receptors (CARs), are also undergoing clinical testing in ovarian cancer patients.

Immune Modulation and Checkpoint Inhibition

Immune modulation is designed to reinstate an existing anti-cancer immune response or elicit novel responses as a result of antigen spreading. This has been achieved through four general strategies: (i) the inhibition of immunosuppressive receptors expressed by activated T lymphocytes, such as cytotoxic T lymphocyte-associated protein 4 (CTLA4) and programmed cell death 1 (PD-1); (ii) the inhibition of the principal ligands of these receptors, such as the PD-1 ligand CD274 (PD-L1 or B7-H1); (iii) the activation of co-stimulatory receptors expressed on the surface of immune effector cells such as tumour necrosis factor receptor superfamily, member 4 (TNFRSF4 or OX40), TNFRSF9 (CD137 or 4-1BB), and TNFRSF18 (GITR); and (iv) the neutralisation of immunosuppressive factors released in the tumour microenvironment, such as transforming growth factor β1 (TGFβ1).

Inhibition of immunosuppressive receptors expressed by activated T lymphocytes is commonly referred to as "checkpoint blockade". This has been shown to induce robust and durable responses in patients with a variety of solid tumours. Antibody blockade of PD1 and PDL1 has demonstrated enhanced anti-tumour immunity in mouse models, with less immune toxicity as compared to CTLA blockade. Initial clinical results have been extremely promising [36] with durable responses in multiple cancers including colon, renal, lung carcinoma and melanoma with significant increases in lymphocyte infiltration into tumour lesions. A number of checkpoint-blocking mAbs were recently approved by the FDA and other international regulatory agencies for use in humans, namely, the anti-CTLA4 mAb ipilimumab (Yervoy™), which was licensed by the US FDA for use in individuals with unresectable or metastatic melanoma; the anti-PD-1 mAb pembrolizumab (Keytruda™), which received accelerated approval by the US FDA for the treatment of advanced or unresectable melanoma patients who fail to respond to other therapies; and nivolumab (Opvido™), another PD-1-targeting mAb licensed by the FDA and Japanese Ministry of Health and Welfare for use in humans. Blockade of additional inhibitory receptors are in various phases of clinical development and include LAG3, B7-H3, B7-H4, and TIM3. Emerging evidence suggests that the clinical efficacy of immunomodulatory mAbs (especially checkpoint blockers) may be profoundly influenced by the mutational burden and "neoantigens" and specific to the neoplasm [37]. The higher neoantigen load leads to recruitment of a diverse repertoire of neoantigen specific T cells, and checkpoint blockade restores a favourable balance of Teff/Treg ratio, leading to more effective tumour control.

Based on the promising results of blockade of the PD-1/PD-L1 pathway, it is important to consider opportunities for combination therapies. These include dual checkpoint blockade, for example, the combination of CTLA-4 and PD-1 blockade. Ipilimumab removes a physiological brake on T cells during activation, whereas anti-PD-1 removes a brake on activation during T-cell effector function. This combination may also overcome resistance to CTLA-4 blockade mediated by tumour PD-L1 expression or resistance to PD-1 blockade mediated by T-cell down-regulation through the co-expression of CTLA-4.

53.3 Endometrial Cancer

The current concept of endometrial cancer integrates histopathology with molecular genetic mechanisms of cancer development. Two major pathogenetic variants of endometrial carcinoma, type I (endometrioid) and type II (serous) evolve via divergent pathways and different precursor lesions, different genetic abnormalities, and ultimately different clinical outcomes parallel their distinct histology.

53.3.1 Type I Cancers

More than 90% of uterine cancers arise in the self-renewing glandular epithelium that lines the uterine cavity. The endometrium epithelium responds to steroid hormones with well-characterised patterns of growth and maturation critical for its role in normal reproduction. Oestrogen is a well-recognised growth factor for the endometrium, promoting glandular proliferation. Subsequent exposure to the progestin-rich environment that follows ovulation results in an arrest of endometrial proliferation accompanied by glandular luteinisation. Several decades of epidemiologic evidence has convincingly demonstrated that continued, unopposed exposure to oestrogen is associated with an increased risk of developing endometrial cancer. These risks are particularly notable among postmenopausal women treated with oestrogen-only hormone replacement. An association between the growth-promoting effects of oestrogen and endometrial carcinomas is thought to underlie the epidemiologic associations found for endometrial cancers, medical conditions such as anovulation, obesity, and other epidemiologically defined risk factors, including early age at menarche and nulliparity. The oestrogen-related endometrioid adenocarcinomas account for 80% of endometrial cancer, demonstrate large number of genetic changes, and appear to arise via a progression pathway. Common genetic changes in this type of endometrial carcinoma include microsatellite instability (MSI), or specific mutations of *PTEN*, *K-ras*, and *βB*-catenin genes.

53.3.1.1 Microsatellite Instability

Microsatellites are short segments of repetitive DNA found predominately in noncoding DNA and scattered through the genome. The MSI phenotype is expressed in the cells with changes in the number of repeat elements as compared with normal tissue because of DNA repair error during replication. Approximately 20% of type I endometrial cancers demonstrate MSI phenotype, while MSI in type II cancers is very rare, present in less than 5% of the cases [38]. MSI is due to inactivation of any of the mismatch repair genes and proteins: *MLH1*, *MSH2*, *MSH3*, and *MSH6*. The most common mechanism of MSI in the endometrium is inactivation of *MLH1* by epigenetic silencing of its promoter through hypermethylation of CpG islands, followed by *MSH6* mutation and *MSH3* frame shift mutations. In contrast, the MSI present in colon cancer is predominantly due to mutations in *MSH2*, followed by *MLH1* and *MSH6* mutations. MSI is an early event in type I cancers and it has been described in precancerous lesions.

Once established, MSI may specifically target or inactivate genes with susceptible repeat elements, such as TGF-β1 receptors and IGFIIR, resulting in new subclones with altered capacity to invade and metastasise.

53.3.1.2 PTEN

Inactivation of *PTEN* (phosphatase and tensin homolog) tumour suppressor gene located at 10q23 is the most common genetic defect in type I endometrial cancers, and it is present in more than 80% of tumours that are preceded by histologically distinct premalignant phase [39]. PTEN protein functions in maintaining G_1 arrest and enabling apoptosis via an AKT-dependent mechanism. *PTEN* inactivation is caused by various mechanisms. The most common *PTEN* defect in endometrial cancer is its complete loss of function through inactivation of both alleles. Mutations or deletions that result in loss of heterozygosity at *PTEN* locus are also observed with high frequency. The *PTEN* mutation pattern is different in microsatellite-stable and MSI cancers. MSI tumours have a higher frequency of deletions, involving three or more base pairs, as compared with the microsatellite-stable tumours. In addition, the mutations in MSI tumours only rarely involve the polyadenine repeat of exon 8, which is the expected target.

KRAS mutations have been found in up to 30% of type I endometrial cancers. The frequency of KRAS mutations is particularly high in MSI-positive tumours [40].

53.3.1.3 β-Catenin

β-catenin (3p21) is a component of the E-cadherin–catenin complex essential for cell differentiation and maintenance of normal tissue architecture, and it also plays a role in signal transduction. The APC protein down-regulates β-catenin levels, inducing phosphorylation of serine-threonine residues coded in exon 3 of the β-catenin and its degradation via ubiquitin-proteosome pathway. Gain-of-function mutations in β-catenin exon 3 are seen in 25% to 38% of type I cancers [41]. These mutations result in protein stabilisation, accumulation, and transcriptional activation. β-catenin mutations have been found also in premalignant endometrial lesions. β-catenin changes may characterise pathways of endometrial cancer separate from PTEN mutations and are characterised by squamous differentiation. Several genes may be targets of dysregulated β-catenin pathway. Although in colon cancer elevated β-catenin levels trigger cyclin D1 expression and uncontrolled progression of tumour cells into the cell cycle, in type I endometrial cancers, β-catenin may regulate expression of MMP-7, which has a role in the establishment of microenvironment necessary for maintenance of tumour growth.

53.3.2 Type II Endometrial Cancer

The more aggressive, non-oestrogen-related, nonendometrioid cancers (predominantly serous and clear cell carcinomas) are characterised by p53 mutations and Her2/neu amplification and bcl-2 changes. These high-grade tumours are known to be associated in some cases with an identifiable intraepithelial neoplasia component. The same pattern of genetic changes is seen in the preneoplastic atrophic endometrium, suggesting that these are early events in type II tumours carcinogenesis [42].

53.4 Cervix, Vaginal, and Vulvar Cancers

53.4.1 Role of Human Papillomavirus

Persistent infections with specific high-risk HPV genotypes (e.g. HPV-16, HPV-18, HPV-31, HPV-33, and HPV-45) have been identified as an essential, although not sufficient, factor in the pathogenesis of majority of cancers of the cervix, vagina, and vulva [43]. The existence of papilloma viruses was first demonstrated by Shope in the 1930s using an ultrafiltrate of warts from rabbits [44]. Since then, papilloma viruses with an epithelial tropism have been demonstrated in nearly every mammalian species, including humans. The HPVs are encapsulated DNA viruses containing a double-stranded DNA genome of approximately 7800 base pairs. After infecting a suitable epithelium, viral DNA replication takes place in the basal cells of the epidermis, where the HPV genome is stably retained in multiple copies, guaranteeing its persistence in the epithelium's proliferative cells. This occurs early in preneoplastic lesions, when the viral genome still persists in an episomal state. In most invasive cancers and also in a few high-grade dysplastic lesions, however, integration of high-risk HPV genomes into the host genome is observed. Integration seems to be a direct consequence of chromosomal instability and an important molecular event in the progression of preneoplastic lesions. HPV integration sites are found to be randomly distributed over the whole genome with a clear predilection for genomic fragile sites. No evidence for targeted disruption or functional alteration of critical cellular genes by the integrated viral sequences could be found [45].

The ability of high-risk HPVs to transform human epithelia relates to the transcription of specific viral gene products. Transcription from the HPV genome occurs in two waves: an early phase with seven to eight gene products and a late phase with two gene products (L1, L2). Early-phase gene products play a critical role in viral DNA replication (E1, E8) and regulation of transcription (E2, E8). In contrast, the L1 and L2 genes code for the capsid's primary and secondary proteins, respectively. The ability of different high-risk HPVs to transform human epithelia has been primarily associated with the expression of two specific viral gene products, E6 and E7. Transformation of human genital tract epithelium likely requires the expression of both E6 and E7; transfection of human keratinocytes in vitro with either is insufficient to accomplish this phenomenon.

At a molecular level, E6 and E7 interfere with important control mechanisms of the cell cycle, apoptosis, and maintenance of chromosomal stability by directly interacting with p53 and pRB, respectively. Moreover, recent studies demonstrated that the two viral oncoproteins cooperatively disturb the mechanisms of chromosome duplication and segregation during mitosis and thereby induce severe chromosomal instability associated with centrosome aberrations, anaphase bridges, chromosome lagging, and breaking [46]. They have also been shown to interact with a number of other cellular proteins whose role in epithelial transformation remains unclear, including transcriptional coactivators, such as p300, and components of junctional complexes, such as hDlg1. Altered expression of hDlg1 has been observed in high-grade cervical dysplasias, consistent with the hypothesis that these gene products play an early role in the HPV-induced progression to cervical cancer. Specific sequence differences have been associated with different levels of risk for ultimately developing cervical cancers. For example, recent evidence demonstrates that the sequence of E6 found in Ashkenazi populations confers a protective advantage against developing cervical cancer, previously attributed to the practice of circumcision. Although much less understood, other early genes, such as E2, have also been implicated in the transformation.

53.4.2 Immune Evasion by Human Papillomavirus

HPV infection has a transitory pattern, whereby most individuals (70% to 90%) eliminate the virus 12 to 24 months after initial diagnosis [47]. HPV has evolved several strategies to evade immune attack. Most obviously, papillomaviruses do not infect and replicate in antigen-presenting cells that are located in the epithelium, nor do they lyse keratinocytes, so there is no opportunity for antigen-presenting cells to engulf virions and present virion-derived antigens to the immune system. Furthermore, there is no blood-borne phase of infection, so the immune system outside the epithelium has little opportunity to detect the virus. Additionally, HPVs have exploited the redundancy of the genetic code to keep the levels of "late" proteins low [48]. Papillomavirus capsid protein production is markedly up-regulated if the "viral" codons are replaced by the ones that are used by mammals, thereby limiting opportunities for the host to mount an effective immune attack. Following viral integration and subsequent malignant change, the local tumour environment at the cervical lesion is immunosuppressive. Thus, antigen-loaded dendritic cells (DCs) fail to mature, and immature DCs transmit a tolerogenic, rather than an immunogenic, signal to T cells bearing antigen-directed T-cell receptors in draining lymph nodes.

53.4.3 Human Papillomavirus Vaccines

The aim of prophylactic vaccination is to generate neutralising antibodies against the HPV L1 and L2 capsid proteins. Prophylactic vaccine development against HPV has focused on the ability of the L1 and L2 virion structural proteins to assemble into virus like particles (VLPs). VLPs mimic the natural structure of the virion and generate a potent immune response. Because the VLPs are devoid of DNA, they are not infectious or harmful. HPV VLPs can be generated by expressing the HPV capsid protein L1 in baculovirus or yeast. They consist of five L1 subunits that multimerise into immunogenic pentamers. Seventy-one L1 pentamers, in turn, multimerise into an HPV VLP. Initial studies have shown that VLPs are capable of inducing high titres of neutralising antibodies to L1 and L2 epitopes [49]. Furthermore, VLPs have proven effective in generating HPV type-specific protection from viral challenge in animal papillomavirus models.

With the approval of preventive HPV vaccines that encompass HPV-16, -18, -6, and -11, large prevention clinical trials targeting the most prevalent HPV types in different regions of the world are warranted. Questions such as the necessity of repeat vaccinations and longevity of protection from HPV infection remain to be determined. It is estimated that if women were vaccinated against all high-risk types of HPV before they become sexually active, there should be a reduction of at least 85% in the risk of cervical cancer, and a decline of 44–70% in the frequency of abnormal Papanicolaou (Pap) smears attributable to HPV [50]. Unfortunately, even after vaccination is implemented, a reduction in the incidence of cervical cancer could not be expected to become apparent for at least a decade [51]. Therefore, therapeutic vaccines are still very much needed to reduce the morbidity and mortality associated with cervical cancer.

The therapeutic approach to patients with pre-invasive and invasive cervical cancers is to develop vaccine strategies that induce specific CD8+ cytotoxic T lymphocyte (CTL) responses aimed at eliminating virus-infected or transformed cells. The majority of cervical cancers express the HPV-16-derived E6 and E7 oncoproteins, which are thus attractive targets for T-cell-mediated immunotherapy. Several HPV vaccine strategies have successfully elicited immune responses against HPV E6 and E7 epitopes and have prevented tumour growth on challenge with HPV-16-positive tumour cells in mice. Early-phase human trials using therapeutic vaccines have shown that they are safe, as no serious adverse effects have been reported.

Low-income countries including African countries face significant difficulties to integrate new vaccines into their national immunisation programmes. In 2006, the programme *HPV Vaccines: Evidence for Impact* project in order to generate evidence to help policymakers and planners worldwide making informed decisions regarding regional HPV vaccination and Uganda is one of the countries chosen as a site for the *HPV Vaccines* project. In Uganda, cervical cancer accounts for 40% of all cancers recorded by the cancer registry, and over 80% of women with cervical cancer are diagnosed with advanced disease. In 2008–2009 in selected districts, HPV vaccine was made available to more than 10,000 girls. The Uganda project was implemented by the Uganda National Expanded Program on Immunisation of the Ministry of Health. The experience of Uganda is, and will be helpful to neighbouring countries and other countries in the African region.

References

1. Dunn GP, Old LJ, Schreiber RD. The immunobiology of cancer immunosurveillance and immunoediting. Immunity. 2004;21:137–48. PMID: 15308095.
2. Karst AM, Drapkin R. Ovarian cancer pathogenesis: a model in evolution. J Oncol. 2010;2010:932371. PMID: 19746182.
3. Levanon K, Crum C, Drapkin R. New insights into the pathogenesis of serous ovarian cancer and its clinical impact. J Clin Oncol. 2008;26:5284–93. PMID: 18854563.
4. Auersperg N, Wong AS, Choi KC, Kang SK, Leung PC. Ovarian surface epithelium: biology, endocrinology, and pathology. Endocr Rev. 2001;22:255–88. PMID: 11294827.
5. Wright JW, Pejovic T, Fanton J, Stouffer RL. Induction of proliferation in the primate ovarian surface epithelium in vivo. Hum Reprod. 2008;23:129–38. PMID: 18000169.
6. Wright JW, Pejovic T, Lawson M, Jurevic L, Hobbs T, Stouffer RL. Ovulation in the absence of the ovarian surface epithelium in the primate. Biol Reprod. 2010;82:599–605. PMID: 19923253.
7. Schlosshauer PW, Cohen CJ, Penault-Llorca F, Miranda CR, Bignon YJ, Dauplat J, Deligdisch L. Prophylactic oophorectomy: a morphologic and immunohistochemical study. Cancer. 2003;98:2599–606. PMID: 14669279.
8. Callahan MJ, Crum CP, Medeiros F, Kindelberger DW, Elvin JA, Garber JE, Feltmate CM, Berkowitz RS, Muto MG. Primary fallopian tube malignancies in BRCA-positive women undergoing surgery for ovarian cancer risk reduction. J Clin Oncol. 2007;25:3985–90. PMID: 17761984.
9. Tone AA, Begley H, Sharma M, Murphy J, Rosen B, Brown TJ, Shaw PA. Gene expression profiles of luteal phase fallopian tube epithelium from BRCA mutation carriers resemble high-grade serous carcinoma. Clin Cancer Res. 2008;14:4067–78. PMID: 18593983.
10. Kurman RJ. Origin and molecular pathogenesis of ovarian high-grade serous carcinoma. Ann Oncol. 2013;24(Suppl 10):x16–21. PMID: 24265397.
11. Ramus SJ. Current status of inherited predisposition to ovarian cancer: lessons from familial ovarian cancer registries in the UK and USA. In: Odunsi K, Pejovic T, editors. Gynaecologic cancer: a multidisciplinary approach to diagnosis and management. New York: Demos Medical; 2013.
12. Ramus SJ, Gayther SA. The contribution of BRCA1 and BRCA2 to ovarian cancer. Mol Oncol. 2009;3:138–50. PMID: 19383375.
13. Miki Y, Swensen J, Shattuck-Eidens D, Futreal PA, Harshman K, Tavtigian S, Liu Q, Cochran C, Bennett LM, Ding W, et al. A strong candidate for the breast and ovarian cancer susceptibility gene BRCA1. Science. 1994;266:66–71. PMID: 7545954.
14. Wooster R, Bignell G, Lancaster J, Swift S, Seal S, Mangion J, Collins N, Gregory S, Gumbs C, Micklem G. Identification of the breast cancer susceptibility gene BRCA2. Nature. 1995;378:789–92. PMID: 8524414.
15. Mazoyer S. Genomic rearrangements in the BRCA1 and BRCA2 genes. Hum Mutat. 2005;25:415–22. PMID: 15832305.
16. Antoniou AC, Easton DF. Risk prediction models for familial breast cancer. Future Oncol. 2006;2:257–74. PMID: 16563094.
17. Sakai W, Swisher EM, Karlan BY, Agarwal MK, Higgins J, Friedman C, Villegas E, Jacquemont C, Farrugia DJ, Couch FJ, Urban N, Taniguchi T. Secondary mutations as a mechanism of cisplatin resistance in BRCA2-mutated cancers. Nature. 2008;451:1116–20. PMID: 18264087.
18. Walsh T, Lee MK, Casadei S, Thornton AM, Stray SM, Pennil C, Nord AS, Mandell JB, Swisher EM, King MC. Detection of inherited mutations for breast and ovarian cancer using genomic capture and massively parallel sequencing. Proc Natl Acad Sci U S A. 2010;107:12629–33. PMID: 20616022.
19. Bradford L, Ambrosio A, Birrer MJ. PARP inhibitors in gyecologic malignancies. In: Odunsi K, Pejovic T, editors. Gynaecologic cancers: a multidisciplinary approach to diagnosis and management. New York: Demos Medical; 2013.
20. Kassim SK, El-Salahy EM, Fayed ST, Helal SA, Helal T, Azzam Eel D, Khalifa A. Vascular endothelial growth factor and interleukin-8 are associated with poor prognosis in epithelial ovarian cancer patients. Clin Biochem. 2004;37:363–9. PMID: 15087251.
21. Jiang H, Feng Y. Hypoxia-inducible factor 1alpha (HIF-1alpha) correlated with tumour growth and apoptosis in ovarian cancer. Int J Gynecol Cancer. 2006;16(Suppl 1):405–12. PMID: 16515634.
22. Zhu G, Saed GM, Deppe G, Diamond MP, Munkarah AR. Hypoxia up-regulates the effects of prostaglandin E2 on tumour angiogenesis in ovarian cancer cells. Gynecol Oncol. 2004;94:422–6. PMID: 15297183.
23. Burger RA, Brady MF, Bookman MA, Fleming GF, Monk BJ, Huang H, Mannel RS, Homesley HD, Fowler J, Greer BE, Boente M, Birrer MJ, Liang SX. Incorporation of bevacizumab in the primary treatment of ovarian cancer. N Engl J Med. 2011;365:2473–83. PMID: 22204724.
24. Zhang L, Conejo-Garcia JR, Katsaros D, Gimotty PA, Massobrio M, Regnani G, Makrigiannakis A, Gray H, Schlienger K, Liebman MN, Rubin SC, Coukos G. Intratumoural T cells, recurrence, and survival in epithelial ovarian cancer. N Engl J Med. 2003;348:203–13. PMID: 12529460.
25. Smyth MJ, Dunn GP, Schreiber RD. Cancer immunosurveillance and immunoediting: the roles of immunity in suppressing tumour development and shaping tumour immunogenicity. Adv Immunol. 2006;90:1–50. PMID: 16730260.
26. Goodell V, Salazar LG, Urban N, Drescher CW, Gray H, Swensen RE, McIntosh MW, Disis ML. Antibody immunity to the p53 oncogenic protein is a prognostic indicator in ovarian cancer. J Clin Oncol. 2006;24:762–8. PMID: 16391298.
27. Odunsi K, Jungbluth AA, Stockert E, Qian F, Gnjatic S, Tammela J, Intengan M, Beck A, Keitz B, Santiago D, Williamson B, Scanlan MJ, Ritter G, Chen YT, Driscoll D, Sood A, Lele S, Old LJ. NY-ESO-1 and LAGE-1 cancer-testis antigens are potential targets for immunotherapy in epithelial ovarian cancer. Cancer Res. 2003;63:6076–83. PMID: 14522938.
28. Old LJ. Cancer/testis (CT) antigens – a new link between gametogenesis and cancer. Cancer Immun. 2001;1:1. PMID: 12747762.
29. Matsuzaki J, Gnjatic S, Mhawech-Fauceglia P, Beck A, Miller A, Tsuji T, Eppolito C, Qian F, Lele S, Shrikant P, Old LJ, Odunsi K. Tumour-infiltrating NY-ESO-1-specific CD8+ T cells are negatively regulated by LAG-3 and PD-1 in human ovarian cancer. Proc Natl Acad Sci U S A. 2010;107:7875–80. PMID: 20385810.
30. Odunsi K, Qian F, Matsuzaki J, Mhawech-Fauceglia P, Andrews C, Hoffman EW, Pan L, Ritter G, Villella J, Thomas B, Rodabaugh K, Lele S, Shrikant P, Old LJ, Gnjatic S. Vaccination with an NY-ESO-1 peptide of HLA class I/II specificities induces integrated

humoral and T cell responses in ovarian cancer. Proc Natl Acad Sci U S A. 2007;104:12837–42. PMID: 17652518.
31. Odunsi K, Matsuzaki J, Karbach J, Neumann A, Mhawech-Fauceglia P, Miller A, Beck A, Morrison CD, Ritter G, Godoy H, Lele S, duPont N, Edwards R, Shrikant P, Old LJ, Gnjatic S, Jager E. Efficacy of vaccination with recombinant vaccinia and fowlpox vectors expressing NY-ESO-1 antigen in ovarian cancer and melanoma patients. Proc Natl Acad Sci U S A. 2012;109:5797–802. PMID: 22454499.
32. Chiang CL, Kandalaft LE, Tanyi J, Hagemann AR, Motz GT, Svoronos N, Montone K, Mantia-Smaldone GM, Smith L, Nisenbaum HL, Levine BL, Kalos M, Czerniecki BJ, Torigian DA, Powell DJ Jr, Mick R, Coukos G. A dendritic cell vaccine pulsed with autologous hypochlorous acid-oxidized ovarian cancer lysate primes effective broad antitumour immunity: from bench to bedside. Clin Cancer Res. 2013;19:4801–15. PMID: 23838316.
33. Kandalaft LE, Chiang CL, Tanyi J, Motz G, Balint K, Mick R, Coukos G. A phase I vaccine trial using dendritic cells pulsed with autologous oxidized lysate for recurrent ovarian cancer. J Transl Med. 2013;11:149. PMID: 23777306
34. Tsuji T, Matsuzaki J, Kelly MP, et al. "Antibody-targeted NYESO-1 to mannose receptor or DEC-205 in vitro elicits dual human CD8+ and CD4+ T cell responses with broad antigen Journal of Drug Delivery 17 specificity", J. Immunol. 2011;186(2):1218–27.
35. van Rooij N, van Buuren MM, Philips D, Velds A, Toebes M, Heemskerk B, et al. Tumor exome analysis reveals neoantigen-specific T-cell reactivity in an ipilimumab-responsive melanoma. J Clin Oncol. 2013;31:e439–42. https://doi.org/10.1200/jco.2012.47.7521.
36. Disis ML, Patel MR, Pant S, et al. Avelumab (MSB0010718C), an anti-PD-L1 antibody, in patients with previously treated, recurrent or refractory ovarian cancer: A phase Ib, open-label expansion trial. J Clin Oncol. 2015;33:5509–81.
37. Snyder A, Makarov V, Merghoub T, et al. Genetic basis for clinical response to CTLA-4 blockade in melanoma. N Engl J Med. 2014;371:2189–99.
38. Mutter GL, Boynton KA, Faquin WC, Ruiz RE, Jovanovic AS. Allelotype mapping of unstable microsatellites establishes direct lineage continuity between endometrial precancers and cancer. Cancer Res. 1996;56:4483–6. PMID: 8813144.
39. Mutter GL, Lin MC, Fitzgerald JT, Kum JB, Baak JP, Lees JA, Weng LP, Eng C. Altered PTEN expression as a diagnostic marker for the earliest endometrial precancers. J Natl Cancer Inst. 2000;92:924–30. PMID: 10841828.
40. Caduff RF, Johnston CM, Frank TS. Mutations of the Ki-ras oncogene in carcinoma of the endometrium. Am J Pathol. 1995;146:182–8. PMID:7856726.
41. Mirabelli-Primdahl L, Gryfe R, Kim H, Millar A, Luceri C, Dale D, Holowaty E, Bapat B, Gallinger S, Redston M. Beta-catenin mutations are specific for colorectal carcinomas with microsatellite instability but occur in endometrial carcinomas irrespective of mutator pathway. Cancer Res. 1999;59:3346–51. PMID: 10416591.
42. Busmanis I, Ho TH, Tan SB, Khoo KS. p53 and bcl-2 expression in invasive and pre-invasive uterine papillary serous carcinoma and atrophic endometrium. Ann Acad Med Singap. 2005;34:421–5. PMID: 16123814.
43. zur Hausen H. Papillomaviruses causing cancer: evasion from host-cell control in early events in carcinogenesis. J Natl Cancer Inst. 2000;92:690–8. PMID:10793105.
44. Shope RE. Serial transmission of vrus of infectious paillomatosis in domestic rabbits. Proc Soc Exp Biol Med. 1935;32:830.
45. Wentzensen N, Vinokurova S, von Knebel Doeberitz M. Systematic review of genomic integration sites of human papillomavirus genomes in epithelial dysplasia and invasive cancer of the female lower genital tract. Cancer Res. 2004;64:3878–84. PMID: 15172997.
46. Duensing S, Munger K. Centrosome abnormalities, genomic instability and carcinogenic progression. Biochim Biophys Acta. 2001;1471:M81–8. PMID: 11342187.
47. Ho GY, Bierman R, Beardsley L, Chang CJ, Burk RD. Natural history of cervicovaginal papillomavirus infection in young women. N Engl J Med. 1998;338:423–8. PMID: 9459645.
48. Zhou J, Liu WJ, Peng SW, Sun XY, Frazer I. Papillomavirus capsid protein expression level depends on the match between codon usage and tRNA availability. J Virol. 1999;73:4972–82. PMID: 10233959.
49. Koutsky LA, Ault KA, Wheeler CM, Brown DR, Barr E, Alvarez FB, Chiacchierini LM, Jansen KU. A controlled trial of a human papillomavirus type 16 vaccine. N Engl J Med. 2002;347:1645–51. PMID: 12444178.
50. Walboomers JM, Jacobs MV, Manos MM, Bosch FX, Kummer JA, Shah KV, Snijders PJ, Peto J, Meijer CJ, Munoz N. Human papillomavirus is a necessary cause of invasive cervical cancer worldwide. J Pathol. 1999;189:12–9. PMID: 10451482.
51. Crum CP. The beginning of the end for cervical cancer? N Engl J Med. 2002;347:1703–5. PMID: 12444186.

Gestational Trophoblastic Disease

54

Clement A. Adepiti and Kunle Odunsi

Learning Objectives

At the end of this chapter, the reader should be able to:

- Understand the terms gestational trophoblastic disease (GTD) and gestational trophoblastic neoplasia (GTN)
- Appreciate the global epidemiology of GTD
- Differentiate between complete mole and partial mole
- Understand the pathology of hydatidiform mole (HM) and GTN
- Appreciate the different clinical presentations of GTD
- Know the different investigations necessary for the diagnosis of GTD
- Understand the basis of management and follow-up of GTD patients
- Appreciate the challenges of GTD management in sub-Saharan Africa and the solutions to these challenges

54.1 Introduction

The term gestational trophoblastic disease (GTD) encompasses a spectrum of abnormal cellular proliferations arising from the placental villous trophoblast with the benign and the malignant components occupying the two extremes. The clinicopathologic types include hydatidiform mole (complete and partial) at the benign end, invasive mole, placental site trophoblastic tumor (PSTT), and choriocarcinoma at the malignant extreme. The term "gestational trophoblastic neoplasia" (GTN) encompasses the latter three conditions, which can progress, invade, metastasize, and lead to death if not properly treated.

GTD was historically associated with significant morbidity and mortality before the development of early detection and effective uterine evacuation techniques. The prognoses of GTN were likewise poor before the introduction of chemotherapy into their management. The mortality rate for invasive mole was as high as 15%, most often because of hemorrhage, sepsis, embolic phenomena, or complications from surgery. Choriocarcinoma had a mortality rate of almost 100% when metastases were present and approximately 60% even when hysterectomy was done for apparent non-metastatic disease. Today, GTN is the most curable of all solid tumors, with cure rates as high as 90% even in the presence of metastatic disease thus allowing affected women to preserve their fertility [1, 2].

54.2 Epidemiology

The incidence and etiologic factors contributing to the development of GTD have been difficult to characterize because of the difficulty in generating and aggregating reliable epidemiologic data [1]. Epidemiologic studies have reported wide regional variations in the incidence of hydatidiform mole [1]. Population-based studies in North America, New Zealand, Australia, and Europe have estimated the incidence of complete mole as between 0.57 and 1.1 per 1000 pregnancies [1]. The risk is increased two to three folds in Saudi Arabia and Japan compared to other populations [3–5]. Though no population-based study has been carried out in Africa, institution-based studies put the incidence as 0.87–4.88 per

C. A. Adepiti
Department of Obstetrics, Gynaecology and Perinatology, Faculty of Clinical Sciences, College of Health Sciences, Obafemi Awolowo University, Ile-Ife, Nigeria

K. Odunsi (✉)
Roswell Park Comprehensive Cancer Centre (Roswell Park), Buffalo, NY, USA

Department of Gynaecologic Oncology, Centre for Immunotherapy, Roswell Park, Buffalo, NY, USA

University of Buffalo, Buffalo, NY, USA
e-mail: Kunle.odunsi@roswellpark.org

F. Okonofua et al. (eds.), *Contemporary Obstetrics and Gynecology for Developing Countries*,
https://doi.org/10.1007/978-3-030-75385-6_54

1000 deliveries in Nigeria, 0.80 per 1000 deliveries in Ghana, and 1.26 per 1000 pregnancies in Tunisia [6–8].

It is not clear as there are several contradictory studies whether these differences in the incidence of molar pregnancy are associated with socioeconomic or dietary factors apart from race. Specifically, it has been reported that the risk of complete molar pregnancy increases with decreased consumption of vitamin A (carotene) and animal fat [9, 10]. Extremes of reproductive ages have also been documented as an associated risk by many studies using both population-based risk estimates and case-control studies [11, 12]. Most of these studies only addressed the maternal age; however, Parezzini and colleagues [8] found that paternal age above 45 years increased the relative risk for the complete mole to 4.9 alone and 2.9 when adjusted for maternal age. However, maternal and paternal age-specific risk factors have not been found in partial mole [13]. Studies have also indicated that a history of previous abnormal pregnancies increased the risk of molar pregnancy [14, 15]. However, it is well recognized that a history of prior molar pregnancy increases the risk of a subsequent mole by ten folds [3].

Like the molar pregnancy, the epidemiology of gestational choriocarcinoma has not been extensively studied because it is relatively rare and clinically difficult to differentiate from the invasive mole. In Europe and North America, choriocarcinoma affects approximately 1 in 40,000 pregnancies, whereas in Southeast Asia and Japan choriocarcinoma rates are higher at 9.2 and 3.3 per 40,000 pregnancies, respectively. However, the incidence of both hydatidiform mole and choriocarcinoma has declined over the past 30 years in all populations [16–18]. The most important risk factor is hydatidiform mole in the previous pregnancy, this increases the incidence of choriocarcinoma 1000–2000 folds compared to prior term pregnancy [3, 19]. Increased risk has also been reported in women older than 45 years and in non-Caucasians [20].

54.3 Cytogenetics of Complete and Partial Moles

The genetic bases of complete and partial moles are established at conception. Complete mole results from diandric diploidy. The egg which is fertilized by a single sperm loses the maternal haploid 23,X genetic component through an unknown mechanism. The paternal haploid set of 23,X is duplicated to reestablish the 46,XX zygote status [21, 22]. This variant accounts for about 90–95% of all complete moles. The YY combination is said to be incompatible with life and so the 46,YY has not been clinically encountered [21]. About 5–10% of complete moles arise from dispermic fertilization of an empty ovum which can either result in 46,XY or 46,XX genotypes [21].

The biparental complete moles have also been described, though rare. Maternal and paternal genes are present but the failure of maternal imprinting causes only the paternal genomes to be expressed [22]. A recurrent, familial form of biparental mole which is inherited as an autosomal recessive trait has been described by Al-Hussaini [23]. Mutations in the *NLRP7* at 19q13.4 have been identified as the cause of recurrent molar pregnancy [24].

Partial moles arise from dispermic fertilization of an egg with the retention of the maternal haploid set, resulting in diandric triploidy [25, 26]. The 69,XXX and the 69,XXY partial moles are seen in ratio 2:3 and the 69,XYY is rarely seen for unknown reasons [27]. The tetraploid partial moles with three paternal and one maternal haploid sets have also been described [27].

Currently, in good laboratories, apart from genotyping and ploidy analysis, immunohistochemistry has been added to the armamentarium for the characterization of the different variants of hydatidiform mole. Staining for p57 a gene product of the paternally imprinted, maternally expressed gene *CDKNIC*, a cyclin-dependent kinase inhibitor gene located on chromosome 11p15.5 has been deployed in delineating moles from androgenetic origins from others [28]. The p57 protein is expressed preferentially off the maternal allele and is therefore not expressed in complete hydatidiform molar villous because it is androgenetic in origin [29]. Thus, when staining for p57 is negative, it is a complete mole, when it is positive it is a partial mole, a mosaic, or a biparental mole.

54.4 Pathology

54.4.1 Hydatidiform Mole

Hydatidiform mole refers to an abnormal pregnancy characterized by varying degrees of trophoblastic proliferation (both cytotrophoblast and syncytiotrophoblast) and vesicular swelling of placental villi associated with an absent or an abnormal fetus/embryo.

54.4.2 Complete Hydatidiform Mole

The classical triad of molar pregnancy includes generalized edema of the chorionic villi, including central cistern formation which is responsible for the macroscopic description of hydatidiform mole as resembling a "bunch of grapes," generalized diffused hyperplasia of both cytotrophoblast and syncytiotrophoblast elements, and absence of an embryo which has resorbed before the development of the cardiovascular system [22, 30, 31].

In complete mole, hCG level is usually above 100,000 mIU/mL [32, 33]. This is usually responsible for the exaggerated symptoms of pregnancy. Some of the associated clinical sequelae are unilateral or bilateral ovarian enlargement produced by theca lutein cysts which is clinically detected in approximately 25–35% of patients with complete mole. There are also increased thyroid hormones but clinical hyperthyroidism is detected in less than 10% of patients with molar pregnancy [34, 35]. Approximately 10–25% of patients with complete molar pregnancy develop "malignant" sequelae after evacuation, the majority develop invasive or persistent mole while about 25–33% of these have gestational choriocarcinoma [33, 36, 37].

54.4.3 Partial Hydatidiform Mole

In contrast with complete mole, the histology of partial mole is characterized by a placenta with focal, variable hydropic villi and also focal, slight cytotrophoblast, and syncytiotrophoblast hyperplasia [22, 31, 38]. Other histologic features are scalloping of the villi with trophoblastic inclusions within the chorionic villi. The embryo survived much longer than in the complete moles, with embryonic death occurring about the eighth week of gestation. Thus, most times, there are macroscopic and microscopic evidence of a fetus [22, 31, 38]. Fetal vessels are usually identified containing nucleated fetal erythrocytes. The histologic features may vary depending on the gestational age of evacuation of a partial mole [22]. Unlike the complete mole, because of the focal nature of the hydropic changes and proliferation, multiple tissue sections must be examined to make the diagnosis. Partial moles are most often clinically diagnosed as a missed abortion because the hydropic changes are not clinically evident and evidence of fetal tissues persists. A recent comparison of retrospective and prospective studies confirmed that partial moles are frequently under-diagnosed [27].

Compared with the complete mole, the level of hCG is usually <100,000 mIU/mL, most of the associated clinical sequelae of elevated levels of hCG are not present and only about 1–5% develop malignant sequelae [38] (Table 54.1).

54.4.4 Invasive Mole

In invasive mole, the pathology is that of the complete mole with invasion beyond the normal placentation site directly into the myometrium, sometimes penetrating into the venous system [22, 39]. Thus occasionally venous metastasis to the lower genital tract and the lungs may occur. The histological diagnosis of the invasive mole is rarely made because myometrial invasion is extremely difficult to ascertain from endometrial curetting [39]. Therefore, noninvasive imaging studies such as arteriogram and magnetic resonance scanning may be more useful in the diagnosis of invasive mole. It causes uterine sub-involution and bleeding, penetration into the myometrium may cause uterine rupture or massive intra-abdominal hemorrhage [39]. Invasive mole though locally invasive should not be considered an intermediate between hydatidiform mole and choriocarcinoma because the natural history of invasive mole includes occasional spontaneous remission.

The hCG levels in invasive mole are usually in the order seen in complete mole and there are also the other associated symptoms of the elevated hCG in affected patients [39].

Table 54.1 Comparison of complete and partial hydatidiform mole

	Complete mole	Partial mole
Cytogenetic analysis	Diploidy; 46,XX most common	Triploidy; 69,XXY most common
Pathology		
Hydropic villi	Diffuse and marked	Focal and variable
Trophoblastic proliferation	Diffuse	Focal, variable
Fetus, amnion, fetal RBCs	Absent	Present
Scalloping of the chorionic villi	Absent	Present
Stroma trophoblast inclusions	Absent	Present
Clinical		
Clinical/ultrasound diagnosis	Common	Rare
Uterus large for date	25–50%	Rare
Theca lutein cysts	25–35%	Rare
Malignant sequelae	10–25%	<5%
	Up to 25% metastatic	>99% non-metastatic

54.4.5 Placenta Site Trophoblastic Tumor (PSTT)

Placenta site trophoblastic tumors are predominantly composed of intermediate trophoblast cells arising from the placenta site [19]. Placenta site trophoblastic tumor can arise from any type of antecedent pregnancy including term pregnancies and are usually locally aggressive, with myometrial invasion. There is only a scanty syncytiotrophoblast component, therefore the production of hCG is usually low and provides a less reliable marker of tumor volume compared to other variants of gestational trophoblastic disease [19]. Surprisingly, PSTT produces human placenta lactogen (hPL) which is a more reliable tumor marker in most patients with this tumor [19].

54.4.6 Choriocarcinoma

Gestational choriocarcinoma arises most times from the malignant transformation of molar tissues or rarely spontaneously from the placenta of a term pregnancy or spontaneous abortion [19]. It contains essentially both cytotrophoblast and syncytiotrophoblast but no chorionic villi [19]. There are also varying degrees of pleomorphism and anaplasia in choriocarcinoma and if villous structures are seen in metastatic deposits, the histologic diagnosis is the invasive mole. Choriocarcinoma is a rapidly growing tumor growing in a centripetal fashion with central necrosis arising from the tumor overgrowing its blood supply [19]. This particularly predisposes to severe hemorrhage when necrosis involves major vessels. It readily invades the blood vessels like the normal and abnormal trophoblasts, producing metastasis via hematogenous routes of dissemination [19]. Disseminations are usually to the lower genital tract as suburethral nodules, the lungs, the liver, the kidneys, and the brain. Similar lesions are seen at the metastatic sites displaying centripetal growth pattern, central necrosis that may produce massive local hemorrhages [19].

Because the tumor is derived from both cytotrophoblast and syncytiotrophoblast, hCG secretion is maintained and it usually corresponds well with the volume of the disease. It is a reliable tumor marker for diagnosis and follow-up of patients with choriocarcinoma [19].

54.5 Clinical Presentation

54.5.1 Hydatidiform Mole

54.5.1.1 Complete Hydatidiform Mole

The most common presentation of the complete mole is vaginal bleeding, usually occurring between 6 and 16 weeks of gestation in most instances. The other classical clinical signs and symptoms are exaggerated symptoms of pregnancy, uterine size greater than expected for gestational age (28%), hyperthyroidism (<10%), hyperemesis gravidarum (8%), and pregnancy-induced hypertension in the first or second trimester (1%). These signs and symptoms occur less frequently now because of earlier diagnosis as a result of widespread use of ultrasonography and accurate quantitative tests for hCG. Bilateral theca lutein cyst enlargement of the ovaries occurs in approximately 15% of cases, hCG levels are often >100,000 mIU/mL, and fetal heart tones are absent [40–44].

54.5.1.2 Partial Mole

Unlike complete mole, more than 90% of patients with partial moles present with symptoms similar to those of incomplete or missed abortion, and the diagnosis is usually made on histological examination of curettage specimens. They usually present with vaginal bleeding. Excessive uterine enlargement, hyperemesis, pregnancy-induced hypertension, hyperthyroidism, and theca lutein cysts are rare associated findings. Pre-evacuation hCG levels are <100,000 mIU/mL in about 90% of patients with partial moles [38, 45–47].

54.5.2 Gestational Trophoblastic Neoplasia (GTN)

The presentation of GTN varies depending on the type of antecedent pregnancy event, extent of disease, and histopathology. Postmolar GTN (invasive mole or choriocarcinoma) most commonly presents as irregular bleeding following the evacuation of a hydatidiform mole. Signs suggestive of postmolar GTN are an enlarged, irregular uterus and persistent bilateral ovarian enlargement. Occasionally, a metastatic vaginal lesion may be noted on evacuation, which may bleed uncontrollably on contact.

Choriocarcinoma associated with nonmolar gestation has no characteristic symptoms or signs, most are related to invasion of tumor into the uterus or at metastatic sites. In patients with postpartum uterine bleeding and subinvolution, GTN should be suspected along with other possible causes, such as retained products of conception or endomyometritis, primary, metastatic tumors of other organ systems, or another pregnancy occurring shortly after the first. Bleeding as a result of uterine perforation or metastatic lesions may result in abdominal pain, hemoptysis, melena, or evidence of increased intracranial pressure from intracerebral hemorrhage leading to headaches, seizures, or hemiplegia. Patients may also exhibit pulmonary symptoms, such as dyspnea, cough, and chest pain, caused by extensive lung metastases [48]. PSTTs most times cause irregular uterine bleeding often distant from a preceding nonmolar gestation, and rarely virilization or nephrotic syndrome. The uterus is usually symmetrically enlarged, and serum hCG levels are only slightly elevated [49, 50]. However, human placenta lactogen (HPL) may be elevated.

54.6 Diagnosis

54.6.1 Ultrasonography

Ultrasonography plays a major role in the diagnosis of both complete and partial mole, and it complements hCG in the preoperative diagnosis [51, 52]. Because of the diffuse hydropic swelling of the chorionic villi in complete moles, a characteristic vesicular ultrasonographic pattern can be observed, consisting of multiples echoes (holes) within the placental mass and usually no fetus. Ultrasonography may also facilitate the early diagnosis of a partial mole by demonstrating focal cystic spaces within the placenta and an increase in the transverse diameter of the gestational sac [51].

54.6.2 Human Chorionic Gonadotropin

Human chorionic gonadotropin is a specific tumor marker produced by hydatidiform moles and gestational trophoblastic neoplasms. It can be quantitatively measured in both blood and urine, and its levels have been shown to correlate closely with the burden of disease. It is a placental glycoprotein composed of two subunits, the α and β subunits. The α subunit resembles the pituitary glycoprotein hormones (LH, TSH) while the β subunit is unique to the placenta [53, 54]. The hCG molecules in GTD are more heterogenous and degraded than those in normal pregnancy, thus, an assay that will detect all main forms of hCG and its multiple fragments should be used to follow-up patients with GTD. The currently available tests use rapid, automated radio-labeled monoclonal antibody sandwich assays that measure different mixtures of hCG-related molecules [41–43]. In molar pregnancy, hCG levels are markedly elevated. The levels are >100,000 mIU/mL in 90% of complete moles and in about 10% of partial moles before evacuation [55].

A clinical suspicion of postmolar GTN should be considered if there is rising or plateauing of hCG levels following the evacuation of a hydatidiform mole. However, choriocarcinoma is usually diagnosed if there is an elevated hCG level, in conjunction with evidence of metastases, following other pregnancy events. PSTT is commonly associated with only slightly elevated hCG levels, the detection of HPL is more in keeping with its diagnosis and it can be used as tumor marker for its follow-up.

Accurate measurements of hCG levels are necessary in the diagnosis and follow-up of GTD; however, some laboratory assays may sometimes yield false-positive hCG results [46]. Such results are called phantom hCG results, with levels reported as high as 800 mIU/mL. This has led to the treatment of healthy patients with unnecessary surgery and chemotherapy [56]. The possible causes of these phantom results are proteolytic enzymes that produce nonspecific protein interference and heterophile (human antimouse) antibodies. Heterophile antibodies are found in 3–4% of healthy people and can mimic hCG immune-reactivity by linking and capturing tracer mouse IgG. There are three ways to determine whether hCG assays are falsely positive when there is a clinical suspicion of phantom hCG: (1) determine a urine hCG level, which should be negative because the interfering substances are not excreted in urine; (2) request serial dilution of the serum, which should not show a parallel decrease with dilution; and (3) send the serum and urine of the patient to an hCG reference laboratory. Additionally, there is some cross-reactivity of hCG with luteinizing hormone (LH), which may lead to falsely elevated low levels of hCG. Measurement of LH to identify this possibility and suppression of LH with oral contraceptive pills will prevent this problem [57].

In other instances, instead of a false-positive test result such as a phantom hCG due to heterophile antibodies, the "hook effect" causes a false-negative hCG value. In the "hook effect," the assay is overwhelmed by very high levels of hCG, generally greater than 1,000,000 mIU/mL. The "hook effect" can be overcome by serial dilution of the serum before using an hCG immunoassay, and this is standard practice in many laboratories; however, if a false-negative hCG is suspected, serial dilution of the patient's serum should be performed [58].

The "quiescent gestational trophoblastic disease" is a term applied to a presumed inactive form of GTN that is characterized by persistent, unchanging low levels (<200 mIU/mL) of "real" hCG for at least 3 months associated with a preceding history of GTD or spontaneous abortion, but without clinical disease. The hCG levels do not change with surgery or chemotherapy. Further analysis of hCG shows the absence of hyperglycosylated hCG, which is associated with cytotrophoblastic invasion. About a quarter of patients with quiescent GTD may develop active GTN on follow-up and this is usually heralded by an increase in both hyperglycosylated hCG and total hCG [59, 60].

54.7 Pathologic Diagnosis

Pathologic diagnosis of complete and partial moles is made by examination of curettage specimens. Immunohistological staining for p57 (a paternally imprinted, maternally expressed gene) can be used to differentiate immunostaining negative complete moles from positively staining hydropic abortuses and partial moles [29].

54.8 Treatment

54.8.1 Hydatidiform Mole

After the diagnosis of molar pregnancy, the patient should be evaluated for the presence of possible medical complications (anemia, preeclampsia, and hyperthyroidism). Baseline investigations such as full blood cell counts, blood chemistry, liver and thyroid functions tests, urinalysis, and chest X-ray should be requested. The preoperative serum hCG level should be determined and blood should be grouped and cross-matched.

Suction evacuation followed by a gentle sharp curettage is the preferred method of evacuation of a hydatidiform mole for patients who wish to retain their fertility [61, 62]. Under appropriate anesthesia, the cervix is dilated to allow a 12–14 mm suction cannula to pass into the lower uterine segment. The cannula is then rotated as the intrauterine contents are removed. It is recommended that an intravenous oxytocin infusion be started at the onset of suction curettage and continued for several hours postoperatively to enhance uterine contraction. Suction evacuation should be followed by gentle sharp curettage. At least two units of blood should be available when the uterus is >16-weeks' gestational size, this is because the risk of bleeding increases with uterine size. Rh negative patients should also receive Rh immunoglobulin at the time of evacuation, as Rh D factor is expressed on trophoblastic cells [60, 63].

When a woman has completed her family size, hysterectomy is an alternative to suction curettage. Hysterectomy apart from eliminating the molar pregnancy additionally provides permanent sterilization and eliminates the risk of invasive mole as a cause of persistent disease. The adnexa may be left intact even in the presence of theca lutein cysts. There is still a 3–5% risk for metastatic disease even after hysterectomy, thereby requiring continued hCG follow-up for GTN [64].

A twin gestation with a complete mole and a coexisting normal fetus is rare, occurring 1: 22,000–100,000 pregnancies [65]. It must be distinguished from a partial mole (triploid pregnancy with fetus). Women with a twin normal fetus/complete mole pregnancy should be counseled that they may be at increased risk for hemorrhage and medical complications as well as the development of persistent GTN. Suction evacuation and curettage are recommended for desired pregnancy termination. However, up to 40% of these pregnancies will result in normal viable fetuses if allowed to continue [65–67].

Prophylactic administration of either methotrexate or actinomycin D chemotherapy at the time of or immediately after evacuation of a hydatidiform mole is associated with a reduction in the incidence of postmolar GTN from approximately 15–20% down to 3–8% [68]. However, the use of prophylactic chemotherapy should be limited to special situations when the risk of postmolar GTN is much greater than normal or where adequate hCG follow-up is not possible, as essentially all patients who are followed up with serial hCG testing after molar evacuation and found to have persistent GTN can be cured with appropriate chemotherapy [68–70].

54.8.2 Follow-Up After Molar Evacuation

Follow-up after the evacuation of a hydatidiform mole is an essential part of the management of the condition to detect trophoblastic sequelae (invasive mole or choriocarcinoma), which develop in approximately 15–20% with complete mole and 1–5% with partial mole [33, 36–38]. The clinical findings of rapid uterine involution, corpus lutein cyst regression, and cessation of bleeding are good reassuring signs of disease resolution. Definitive follow-up, however, requires serial serum quantitative hCG measurements fortnightly until three normal consecutive tests (hCG level < 5 mIU/mL), after which hCG levels should be measured 3-monthly for 6 months. More than half of all the patients will have complete regression of hCG to normal within 2 months of evacuation.

Contraception is recommended for 6 months after the first normal hCG result, to differentiate between a rising hCG as a result of persistent or recurrent disease from a rising hCG associated with a current pregnancy. Oral contraceptive pills are the preferable contraceptive method because they have the advantage of suppressing endogenous LH, which may interfere with the measurement of hCG at low levels and studies have shown conclusively that they do not increase the risk of postmolar GTN [62, 71, 72]. In all future pregnancies in women managed for molar pregnancy, it is recommended that the placenta and other products of conception be pathologically examined and the hCG level should also be measured 6 weeks postpartum.

The risk of persistent disease after the evacuation of a complete mole increases if the pre-evacuation hCG level >100,000 mIU/mL, the uterine size (>20 weeks), and theca lutein cysts >6 cm in diameter. Patients with ≥1 of these signs have approximately a 40% incidence of persistent disease compared to 4% for those without any of these signs. Patients older than 40 years, with a repeat molar pregnancy, aneuploidy, and with medical complications of molar pregnancy, such as toxemia, hyperthyroidism, and trophoblastic embolization, are also at increased risk for persistent disease [73].

54.8.3 Gestational Trophoblastic Neoplasia (GTN)

The International Federation of Gynecology and Obstetrics (FIGO) defined a set of criteria for diagnosing persistent GTD in 2000 [40]. Postmolar GTN is usually diagnosed when hCG levels plateau or rise during follow-up after molar evacuation, without histologic diagnosis. An hCG plateau is defined as a less than 10% decline in four measurements taken over 3 weeks. A rise is defined as a greater than 20% increase in three measurements taken over 2 weeks. The presence of elevated hCG in addition to metastases is usually diagnostic of choriocarcinoma, whereas with PSTT serum hCG levels are only slightly elevated, making diagnosis particularly difficult [48, 74]. Although a diagnosis of GTN can be confirmed histologically by examination of the curettage, or hysterectomy specimens, or the placenta, or biopsy of metastatic lesions, the risk of hemorrhage is too high making these procedures too risky and unnecessary [75]. When there is a suspicion GTN in any patient, a metastatic workup and evaluation of risk factors should be performed.

A good history, physical examination, and laboratory work-up (full blood cell count, coagulation studies, serum chemistries, blood grouping and cross-matching, and quantitative serum hCG level) should be done. Radiologic studies should start with a chest X-ray; if abnormal, a CT or MRI of the chest should be requested to detect pulmonary metastases. CT scans of the abdomen and pelvis and MRI of the brain should also be performed. Majority of patients with brain metastases (94%) have associated lung involvement; conversely, 20% of patients with lung metastases also have brain involvement [74].

GTN usually spreads mainly by the hematogenous route. Venous metastasis can occur in the subvaginal venous plexus, resulting in vaginal metastases, or in the main uterine venous system with metastases to the parametrium and lungs [75]. Also, direct shunting into the systemic circulation may occur; the majority of disseminated metastases develop only after pulmonary metastases had occurred. The brain, liver, GI tract, and kidneys are the distant organs most often affected, but metastases to virtually every organ have been reported, lymphatic spread can also occur though this is relatively uncommon [76, 77].

54.8.4 Staging and Risk Scoring

FIGO adopted a combined anatomic staging system and a modified version of the WHO risk factor scoring system for GTN in 2000 [78]. In this 2000 FIGO revised system, the original anatomic stages were retained (Table 54.2), but the 1992 risk factors were replaced by a risk factor score that used a modification of the WHO prognostic index score. This risk score takes into consideration eight criteria, each of which is given a score from 0 to 4. The changes to the WHO classification included the elimination of ABO blood group risk factors and a change in the risk score for liver metastasis from 2 to 4, reflecting a worse prognosis for patients with liver metastasis (Table 54.3). Radiographic staging studies were standardized and the three risk groups of the WHO prognostic index score were consolidated into two groups: low risk with a score of 6 or less and high risk with a score of 7 or more. In this current FIGO system, pulmonary metastases are only counted and measured if they are visible on a chest radiograph. Other recommended studies include CT scan of the abdomen and pelvis, ultrasonography of the uterus, and MRI or contrasted CT scan of the brain. It must be noted that the hCG level used to generate the risk score is that recorded at the time the GTN is diagnosed and not the hCG at the time of molar evacuation.

Thus using the new FIGO system, the classification of patients includes both anatomic stage and FIGO risk score.

Table 54.2 FIGO 2000 anatomic staging for gestational trophoblastic neoplasia

Stage	Criteria
I	Disease confined to uterus
II	Disease extends outside uterus but is limited to genital structures (adnexa, vagina, broad ligament)
III	Disease extends to lungs with or without genital tract involvement
IV	Disease involves other metastatic sites

Table 54.3 The revised FIGO 2000 scoring system for gestational trophoblastic neoplasia

FIGO score	0	1	2	4
Age (years)	<40	≥40	–	–
Antecedent pregnancy	Hydatidiform mole	Abortion	Term pregnancy	–
Interval from index pregnancy (months)	<4	4–6	7–12	≥13
Pretreatment hCG (mIU/mL)	<1000	1000–<10,000	10,000–100,000	>100,000
Largest tumor size including uterus (cm)	<3	3–5	>5	–
Site of metastases	–	Spleen, kidney	Gastrointestinal	Brain, liver
Number of metastases identified	0	1–4	5–8	>8
Previous failed chemotherapy	–	–	Single drug	≥2 drugs

For instance, a 32-year-old patient with nonmetastatic GTN diagnosed 4 months after molar evacuation with an hCG level of 6000 mIU/mL would be recorded as a FIGO stage I: 2. Also, a 45-year-old patient with index term pregnancy 13 months previously, hCG of 100,000 mIU/mL, two brain metastases, six lung lesions, uterine tumor measuring 6 cm, and a previous methotrexate use failure would be FIGO stage IV: 19. The FIGO system is essential for selecting initial therapy for patients with GTN that will ensure the best possible outcomes with the fewest side effects [79].

54.8.5 Nonmetastatic and Metastatic Low-Risk GTN

This category of patients is those with Stage I disease (nonmetastatic) or Stage II and III disease (metastatic) with a risk score of less than 7. The treatment outcomes of patients treated for nonmetastatic or metastatic low-risk GTN are similar using a variety of chemotherapy regimens. Basically, majority can be cured without recourse to hysterectomy with initial single-agent chemotherapy regimens of methotrexate or dactinomycin (Table 54.4). Methotrexate 0.4 mg/kg/day given by intramuscular (IM) injection for 5 days, with cycles repeated every 12–14 days was the earliest regimen used in treating low-risk GTN [80]. However, about 7–10% of patients initially treated with 5-day IM methotrexate therapy will require a second agent, 1.2% will need multiagent chemotherapy, and only 0.8% require a hysterectomy to achieve a complete remission [81]. Factors significantly associated with methotrexate resistance include pretreatment serum

Table 54.4 Agent and schedule dosage methotrexate

5 day/every 2 weeks	0.4 mg/kg IM or IV (maximum, 25 mg/day total dose)
Weekly	30–50 mg/m^2 IM
Methotrexate–folinic acid rescue	MXT 1 mg/kg IM/ IV, days 1, 3, 5, 7; and folinic acid 0.1 mg/kg IM, days 2, 4, 6, 8
Every 2 weeks methotrexate infusion-	
Folinic acid	MXT 100 mg/m^2 IV bolus; and MXT 200 mg/m^2 12 h infusion with 15 mg PO every 6 h for four doses
Dactinomycin	5 day/every 2 weeks 9–13 mcg/kg/day IV (maximum dose, 500 mcg/day) bolus every 2 weeks 1.25 mg/m^2 IV bolus
Etoposide	5 day/every 2 weeks 200 mg/m^2/day PO
Methotrexate/ dactinomycin	Alternating MTX 0.4 mg/kg (max 25 mg)/day IV or IM for 5 days and Act D 10–13 mg/kg IV every day for 5 days

hCG >50,000 mIU/mL, nonmolar antecedent pregnancy, and histopathologic diagnosis of choriocarcinoma. Methotrexate toxicity is however frequently seen in patients receiving the 5-day methotrexate regimen. Bagshawe and Wilde first reported the use of alternating daily doses of IM methotrexate (1 mg/kg) and leucovorin factor or folinic acid (0.1 mg/kg) for four doses of each agent in an attempt to reduce the toxicity of daily methotrexate regimens [82]. Evaluation of this regimen showed that whereas patients on the methotrexate-folinic acid regimen had higher peak methotrexate levels after treatment with the higher methotrexate dose, trough levels were both subtoxic and subtherapeutic 24 h after methotrexate administration showing the superiority of the lower daily dose regimen [83]. Various other studies suggest that the 5-day methotrexate or dactinomycin protocols or the 8-day methotrexate-folinic acid protocol are more effective than either weekly intramuscular (IM) or intermittent intravenous (IV) infusion of methotrexate or the biweekly single-dose dactinomycin protocols [84, 85].

The need to preserve fertility must be assessed early in the management plan of patients with nonmetastatic and low-risk GTN because early hysterectomy will shorten the duration and amount of chemotherapy needed to produce remission. Hysterectomy may be performed during the first cycle of chemotherapy and chemotherapy should be continued after the hysterectomy until hCG values are normal.

Patients managed with chemotherapy should have weekly hCG values monitored during treatment and there should be hematologic, liver, and renal functions monitoring for toxicity. Chemotherapy should be repeated until hCG levels is normal, and thereafter, at least one cycle of chemotherapy should be given as maintenance chemotherapy to prevent recurrence. Effective contraception is necessary to prevent a new pregnancy while patients are on chemotherapy and hCG monitoring after remission. Oral contraceptives are preferable, given the effect of the LH surge on hCG assay measurement [71]. The overall cure rate for patients with nonmetastatic and low-risk GTN is near 100% and majority of women who wish to preserve fertility can be cured without hysterectomy [86].

54.8.6 High-Risk GTN

54.8.6.1 Chemotherapy

Patients in the high-risk group have metastatic GTN, either Stage II or III disease with a risk factor score greater than 7 or Stage IV disease. A more aggressive treatment with multidrug chemotherapy is the standard of care for high-risk GTN. With appropriate regimens, cure rates up to 90% can be achieved. Treatment failure may arise if treatment is delayed or there is dose reduction due to side effects which may increase the likelihood of tumor resistance. The combination of methotrexate, dactinomycin, and either chlorambucil or cyclophosphamide (MAC) was the standard regimen for many years with remission rates of 63–73% [87, 88]. The Charing Cross group developed in the late 70s, a complex alternating regimen using cyclophosphamide, hydroxyurea, actinomycin D, methotrexate–folinic acid, vincristine, and doxorubicin (CHAMOCA) [89]. The reported sustained remissions with this regimen were 56–83% of patients with high-risk GTN with an overall impression of reduced toxicity compared to MAC. However, a subsequent randomized trial comparing MAC and CHAMOCA found that the primary remission rate and the cure rate were better with MAC compared with CHAMOCA, which also had a more toxic side effect profile [90].

Etoposide has been added to recent regimens of primary combination chemotherapy for GTN. This regime alternate weekly chemotherapy with etoposide, methotrexate-folinic acid rescue, dactinomycin, cyclophosphamide, and vincristine (EMA/CO) and was first developed by the Charing Cross group. The efficacy of the EMA-CO regimen for high-risk GTN has been reported to achieve complete response rates between 71% and 78% and long-term survival rates of 85–94% [91–93]. Today, EMA/CO regimen has become the most widely used first-line choice for the treatment of patients with high-risk GTN (Table 54.5). Toxicity of EMA/CO includes universal alopecia and rarely mucositis/stomatitis, nausea, and vomiting. Myelosuppression is often the acute dose-limiting toxicity. Currently, stem cell support with granulocyte colony-stimulating factor (GC-SF) is being used to avoid dose reductions or treatment delays during EMA/CO therapy arising from myelosupression [94, 95].

The platinum-containing regimens have also been found to be active in treating GTN. Some centers use the EMA-EP regimen for patients with scores greater than 12. The EMA-EP is also the appropriate second-line or Salvage therapy in patients with high-risk metastatic GTN with poor response to EMA/CO or with relapse. Chemotherapy should

Table 54.5 EMA-CO chemotherapy for high-risk GTN

Treatment	Regimen	
Day 1	Etoposide	100 mg/m² IV over 30 min
	Act D	0.5 mg IV
	MTX	100 mg/m² IV, then 200 mg/m² in 500 mL D5W over 12 h
Day 2	Etoposide	100 mg/m² IV over 30 min
	Act D	0.5 mg IV
	Folinic acid	15 mg IM or PO every 12 h for four doses starting 24 h after start of MTX (on day 1)
Day 8	Cyclophosphamide	600 mg/m² IV
	Vincristine	1.0 mg/m² IV

Cycle repeats every 2 weeks (i.e., days 15, 16, and 22)

be continued for at least 2–3 courses after the first normal hCG level is achieved [96].

54.8.6.2 Radiotherapy

Radiotherapy has a limited role generally in the treatment of metastatic GTN but it is deplored most frequently to treat patients with brain or liver metastases in an effort to minimize hemorrhagic complications from disease at these sites.

Brain and liver metastases occur in 8–15% and 2–8% of patients with metastatic GTN respectively and are associated with a worse prognosis than vaginal or pulmonary metastases.

In patients with brain metastases, whole brain radiation (3000 cGy in 200 cGy fractions) is indicated and is usually performed at the start of chemotherapy to reduce the risk of hemorrhage [97]. The EMA-CO regimen is modified such that methotrexate is increased to 1 g/m² with 30 mg of folinic acid every 12 h for 3 days, starting 32 h after the start of infusion. Intrathecal methrotrexate has also been used in patients with brain metastases. Convulsions and cerebral edema should be controlled with anticonvulsants and dexamethasone respectively. The brain lesion should also be monitored with serial CT scan or MRI [98].

54.8.6.3 Surgery

A good number of patients with high-risk metastatic GNT will require some form of adjuvant surgery such as hysterectomy and pulmonary resection for chemotherapy-resistant disease and to control hemorrhage and sepsis [99]. As a general rule, it is important to exclude active disease elsewhere before attempting surgical resection.

54.8.6.4 PSTT

PSTT has slightly different clinicopathological behavior from the other GTNs and thus requires some modification in the way it is managed. It is relatively resistant to chemotherapy with a high risk of lymphatic spread. Therefore, hysterectomy with lymph node dissection is the recommended treatment of choice. Before surgery, histologic diagnosis of PSTT with endometrial biopsy or curettage specimen should be confirmed with immunohistochemical staining for the presence of human placental lactogen and the absence of hCG. Chemotherapy may be used in patients with metastatic disease and in patients with nonmetastatic disease and poor prognostic factors. These poor prognostic factors include: a long interval between antecedent pregnancy and diagnosis (>2 years), deep myometrial invasion, tumor necrosis, and mitotic count greater than 5/10 high-power fields [100]. Hysterectomy should be combined with platinum-containing chemotherapy regimen, such as EMA-EP or a paclitaxel/cisplatin-paclitaxel/etoposide (TP/TE) doublet in patients with poor prognostic factors. This modality of treatment has a survival rate of approximately 100% for nonmetastatic disease and 50–60% for metastatic disease [101, 102].

54.8.7 Follow-Up of Patients with GTN

When hCG has returned to normal levels and treatment has been completed, serum hCG levels should be monitored monthly for 12 months and physical clinical examinations should be performed at intervals of 6–12 months. Most women resume normal ovarian function after chemotherapy with no alteration in fertility even though menopause may occur earlier [103]. Therefore, contraception should be maintained during treatment and for 1 year after completion of chemotherapy, preferably using oral contraceptives, to allow for uninterrupted hCG follow-up. Successful pregnancies and deliveries have been reported after GTN, without an increased rate of abortion, stillbirth, congenital anomalies, prematurity, or major obstetric complications [104–106].

Even though there is no evidence for reactivation of disease in subsequent pregnancies, there is a 1–2% risk of a second GTD event in patients who have had one trophoblastic disease episode independent of previous chemotherapy [105, 106]. Therefore, pelvic ultrasound is recommended in the first trimester of any post-GTN pregnancy to confirm a normal gestation. The products of conception or placentas from subsequent pregnancies should also be carefully examined histopathologically, and a serum quantitative hCG level should be determined 6 weeks after all pregnancies.

54.9 Challenges in Management of GTD in Sub-Saharan Africa

The general challenges in the health systems of most countries in sub-Saharan Africa affect every aspect of prognoses of diseases and engender health inequalities. Some of these challenges are dearth of appropriate health personnel, ill-equipped hospitals, counterfeit and substandard drugs, and out of pocket health financing. Even though the outcome of

GTD management in most developed countries has improved drastically, the case fatality is still very high in sub-Saharan Africa because apart from deficiencies in the health systems, patients also present to the hospitals very late perhaps because of poverty and ignorance [107]. Compliance with follow-up instructions is also very poor.

54.10 Conclusion

Globally, with the advent of early detection and effective uterine evacuation techniques, the serious bleeding and other medical complications associated with molar pregnancy have drastically reduced. The prognoses of GTN which were likewise poor before the advent of chemotherapy, have also improved, even metastatic GTN are no longer death sentences. However, mortality from gestational trophoblastic disease is still relatively high in sub-Saharan Africa because of the peculiar health systems' challenges in this region. The most pragmatic ways to improve the care outcome of GTD in this region are the establishment of dedicated regional referral centers for GTD and the establishment of health insurance schemes to foster universal access to all components of qualitative care including chemotherapy.

54.11 Summary

1. The term gestational trophoblastic disease (GTD) encompasses a spectrum of abnormal cellular proliferations arising from the placental villous trophoblast with the benign and the malignant components occupying the two extremes.
2. The term "gestational trophoblastic neoplasia" (GTN) encompasses the latter three conditions, which can progress, invade, metastasize, and lead to death if not properly treated.
3. Complete hydatidiform moles are derived from the paternal genome and most frequently have a diploid 46XX karyotype.
4. Partial moles are derived from both paternal and maternal genomes, resulting in triploidy, and 69XXX is the commonest karyotype. Partial moles have evidence of fetal development, which differentiates them from complete moles.
5. Malignant GTN is commoner after a complete molar pregnancy than a partial molar pregnancy.
6. Human chorionic gonadotropin (hCG) values should be monitored for 6 months after molar pregnancy evacuation to detect postmolar GTN.
7. GTN is defined by a plateaued, rising, or prolonged persistence of elevated hCG values after molar evacuation; histologic diagnosis of choriocarcinoma, invasive mole, PSTT, or identification of metastatic disease after molar evacuation.
8. GTN is staged based on both the anatomic and the World Health Organization prognostic score as either low risk (<7) or high risk (≥7).
9. Low-risk GTN is treated with methotrexate or dactinomycin. Cure rates are near 100%.
10. High-risk GTN is treated with EMA/CO (etoposide, methotrexate, dactinomycin, cyclophosphamide, and vincristine/oncovin) chemotherapy. Cure rates are >90%.
11. The case fatality of GTD is still high in sub-Saharan Africa due to inefficient health systems and late presentation.

References

1. Soper JT. Gestational trophoblastic disease. Obstet Gynecol. 2006;108:176–87.
2. Berkowitz RS, Goldstein DP. Current management of gestational trophoblastic disease. Gynecol Oncol. 2009;112:654–62.
3. Palmer JR. Advances in the epidemiology of gestational trophoblastic disease. J Reprod Med. 1994;39:155.
4. Chattopadhyay SK, Sengupta BS, Al-Ghreimi M, et al. Epidemiologic study of gestational trophoblastic diseases in Saudi Arabia. Surg Gynecol Obstet. 1988;167:393.
5. Takeuchi S. Incidence of gestational trophoblastic disease by regional registration in Japan. Hum Reprod. 1987;2:729.
6. Chechia A, Koubaa A, Makhlouf T, Anis B, Terras K, Hamouda B, et al. Molar pregnancy retrospective study of 60 cases in Tunisia. Tunis Med. 2001;79:441–6.
7. Osamor JO, Oluwasola AO, Adewole IF. A clinicopathological study of complete and hydatidiform mole in a Nigerian population. J Obstet Gynaecol. 2002;22:423–4.
8. Akosa AB, Mpadu FO, Gyasi RK. A review of complete hydatidiform mole in Ghana. Ghana Med J. 2001;35:85–9.
9. Parazzini F, LaVecchia C, Pampallona S. Parental age and risk of complete and partial hydatidiform mole. Br J Obstet Gynaecol. 1986;93:582–5.
10. Sebire NJ, Foskett M, Fisher RA, et al. Risk of partial and complete molar pregnancy in relation to maternal age. Br J Obstet Gynaecol. 2002;109:99–102.
11. Mazzanti P, LaVecchia C, Parazzini F, et al. Frequency of hydatidiform mole in Lombardy, Italy. Gynecol Oncol. 1986;24:337.
12. Bagshawe KD, Dent J, Webb J. Hydatidiform mole in England and Wales 1973-1983. Lancet. 1986;2:673.
13. Parazzini F, LaVecchia C, Mangili G, et al. Dietary factors and risk of trophoblastic disease. Am J Obstet Gynecol. 1988;158:93.
14. Acaia B, Parazzini F, LaVecchia C, et al. Increased frequency of complete hydatidiform mole in women with repeated abortion. Gynecol Oncol. 1988;31:310.
15. Brinton LA, Wu BZ, Wang W, et al. Gestational trophoblastic disease: a case-control study from the People's Republic of China. Am J Obstet Gynecol. 1989;161:121.
16. Atrash HK, Hogue CJ, Grimes DA. Epidemiology of hydatidiform mole during early gestation. Am J Obstet Gynecol. 1986;154:906.
17. Brinton LA, Bracken MB, Connelly RR. Choriocarcinoma incidence in the United States. Am J Epidemiol. 1986;123:1094–100.

18. Smith HO, Qualls CR, Prairie BA, et al. Trends in gestational choriocarcinoma: a 27-year perspective. Obstet Gynecol. 2003;102:978–87.
19. Mazur MT, Kurman RJ. Choriocarcinoma and placenta site tumour. In: Szulman AE, Buchsbaum HJ, editors. Gestational trophoblastic disease. New York: Springer-Verlag; 1987. p. 45.
20. McAna JF. Gestational choriocarcinoma in New York state. Diss Abstr Int. 1987;48:694.
21. Kajii T, Ohama K. Androgenetic origin of hydatidiform mole. Nature. 1977;268:633.
22. Surti U, Szulma AE, O'Brien S. Dispermic origin and clinical outcome of three complete hydatidiform moles with 46,XY karyotype. Am J Obstet Gynecol. 1982;144:84.
23. Fisher RA, Hodges MD. Genomic imprinting in gestational trophoblastic disease: a review. Placenta. 2003;24:111–8.
24. Al-Hussaini TK, Abd el-Aal DM, Van den Veyver IB. Recurrent pregnancy loss due to familial and non-familial habitual molar pregnancy. Int J Gynaecol Obstet. 2003;83(2):179–86.
25. Hodges MD, Rees HC, Seckl MJ, et al. Genetic refinement and physical mapping of a biparental complete mole locus on chromosome 19q13.4. J Med Genet. 2003;40(8):95.
26. Jacobs PA, Szulman AE, Funkhouser J, et al. Human triploidy: relationship between paternal origin of the additional haploid component and development of partial hydatidiform mole. Ann Hum Genet. 1982;46:223.
27. Lawler SD, Fisher RA, Pickhall VJ, et al. Genetic studies on hydatidiform moles: the origin of partial moles. Cancer Genet Cytogenet. 1982;5:309.
28. Szulman AE. Trophoblastic disease: clinical pathology of hydatidiform moles. Obstet Gynecol Clin N Am. 1988;15:433.
29. Lewis GH, DeScipio K, Murphy M, et al. Characterization of androgenetic/biparental mosaic/chimeric conceptions, including those with a molar component: morphology, p57 immunohistochemistry, molecular genotyping, and risk of persistent gestational trophoblastic disease. Int J Gynecol Pathol. 2013;32(2):199–214.
30. Szulman AE, Surti U. The syndromes of hydatidiform moles. 1: Cytogenetic and morphologic correlations. Am J Obstet Gynecol. 1978;131:665.
31. Szulman AE, Surti U. The syndromes of hydatidiform moles. 2: Morphologic evolution of the complete and partial mole. Am J Obstet Gynecol. 1978;132:20.
32. Berkowitz RS, Goldstein DP, DuBeshter B, et al. Management of complete molar pregnancy. J Reprod Med. 1987;32:634.
33. Curry SL, Harmond CG, Tyrey L, et al. Hydatidiform mole. Diagnosis, management and long term follow up of 347 patients. Obstet Gynecol. 1975;45:1.
34. Montz FJ, Schaerth JB, Morrow CP. The natural history of theca lutein cysts. Obstet Gynecol. 1988;72:247.
35. Amir SM, Osathanoudh R, Berkowitz RS, et al. Human chorionic gonadotropin and thyroid function in patients with hydatidiform mole. Am J Obstet Gynecol. 1984;150:723.
36. Brewer JI, Torok EE, Webster A, et al. Hydatidiform mole: a follow up regime for identification of invasive mole and choriocarcinoma and for selection of patients for treatment. Am J Obstet Gynecol. 1968;101:557.
37. Lurain JR, Brewer JI, Torok EE, et al. Natural history of hydatidiform mole after primary evacuation. Am J Obstet Gynecol. 1983;145:591.
38. Szulman AE, Surti U. The clinicopathologic profile of the partial hydatidiform mole. Obstet Gynecol. 1982;59:597–602.
39. Lurain J, Brewer JL. Invasive mole. Semin Oncol. 1982;9:174.
40. Allison KH, Love JE, Garcia RL. Epithelioid trophoblastic tumor: review of a rare neoplasm of the chorionic-type intermediate trophoblast. Arch Pathol Lab Med. 2006;130(12):1875–7.
41. Curry SL, Hammond CB, Tyrey L, et al. Hydatidiform mole: diagnosis, management, and long-term follow-up of 347 patients. Obstet Gynecol. 1975;45:1–8.
42. Kohorn EI. Molar pregnancy: presentation and diagnosis. Clin Obstet Gynecol. 1984;27:181–9.
43. Soto-Wright V, Bernstein MR, Goldstein DP, et al. The changing clinical presentation of complete molar pregnancy. Obstet Gynecol. 1995;86:775–9.
44. Hou JL, Wan XR, Xiang Y, et al. Changes in clinical features in hydatidiform mole: analysis on 113 cases. J Reprod Med. 2008;53:629–33.
45. Czernobilsky B, Barash A, Lancet M. Partial moles: a clinicopathologic study of 25 cases. Obstet Gynecol. 1982;59:75–7.
46. Berkowitz RS, Goldstein DP, Bernstein MR. Natural history of partial molar pregnancy. Obstet Gynecol. 1985;66:677–81.
47. Lurain JR. Gestational trophoblastic tumors. Semin Surg Oncol. 1990;6:347–53.
48. Baergen RN, Rutgers JL, Young RH, et al. Placental site trophoblastic tumor: a study of 55 cases and review of the literature emphasizing factors of prognostic significance. Gynecol Oncol. 2006;100(3):511–20.
49. Shih IM, Kurman RJ. Epithelioid trophoblastic tumor: a neoplasm distinct from choriocarcinoma and placental site trophoblastic tumor simulating carcinoma. Am J Surg Pathol. 1998;22:1393–403.
50. Santos-Ramos R, Forney JP, Schwarz BE. Sonographic findings and clinical correlations in molar pregnancy. Obstet Gynecol. 1980;56:186–92.
51. Benson CB, Genest DR, Bernstein MR, et al. Sonographic appearance of first trimester complete hydatidiform moles. Ultrasound Obstet Gynecol. 2000;16:188–91.
52. Cole LA. hCG, its free subunits and its metabolites: roles in pregnancy and trophoblastic disease. J Reprod Med. 1998;43:3–10.
53. Berkowitz RS, Ozturk M, Goldstein D, et al. Human chorionic gonadotropin and free subunits' serum levels in patients with partial and complete hydatidiform moles. Obstet Gynecol. 1989;74:212–6.
54. Ozturk M, Berkowitz R, Goldstein D, et al. Differential production of human chorionic gonadotropin and free subunits in gestational trophoblastic disease. Am J Obstet Gynecol. 1988;158:193–8.
55. Rotmensch S, Cole LA. False diagnosis and needless therapy of presumed malignant disease in women with false-positive human chorionic gonadotropin concentrations. Lancet. 2000;355:712–5.
56. Hancock BW. hCG measurement in gestational trophoblastic neoplasia: a critical appraisal. J Reprod Med. 2006;51:859–60.
57. Winder AD, Mora AS, Berry E, Lurain JR. The "hook effect" causing a negative pregnancy test in patient with an advanced molar pregnancy. Gynecol Oncol Rep. 2017;21:34–6.
58. Cole LA, Butler SA, Khanlian SA, et al. Gestational trophoblastic diseases, hyperglycosylated hCG as a tumor marker of active neoplasia. Gynecol Oncol. 2006;102:151–9.
59. Khanlian SA, Cole LA. Management of gestational trophoblastic disease and other cases with low serum levels of human chorionic gonadotropin. J Reprod Med. 2006;51:812–8.
60. Soper JT. Surgical therapy for gestational trophoblastic disease. J Reprod Med. 1994;39:168–74.
61. Tidy JA, Gillespie AM, Bright N, et al. Gestational trophoblastic disease: a study of mode of evacuation and subsequent need for treatment with chemotherapy. Gynecol Oncol. 2000;78:309–12.
62. Berkowitz RS, Goldstein DS. Clinical practice: molar pregnancy. N Engl J Med. 2009;360:1639–45.
63. Hancock BW, Tidy JA. Current management of molar pregnancy. J Reprod Med. 2002;47:347–54.
64. Fishman DA, Padilla LA, Keh P, et al. Management of twin pregnancies consisting of a complete hydatidiform mole and normal fetus. Obstet Gynecol. 1998;91:546–50.
65. Matsui H, Sekiya S, Hando T, et al. Hydatidiform mole coexistent with a twin live fetus: a national collaborative study in Japan. Hum Reprod. 2000;15:608–11.

66. Sebire NJ, Foskett M, Paradinas FJ, et al. Outcome of twin pregnancies with complete hydatidiform mole and healthy co-twin. Lancet. 2002;359:2165–6.
67. Kashimura Y, Kashmira M, Sugimori H, et al. Prophylactic chemotherapy for hydatidiform mole: 5-15 years follow-up. Cancer. 1986;58:624–9.
68. Kim DS, Moon H, Kim KT, et al. Effects of prophylactic chemotherapy for persistent trophoblastic disease in patients with complete hydatidiform mole. Obstet Gynecol. 1986;67:690–4.
69. Limpongsanurak S. Prophylactic actinomycin D for high-risk complete hydatidiform mole. J Reprod Med. 2001;46:110–6.
70. Berkowitz RS, Goldstein DP, Marean AR, et al. Oral contraceptives and postmolar gestational trophoblastic disease. Obstet Gynecol. 1981;58:474–7.
71. Curry SL, Schlaerth JB, Kohorn EI, et al. Hormonal contraception and trophoblastic sequelae after hydatidiform mole (a gynecologic oncology group study). Am J Obstet Gynecol. 1989;160:805–11.
72. Deicas RE, Miller DS, Rademaker AW, et al. The role of contraception in the development of postmolar gestational trophoblastic tumor. Obstet Gynecol. 1991;78:221–6.
73. FIGO Oncology Committee. FIGO staging for gestational trophoblastic neoplasia 2000. FIGO Oncology Committee. Int J Gynaecol Obstet. 2002;77(3):285–7.
74. Berry E, Hagopian GS, Lurain JR. Vaginal metastases in gestational trophoblastic neoplasia. J Reprod Med. 2008;53(7):487–92.
75. Athanassiou A, Begent RH, Newlands ES, et al. Central nervous system metastases of choriocarcinoma: 23 years' experience at Charing Cross Hospital. Cancer. 1983;52(9):1728–35.
76. Kumar J, Ilancheran A, Ratnam SS. Pulmonary metastasis in gestational trophoblastic disease: a review of 97 cases. Br J Obstet Gynaecol. 1988;95(1):70–4.
77. Ngan HY, Bender H, Benedet JL, et al. Gestational trophoblastic neoplasia, FIGO 2000 staging and classification. Int J Gynaecol Obstet. 2003;83(suppl. 1):175–7.
78. Lurain JR, Casanova LA, Miller DS, et al. Prognostic factors in gestational trophoblastic tumors: a proposed new scoring system based on multivariate analysis. Am J Obstet Gynecol. 1991;164(2):611–6.
79. Hammond CB, Hertz R, Ross GT, et al. Primary chemotherapy for nonmetastatic gestational trophoblastic neoplasms. Am J Obstet Gynecol. 1967;98:71.
80. Homesley HD. Single agent therapy for nonmetastatic and low-risk gestational trophoblastic disease. J Reprod Med. 1998;43(1):69–74.
81. Bagshawe KD, Wilde CE. Infusion therapy for pelvic tumours. Br J Obstet Gynaecol. 1964;71:565.
82. Smith EB, Weed JC Jr, Tyrey L, et al. Treatment of nonmetastatic gestational trophoblastic disease: results of methotrexate alone versus methotrexate-folinic acid. Am J Obstet Gynecol. 1982;144:88.
83. Lurain JR. Pharmacotherapy of gestational trophoblastic disease. Expert Opin Pharmacother. 2003;4(11):2005–17.
84. Alazzam M, Tidy J, Hancock BW, et al. First line chemotherapy in low risk gestational trophoblastic neoplasia. Cochrane Database Syst Rev. 2009;(1):CD007102.
85. Berkowitz RS, Goldstein DP, Bernstein MR. Ten year's experience with methotrexate and folinic acid as primary therapy for gestational trophoblastic disease. Gynecol Oncol. 1986;23:111.
86. Hammond CB, Borchert LG, Tyrey L, et al. Treatment of metastatic trophoblastic disease: good and poor prognosis. Am J Obstet Gynecol. 1973;115:4.
87. Lurain JR, Brewer JI. Treatment of high-risk gestational trophoblastic disease with methotrexate, actinomycin D and cyclophosphamide chemotherapy. Obstet Gynecol. 1985;65:830.
88. Bagshawe KD. Treatment of trophoblastic tumours. Ann Acad Med Singap. 1976;5:273.
89. Curry SL, Blessing JA, DiSaia PJ, et al. A prospective randomized comparison of methotrexate, dactinomycin, and chlorambucil versus methotrexate, dactinomycin, cyclophosphamide, doxorubicin, melphalan, hydroxyurea, and vincristine in "poor prognosis" metastatic gestational trophoblastic disease: a Gynecologic Oncology Group study. Obstet Gynecol. 1989;73(3 Pt 1):357–62.
90. Bolis G, Bonazzi C, Landoni F, et al. EMA/CO regimen in high-risk gestational trophoblastic tumor (GTT). Gynecol Oncol. 1988;31(3):439–44.
91. Bower M, Newlands ES, Holden L, et al. EMA/CO for high-risk gestational trophoblastic tumors: results from a cohort of 272 patients. J Clin Oncol. 1997;15(7):2636–43.
92. Lurain JR, Singh DK, Schink JC. Primary treatment of metastatic high-risk gestational trophoblastic neoplasia with EMA-CO chemotherapy. J Reprod Med. 2006;51(10):767–72.
93. Turan T, Karacay O, Tulunay G, et al. Results with EMA/CO (etoposide, methotrexate, actinomycin D, cyclophosphamide, vincristine) chemotherapy in gestational trophoblastic neoplasia. Int J Gynecol Cancer. 2006;16(3):1432–8.
94. Lu WG, Ye F, Shen YM, et al. EMA-CO chemotherapy for high-risk gestational trophoblastic neoplasia: a clinical analysis of 54 patients. Int J Gynecol Cancer. 2008;18(2):357–62.
95. Newlands ES, Bagshawe KD, Begent RHJ, et al. Developments in chemotherapy for medium- and high-risk patients with gestational trophoblastic tumours (1979–1984). Br J Obstet Gynaecol. 1986;93:63.
96. Small W Jr, Lurain JR, Shetty RM, et al. Gestational trophoblastic disease metastatic to the brain. Radiology. 1996;200(1):277–80.
97. Rustin GJ, Newlands ES, Begent RH, et al. Weekly alternating etoposide, methotrexate, and actinomycin/vincristine and cyclophosphamide chemotherapy for the treatment of CNS metastases of choriocarcinoma. J Clin Oncol. 1989;7(7):900–3.
98. Lurain JR, Singh DK, Schink JC. Role of surgery in the management of high-risk gestational trophoblastic neoplasia. J Reprod Med. 2006;51(10):773–6.
99. Bower M, Paradinas FJ, Fisher RA, et al. Placental site trophoblastic tumor: molecular analysis and clinical experience. Clin Cancer Res. 1996;2(5):897–902.
100. Chang YL, Chang TC, Hsueh S, et al. Prognostic factors and treatment for placental site trophoblastic tumor-report of 3 cases and analysis of 88 cases. Gynecol Oncol. 1999;73(2):216–22.
101. Hassadia A, Gillespie A, Tidy J, et al. Placental site trophoblastic tumour: clinical features and management. Gynecol Oncol. 2005;99(3):603–7.
102. Schmid P, Nagai Y, Agarwal R, et al. Prognostic markers and long-term outcome of placental-site trophoblastic tumours: a retrospective observational study. Lancet. 2009;374(9683):48–55.
103. Bower M, Rustin GJ, Newlands ES, et al. Chemotherapy for gestational trophoblastic tumours hastens menopause by 3 years. Eur J Cancer. 1998;34(8):1204–7.
104. Garrett LA, Garner EI, Feltmate CM, et al. Subsequent pregnancy outcomes in patients with molar pregnancy and persistent gestational trophoblastic neoplasia. J Reprod Med. 2008;53(7):481–6.
105. Woolas RP, Bower M, Newlands ES, et al. Influence of chemotherapy for gestational trophoblastic disease on subsequent pregnancy outcome. Br J Obstet Gynaecol. 1998;105(9):1032–5.
106. Matsui H, Iitsuka Y, Suzuka K, et al. Early pregnancy outcomes after chemotherapy for gestational trophoblastic tumor. J Reprod Med. 2004;49(7):531–4.
107. Iyoke CA, Ugwu GO, Ezugwu EC, et al. Challenges associated with the management of gynecological cancers in a tertiary hospital in South East Nigeria. Int J Womens Health. 2014;6:123–30.

Cancers of the Vagina and Vulva

55

Rakiya Saidu and Lynette Denny

Learning Objectives

After studying this chapter, the student should be able to:

- Demonstrate an understanding the aetio-pathogenesis of cancers of the vagina and vulva
- Discuss the clinical features, diagnosis and staging of vaginal and vulvar cancers
- Discuss the management, treatment and prognosis of vaginal and vulvar cancers

55.1 Overview

Cancers of the vagina and vulva are not common and make up about 6% (vulva) and about 1–2% (vagina) of all malignancies of the female genital tract. They are however significant cancers to women's health because of the distressing disease and treatment-related morbidities, including reduced quality of life and sexual functionality, leg oedema, bleeding and foul odour [1, 2].

55.2 Cancer of the Vagina

About 80% of tumours involving the vagina are secondary from direct extension (from the cervix, endometrium, vulva, bladder and rectum) or metastatic by lymphatic or haematogenous spread (from the ovaries, choriocarcinoma, renal, breast and colon) [3]. Primary cancer of the vagina is rare.

In 2008 about 13,000 new cases of primary vaginal cancer were diagnosed worldwide, accounting for 1–3% of all gynaecologic malignancies [3, 4]. According to estimates, there will be 5170 new cases and 1330 deaths from vaginal cancer in the United States, in 2018 [5].

Vaginal cancer is a disease of the elderly, diagnosed after the age of 60 in more than half of the cases, with the median age at diagnosis of 65 years. It is rarely diagnosed in women under 45 years, although there are reports of cases in young women in their 20s and 30s [4, 6].

55.2.1 Aetiology of Vaginal Cancer

Vaginal cancer is believed to have risk factors similar to cervical cancer. Like cervical cancer, it has a premalignant disease called vaginal intra-epithelial neoplasia (VAIN), but unlike in the case of cervical cancer, the natural history and true malignant potential of VAIN is not fully understood. Between 3% and 7% of patients with VAIN will progress to invasive disease despite treatment [4, 7, 8]. VAIN and invasive vaginal cancer have a strong relationship to infection with human papilloma virus (HPV). Studies have shown that HPV DNA was detected in about 70% of invasive vaginal cancer (91% of VAIN 2/3, 100% in VAIN 1) and HPV 16 was the most frequent HPV type identified in 50–70% of the HPV-positive cancers [4, 9–12].

Women with a history of prior anogenital cancer, particularly cervical cancer have a relatively increased risk of developing vaginal cancer. About 30% of patients with primary vaginal cancer patients have a history of in situ or invasive cervical cancer 5 years earlier [4, 8, 13]. Radiation-induced tumourigenesis is a possible aetiology of vaginal cancer. Chronic vaginal irritation from the long-term use of vaginal pessaries has been suggested to cause vaginal cancer, but the mechanism by which this promotes carcinogenesis is not well understood [4, 8].

R. Saidu (✉)
College of Health Sciences, University of Ilorin, Ilorin, Nigeria

University of Cape Town, Cape Town, South Africa

L. Denny
Obstetrics and Gynaecology, University of Cape Town, Cape Town, South Africa

Gynaecological Cancer Research Centre, Cape Town, South Africa
e-mail: lynette.denny@uct.ac.za

F. Okonofua et al. (eds.), *Contemporary Obstetrics and Gynecology for Developing Countries*,
https://doi.org/10.1007/978-3-030-75385-6_55

55.2.2 Screening for Vaginal Cancer

The incidence of vaginal cancer is very low. Therefore, routine screening in all women is not cost effective. Pap smear is used to monitor women who had previous cervical dysplasia or invasive disease and also those who had a hysterectomy for non-benign indications.

55.2.3 Symptoms and Signs of Vaginal Cancer

Painless vaginal bleeding is the most common symptom reported by patients with vaginal cancer. The bleeding is usually postcoital or postmenopausal. A watery, blood-stained and malodorous vaginal discharge may be the presenting symptom. A vaginal mass may be noticed by the patient [7, 13, 14]. Some women may be asymptomatic, and diagnosis in these patients may be by routine clinical examination or abnormal cytology. Other potential symptoms include urinary (dysuria, frequency) or gastrointestinal (tenesmus, melena stools) that may be related to direct extension of the disease to the surrounding organs. There may be a pelvic pain when the disease extends beyond the vagina [4, 14, 15].

The majority of vagina cancer is in the upper vagina in the posterior wall, usually exophytic lesions [4, 16].

If the patient has an abnormal pap smear, but no visible lesion, a thorough vaginal colposcopic examination is necessary, and an upper vaginectomy may be required to make a diagnosis of early vaginal cancer [8, 13, 14].

55.2.4 Pathology

The vagina extends from the vulva upward to the uterine cervix lined by squamous epithelium. The lymphatic drainage of the vagina is towards the pelvic nodes from its upper two-thirds and towards the inguinal nodes from its lower third.

55.2.4.1 Pathological Types of Vaginal Cancer

Squamous cell carcinoma is the most common type of vaginal cancer, comprising about 80%. Other pathological types of vaginal cancers include adenocarcinoma (10%), malignant melanoma (less than 2%), sarcoma that present as leiomyosarcomas in adults and sarcoma botryoides in children (2%) other rarer pathologies include while carcinoid, undifferentiated and lymphomas form about 1.5% [4, 14, 17]. Diethylstilbesterol (DES) associated clear cell carcinoma of the vagina and other genital tract abnormalities have been reported in young women exposed to DES in utero in the 1970s. DES-associated clear cell carcinoma is now rare since the drug was discontinued in the 1970s [14].

55.2.4.2 Histologic Grading of Vulvar Cancer

The histopathologic grading of squamous cell carcinoma of the vagina is as follows [8]:

1. GX where the grade cannot be assessed
2. G1: Well differentiated
3. G2: Moderately differentiated
4. G3: Poorly or undifferentiated

55.2.4.3 Patterns of Spread of Vaginal Cancer

Vaginal cancer spread by direct invasion of pelvic soft tissues including parametria, bladder, urethra, rectum and eventually the bony pelvis. It also spreads by lymphatics to the pelvic nodes and the para-aortic nodes when the lesion is in the upper vagina. When the lesion is in the distal third of the vagina, it spreads to the inguinal nodes first then to the pelvic lymph nodes. Late in the disease, it can spread by the haematogenous route to distant organs like the lungs, liver and bone [4, 8, 14, 16].

55.2.5 Staging of Vaginal Cancer

Staging vaginal cancer is currently based on the 2009 International Federation of Gynaecology and Obstetrics (FIGO) staging system as shown in Table 55.1 [18].

The FIGO staging is clinical and based on clinical examination, cystoscopy, proctoscopy and chest x-ray. Additional information obtained from resected vaginal tissue, pelvic and peritoneal lymph nodes at surgery should not alter the FIGO staging but should be noted as pathological staging using the tumour, nodes and metastases (TNM) classification of the American Joint Committee on Cancer (AJCC) as described in Tables 55.2 and 55.3 [19].

Table 55.1 Carcinoma of the vagina: FIGO nomenclature

Stage I	The carcinoma is limited to the vaginal wall
Stage II	The carcinoma has involved the subvaginal tissue but has not extended to the pelvic wall
Stage III	The carcinoma has extended to the pelvic wall
Stage IV	The carcinoma has extended to the beyond the true pelvis or has involved the mucosa of the bladder or rectum; bullous oedema as such does not permit a case to be allotted stage IV
IVA	Tumour invades bladder and/or rectal mucosa and/or direct extension beyond the true pelvis
IVB	Spread to distant organs

Table 55.2 Carcinoma of the vagina: the definitions of TNM staging

Definition	
Primary Tumour	
Tx	Primary tumour cannot be assessed
T0	No evidence of primary tumour
Tis[a]	Carcinoma in situ (preinvasive carcinoma)
T1	Tumour confined to vagina
T2	Tumour invades paravaginal tissues but not to pelvic wall
T3	Tumour extends to pelvic wall[b]
T4	Tumour invades mucosa of the bladder or rectum and/or extends beyond the true pelvis (bullous oedema is not sufficient evidence to classify a tumour as T4)
Regional Lymph Nodes	
Nx	Regional lymph nodes cannot be assessed
N0	No regional lymph node metastasis
N1	Pelvic or inguinal lymph node metastasis
Metastasis	
M0	No distant metastasis
M1	Distant metastasis

[a]FIGO no longer includes Stage 0 (Tis)
[b]Pelvic wall is defined as muscle, fascia, neurovascular structures or skeletal portions of the bony pelvis. On rectal examination, there is no cancer-free space between the tumour and pelvic walls

Table 55.3 FIGO staging and its corresponding TNM staging

FIGO	TNM		
	T	N	M
0	Tis	N0	M0
I	T1	N0	M0
II	T2	N0	M0
III	T1	N1	M0
	T2	N1	M0
	T3	N0	M0
	T3	N1	M0
Iva	T4	Any N	M0
IVb	Any T	Any N	M1

55.2.6 Diagnosis of Vaginal Cancer

A full work-up including adequate history, physical examination and relevant investigations are needed to determine the extent of the disease and prepare the patient towards therapy. It is essential to carry out a detailed pelvic examination, if necessary, under anaesthesia to determine the stage of the disease and to take biopsies for definitive diagnosis.

To make a diagnosis of vaginal cancer, the primary site of the growth must be in the vagina. The growth should not involve the cervix, urethra or vulva. Tumours that extend to the portio and reached the external os should be considered cervical cancers, those tumours limited to the urethra should be considered urethral cancers, while those involving the vulva should be classified as vulvar cancers [8, 13].

55.2.7 Treatment of Vaginal Cancer

The patients diagnosed with vaginal cancer should be managed in a specialist centre. Treatment is individualised, varying, depending on the stage of disease and the site of vaginal involvement and whenever possible, an effort should be made to maintain a functional vagina [8, 16, 20].

55.2.7.1 Chemoradiation

The concurrent use of radiation with chemotherapy (5-fluorouracil and cisplatin) is the standard treatment of locally advanced vaginal cancer [27]. A recent National Cancer Database study reported an increase in the use of chemoradiation from 20.8% in 1998 to 59.1% in 2011 [27]. Chemoradiation has been reported by several studies to improve survival and well tolerated by the patients [24].

55.2.7.2 Radiation Therapy

Radiation therapy involves using external beam radiation (EBRT) supplemented with intracavitary (for lesions <5 mm thick) or interstitial brachytherapy (for thicker lesions). Carefully selected patients with stages I and II lesions can be treated with brachytherapy alone. The total radiation dose should range between 70 and 85 Gy [4, 8, 15, 16, 24–26].

55.2.7.3 Surgery

Surgery has a limited role in the management of vaginal cancer due to the very close relationship of the vagina to the other organs in the pelvis particularly the bladder and the rectum. In carefully selected patients, the role of surgery includes the following situations [4, 8, 16, 20–23]:

1. Stage 1 disease in the upper posterior vagina and the procedure involves a radical hysterectomy, partial vaginectomy and pelvic lymphadenectomy. If the patient has had a hysterectomy, then radical upper vaginectomy and pelvic lymphadenectomies should be done.
2. Pelvic exenteration with vaginal reconstruction for women with stage IV disease with rectovaginal or vesicovaginal fistula. Bilateral inguino-femoral lymphadenectomy should be included if the distal vagina is involved in the disease.
3. Pelvic exenteration may be required women with central recurrence the after irradiation.

55.2.8 Prognosis

The 5-year survival rate for vaginal cancer has been reported to be 52%, which is lower than that of cervical cancer [4]. Other reports have indicated survival rates close to that of the cervix.

Beller et al. in the 26th Annual Report on the Results of Treatment in Gynaecological Cancer reported that the 5-year survival rate of vaginal cancer was 77.6% in stage I, 52.2% in stage II, 42.5% in stage III, 20.5% in stage IVa and 12.9% in stage IVb. Frank et al. from the University of Texas MD Anderson Cancer Centre reported a 5-year survival rate of 85% for stage I, 78% for stage II and 58% for stages III and IV [17, 28].

55.3 Cancer of the Vulva

Cancer of the vulva is rare among women worldwide, accounting for 3–5% of cancers of the female genital tract. In 2008, it there was approximately 27,000 new cases worldwide [3] and more than half of these occurred in developed countries. Traditionally, it is a disease predominantly found in elderly women, with a median age of diagnosis of 65–70 years [29]. In recent decades, the incidence of both vulva intraepithelial neoplasia (VIN), the precursor lesion to invasive vulvar cancer and invasive vulvar cancer has increased worldwide, and the median age of onset has reduced [2, 30–33]. The median age was reported to be 10–15 years younger in women in South Africa [36]. The overall increasing incidence of vulvar cancer has been attributed to increasing diagnosis of vulvar cancer in young women, presumably as a result of increasing human papillomavirus (HPV) associated VIN in this group of women [2, 30, 34, 35].

55.3.1 Aetiopathogenesis of Vulvar Cancer

There are two different etiological pathways for the development of squamous cell carcinoma of the vulva.

The first type, the HPV-related vulva squamous cell carcinoma mainly occurs in relatively younger women, related to HPV infection, smoking, impaired immunological status and it is commonly associated with the usual type (undifferentiated) VIN [4, 39, 40, 41].

The second type and more common HPV-independent vulva squamous cell carcinoma are mainly found in elderly patients, not related to HPV or smoking. Concurrent VIN is uncommon in this group of patients, and when VIN is present, it is of differentiated type and situated adjacent to the tumour. It frequently occurs in women with chronic dystrophic diseases, especially lichen sclerosis [4, 30, 40, 41].

There are three histological subtypes of squamous cell carcinoma of the vulva [37, 42]:

1. Basaloid squamous cell carcinoma is composed of cells similar to the cells of the basal layer of the epidermis with scanty cytoplasm and little keratinisation.
2. Warty squamous cell carcinoma is composed of cells that form irregular nests, often keratinised and with prominent koilocytic changes.
3. Keratinising squamous cell carcinoma is composed of differentiated cells with abundant keratin pearls and no koilocytosis. This is the most common type of vulva cancer.

Basaloid and warty squamous cell carcinoma of the vulva have been associated with HPV infection, and the keratinising squamous cell carcinoma are usually HPV negative. However, predicting the HPV association by histologic type of tumour is of limited reliability because studies have shown an overlap with some keratinising tumours being HPV positive. The type of abnormality found in the skin adjacent to the tumour is more reliable; when there is differentiated VIN and/or lichen sclerosus in the skin adjacent to the tumour is strong evidence that the tumour is HPV-independent, while the presence of usual-type VIN strongly indicates an HPV-related disease [37, 38].

55.3.2 Clinical Features

Most women present with a vulval mass or lump or ulcer, usually in the background of long-standing vulvar pruritus. Other symptoms include vulvar bleeding, discharge or dysuria. In some patients, a groin mass may be the presenting symptom [4, 42, 43].

In about 50% of cases, the labia majora are the most common site of vulvar carcinoma while the labia minora account for 15–20% of vulvar carcinoma cases. Less frequently, vulvar cancer may arise from the clitoris, and in some cases, the lesion may be too extensive to determine the area of origin. The lesions are unifocal in about 95% of cases and multifocal in 5% therefore, it is essential to carefully examine all vulvar and perianal skin surfaces, as well as the cervix and vagina in cases of vulvar cancer [4, 14, 43–45].

55.3.3 Pathology

55.3.3.1 Histological Types

- Squamous cell carcinoma accounts for about 80% of vulva cancers
- Melanoma is rare but the second most common type of vulva cancer
- Bartholin's gland carcinoma
- Basal cell carcinoma
- Paget's disease of the vulva
- Verrucous carcinoma

55.3.3.2 Histopathologic Grades

A three-grade system is used for pathologic grading of the tumour:

- Gx: grade cannot be assessed
- G1: well differentiated
- G2: moderately differentiated
- G3: poorly differentiated

55.3.3.3 Mode of Spread

Vulvar cancer spread mainly by direct spread to adjacent structures (urethra, anus and vagina) and by lymphatic spread. Haematogenous spread is rare.

Embolisation to regional lymph nodes can occur early in the disease, even in those with small lesions. The superficial inguinal nodes are usually the first group of nodes to be affected from where the disease spreads to the femoral lymph nodes. From the inguinofemoral nodes, the pelvic lymph nodes mainly external iliac nodes may become involved.

In general, lateral tumours drain primarily to the ipsilateral lymph nodes whereas, central tumours drain bilaterally in 25% of cases. Overall lymphatic involvement is reported to be 30% and varies based on the stage of the disease and depth of invasion of the tumour [4, 46, 47].

55.3.4 Staging of Cancer of the Vulva

Since 1994, vulvar cancer has been staged surgicopathologically using the International Federation of Gynaecology and Obstetrics (FIGO) staging system. The FIGO surgical staging system has undergone several revisions, with the latest in 2009 (Table 55.4). The TNM staging system is the alternative staging system based on clinical/pathological classification (Table 55.5). Like in other organs, the TNM staging comprises of the assessment of the primary tumour, nodal and metastatic status of the disease. Table 55.6 shows the 2009 FIGO stages with the corresponding TNM stages.

55.3.5 Diagnosis

It is essential to carry out a complete clinical assessment of the patient, including a careful examination of the groins and a pelvic examination. On vulva examination, the lesion may be raised, fleshy, ulcerated or warty. In advanced stages, it could be large irregular fungating mass, an ulcer or a large groin mass [4, 8, 46]. Most squamous cell carcinomas of the vulva occur in the labia majora. However, they may occur in other parts of the vulva as well.

Table 55.4 Carcinoma of the vulva: 2009 FIGO nomenclature [49]

Stage I	The carcinoma is confined to the vulva
IA	Lesions ≤2 cm in size, confined to the vulva or perineum and with stromal invasion ≤1.0 mm,[a] no nodal metastasis
IB	Lesions >2 cm in size or with stromal invasion >1.0 mm,[a] confined to the vulva or perineum, with negative nodes
Stage II	Tumour of any size with extension to adjacent perineal structures (one-third lower urethra, one-third lower vagina, anus) with negative nodes
Stage III	Tumour of any size with or without extension to adjacent perineal structures (one-third lower urethra, one-third lower vagina, anus) with positive inguinofemoral lymph nodes
IIIA	(i) One lymph node macrometastasis (≥5 mm) or (ii) One to two lymph node micrometastases (<5 mm)
IIIB	(i) Two or more lymph node macrometastases (≥5 mm), or (ii) Three or more lymph node micrometastases (<5 mm)
IIIC	With positive nodes with extracapsular spread
Stage IV	Tumour invades other regional (two-thirds upper urethra, two-thirds upper vagina) or distant structures
IVA	Tumour invades any of the following: (i) Upper urethral and/or vaginal mucosa, bladder mucosa, rectal mucosa, or fixed to the pelvic bone or (ii) Fixed or ulcerated inguinofemoral lymph nodes
IVB	Any distant metastasis including pelvic lymph node

[a]The depth of invasion is defined as the measurement of the tumour from the epithelial-stromal junction of the adjacent most superficial dermal papilla to the deepest part of invasion

Table 55.5 Carcinoma of the vulva: the definitions of TNM staging [19]

T1	Confined to the vulva/perineum
T1a	2 cm with stromal invasion 1.0 mm
T1b	2 cm or stromal invasion >1.0 mm
T2	Lower urethra/vagina/anus
T3	Upper urethra/vagina, bladder, rectal mucosa, bone, fixed to the pelvic bone
N1a	One or two nodes <5 mm
N1b	One node 5 mm
N2a	Three or more nodes <5 mm
N2b	Two or more nodes 5 mm
N2c	Extracapsular spread
N3	Fixed, ulcerated
M1	Distant

Table 55.6 Vulvar cancer FIGO staging and its corresponding TNM staging [50]

Stage 0	Tis	N0	M0
Stage I	T1	N0	M0
Stage IA	T1a	N0	M0
Stage IB	T1b	N0	M0
Stage II	T2	N0	M0
Stage IIIA	T1, T2	N1a, N1b	M0
Stage IIIB	T1, T2,	N2a, N2b	M0
Stage IIIC	T1, T2	N2c	M0
Stage IVA	T1, T2,	N3	M0
	T3	Any N	M0
Stage IVB	Any T	Any N	M1

All cases with suspected vulvar cancer should have a diagnostic biopsy to confirm malignancy. The biopsy is usually done in the office under local anaesthesia using the Keyes punch biopsy forceps. The biopsies should include underlying stroma (more than 1 mm depth) for adequate histological assessment. It is important to avoid removing the whole primary lesion so that the treating surgeon can plan to get adequate margins at the definitive surgery [4, 8, 12, 46].

55.3.6 Investigations

Proper work-up of patients diagnosed with vulvar cancer is an essential component of the management of these patients. Baseline tests to be done include blood tests (full blood count and biochemical profile) and chest X-ray. Imaging (computed tomography [CT] or magnetic resonance imaging [MRI] scans] of the pelvis and the groin may be done to detect lymph nodes or the presence of other metastatic disease [42].

55.3.7 Management of Cancer of the Vulva

Management of vulvar cancer has become more individualised and requires a multidisciplinary team approach. The primary tumour and the status of the lymph nodes must be assessed separately before deciding overall management of the patient.

Overall, the management of vulva cancer has been evolving over the decades, from the classic traditional "*en bloc*" (butterfly incision) radical vulvectomy to more conservative and surgical approaches introduced in the 1980s, together with the development of other modalities of treatment (radiotherapy and chemotherapy) with the aim of decreasing complications without compromising standards [4, 51, 52].

55.3.7.1 Management of Early Vulvar Cancer (FIGO I and II)

- Stage 1A:

The modality of treatment is surgery. The procedure commonly employed is radical wide local excision. Studies have shown that local recurrence and lymph node metastasis are very rare in this stage and groin node dissection is not necessary if adequate margins of disease-free tissue are at least 1 cm [14, 32, 42, 53].

- Stage 1B and II:

Management of the Primary Tumour

The management of tumours with depth more than 1 mm is historically the radical vulvectomy with bilateral inguino-femoral lymphadenectomy (the classic 'en bloc' or 'butterfly' incision). This procedure improved survival, resulting in 5-year survival rates of 60–70% compared to rates of 20–25% before the introduction of radical vulvectomy. However, this operation was associated with high rates of post-operative complications including leg oedema, wound breakdown, pelvic organ prolapse, urinary incontinence, psychosexual impairment and prolonged hospital stay [4, 32, 42, 44]. Radical wide local excision, a more conservative procedure is as effective as radical vulvectomy. This procedure should achieve at least 1 cm lateral tumour-free margins, and the depth should be up to the inferior fascial of the urogenital diaphragm. The Royal College of Obstetricians and Gynaecologists (RCOG) recommends at least 1.5 cm of disease-free margin after a radical wide local excision [46]. Where the margins are inadequate, a re-excision or postoperative radiation may be used as close surgical margins have been recognised as a risk factor for local recurrence of a tumour [42, 44, 54–56].

Management of the lymph nodes is important because groin recurrence carries a high mortality. Patients with early disease (stages IB and II) should have at least unilateral inguinal lymphadenectomy in lateral tumours. Bilateral inguinal lymphadenectomy should be done in large tumours and when the tumour is located in the midline. This procedure should be carried out through separate incisions to reduce morbidity. However, there are still some associated morbidities, including leg oedema, lymphocysts, wound breakdown, and erysipelas [4, 42, 56, 57].

Sentinel Node Excision

A sentinel lymph node (SLN) is the first lymph node that receives drainage from a tumour. An SLN biopsy (SNLB) provides information about lymph node involvement. It is performed by pre-operative injection of radioactive tracer and intra-operative injection of blue dye. At surgery, the SLN is identified and removed with limited surgery and then sent for pathologic evaluation. The findings at this evaluation determine whether full groin node dissection is required or not [42, 53, 58]. Based on the results from the two major clinical studies, GROINSSV [59] and GOG173 [60], that demonstrated the feasibility and reproducibility of SLN biopsy, women with unifocal, primary tumours smaller than 4 cm, with no clinical or radiological evidence of suspect lymph node metastasis should be offered SLN biopsy procedure [42, 46, 58]. This procedure has now become part of the standard management of vulvar cancer in many centres. SNL biopsy reduces the morbidity associated with full groin node dissection, thus improved quality of life. It is also cost effective and allows for improved pathologic evaluation of the lymph node [4, 14, 42, 58, 61].

Management of Positive Groin Nodes Adjuvant radiation directed at the groins and pelvis has replaced pelvic lymphadenopathy, the traditional treatment for patients with positive inguinal nodes. Several studies have also shown that the morphology of the positive lymph nodes is of prognostic importance, particularly the size of the metastasis and the presence or absence of extracapsular spread [4, 42, 62–64]. The management of patients with positive groin nodes is as follows [4, 42]:

- Patients with micrometastasis (metastatic deposit less than 5 mm) should be observed because the prognosis in this group of patients is excellent without further treatment
- Bilateral pelvic and groin irradiation is indicated in patients with
  - two or more positive nodes
  - extracapsular spread

Patients with one or more positive lymph node at sentinel node procedure should be treated with full groin node dissection

55.3.7.2 Management of Advanced Vulvar Cancer (FIGO III and IV)

This group includes patients with large bulky tumours or bulky positive nodes who require careful pre-operative planning. Multimodality treatment planning is crucial in these patients, including involving the plastic surgeons where they are required. As with the early disease, the primary tumour and the state of the lymph nodes must be assessed separately before deciding overall management of the patient [4, 14, 42, 56, 65–67].

Management of the Primary Tumour [4, 42, 66, 68–70]
Primary surgical excision is preferred if the tumour is resectable with adequate margins (more than 1 cm tumour-free margin) and without compromising the sphincters (causing urinary or faecal incontinence and sometimes requiring a bowel or urinary stoma).

Primary radiation is preferred if a tumour cannot be excised without compromising the sphincters. The radiation is sometimes given to reduce the size of the tumour, in which case, surgical resection of the smaller tumour follows it. The groin and pelvic lymph nodes may be included in the radiation field.

Chemoradiation has also been extensively used, and complete responses without the need for post-treatment surgery have been well established. Mitomycin C, 5-FU, cisplatin, Ifosfamide and paclitaxel are the most commonly used chemotherapeutic drugs (usually in a combination of two drugs) in chemoradiation for vulvar cancer.

Patients with advanced disease and distance metastasis may be offered radiation or chemotherapy for palliative purposes.

Management of Groin Lymph Nodes
Determining the status of the lymph nodes by pelvic CT scan or an MRI is essential before planning the overall treatment of the patient. Patients with no clinically or radiologically suspicious nodes should have full bilateral groin node dissection. If the groin nodes are confirmed positive by histology, the patient should have adjuvant radiotherapy to the groins and pelvis. If the nodes are negative by histology, the groins and the pelvis can be excluded from any subsequent radiotherapy.

In patients with clinically positive nodes, only the enlarged nodes should be removed if feasible followed by postoperative pelvic and groin radiotherapy.

In patients that present with fixed or ulcerated groin lymph nodes, the diagnosis should be made either by resecting the node if feasible or by biopsy (if they are not resectable) followed by radiotherapy with or without chemotherapy.

55.3.7.3 Prognosis Vulvar Cancer

Survival in vulvar cancer depends on the stage of the disease. The 5-year survival according to the stage of disease was reported to be up to 98% in stage I disease and drops gradually to 31% in stage IV disease [4].

The status of the lymph nodes is perhaps the most important prognostic factor in vulvar cancer. Number of positive lymph nodes is the single most important prognostic factor in vulvar cancer. Regardless of the stage of the disease, the presence of one microscopically positive node has a better prognosis than the presence of three or more lymph nodes. The 5-year survival rate in vulvar cancer was reported in the 26th FIGO annual report as 80.7% in node-negative patients which plummeted to 13% in those with four or more involved lymph nodes. Extracapsular spread of the tumour is also a poor prognostic sign [4, 14, 29, 42].

Other prognostic pathological factors include size of the lesion, depth of invasion and lymph vascular space involvement [47, 48, 71–73].

55.3.8 Other Histologic Types of Vulvar Cancer [4, 14, 42, 48]

Malignant melanoma is the second most common type of vulva cancer, occur predominantly in post-menopausal women and it may arise de novo or from a pre-existing junctional or compound naevus. Any pigmented lesion on the vulva must be excised for histology. These tumours are treated with radical local excision usually combined with groin node dissection. The 5-year survival is usually 21–54%.

Bartholin gland carcinoma accounts for 5% of vulvar cancers. It may be adenocarcinomas, squamous cell carcinomas or rarely transitional cell carcinoma. Treatment of Bartholin's gland carcinoma is be hemi-vulvectomy and ipsilateral groin node dissection. Post-operative radiation reduces the rate of local recurrence.

Basal cell carcinoma accounts for 2–4% of vulvar cancers and present as "rodent" ulcer. As they are locally malignant and do not metastasise, wide local; excision is adequate treatment.

Verrucous carcinomas are commonly found in the oral cavity. They do also occur in other moist membranes. They appear like cauliflower and found in post-menopausal women. They are locally aggressive but very slow growing and hardly metastasise to the lymph nodes. Radical wide local excision is the treatment of choice.

Vulvar sarcomas are very rare and account for 1–2% of vulvar cancers. Leiomyosarcomas are the most common types, other types being fibrosarcomas, neurofibrosarcomas, liposarcomas, rhabdomyosarcomas, angiosarcormas and malignant schwannomas. They are treated by wide local excision.

55.4 Summary

Cancer of the vagina and the vulva are not common but have significant social and psychosexual effects especially when they occur in young women. Some of these cancers are HPV related, particularly in young women. Management is primarily surgical but has attendant physical and sexual long-term complications. Management should, therefore, be multidisciplinary and individualised to the specific patient needs. There is no evidence-based screening method for vulva or vaginal cancers.

References

1. Wills A, Obermair A. A review of complications associated with the surgical treatment of vulvar cancer. Gynecol Oncol. 2013;132(2):467–79.
2. Lai J, Elleray R, Nordin A, Hirschowitz L, Rous B, Gildea C, et al. Vulval cancer incidence, mortality and survival in England: age-related trends. BJOG. 2014;121(6):728–38.
3. De Martel C, Ferlay J, Franceschi S, Vignat J, Bray F, Forman D, et al. Global burden of cancers attributable to infections in 2008: a review and synthetic analysis. Lancet Oncol. 2012;13(6):607–15.
4. Berek JS, Hacker N. Berek and Hacker's gynaecologic oncology. Philadelphia: Lippincott Williams & Wilkins; 2010.
5. Siegel R, Miller K, Jemal A. Cancer statistics, 2018. CA Cancer J Clin. 2018;68(1):7–30.
6. Shah C, Goff BA, Lowe K, Peters WA, Li CI. Factors affecting risk of mortality in women with vaginal cancer. Obstet Gynecol. 2009;113(5):1038–45.
7. Pingley S, Shrivastava SK, Sarin R, Agarwal JP, Laskar S, Deshpande DD, et al. Primary carcinoma of the vagina: Tata Memorial Hospital experience. Int J Radiat Oncol Biol Phys. 2000;46(1):101–8.
8. Hacker NF, Eifel PJ, van der Velden J. Cancer of the vagina. Int J Gynaecol Obstet. 2015;131(Suppl):S84–7.
9. De Vuyst H, Clifford GM, Nascimento MC, Madeleine MM, Franceschi S. Prevalence and type distribution of human papillomavirus in carcinoma and intraepithelial neoplasia of the vulva, vagina and anus: a meta-analysis. Int J Cancer. 2009;124(7):1626–36.
10. Alemany L, Ordi J, Tous S, Alejo M, De Sanjose S, Bigby SM, et al. Worldwide human papillomavirus genotype attribution in over 2000 cases of intraepithelial and invasive lesions of the vulva. Eur J Cancer. 2013;49:3450–61.
11. Daling JR, Madeleine MM, Schwartz SM, Shera KA, Carter JJ, McKnight B, et al. A population-based study of squamous cell vaginal cancer: HPV and cofactors. Gynecol Oncol. 2002;84(2):263–70.
12. Madsen BS, Jensen HL, van den Brule AJC, Wohlfahrt J, Frisch M. Risk factors for invasive squamous cell carcinoma of the vulva and vagina--population-based case-control study in Denmark. Int J Cancer. 2008;122(12):2827–34.
13. Siu SSN, Luesley D. Malignant disease of the vulva and vagina. In: Gynaecology. 4th ed. London: Elsevier Ltd; 2011. p. 613–28.
14. Hacker NF. Vulvar and vaginal cancer. In: Hacker NF, Gambone JC, Hobel C, editors. Hacker & Moore's essentials of obstetrics and gynaecology. 6th ed. Philadelphia: Elsevier Inc.; 2016. p. 449–56.
15. Hellman K, Lundell M, Silfverswärd C, Nilsson B, Hellström A-C, Frankendal B. Clinical and histopathologic factors related to prognosis in primary squamous cell carcinoma of the vagina. Int J Gynecol Cancer. 2006;16(3):1201–11.
16. Gadducci A, Fabrini MG, Lanfredini N, Sergiampietri C. Squamous cell carcinoma of the vagina: natural history, treatment modalities and prognostic factors. Crit Rev Oncol Hematol. 2015;93(3):211–24.
17. Beller U, Benedet JL, Creasman WT, Ngan HYS, Quinn MA, Maisonneuve P, et al. Carcinoma of the vagina. Int J Gynaecol Obstet. 2006;95(Suppl 1):29–42.
18. FIGO Committee on Gynaecologic Oncology. Current FIGO staging for cancer of the vagina, fallopian tube, ovary, and gestational trophoblastic neoplasia. Int J Gynaecol Obstet. 2009;105(1):3–4.
19. Compton CC, Byrd DR, Garcia-Aguilar J, Kurtzman SH, Olawaiye A, Washington MK. Vagina. In: Compton CC, Byrd RD, Garcia-Aguilar J, Kurtzman HS, Olawaiye A, Washington KM, editors. AJCC cancer staging atlas: a companion to the seventh editions of the AJCC cancer staging manual and handbook. New York: Springer; 2012. p. 455–61.
20. Di Donato V, Bellati F, Fischetti M, Plotti F, Perniola G. Vaginal cancer. Crit Rev Oncol Hematol. 2012;81(3):286–95.
21. Yin D, Wang N, Zhang S, Huo N, Xiao Q, Ling O, et al. Radical hysterectomy and vaginectomy with sigmoid vaginoplasty for stage I vaginal carcinoma. Int J Gynaecol Obstet. 2013;122(2):132–5.
22. Tjalma WA, Monaghan JM, de Barros Lopes A, Naik R, Nordin A, Weyler J. The role of surgery in invasive squamous carcinoma of the vagina. Gynecol Oncol. 2001;81:360–5.
23. Mclean KA, Zhang W, Dunsmoor-su RF, Shah CA, Gray HJ, Swensen RE, et al. Pelvic exenteration in the age of modern chemoradiation. Gynecol Oncol. 2011;121(1):131–4.
24. Hiniker SM, Roux A, Murphy JD, Harris JP, Tran PT, Kapp DS, et al. Primary squamous cell carcinoma of the vagina: prognostic factors, treatment patterns, and outcomes. Gynecol Oncol. 2013;131(2):380–5.
25. Lian J, Dundas G, Carlone M, Ghosh S, Pearcey R. Twenty-year review of radiotherapy for vaginal cancer: an institutional experience. Gynecol Oncol. 2008;111(2):298–306.
26. Peters W, Kumar N, Morley GW. Microinvasive carcinoma of the vagina: a distinct clinical entity? Am J Obstet Gynecol. 1985;153(5):505–7.
27. Rajagopalan MS, Xu KM, Lin JF, Sukumvanich P, Krivak TC, Beriwal S. Adoption and impact of concurrent chemoradiation therapy for vaginal cancer: a National Cancer Data Base (NCDB) study. Gynecol Oncol. 2014;135(3):495–502.
28. Frank S, Jhingran A, Levenback C, Eifel PJ. Definitive radiation therapy for squamous cell carcinoma of the vagina. Int J Radiat Oncol Biol Phys. 2005;62(1):138–47.

29. Beller U, Quinn MA, Benedet JL, Creasman WT, Ngan HYS, Maisonneuve P, et al. Carcinoma of the vulva. FIGO 26th annual report on the results of treatment in gynaecological cancer. Int J Gynaecol Obstet. 2006;95(Suppl 1):S7–S27.
30. Judson PL, Habermann EB, Baxter NN, Durham SB, Virnig BA. Trends in the incidence of invasive and in situ vulvar carcinoma. Obstet Gynecol. 2006;107(5):1018–22.
31. Akhtar-Danesh N, Elit L, Lytwyn A. Trends in incidence and survival of women with invasive vulvar cancer in the United States and Canada: a population-based study. Gynecol Oncol. 2014;134(2):314–8.
32. Dittmer C, Fischer D, Diedrich K, Thill M. Diagnosis and treatment options of vulvar cancer: a review. Arch Gynecol Obstet. 2011;285(1):183–93.
33. Somoye GO, Mocroft A, Olaitan A. Analysis of the incidence and mortality of vulval cancer in women in South East England 1960–1999. Arch Gynecol Obstet. 2009;279(2):113–7.
34. Tans L, Ansink AC, van Rooij PH, Kleijnen C, Mens JW. The role of chemo-radiotherapy in the management of locally advanced carcinoma of the vulva. Am J Clin Oncol. 2011;34(1):22–6.
35. Rumbold AR, Tan SE, Condon JR, Taylor-Thompson D, Nickels M, Tabrizi S, et al. Investigating a cluster of vulvar cancer in young women: a cross-sectional study of genital human papillomavirus prevalence. BMC Infect Dis. 2012;12:243.
36. Butt JL, Botha MH. Vulvar cancer is not a disease of the elderly: treatment and outcome at a tertiary referral centre in South Africa. S Afr Med J. 2017;107(11):1000–4.
37. Del Pino M, Rodriguez-Carunchio L, Ordi J. Pathways of vulvar intraepithelial neoplasia and squamous cell carcinoma. Histopathology. 2013;62(1):161–75.
38. Ueda Y, Enomoto T, Kimura T, Yoshino K, Fujita M, Kimura T. Two distinct pathways to development of squamous cell carcinoma of the vulva. J Skin Cancer. 2011;2011:951250.
39. Madeleine MM, Daling JR, Carter JJ, Wipf GC, Schwartz SM, McKnight B, et al. Cofactors with human papillomavirus in a population-based study of vulvar cancer. J Natl Cancer Inst. 1997;89(20):1516–23.
40. van de Nieuwenhof HP, Bulten J, Hollema H, Dommerholt RG, Massuger LFAG, van der Zee AG, et al. Differentiated vulvar intraepithelial neoplasia is often found in lesions, previously diagnosed as lichen sclerosus, which have progressed to vulvar squamous cell carcinoma. Mod Pathol. 2011;24(2):297–305.
41. Jones RW, Baranyai J, Stables S. Trends in squamous cell carcinoma of the vulva: the influence of vulvar intraepithelial neoplasia. Obstet Gynecol. 1997;90(3):448–52.
42. Hacker NF, Eifel PJ, van der Velden J. Cancer of the vulva. Int J Gynecol Obstet. 2015;131(Suppl):S76–83.
43. Canavan TP. Vulvar cancer. Am Fam Physician. 2002;66(7):1269–74.
44. Hacker NF, Barlow EL. Staging for vulvar cancer. Best Pract Res Clin Obstet Gynecol. 2015;29(6):802–11.
45. de Hullu JA, van der Avoort IAM, Oonk MHM, van der Zee AGJ. Management of vulvar cancers. Eur J Surg Oncol. 2006;32(8):825–31.
46. Crowley T. Guidelines for the diagnosis and management of vulval carcinoma. RCOG. 2014;(May):1–35.
47. Homesley HD, Bundy BN, Sedlis A, Yordan E, Berek JS, Jahshan A, et al. Assessment of current International Federation of Gynaecology and Obstetrics staging of vulvar carcinoma relative to prognostic factors for survival (A Gynaecologic Oncology Group study). Am J Obstet Gynecol. 1991;164(4):997–1004.
48. Lesley D. Malignant diseases of the vulva and the vagina. In: Edmond KD, editor. Dewhurst's textbook of obstetrics and gynaecology. 7th ed. Malden: Blackwell Publishing Ltd; 2007. p. 591–608.
49. Pecorelli S, Zigliani L, Odicino F. Revised FIGO staging for carcinoma of the cervix. Int J Gynecol Obstet. 2009;105(2):107–8.
50. Hacker NF, Eifel PJ, van der Velden J. Cancer of the vulva. Int J Gynecol Obstet. 2012;119:S90–6.
51. Viswanathan AN, Pinto AP, Schultz D, Berkowitz R, Crum CP. Relationship of margin status and radiation dose to recurrence in post-operative vulvar carcinoma. Gynecol Oncol. 2013;130(3):545–9.
52. van Doorn HC, Ansink A, Verhaar-Langereis M, Stalpers L. Neoadjuvant chemoradiation for advanced primary vulvar cancer. Cochrane Database Syst Rev. 2006;(3):CD003752.
53. de Hullu JA, van der Zee AG. Sentinel node techniques in cancer of the vulva. Curr Womens Health Rep. 2003;3(1):19–26.
54. Woelber L, Choschzick M, Eulenburg C, Hager M, Jaenicke F, Gieseking F, et al. Prognostic value of pathological resection margin distance in squamous cell cancer of the vulva. Ann Surg Oncol. 2011;18(13):3811–8.
55. Iacoponi S, Zapardiel I, Diestro MD, Hernandez A, De Santiago J. Prognostic factors associated with local recurrence in squamous cell carcinoma of the vulva. J Gynecol Oncol. 2013;24(3):242–8.
56. Deppe G, Mert I, Winer IS. Management of squamous cell vulvar cancer: a review. J Obstet Gynaecol Res. 2014;40:1217–25.
57. Woelber L, Kock L, Gieseking F, Petersen C, Trillsch F, Choschzick M, et al. Clinical management of primary vulvar cancer. Eur J Cancer. 2011;47(15):2315–21.
58. Slomovitz BM, Coleman RL, Oonk MHM, Van Der Zee A, Levenback C. Update on sentinel lymph node biopsy for early-stage vulvar cancer. Gynecol Oncol. 2015;138(2):472–7.
59. Van Der Zee AGJ, Oonk MH, De Hullu JA, Ansink AC, Vergote I, Verheijen RH, et al. Sentinel node dissection is safe in the treatment of early-stage vulvar cancer. J Clin Oncol. 2008;26(6):884–9.
60. Levenback CF, Ali S, Coleman RL, Gold MA, Fowler JM, Judson PL, et al. Lymphatic mapping and sentinel lymph node biopsy in women with squamous cell carcinoma of the vulva: a Gynaecologic Oncology Group study. J Clin Oncol. 2012;30(31):3786–91.
61. Oonk MHM, de Hullu JA, van der Zee AGJ. Current controversies in the management of patients with early-stage vulvar cancer. Curr Opin Oncol. 2010;22(5):481–6.
62. van der Velden J, Hacker NF. Prognostic factors in squamous cell cancer of the vulva and the implications for treatment. Curr Opin Obstet Gynecol. 1996;8(1):3–7.
63. Heaps JM, Fu YS, Montz FJ, Hacker NF, Berek JS. Surgical-pathologic variables predictive of local recurrence in squamous cell carcinoma of the vulva. Gynecol Oncol. 2015;38(3):309–14.
64. Woelber L. Clinicopathological prognostic factors and patterns of recurrence in vulvar cancer. Anticancer Res. 2009;29(2):545–52.
65. Aragona AM, Soderini AH, Cuneo NA. Defining the concept of locally advanced squamous cell carcinoma of the vulva: a new perspective based on standardisation of criteria and current evidence. J Gynecol Oncol. 2014;25(4):272–8.
66. Sharma C, Deutsch I, Herzog TJ, Lu Y-S, Neugut AI, Lewin SN, et al. Patterns of care for locally advanced vulvar cancer. Am J Obstet Gynecol. 2013;209(1):60.
67. Hoffman MS, Greenberg H, Roberts WS, Fiorica JV, LaPolla JP, Barton DP, et al. Management of locally advanced squamous cell carcinoma of the vulva. J Gynecol Surg. 1991;7(3):175–82.
68. Shylasree TS, Bryant A, Howells RE. Chemoradiation for advanced primary vulval cancer. Cochrane Database Syst Rev. 2011;(4):CD003752.
69. Gaudineau A, Weitbruch D, Quetin P, Heymann S, Petit T, Volkmar P, et al. Neoadjuvant chemoradiotherapy followed by surgery in locally advanced squamous cell carcinoma of the vulva. Oncol Lett. 2012;4(4):719–22.
70. Aragona AM, Cuneo ÞN, Soderini AH, Alcoba E, Greco A, Reyes C, et al. Tailoring the treatment of locally advanced squamous cell carcinoma of the vulva: neoadjuvant chemotherapy followed by radical surgery: results from a multicentre study. Int J Gynecol Cancer. 2012;22(7):1258–63.

71. Aragona AM, Cuneo NA, Soderini AH, Alcoba EB. An analysis of reported independent prognostic factors for survival in squamous cell carcinoma of the vulva: is tumour size significance being underrated? Gynecol Oncol. 2014;132(3):643–8.
72. Ayhan A, Velipasaoglu M, Salman MC, Guven S, Gultekin M, Bayraktar O. Prognostic factors for recurrence and survival in primary vulvar squamous cell cancer. Acta Obstet Gynecol Scand. 2008;87(11):1143–9.
73. Chan JK, Sugiyama V, Pham H, Gu M, Rutgers J, Osann K, et al. Margin distance and other clinico-pathologic prognostic factors in vulvar carcinoma: a multivariate analysis. Gynecol Oncol. 2007;104(3):636–41.

Cervical Cancer Screening and Prevention

56

Adeola Olaitan and Michael Chudi Ezeanochie

Learning Objectives
At the end of this chapter, the reader should be able to:

- Discuss the burden of cervical cancer in developing countries
- Explain the role of human papilloma virus (HPV) as a causal factor for cervical cancer
- Identify the risk factors for cervical cancer
- Describe the common symptoms and signs of cervical cancer
- Discuss the treatment options that are available for cervical cancer
- Understand the challenges associated with the management of cervical cancer in developing countries
- Identify the role of vaccination against HPV in the prevention of cervical cancer
- Describe the available screening methods in the prevention of cervical cancer

56.1 Introduction

Cervical cancer remains an important health problem worldwide. It is the fourth most common cancer in women, after breast, colorectal and lung cancers. Over half a million cases occur every year, with the majority of cases occurring in less well-resourced countries, particularly in sub-Saharan Africa. A fifth of all cases occur in India. Cervical cancer is the fourth most common cause of cancer deaths: 266,000 women died of this disease in 2012, of which over 25% of deaths occurred in India. African countries such as Kenya, Uganda and Nigeria also rank high in the mortality stakes [1]. In sub-Saharan Africa, 34.8 new cases of cervical cancer are diagnosed per 100,000 women annually, and 22.5 per 100,000 women die from the disease. By contrast, 6.6 new cases are diagnosed annually, while only 2.5 per 100,000 women die from the disease in North America. These figures from developing countries may indeed be worse than reported. They are confounded by the lack of accurate data which are in part due to a dearth of cancer registries in the worst-affected countries and also because a significant number of women do not seek healthcare or lack access to proper diagnostic facilities. Poor access to effective treatment or palliative care leads to much suffering before death.

The observed differences in the prevalence and mortality from cervical cancer between developed and developing countries can be largely explained by lack of access to effective screening and to services that facilitate early detection and treatment in many developing countries [2]. In order to design effective strategies for prevention and early detection of cervical cancer, it is important to understand the causes and risk factors for this disease.

56.2 Predisposing Factors for Cervical Cancer

The vast majority of cervical cancer cases are caused by infection with the high-risk human papilloma virus (HRHPV). Human papillomavirus (HPV) is a group of viruses that are extremely common worldwide. There are more than 100 types of HPV, of which at least 20 are oncogenic and these are known as high-risk types (HRHPV). The majority of HPV types are associated with benign conditions such as skin warts.

A. Olaitan (✉)
UCLH Gynaecological Cancer Centre, London, UK

North London Gynaecological Cancer Network, London, UK
e-mail: adeola.olaitan@nhs.net

M. C. Ezeanochie
University of Benin Teaching Hospital, Benin City, Nigeria

Department of Obstetrics & Gynaecology, University of Benin, Benin City, Nigeria

F. Okonofua et al. (eds.), *Contemporary Obstetrics and Gynecology for Developing Countries*,
https://doi.org/10.1007/978-3-030-75385-6_56

Human papillomavirus (HPV) is the most common viral infection of the reproductive tract. Most sexually active women and men will be infected at some point in their lives and some may be repeatedly infected. The peak time for acquiring infection for both women and men is shortly after becoming sexually active. HPV is sexually transmitted, but penetrative sex is not required for transmission. Skin-to-skin genital contact is a well-recognised mode of transmission [3].

HPV infections usually resolve without any intervention within a few months after acquisition, and about 90% resolve within 2 years. Persistent infection with HRHPV increases the risk of cervical cancer.

Cervical cancer is by far the most common HRHPV-related disease. Nearly all cases of cervical cancer can be attributable to HPV infection. Though data on ano-genital cancers other than cancer of the cervix are limited, there is an increasing body of evidence linking HPV with cancers of the anus, vulva, vagina, and penis. Although these cancers are less frequent than cancer of the cervix, their association with HPV makes them potentially preventable using similar primary prevention strategies as those for cervical cancer.

Risk factors for the development of cervical cancer are therefore centred on risk factors for acquiring persistent HPV infection (a sexually transmitted infection). Multiple sexual partners increase the chance of acquiring HPV infection and the development of cervical cancer. Other risk factors include early initiation of sexual activity, smoking, high number of childbirth (parity), age over 40 years, weak immune system (HIV/AIDS) and prolonged use of the combined oral contraceptive pill [4].

56.3 Staging of Cervical Cancer

The revised FIGO 2009 staging for cervical cancer is presented [5]:

- Stage I: The carcinoma is strictly confined to the cervix (disregard extension to the corpus)
  - IA: Microscopic invasive carcinoma
    IA1: Measured stromal invasion of ≤3.0 mm in depth and extension of ≤7.0 mm
    IA2: Measured stromal invasion of >3.0 mm and not >5.0 mm in depth and extension of >7.0 mm
  - IB: Clinically visible lesions limited to the cervix uteri or pre-clinical cancers greater than stage IA
    IB1: Clinically visible lesion ≤4.0 cm in greatest dimension
    IB2: Clinically visible lesion >4.0 cm in greatest dimension
- Stage II: Carcinoma spreads beyond the cervix, but not to the pelvic wall or lower third of the vagina
  - IIA: Without parametrial invasion
    IIA1: Clinically visible lesion ≤4.0 cm in greatest dimension
    IIA2: Clinically visible lesion N4 cm in greatest dimension
  - IIB: With obvious parametrial invasion
- Stage III: The tumour extends to the pelvic wall and/or involves lower third of the vagina and/or causes hydronephrosis or non-functioning kidney
  - IIIA: Tumour involves lower third of the vagina, with no extension to the pelvic wall
  - IIIB: Extension to the pelvic wall and/or hydronephrosis or non-functioning kidney
- Stage IV: The carcinoma has extended beyond the true pelvis
  - IVA: Spread of the growth to adjacent pelvic organs
  - IVB: Spread to distant organs

56.4 Clinical Presentation

Women who have invasive cervical cancer commonly present with abnormal vaginal bleeding which can be postcoital or postmenopausal. Other symptoms may include back ache, offensive vaginal discharge, haematuria, tumour bulk pressure effects leading to changes in urinary or bowel habits, weight loss, renal impairment and malaise. Majority of patients in Nigeria and many developing countries present with advanced disease unlike women in developed countries where an organised screening service makes early detection more likely.

On examination, they may be chronically ill-looking with a characteristic fetor around them. Pelvic examination will reveal an ulcerative exophytic craggy mass on the ecto-cervix that bleeds easily on contact. The mass can extend into the vaginal and adjacent parametrium. Occasionally, a barrel-shaped ballooned cervix with normal ecto-cervix but an endophytic (endocervical) growth may be seen and this is suggestive of an adenocarcinoma. Smaller tumours may present as an abnormal-looking friable ectropion with irregular margins and copious contact bleeding.

There are different histological types of cervical cancer. The majority are squamous cell carcinoma and adenocarcinoma which comprise about 80% and 10%, respectively, while rare variants include neuroendocrine cancer, glassy cell carcinoma, verrucuous carcinoma, adenoma malignum, sarcomas and lymphomas.

56.5 Investigation and Diagnosis

The diagnosis of cervical cancer is confirmed on histological examination of an incisional biopsy of the mass. At this same procedure, a clinical staging is performed to evaluate the mass and its extent of infiltration into adjacent tissues.

Other investigative modalities will assess the overall state of well-being of the patient and fitness for the various treatment modalities. This may include a complete blood count to detect anaemia or markers of infection, renal function tests (serum electrolytes, urea and creatinine), liver function tests and urine microscopy, culture and sensitivity.

Ultrasound of the abdomen and pelvis will assist to evaluate the mass and its relationship to the uterus and bladder. Obstructive uropathy from spread to the ureters will be detected, while metastasis to the liver can also be demonstrable. A chest X-ray can help in detecting metastasis to the lungs, while an intravenous urogram assesses renal excretory function and outlines its anatomy.

In centres where resources are available, a magnetic resonance imaging (MRI) of the pelvis provides excellent soft-tissue contrast resolution (superior to ultrasound and computed tomography [CT] scan) that is helpful in assessment of the size of the mass, loco-regional extent of the disease and assessing lymph node involvement [6].

56.6 Management

Following a diagnosis of invasive cervical cancer, the main treatment option includes surgery (radical hysterectomy), radiotherapy, chemotherapy and combinations of any of these treatment modalities. The choice of treatment is influenced by the stage of the disease and objective of therapy (whether curative or palliative), the clinical state of the patient and the resources available. It is important to decide at the outset, by careful assessment, which modality is most likely to cure the patient. Radical hysterectomy followed by chemoradiation does not improve cure rates but has been shown to increase complication rates.

Using the 2009 revised Federation of Gynecology and Obstetrics (FIGO) staging for cervical cancer, early disease (stage IA–2A) can be treated by radical hysterectomy with good 5-year survival outcomes. The components of this procedure may include removal of the uterus, upper vagina, the parametrial tissues and lymphadenectomy. Occasionally, cancers in very early stages (1A1) in patients who want their fertility preserved may be treated with conservative surgery such as cone biopsy and trachelectomy. Also, a simple hysterectomy may be appropriate for a woman with early stage tumour who does not desire to have her fertility preserved.

Radiation therapy is preferable in treating advanced disease (stage 2B–4) and tumours larger than 4 cm in diameter. Radiotherapy for cervical cancer is usually a combination of external beam therapy (Teletherapy) and internal radiotherapy (Brachytherapy). Teletherapy is designed to treat the primary tumour and adjacent tissues including lymph nodes. It is preferably delivered using high-energy beams with a linear accelerator. The Cobalt-60 machine which delivers low-energy beam for teletherapy, and is becoming obsolete in the developed world, is still, however, widely used in many developing countries. Low-energy beams are less penetrating and associated with more side effects.

Brachytherapy involves the administration of radiation through radioactive sources in close proximity (intracavitary) or within (interstitial) the tumour. It may be delivered as high-dose rate (HDR) over a short period as outpatient or low-dose rate (LDR) over a longer period usually as inpatients. Evidence has shown that the addition of concomitant chemotherapy with Cisplatin improves outcome [7].

Early complications following radiotherapy includes diarrhoea, urinary symptoms (from radiation cystitis) nausea, malaise, vagina bleeding, dermatitis and soreness around the vulva. Late complications may include loss of ovarian function, bone marrow suppression, osteo-dystrophy and acquired gynaetresia with sexual dysfunction.

56.7 Follow-Up Plans

Following treatment, there is risk of recurrence of cervical cancer usually within 3 years. Follow-up regimen usually is consensus-based depending on a centre's protocol as there is no high-quality evidence on the preferred frequency of visits. It is important that the patient is closely followed up every 3 months for the first year and subsequently every 6 months over the next 2 years. At each visit, history and physical examination for features of recurrence are essential. Investigative modalities may include ultrasound scans, MRI imaging and vaginal vault cytology where appropriate.

56.8 Special Issues

Cervical cancer is best managed in a multidisciplinary setting involving gynaecological oncologists, medical oncologists, pathologists, radiation oncologists, and other healthcare workers who are needed for cancer care. This spectrum of manpower is clearly lacking in many developing countries and this has an impact on the quality of care patients receive. Although developing countries make up about 85% of the world's population and 60% of the global cancer burden, data from the Directory of Radiotherapy Centres (DIRAC) of the International Atomic Energy Agency (IAEA) reveal that over 60% of the cancer treatment centres are located in developed countries. Furthermore, it has been reported that of 52 African countries, only 23 are known to have teletherapy facilities while Brachytherapy resources (high-dose rate or low-dose rate) were only available in 20 countries [8]. Indeed, it has been estimated that between 50% and 90% of cancer patients in middle-income and low-income countries, respectively, lack access to optimal cancer care [9].

Clearly, it is obvious that developing countries who have the largest proportion of cervical cancer patients who often come with advanced disease requiring highly skilled manpower and expensive infrastructure for treatment are not receiving it. Faced with the burden of communicable diseases, widespread poverty and competing needs, the situation seems unlikely to change in the near future unless there is a paradigm shift. The prevention of cervical cancer using currently available technology (screening with prompt treatment of premalignant lesions) that has demonstrably reduced the burden of cervical cancer in many developed countries becomes imperative.

56.9 Cervical Cancer Prevention

Cervical cancer is a potentially preventable disease. Knowledge of its aetiology and natural history has enabled the development of strategies to protect against the disease and to screen for its precursors. The prevention strategy can be broadly divided into primary prevention which involves administering prophylaxis against HRHPV and secondary prevention which comprises screening for and where appropriate, treating the precursor lesions of cervical cancer.

56.10 Vaccination Against HRHPV

56.10.1 Vaccine Development

From as far back as the nineteenth century, epidemiological evidence suggested that a sexually transmissible agent played a role in the development of cervical cancer. In the 1980s, researchers at the German Cancer Research Centre identified the presence of HPV types in cervical tumours. Consequently, research focused on whether HPV could cause cancer and on developing an understanding of the pathway. An important milestone was achieved when a team of researchers, supported by the National Cancer Institute (NCI) USA led by J DiPaolo, and Donniger, showed that DNA from HPV 16, the type of HPV found most often in cervical cancer cells, was able to induce cell transformation in vitro.

The discovery was made in the early 1990s that the proteins that form the outer shell of HPV could form particles that closely resemble the original virus could induce an antibody immune response to the virus. These virus-like particles (VLPs) became the basis of two HPV vaccines: a quadrivalent vaccine that protects against HPV 16 & 18 as well as the low risk 6 & 11, licensed by the Food and Drug Administration (FDA) for prevention of cervical cancer in 2006; and the bivalent vaccine that protects against HPV 16 & 18, approved 3 years later. These vaccines now form part of the national vaccination programmes in most developed countries.

It has remained a challenge to make these vaccines accessible to countries in the developing world that incidentally carry the greatest burden of cervical cancer. Policymakers debating the use of HPV vaccine in any particular country will have to consider the country's disease burden, its healthcare infrastructure and its capacity for initiating and sustaining an immunisation programme for adolescents. Other considerations include the affordability and cost-effectiveness of vaccination relative to other programmes competing for resources and the likelihood of cultural acceptability, political will, and public support [10].

56.11 Screening for Cervical Cancer as a Prevention Strategy

Screening aims to detect precancerous changes on the cervix induced by HPV infection, which if not treated may lead to cancer.

Cytology-based screening methods basically involve obtaining exfoliated cells from the transformation zone of the cervix using a wooden spatula or special brushes for cytological analysis. The majority of established screening programmes rely on visual assessment, under the microscope of these exfoliated cervical epithelial cells to classify them as normal or abnormal (dysplastic lesions). This was made possible by the discovery by George Papanicolau in 1928 that cervical cancer could be diagnosed by means of a vaginal smear. Modifications of this initial concept have for several years formed the basis of population screening for cervical cancer for over 50 years.

These clearly defined abnormal cervical lesions known as cervical intraepithelial neoplasia (CIN) are graded as 1, 2 and 3. CIN 1 carries a low risk of malignancy while CIN2 & 3, otherwise known as high-grade CIN carry a risk of progression to cervical cancer if undetected and untreated.

Screening programmes rely on identifying these lesions and having a defined strategy for managing them. Cervical cytology is used to identify women at risk of having the precursor lesions of cervical cancer and referring such women for a diagnostic test, usually in a colposcopy clinic where suspicious lesions are biopsied and then treatment undertaken only when high-grade lesions have been histologically confirmed.

The treatment options may involve either ablative treatment using cryotherapy, excisional treatment with either the Loop electrosurgical excision procedure (LEEP) or the cold knife biopsy. Cryotherapy involves applying a highly cooled metal disc (cryoprobe) to the cervix, and freezing its surface using carbon dioxide or nitrous oxide gas. Ablative treatment provides no specimen for histological assessment. LEEP is the removal of abnormal areas from the cervix using a thin heated wire. It requires an electrosurgical unit that produces a constant low voltage and transmits it to the wire loop device, which is used to remove the abnormal tissue. Cold knife conisation is the removal of a cone-shaped volume of tissue from the cervix (portions of the ecto-cervix and the endocervix) with a scalpel. It is a more invasive treatment for dysplasia in theatre that requires anaesthesia to rule out invasive cancer. Excisional treatments provide histological specimens for further evaluation. Organised and effective screening programmes in many developed countries have reduced the incidence of invasive cervical by about 80% using this method [11].

The World Health Organisation (WHO) recognises that this traditional screening method requires highly trained human resources and substantial amount of laboratory equipment, which makes it expensive. The high cost means that coverage of screening is very low in low- and middle-income countries, and that alternative screening methods are needed.

The WHO, in the 2013 guidelines, proposed an alternative approach using a 'screen-and-treat' protocol in which the treatment decision is based on a screening test, and not on a histologically confirmed diagnosis of high-grade disease and treatment is provided soon or, ideally, immediately after a positive screening test [12].

Depending on the country's resources, the initial screen can be visual inspection with acetic acid (VIA), HPV testing or cytology. There are algorithms for deciding on strategies that reduce the risk of cervical cancer with minimal morbidity to the woman screened [13]. Most African countries currently lack effective screening programmes and would benefit from implementing one of the strategies proposed by the WHO.

Visual inspection of the cervix is aided with either acetic acid (VIA) or Lugol's iodine (VILI) without the use of magnification to help in detecting abnormal precancerous lesions of the cervix. VIA is premised on premalignant lesions of the cervix producing a positive 'aceto-white' reaction after staining with 3–5% acetic acid while in VILI they give 'iodine-negative areas' which fail to produce the blue-black reaction to Lugol's iodine by normal cervical epithelial cells.

There is increasing evidence that VIA or VILI linked with immediate treatment of abnormal lesions (see and treat model) is a viable option for reducing the incidence of cervical cancer in developing countries [13, 14]. HPV testing is based on the detection of high-risk HPV DNA (either DNA or mRNA) in vaginal or cervical smears. It is also currently been evaluated as a primary screening tool for preventing cervical cancer and may play an increasing role in screening programmes in the near future as the tests become more affordable.

56.12 Conclusion

Cervical cancer remains a major health challenge globally and is a leading cause of cancer-related deaths in many developing countries. It develops from abnormal cells on the endocervix following persistent infection with HRHPV serotypes. This usually occurs following a long period of latency lasting several years. This has created a window of opportunity for organised screening of asymptomatic women to detect these abnormal cellular lesions for prompt treatment. This has markedly reduced the prevalence of the disease in many developed countries. Invasive cervical cancer is best managed in a multidisciplinary setting with gynaecological oncologists, medical oncologists, pathologists, radiation oncologists, and other healthcare workers. Early disease can be treated successfully with surgery, while radiation therapy is an acceptable alternative for all stages of the disease. However, the manpower and infrastructure necessary for successful screening and treatment of cervical cancer are not readily available in many developing countries which still struggle with other challenges; hence, cervical cancer morbidity and mortality profile remains poor in these settings. Primary prevention of cervical cancer using HPV vaccines to prevent the acquisition of HPV infections offers a novel opportunity for the cervical cancer control in developing countries. Most African countries, currently lacking effective screening programmes, would benefit from implementing one of the strategies proposed by the WHO in the 'see and treat' protocol in which prompt treatment decision is offered following a screening test involving VIA, HPV testing or cytology.

56.13 Summary

Cervical Cancer is a public health problem, especially for developing countries. The causal factor, persistent infection with HRHPV, and the pathway to invasive cancer have been clearly described. Widespread use of organised screening, treatment of premalignant disease of the cervix and more recently vaccination against HRHPV has substantially reduced the prevalence of the disease in developed countries. Many developing countries have not been able to replicate organised screening services and vaccination against HRHPV for the prevention of cervical cancer. There is a need for increased political will by governments and the use of appropriate technology to successfully control cervical cancer in developing countries.

References

1. Bray F, Ren JS, Masuyer E, Ferlay J. Global estimates of cancer prevalence for 27 sites in the adult population in 2008. Int J Cancer. 2013;132(5):1133–45.
2. Ferlay J, Soerjomataram I, Ervik M, Dikshit R, Eser S, Mathers C, Rebelo M, Parkin DM, Forman D, Bray F. GLOBOCAN 2012 v1.1. Cancer incidence and mortality worldwide: IARC CancerBase No. 11 [Internet]. Lyon: International Agency for Research on Cancer; 2014. Available from: http://globocan.iarc.fr. Accessed on 16 Jan 2015.
3. WHO. Human papillomavirus (HPV) and cervical cancer. Fact sheet N°380. Geneva: WHO; 2015. Reviewed March 2015.
4. Bosch FX, Muñoz N, de Sanjosé S, Izarzugaza I, Gili M, Viladiu P, et al. Risk factors for cervical cancer in Colombia and Spain. Int J Cancer. 1992;52(5):750–8.
5. Pecorelli S. Revised FIGO staging for carcinoma of the vulva, cervix and endometrium. Int J Gynaecol Obstet. 2009;105(2):103–4.
6. Scheidler J, Heuck AF. Imaging of cancer of the cervix. Radiol Clin N Am. 2002;40(3):577–90.
7. Rose PG. Chemoradiotherapy: the new standard care for invasive cervical cancer. Drugs. 2000;60(6):1239–44.
8. Abdel-Wahab M, Bourque JM, Pynda Y, Iżewska J, Van der Merwe D, Zubizarreta E, et al. Status of radiotherapy resources in Africa: an International Atomic Energy Agency analysis. Lancet Oncol. 2013;14(4):e168–75.
9. Zubizarreta EH, Fidarova E, Healy B, Rosenblatt E. Need for radiotherapy in low and middle income countries – the silent crisis continues. Clin Oncol (R Coll Radiol). 2015;27(2):107–14.
10. Agosti JM, Goldie SJ. Introducing HPV vaccine in developing countries – key challenges and issues. N Engl J Med. 2007;356:1908–10.
11. Läärä E, Day NE. Hakama M Trends in mortality from cervical cancer in the Nordic countries: association with organised screening programmes. Lancet. 1987;1(8544):1247–9.
12. WHO. Guidelines for screening and treatment of precancerous lesions for cervical cancer prevention. Geneva: WHO; 2013.
13. Chen C, Yang Z, Li Z, Li L. Accuracy of several cervical screening strategies for early detection of cervical cancer: a meta-analysis. Int J Gynecol Cancer. 2012;22(6):908–21.
14. Deodhar K, Sankaranarayanan R, Jayant K, Jeronimo J, Thorat R, Hingmire S, et al. Accuracy of concurrent visual and cytology screening in detecting cervical cancer precursors in rural India. Int J Cancer. 2012;131(6):E954–62.

57 Cancer of the Uterine Corpus

Peter Adefuye and Alex Olawaiye

Learning Objectives
After studying this chapter, the reader should be able to:

- Discuss the epidemiology of the cancers of the uterine corpus
- Describe the different cancers of the uterine corpus
- Describe the histopathologic characteristics of the endometrial cancers
- Discuss the etiopathologic characteristics of endometrial cancer and other cancers of the uterine corpus
- Understand the clinical presentation of the endometrial cancer and other cancers of the uterine corpus
- Discuss the investigations and treatment for different types of cancers of the uterine corpus

57.1 Introduction

Globally, cancer of the uterine corpus constitutes 6% of all malignancies in women [1, 2]. It is the most common gynecologic malignancy in the United States and other advanced countries of the world where there are effective population-based screening programs for cervical cancer prevention [3]. However, in low- and medium-income countries (LIMC) the incidence remains very low with cervical and ovarian cancers being more prevalent [4, 5]. This disparity in burden of the disease has been ascribed to higher levels of affluence due to high level of industrialization in the United States and other advanced countries of the world [2, 3].

Cancers from the uterine corpus arise largely (85–90%) from the endometrial lining of the uterus, and less commonly (10–15%) from the mesenchyme [3]. Cancers from the endometrial lining of the uterus are referred to as *endometrial cancers (EC)* and they are commonly related to effects of estrogen in the woman. *Mesenchymal cancers*, on the other hand, have no bearing with the effects of estrogen.

57.2 Endometrial Cancer

Endometrial cancer (EC) constitutes over 90% of all cancers arising from the corpus uteri [3]. It is the commonest gynecological cancer in the developed world. The disease is common in western than eastern countries. In the United States alone, it was estimated in the year 2015 that 54,870 new cases would be diagnosed and 10,170 women would die of the disease [6]. Factors influencing this prominence are declining incidence of cervical cancer, longer life expectancy, and earlier diagnosis. Within the cultures of the United States and similar advanced countries of the world, rates are highest in Whites than Black women, being twice as common in the Whites as Blacks [2, 3].

EC is primarily a disease of postmenopausal women, the peak age incidence of occurrence being between 50 and 65 years. About 25% of EC occurs in the peri-menopausal women and about 5% occurs under the age of 40 years [7, 8].

57.2.1 Etiology and Risk Factors

The precise causes of EC are still far from being understood. There are, however, number of epidemiological observations linking occurrence of EC with hyper-estrogenism resulting

P. Adefuye (✉)
Department of Obstetrics and Gynaecology, Olabisi Onabanjo University Teaching Hospital, Sagamu, Nigeria

A. Olawaiye
Gynaecologic Cancer Research, Mage Women's Hospital, University of Pittsburgh Medical Centre, Pittsburgh, PA, USA

Gynaecologic Oncology, University of Pittsburgh Cancer Institute, Pittsburgh, PA, USA
e-mail: olawaiyea@mail.magee.edu

F. Okonofua et al. (eds.), *Contemporary Obstetrics and Gynecology for Developing Countries*,
https://doi.org/10.1007/978-3-030-75385-6_57

in direct or indirect unopposed estrogen stimulation of the endometrium.

Risk factors implicated in the development of EC include:

(a) Unopposed estrogen stimulation

Following epidemiological observations, it has been postulated that long-term unopposed estrogen stimulation of the endometrium will result in endometrial hyperplasia that commonly progress into EC, the type I form of the disease [9]. Unopposed estrogen stimulation of the endometrium can arise from within (endogenous) and without (exogenous). Endogenous causes of unopposed estrogen stimulation include obesity, infertility arising from anovulation and cases of polycystic ovary syndrome, early attainment of menarche and late menopause (after the age of 52). Another known cause of excessive stimulation from estrogen is estrogen-producing tumor of the ovary, that is, the granulosa cell cancer of the ovary. EC arising from excessive estrogen stimulation begin as endometrial hyperplasia. This type of EC is classified as type I EC; it is better differentiated and has a more favorable prognosis than tumors that are unrelated to estrogen stimulation [10]. Endometrial hyperstimulation can also occur in women who are overweight and have elevated blood pressure [1, 2].

Exogenous causes of hyper-estrogenism are found in women taking anti-estrogen tamoxifen for treatment of breast cancer in the presence of intact uterus [11–13]. Unopposed estrogen stimulation will also arise from long-term use of hormone replacement therapy without addition of progestogens in the presence of intact uterus. Studies have demonstrated that the risk of EC is increased 4- to 15-fold in long-term users of estrogen when compared to age-matched controls.

It has equally been established that past use of oral contraceptives (OCs) with either high- or low-potency progestins is protective against development of EC [6].

(b) Obesity

Obesity is a major risk factor in EC, and epidemiological observations have shown that majority of women who develop EC tend to be obese [14]. Commonly women weighing 15 kg (30 lb) over ideal weight for height have a threefold increased risk of developing EC, and those weighing 25 kg (50 lb) or more over ideal weight for height have a 10-fold increased risk [6]. Weight closer to the time of diagnosis appears more relevant than weight at younger age and weight gain over the adult life period is a strong predictor of risk. The obese woman, especially postmenopause, is in a state of hyper-estrogenism arising from peripheral conversion of androstenedione to estrone. Also in the adipose tissue, androgens are aromatized to estradiol. Both mechanisms lead to high levels of unopposed estrogen in the obese woman, resulting in complex hyperplasia and atypia that may result in type I endometrial cancer.

(c) Diets

Diets, perhaps, account for high rate of occurrence of endometrial cancers in western societies and very low in low- and medium-income countries such as Eastern Europe, Asia, and sub-Saharan Africa [2, 3].

Diets in affluent countries are rich in animal fats and observations have suggested a direct relationship between high-fat diets and higher incidence of endometrial carcinoma in women [14, 15]. As in obesity, high-fat diets result in a state of hyper-estrogenism. Fatty diets result in fat deposition leading to increased adipose tissue. Within the adipose tissue, androgens are aromatized to estradiol [15].

(d) Diabetes mellitus and hypertension

Diabetes mellitus and hypertension are expressions of obesity in individuals, be it man or woman. That they could, however, be risk factors for endometrial cancer are still inconclusive [3]. Diabetes mellitus and hypertension in the presence of obesity and overweight women are important risk factors in the development of endometrial cancer [3, 6]. The non-insulin-dependent type of diabetes mellitus is more implicated in the development of endometrial cancer. Non-insulin-dependent diabetes mellitus is associated with elevation in the estrogen levels, hyperinsulinemia, and insulin-like growth factor 1 (IGF-1) [16, 17]. The resulting elevation in estrogen leads to complex endometrial hyperplasia with atypia leading to the development of type I form of endometrial carcinoma.

(e) Endogenous estrogens

Persistent or recurrent anovulation in women leads to deprivation of progesterone that is required to oppose ever-increasing estrogen levels in such women. An ovulation arising from polycystic ovary disease (PCO) does not only deprive the woman needed progesterone to oppose effects of estrogen on the endometrium [9], the condition is associated with elevated levels of the androgen *androstenedione* that is aromatized peripherally to estradiol. The hyper-estrogenic state does not only lead to endometrial hyperplasia and abnormal uterine bleeding but that the hyperplasia can progress to complex hyperplasia with atypia and endometrial hyperplasia.

Other condition leading to increased and opposed estrogen secretion in women is the development of granulosa cell tumor of the ovary. This resulting estrogen secretion results in state of hyper-estrogenism that is frequently associated with complex endometrial hyperplasia with atypia and endometroid type of endometrial cancer [3].

(f) Exogenous estrogens

Climacteric women or postmenopausal women with discomforting symptoms, such as flushes, dyspareunia, vaginitis., may seek relief with administration of hormone replacement therapy (HRT). The hormone being replaced to ameliorate symptoms is estrogen. This treatment leads to a state of hyper-estrogenism in women, and when given unopposed by progestins for a long time in the presence of intact uterus could lead to endometrial hyperplasia that may progress into complex hyperplasia with atypia and type I endometrial hyperplasia [9]. Every user of estrogen has a 2.3 relative risk of developing endometrial cancer. The risk increases to 9.5 where such use has been 10 and more. It is therefore advised that when estrogen is to be administered to woman with intact uterus, a progestogen be administered concurrently to prevent endometrial hyperplasia.

Another exogenous estrogen that may lead to rise in the incidence of endometrial cancer and probably carcinosarcoma is prolonged treatment with *tamoxifen.* Tamoxifen belongs to a group of drugs referred to as selective estrogen receptor modulators (SERM) with anti-estrogenic effects on the breast and estrogenic effects on tissues such as the bone, the cardiovascular system, and the uterus [3]. It is widely used as an adjuvant therapy in the management of breast cancer. This medication has estrogenic effect on the endometrium. When tamoxifen is used for 5 years and longer, it induces a relative risk of about 6.0 of developing endometrial cancer [6, 12, 13]. The protective effect of tamoxifen from recurrent breast cancer far outweighs any potential mortality from endometrial cancer. In order to prevent rise in the incidence of endometrial cancer while treating to prevent recurrent breast cancer disease, newer generation of SERMs with wider range of anti-estrogenic effect on breast and other tissues that include bone and uterus (such as raloxifene, anastrozole, letrozole, exemestane.) are now replacing tamoxifen to treat or prevent recurrent disease in breast cancer [18, 19].

(g) Parity

The less parous a woman, the greater is her risk of developing endometrial cancer. Nulliparous women have two times greater risk for developing endometrial cancer than parous women. In nulliparous women there is incessant ovulation with resultant states of hyper-estrogenism and endometrial hyperplasia [2, 6].

(h) Hereditary

Most cases of endometrial cancers are sporadic; however, some of them clearly have a hereditary basis. A family history of endometrial, breast, and colon cancer suggests possible hereditary factor arising from defective genes. This group of endometrial cancer is not preceded by risk factor of unopposed estrogen stimulation, occurs in younger age, less differentiated, and has poorer prognosis. Commonest defective gene resulting in endometrial cancer is hereditary nonpolyposis colorectal cancer (HNPCC) gene. HNPCC is an autosomal dominant condition characterized by colorectal cancer occurring at younger age than is found in the general population. The extra-colonic malignancies of this genetic mutation include carcinoma of the stomach, small intestines, renal and biliary tracts, ovary, and endometrium. Endometrial cancer is the second most common cancer seen in HNPCC gene mutation. Controversies exist regarding the relationship of BRCA1 and BRCA2 and incidence of endometrial cancer [6, 20–23].

57.2.2 Protective Factors

(a) Combined oral contraceptives (OCP) and progesterone administration

Observations have revealed that women who use low-dose combined oral contraceptive pills have lower risk of endometrial cancer than women in the general population. The protective effect can be as long as 20 years or more after discontinuation in women who have used OCP for long.

In women receiving estrogen for hormone replacement administration of progesterone protects against development of endometrial cancer. The progesterone must be administered cyclically for at least 10 days per cycle. Administration of progesterone opposes the stimulation of the endometrium by estrogen and consequent incomplete shedding. It exerts this effect by reducing the estrogen receptors in the endometrium. In addition, the progesterone increases the activity of the enzymes *estradiol-17β dehydrogenase* that metabolizes estradiol to less potent metabolites [24, 25].

The protective effect of administration of progestins as used in OCP is dose related. OCPs with higher dose progestin may be more protective than OCs with lower progestin, however, the progestin as in most OCPs appears adequate to provide a protective effect against endometrial cancer [25].

(b) Smoking and alcohol

It has been observed that there is reduction in circulating levels of estrogen in women who smoke than non-smokers. The reason for this association has, however, not been fully elucidated. As protective as this habit is, it could not, however, be advised as a mean or routine to preventing endometrial cancer as deadly consequences of smoking outweigh this apparent advantage. On the other hand, no similar correlation has been observed between alcohol and endometrial cancer [24].

(c) Lifestyle

Other protective habits include active lifestyles than sedentary nature or job occupation. Consumption of vegetables and some dairy products are also protective [24].

57.2.3 Pathology of Endometrial Cancer

Endometrial carcinoma is a heterogeneous disease characterized by a number of histologic subtypes, each having its distinct clinical course and behaviors. The disease can broadly be divided into endometrioid, mucinous, and non-endometrioid subtypes. The non-endometrioid subtype is further divided into serous carcinoma, clear-cell carcinoma, and carcinosarcoma.

(a) Endometrioid endometrial adenocarcinoma

It constitutes about 85% of all types of endometrial cancer and arise chiefly from endometrial hyperplasia in pre- and postmenopausal women as a result of estrogen excess that may arise from obesity and other clinical conditions associated with hyper-estrogenism.

Microscopically composed of crowded, back-to-back, and fused glands and solid nests of tumor. The nuclei are pseudostratified and atypical, but generally maintain intraepithelial polarity. Morular, squamous, or mucinous is often present.

Histologic diagnostic criteria include:

I. Back tobacco proliferation of endometrial glands occupying an area of at least 2 × 2 mm
II. Extensive papillary pattern
III. Desmoplastic or fibroblastic stroma infiltrated by irregular glands

The tumor is graded by FIGO on a scale of 1–3, based on the amount of solid tumor component:

- Grade 1: made up of 6% solid tumor component
- Grade 2: consists of between 6% and 50% solid tumor components
- Grade 3: made of more than 50% solid tumor components

Grades 1 and 2 constitute the low-grade tumor types and are associated with good prognosis. Grade 3 tumors have intermediate to poor prognosis.

Endometrioid endometrial adenocarcinoma has several microscopic morphological variant that include squamous, villoglandular, and secretory or ciliated variants [3]. These variants are merely for histologic expression and have little or no known clinical significance.

(b) Mucinous endometrial adenocarcinoma

This tumor represents approximately 1% of endometrial cancers. It is composed predominantly of mucinous glands [26]. WHO criteria define the mucinous adenocarcinoma as tumor having more than 90% of cells with intracytoplasmic mucin [27, 28]. However, other investigators define the tumor with 50% and more of cells with intracytoplasmic mucin.

Mucinous endometrial adenocarcinoma are graded in the same manner, has comparable prognosis, as endometrioid adenocarcinoma. It is, however, found to have a slightly higher association with lymph node metastasis than endometrioid adenocarcinoma [28]. The tumors appear, on histology, like primary endocervical carcinoma or metastasis from GI tract.

(c) Non-endometrioid endometrial carcinoma

Unlike endometrioid type, the pathogenesis of this tumor is independent of estrogen and has no known precursor. It occurs typically in older postmenopausal women.

Non-endometrioid tumor constitutes about 10–15% of all endometrial cancers. It includes serous, clear-cell, and carcinosarcoma subtypes. These histotypes are associated with high-grade cytologic features and are not graded [28].

I. Uterine serous carcinoma

Uterine serous carcinoma accounts for 5–13% of all endometrial cancers. The hallmark of this disease is the loss of intraepithelial polarity in combination with pronounced cytological atypia that include prominent nucleoli and a large variation in nuclear size and shape. Its microscopic architectural configuration ranges from intraepithelial carcinoma to invasive forms consisting of glandular, papillary, or solid patterns. The disease has a poor prognosis with the presence of extra-uterine disease in as many as 37% of patients at presentation despite no evidence of endometrial stromal or myometrial invasion [3].

II. Clear-cell uterine carcinoma

The clear-cell variant of non-endometrioid disease constitutes between 1% and 7% of all endometrial cancers [28]. The tumor cells are typically polygonal with clear to eosinophilic cytoplasm and eccentrically placed atypical nuclei, arranged in solid sheets, papillae, or glands. The papillary forms exhibit hyalinized cores and a single-cell layer with hobnail nuclei typically lines. In addition, the tumor may contain hyaline globules. The prognosis is poor and comparable with uterine serous carcinoma.

III. Uterine carcinosarcoma

This disease is also known as *malignant mixed Müllerian* tumors. It is histologically composed of distinct malignant epithelial (carcinomatous) and malignant mesenchymal (sarcomatous) components. In the current WHO classification, it is described as sarcoma rather than carcinoma [27]. It is, however, being increasingly regarded by pathologists as a high-grade metaplastic carcinoma. It has recurrence and metastasis patterns that mirror that of carcinoma rather than sarcoma. Clonality and mutational studies have shown that the carcinomatous and sarcomatous components derive from same precursor [28].

Uterine carcinosarcoma have poor prognosis with worse outcome than the endometrioid, serous, and clear-cell carcinomas. The tumors with polypoid shapes are associated with lower rates of myometrial and lymphovascular invasion as well as with longer patient survival compared with non-polypoid counterparts [28].

(d) Unclassified uterine carcinoma

This is a recently described entity in the classification of uterine malignancies. It constitutes about 9% of endometrial carcinoma. It does not exhibit any gland or solid nest configuration but rather monotonous discohesive cells arranged in solid sheets with focal evidence of epithelial differentiation. About 5–10% of cells express keratin markers by immunochemistry and very minimal expression of the estrogen and progesterone receptors. The disease is commonly underdiagnosed due to diagnostic confusion with the FIGO Grade 3 endometrioid adenocarcinoma that has a significantly better prognosis.

Undifferentiated carcinoma may appear as a mixed carcinoma in combination with endometrioid adenocarcinoma, giving a hypothesis of a probable common origin with dedifferentiation of endometrioid adenocarcinoma [28]. However, controversies still exist on whether the tumor should be classified as an endometrioid or a non-endometrioid uterine carcinoma.

(e) Mixed endometrial carcinoma

WHO describes these group of endometrial cancers as tumors consisting of one endometrioid or mucinous carcinoma component and another non-endometrioid carcinoma component, each representing at least 10% of the overall tumor [27, 29].

Experience with mixed endometrial tumors is limited and the most studied of its subtypes is the endometrioid serous type whose components is 50% or more of serous carcinoma. Mixed endometrial carcinoma has behaviors comparable to that of pure serous carcinoma. The endometrioid clear-cell variant has poor prognosis [29].

(f) Other rare endometrial carcinomas

These histotypes include pure *squamous cell carcinoma, transitional-cell carcinoma, and small-cell carcinoma.* These three histotypes of endometrial cancers are so rare and regarded as endometrioid-type endometrial carcinoma that has undergone extensive metaplastic changes.

57.2.4 Spread of Endometrial Cancer

Endometrial cancer can spread by any of the four common channels through which tumors spread, the direct spread to contiguous structures or space, hematogenous and lymphatic channels, and peritoneal implants after transtubal spread [24, 29].

(a) Local spread

This is spread by direct invasion through the myometrium to the serous covering of the uterus into the peritoneal cavity. Another route of spread to the peritoneum is spread through the fallopian tube lumen.

(b) Hematogenous spread

Hematogenous metastases are most commonly to the liver in endometrial cancer. Spread to the liver may also occur from interchange between the para-aortic and portal vein lymphatic. Hematogenous spread to the lungs is rare in primary endometrial cancer. Other site of hematogenous spread is the bone.

(c) Lymphatic spread

The lymphatic drainage of the uterus appears somewhat complex and therefore determines the complex pattern of lymphatic spread in uterine cancers. From the subperitoneal plexus, the collecting lymphatics in the lower uterine segment may drain through the cervix to the external iliac lymph nodes. This plexus can also drain by way of the isthmus to the lateral sacral node. The plexus of lymphatic at the base of the broad ligament drain into the internal iliac lymph nodes. Tubal and ovarian pedicles (the infundibulo-pelvic ligament) drain into para-aortic lymph nodes. Through the left ovary that drains into the left renal vein and its lymphatic channel distant metastases can occur directly to the upper abdomen. Drainage along the round ligament progresses to the superficial inguinal nodes, then the femoral and finally to external iliac nodes.

Risk of nodal involvement is negligible for endometrial cancer confined only to endometrium. Even with the invasion of inner third of the myometrium, and the tumor is Grade 1 or 2, the risk is still negligible. With invasion of the outer third of the myometrium, the risk of nodal invasion becomes increased. Pelvic nodes are valid indicators of the risk of para-aortic node metastases. When there are metastases to the pelvic nodes, more than 50% of the cases would have para-aortic nodes involvement.

Metastasis to the pelvic nodes is related to tumor extension into the cervical canal. The paracervical tissue is rich in lymphatic; hence, spread to the cervix increases the potential for dissemination to pelvic nodes. The frequency of extension of endometrial cancer to the isthmus and cervical canal increases with the extent of myometrial invasion.

In about 3–8% of patients with clinical Stage I disease vaginal metastases are found. These metastases are more through submucosal lymphatic or vascular spread than by spillage at the time of surgery as reasoned by some [3, 24, 29]. However, metastases to the vagina are more common with higher histologic grade, lower uterine segment or cervical involvement of the disease.

57.2.5 Staging and Prognosis of Endometrial Cancer

The recommended staging procedure for uterine corpus cancers now is surgical staging as described by FIGO in 1988. Before this time, in 1971, FIGO introduced the clinical method of staging the disease. This clinical staging remains relevant where resources are limited, as obtainable in most low- and middle-income countries, and when the patient's clinical condition may not allow for surgical staging [3, 30]. Components of clinical staging as proposed by FIGO in 1971 are as shown in Table 57.1. To complement clinical staging are the needs to clinically examine the woman for superficial lymph node such as supra-clavicular, inguinal, and/or anterior abdominal wall lymph nodes. In addition, clinical evidence of pleural effusion, ascites, and omental caking are suggestions of extra-pelvic and distance metastases of the disease. Pelvic examination will reveal cervical, vaginal, or adnexal spread. Assessment of the uterine size and its mobility is important especially for patient that is being considered for vaginal hysterectomy. Imaging, that is chest radiograph, will be of value in assessing extent of spread to the lungs and cardiopulmonary compromise. In addition, computed tomographic scan (CT scan) and magnetic resonance imaging (MRI) are valuable in detecting early metastases to the abdomen, the cervix and other distant sites. Cystoscopy and proctoscopy will conform or rule out spread to urinary bladder and rectum respectively [3].

In highly resourceful settings, surgical staging is undertaken, in addition to ancillary investigations as mentioned above, at the time of instituting the primary treatment of the disease. The technique of surgical staging involves the application of desirable incision, peritoneal washing for needed specimen for cytological examination, intra-peritoneal inspection, removal of the uterus, ovaries, and the tubes, the adnexa, upper cuff of the vagina, and lymph node sampling [3, 24].

It is generally recommended that the abdomen should be opened with a midline vertical *incision* extending from just above the symphysis pubis to a point para-umbilical or above the umbilicus good enough to allow for intra-abdominal inspection. *Peritoneal washings* must be immediately taken upon entry into the abdomen from the abdomen and pelvis. This is then followed by careful exploration of the intra-abdominal contents; the peritoneal, liver, diaphragmatic, omental, adnexal, and cul-de-sac surfaces must be palpated for multiple metastases [1–3, 24, 29]. In addition the surgeon must palpate for suspicious or enlarged lymph nodes in the pelvis (internal and external iliac groups) and para-aortic in the abdomen [3, 24]. Table 57.2. and 57.3. are surgical staging as introduced by FIGO in 1988, and later revised in 2009 and histopathologic grading respectively.

In order for the patient to have best outcome from management of endometrial cancer, some factors are necessary for consideration to be able to categorize patients into high- and low-risk groups. The classification is necessary to guide the use of adjuvant therapies. Understanding these factors also allows for the development of novel strategies to reduce risk of recurrence or alter patterns of disease failure. Patients at highest risk for recurrence and death are those with spread of disease outside of the uterus as reflected by FIGO staging. The stage of the disease as described by FIGO surgical staging is the single strongest predictor of outcome for women with endometrial carcinoma. Patients with surgical

Table 57.1 FIGO staging of uterine sarcomas (excluding carcinosarcoma)

Stage	Description
Leiomyosarcoma (uLMS) and endometrial stromal sarcoma (ESS)	
I	Tumor limited to the uterus
IA	Tumor less than 5 cm
IB	Tumor more than 5 cm
II	Tumor extends beyond the uterus but within the pelvis
IIA	Adnexal involvement
IIB	Involvement of other pelvic tissues
III	Tumor invades abdominal tissues (not just protruding into the abdomen)
IIIA	One site
IIIB	More than one site
IIIC	Metastasis to pelvic and/or para-aortic lymph node
IVA	Tumor invades bladder and/or rectum
IVB	Distant metastasis
Adenosarcoma	
I	Tumor limited to uterus
IA	Limited to endometrium/endocervix with no myometrial invasion
IB	Less, or equal, half myometrial invasion
IC	More than half myometrial invasion
II	Tumor extends to the pelvis
IIA	Adnexal involvement
IIB	Tumor extends to extra-uterine pelvic tissue
III	Tumor invades abdominal tissues (not just protruding into the abdomen)
IIIA	One site
IIIB	More than one site
IIIC	Metastasis to pelvic and/or para-aortic lymph node
IVA	Tumor invades bladder and/or rectum
IVB	Distant metastasis

Table 57.2 1988 FIGO staging of endometrial cancer

Stage	Description
I	Cancer that is confined to the uterus
II	Cancer that has spread to the cervix
III	Cancer that has spread to the vagina, ovaries and/or lymph nodes
IV	Cancer that has spread to the urinary bladder, rectum or organs located far from the uterus, such as the lungs or bones

Table 57.3 2009 FIGO staging system for endometrial cancer

Stage	Description
IA	Tumour confined to uterus, <50% myometrial invasion
IB	Tumour confined to uterus, ≥50% myometrial invasion
II	Cervical stromal invasion
IIIA	Tumour invasion into serosa or adnexa
IIIB	Vaginal and parametrial involvement
IIIC1	Pelvic node involvement
IIIC2	Para-aortic node involvement
IVA	Tumour invasion into bladder or bowel mucosa
IVB	Distant metastases (including abdominal metastases) or inguinal lymph node involvement

Stage IV disease have the poorest prognosis with 5-year survival ranging from 20% to 25%. In cytology-negative patients, 5-year survival can be as high as 97%. Factors determining prognosis in endometrial carcinoma include the histologic cell type of the disease, the grade of differentiation, depth of myometrial invasion, extent of lymphovascular space invasion, age, race, and presence of steroid hormones (estrogen and progesterone) receptors [2, 3].

(a) *Histologic cell types*

The cell type of the endometrial carcinoma has consistently appeared to be important in predicting the biologic behavior and probability of survival in a patient with endometrial carcinoma. Endometrioid adenocarcinoma, with the majority of the tumors located in the uterine corpus carries a relatively favorable prognosis. Other histological types that have comparable biologic behavior and patients survival with endometrioid adenocarcinoma are adenocarcinoma with squamous differentiation and villoglandular carcinoma. Serous carcinoma and clear-cell carcinoma, on the other hand, tend to have more aggressive behavior with about 40–70% of them having extra-uterine spread at presentation and poorer prognosis [3].

(b) *Grade (histologic differentiation)*

Histologic differentiation is an important indicator of spread. The less differentiated a tumor is, the more the tendency for deep myometrial invasion and, subsequently, higher rates of pelvic and para-aortic lymph node involvement and lesser the rate of 5-year survival.

(c) *Myometrial invasion*

Myometrial invasion directly correlates with risk of extra-uterine tumor spread, treatment failure and disease recurrence and inversely for probability of patient survival. Myometrial invasion is an independent predictor for recurrence and survival even in node-negative patients.

(d) *Lymphovascular space invasion (LVSI)*

This is another strong predictor of recurrence and death in endometrial carcinoma, and it is independent of myometrial invasion and histologic differentiation. LVSI is found in 35–95% of patients with serous-type carcinoma, giving increased risk of tumor recurrence or death from the disease.

(e) *Age and race*

As the mean age at diagnosis rises, other prognostic factors tend to accelerate with increasing age. Women aged between 70 and 90 years tend to present with tumors that are more invasive and at advanced stage. The younger woman tends to have better prognosis. Caucasian women also tend to have higher survival rate than Black patients who tend to have poorer differentiated tumors.

(f) *Presence and extent of steroid hormone receptors*

Normal endometrium is richer in steroid hormone (estrogen and progesterone) receptors than endometrial cancers. The highest levels of estrogen and progesterone receptors are found in well-differentiated (Grade 1) tumors and lowest in Grade 3 tumors.

Survival rate with each stage of the disease is noted to be better for patients with receptor-rich tumors than those with receptor-poor or receptor-negative tumors. Progesterone receptor status has been found to be the most significant prognostic factor after clinical stage. Progesterone receptor status is a more determinant factor for response to progestational treatment than estrogen receptor.

57.2.6 Clinical Presentation

Virtually all variant and histotypes of endometrial cancers have similar patterns of clinical presentation.

(a) *Abnormal uterine bleeding*

Abnormal bleeding from the uterus is the classic symptom of endometrial carcinoma, especially when the bleeding occurs in postmenopausal women or in women aged 40 years and more and with risk factors. Eighty percent of patients will present with abnormal uterine bleeding and approximately 10% of the symptomatic postmenopausal patients will be found to have cancer on biopsy [2, 3]. Benefits of abnormal uterine bleeding in endometrial carcinoma is its propensity to occur or present early in the disease and account for its early presentation and high survival rate. It is an alerting symptom of endometrial carcinoma, alerting the practitioner to rule out endometrial carcinoma regardless of age.

Differential diagnosis of abnormal uterine bleeding will include cervical cancer, endometrial polyps, endometritis, degenerating sub-mucous uterine fibroid, vaginal and vulval lesion, and ovarian tumors (granulosa cell tumor). In the early stage of the disease, the patient looks well clinically and the only physical finding may just be the uterine bleeding.

(b) *Vaginal discharge*

Abnormal vaginal discharge may be a reflection of severe endometrial hyperplasia or early invasive stage of the disease that is usually detected incidentally on routine examinations for other reasons. Presence of vaginal discharge in association with thickened endometrium in a postmenopausal woman arouses a suspicion of endometrial malignancy.

(c) *Other modes of presentation*

About 10% of patients will complain of lower abdominal cramps and pain, and they may be secondary to uterine contractions caused distension and blood trapped behind a stenotic cervix. Abscesses, and systemic infection, may arise following secondary bacterial infection of the trapped blood or secretion. Systemic signs of infection will include fever and offensive vaginal discharge.

In the late stage of the disease there may be weight loss.

57.2.6.1 Physical Findings

In the early stage of the disease, the patient usually appears clinically well. Bleeding from the uterus is early symptom and its sequelae is anemia, which may be detected clinically. Other detectable physical presentations are common with advanced stage of the disease and they include weight loss, lower abdominal uterine mass from hematometra, or tender lower abdominal mass which is a reflection of superimposed infection of the uterine content. Findings of supra-clavicular, peri-umbilical, and inguinal lymph nodes are pointers to late stages of the disease.

57.2.7 Diagnosis

Routine laboratory findings are normal in most patients with endometrial carcinoma. However, in long-standing disease, laboratory findings are evident or suggestive of endometrial carcinoma and its complications.

(a) *Complete blood count (CBC), blood chemistry, urine and stool analyses*

These are useful ancillary diagnostic tests in patients with endometrial carcinoma. CBC may reveal low hematocrit and/or hemoglobin concentration (anemia) following prolonged bleeding. Elevation in the number of white cells count may be pointer to infection. Liver function test, blood chemistry, urea and nitrogen, liver enzymes, creatinine, and other findings may be normal or deranged in early and late stages respectively. In advanced stage, micro- or macrohematuria may be found on urinalysis, and there may be occult blood or frank blood on stool analysis.

(b) *Cytological study*

Smears taken from the cervix and vaginal fornices can reveal endometrial carcinoma by the presence of endometrial cells in cervical or vaginal smears of a menopausal or postmenopausal woman.

(c) *Endometrial biopsy and histology*

Endometrial biopsy provides histologic diagnosis of endometrial carcinoma and can, in addition, identify other etiologies of abnormal uterine bleeding and these include chronic endometritis, endometrial atrophy, endometrial polyps, or endocervical carcinoma. The accuracy of diagnosis of endometrial carcinoma with this method becomes higher in postmenopausal woman than premenopausal woman.

Fractional dilation and curettage allows for endocervical curettage and differentiates endometrial carcinoma from primary disease of the endocervical carcinoma.

(d) *Endoscopic studies*

I. Hysteroscopy

Hysteroscopy is an important adjuvant to D&C to improve detection of pathology in the evaluation of postmenopausal bleeding. Drawbacks of this procedure include transtubal migration of tumor cells that may become detectable as malignant cells in the peritoneal washing during surgical staging of the disease.

II. Cystoscopy and sigmoidoscopy

These endoscopic studies are ancillary adjuvant investigation to complement diagnosis and detect disease progression. Cystoscopy and proctoscopy are necessary tools that clinically evaluate Stage IV disease. Sigmoidoscopy and colonoscopy are of value in screening, or diagnosis, of patients with HNPCC (Lynch syndrome) in young and middle-aged women or patients.

III. Ultrasonogram

Pelvic ultrasonography is of value in surveillance of asymptomatic high-risk women. It provides information regarding the size and shape of the uterus and the thickness of the endometrium. Endometrial thickness of >5 mm in postmenopausal woman is suspicious of endometrial carcinoma or hyperplasia. Trans-vaginal scan is more specific than the trans-abdominal scan. The cut-off of 5 mm endometrial thickness depends on the postmenopausal status of the woman and/or whether on HRT or not. For women on HRT, finding of endometrial thickness of 2–3 mm is more significant than endometrial thickness of more than 5 mm.

IV. Imaging techniques

Metastases to the chest and assessment of cardiopulmonary compromise in the disease can be revealed by chest X-ray. This is, however, rarely positive in the early stages.

Computed tomography scan (CT scan) is useful in the evaluation of enlarged pelvic and para-aortic lymph nodes, and establishing distant metastases to the liver and lungs.

Magnetic resonance imaging (MRI) is particularly helpful in identifying myometrial invasion and extending same to the lower uterine segment and the cervix.

57.2.8 Treatment

Primary treatment of both primary and recurrent endometrial carcinoma is surgery [2, 3, 24, 31]. Other adjunctive methods of treatment are irradiation and chemotherapy.

(a) *Surgery*

Because of early presentation of endometrial carcinoma, most patients can be adequately and completely treated by surgery.

The surgical procedures in the primary surgery for endometrial carcinoma are extrafascial total hysterectomy (abdominal or vaginal), bilateral salpingo-oophorectomy, peritoneal washing for cytology and pelvic and para-aortic lymph node removal and surgical staging.

Patient should be brought to operating room after appropriate bowel preparation. Prophylactic heparin should be administered, especially in fat patients, to prevent risk of venous thrombosis and preoperative broad spectrum (and with good anaerobic coverage) antibiotics be given.

Lower midline incision is used to enter the abdominal cavity and peritoneal washings are obtained by injecting 50–100 ml of saline solution into the pelvis (if there is no ascites). Washings are aspirated and placed in sterile container with dilute heparin and sent for cytological studies.

The peritoneal cavity is then thoroughly explored by palpating and inspecting the following: uterus and the tubes, ovaries, retroperitoneal spaces and the para-aortic area up to the level of renal vessels. Thorough palpation of the hemidiaphragm, omentum, liver, kidneys, and peritoneal gutters should be undertaken. The intestines are then packed away and the pelvis exposed. Adhesiolysis is performed as necessary. Vagina cuff is closed with interrupted sutures. The peritoneal cavity is thoroughly irrigated before and after closure of the vaginal cuff.

Novel in the surgical management of endometrial carcinoma is the minimally invasive methods such as laparoscopic-assisted and robotic-assisted surgeries that have been successfully performed in highly resourceful settings of Western Europe and North America. The uses of these methods are still non-existent or very limited in resource poor settings of LMIC. The outcome of management in laparoscopic surgery is equivalent to outcome in open surgery. In addition, length of hospitalization and recovery from surgery are both short.

Gross pathologic assessment of the uterus should be performed during the operation to determine the need for lymphadenectomy in the surgical staging, especially in patient with Grade 1 or 2 endometrioid endometrial carcinoma. Patient requiring lymphadenectomy for surgical staging at the time of surgery will include: (i) Stage I disease with Grade 3 lesion, (ii) tumor greater than 2 cm in maximum dimension, (iii) tumors with more than 50% myometrial invasion, (iv) cervical extension, (v) evidence of extra-uterine spread and (vi) clear-cell and papillary serous carcinoma because of high incidence of lymphatic spread in them. Criteria for lymphadenectomy are not universally accepted and are subject of repeated reviews and investigation. Bulky positive nodes that are unlikely to respond to external beam radiation therapy (EBRT) should be removed during the surgery.

Radical hysterectomy is indicated in patients with Stage II tumors and in patients with recurrence following primary treatment with radiotherapy alone or for those who have received therapeutic doses of pelvic radiation treatment for other pelvic cancers. Risks of bowel or urinary tract injury in this setting must be understood and accepted by both patient and physician. Exploratory laparotomy should be considered in-patient whose disease seems resectable.

Debulking surgery is an added procedure in patients with extra-pelvic spread of the disease and it includes resection and appropriate biopsies of visible tumor and omentectomy (infra-colic) in addition to standard surgical procedure.

Postoperatively and surgico-pathologic findings, 50–60% of the patients will not need further therapy. Further treatment depends on clinical stage and grade of the disease.

(b) *Radiotherapy*

Radiotherapeutic methods employed in the treatment of endometrial carcinoma are largely teletherapy, external beam radiation treatment, using cobalt machine or linear accelerator and brachytherapy intracavitary. Radiation treatment is employed chiefly as adjuvant to surgery. Primary radiation treatment is used only in patients with medical co-morbidity that contraindicates surgery (laparotomy), or when there is advanced pelvic disease. Primary radiation treatment has been demonstrated to cure endometrial carcinoma; the cure rate, however, is about 20% lower than that of surgery in Stage I disease. Adjuvant treatment is dependent on the result of surgical staging and histology. Adjuvant radiotherapy is frequently required in high-risk endometrial carcinoma of endometrioid histotype to prevent pelvic recurrence. Advanced pelvic disease may be treated with radiation followed by chemotherapy. Biology of serous variant of endometrial carcinoma behaves similarly to ovarian cancer and is treated with adjuvant platinum-based chemotherapy in conjunction with radiation treatment. Where the patient presents with gross cervical involvement, radiation may be employed preoperatively. Relative contraindications to preoperative radiotherapy include pelvic mass, pelvic kidney, pyometria, pelvic abscess, prior pelvic radiation and history of previous laparotomies.

Adjuvant radiotherapy improves locoregional control in early and high-risk disease. External beam radiation therapy (EBRT) in early-stage, high-risk endometrial carcinoma decreases the rate of vaginal and pelvic recurrences than when only surgery is employed. Adjuvant radiotherapy is also recommended in disease with extra-uterine extension, lower uterine segment or cervical involvement, poor histologic differentiation (papillary serous or clear-cell histology), or myometrial invasion greater than one-third of the full thickness. Palliative radiation (to bone or brain metastases) is beneficial for symptomatic relief. In the absence of the above-mentioned risk, it is difficult to justify the risk and morbidity of any additional treatment method beyond total hysterectomy and bilateral salpingo-oophorectomy. In Stages III and IV disease, radiotherapy could be employed as primary treatment method, and complemented by adjuvant chemotherapy to improve locoregional control. Overall, consideration for radiation treatment as adjuvant treatment in patients with early-stage, high-risk endometrioid endometrial carcinoma should be individualized based on stage and grade, and on whether surgical lymph node staging was performed or not. Risk of nodal and vaginal recurrence is also a consideration for employing radiation treatment as adjuvant to surgery.

(c) *Chemotherapy*

Anti-cancer chemotherapeutic agents are commonly employed as adjuvant to primary treatment by surgery or radiotherapy. Most common combination treatment is with doxorubicin and cisplatin. They can also be employed as single agent in the treatment of the disease. Doxorubicin when used alone has an overall response rate of 38%, and 26% of these patients can achieve complete response. Combination of cisplatin and doxorubicin shows slightly longer survival rates than either agent alone. Addition of paclitaxel to cisplatin and doxorubicin shows overall response rate of 57% with little improved long-term survival compared to the same regimen without paclitaxel. A novel approach to chemotherapy in the management of the disease is the combination of paclitaxel and carboplatin, which has shown comparable response rates and fewer side effects. Other agents with anti-tumor activities against endometrial carcinoma include cyclophosphamide, hexamethylmelamine, and 5-fluorouracil.

(d) *Hormone therapy*

The presence of steroid hormone receptors in endometrial carcinoma is indicative of their modulations and responses when these hormones are administered as treatment modalities. While therapeutic benefits of estrogen remains controversial considering its role in the pathogenesis of the disease, progesterone has shown efficacy in the treatment of recurrent endometrial carcinoma that are not amenable to irradiation or surgery.

Progesterone can be administered orally or parenterally. Oral medications include medroxyprogesterone acetate suspension and hydroxyprogesterone caproate. Oral megesterol and parenteral medroxyprogesterone acetate and hydroxyprogesterone caproate have similar effectiveness with response rates of approximately 25%. Approximately 13% of patients with recurrent disease appear to achieve long-term remission with progesterone treatment. The average duration of response is 20 months and up to 30% responders survive for 5 years.

With use of hormonal treatment, clinical response is better in patients with localized recurrence, well-differentiated tumor, long disease-free interval and positive estrogen and progesterone receptors status.

With hormone therapy some patients may not achieve remission until after 10–12 weeks of treatment with hormones, hence, the minimum duration of treatment should be longer than 3 months. While progesterone is of immense benefit and efficacy in the treatment of recurrent endometrial carcinoma, it is, however, of disappointing results when employed prophylactically.

Tamoxifen, when used alone or in combination with progesterone, has been of benefits in advanced or recurrent endometrial carcinoma. Patients with well-differentiated, estrogen-receptor-positive tumor and with long disease-free intervals tend to have better response to tamoxifen. Tamoxifen is administered orally at 10–20 mg twice daily. Overall response rate for single-agent tamoxifen is approximately 15–20%. Studies on combination of tamoxifen-progestin treatment have shown good clinical response of up to 40%.

(e) *Treatment by stages*

I. *Stage I disease*

At Stage I disease, the tumor is limited to the uterus. The degree of nodal spread will depend on the grade of tumor differentiation that also determines largely the adjuvant treatment for the disease.

The clinical state of the patient will determine the treatment modality.

Medically operable patient: The primary treatment is total hysterectomy, bilateral salpingo-oophorectomy and surgical staging.

Fertility-sparing treatment is considered in patient who still desires childbearing. Indication for this mode of treatment include:

(i) Well-differentiated (Grade 1) endometrioid endometrial carcinoma
(ii) Disease that is limited to the endometrium as confirmed by MRI
(iii) Absence of suspicious or metastatic disease on imaging
(iv) Absence of contraindication to medical treatment, or pregnancy
(v) Patient's consent following counseling that fertility sparing is *not* standard care for the treatment of the disease

Recommended primary treatment for this class of patient is continuous progestin-based treatment using any of the recommended progestins: megestrol, medroxyprogesterone, or levonorgestrel IUD.

The patient is followed up using 3–6 monthly endometrial sampling and histology. If findings show complete response, patient is encouraged to complete her childbearing and then ultimately treated by total hysterectomy and bilateral salpingo-oophorectomy.

If, however, there is disease progression while still on progestin patient should be treated with total hysterectomy and bilateral salpingo-oophorectomy.

Medically inoperable/unfit patient: This group of patient is managed by tumor-directed radiation treatment. In a select group of patient, hormone therapy is considered.

II. *Stage II disease*

At this stage of the disease, tumor has extended to the cervix with increased risk of spread to pelvic and para-aortic nodes. Three therapeutic options have been proposed as primary treatment options: radical hysterectomy and pelvic node dissection, external beam radiation treatment, and chemotherapy.

Clinical Stage II but negative cervical stromal involvement (Table 57.1): The treatment is total hysterectomy, bilateral salpingo-oophorectomy and surgical staging.

Biopsy or MRI confirmed cervical stromal involvement: If the patient is medically operable, the treatment is radical hysterectomy, bilateral salpingo-oophorectomy and surgical staging. Alternatively patient could be initially treated with radiation treatment using brachytherapy and giving between 75 and 80 Grays to point A. Following the radiation treatment, patient should then have hysterectomy, bilateral salpingo-oophorectomy and surgical staging.

If the patient is medically inoperable (or unfit for surgery), treatment options include tumor-directed radiation treatment and with or without chemotherapy and then followed with surgical resection or initial treatment with chemotherapy and then surgical resection when chemotherapy has rendered the patient operable.

III. *Stages III and IV disease*

These stages of the disease are commonly found in older patients who are commonly less able to withstand surgery. The management options at these stages of disease include surgery, irradiation, and chemotherapy. The patients are classified into three groups based on tumor spread and resectability as may be revealed by findings of CA-125 levels and imaging evidence from CT scan, MRI, and PET scan.

Resectable patients (but with ascites, spread to the omentum, abdominal nodes, ovaries, and the peritoneum) will be treated with total hysterectomy, bilateral salpingo-oophorectomy and surgical staging or debulking surgery.

Unresectable patients (with extra-uterine pelvic disease to the vagina, bladder, bowel/rectum, and parametria) would best be treated with external beam radiation treatment and brachytherapy, with or without chemotherapy, or chemotherapy to make the patient resectable for surgery.

Extensive tumor spread including liver metastasis. Treatment options include chemotherapy and/or radiotherapy or hormone treatment. In operable patient, palliative total hysterectomy and bilateral salpingo-oophorectomy is a treatment option.

Stage		Risk assessment	Grade 1	Grade 2	Grade 3
Stage I	Stage IA	Low-risk patients	Observe	Observe or vaginal brachytherapy	Observe or vaginal brachytherapy
		High-risk patients	Observe or vaginal brachytherapy	Observe or vaginal brachytherapy and/or EBRT	Observe or vaginal brachytherapy and/or EBRT
	Stage IB	Low-risk patients	Observe or vaginal brachytherapy	Observe or vaginal brachytherapy	Vaginal brachytherapy and/or EBRT
		High-risk patients	Observe or vaginal brachytherapy and/or EBRT	Observe or vaginal brachytherapy and/or EBRT	EBRT and/or vaginal brachytherapy ± chemotherapy
Stage II			Vaginal brachytherapy and/or EBRT	Vaginal brachytherapy and/or EBRT	EBRT ± vaginal brachytherapy ± chemotherapy
Stage III	Stage IIIA		(i) Chemotherapy ± radiotherapy (ii) Tumor-directed radiotherapy (iii) EBRT ± vaginal brachytherapy		
	Stage IIIB		Chemotherapy and/or tumor-directed radiotherapy		
	Stage IIIC1	Pelvic node positive	Chemotherapy and/or tumor-directed radiotherapy		
	Stage IIIC2	Para-aortic node positive ± pelvic node positive			
Stage IV	Stage IVA	Debulked and with no gross residual disease or microscopic abdominal disease	Chemotherapy ± radiotherapy		
	Stage IVB				

57.2.9 Adjuvant Treatment for Endometrial Carcinoma

57.2.9.1 Management of Recurrent Disease

Following initial treatment, the disease may progress and this necessitate periodic evaluation that include detailed history, physical examination and pelvic examination at regular 3–6 monthly intervals for the first 5 years and then yearly thereafter [6]. More costly evaluation procedures such as chest radiograph, CT scan and tumor markers would be of value more in symptomatic than asymptomatic patients [2, 6, 32].

Endometrial carcinoma recurrent disease commonly present as central disease, confined to the vagina, especially in non-irradiated patient in about 50% of the patients [6]. Other sites of recurrent disease could be the pelvic sidewall, abdominal cavity, liver, and the lungs [6, 33]. Locoregional recurrence can develop in isolation without distant metastasis [3, 6].

57.2.10 Pelvic Recurrence

Treatment prescriptions for recurrent disease confined to the pelvis include irradiation, surgery, chemotherapy, and hormone treatment [6, 28].

57.2.10.1 Radiation Treatment

Treatment of pelvic recurrence disease with irradiation has recorded 5-year disease-specific survival rate as high as 51%. Factors that may militate against this outcome include increased tumor volume, young age, pelvic versus vaginal involvement, and treatment with EBRT versus vaginal brachytherapy [28, 33].

Radiation treatment for pelvic recurrence consists of EBRT with vaginal brachytherapy using colpostats, cylinder, interstitial needle, or seeds [6]. Treatment must be individualized based on tumor size and location, and tolerance of normal tissue must be respected. Combined doses greater than 60 cGy have improved local tumor control [6, 28].

57.2.10.2 Surgery

Isolated pelvic central recurrence after irradiation is rare. If it, however, occurs in select few pelvic exenteration is surgery of choice. Long-term survivors have been reported in 20% of patients managed with this method [28, 34].

57.2.11 Extra-Pelvic Recurrence

57.2.11.1 Irradiation

Radiation treatment in extra-pelvic recurrence may be of value in localized symptomatic lesions. It will also be of value in palliation treatment of recurrences in the lymph nodes, brain, or bones; doses and protocols would be determined by site of tumor recurrence.

57.2.11.2 Endocrine Therapy

Use of progestins produces complete and partial response rates in 15–25% of patients with locoregional recurrence or distant metastasis. The route, types, and dose of progestins do not appear to be related to response, hence, oral therapy is preferred [6, 35, 36]. Factors that are predictive of favorable response to progestin treatment include tumor differentiation and grade [6]. Well-differentiated lesions are more likely to respond than those with poorly differentiated tumors. Much of the Grade 1 tumors have significant levels of estrogen and progestin receptors, and the higher the receptor levels, the more the response to progestins [6, 37].

Tamoxifen is another drug of choice in the management of recurrent disease. It has between 0% and 30% response rate and it is not as active as progestins and may be of little value as second-line treatment in patients who do not respond to progestins [6, 36–39].

57.2.11.3 Chemothearpy

Chemotherapeutic options for the management of recurrent disease can either be by single-agent medication or combination therapy. Three groups of medications have been found to be of value and have encouraging activities. They are anthracyclines, platinum compounds, and taxanes [6]. Anthracyclines include doxorubicin and epirubicin, with doxorubicin having the higher activity than epirubicin. Platinum compounds are cisplatin and carboplatin, with carboplatin having a higher activity. The taxanes include paclitaxel and docetaxel, with paclitaxel having a higher activity. Other single agents with modest activity in the management of endometrial carcinoma recurrent disease are ifosfamide, topotecan, and bevacizumab (Avastin) [6].

Combination regimens include carboplatin + paclitaxel, carboplatin + doxorubicin, and cisplatin + doxorubicin + paclitaxel.

Carboplatin and paclitaxel have a response rate of 50–60% [38, 40]. Cisplatin + doxorubicin + paclitaxel combination appear to have a greater response rate over cisplatin + paclitaxel. Other combination treatments in consideration and trials included (1) cyclophosphamide + doxorubicin + cisplatin + megestrol, (2) melphalan + fluorouracil + megestrol. Pilot studies have demonstrated response rates of 75% and 94% and randomized studies demonstrated response rates of 36% and 38% respectively [6].

Therefore, treatment recommendations for recurrence disease should be as follows:

(a) Patient with Grade 1 (and/or well-differentiated) and known progestin-receptor-positive tumors will benefit from progestin treatment.
(b) Patients with Grades 2–3 (or known progestin-receptor-negative) disease should be considered initially with

single-agent chemotherapy (e.g. paclitaxel, doxorubicin, or carboplatin), or a combination of regimens such as cisplatin + doxorubicin, or cisplatin + doxorubicin + paclitaxel, or carboplatin + paclitaxel.

Any of the treatments mentioned above can also be considered for patients who do not respond to initial hormonal therapy.

57.3 Summary

Corpus uterine cancers constitute about 6% of all malignancies in women. Incidence in low- and medium-income countries is very low with cervical and ovarian cancers being more common. Endometrial cancers are the most common varieties of cancers of the uterine corpus. Obesity, unexplained estrogen stimulation, diabetes, and hypertension are known common risk factors. Exogenous use of estrogen, low parity and family history are also recognized risk factors. Most common histopathological type is endometrioid endometrial adenocarcinoma and the rare varieties are sarcomas.

Abnormal uterine bleeding, most commonly postmenopausal, and abnormal vaginal discharge remain most common presentation. Treatment consists of primary surgery, chemotherapy, and radiation therapy.

57.4 Uterine Sarcoma

Uterine sarcomas are malignant histotypes of mesenchymal tumors that include *endometrial stromal sarcoma* (ESS), *undifferentiated uterine sarcoma* (UUS) and *uterine leiomyosarcoma* (uLMS) [27, 41]. They are uncommon tumors and accounts for 3–7% of all cancers of the uterine corpus and about 1% of all female genital tract malignancies [42]. Carcinosarcomas were previously considered among the uterine sarcomas, but has been dropped since early 2000 and now considered and treated as high-grade epithelial tumor [43]. Until re-classification, carcinosarcomas constitutes about 50% of the uterine sarcomas [42, 43]. Of the other sarcomas, uLMS constitutes the most common subtype (63%), followed by ESS [6]. Other rare types of malignant mesenchymal tumors include adenocarcinoma, rhabdomyosarcoma, and perivascular epithelioid cell neoplasm [6]. uLMS and ESS are characterized by differentiation toward one or more stromal tissues. The ESS are composed of cells resembling the endometrial stroma in the proliferative phase and are of three distinct subtypes: low grade, high grade, and undifferentiated types based on their histopathology, clinical behavior, and patient outcome. All uterine sarcomas are characterized by aggressive growth with early lymphatic or hematogenous spread. The survival rate is poor and majority of the patients will die within 2 years of diagnosis [44].

57.4.1 Staging

The stage of the disease in uterine sarcomas is the single most important prognostic factor in the management of uterine sarcoma [45, 46]. In FIGO staging of uterine cancers in 1988, staging for uterine sarcomas was considered along with endometrial carcinoma but was, on application, found to be unsatisfactory [46]. In 2009, FIGO developed staging for uterine sarcomas with two parts, one for uLMS and ESS and the other for adenocarcinoma (Table 57.1) [46].

57.4.1.1 Treatment of Uterine Sarcomas

Uterine Leiomyosarcoma

Primary treatment for uLMS is total abdominal hysterectomy and bilateral salpingo-oophorectomy, and debulking of the tumor if present outside the uterus and pelvis. Ovarian preservation may be considered in early-stage tumor in premenopausal woman who desires hormonal function [6]. Radiotherapy may be useful in controlling local recurrence and chemotherapy with doxorubicin or docetaxel/gemcitabine combination is now employed in advance or recurrence disease with response rate ranging from 27% to 36% [47].

Endometrial Stromal Sarcoma

It is the second most common uterine sarcoma [41]. It is divided into benign and malignant types based on type of tumor margin; those with well-circumscribed are benign, and those with exhibiting myometrial invasion and permeation of the myometrial lymphovascular spaces are sarcomas [42]. They are further classified by the latest WHO classification based on resemblance to (or lack of) proliferative-type endometrial stroma into three main categories: low grade, high grade, and undifferentiated type [42].

Low-Grade Endometrial Stromal Sarcoma

Occurs frequently in women aged 40–55 years and more than 50% of patients are premenopausal [48]. The disease had been reported in association with polycystic ovary, and after estrogen use and tamoxifen treatment [48].

Common clinical features include uterine bleeding, pelvic pain, and dysmenorrhea. About 25% are asymptomatic [49]. Extra-uterine pelvic extension to the ovaries is found in about a third of the patients [49].

Low-grade ESS microscopically consists of well-differentiated endometrial stromal cells exhibiting only mild nuclear atypia and characteristically invades the lymphovascular spaces of the myometrium. Tumor cell necrosis is rarely seen and it is usually positive for estrogen, progestin, and androgen receptors. They are indolent tumors with favorable prognosis [50]. Five-year survival with Stages I and II tumors is 90% and 50% for Stages III and IV disease [51].

Primary treatment is largely total hysterectomy and bilateral salpingo-oophorectomy and lymph node dissection does not seem to have a role in the treatment. Following surgery, patient may receive adjuvant radiotherapy or hormonal treatment with progestational agents or aromatase inhibitor.

High-Grade Endometrial Stromal Sarcoma

Microscopically, the features of high-grade ESS are intermediate between low-grade ESS and undifferentiated ESS [52]. The mean age of occurrence is 50 years, the range being 28 and 67 years [53]. The disease present usually with abnormal vaginal bleeding, enlarged uterus, and/or pelvic mass can appear as intracavitary polypoid or mural masses with sizes up to 9 cm. The tumor is estrogen and progestin receptors negative. High-grade ESS has more frequent recurrences, with the patient more likely to die of the disease than low-grade ESS [53].

Advance or recurrent tumor should be treated aggressively with combination of radiation and chemotherapy [54, 55].

Undifferentiated Endometrial Stromal Sarcoma

Undifferentiated ESS is a rare tumor occurring typically in postmenopausal women. The mean age of occurrence is 60 years. Its clinical features include vaginal bleeding, pelvic pain, and/or pelvic mass. There may also be symptoms and signs secondary to extra-uterine spread of the disease [43, 56]. Approximately 60% of the patients present in advance stages, Stages III and IV. Undifferentiated ESS is typically estrogen receptor positive and progesterone receptor negative, or weakly positive for progesterone receptor. It is a highly aggressive tumor with very poor prognosis with less than 2 years survival [56].

Primary treatment approach is total hysterectomy and bilateral salpingo-oophorectomy. Adjuvant treatment includes radiotherapy and/or chemotherapy.

57.4.2 Adenosarcoma

Adenosarcoma of the uterus constitute about 5% and 10% of all uterine sarcoma and occurs mainly in postmenopausal women [57]. The mean age of occurrence is 58 years, but can also occur in the adolescent and young adults [57]. This is a mixed Müllerian tumor of low malignant potential. Microscopically, there is intimate admixture of benign glandular epithelium and low-grade sarcoma, usually of endometrial stromal type. The tumor most commonly arises from the endometrium, including the lower uterine segment, and rarely (5–10% of cases) in the endocervix and extra-uterine locations [58].

Adenosarcoma is a fleshy hemorrhagic and necrotic tumor on cut surface and invades the myometrium more often than other uterine sarcomas [58]. Vaginal or pelvic recurrence occurs in approximately 25% and 30% of cases at 5 years [58].

Except when associated with myometrial invasion or sarcomatous overgrowth, the prognosis is far more favorable than that of carcinosarcoma [57]. About 25% of patients with adenosarcoma ultimately die of the disease.

Primary treatment measures are total hysterectomy and bilateral salpingo-oophorectomy [57, 58].

57.4.2.1 Carcinosarcoma

Carcinosarcoma comprises less than 5% of malignant neoplasm of the uterine corpus. Typically a disease in postmenopausal women, median age of patients at presentation is 65 years, but may occur in young and even children [59]. It is common in Blacks than Whites [59, 60].

Risk factors for developing carcinosarcoma include excessive weight, exogenous estrogen use, and nulliparity [60]. Some cases result from prior pelvic radiation and have also been found to be associated with long-term tamoxifen treatment [60–62]. Oral contraceptives and smoking are thought to be protective [63].

Carcinosarcoma of the uterus is a biphasic neoplasm composed of malignant epithelium and mesenchymal element. While carcinosarcoma remains the preferred term, the WHO and International Society of Gynaecological Pathologist (ISGP) refer to it as malignant Müllerian mixed tumor [64]. Various synonyms for its subtypes are carcinosarcoma for those with only homologous mesenchymal element and malignant mesodermal mixed tumor (or malignant Müllerian mixed tumor) for those with heterologous mesenchymal elements [65]. Epithelial component is serous (or high-grade carcinoma not otherwise specified) in about two-third of cases and endometrioid carcinoma in approximately one-third of the patients [66]. The homologous components are usually spindle cell sarcoma without obvious differentiation, many resembling fibrosarcomas or pleomorphic sarcomas [65, 66]. Most common heterologous elements are malignant cartilage or skeletal muscle, resembling either pleomorphic rhabdomyosarcoma or embryonal rhabdomyosarcoma [64, 67]. Carcinosarcoma are highly aggressive tumor, far more aggressive than usual endometrial carcinoma.

Overall 5-year survival ranges from 60% to 75% for uterine-defined disease, 40% to 60% for early-stage disease (Stages I and II), and 15% to 30% for late-stage disease with a median survival of less than 2 years [57, 68, 69]. Presence of heterologous element is a poor prognostic factor even in patient with Stage I tumor [57]. Other prognostic factors include histologic grade, the percentage of tumor with sarcomatous differentiation, depth of myometrial invasion, and presence of lymphovascular invasion [68–70]. Black (or non-White) race and advanced age of patients have been linked with decreased survival [69, 71, 72]. Disease confined to polyp is thought to have a better prognosis [73–75].

Clinical features of carcinosarcoma include abnormal vagina bleeding, pelvic or lower abdominal pain, bloody or watery vaginal discharge, and/or abdominal mass. A polypoid tumor protruding from the external cervical os may be found on examination. In about one-third of cases, patients present with symptoms of extra-uterine spread to the gastrointestinal and genitourinary systems [65].

Treatment of carcinosarcoma includes primary surgery of total hysterectomy and bilateral salpingo-oophorectomy, pelvic node dissection and omentectomy. Complete cytoreduction should be the aim of the surgery as this would be associated with an overall survival benefit [65, 76]. Postoperative adjuvant treatment with combination regimens with ifosfamide/paclitaxel or carboplatin/paclitaxel results in fewer recurrences than whole-body radiation treatment [77, 78].

References

1. Robboy SJ, Anderson MC, Rusell P. Cancer of the Uterine corpus. In Blaustein's pathology of the reproductive tract, Kurman RJ. (Ed). Churchill Livingstone; 2002:1125–188.
2. Tropé CG, Abeler VM, Kristensen GB. Diagnosis and treatment of sarcoma of the uterus: a review. Acta Oncol. 2012;51(6):694–705.
3. D'Angelo E, Prat J. Uterine sarcoma: a review. Gynecol Oncol. 2010;116(1):131–9.
4. OLiva E, Carcangiu MI, Carinelli SG, Ip P, Loening T, Longacre TA, et al. Mesenchymal tumours. In: Kurman RJ, Carcangiu MI, Herrington CS, Young RH, editors. WHO classification of tumours of female reproductive organs. 4th ed. Lyon: IARC; 2014. p. 135–47.
5. Giuntoli RL, Metzinger DS, DiMarco CS, Cha SS, Sloan JA, Keeney GL, et al. Retrospective review of 208 patients with leiomyosarcoma of the uterus: prognostic indicators, surgical management, and adjuvant therapy. Gynecol Oncol. 2003;89(3):460–09.
6. Greven KM, Markman M, Miller DS. Uterine corpus tumours. In: Cancer Management: a multidisciplinary approad (Eds. Haller DG, Wagman LD, Camphausen KA and Hoskin WJ), 2009; Ch.18: 475–504.
7. Murphy KT, Rotmenschi J, Yamada SD, Mundt AJ. Outcome and pattern of failure in pathologic stages I–IV clear cell carcinoma of the endometrium: implications for adjuvant radiation therapy. Int J Radiat Oncol Biol Phys. 2003;55(5):1272–6.
8. Prat J. FIGO staging for uterine sarcomas. Int J Gynecol Obstet. 2009;104(3):177–8.
9. Hardman MP, Roman JJ, Burnett AF, Santin AD. Metastatic uterine leiomyosarcoma regression using an aromatase inhibitor. Obstet Gynecol. 2007;110(2Pt2):518–20.
10. Chang KL, Grabtree GS, Lim-Tan SK, Kempson RL, Hendrickson MR. Primary uterine endometrial stromal neoplasms. A clinicopathologic study of 117 cases. Am J Surg Pathol. 1990;4(5):415–38.
11. Baker P, Oliva E. Endometrial stromal tumours of the uterus: a practical approach using conventional morphology and ancillary techniques. J Clin Pathol. 2007;60(3):235–43.
12. Nucci MR, Harburger D, Koontz J, Dal Cin P, Sklar J. Molecular analysis of the JAZF1-JJAZ1 gene fusion by RT-PCR and fluorescence in situ hybridization in endometrial stromal neoplasm. Am J Surg Pathol. 2007;31(1):65–70.
13. Chan JK, Kawar NM, Shin JY, Osann K, Chen LM, Powell CB, et al. Endometrial stromal sarcoma: a population-based analysis. Br J Cancer. 2008;99(8):1210–5.
14. Kurihara S, Oda Y, Ohishi Y, Iwasa A, Takahira T, Kaneki E, et al. Endometrial stromal sarcomas and related high-grade sarcomas: immunohistochemical and molecular genetic study of 31 cases. Am J Surg Pathol. 2008;32(8):1228–38.
15. Lee CH, Marino-Enriquez A, Ou W, Zhu M, Ali RH, Chiang S, et al. The clinicopathologic features of YWHAE-FAMZZ. Endometrial stromal sarcomas: a histologically high-grade and clinically aggressive tumour. Am J Surg Pathol. 2012;36(5):641–53.
16. Ricci S, Giuntoli RL, Eisenhauer E, Lopez MA, Krill L, Tanner EJ, Gehrig PA, Havrilesky LJ, Secord AA, Levinson K, Frasure H, Celano P, Fader AN. Does adjuvant chemotherapy improve survival for women with early-stage uterine leiomyosarcoma? Gynecol Oncol. 2013;131(3):629–33.
17. Hensley ML, Wathen JK, Maki RG, Araujo DM, Sutton G, Priebat DA, George S, Soslow RA, Baker LH. Adjuvant therapy for high-grade uterus-limited leiomyosarcoma; result of phase 2 trial (SARC 005). Cancer. 2013;119(8):1555–61.
18. Tanner EJ, Garg K, Leitao MM Jr, Soslow RA, Hensley ML. High grade undifferentiated uterine sarcoma: surgery, treatment, and survival outcomes. Gynecol Oncol. 2012;127(1):27–31.
19. Clement PB, Scully RE. Mullerian adenosarcoma of the uterus: a clinicopathologic analysis of 100 cases with a review of the literature. Hum Pathol. 1990;21(4):363–81.
20. Gallardo A, Prat J. Mullerian adenosarcoma: a clinicopathologic and immunohistochemical study of 55 cases challenging the existence of adenofibroma. Am J Surg Pathol. 2009;33(2):278–88.
21. Silverberg SG, Major FJ, Blessing JA, Fetter B, Askin FB, Liao SY. Carcinosarcoma (malignant mixed mesodermal tumour) of the uterus. A Gynaecologic Oncology Group pathologic study of 203 cases. Int J Gynecol Pathol. 1990;9(1):1–9.
22. Major FJ, Blessing JA, Silverberg SG, Morrow CP, Creasman WT, Currie JL, Yordan E, Brady MF. Prognostic factor in early-stage uterine sarcoma. A Gynaecologic Oncology Group study. Cancer. 1993;71(4 Suppl):1702–9.
23. Ali S, Wells M. Mixed Mullerian tumours of the uterine corpus: a review. Int J Gynecol Cancer. 1993;3(1):1–11.
24. Pothuri B, Ramondetta L, Martino M, Alektiar K, Eifel PJ, Deavers MT. Development of endometrial cancer after radiation treatment for cervical carcinoma. Obstet Gynecol. 2003;101(5Pt1):941–5.
25. Zelmanowicz A, Hildesheim A, Sherman ME, Sturgeon SR, Kurman RJ, Barret RJ. Evidence for a common etiology for endometrial carcinomas and malignant mixed Mullerian tumours. Gynecol Oncol. 1998;69(3):253–7.
26. McCluggage WG, Haller U, Kurman RJ, et al. Mixed epithelial and mesenchymal tumours. In: Tavassoli FA, Devilee P, editors. World Health Organisation classification of tumours. Pathology and genetics of tumours of the breast and female genital organs. Lyon: IARC Press; 2003. p. 247–8.
27. Fleming ND, Dorigo O. Sarcoma of the uterus. In: Decherney AH, Nathan L, Laufer N, Roman AS, editors. Current diagnosis and treatment in obstetrics and gynaecology. New York: McGraw-Hill; 2013. p. 841–7.
28. Ferguson SE, Tornos C, Hummer A, Barakat RR, Soslow RA. Prognostic feature of surgical stage 1 uterine carcinosarcoma. Am J Surg Pathol. 2007;3(11):1653–61.
29. Reymundo C, Toro M, Morales C, López-Beltrain A, Nogales F, Nogales F Jr. Hyaline globules in uterine malignant mixed Müllerian tumours. A diagnostic aid? Pathol Res Pract. 1993;189(9):1063–6.
30. George E, Lillemoe TJ, Twiggs LB, Perrone T. Malignant mixed Müllerian tumour versus high-grade endometrial carcinoma and aggressive variants of endometrial carcinoma: a comparative analysis of survival. Int J Gynecol Pathol. 1995;14(1):39–44.

31. Ronnett BM, Zaino RJ, Ellenson LH, Kurman RJ. Endometrial carcinoma. In: Kurman RJ, editor. Blaustein's pathology of the female genital tract, vol. 5. New York: Springer-Verlag; 2002. p. 538–41.
32. Bansal N, Herzog TJ, Seshan VE, Schiff PB, Burke WM, Cohen CJ, Wright JD. Uterine carcinosarcoma and grade 3 endometrial cancers: evidence for distinct tumour behaviour. Obstet Gynecol. 2008;112(1):64–70.
33. Arend R, Bagaria M, Lewin SN, Sun X, Deutsch I, Burke WM, Herzog TJ, Wright JD. Long-term outcome and natural history of uterine adenosarcomas. Gynecol Oncol. 2010;119(2):305–8.
34. Smotkin D, Nevadunsky NS, Harris K, Enstein MH, Yu Y, Goldberg GL. Histopathologic differences account for racial disparity in uterine cancer survival. Gynecol Oncol. 2012;127(3):616–9.
35. Barwick KW, LiVolsi VA. Heterologous mixed Müllerian tumour confined to an endometrial polyp. Obstet Gynecol. 1979;53(4):512–4.
36. Kahner S, Ferenczy A, Richart RM. Homologous mixed Müllerian tumours (carcinosarcomal) confined to endometrial polyps. Am J Obstet Gynecol. 1975;121(2):278–9.
37. Djordjevic B, Gien LT, Covens A, Malpica A, Khalifa MA. Polypoid or non-polypoid? A novel dichotomous approach to uterine carcinosarcoma. Gynecol Oncol. 2009;115(1):32–6.
38. Kitchener HC. Cancer of the uterine corpus. In: Edmonds KD, editor. Dewhurst's textbook of obstetrics and gynaecology. Malden: Blackwell; 2007. p. 645–50.
39. Callister M, Ramondetta LM, Jhingran A, Burke TW, Eifel PJ. Malignant mixed Müllerian tumours of the uterus: analysis of patterns of failure, prognostic factors, and treatment outcome. Int J Radiat Oncol Biol Phys. 2004;58(3):786–96.
40. Reed NS, Mangioni C, Malmstrom H, Scarfone G, Poveda A, Pecorelli S, et al. Phase III randomised study to evaluate the role of adjuvant pelvic radiotherapy in the treatment of uterine sarcomas stages I and II: an European organisation for research and treatment of cancer. Gynaecological Cancer Group study (protocol 55874). Eur J Cancer. 2008;44(6):808–18.
41. McMeekins DS, Yasha C, Campos S, Zaino RJ. Corpus: epithelial tumours. In: Principle and practice of gynaecologic oncology. Barakat RR, Berchuk A, Markman M, Randall M. (Eds). Philadelphia: Lippincott Williams & Wilkins, 2013, 661–714.
42. Mordi VP, Nnatu SN. Endometrial carcinoma in Nigeria. A pathologic study. Cancer. 1986;57(9):1840–1.
43. Adefuye PO, Adefuye BO, Oluwole AA. Female genital tract cancers in Sagamu, southwest Nigeria. East Afr Med J. 2014;19(11):398–406.
44. Norris HJ, Tavassoli FA, Kurman RJ. Endometrial hyperplasia and carcinoma: diagnostic consideration. Am J Surg Pathol. 1983;7:838–47.
45. Parkin DM, Whalan SL, Ferlay J, et al. Cancer incidence in five continents. Vol VII IARC Scientific. Publications No. 143. Lyon: IARC; 1997.
46. Akhmedkhanov A, Zeleniuch-Jaquotte A, Toniolo P. Role of exogenous and endogenous hormones in endometrial cancer. Ann N Y Acad Sci. 2001;943:296–315.
47. Ziel HK, Finkle WD. Increased risk of endometrial carcinoma among users of conjugated estrogens. N Engl J Med. 1975;293:1167–70.
48. Killackey MA, Hakes TB, Pierce VK. Endometrial adenocarcinoma in breast cancer patients receiving anti-estrogen. Cancer Treat Rep. 1985;69:237–8.
49. Fisher B, Constantino JP, Redmond CK, et al. Endometrial cancer in tamoxifen-treated breast cancer patient: findings from National Surgical Adjuvant Breast and Bowel Project (NSABP) B-14. J Natl Cancer Inst. 1994;86:527–37.
50. Abudu FK, Musa O, Adefuye PO, Abdul-Kareem FB, Agboola AOJ, Banjo AAF. Endometrial carcinoma following treatment for breast carcinoma in a Nigerian female. A case report and review of literature. Niger Postgrad Med J. 2007;14(4):335–7.
51. Weiss JM, Saltzman BS, Doherty JA, Voigt LF, Chen C, Beresford SA, Hill DA, Weiss NS. Risk factors for the incidence of endometrial cancer according to the aggressiveness of disease. Am J Epidemiol. 2006;164(1):56–62.
52. Olson SH, Trevisan M, Marshall JR, Graham S, Zielezny M, Vena JE, Hellmann R, Freudenheim JL. Body mass index, weight gain, and risk of endometrial cancer. Nutr Cancer. 1995;23(2):144–9.
53. O'Mara BA, Byers T, Schoenfeld E. Diabetes mellitus and cancer risk: a multisite case-control study. J Chronic Dis. 1985;38(5):435–41.
54. Parazzini F, La Vecchia C, Negri E, Riboldi GL, Surace M, Benzi G, Maina A, Chiaffarino F. Diabetes and endometrial cancer: an Italian case-control study. Int J Cancer. 1999;81(4):539–42.
55. Fornander T, Hellstrom AC, Moberger B. Descriptive clinicopathologic study of 17 patients with endometrial cancer during or after adjuvant tamoxifen in early breast cancer. J Natl Cancer Inst. 1993;85(22):1850–5.
56. DeMichele A, Troxel A, Berlin JA, Weber AL, Bunin GR, Turzo E, Schnnar R, Burgh D, Berlin M, Rubin SC, Rebbeck TR, Strom BL. Impact of raloxifiene or tamoxifen use on endometrial cancer risk: a population based case-control study. J Clin Oncol. 2008;26(25):4151–9.
57. Lynch HT, Lanspa SJ, Boman BM, Smyrk T, Watson P, Lynch JF, Lynch PM, Cristofaro G, Bufo P, Tauro AV, et al. Hereditary nonpolyposis colorectal cancer – Lynch syndrome I and II. Gastroenterol Clin N Am. 1988;17(4):679–712.
58. Berends MJ, Wu Y, Sijmons RH, van der Sluis T, Ek WB, Ligtenberg MJ, Arts NJ, ten Hoor KA, Kleibeuker JH, de Vries EG, Mourits MJ, Hollema H, Buys CH, Hofstra RM, van der Zee AG. Toward new strategies to select young endometrial cancer patients for mismatch repair gene mutation analysis. J Clin Oncol. 2003;21(23):4364–70.
59. Hornreich G, Beller U, Lavie O, Renbaum P, Cohen Y, Levy-Lahad E. Is uterine serous papillary carcinoma a BRCA1-related disease? Case report and review of the literature. Gynecol Oncol. 1999;75(2):300–4.
60. Levine DA, Lin O, Barakat RR, Robson ME, McDermott D, Cohen L, Satagopan J, Offit K, Boyd J. Risk of endometrial carcinoma associated with BRCA mutation. Gynecol Oncol. 2001;80(3):395–8.
61. Kwawukume EY, Laryea HND. Endometrial cancer. In: Kwawukume EY, Emuveyan EE, editors. Comprehensive gynaecology in the tropics. Dansoman: Asante & Hittsher; 2005. p. 434–48.
62. Weiderpass E, Adami HO, Baron JA, Magnusson C, Lindgren A, Persson I. Use of oral contraceptives and endometrial cancer risk (Sweden). Cancer Causes Control. 1999;10(4):277–84.
63. Melhem MF, Tobon H. Mucinous adenocarcinoma of the endometrium: a clinico-pathological review of 18 cases. Int J Gynecol Pathol. 1987;6(4):347–55.
64. Baak JP, Mutter GL, Robboy S, van Diest PJ, Uyterlinde AM, Orbo A, Palazzo J, Fiane B, Løvslett K, Burger C, Voorhorst F, Verheijen RH. The molecular genetics and morphometry-based endometrial intraepithelial neoplasia classification system predicts disease progression in endometrial hyperplasia more accurately than the 1994 World Health Organization classification system. Cancer. 2005;103(11):2304–12.
65. Amant F, Mirza MR, Koskas M, Creutzberg CL. Cancer of the corpus uteri. Int J Gynaecol Obstet. 2015;131(Suppl 2):S96–104.
66. Djordjevic B, Broaddus RR. Surgical-pathologic features of uterine cancers. In: Odunsi K, Pejovic T, editors. Gynaecologic cancers. A multidisciplinary approach to diagnosis and management. New York: Demos Medical; 2014. p. 53–9.
67. Pecorelli S. Revised FIGO staging for carcinoma of the vulva, cervix, and endometrium. Int J Gynaecol Obstet. 2010;108(2):176.
68. Ackerman I, Malone S, Thomas G, Franssen E, Balogh J, Dembo A. Endometrial carcinoma--relative effectiveness of adjuvant

irradiation vs therapy reserved for relapse. Gynecol Oncol. 1996;60(2):177–83.
69. Fung-Kee-Fung M, Dodge J, Elit L, Lukka H, Chambers A, Oliver T. Follow-up after primary therapy for endometrial cancer: a systematic review. Gynecol Oncol. 2006;101(3):520–9.
70. Fanning J, Kesterson JP. Multidisciplinary approach to treatment of endometrioid uterine carcinoma. In: Odunsi K, Pejovic T, editors. Gynaecologic cancers. A multidisciplinary approach to diagnosis and management. New York: Demos Medical; 2014. p. 61–5.
71. Barakat RR, Goldman NA, Patel DA, Venkatraman ES, Curtin JP. Pelvic exenteration for recurrent endometrial cancer. Gynecol Oncol. 1999;75(1):99–102.
72. Fiorica JV, Brunetto VL, Hanjani P, Lentz SS, Mannel R, Andersen W. Phase II trial of alternating courses of megestrol acetate and tamoxifen in advanced endometrial carcinoma: a Gynaecologic Oncology Group study. Gynecol Oncol. 2004;92(1):10–4.
73. Whitney CW, Brunetto VL, Zaino RJ, Lentz SS, Sorosky J, Armstrong DK, Lee RB. Phase II study of medroxyprogesterone acetate plus tamoxifen in advanced endometrial carcinoma: a Gynaecologic Oncology Group study. Gynecol Oncol. 2004;92(1):4–9.
74. Singh M, Zaino RJ, Filiaci VJ, Leslie KK. Relationship of estrogen and progesterone receptors to clinical outcome in metastatic endometrial carcinoma: a Gynaecologic Oncology Group study. Gynecol Oncol. 2007;106(2):325–33.
75. Quinn MA, Campbell JJ. Tamoxifen therapy in advanced/recurrent endometrial carcinoma. Gynecol Oncol. 1989;32(1):1–3.
76. Thigpen T, Brady MF, Homesley HD, Soper JT, Bell J. Tamoxifen in treatment of advanced or recurrent endometrial carcinoma: a Gynaecologic Oncology Group study. J Clin Oncol. 2001;9(2):364–7.
77. Randall ME, Filiaci VL, Muss H, Spirtos NM, Mannel RS, Fowler J, Thigpen JT, Benda JA, Gynecologic Oncology Group Study. Randomised phase III trial of whole-abdominal irradiation versus doxorubicin and cisplatin chemotherapy in advanced endometrial carcinoma: a Gynaecologic Oncology Group study. J Clin Oncol. 2006;24(1):36–44.
78. Akram T, Maseelall P, Fanning J. Carboplatin and paclitaxel for the treatment of advanced or recurrent endometrial cancer. Am J Obstet Gynecol. 2005;192(5):1365–7.

Epithelial Ovarian Cancer

58

Olusegun Kayode Ajenifuja and Kunle Odunsi

Learning Objectives

After studying this chapter, the reader should be able to:

- Understand the epidemiology clinical presentations of Epithelial Ovarian Cancer (EOC)
- Investigate and carry out clinical work up of patients with ovarian cancer
- Carry out definitive management of patients with EOC
- Understand the rationale for the use of adjuvant and neo-adjuvant chemotherapy in patients with EOC
- Risk reduction procedure and screening for ovarian cancer in high-risk population

58.1 Introduction

Ovarian cancer is not a single disease but composed of heterogeneous group of malignancies with epithelial ovarian cancer (EOC) being the most common ovarian malignancy comprising about 85% of cases [1]. EOC is the most lethal of all gynaecological malignancies. In the Caucasian population, a woman risk of developing ovarian cancer is 1 in 70, while her risk of dying from the disease is 1 in 100 [2].

Globally, 239,000 new cases were diagnosed in 2012, which constitute 1.7% of all cancers leading to premature death of 152,000 women [3]. It is the seventh most common cancer in women and is the eighth most common cause of cancer deaths among women. There is a global disparity in incidence of EOC between developed and developing countries. Higher incidences are found in developed countries with the exception of Japan than in developing countries. Caucasians have higher incidences than Asians and Negroid races while low incidence of the disease was reported in sub-Saharan Africa. The low incidence in sub-Saharan African may be due to lower life expectancy because EOC is a disease of post-menopausal women. Other reasons for the low incidence may be due to high parity seen in this region and poor data collection. Other reasons may be due to larger family sizes seen in Africa and the higher incidence of breastfeeding in the African population.

58.2 Classification

EOC is the general term used for a highly heterogeneous group of cancers [4–6].

It has traditionally been classified into five different histologic subtypes: serous, mucinous, endometrioid, clear cell and transitional cell tumours [7]. With increasing understanding of the tumour biology, genetic and results from immuno-histochemical techniques, it has been widely known that EOC is not a single disease entity [1].

A dualistic classification which classified EOC into two groups, Types 1 and 11 tumours, has been proposed based on origin, pathogenesis and survival [8].

Type 1 tumours are low-grade serous, endometrioid, mucinous, clear cell carcinomas and malignant Brenner tumours [9].

Low-grade tumours are believed to arise from benign lesions in the ovary and surrounding structures and are generally genetically stable, do not exhibit P53 mutations but have mutations of KRAS, BRAF or ERBB2 genes [10]. They run an indolent course and tend to present in stage 1 when they are still confined to the ovaries. Apart from endo-

O. K. Ajenifuja
College of Health Sciences, Obafemi Awolowo University, Ile-Ife, Nigeria

Obafemi Awolowo University Teaching Hospitals, Ile-Ife, Nigeria

K. Odunsi (✉)
Roswell Park Comprehensive Cancer Centre (Roswell Park), Buffalo, NY, USA

Department of Gynaecologic Oncology, Centre for Immunotherapy, Roswell Park, Buffalo, NY, USA

University of Buffalo, Buffalo, NY, USA
e-mail: Kunle.odunsi@roswellpark.org

F. Okonofua et al. (eds.), *Contemporary Obstetrics and Gynecology for Developing Countries*,
https://doi.org/10.1007/978-3-030-75385-6_58

metrioid and clear cell tumours which originate from endometriosis, low-grade serous tumours are thought to originate from ovarian surface epithelium [11].

Type 11 or high-grade tumours comprise high-grade serous, undifferentiated carcinomas and carcinosarcomas. They are genetically unstable and very aggressive and in majority of cases have P 53 mutations.

58.3 Risk Factors

58.3.1 Family History

A family history of ovarian cancer is the strongest risk factor. Though most cases of EOC are sporadic in about 85–90% of cases, about 10–15% of EOC are inherited. Majority of the hereditary EOC are associated with mutations of the tumour suppressor genes BRCA 1 and BRCA2, while 10–15% of cases are associated with HNPCC syndrome [12]. The BRCA genes are a pair of genes whose functions include tumour suppression. Loss of both alleles leads to development of ovarian cancer. There are two distinct forms of the BRCA genes: BRCA 1 and BRCA 2. The commoner is BRCA 1 that is located on chromosome 17 and is associated with most forms of hereditary ovarian cancer, while the less common form is BRCA 2 located on chromosome 13. In addition to ovarian cancer, mutations of BRCA genes also predispose to development of breast cancer [13].

The inherited forms of EOC tend to occur in younger aged women and the tumours are likely to be of high-grade serous subtypes and in minority of cases endometrioid and clear cell tumours. Mucinous tumours are less likely in patients with BRCA mutations. Patients with mutations in BRCA1 are more susceptible to EOC than those with BRCA2 mutations. The incidence of BRCA mutations are higher in certain populations such as Ashkenazi Jewish and women from Island. The life time risk of developing ovarian cancer from BRCA1 and BRCA2 mutations was calculated to be 39% and 11% by Antonious et al. [14].

Endometriosis This is a condition in which ectopic endometrial glands and stroma are found in structures other than the endometrial linings of the uterus. It is found in about 10% of women and in majority of cases are located in the ovaries [15].

Endometriosis has been recognised as a precursor lesion for endometrioid cancer. Various epidemiologic studies have linked endometriosis to the development of ovarian cancer. In fact, the term 'Endometriosis Associated Ovarian Cancer' or EAOC has been coined [16].

Ovarian cancers associated with endometriosis are clear cells carcinoma and endometrioid subtypes.

Pelvic Inflammatory Disease (PID) This is a common condition among sexually active women, which has also been implicated as a risk factor for ovarian cancer. Women with PID often have impaired fertility principally due to tubal blockage, have reduced chances of spontaneous pregnancy and, thus, have low parity which is also a risk factor for EOC. In a case-control study involving 67,936 women with PID and 135,872 controls, Lin et al. (2011) discovered that the hazard ratio for development of EOC was almost double in women with PID compared with controls [17]. They also discovered that the more the episodes of PID, the more the risk of developing EOC.

58.4 Use of Ovulation-Inducing Agents

The theory linking ovulation and ovarian cancer was first proposed by Fathalla in 1971, the so-called 'incessant ovulation' [18]. Fathalla suggested that the risks of developing ovarian cancer has been linked to repeated ovulation. According to this theory, ovulation creates a disruption on the ovarian surface epithelium which is healed by epithelial proliferation and may lead to inclusion of epithelial cells into the ovarian stroma. The more ovulatory cycles a woman has the higher her risk of developing ovarian cancer. Repeated cycles of ovulation and repair process may lead to DNA damage and deviate the repair process along neoplastic transformation leading to development of EOC [19, 20].

The age at which a woman attained menarche has no statistical relationship with the risk of developing ovarian cancer; however, there was a weak relation with increased risk in women with late menopause [21].

The incessant ovulation theory was supported by findings that certain reproductive factors, such as increasing numbers of live births, with increasing numbers of incomplete pregnancies and with the use of oral contraceptives which suppress ovulation decrease the risk of ovarian cancer [22].

This findings have led to concerns that ovulation-inducing drugs such as clomiphene citrate and gonadotrophins may increase a woman's chance of developing ovarian cancer. Studies have shown that though women on ovulation-inducing agents may show slight increased risk of developing EOC, this, however, does not reach statistical significance. The apparent increase may be due to increased surveillance that these women were subjected to [23]. In a retrospective study of over 12,000 patients, Brinton et al. [24] reported a slight but not significant increased risk of ovarian cancer among infertile women on ovulation induction. The risk was higher for Gonadotrophins usage than for Clomiphene citrate.

58.4.1 Protective Factors

A number of reproductive and behavioural factors have been shown to be protective against the development of ovarian cancer.

Parity Among the protective factors against the development of ovarian cancer is parity; results from several studies have shown that the more children a woman has the more she is protected from EOC. Negri et al. [25] reported that women with four or more children had a 40% reduction in the risk of ovarian cancer than nulliparous women. In that study, nulliparous per se was not associated with increased risk but delay in getting pregnant above the age of 35 years.

Combined Oral Contraceptive Pill It has long been known that one of the non-contraceptive benefits of the combined oral contraceptive pill is the reduction in the risk of developing ovarian cancer and ever user of the pills compared with non-user, about 30% protection [26]. The protective effect of oral contraceptive pill on the risk of developing ovarian cancer is cumulative. A 5 years of use is associated with a 50% reduction, and the protective effect continues even after cessation of the pill for up to 10 years.

Breastfeeding Breastfeeding has been widely claimed to reduce the incidence of ovarian cancer; however, data regarding the effects of breastfeeding on the development of ovarian cancer have been conflicting. Danforth et al. found non-significant reduction in the incidence of ovarian cancer between ever breastfeeding women and never breastfeeding mothers [27]. The protective effects of breastfeeding seem related to the pattern of breastfeeding. There are, however, conflicting reports of the effects duration of breastfeeding and number of children breastfed [28]. Titus-Ernstoff et al. in a case-control study reported that protective effects of breastfeeding are related to breastfeeding the last child.

58.4.2 Hysterectomy Tubal Ligation and Oophorectomy

Hysterectomy with tubal ligation with or without the removal of the ovaries is associated with reduced risk of developing ovarian cancer. The magnitude of the protection depends on the histological type of the ovarian tumour being greater for non-serous tumours. Hysterectomy with tubal ligation had greater protective effective than tubal ligation alone, OR = 0.65, 95% CI: 0.45–0.94 vs. OR, 0.76; 95% CI 0.64–0.90, respectively. Hysterectomy alone does not protective against ovarian cancer [29].

58.4.3 Clinical Presentations

EOC is a disease of post-menopausal women. In the UK, though incidence of ovarian cancer starts rising after 35 years of age, however, more than half of the women diagnosed with ovarian cancer in the UK are more than 65 years [25, 30].

One of the reasons for the high mortality associated with ovarian cancer is that in majority of cases there are no specific symptoms attributed to the disease that could alert either the patient or the physician. Despite the lack of specific symptoms, most patients usually have symptoms at least 1 year before diagnosis. In an Australian study, Olsen et al. reported that 92% of patients had symptoms at the time of their diagnosis [31]. Women with invasive lesions had more symptoms than women with benign lesion.

In a retrospective analysis of symptoms matched with controls in 100 women with diagnosis of ovarian cancer, Behtash et al. reported that the commonest symptoms in more than half of the cases were abdominal or low back pain followed by abdominal bloating, fullness and pressure in the abdomen in 37% and gastro-intestinal problems in 36% of the cases [32]. Other symptoms may include early satiety and loss of weight. The challenge, therefore, is for physicians to recognise the symptoms and order appropriate investigations.

This view has been challenged in a study that showed women who presents early may have different disease from women with late presentations [31].

Any woman suspected of having an ovarian cancer should have a detailed personal and family history taken including history of breast and ovarian cancer. Physical examination should be thorough, one of the commonest physical findings is the presence of pelvic mass and/or ascites in advanced cases. The probability that adnexal mass in a pre-menopausal women being benign is low, while the chances of it being malignant are high in post-menopausal women. The risk of adnexal mass being malignant in a pre-menopausal women is 13% rising to 45% in a post-menopausal woman [33].

Adnexal masses could be benign ovarian, benign non-ovarian, primary malignant ovarian and secondary malignant ovarian [34]. The risk of malignant index (RMI) described by Jacob and co-workers has been developed to assist physicians to distinguish between benign and malignant adnexal masses [35]. There are various versions of the RMIs but they all utilise three parameters: menopausal status, ultrasound score and serum CA-125 level. The product of the three parameters is used to detect if the adnexal mass is malignant or not. In the RMI 1, a cut-off score of 200 was demonstrated to have a sensitivity of 78% (95% CI 71–85%) and specificity of 87% (95% CI 83–91%) [36].

The International Ovarian Tumour Analysis group (IOTA) has designed simple rules using ultrasound to differentiate benign from malignant adnexal masses. The rules are used to classify ovarian masses as benign and those used for malignant masses known as B rules and M rules, respectively [37].

58.5 Laboratory Investigations

Detailed pre-operative investigations should be carried out before surgical exploration of the patient. This should include complete blood count and complete evaluation of the renal and hepatic functions. Radiological tests should be carried out including chest X-ray, pelvic ultrasound scanning and CT scan of the abdomen and serum. Upper and lower gastro-intestinal endoscopic evaluation should be done to exclude metastatic tumours. The usefulness of mechanical bowel preparation is questionable. It is desirable to determine the pre-operative serum level of CA-125, which is the principal tumour marker in epithelial ovarian cancer, especially the serous subtype. This is a glycoprotein which is elevated in more than 80% of patients with EOC, especially serous tumours. Moderate elevations are seen in mucinous tumours. A cut-off value of 35 units/ml is used as the upper limit of normal. A grossly elevated serum CA-125 level in a post-menopausal woman with adnexal mass is highly suggestive of EOC. Other tumour markers such as alpha foetoprotein and serum human chorionic gonadotrophins (HCG) should be done especially in younger age women.

The definitive diagnosis of ovarian cancer is made by histopathological examination of specimens removed at staging laparotomy. Surgery for ovarian when performed by gynaecological oncologist in a dedicated cancer centre has been proven to give better outcomes than when performed by general gynaecologists or surgeons. It is preferable that patients with suspected EOC should be referred to oncology centres from peripheral hospitals for better patients' outcome, though this may not be possible in many developing countries.

In performing surgery for suspected ovarian cancer, the incision should be wide enough to permit detailed exploration of both the lower and upper abdomen. This is best achieved by a midline incision which may initially end at the sub-umbilical region but which can be extended as the need arises.

On gaining entry into the abdomen, the surgeon should take sample of ascitic fluid for cytology and where there is none, about 100–200 ml of normal saline should be instilled into both the paracolic gutters and the pouch of Douglas, withdrawn and sent for cytology.

The general peritoneal surfaces should be inspected in a careful and systematic way including the liver surfaces, the sub-diaphragmatic surface and all the intra-abdominal organs. All suspicious areas should be biopsied, well-labelled and sent separately for frozen section.

Surgery for ovarian cancer with the exception of early-stage disease where preservation of fertility is a concern involves total abdominal hysterectomy, bilateral oophorectomy, bilateral pelvic lymphadenectomy, bilateral pelvic lymph node dissection and infracolic omentectomy. The appendix should be inspected and removed if involved in the disease process and if the ovarian tumour is of mucinous type. In early-stage disease, it is important that the ovarian tumour should be removed intact because rupture during surgical manipulation may lead to dissemination of tumour cells in the peritoneal cavity and, thus, upstage the disease. All visible tumours should be removed as the volume of residual tumour is an important prognostic factor. Surgical removal of malignant ovarian cancer has the advantages of removing bulky tumours that are poorly vascularised, reduce the tumour burden, thereby eliminating clone of resistance tumour, and it enhances the immune status of the patient. Drainage of ascitic fluid at surgery improves the nausea and early satiety and increase the appetite, thereby enhancing the performance status of the patient [38].

Optimal cytoreductive surgery for EOC has undergone several definitions when it was first proposed by Griffiths, who defined it as residual less than 1.5 cm after initial surgery. Since then, Berek and Hacker further reduced it to less than 5 mm of residual tumour. Currently, optimal cytoreductive surgery is defined as no visible tumour at the end of the initial surgery [39].

Often patients in developing countries presenting with advanced EOC have other comorbidities and as such are poor candidates' for immediate cytoreductive surgery. Such patient may be given three cycles of neo-adjuvant chemotherapy before definitive surgery. In a randomised control trial of 670 patients with advanced EOC, Vergote et al. and others showed that overall median survival was comparable between primary debulking surgery and neo-adjuvant chemotherapy and the progression-free survival was the same in both arms, though patients in the neo-adjuvant arm of the study had fewer post-operative surgical morbidities [40].

58.6 2014 FIGO Staging for Ovarian Cancer

- Stage I: Tumour confined to ovaries or fallopian tube(s).
  - IA: Tumour limited to 1 ovary (capsule intact) or fallopian tube; no tumour on ovarian or fallopian tube surface and no malignant cells in the ascites or peritoneal washings
  - IB: Tumour limited to both ovaries (capsules intact) and fallopian tubes; no tumour on ovarian or fallopian tubes surface and no malignant cells in the ascites or peritoneal washings
  - IC: Tumour limited to 1 or both ovaries or fallopian tubes, with any of the following:
    IC1: Surgical spill
    IC2: Capsule ruptured before surgery or tumour on ovarian or fallopian tube surface
    IC3: Malignant cells in the ascites or peritoneal washings

- Stage II: Tumour involves 1 or both ovaries or fallopian tubes with pelvic extension (below pelvic brim) or primary peritoneal cancer
  - IIA: Extension and/or implants on uterus and/or fallopian tubes and/or ovaries
  - IIB: Extension to other pelvic intraperitoneal tissues
- Stage III: Tumour involves 1 or both ovaries or fallopian tubes, or primary peritoneal cancer, with cytologically or histologically confirmed spread to the peritoneum outside the pelvis and/or metastasis to the retroperitoneal lymph nodes
  - IIIA1: Positive retroperitoneal lymph nodes only (cytologically or histologically proven):
    IIIA1(i) Metastasis up to 10 mm in greatest dimension
    IIIA1(ii) Metastasis more than 10 mm in greatest dimension
  - IIIA2: Microscopic extra-pelvic (above the pelvic brim) peritoneal involvement with or without positive retroperitoneal lymph nodes
  - IIIB: Macroscopic peritoneal metastasis beyond the pelvis up to 2 cm in greatest dimension, with or without metastasis to the retroperitoneal lymph nodes
  - IIIC: Macroscopic peritoneal metastasis beyond the pelvis more than 2 cm in greatest dimension, with or without liver and spleen (without parenchymal involvement of either organ)
- Stage IV: Distant metastasis excluding peritoneal metastases:
  - Stage IVA: Pleural effusion with positive cytology

58.6.1 Adjuvant Chemotherapy

Surgery is the primary treatment for EOC, however, surgery alone rarely leads to cure due mainly to the presence of micro-metastases that are widely distributed throughout the peritoneal surfaces. Therefore, surgery is often combined with adjuvant chemotherapy. The use of adjuvant chemotherapy, however, takes into consideration the stage of the disease and the histological grade of the tumour.

The role of adjuvant chemotherapy versus observation for early-stage, high-risk EOC was initially the subject of controversy. Mortality is high in early-stage ovarian cancer about 20–30%. Early-stage ovarian cancer is further divided into early stage, low risk defined as stage 1A, grade 1 non-serous tumour and early stage, high risk defined as stage 1B, 1C grade 2 or 3 or serous tumour. In early-stage low-risk disease defined as stage 1A cancer and non-serous tumour, there was equal survival between observation and adjuvant chemotherapy in this group. A meta-analysis, however, showed that except where patients were adequately staged, the use of chemotherapy was beneficial in terms of overall survival and disease-free survival [41].

There is no controversy when it comes to the use of adjuvant chemotherapy in late stages of EOC. The acceptable standard therapy after surgery was platinum-based chemotherapy often combined with an alkylating agent such as cyclophosphamide. Paclitaxel was added to the combination after the land mark study of McGuire et al. (1996), who demonstrated that the addition of paclitaxel was associated with a longer survival of 37.5 vs. 24.4 months ($p < 0.001$) with Cis-platinum cyclophosphamide combination and longer progression-free survival of 12.9 vs. 17.9 months ($p < 0.001$). Carboplatin could effectively be substituted for Cis-platinum because of better tolerated toxicity [42]. Carboplatin could be used as a single agent in resource-constraints region [43]. Likewise, Docetaxel could be substituted for paclitaxel in elderly patients with neuropathy.

Despite initial response to combination first-line chemotherapy, majority of patients with EOC will experience relapse. The choice of chemotherapy for patients who relapse after an initial treatment for EOC depends on if the patient was platinum sensitive, resistant or refractory. Patients who showed an initial sensitivity to platinum-based chemotherapy defined as relapse more than 6 months after completing the initial platinum-based regimen can be given platinum-based chemotherapy. Patients who relapsed within 6 months after the initial platinum-based treatment or who progressed while on platinum-based chemotherapy are classified as platinum resistant or refractory, respectively. Patients who responded to initial platinum-based combination chemotherapy may also be given weekly paclitaxel, topotecan or monthly pegylated liposomal doxorubicin. In a recent study, weekly paclitaxel has been shown to have better median progression-free survival and overall survival in patients with platinum-resistant EOC [44].

58.6.2 Intraperitoneal Chemotherapy

The idea of administering intraperitoneal chemotherapeutic drugs in EOC patients appears very attractive for the following reasons: it enables higher local concentration of chemotherapeutic agents and a longer half-life of the administered agents leading to prolonged exposure to the drugs. One of the earliest studies to demonstrate the improved survival of IP chemotherapy over the IV route was the joint study by the SWOG and the GOG involving 546 patients, in which patients with advanced ovarian cancer were randomised to receive either IP Cisplatin or IV Cisplatin. The IP arm had better overall median survival of 49 months compared with 41 months for the IV arm of the study [45]. In another phase, 111 trial by the Gynaecological Oncology Group (GOG

172), intraperitoneal chemotherapy was shown to have a higher median survival compared with intravenous chemotherapy 65.6 vs. 49.7 months [46]. The improved survival of IP chemotherapy is, however, associated with increased toxicities and short-term reduced quality of life when compared with IV chemotherapy. The toxicities associated with IP chemotherapy includes more pain, leucopaenia, gastro-intestinal side effects, neuropathy and catheter-related complications. The completion rate for patients in the IP arm of most studies comparing IP and IV chemotherapy was lower than in the IV due to increased toxicities in the IP arm. Most of the toxicities are, however, short term and were not associated with increased mortality [47].

A Cochrane review concluded that women receiving primary treatment for ovarian cancer are less likely to die if they received IP chemotherapy and that IP prolonged disease-free survival. Patients who are maximally cytoreduced tends to benefit the most from IP chemotherapy compared with patients with bulky disease [48].

Better understanding of the molecular biology of tumour has led to the development of agents that targets specific pathways in malignant cells. Two of these agents are the anti-angiogenetic drug, bevacizumab, a humanised monoclonal antibody with affinity for VEGF receptors, and the oral anti-PARP drug, olaparib. Bevacizumab has demonstrated increased activity in EOC but is associated with increased incidence of elevated blood pressure and bowel perforation [49]. Both Bevacizumab and Olaparib have activities against platinum-resistant tumours.

58.7 Prevention and Screening of EOC

Ovarian cancer, despite being the fourth most common gynaecological cancer, is associated with the highest case fatality ratio mainly due to late presentations of most patients. By the time most patients are diagnosed, the tumour has metastasised to the general peritoneal cavity. Other reason being that the ovary is an intraperitoneal organ, it is not easily accessible except with imaging studies.

58.7.1 Screening for Epithelial Ovarian Cancer

The high mortality associated with EOC has prompted a search for screening of ovarian cancer. The greatest risks of developing EOC are related to increasing age and family history. EOC is a disease of post-menopausal women and is sporadic in majority of cases and the risk increases with increasing age. About 5–10% of EOC are hereditary with most being associated with mutations of BRCA 1 and 2.

A number of tests have been developed to screening for EOC in the general population. Among these is serum CA-125, which is a glycoprotein secreted by the coelomic epithelium first discovered by Bast et al. [50]. It was found to be elevated in many patients with advanced EOC and the serum levels correlates with the stage of the disease and response to either surgery of chemotherapy. What limits the use of serum CA-125 as a stand-alone screening biomarker is that elevated levels are also seen in many pre-menopausal women and in women with benign conditions such as endometriosis, pelvic inflammatory disease and physiological states like pregnancy and menstruation. In addition, not all EOC have elevated serum levels of CA-125 [51]. Jacobs et al. have shown that serial measurement of serum CA-125 improves the specificity than a single measurement. When measured serially, levels of CA-125 increase with time in patients with ovarian cancer in the absence of therapy, while in non-malignant conditions, the level decreases with time [52]. Nevertheless a cut-off value of 35 kU/l is widely used as a risk factor for EOC especially in post-menopausal women. CA-125 is more useful to monitor response to therapy than being used alone to screen for ovarian cancer.

Human epididymal secretory protein (He 4) is an up-regulated gene found in EOC. Serum level of this glycoprotein has been shown to be an effective biomarker of EOC especially the serous subtype [53]. A particular advantage of He4 over CA-125 is that He4 is able to distinguish benign from malignant ovarian masses in pre-menopausal women, a significant drawback using serum CA-125. Combining both serum CA-125 and He4 increases the accuracy of screening for EOC. Serum levels of HE4 and CA-125 are combined in the risk of malignant algorithm (ROMA) score in order to increase the sensitivity and specificity of early detection of ovarian cancer. In a study of 104 women with adnexal masses scheduled for surgery, using the ROMA score, Montagnana et al. [54] were able to correctly identify 8 pre-menopausal women out of 15 with EOC and 29 pre-menopausal women with benign adnexal masses out of 33 specificity of 80.6%; 95% CI: 64.0–91.8%, and sensitivity of 53.3%; 95% CI: 26.6–78.7%, respectively. While in post-menopausal women, 11 of 13 benign cases were correctly classified as high-risk specificity of 84.6%; 95% CI: 54.6–98.0%, and 33 of 40 cases of EOC were classified as high-risk sensitivity of 82.5%; 95% CI: 67.2–92.7%. In their pre-operative of 224 women, 128 with benign adnexal masses and 96 with ovarian malignancy, Terlikowska et al. found that the ROMA algorithm has better diagnostic accuracy in distinguishing benign from malignant adnexal conditions [55].

58.7.2 Imaging

Pelvic ultrasonography has been used extensively in various studies as screening methods either alone or in combination with serum levels of biomarkers. Ultrasonography is more sensitive than pelvic examination at detecting ovarian malignancy. Transvaginal ultrasound approach is mainly employed for this purpose due to closeness to the ovaries, an advantage in obese patients and also due to better image resolution and discards the discomfort of a full bladder. To increase the diagnostic accuracy, Bourne et al. introduce the colour Doppler flow. Ultrasound features that have been shown to be highly suggestive of ovarian malignancy are volume of mass, type of mass, presence and thickness of septae, presence and length of papillary projections, location of vessels at colour Doppler and colour score [56]. However, despite the initial hope and enthusiasm of pelvic ultrasound for the screening of EOC, results from various studies have not been encouraging [57]. In view of this shortcoming, ultrasonography is often combined with parameters to screening for ovarian malignancy. This was first introduced into clinical medicine by Jacob et al., when he introduced the risk of malignant index (RMI) using a combination of serum CA-125 level, menopausal status and ultrasonographic features.

Despite the improvement in imaging techniques and identification of novel biomarkers with the use of multi-model screening methods, large-scale screening studies showed at best moderate non-significant reduction in the mortality of ovarian cancer [58].

58.7.3 Screening in High-Risk Group

Individuals with family histories suggestive of BRCA 1 and 2 mutations are at increased risk of developing ovarian cancer than the general population. Initial suggestion of annual pelvic transvaginal ultrasound with Doppler flow with regular CA-125 estimation has not shown any reduction in cancer-related deaths in high-risk women for ovarian cancer. What is globally recommended was this group of women should be offered genetic counselling before undergoing genetic test to determine their risk of developing ovarian cancer. A positive test result is indicative of a higher probability of developing ovarian cancer. Women in this category are offered two choices: to have prophylactic of the ovaries and fallopian tubes (salpingo-oophorectomy), the so-called risk-reducing salpingo-oophorectomy (RRSO), after completion of family size and chemoprevention with the use of combined oral contraceptive pills. RRSO does not totally eliminate the risk of ovarian cancer but it significantly reduces the risk. Women undergoing this procedure should be counselled that there is a small risk of about 0.2% of primary peritoneal carcinomatosis and the attendant effects of premature surgically induced menopause.

References

1. Ramalingam P. Morphologic, immunophenotypic, and molecular features of epithelial ovarian cancer. Oncology (Williston Park). 2016;30(2):166–76.
2. Howlader N, Noone AM, Krapcho M, et al. SEER cancer statistics review, 1975–2013. Bethesda: National Cancer Institute. http://seer.cancer.gov/csr/1975_2013/, based on November 2015 SEER data submission, posted to the SEER website, April 2016.
3. Ferlay J, Soerjomataram I, Dikshit R, Eser S, Mathers C, Rebelo M, Parkin DM, Forman D, Bray F. Cancer incidence and mortality worldwide: sources, methods and major patterns in GLOBOCAN 2012. Int J Cancer. 2015;136:E359–86.
4. Rescigno P, Cerillo I, Ruocco R, Condello C, De Placido S, Pensabene M. New hypothesis on pathogenesis of ovarian cancer leads to future tailored approaches. Biomed Res Int. 2013;2013:852839.
5. Lalwani N, Prasad SR, Vikram R, et al. Histologic, molecular, and cytogenetic features of ovarian cancers: implications for diagnosis and treatment. Radiographics. 2011;31:625–46.
6. Lee K, Young R. The distinction between primary and metastatic mucinous carcinomas of the ovary: gross and histologic findings in 50 cases. Am J Surg Pathol. 2003;27:281–92.
7. Ioka A, Tsukuma H, Ajiki W, Oshima A. Ovarian cancer incidence and survival by histologic type in Osaka, Japan. Cancer Sci. 2003;94(3):292–6.
8. Meinhold-Heerlein I, Fotopoulou C, Harter P, Kurzeder C, Mustea A, Wimberger P, Hauptmann S, Sehouli J. The new WHO classification of ovarian, fallopian tube, and primary peritoneal cancer and its clinical implications. Arch Gynecol Obstet. 2016;293(4):695–700.
9. Kurman RJ, Shih IM. Pathogenesis of ovarian cancer: lessons from morphology and molecular biology and their clinical implications. Int J Gynecol Pathol. 2008;27:151–60.
10. Vang R, Shih I-M, Kurman RJ. Ovarian low-grade and high-grade serous carcinoma: pathogenesis, clinicopathologic and molecular biologic features, and diagnostic problems. Adv Anat Pathol. 2009;16(5):267–82.
11. Kurman RJ, Shih IM. Molecular pathogenesis and extraovarian origin of epithelial ovarian cancer--shifting the paradigm. Hum Pathol. 2011;42(7):918–31.
12. Prat J, Ribe A, Gallardo A. Hereditary ovarian cancer. Hum Pathol. 2005;36:861–70.
13. Toss A, Tomasello C, Razzaboni E, Contu G, Grandi G, Cagnacci A, Schilder RJ, Cortesi L. Hereditary ovarian cancer: not only BRCA 1 and 2 genes. Biomed Res Int. 2015;2015:341723.
14. Antoniou A, et al. Average risks of breast and ovarian cancer associated with BRCA1 or BRCA2 mutations detected in case Series unselected for family history: a combined analysis of 22 studies. Am J Hum Genet. 2003;72(5):1117–30.
15. Krawczyk N, Banys-Paluchowski M, Schmidt D, Ulrich U, Fehm T. Endometriosis-associated malignancy. Geburtshilfe Frauenheilkd. 2016;76(2):176–81.
16. Chene G, Caloone J, Moret S, Le Bail-Carval K, Chabert P, Beaufils E, Mellier G, Lamblin G. Is endometriosis a precancerous lesion? Perspectives and clinical implications. Gynecol Obstet Fertil. 2016;44(2):106–12.
17. Lin HW, Tu YY, Lin SY, Su WJ, Lin WL, Lin WZ, Wu SC, Lai YL. Risk of ovarian cancer in women with pelvic inflammatory disease: a population-based study. Lancet Oncol. 2011;12(9):900–4.
18. Fathalla MF. Incessant ovulation--a factor in ovarian neoplasia? Lancet. 1971;2(7716):163.
19. Cramer DW, Welch WR. Determinants of ovarian cancer risk. II. Inferences regarding pathogenesis. J Natl Cancer Inst. 1983;71(4):717–21.
20. Preston-Martin S, Pike MC, Ross RK, Jones PA, Henderson BE. Increased cell division as a cause of human cancer. Cancer Res. 1990;50(23):7415–21.
21. Franceschi S, La Vecchia C, Booth M, Tzonou A, Negri E, Parazzini F, Trichopoulos D, Beral V. Pooled analysis of 3 European case-control studies of ovarian cancer: II. Age at menarche and at menopause. Int J Cancer. 1991;49(1):57–60.

22. Casagrande JT, Louie EW, Pike MC, Roy S, Ross RK, Henderson BE. "Incessant ovulation" and ovarian cancer. Lancet. 1979;2(8135):170–3.
23. Sallam HN, Abdel-Bak M, Sallam NH. Does ovulation induction increase the risk of gynaecological cancer? Facts Views Vis Obgyn. 2013;5(4):265–73.
24. Brinton LA, Lamb EJ, Moghissi KS, Scoccia B, Althuis MD, Mabie JE, Westhoff CL. Ovarian cancer risk associated with varying causes of infertility. Fertil Steril. 2004;82(2):405–14.
25. Negri E, Franceschi S, Tzonou A, Booth M, La Vecchia C, Parazzini F, Beral V, Boyle P, Trichopoulos D. Pooled analysis of 3 European case-control studies: I. Reproductive factors and risk of epithelial ovarian cancer. Int J Cancer. 1991;49:50–6.
26. Riman T, Persson I, Nilsson S. Hormonal aspects of epithelial ovarian cancer: review of epidemiological evidence. Clin Endocrinol (Oxf). 1998;49(6):695–707.
27. Danforth KN, Tworoger SS, Hecht JL, Rosner BA, Colditz GA, Hankinson SE. Breastfeeding and risk of ovarian cancer in two prospective cohorts. Cancer Causes Control. 2007;18(5):517–23.
28. Titus-Ernstoff L, Rees JR, Terry KL, Cramer DW. Breast-feeding the last born child and risk of ovarian cancer the last child. Cancer Causes Control. 2010;21(2):201–7.
29. Rice MS, Murphy MA, Vitonis AF, Cramer DW, Titus LJ, Tworoger SS, Terry KL. Tubal ligation, hysterectomy and epithelial ovarian cancer in the New England Case-Control Study. Int J Cancer. 2013;133(10):2415–21.
30. Ovarian cancer statistics. Available on line from https://www.cancerresearchuk.org/health-professional/cancer-statistics/statistics-by-cancer-type/ovarian-cancer. Accessed 3 June 2019.
31. Olsen CM, Cnossen J, Green AC, Webb PM. Comparison of symptoms and presentation of women with benign, low malignant potential and invasive ovarian tumours. Eur J Gynaecol Oncol. 2007;28(5):376–80.
32. Behtash N, Ghayouri Azar E, Fakhrejahani F. Symptoms of ovarian cancer in young patients 2 years before diagnosis, a case-control study. Eur J Cancer Care (Engl). 2008;17(5):483–7.
33. Koonings PP, Campbell K, Mishell DR Jr, Grimes DA. Relative frequency of primary ovarian neoplasms: a 10-year review. Obstet Gynecol. 1989;74:921–6.
34. RCOG. Management of suspected ovarian masses in premenopausal women. Green-top guideline no. 62. London: RCOG; 2011. Available online from https://www.rcog.org.uk/globalassets/documents/guidelines/gtg_62.pdf. Accessed 2 June 2019.
35. Jacobs I, Oram D, Fairbanks J, Turner J, Frost C, et al. A risk of malignancy index incorporating CA 125, ultrasound and menopausal status for the accurate preoperative diagnosis of ovarian cancer. Br J Obstet Gynaecol. 1990;97(10):922–9.
36. Mol BW, Boll D, De Kanter M, Heintz AP, Sijmons EA, Oei SG, et al. Distinguishing the benign and malignant adnexal mass: an external validation of prognostic models. Gynecol Oncol. 2001;80:162–7.
37. Timmerman D, Ameye L, Fischerova D, Epstein E, Melis GB, Guerriero S, Van Holsbeke C, Savelli L, Fruscio R, Lissoni AA, Testa AC, Veldman J, Vergote I, Van Huffel S, Bourne T, Valentin L. Simple ultrasound rules to distinguish between benign and malignant adnexal masses before surgery: prospective validation by IOTA group. BMJ. 2010;341:c6839.
38. Bookman M, Berek J. Biologic and immunologic therapy of ovarian cancer. Hematol Oncol Clin North Am. 1992;6:941–65.
39. Eisenkop SM, Friedman RL, Wang H-J. Complete cytoreductive surgery is feasible and maximises survival in patients with advanced epithelial ovarian cancer: a prospective study. Gynecol Oncol. 1998;69:103–8.
40. Vergote I, Tropé CG, Amant F, et al. Neoadjuvant chemotherapy or primary surgery in stage IIIC or IV ovarian cancer. N Engl J Med. 2010;363:943–53.
41. Winter-Roach B, Hooper L, Kitchener H. Systematic review of adjuvant therapy for early stage (epithelial) ovarian cancer. Int J Gynecol Cancer. 2003;13(4):395–4.
42. McGuire WP, Hoskins WJ, Brady MF, Kucera PR, Partridge EE, Look KY, Clarke-Pearson DL, Davidson M. Cyclophosphamide and cisplatin versus paclitaxel and cisplatin: a phase III randomised trial in patients with suboptimal stage III/IV ovarian cancer (from the Gynaecologic Oncology Group). Semin Oncol. 1996;23(5 Suppl 12):40–7.
43. International Collaborative Ovarian Neoplasm Group. Paclitaxel plus carboplatin versus standard chemotherapy with either single-agent carboplatin or cyclophosphamide, doxorubicin, and cisplatin in women with ovarian cancer: the ICON3 randomised trial. Lancet. 2002;360(9332):505–15.
44. Osman MA, Elkady MS, Nasr KE. Weekly paclitaxel versus three-weekly paclitaxel in recurrent platinum-resistant epithelial ovarian and peritoneal cancers: a phase III study. Clin Med Insights Oncol. 2016;10:35–1.
45. Alberts DS, Liu PY, Hannigan EV, et al. Intraperitoneal cisplatin plus intravenous cyclophosphamide versus intravenous cisplatin plus intravenous cyclophosphamide for stage III ovarian cancer. N Engl J Med. 1996;335:1950–5.
46. Markman M, Bundy BN, Alberts DS, et al. Phase III trial of standard-dose intravenous cisplatin plus paclitaxel versus moderately high-dose intravenous carboplatin followed by intraperitoneal paclitaxel and intraperitoneal cisplatin in small-volume stage III ovarian cancer: an intergroup study of the Gynaecologic Oncology Group, Southwestern Oncology Group, and the Eastern Cooperative Oncology Group. J Clin Oncol. 2001;19:1001–7.
47. Chan DL, Morris DL, Rao A, Chua TC. Intraperitoneal chemotherapy in ovarian cancer: a review of tolerance and efficacy. Cancer Manag Res. 2012;4:413–22.
48. Jaaback K, Johnson N. Intraperitoneal chemotherapy for the initial management of primary epithelial ovarian cancer. Cochrane Database Syst Rev. 2006;25(1):CD005340. https://doi.org/10.1002/14651858.CD005340.pub2.
49. Zhang W, Shen Z, Luo H, Hu X, Zheng L, Zhu X. The benefits and side effects of bevacizumab for the treatment of recurrent ovarian cancer. Curr Drug Targets. 2017;18(10):1125–31. https://doi.org/10.2174/1389450117666160502150237.
50. Bast RC Jr, Feeney M, Lazarus H, et al. Reactivity of a monoclonal antibody with human ovarian carcinoma. J Clin Invest. 1981;68(5):1331–7.
51. Cohen JG, White M, Cruz A, Farias-Elsner R. In 2014, can we do better than CA-125 in the early detection of ovarian cancer ? World J Biol Chem. 2014;5(3):286–300.
52. Jacobs IJ, Skates S, Davies AP, et al. Risk of diagnosis of ovarian cancer after raised serum CA 125 concentration: a prospective cohort study. BMJ. 1996;313(7069):1355–8.
53. Huhtinen K, Suvitie P, Hiissa J, et al. Serum HE4 concentration differentiates malignant ovarian tumours from ovarian endometriotic cysts. Br J Cancer. 2009;100:1315–9.
54. Montagnana M, Danese E, Ruzzenente O, Bresciani V, Nuzzo T, Gelati M, Salvagno GL, Franchi M, Lippi G, Guidi GC. The ROMA (Risk of Ovarian Malignancy Algorithm) for estimating the risk of epithelial ovarian cancer in women presenting with pelvic mass: is it really useful? Clin Chem Lab Med. 2011;49(3):521–5. https://doi.org/10.1515/CCLM.2011.075.
55. Terlikowska KM, Dobrzycka B, Witkowska AM, Mackowiak-Matejczyk B, Sledziewski TK, Kinalski M, Terlikowski SJ. Preoperative HE4, CA125 and ROMA in the differential diag-

nosis of benign and malignant adnexal masses. J Ovarian Res. 2016;9(1):43.
56. Abbas AM, Zahran KM, Nasr A, Kamel HS. A new scoring model for characterisation of adnexal masses based on two-dimensional gray-scale and colour Doppler sonographic features. Facts Views Vis Obgyn. 2014;6(2):68–74.
57. Bourne T, Campbell S, Reynolds KM, et al. Screening for early familial ovarian cancer with transvaginal ultrasonography and color blood flow imaging. BMJ. 1993;306:1025–9.
58. Jacobs IJ, et al. Ovarian cancer screening and mortality in the UK Collaborative Trial of Ovarian Cancer Screening (UKCTOCS): a randomised controlled trial. Lancet. 2016;387(10022):945–56.

59 Germ Cell Tumours of the Ovary

Okechukwu A. Ibeanu

Learning Objectives

After studying this chapter, the reader should be able to:

- Understand the current classification and epidemiologic risk factors of ovarian germ cell tumours.
- Discuss the most common clinical presentations of ovarian germ cell tumours.
- Appreciate the epidemiological and clinical-pathological differences between ovarian germ cell tumours and epithelial ovarian cancers.
- Recognise the pathognomonic histologic features, as well as the clinical behaviours of the various subtypes of ovarian germ cell tumours.
- Describe the current treatment strategies for ovarian germ cell tumours, with emphasis on the indications for fertility preservation.
- Discuss the indications for the use of chemotherapy in the treatment of ovarian germ cell malignancies.
- Understand the evaluation of patients who have completed treatment for ovarian germ cell malignancy, and know when to use investigational tests appropriately.

59.1 Introduction

Ovarian germ cell tumours represent a group of histologically diverse neoplasms that arise from primitive pluripotent gonadal germ cells, and undergo differentiation into either embryonic or extra-embryonic type tissue. These tumours give rise to a variety of clinical presentations ranging from indolent benign cysts to frankly aggressive malignancies. Many practitioners will encounter these tumours in the course of evaluation of patients with adnexal masses. Germ cell tumours should be suspected in peri-pubertal and young reproductive age females. In recent decades, better understanding of the clinical behaviours of malignant ovarian germ cell tumours has resulted in the adoption of fertility sparing surgery for initial management in suitable patients. Also, early experience with testicular germ cell cancers partly contributed to the development of current chemotherapy regimens for post-surgery management of ovarian germ cell cancers. Cure rates have significantly improved, notably in patients with advanced disease, who previously had unfavourable prognoses.

This chapter reviews the epidemiology, classification, clinical features, and management of ovarian germ cell tumours. Detailed descriptions of surgical techniques, as well as pharmacologic information on chemotherapy drugs, are beyond the scope of discussion, and the reader should refer to standard texts and review articles. Where applicable, management suggestions for resource challenged settings are provided by the author.

59.2 Classification, Epidemiology, and Risk Factors

The most current classification illustrates the diverse histologic variants derived from ovarian germ cell elements. A classification of germ cell tumours of the ovary based on the World Health Organization scheme is shown in Table 59.1 [1].

Malignant ovarian germ cell tumours are rare, and make up less than 2% of all malignant ovarian cancers. Taken as a whole, germ cell tumours represent approximately one-quarter of all ovarian neoplastic lesions. The majority of germ cell tumours are benign; only 5% are considered malignant [2, 3]. Incidence data for developing countries is sparse. Population data from the United States reports an approximate incidence of 0.4 per 100,000 women, with higher

O. A. Ibeanu (✉)
Gynaecologic Oncology, John Hopkins University, Baltimore, MD, USA

Alvin & Lois Lapidus Cancer Institute, Sinai and Northwest Hospital, Baltimore, MD, USA
e-mail: oibeanu1@jhmi.edu

F. Okonofua et al. (eds.), *Contemporary Obstetrics and Gynecology for Developing Countries*,
https://doi.org/10.1007/978-3-030-75385-6_59

Table 59.1 Classification of germ cell tumours

Ovarian germ cell tumours
I – Primitive germ cell tumours
Dysgerminoma
Yolk sac tumour (endodermal sinus tumour)
Embryonal carcinoma
Polyembryoma
Choriocarcinoma (non-gestational)
Mixed germ cell tumour
II – Teratoma
Immature teratoma
Mature teratoma
Cystic
Cystic with malignant change
Solid
III – Monodermal teratoma, specialised somatic type elements
Struma ovarii (thyroid)
Carcinoid (neuroendocrine)
Mixed struma ovarii, carcinoid
Others – neural, sarcoma, carcinoma, melanoma, etc.

incidence among non-white compared to white females. Adjusted for histology, white women have a higher rate of dysgerminomas, and a lower rate of malignant teratomas compared to non-whites. The highest incidence of germ cell tumours occurs in the 15–19 years age group, in which approximately 60% of all ovarian neoplasms are of germ cell derivation; and of these, roughly one-third are malignant [3]. Race has not been consistently shown to independently affect disease survival when other factors such as histology and stage are controlled for multivariate analyses [4, 5]. Advanced stage disease, non-dysgerminoma histology, and older age have been identified as risk factors for less favourable survival outcomes following treatment. Genetic factors have not yet been implicated as a cause of ovarian germ cell tumours.

59.3 Clinical Features and Presentation

The classic presentation of ovarian germ cell tumour is that of a rapidly enlarging, painful pelvic or abdominal mass in a young woman, diagnosed after surgical removal, and usually confined to one ovary.

Abdominal pain is the main symptom in over 60% of patients; combination of pain with abdominal mass or swelling is seen in over 80%. Acute abdominal presentation requiring hospital admission can be seen in 15% of patients if torsion or tumour rupture with peritonitis occurs. Such presentation can be mistaken for an ectopic pregnancy, ruptured haemorrhagic cyst or tubo-ovarian abscess, and can lead to surgical under-treatment if specialist consultation is not sought or available at the time of surgery. Fever, abdominal swelling, incidental finding of ascites, or asymptomatic pelvic mass are less common presentations (less than 20% of patients). Abnormal vaginal bleeding may be a presenting issue in patients with germ cell tumours that secrete human chorionic gonadotropin (hCG). Abnormal hCG secretion can be associated with signs of sexual precosity [6–8]. The tumour marker secretion profile of germ cell tumours is shown in Table 59.2.

Table 59.2 Germ cell histology and tumour marker profile

Tumour	AFP	hCG	LDH
Dysgerminoma	–	+/–	+/–
Yolk sac tumour	+	–	–
Immature teratoma	+/–	–	–
Choriocarcinoma	–	+	–
Embryonal cell carcinoma	+/–	+	–
Polyembryoma	+/–	+	–
Mixed tumour	+/–	+/–	+/–

Tumour marker levels should be assayed in young patients with pelvic pain and mass, to aid diagnosis, assess treatment response, and evaluate disease recurrence. Tumour markers have been shown in some cases to be elevated significantly earlier than reported symptoms or appearance of radiologic lesions in the recurrent disease setting. Other initial evaluation measures for patients with suspected germ cell ovarian tumours are shown in Table 59.3.

Table 59.3 Initial evaluation of patients with suspected germ cell tumour

History and examination
Blood studies
Complete blood count
Metabolic profile
Serum tumour markers
Type and screen, clotting profile
Karyotype[a]
Radiologic studies
Pelvic ultrasound
Chest X-ray
Computed tomography of abdomen and pelvis[b]
Magnetic resonance imaging of abdomen and pelvis[b]

[a]See Sect. 59.5.2

[b]Indicated in patients with abdominal signs suggestive of disseminated disease

Unlike their epithelial ovarian counterpart, malignant germ cell tumours are diagnosed in early stage in 60–70% of patients, and are associated with favourable prognosis following surgery and adjuvant treatment (Table 59.4).

Most germ cell tumours show unilateral ovarian involvement [9], and are amenable to unilateral salpingo-oophorectomy in patients who desire fertility. Note that dysgerminoma and mature teratoma are bilateral in up to 15% of cases. Dissemination of malignant germ cell tumours occurs through direct peritoneal invasion and implantation, as well as by lymphatic and haematogenous metastasis to intra-peritoneal extrapelvic sites. Unlike epithelial ovarian cancer, lymphatic dissemination occurs more frequently in malignant germ cell tumours [10] (Table 59.5). As a general rule, germ cell malignancies are chemosensitive, given the

Table 59.4 Comparison of germ cell and epithelial ovarian cancers

Feature	Malignant ovarian germ cell tumour	Epithelial ovarian cancer
Peak age incidence	Second and third decade	Sixth and seventh decade
Pathogenesis	Malignant transformation of ovarian germ cells	Fallopian tubal serous intra-epithelial carcinomatous change Ovarian surface epithelial invagination with incessant ovulation Genetic
Genetics	Not determined	Established genetic aetiology in at least 10% of cases; BRCA 1 and 2 mutation Lynch syndrome
Tumour spread	Lymphatic dissemination mainly; haematogenous, peritoneal	Peritoneal dissemination mainly; lymphatic, haematogenous
Stage at presentation	I–II (70% of cases)	III–IV (70% of cases)
Prognostic factors	Stage, histology	Stage, post-surgical residual disease, grade
Primary treatment	Surgery	Surgery
Fertility sparing surgery	Yes	Yes; stage I; not standard treatment
Chemosensitivity	Yes	Yes
Adjuvant chemotherapy	Yes; platinum based	Yes; platinum based

Table 59.5 Frequency of lymphatic spread in germ cell malignancies

Tumour	Lymph node metastasis (%)
Dysgerminoma	28
Yolk sac tumour	16
Immature teratoma	8

fast doubling times. In the era of platinum-based chemotherapy, favourable response rates have been noted even in patients with advanced stage disease.

59.4 Clinical Pathology: Benign Germ Cell Tumours

59.4.1 Mature Cystic Teratoma

Also referred to as 'dermoid cyst' or 'benign cystic teratoma'.

This is the most common type of ovarian germ cell neoplasm, accounting for over 95% of all ovarian teratomas diagnosed in clinical practice. Dermoid cysts are benign tumours with well-differentiated or 'mature' tissue derived from endoderm, mesoderm, and ectoderm cells [11]. As such, on gross inspection, these tumours can contain any combination of well-formed skin, hair, cheesy malodorous sebaceous fluid, nerve, eye, teeth, muscle, urinary, and gastrointestinal epithelium. These tumours are seen in reproductive age and post-menopausal women, and can grow quite large before becoming symptomatic. Bilateral ovarian involvement is seen in 10–15% of cases [12], and malignant transformation is a rare event, observed in less than 1% of dermoids. Pathologic examination usually reveals a solid nodularity in the tumour, which represents 'Rokitansky's tubercle or protuberance', and is the typical site for malignant transformation to occur [13] (cell interface between normal ovary and tumour tissue). Such malignant transformation usually involves ectodermal cells, specifically, neural tissue or squamous cells, but can arise from any cell types contained in the tumour (mature cystic teratoma with malignant transformation). Risk factors for malignant change include older age (>40 years), large tumour (>10 cm), and rapid increase in tumour size. Ultrasound appearance of calcifications is highly specific for dermoid cysts [12, 14, 15]. Ovarian cystectomy or unilateral oophorectomy is the recommended treatment for dermoid cysts.

Dermoid Cysts and Pregnancy This is a rare clinical scenario, however, it is important to note that dermoid cysts are also the most common benign tumours encountered in pregnant women. This is hardly surprising, given the peak incidence of germ cell tumours in young women in their reproductive prime. Dermoid cysts in pregnancy are not hormonally driven, are typically asymptomatic, and are diagnosed incidentally in the first or early second trimesters in pregnancy when ultrasound is typically used for various reasons. Acute presentations can occur as the uterus enlarges, with rupture or torsion. Asymptomatic, stable cysts <10 cm, can be managed expectantly. If intervention is necessary due to pain, torsion, progressive or rapid growth, surgical removal can be safely performed in the second or early third trimester, using a laparoscopic or open abdominal approach as determined by tumour size and availability of endoscopic expertise and facilities. Ovarian cystectomy is acceptable and preferred over oophorectomy if technically feasible. Intra-operative pathology consultation is ideal to guide management. Spilled sebaceous cyst contents can irritate the peritoneum, and should be washed out of the peritoneal cavity by irrigating with water or saline.

59.4.2 Mature Solid Teratoma

Rarely, a mature teratoma may consist of mostly solid tissue [16]. The majority of such tumours are benign, given the mature differentiation of the contained elements. Unilateral ovarian disease is the norm, however, in few cases, the gross clinical picture may suggest disseminated malignancy in the form of solid peritoneal implants. Pathologic evaluation usually confirms the benign nature of the primary lesion and implants, such that conservation of the contralateral ovary is usually possible at the time of unilateral oophorectomy. In rare cases, this tumour may be difficult to distinguish from immature teratoma, and a detailed pathology review is necessary to guide post-surgical management.

59.4.3 Monodermal Teratoma

Also referred to as 'specialised teratoma'.

These are rare, mostly benign neoplasms that are composed of usually one predominant tissue type. Clinical presentation is similar to other germ cell tumours, and unilateral ovarian involvement is commonly encountered. The most common varieties of monodermal teratomas are thyroid tissue-predominant 'struma ovarii', and neuroendocrine tissue-predominant 'ovarian carcinoid' tumours.

59.4.4 Struma Ovarii:

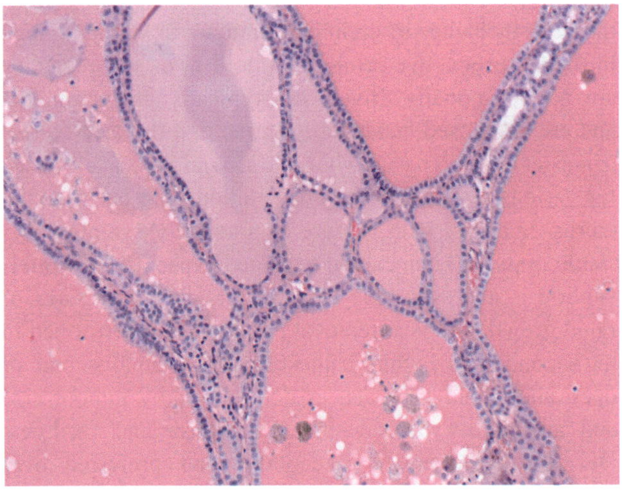

Struma ovarii. (Courtesy of Dr. Ander J. Pindzola, Department of Pathology, York Hospital, Pennsylvania, USA)

This tumour is essentially a teratoma with predominantly mature thyroid tissue differentiation. Struma ovarii are very rare tumours, representing only 3% of ovarian teratomas. Thyroid hormone secretion with symptoms is seen in approximately one-third of patients, and symptoms resolve after oophorectomy [17, 18]. A minority of patients may present with thyrotoxic clinical features. Majority of patients have minimal if any symptoms, and diagnosis is made after routine pathology analysis following surgery for an adnexal mass.

Ovarian Carcinoid Tumour This is a rare neoplasm seen in post-menopausal females, in which tumour secretion of peptides and vasoactive amines leads to clinical manifestation of carcinoid syndrome. The most frequent symptoms are skin flushing and diarrhoea. Telangiectasias, cardiac murmurs from valve disease, tachycardia, and bronchospasm are less common presentations. Florid carcinoid syndrome is seen in approximately one-third of patients. These tumours can be quite vascular, however, are usually confined to one ovary at diagnosis, and tend to be cured with unilateral oophorectomy. Assay of urinary 5-hydroxy indoleacetic acid is useful for diagnosis, and assessment of treatment response [19, 20].

Mixed monodermal teratomas: Mixed specialised tissue types are rare, and most frequently consist of struma ovarii and carcinoid combination. Other specialised or monodermal teratomas containing sarcoma, melanoma, pituitary, and other tissue elements have been described.

59.5 Clinical Pathology: Malignant Germ Cell Tumours

59.5.1 Immature Teratoma

Also referred to as 'malignant teratoma' or 'teratoblastoma'.

Immature teratoma is a rare, malignant tumour, accounting for 1% of ovarian teratomas, and, up to a third of germ cell malignancies. The defining histologic feature of an immature teratoma is the predominance of immature neural tissue elements [21], seen as sheets of small rounded cells with atypia and high mitotic activity. The most currently used grading system for this tumour is Norris' system which assigns grade based on the amount of immature (poorly dif-

Table 59.6 Norris grading system for immature teratoma

Grade	Description
0	No immature neural tissue elements present, rare mitoses
1	Rare foci of immature neural tissue elements present in 1 low power field in any slide
2	Immature neural tissue elements present in 1–3 low power fields in any one slide
3	Immature neural tissue elements present in more than 3 low power fields in any one slide

ferentiated or undifferentiated) neural tissue present in the tumour (Table 59.6).

Immature teratomas are typically diagnosed in women less than 20 years of age (contrast with well-differentiated mature teratomas seen in all age groups). The usual presentation is a unilateral adnexal mass with worsening abdominal pain of recent onset. Bilateral lesions occur rarely, and it is not uncommon to have a contralateral mature teratoma in such cases. Serum AFP levels may be elevated with immature teratoma. Seventy to ninety per cent of patients are diagnosed with stage I disease. Surgery (unilateral salpingo-oophorectomy) is the initial treatment. Adjuvant chemotherapy for stage I patients is usually reserved for tumours that are grade 2 or 3. Multi-agent chemotherapy has favourably altered the survival outcomes for patients with this cancer. Prognosis is related to stage and grade, with several investigators reporting over 85% survival rates for patients with grade 1 lesions that are early stage. Clinical studies by the Gynaecologic Oncology Group (GOG) in the United States have confirmed similar rates of disease control in patients treated with surgery and combination chemotherapy for completely resected early stage tumours. Given concerns regarding the gonadotoxicity and other effects of chemotherapy on young patients, an issue of debate is the use of surgery alone for patients with stage 1A grade 2 tumours. This approach has been in use among paediatric oncology groups for years, based on clinical studies that have shown overall survival rates of 90–100% even in patients with grade 2, 3 tumours. Furthermore, patients who subsequently had recurrent disease achieved favourable remission rates with salvage chemotherapy [22–24].

Growing Teratoma Syndrome (GTS) In 1982, a description of this clinical entity was published by Logothetis and colleagues on a subset of patients with non-seminoma testicular germ cell cancers, who developed rapidly enlarging tumours during or shortly after chemotherapy [25, 26]. The tumours were noted to contain (benign) mature tissue elements on histological sectioning. Interestingly, in 1977, DiSaia had described a similar phenomenon of 'chemotherapeutic retroconversion' in patients treated for ovarian immature teratomas. Current accepted hypotheses for GTS are: (1) De-differentiation theory; immature elements in treated malignant germ cell tumour undergo (retrograde) differentiation into mature tissue elements which then proliferate from (microscopic) disease residuum to clinically significant tumour mass. (2) Chemotherapy-induced selective cell death theory; chemotherapy targets the immature elements in primary germ cell cancer, which allows pre-existing mature elements to proliferate into a growing tumour mass. GTS should be suspected with any post-treatment mass in a patient being treated for germ cell malignancy.

Three conditions must be met for a diagnosis of GTS [27]:

1. Normalisation of any elevated pre-treatment tumour marker levels
2. Increasing size of tumour mass during chemotherapy
3. Histologic confirmation of mature teratoma elements (imaging-guided needle biopsy can be used pre-operatively).

The reported incidence of GTS varies between 2% and 12% based on available case series of testicular cancer patients. Based on the few reports on patients with GTS of the ovary, recurrences tend to occur within 2 years of primary treatment, usually do not involve extra-abdominal sites, and can be associated with secondary recurrences years after surgery. Most recurrences occur in the retroperitoneum, and may be associated with pain, visceral compression, bowel or urinary obstruction, neuropathy, and venous thromboembolism. Surgery is the accepted initial approach for GTS lesions for several reasons. Firstly, the mature teratoma is mostly benign and potentially curable with resection. Secondly, surgical resection provides histologic confirmation of the mass as a mature teratoma. Thirdly, surgery is needed for symptom control. Finally, the mature cell elements are potentially less responsive to cytotoxic chemotherapy compared to immature cells with faster doubling times. Complete surgical resection is associated with a reduced likelihood of a malignant secondary recurrence that may arise out of the teratoma mass [27, 28].

59.5.2 Dysgerminoma

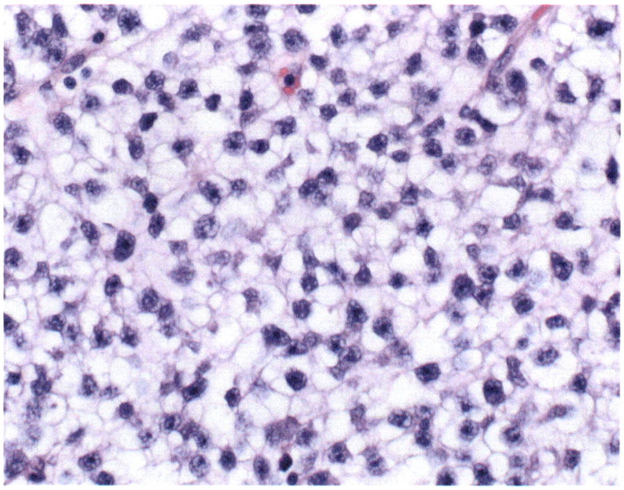

Dysgerminoma. (Courtesy: Dr. Ander J. Pindzola)

Dysgerminoma is a rare, malignant neoplasm representing approximately one-third of ovarian germ cell tumours, but less than 2% of all ovarian neoplasms. Majority (approximately 75%) of dysgerminomas occur in young women under 30 years old. Dysgerminoma is the commonest malignant ovarian germ cell tumour, and also the commonest malignant ovarian neoplasm in pregnant women. In contrast to other malignant germ cell tumours, dysgerminoma has the highest incidence of bilateral disease (10–15%), and also is radiosensitive [2, 29]. Histologically, the tumour cells have a 'fried egg appearance', with clear cytoplasm and centric nuclei. Dysgerminoma on a histologic slide is virtually indistinguishable from seminoma of the testis. Certain pre-pubertal patients with dysgenetic gonads which can develop into (malignant) gonadoblastomas, can have co-existent dysgerminoma [30, 31]. Therefore, karyotype analysis is recommended in patients with suspected germ cell tumours who also have primary amenorrhea, in which case, bilateral salpingo-oophorectomy is the recommended treatment for confirmed dysgenetic gonads. Clinically, dysgerminomas grow rapidly, and the initial presentation can be in the acute setting, following torsion, or spontaneous tumour rupture with hemoperitoneum. A minority of patients may have elevated LDH, hCG, or human placental lactogen (hPl). In cases of mixed histology with yolk sac elements (see below), AFP levels may be elevated [32]. Up to 75% of patients who have dysgerminoma present with stage IA disease, with an additional 10–15% of cases diagnosed in stage IB. Patients with stage I disease have 5-year survival rates approaching 95% following conservative surgery [33], and approximately 75% 5-year survival rate for stage II and III disease (see Table 59.7 for treatment recommendations by stage).

Table 59.7 Summary of treatment recommendations for malignant ovarian germ cell tumours

Histology	Stage/grade	Treatment
Dysgerminoma	Stages IA, IB	Surgery
	Stages IC, II–IV	Surgery + chemotherapy
Immature teratoma	Stage I; intact ovary, grade 1	Surgery
	Stage I; ruptured ovary Any grade 2 or 3 tumour Stages II–IV	Surgery + chemotherapy
Other histologies Embryonal carcinoma Polyembryoma Choriocarcinoma	Stages I–IV	Surgery + chemotherapy
Recurrent disease		Chemotherapy (surgical resection in select cases with isolated, resectable lesion)

59.5.3 Endodermal Sinus Tumour

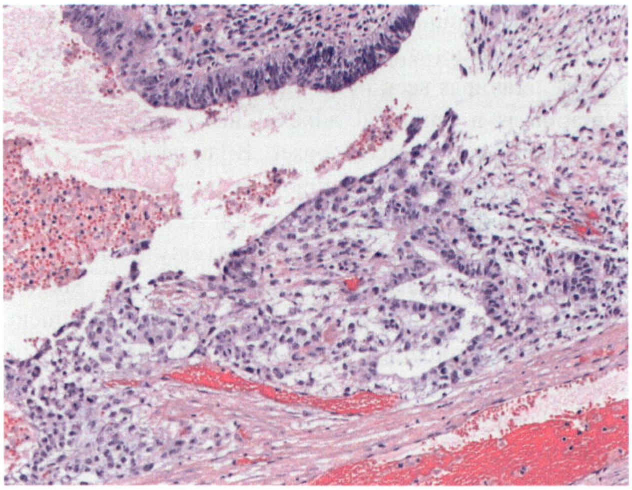

Yolk sac tumour (a). (Courtesy of Dr. Ander J. Pindzola)

Also traditionally referred to as 'yolk sac tumour'.

This is a malignant tumour, representing 15–20% of germ cell tumours. Histologically, yolk sac tumour consists of clear spaces or sinuses lined by single layers of cuboidal cells. Tubular or reticular growth patterns can exist. Within the spaces mentioned above, a papillary structure may be seen, with a central vessel, and is known as a 'Schiller-Duval body' [34].

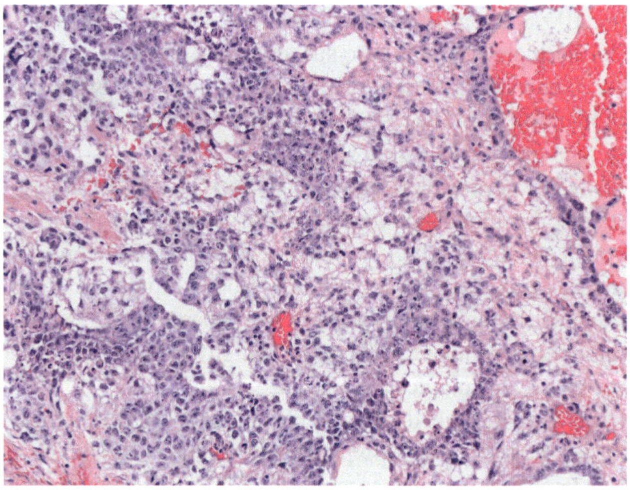

Yolk sac tumour (b). (Courtesy of Dr. Ander J. Pindzola)

Clinical presentation is similar to other germ cell tumours. Most tumours are seen in patients less than 20 years of age, tend to be unilateral and around 10 cm in diameter on average. Yolk sac tumours can be aggressive, with a propensity for early lymphatic dissemination, as well as direct invasion of adjacent pelvic structures [35, 36]. An elevated serum level of AFP is characteristic of this tumour, and serves as a useful diagnostic and surveillance tool [37]. Historically, the prognosis for patients with this tumour was unfavourable even with early stage disease, until the use of modern combination chemotherapy. The GOG as well as several other investigators have reported short-term remission rates ranging from 60% to 73% for patients with stages I–III disease [33, 38, 39].

59.5.4 Choriocarcinoma

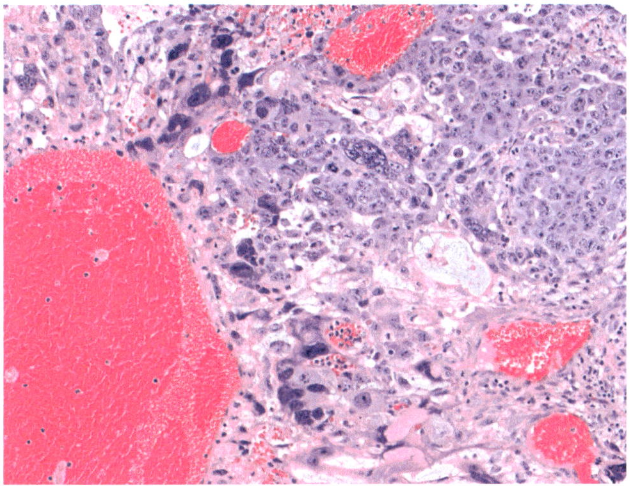

Choriocarcinoma. (Courtesy of Dr. Ander J. Pindzola)

Also referred to as 'non-gestational choriocarcinoma' or 'primary ovarian choriocarcinoma'.

This is a rare malignancy, accounting for less than 2% of germ cell tumours of the ovary. Unlike gestational choriocarcinoma, primary ovarian choriocarcinoma is devoid of paternal DNA; a useful diagnostic feature. Histologically, this tumour is similar to gestational choriocarcinoma, and hCG production is also characteristic. Clinically, the tumour can be seen in children and may present with abnormal vaginal bleeding or other signs of precocious development due to hCG secretion [38]. Pure non-gestational choriocarcinoma is quite rare, such that, it is typically diagnosed in the context of a mixed germ cell tumour. Hematogenous dissemination to distant sites is the favoured route of spread [40]. Unlike gestational choriocarcinoma, this tumour is not as chemosensitive, and is associated with low survival rates in patients with metastatic disease [41–43]. Data on remission rates is limited due to the rarity of the tumour; however, modest increases in short-term survival have been reported with a variety of single-agent and combination regimens.

59.5.5 Embryonal Carcinoma

Embryonal carcinomas are rare, clinically aggressive malignant tumours that represent approximately 4–5% of malignant germ cell tumours. Histologically, the tumour consists of multinucleated giant cells with the appearance of syncytial cells that show atypia and high mitotic rates. Not much is known about the clinical behaviour of this disease due to the rare incidence. Patients tend to be, on average, around 15 years of age at the time of diagnosis, and may also show signs of precocious sexual development, or abnormal vaginal bleeding, due to hCG secretion [44]. AFP secretion is also seen in over half of cases. The optimal chemotherapy regimen following primary surgery remains undetermined, and few reported series exist in the literature. Older data from a single source showed about 50% survival rate in patients with early stage disease [34].

59.5.6 Polyembryoma

This is a malignant germ cell tumour with few reported cases in the literature. Histologically, the tumour consists of numerous cells that have the appearance of very early developing embryos. Early, distant metastatic spread has been described, as well as locally invasive spread. Little is known about clinical behaviour or chemosensitivity of this disease [2, 3, 45].

59.5.7 Mixed Germ Cell Tumour

Mixed germ cell tumour is defined by the presence of at least two germ cell tumour types in the same tumour mass or peritoneal implant. Any combination or number of tumour types can occur, including benign teratoma; however, the most common tumour combination usually diagnosed is dysgerminoma and yolk sac tumour. Tumour marker assays may suggest the presence of mixed cell populations, and a thorough pathologic review of the tumour is essential in establishing diagnosis and guiding management. Following surgery, the use of adjuvant treatment should be decided based on the most malignant subtype. It is also important to know the most prevalent cell type. Bilateral ovarian involvement may be seen with the presence of dysgerminoma [2, 3, 46].

59.6 Treatment Modalities: Surgery

The clinical features of ovarian germ cell tumours are summarised in Table 59.8. Pursuant to our understanding of these features, surgery has become the accepted primary treatment modality in the management of these tumours. Given the incidence of these lesions in young women, preservation of fertility is a major consideration in management. There is clinical data supporting equivalent survival outcomes in

Table 59.8 Summary of clinical features of malignant ovarian germ cell tumours

Incidence in younger age women
Unilateral ovarian involvement
Secrete tumour markers
Predilection for lymphatic spread
Majority are stage I at diagnosis
Most primary and recurrent tumours are platinum-sensitive

patients who undergo unilateral versus bilateral salpingo-oophorectomy. Laparoscopy can be used for small adnexal masses, and even for staging surgery [47–49].

Laparotomy through a midline vertical incision should be used in situations where expertise with laparoscopy is not available, in patients with advanced bulky disease, and for large ovarian tumours (to avoid up-staging from iatrogenic cyst rupture and tumour spillage in the abdomen).

Surgery for Disease Confined to the Ovaries In patients who desire fertility, unilateral salpingo-oophorectomy is an appropriate treatment. Intra-operative pathology analysis can be useful in deciding surgical management. In all patients with malignant germ cell neoplasms, surgical staging should be performed because of the known risk of lymphatic spread, in order to accurately map the extent of disease, and to tailor the use of adjuvant treatment.

In emergency or other situations where intra-operative pathology analysis or staging surgery is not available, for young patients, unilateral salpingo-oophorectomy should be performed to preserve fertility. An accurate description of the findings at surgery should be documented. Further treatment decisions can be made after a pathology report becomes available.

Such patients in whom a presenting adnexal mass was completely removed may be managed expectantly. Chemotherapy can be used in patients who have unresected bulky disease or implants that have been biopsied and confirmed to be malignant, if there is no available surgeon trained to perform radical tumour resection.

The recommended surgical protocol for germ cell tumours is shown in Table 59.9.

The FIGO staging system for ovarian cancer is shown in Table 59.10.

Patients who have completed childbearing should undergo bilateral salpingo-oophorectomy, total hysterectomy, pelvic and para-aortic lymphadenectomy, and omentectomy. Thorough abdominal and pelvic inspection and palpation, pelvic washings, and peritoneal biopsies should be performed prior to commencing the surgical resections.

In resource challenged settings where expertise for staging lymphadenectomy and omentectomy may not be available, bilateral salpingo-oophorectomy and hysterectomy

Table 59.9 Staging protocol for malignant ovarian germ cell tumours

	Stage I disease	Stages II–IV disease
Fertility sparing	Pelvic washings Peritoneal biopsies Unilateral salpingo-oophorectomy[a] Bilateral pelvic and para-aortic lymphadenectomy Omentectomy	Pelvic washings Peritoneal biopsies Unilateral salpingo-oophorectomy[b] Bilateral pelvic and para-aortic lymphadenectomy Omentectomy OR Optimal cytoreductive surgery[c]
Completed childbearing	Pelvic washings Peritoneal biopsies Total hysterectomy Bilateral salpingo-oophorectomy Bilateral pelvic and para-aortic lymphadenectomy Omentectomy	Optimal cytoreductive surgery[c]

[a]Bilateral salpingo-oophorectomy advised for bilateral ovarian involvement when contralateral ovarian cystectomy is not feasible
[b]Unilateral salpingo-oophorectomy acceptable if contralateral ovary and uterus are not grossly involved with tumour infiltration
[c]Surgical resection to no gross visible disease using radical surgical techniques as necessary

should be performed. Pelvic washings and random peritoneal biopsies should also be performed. Any suspicious bulky or implant lesions should be biopsied for confirmation of malignancy, to guide the use of adjuvant chemotherapy.

In general practice, some patients with germ cell tumours may undergo surgery for suspected ectopic pregnancy, or other acute presentations, without the availability of oncologic consultation. The decision to re-operate on such patients to complete surgical staging may depend on completeness of the initial tumour resection, presence of gross unresected disease, histology, grade, known chemosensitivity, and the patient's wishes.

Management of the contralateral ovary remains a subject of debate. Most clinicians agree that normal-appearing contralateral ovaries should be left alone. Wedge excisional biopsy of the normal-appearing contralateral ovary has fallen out of favour, because of low yield for malignancy, and the risk of compromising fertility due to adhesion formation. Grossly abnormal ovaries should be subjected to simple biopsy or cystectomy, with intra-operative pathology analysis. If malignancy is confirmed, contralateral salpingo-oophorectomy should be performed. Fertility sparing surgery should be avoided when there is gross bilateral involvement of the ovaries with tumour masses.

Surgery for Bulky or Metastatic Disease Following an appropriate work-up, surgical resection to 'no gross visible residual disease' is the recommended initial treatment for germ cell tumours with bulky intra-peritoneal dissemination, whenever feasible. This is based on GOG study data in patients treated with surgery and adjuvant chemotherapy, with observation of higher disease recurrence rates in patients who underwent incomplete initial surgeries compared to patients with complete resections prior to receiving chemotherapy. In cases of germ cell tumour where the uterus and one ovary are grossly unaffected, these can be left in-situ to preserve fertility if desired by the patient [50, 51]. Single institution data suggest that this approach is feasible, with comparable overall survival rates in a small group of patients with advanced bulky disease subjected to fertility sparing surgery versus radical tumour debulking surgery.

Recurrent disease With the development of effective chemotherapy regimens and the observed favourable response rates even in patients with recurrent tumours, surgery now has limited use in the treatment of recurrent germ cell malignancies. Please see the section on 'Growing Teratoma Syndrome'.

Table 59.10 FIGO staging of malignant ovarian germ cell tumours

Stage	Description
I	Tumour confined to the ovary
IA	Tumour limited to one ovary; capsule intact, no tumour on ovarian surface, no malignant ascites or pelvic washings
IB	Tumour limited to both ovaries; capsule intact, no tumour on ovarian surface, no malignant ascites or pelvic washings
IC	Tumour limited to one or both ovaries, with any of:
IC 1	Surgical spill
IC 2	Rupture of ovarian capsule, tumour on ovarian surface
IC 3	Malignant ascites or pelvic washings
II	Tumour involves one or both ovaries with involvement of pelvic tissues (below the pelvic brim)
III	Tumour involves one or both ovaries with pathologically confirmed metastasis to peritoneum outside the pelvic cavity, or to retroperitoneal lymph nodes
IIIA	Microscopic metastases in retroperitoneal lymph nodes or outside pelvis
IIIA 1	Microscopic metastases in retroperitoneal lymph nodes
IIIA 2	Microscopic metastases in extrapelvic peritoneum (above pelvic brim); with or without retroperitoneal lymph node involvement
IIIA 2 i	Metastases up to 10 mm in greatest dimension
IIIA 2 ii	Metastases more than 10 mm in greatest dimension
IIIB	Macroscopic metastases in extrapelvic peritoneum up to 2 cm size; with or without retroperitoneal lymph node involvement
IIIC	Macroscopic metastases to extrapelvic peritoneum more than 2 cm in size; capsular involvement of liver and/or spleen without parenchymal involvement; with or without retroperitoneal lymph node involvement
IV	Distant metastases; does not include peritoneal metastases Pleural effusion with malignant cytology Parenchymal metastases (liver, lung), metastases to extra-abdominal lymph nodes (inguinal, mediastinal)

Taken from: Prat [62]

59.7 Treatment Modalities: Chemotherapy

The most commonly encountered germ cell malignancies are chemosensitive, and the main role of chemotherapy is in the post-surgical treatment of patients with high-risk tumours (see Table 59.7 for treatment recommendations).

In the 1970s, combination chemotherapy with vincristine, actinomycin D, and cyclophosphamide (VAC) for testicular germ cell cancers was adapted for use in patients with malignant ovarian germ cell tumours [52]. Subsequent advances in platinum drug therapy led to the use of cisplatin, vinblastine, and bleomycin (PVB) [53, 54]. Subsequently, the efficacy of etoposide and cisplatin in testicular germ cell cancers was also observed in GOG studies of ovarian germ cell tumours. This resulted in the emergence of bleomycin, etoposide, and cisplatin (BEP) as the current standard regimen for adjuvant treatment of ovarian germ cell malignancies. The use of BEP has been associated with at least 90% and 80% overall survival rates for early and advanced stage disease respectively [38]. Patients with dysgerminoma have a more favourable 5-year overall survival rate compared to non-dysgerminoma cancers (95–100% vs. 75–80%) [55, 56]. Current guidelines advise the use of three cycles of BEP as standard adjuvant chemotherapy for malignant ovarian germ cell tumours (see Table 59.11 for BEP regimen).

Other active chemotherapy agents, used singly or in combination for recurrent disease, include ifosfamide, paclitaxel, gemcitabine, oxaliplatin, vincristine, and actinomycin D.

Neoadjuvant Chemotherapy Few recent reports in the literature describe the upfront use of chemotherapy in patients with unresectable initial disease presentations. These non-randomised series indicate that this is probably a reasonable consideration in circumstances where patients cannot undergo upfront surgery. Long-term survival rates are unknown with this approach; however, in one report on 23 patients who received four cycles of BEP prior to surgery, 18

Table 59.11 BEP chemotherapy regimen

Drug	Dose	Route	Frequency
Bleomycin	20 units/m^2	Intravenous	Day 1; give weekly for 9 cycles
Etoposide	100 mg/m^2	Intravenous	Days 1–5; give every 4 weeks for 3 cycles
Cisplatin	20 mg/m^2	Intravenous	Days 1–5; give every 4 weeks for 3 cycles

patients were able to receive interval surgery followed by two further cycles of BEP. The reported 10-year survival was 87% of patients [57].

Gonadotoxicity and Post-Treatment Fertility Premature ovarian failure is a serious concern in young patients who undergo chemotherapy for germ cell tumours. Fortunately, available clinical data from the paediatric oncology and adult literature have shown that patients treated with BEP appear to recover ovarian function without significant diminution in fecundity. The incidence of congenital foetal malformations is not significantly elevated over that of the general population, and normal pregnancy and miscarriage rates have been observed in most treated patients [58–60].

59.8 Post-Treatment Surveillance

The median time for disease recurrence in patients treated with surgery and adjuvant chemotherapy is 2 years, and approximately 25% of patients will experience this. Close follow-up is recommended following completion of therapy beginning with 3-monthly evaluations for the first 2 years, then yearly visits thereafter. Each surveillance visit evaluation should consist of symptom evaluation, complete physical examination, and tumour marker assay if tumour marker values were elevated pre-operatively. Imaging studies are typically reserved for symptomatic patients, assessment of abnormal examination findings, or abnormal tumour marker levels. In patients with no tumour marker elevations at diagnosis, imaging studies are indicated 6-monthly in the first 2 years, since the peak incidence of recurrence is highest during this interval [61].

59.9 Summary

The successful management of patients with ovarian germ cell tumours requires understanding of the presentation and clinical behaviour of these lesions. General practitioners and gynaecologists involved in the evaluation of patients with adnexal masses should maintain a high index of suspicion for germ cell tumours especially in young females. Referral for specialist consultation is ideal, however, in situations where such resources are unavailable, safe management is still feasible with prudent surgical decision-making. Given the rarity of these lesions, the establishment of modern tumour registries in developing countries could enhance current knowledge, and help to formulate tailored management protocols.

Glossary of Terms

Adjuvant treatment A treatment modality that is used following intended primary treatment. Chemotherapy is the adjuvant treatment of choice following (primary) surgery for malignant germ cell tumours.

Neoadjuvant treatment A treatment modality that is used prior to the intended primary treatment. Chemotherapy has been used as neoadjuvant treatment for malignant germ cell tumours; as part of non-standard management.

Optimal cytoreduction Often used in the context of surgery for intra-peritoneal peritoneal cancer dissemination. In ovarian cancer, the GOG has re-defined optimal surgical cytoreduction as residual disease comprising lesions no more than 1 cm in greatest diameter, at the end of surgical resection in the peritoneal cavity. In practice, surgical resection to no gross visible lesions (microscopic disease) is the goal for optimal cytoreductive surgery.

Primary treatment The intended definitive treatment modality. As described in this chapter, surgery is the primary treatment for germ cell tumours.

References

1. Quirk JT, Natarajan N, Mettlin CJ. Age specific ovarian cancer rate patterns in the United States. Gynecol Oncol. 2005;99(1):248–50.
2. Tewari K, Cappucini F, Disaia P, et al. Malignant germ cell tumours of the ovary. Obstet Gynecol. 2000;95(1):128–33.
3. Smith HO, Berwick M, Verschraegen CF, et al. Incidence and survival rates for female malignant germ cell tumours. Obstet Gynecol. 2006;107:1075–85.
4. Bryant CS, Kumar S, Shah JP, et al. Racial disparities in survival among patients with germ cell tumours of the ovary – United States. Gynecol Oncol. 2009;114:437–41.
5. Hinchcliff E, Rauh-Hain A, Clemmer J, et al. Racial disparities in survival in malignant germ cell tumours of the ovary. Gynecol Oncol. 2016;140:463–9.
6. Kurman R, Norris H. Malignant germ cell tumours of the ovary. Hum Pathol. 1977;8(5):551–64.
7. Talerman A. Germ cell tumour of the ovary. Curr Opin Obstet Gynecol. 1997;9(1):44–7.
8. Pectasides D, Pectasides E, Kassanos D. Germ cell tumours of the ovary. Cancer Treat Rev. 2008;34:427–41.
9. Zalel Y, Piura B, Elchalal U, et al. Diagnosis and management of malignant germ cell ovarian tumours in young females. Int J Gynaecol Obstet. 1996;55:1.
10. Kumar S, Shah J, Bryant C, et al. The prevalence and prognostic impact of lymph node metastasis in malignant germ cell tumours of the ovary. Gynecol Oncol. 2008;110:125.
11. Ayhan A, Bukulmez O, Genc C, et al. Mature cystic teratomas of the ovary: case series from one institution over 34 years. Eur J Obstet Gynecol Reprod Biol. 2000;88:153–7.
12. Hackethal A, Brueggmann D, Bohlmann M, et al. Squamous cell carcinoma in mature cystic teratoma of the ovary: systematic review and analysis of published data. Lancet Oncol. 2008;9:1173–80.

13. Dos Santos L, Mok E, Iasonos A, et al. Squamous cell carcinoma arising in mature cystic teratoma of the ovary: a case series and review of the literature. Gynecol Oncol. 2007;105:321–4.
14. Patel M, Feldstein V, Lipson S, et al. Cystic teratomas of the ovary: diagnostic value of sonography. Am J Roentgenol. 1998;171:1061–5.
15. Tongsong T, Luewan S, Phadungkiatwattana P, et al. Pattern recognition using transabdominal ultrasound to diagnose ovarian mature cystic teratoma. Int J Gynaecol Obstet. 2008;103:99–104.
16. Westhoff C, Pike M, Vessey M. Benign ovarian teratomas: a population based case-control study. Br J Cancer. 1988;58:93–8.
17. Robboy S, Shaco-Levy R, Peng R, et al. Malignant struma ovarii: an analysis of 88 cases, including 27 with extraovarian spread. Int J Gynecol Pathol. 2009;28:405–22.
18. Shaco-Levy R, Bean S, Bentley R, et al. Natural history of biologically malignant struma ovarii: analysis of 27 cases with extraovarian spread. Int J Gynecol Pathol. 2010;29:212–27.
19. Davis K, Hartmann L, Keeney G, et al. Primary ovarian carcinoid tumours. Gynecol Oncol. 1996;61:259–65.
20. Strosberg J, Nasir A, Cragun J, et al. Metastatic carcinoid tumour to the ovary: a clinicopathologic analysis of seventeen cases. Gynecol Oncol. 2007;106:65–8.
21. Norris HJ, Zirkin HJ, Benson WL. Immature (malignant) teratoma of the ovary: a clinical and pathological study of 58 cases. Cancer. 1976;37:2359–72.
22. Patterson D, Murugaesu N, Holden L, et al. A review of the close surveillance policy for stage I female germ cell tumours of the ovary and other sites. Int J Gynecol Cancer. 2008;18:43–50.
23. Billmire D, Cullen J, Rescoria F, et al. Surveillance after initial surgery for paediatric and adolescent girls with stage I ovarian germ cell tumours: a report from the Children's Oncology Group. J Clin Oncol. 2014;95:465–70.
24. Mangili G, Scarfone G, Gadducci A, et al. Is adjuvant chemotherapy indicated in stage I pure immature ovarian teratoma (IT)? A multicentre Italian trial in ovarian cancer (MITO-9). Gynecol Oncol. 2010;119:48–52.
25. Logothetis CJ, Samuels M, Trindade A, Johnson D. The growing teratoma syndrome. Cancer. 1982;50:1629–35.
26. DiSaia PJ, Saltz A, Kagan AR, et al. Chemotherapeutic retroconversion of immature teratoma of the ovary. Obstet Gynecol. 1977;49:346–50.
27. Djordjevic B, Euscher E, Malpica A. Growing teratoma syndrome of the ovary: review of literature and first report of a carcinoid tumour arising in a growing teratoma of the ovary. Am J Surg Pathol. 2007;31(12):1913–8.
28. Andre F, Fizazi K, Culine S, et al. The growing teratoma syndrome: results of therapy and long-term follow-up of 33 patients. Eur J Cancer. 2000;36:1389–94.
29. Gordon A, Lipton D, Woodruff J. Dysgerminoma: a review of 158 cases from the Emil Novak Ovarian Tumour Registry. Obstet Gynecol. 1981;58:497–504.
30. Krasna I, Lee M, Smilow P, et al. Risk of malignancy in bilateral streak gonads: the role of the Y chromosome. J Pediatr Surg. 1992;27:1376–80.
31. De Arce M, Costigan C, Gosden J, et al. Further experience consistent with Yqh as an indicator of risk of gonadal blastoma in Y-bearing mosaic Turner syndrome. Clin Genet. 1992;41:28–32.
32. Schwartz PE, Morris JM. Serum lactate dehydrogenase: a tumour marker for dysgerminoma. Obstet Gynecol. 1988;72:511–5.
33. Williams SD, Blessing JA, Moore DH, et al. Cisplatin, vinblastine, and bleomycin in advanced and recurrent ovarian germ cell tumours. A trial of the Gynaecologic Oncology Group. Ann Intern Med. 1989;111:22–7.
34. Kurman R, Norris H. Endodermal sinus tumour of the ovary: a clinical and pathologic analysis of 71 cases. Cancer. 1976;38:2404–19.
35. Shah JP, Kumar S, Bryant S, et al. A population-based analysis of 788 cases of yolk sac tumours: a comparison of males and females. Int J Cancer. 2008;123:2671–5.
36. Gershenson D, Del Junco G, Herson J, et al. Endodermal sinus tumour of the ovary: the M D Anderson experience. Obstet Gynecol. 1983;61:194–202.
37. Talerman A, Haije WG, Baggerman L. Serum alphafoetoprotein (AFP) in diagnosis and management of endodermal sinus (yolk sac) tumour and mixed germ cell tumour of the ovary. Cancer. 1978;41:272–8.
38. Williams S, Blessing JA, Liao S, et al. Adjuvant therapy of ovarian germ cell tumours with cisplatin, etoposide and bleomycin: a trial of the Gynaecologic Oncology Group. J Clin Oncol. 1994;12:701–6.
39. Williams SD, Kauderer J, Burnett A, et al. Adjuvant therapy of completely resected dysgerminoma with carboplatin and etoposide: a trial of the Gynaecologic Oncology group. Gynecol Oncol. 2004;95:496–9.
40. Steigrad S, Cheung A, Osborn R. Choriocarcinoma co-existent with an intact pregnancy: case report and review of the literature. J Obstet Gynaecol Res. 1999;25:197–203.
41. Abu-Rustum N, Aghajanian C. Management of malignant germ cell tumours of the ovary. Semin Oncol. 1998;25:235–42.
42. Fisher RA, Newlands E, Jeffreys A, et al. Gestational and non-gestational trophoblastic tumours distinguished by DNA analysis. Cancer. 1992;69:839–45.
43. Wheeler C, Davis S, Degefu S, et al. Ovarian choriocarcinoma: a difficult diagnosis of an unusual tumour and a review of the hook effect. Obstet Gynecol. 1990;75:547–9.
44. Ueda G, Abe Y, Yoshida M, et al. Embryonal carcinoma of the ovary: a six year survival. Int J Gynaecol Obstet. 1990;31:287–92.
45. Roth L, Talerman A. Recent advances in the pathology and classification of ovarian germ cell tumours. Int J Gynecol Pathol. 2006;25:305–20.
46. Gershenson DM. Management of ovarian germ cell tumours. J Clin Oncol. 2007;25(20):2938–43.
47. Thomas G, Dembo A, Hacker N, et al. Current therapy for dysgerminoma of the ovary. Obstet Gynecol. 1987;70:268–75.
48. Shim S, Kim D, Lee S, et al. Laparoscopic management of early stage malignant non-epithelial ovarian tumours: surgical and survival outcomes. Int J Gynecol Cancer. 2013;23:249–55.
49. Lu K, Gershenson D. Update on the management of ovarian germ cell tumours. J Reprod Med. 2005;50:417–25.
50. Slayton R, Park R, Silverberg S, et al. Vincristine, dactinomycin, and cyclophosphamide in the treatment of malignant germ cell tumours of the ovary. A Gynaecologic Oncology Group Study (a final report). Cancer. 1985;56:243–8.
51. Low J, Perrin L, Crandon A, et al. Conservative surgery to preserve ovarian function in patients with malignant ovarian germ cell tumours. A review of 74 cases. Cancer. 2000;89:391–8.
52. Smith J, Rutlegde F. Advances in chemotherapy for gynaecologic cancer. Cancer. 1975;36:669–74.
53. Gershenson D, Kavanagh J, Copeland L, et al. Treatment of malignant non-dysgerminomatous germ cell tumours of the ovary with vinblastine, bleomycin, and cisplatin. Cancer. 1986;57:1731–7.
54. Carlson R, Sikic B, Turbow M, et al. Combination cisplatin, vinblastine, and bleomycin chemotherapy (PVB) for malignant germ cell tumours of the ovary. J Clin Oncol. 1983;1:645–51.
55. Murugaesu N, Schmid P, Dancey G, et al. Malignant ovarian germ cell tumours: identification of novel prognostic markers and long-term outcome after multi-modality treatment. J Clin Oncol. 2006;24:4862–6.

56. Rogers P, Olson T, Cullen J, et al. Treatment of children and adolescents with II testicular and stages I and II ovarian malignant germ cell tumours: a Paediatric Intergroup Study – Paediatric Oncology Group 9048 and Childrens Cancer Group 8891. J Clin Oncol. 2004;22:3563–9.
57. Talukdar S, Kumar S, Bhatia N, et al. Neo-adjuvant chemotherapy in the treatment of advanced malignant germ cell tumours of the ovary. Gynecol Oncol. 2014;132:28–32.
58. Brewer M, Gershenson D, Herzog C, et al. Outcome and reproductive function after chemotherapy for ovarian dysgerminoma. J Clin Oncol. 1999;17:2670–5.
59. Zanetta G, Bonazzi C, Cantu M, et al. Survival and reproductive function after treatment of malignant germ cell ovarian tumours. J Clin Oncol. 2001;19:1015–20.
60. Gershenson DM, Miller AM, Champion V, et al. Reproductive and sexual function after platinum based chemotherapy in long-term ovarian germ cell tumour survivors: a Gynaecologic Oncology Group Study. J Clin Oncol. 2007;25:2792–7.
61. Salani R, Backes F, Fung M, et al. Post-treatment surveillance and diagnosis of recurrence in women with gynaecologic malignancies: Society of Gynaecologic Oncologists recommendations. Am J Obstet Gynecol. 2011;204:46.
62. Prat J. Staging classification for cancer of the ovary, fallopian tube and peritoneum. Int J Gynaecol Obstet. 2014;124:1.

Principle of Radiation Therapy for Gynaecologic Cancers

60

Shushan Rana, Sophia Bornstein, and Jerry J. Jaboin

Learning Objectives

After studying this chapter, the reader should be able to:

- Highlight the factors characterising the global burden of cervical cancer
- Contrast the differences in incidence and mortality of cervical cancer between developing and developed nations
- Identify the major signs and symptoms of early- versus late-stage cervical cancer
- Define the components of formal FIGO cervical cancer staging
- Discuss the therapeutic paradigm of early- and late-stage cervical cancer
- Define the radiation treatment volumes and techniques
- Evaluate the role and efficacy of brachytherapy in cervical cancer
- Identify the components of post-treatment surveillance
- Highlight the factors characterising the global burden of endometrial cancer
- Contrast the differences in incidence and mortality of endometrial cancer between developing and developed nations
- Identify the major signs and symptoms of early- versus late-stage endometrial cancer
- Define the components of formal FIGO endometrial cancer staging
- Discuss the therapeutic paradigm of early and late endometrial cancer
- Define the radiation treatment volumes and techniques in the management of endometrial cancer
- Evaluate the role and efficacy of brachytherapy in endometrial cancer
- Identify the components of post-treatment surveillance

60.1 Cervical Cancer

60.1.1 Introduction

Cervical cancer is a globally prevalent malignancy with the highest mortality rate among gynaecological malignancies. Lack of disease screening resources and accessibility has largely contributed to the higher incidence of mortality in developing nations. Formal staging of cervical cancer is confined to clinical staging as the resources for surgical staging are limited. Most patients in developing patients present with locally advanced or metastatic disease. Treatment strategies for non-bulky localised disease are confined to surgical resection potentially followed by adjuvant external beam radiation or vaginal brachytherapy and/or chemoradiation. The remaining patient with bulky or locally advanced disease undergoes chemoradiation alone consisting of a platinum-based chemotherapy and conventional external beam radiation therapy techniques followed by vaginal brachytherapy. Post-treatment surveillance is essential in the early detection of potential recurrent disease as well as management of therapeutic adverse effects.

Cervical cancer remains a prominent global burden with an estimated 527,600 cases reported in 2012 ranking it as the fourth most common cancer among women and seventh overall. Less developed nations, as defined by the United Nations, account for approximately 85% of cases. Among

S. Rana · S. Bornstein · J. J. Jaboin (✉)
Department of Radiation Medicine, Oregon Health and Science University, Portland, OR, USA
e-mail: ranas@ohsu.edu; jaboin@ohsu.edu

F. Okonofua et al. (eds.), *Contemporary Obstetrics and Gynecology for Developing Countries*,
https://doi.org/10.1007/978-3-030-75385-6_60

gynaecological malignancies, it possesses the highest incidence of mortality with approximately 265,700 deaths annually with the average risk of death three times higher in less developed nations compared to their more developed counterparts [1, 2]. Areas with highest incidence and mortality include sub-Saharan Africa, Southeast Asia, Latin America and the Caribbean, and Central and Eastern Europe. This disparity is attributable to a variety of factors, including but not limited to, inadequate access to screening, patient education, and access to medical resources. The importance of cytological screening has been evident for several decades in developed nations as Western European nations have observed a 4% annual decline in cervical cancer and 70% overall since the adoption of routine cervical cancer screening [3]. Though screening has exhibited proven clinical benefit, many women in developed nations do not undergo screening. In the United States, women who never underwent a Pap smear in their lifetime account for 50% of women with newly diagnosed cervical cancer [4]. In some developing nations, alternative cost-effective screening methods have shown benefit in reducing cervical cancer incidence. A randomised controlled trial in India compared cancer education and visual inspection with acetic acid (VIA) to cancer education alone among 150,000 women. At 12-year follow-up, VIA and cancer education led to a statistically significant reduction in mortality compared to cancer education alone (RR = 0.69; $p = 0.003$).

Clinical manifestations of cervical cancer are also reflective of the impact in screening and access to health care. Developing nations with more robust screening detect precancerous lesions or minimally invasive cervical cancers well before growth to symptomatic disease. More advanced disease can present with abnormal clear or foul-smelling vaginal bleeding. Sciatica, lower extremity oedema, and hydronephrosis portend pelvic sidewall involvement, and bladder and rectal symptoms further suggest locally advanced pelvic disease. With the paucity of healthcare providers and their accessibility, patients in developing nations present late in the course of their disease. Approximately 60–80% of patients in sub-Saharan Africa, Nepal, and India present with Stage III or IV disease [5–8].

Treatment recommendations are contingent on clinical staging as designated by the International Federation of Gynaecology and Obstetrics (FIGO). Although clinical staging is less accurate than surgical staging, cervical cancer remains primarily a localised pelvic disease. Additionally, late presentation and poor surgical access precludes adequate implementation of surgical staging. Diagnostic evaluation and procedures in FIGO staging include inspection, pelvic examination under anaesthesia, cystoscopy, hysteroscopy, proctoscopy, intravenous pyelogram, and biopsy of suspected bladder or rectal lesions. Lymphangiography and routinely obtained imaging studies in developed nations such as CT, MRI, or PET are not included in FIGO staging as these modalities are not readily available in developing nations of high incidence. An exception lies within CT findings if there is presence of hydronephrosis, and these data can be incorporated into final FIGO staging. Despite the exclusion of modern imaging from FIGO staging, they can be utilised for prognostication and in final treatment recommendations. Additional prognostic features incorporated into overall patient evaluation include lymphovascular space invasion and lymph node status [9, 10].

Therapeutic management of cervical cancer is largely dependent on the FIGO tumour stage. Patients with either microscopic disease or small grossly visible non-bulky (<4 cm) tumours confined to the cervix can be adequately treated with surgery alone. Cervical conisation or extrafascial hysterectomy is pursued in FIGO Stage IA1, described as microinvasive disease, with some younger women eligible from radical trachelectomy for fertility sparing. Disease more extensive though confined to the cervix is managed with modified radical hysterectomy with pelvic lymph node dissection. In FIGO IA1 and IA2 non-surgical candidates or those who decline surgery, vaginal brachytherapy yields excellent local control and progression-free survival exceeding 95% [11, 12]. Alternatively, combination external beam radiation followed by low-dose brachytherapy is also a suitable treatment regimen as supported by Landon et al. Among 337 women with FIGO IB-IIA cervical cancer, radical hysterectomy followed by pelvic lymph node dissection was compared to whole pelvis external beam radiation followed by low-dose brachytherapy to a cumulative dose of 76 Gy. Five-year overall survival and disease-free survival were similar between the two groups at 83% and 74%, respectively [13].

In the post-operative setting, distinct pathological findings dictate the provision of adjuvant therapy. The Gynaecology Oncology Group's (GOG) study GOG 92 highlighted the benefit of post-operative radiation in patients who met intermediate-risk disease criteria also referred to as the Sedlis criteria and commonly simplified as presence of LVSI, tumour greater than 4 cm, and greater than 1/3rd stromal invasion in the setting of negative surgical margins and uninvolved pelvic lymph nodes. These criteria were extrapolated from GOG 49 which found higher depth of invasion, larger tumour size, and presence of LVSI led to inferior disease-free interval [14]. In GOG 92, 277 FIGO Stage IB cervical cancer patients who underwent radical hysterectomy and pelvic lymphadenectomy and met the aforementioned Sedlis criteria were randomised to observation versus post-operative radiation to 46–50.4 Gy. Local recurrence was significantly reduced when administering adjuvant RT at 14% vs 21% (HR 0.54, $p = 0.007$) with a trend towards overall survival benefit 81% vs 71% (HR 0.70, $p = 0.074$) [15]. A 2012 meta-analysis further validated the beneficial role of adjuvant RT as it significantly reduced the 5-year risk of disease progression (RR 0.58) though at increased risk of serious grade 3/4 haematological toxicity and gastrointestinal toxicity (RR 2.38 and 7.32, respectively) [16]. In regard to post-operative chemoradiation for intermediate-risk disease, randomised evidence supporting its use is currently ongoing in the setting of GOG 263 randomising FIGO Stage I–IIA post-operative intermediate-risk cervical cancer patients to adjuvant radiation versus adjuvant chemoradiation with weekly cisplatin.

Among high-risk patients, referred to as Peters' criteria and defined as having positive surgical margins, positive lymph nodes, and microscopic involvement of the parametrium, post-operative chemoradiation has been shown to decrease local recurrence and improve overall survival. This was elucidated in phase III randomised clinical trial GOG 109 which randomised 268 FIGO Stage IA2, IB, and IIA high-risk patients to radiation vs chemoradiation with cisplatin and 5-fluorouracil. ChemoRT was found to improve 4 year PFS, 80% vs 63% ($p = 0.003$), and OS (81% vs 71%, $p = 0.007$) [17]. A subset analysis did reveal, however, patients with tumour ≤2 cm or only one positive lymph node did not benefit from chemoradiation [18].

Radiation in the adjuvant setting is typically delivered using a four-field box technique with equally weighted AP/PA fields with opposed laterals. Three-dimensional conformal radiation planning objective includes adequate coverage of the at-risk post-operative region including the parametrium, vagina, and adjacent pelvic nodes. In recent years, there has been progressive implementation of intensity-modulated RT which has been shown to decrease toxicity while preserving disease control in the phase II trial RTOG 0418 in patients treated with post-operative chemoradiation [19, 20].

In locally advanced disease, surgery alone is insufficient treatment associated with high rates of relapse [14, 15]. Primary chemoradiation was established as a standard of care upon a 1999 National Cancer Institute meta-analysis which demonstrated its superiority over radiation alone amongst 5 RCTs (GOG 85, GOG 120, GOG 123, SWOG 8797, and RTOG 90-01) [21]. A more recent 2010 meta-analysis which compared CRT versus RT alone among 13 RCTs demonstrated a 19% relative reduction in risk of death translating to an absolute overall survival benefit of 6% (60–66%) at 5 years. There were also significant absolute benefits in DFS, locoregional DFS, time to locoregional recurrence/progression, and metastasis-free survival of 8%, 9%, 6%, and 7%, respectively [22]. The optimal chemotherapy regimen is defined as either weekly cisplatin at 40 mg/m^2 or cisplatin 75 mg/m^2 and 5-FU, 1000 mg/m^2/day for 4 days delivered every 3 weeks per GOG 120 and RTOG 90-01 [23, 24].

The efficacy of radiation therapy is greatly enhanced with the use of vaginal brachytherapy after EBRT in order to maximise dose while sparing adjacent normal tissue, and this has been established as a standard component in cervical cancer management. A recent Surveillance, Epidemiology, and End Results (SEER) database analysis demonstrated that among patients with FIGO Stage IB2-IVA cervical cancer, combination EBRT and brachytherapy improved 4-year cause-specific survival (64.3% vs 51.5%, $p < 0.01$) and OS (58.2% vs 46.2%, $p < 0.001$) over brachytherapy alone [25]. Either low-dose or high-dose brachytherapy can be administered to achieve a cumulative point A dose, to ensure coverage of the parametrium, of 80–90 Gy LDR equivalent [26].

Post-treatment surveillance is essential in the early detection of potential recurrent disease as well as management of therapeutic adverse effects. Guidelines have been well established by several major medical professional societies including the National Comprehensive Cancer Network, American College of Obstetrics and Gynaecology, and the Society of Gynaecology Oncology. In general, history and physical is recommended every 3–6 months in the first 2 years, every 6–12 months during years 3–5, and annually thereafter based on the risk of recurrence. Cervical and vaginal cytology is usually recommended on annual basis. Further imaging and lab assessment is obtained if the history and physical exam indicate possible recurrence [27].

Summary Globally, cervical cancer is associated with a high incidence and mortality in developing nations due to the lack of readily accessible screening. The treatment paradigm is largely based on tumour size in relation to FIGO Staging with radiation and chemoradiation generally reserved for bulky and locally advanced tumours. Definitive treatment recommendations are highlighted in Table 60.1.

Table 60.1 Treatment overview of cervical cancer by FIGO Stage

FIGO stage	Treatment
HGSIL CIN III	Colposcopy followed by conisation, LEEP, cryotherapy, or simple hysterectomy
IA1	Cervical conisation or extrafascial hysterectomy Consider vaginal trachelectomy for fertility sparing Brachytherapy alone – LDR 65–75 Gy or HDR 7 Gy × 5–6 fx
IA2 IB1	MRH & PLND Consider vaginal trachelectomy for fertility sparing (select cases) Definitive RT EBRT Brachytherapy
IB2	MRH & PLND only in well-selected patients Definitive RT EBRT Brachytherapy
IIA1–IVA	Definitive CRT EBRT + weekly cisplatin Brachytherapy boost
IVB	Chemotherapy +/− palliative RT

Abbreviation: *LEEP*, loop electrosurgical excisional procedure; *LDR*, low-dose rate; *HDR*, high-dose rate; *PLND*, pelvic lymph node dissection; *EBRT*, external beam radiation therapy; *CRT*, chemoradiation

60.2 Endometrial Cancer

Endometrial cancer is less prevalent in developing nations than in developed nation often associated with obesity and related co-morbidities. This cancer is more prevalent in post-menopausal women and older pre-menopausal women thought largely due to a longer period of oestrogen exposure. Endometrial cancer is staged surgically with total extrafascial hysterectomy with bilateral salpingo-oophorectomy and pelvic and para-aortic lymph node dissection. Early-stage operable disease is managed with observation and/or radiation therapy. Chemoradiation is reserved for medically inoperable and locally advanced disease with treatment volumes confined to either the pelvis or extending up the para-aortic lymph node chain. Post-treatment surveillance is warranted for management of treatment sequelae, such as vaginal stenosis and/or lymphedema, and treatment recurrence.

Endometrial cancer incidence is typically higher in developed nations attributable to an ageing population and concurrent increase in obesity among their populations. Worldwide, 319,600 new cases of endometrial cancer were diagnosed with 76,200 recorded deaths in 2012. The estimated age-standardised rates (per 100,000 person-years) were noticeably higher in more developed nations than less developed nations at 14.7 vs 5.5, respectively [1].

Presentation of endometrial cancer is characterised by abnormal uterine bleeding in 75–90% cases and more commonly in post-menopausal women and older pre-menopausal women. Designation of bleeding is further delineated based on menopausal status. Any quantity of bleeding in post-menopausal warrants further evaluation for endometrial cancer as 5–20% of these patients are found to have endometrial carcinoma. In pre-menopausal women age 45 or greater, intermenstrual bleeding in ovulatory women, frequent bleeding with intervals less than 3 weeks, volume greater than 80 cc, or persistent bleeding greater than 7 days should elicit further work-up [28–30]. A smaller subset of patients may also present with profuse watery discharge. Although the majority of women in developed nations present with early-stage disease, lack of easily accessible health care in developing nations translates to delayed diagnosis and presentation of advanced disease. Disease progression with advanced-stage disease can manifest with abdominal compression symptoms with associated gastrointestinal manifestations, back pain, or lymphedema [31].

Evaluation of suspected endometrial cancer in patients with the aforementioned symptoms begins with further history and focused physical examination. Risk factors of obesity, hypertension, diabetes mellitus, exogenous oestrogen or tamoxifen use, nulliparity, early menarche, late menopause, and family history should be elicited on history [32–39]. Complete pelvic examination includes vaginal inspection and bimanual exam to ascertain cervical involvement, adnexal disease, and vaginal metastases. Lab assessment of urine or serum human chorionic gonadotropin is obtained to prevent further invasive diagnostic procedures from disrupting a pregnancy. First-line imaging is transvaginal ultrasound with focus to endometrial thickness. If this measures <4 mm in post-menopausal with temporal cessation of bleeding, pathological sampling can be deferred. Endometrial biopsy is generally performed in the outpatient with no to minimal anaesthesia. In settings of high clinical suspicious despite equivocal pathology, dilation and curettage is pursued. The addition of hysteroscopy permits direct visual guidance of lesions of the endocervix and endometrial cavity amenable to biopsy [40].

Diagnostic confirmation of endometrial cancer is preceded by surgical staging according to the FIGO classification. Standard surgery consists of total extrafascial hysterectomy with bilateral salpingo-oophorectomy and pelvic and para-aortic lymph node dissection. Peritoneal washings are often obtained from regions of suspected metastases. Locoregional spread of disease is dependent upon tumour stage and grade. In an early GOG study, approximately 11% of patients with FIGO Stage I or II uterine cancer had either pelvic or para-aortic nodal metastases [41]. Twenty-two per cent of patients with higher grade tumours, greater than 50% myometrial invasion, or tumours larger than 2 cm are found to harbour regional nodal metastases after pelvic lymphadenectomy. Furthermore, non-endometroid uterine carcinoma is associated with higher rates of nodal metastases at around 40% [42]. Given nodal involvement rates among historic and recent studies and surgical morbidity, particularly lymphedema and associated cellulitis, of extensive lymph node dissection, controversy remains on whether to perform pelvic and/or para-aortic nodal sampling versus directly proceeding to complete node dissection. Sampling entails inspection and palpation of clinically suspicious appearing nodes with an intrinsically higher risk of missing involved nodes when compared to pelvic lymphadenectomy. The therapeutic efficacy of systematic pelvic lymphadenectomy was further defined in the ASTEC trial which randomised 1408 women with endometrial cancer to pelvic lymphadenectomy versus no further resection after standard surgery. At median follow-up of 37 months, pelvic lymphadenectomy did not confer an overall (85.7% vs 87.5%) or recurrence-free survival benefit (79.5% vs 84.9%) [43]. This trial should, however, be interpreted with caution as 45% of patient were considered to have low-risk intrauterine features and thus low risk of nodal involvement. Despite the lack of therapeutic benefit, complete node dissection ensures adequate classification of advanced-stage disease to guide appropriate adjuvant therapy [44].

Post-operative management of endometrial cancer is guided by stratification of pathological and clinical features based on their risk of recurrence. Adjuvant therapy may include observation, radiation therapy in the form of vaginal brachytherapy (VBT) and/or external beam radiation therapy, and/or systemic chemotherapy. Post-operative radiation therapy targets residual gross or potential microscopic disease in the pelvic lymph node as well as the vaginal cuff. Three randomised trials have demonstrated the efficacy of EBRT to decrease locoregional recurrence when compared to observation alone. PORTEC-1 found EBRT reduced 10-year LRR from 14% to 5% over observation. Among those who recurred, 75% experience vaginal recurrence. In this trial, 714 patients were enrolled who underwent TAH/BSO with washings however, pelvic lymphadenectomy was not performed [45]. GOG 99 randomised 392 patients after TAH/BSO, pelvic and para-aortic lymph node sampling, and peritoneal cytology, to observation versus 50.4 Gy whole pelvis EBRT. This trial further defined high-intermediate risk endometrial cancer upon age and the following risk factors of grade 2 or higher, LVSI, and outer 1/3rd myometrial invasion. Patients 70 years or older with one risk factor, 50 years or older with two risk factors or any age with three risk factors were designated as possessing high-intermediate risk disease. EBRT decreased LR at 2 years from 12% to 3% with the greatest benefit in the high-intermediate risk group with LR decreased from 26% to 6% [46]. The role of VBT as alternative to EBRT was addressed in PORTEC-2 which randomised 427 patients with intermediate high-risk disease status-post TAH/BSO with no pelvic LND to 46 Gy EBRT versus vaginal brachytherapy alone with either HDR 21 Gy in 3 fx or LDR 30 Gy. Five-year vaginal relapse and isolated pelvic relapse rates were similar between EBRT and VBT at 1.8% vs 1.5% and 1.5% vs 0.5%, respectively. LRR was improved from 5.1% to 2.1% with EBRT compared to VBT however, this did not translate into a survival benefit [47].

The utility of chemotherapy is generally reserved for advanced-stage disease. With focus to treating larger disease burden, chemotherapy has been shown to confer a survival in this setting. GOG 122 randomised 388 patients with Stage III–IV endometrial cancer to either whole abdominal irradiation, consisting of 30 Gy in 20 fx AP/PA followed by boost to the pelvic and/or para-aortic LNs to 15 Gy in 8 fx versus chemotherapy, consisting of doxorubicin + cisplatin q3 weekly × 8 cycles. Although recurrence was similar between the two arms, 5-year OS was improved to 55% with chemotherapy compared to 42% with WAI. Five-year PFS was also significantly improved in the chemotherapy arm at 50% vs 38% [48]. In contrast, the Japanese GOG (JGOG) 2033 which enrolled 385 patients with Stage I–III endometrial cancer found no LC, PFS, or OS advantage when comparing whole pelvis RT to 40–50 Gy vs chemotherapy of cyclophosphamide, doxorubicin, and cisplatin [49].

Combined modality chemoradiation has been shown to be tolerable in advanced-stage disease with small number of trials defining its efficacy. A Finnish trial compared 156 patients with FIGO IA grade 3 and/or IIB-IIIA grade 1–3 disease between adjuvant split-course EBRT 56 Gy in 28 fx to interdigitated, or "sandwich", chemoradiation described as radiation to 28 Gy followed by cisplatin, epirubicin, and cyclophosphamide chemotherapy followed by radiation to 28 Gy and completed with an additional cycle of chemotherapy. This study did not demonstrate a survival or local control benefit with the addition of chemotherapy [50]. Sequential chemoradiation was analysed among 382 patients in the NSGO-EC-9501/EORTC-55991 trial which compared sequential chemotherapy and radiation to pelvic EBRT alone. Preliminary results at 5 years demonstrated an improvement in PFS (79% vs 72%, p = 0.03). This trial published its final data in a pooled analysis with the MaNGO ILIADE-IIII trial and found 5-year PFS was improved with combined modality treatment (78% vs 69%, HR 0.63 p = 0.009) with a trend towards benefit in 5-year OS (82% vs 75%, HR 0.69, p = 0.07) [51]. The role of chemoradiation remains under further investigation in a number of ongoing trials. PORTEC-3 is evaluating chemoradiation followed by adjuvant chemotherapy compared to radiation alone, while GOG 258 is comparing chemotherapy alone to chemoradiation followed by adjuvant chemotherapy [52, 53].

Follow-up priorities post-treatment are highlighted to be management of treatment sequel management and surveillance for disease recurrence. Per the NCCN and SGO, history and physical is recommended every 3–6 months in the first 2 years, every 6–12 months during years 3–5, and annually thereafter based on the risk of recurrence. Cervical and vaginal cytology is usually recommended on annual basis per the NCCN. Further imaging with CT and lab assessment with CA-125 is obtained if the history and physical exam indicate possible recurrence [27].

Summary Globally, endometrial cancer is less prevalent in developing nations than in developed counterparts. Treatment is largely dictated by surgical findings with adjuvant therapy of active surveillance, external beam radiation, and/or vaginal brachytherapy for early-stage patients. Locally advanced patients are offered platinum-based chemoradiation therapy. Treatment recommendations are outlined in Table 60.2.

Table 60.2 Treatment overview of endometrial cancer by FIGO stage

FIGO Stage	Treatment
All medically operable patients	Surgery TAH/BSO or radical hysterectomy PLND or para-aortic node dissection Peritoneal cytology Adjuvant treatment
Endometrioid adenocarcinoma	
I–II	If confined to endometrium and grade 1–2, no further therapy If deep myometrial invasion, grade 2–3, or +LVSI VBT Pelvic EBRT
III	Chemotherapy: carboplatin/paclitaxel Chemoradiation
IV	Chemotherapy +/− palliative RT
Serous carcinoma Clear cell carcinoma	
I–III	Adjuvant chemotherapy: carboplatin/paclitaxel +/− VBT Pelvic EBRT
IV	Chemotherapy +/− palliative RT

Abbreviation: *TAH*, total abdominal hysterectomy; *BSO*, bilateral salpingo-oophorectomy; *PLND*, pelvic lymph node dissection; *VBT*, vaginal brachytherapy; *EBRT*, external beam radiation therapy; *LVSI*, lymphovascular space invasion

References

1. Ferlay J, Soerjomataram I, Dikshit R, et al. Cancer incidence and mortality worldwide: sources, methods and major patterns in GLOBOCAN 2012. Int J Cancer. 2015;136(5):E359–86.
2. Torre LA, Siegel RL, Ward EM, et al. Global cancer incidence and mortality rates and trends--an update. Cancer Epidemiol Biomark Prev. 2016;25(1):16–27.
3. Bray F, Loos AH, McCarron P, et al. Trends in cervical squamous cell carcinoma incidence in 13 European countries: changing risk and the effects of screening. Cancer Epidemiol Biomark Prev. 2005;14(3):677–86.
4. Munoz N, Bosch FX, de Sanjose S, et al. The role of HPV in the etiology of cervical cancer. Mutat Res. 1994;305(2):293–301.
5. Mlange R, Matovelo D, Rambau P, et al. Patient and disease characteristics associated with late tumour stage at presentation of cervical cancer in northwestern Tanzania. BMC Womens Health. 2016;16:5.
6. Eze JN, Emeka-Irem EN, Edegbe FO. A six-year study of the clinical presentation of cervical cancer and the management challenges encountered at a state teaching hospital in southeast Nigeria. Clin Med Insights Oncol. 2013;7:151–8.
7. Mishra K, Desai A, Patel S, et al. Role of percutaneous nephrostomy in advanced cervical carcinoma with obstructive uropathy: a case series. Indian J Palliat Care. 2009;15(1):37–40.
8. Gyenwali D, Pariyar J, Onta SR. Factors associated with late diagnosis of cervical cancer in Nepal. Asian Pac J Cancer Prev. 2013;14(7):4373–7.
9. Pecorelli S, Zigliani L, Odicino F. Revised FIGO staging for carcinoma of the cervix. Int J Gynaecol Obstet. 2009;105(2):107–8.
10. Tsikouras P, Zervoudis S, Manav B, et al. Cervical cancer: screening, diagnosis and staging. J BUON. 2016;21(2):320–5.
11. Grigsby PW, Perez CA. Radiotherapy alone for medically inoperable carcinoma of the cervix: stage IA and carcinoma in situ. Int J Radiat Oncol Biol Phys. 1991;21(2):375–8.
12. Hamberger AD, Fletcher GH, Wharton JT. Results of treatment of early stage I carcinoma of the uterine cervix with intracavitary radium alone. Cancer. 1978;41(3):980–5.
13. Landoni F, Maneo A, Colombo A, et al. Randomised study of radical surgery versus radiotherapy for stage IB–IIA cervical cancer. Lancet. 1997;350(9077):535–40.
14. Delgado G, Bundy B, Zaino R, et al. Prospective surgical-pathological study of disease-free interval in patients with stage IB squamous cell carcinoma of the cervix: a Gynaecologic Oncology Group study. Gynecol Oncol. 1990;38(3):352–7.
15. Rotman M, Sedlis A, Piedmonte MR, et al. A phase III randomised trial of postoperative pelvic irradiation in stage IB cervical carcinoma with poor prognostic features: follow-up of a Gynaecologic Oncology Group study. Int J Radiat Oncol Biol Phys. 2006;65(1):169–76.
16. Rogers L, Siu SS, Luesley D, et al. Radiotherapy and chemoradiation after surgery for early cervical cancer. Cochrane Database Syst Rev. 2012;(5):CD007583.
17. Peters WA 3rd, Liu PY, Barrett RJ 2nd, et al. Concurrent chemotherapy and pelvic radiation therapy compared with pelvic radiation therapy alone as adjuvant therapy after radical surgery in high-risk early-stage cancer of the cervix. J Clin Oncol. 2000;18(8):1606–13.
18. Monk BJ, Wang J, Im S, et al. Rethinking the use of radiation and chemotherapy after radical hysterectomy: a clinical-pathologic analysis of a Gynaecologic Oncology Group/Southwest Oncology Group/Radiation Therapy Oncology Group trial. Gynecol Oncol. 2005;96(3):721–8.
19. Folkert MR, Shih KK, Abu-Rustum NR, et al. Postoperative pelvic intensity-modulated radiotherapy and concurrent chemotherapy in intermediate- and high-risk cervical cancer. Gynecol Oncol. 2013;128(2):288–93.
20. Klopp AH, Moughan J, Portelance L, et al. Haematologic toxicity in RTOG 0418: a phase 2 study of postoperative IMRT for gynaecologic cancer. Int J Radiat Oncol Biol Phys. 2013;86(1):83–90.
21. Thomas GM. Improved treatment for cervical cancer--concurrent chemotherapy and radiotherapy. N Engl J Med. 1999;340(15):1198–200.
22. Chemoradiotherapy for Cervical Cancer Meta-Analysis Collaboration. Reducing uncertainties about the effects of chemoradiotherapy for cervical cancer: individual patient data meta-analysis. Cochrane Database Syst Rev. 2010;(1):CD008285.
23. Rose PG, Ali S, Watkins E, et al. Long-term follow-up of a randomised trial comparing concurrent single agent cisplatin, cisplatin-based combination chemotherapy, or hydroxyurea during pelvic irradiation for locally advanced cervical cancer: a Gynaecologic Oncology Group study. J Clin Oncol. 2007;25(19):2804–10.
24. Eifel PJ, Winter K, Morris M, et al. Pelvic irradiation with concurrent chemotherapy versus pelvic and para-aortic irradiation for high-risk cervical cancer: an update of radiation therapy oncology group trial (RTOG) 90-01. J Clin Oncol. 2004;22(5):872–80.
25. Han K, Milosevic M, Fyles A, et al. Trends in the utilisation of brachytherapy in cervical cancer in the United States. Int J Radiat Oncol Biol Phys. 2013;87(1):111–9.
26. Viswanathan AN, Beriwal S, De Los Santos JF, et al. American Brachytherapy Society consensus guidelines for locally advanced carcinoma of the cervix. Part II: high-dose-rate brachytherapy. Brachytherapy. 2012;11(1):47–52.
27. Salani R, Backes FJ, Fung MF, et al. Posttreatment surveillance and diagnosis of recurrence in women with gynaecologic malignancies: Society of Gynaecologic Oncologists recommendations. Am J Obstet Gynecol. 2011;204(6):466–78.

28. American College of Obstetricians and Gynaecologists. ACOG practice bulletin, clinical management guidelines for obstetrician-gynaecologists, number 65, August 2005: management of endometrial cancer. Obstet Gynecol. 2005;106(2):413–25.
29. Espindola D, Kennedy KA, Fischer EG. Management of abnormal uterine bleeding and the pathology of endometrial hyperplasia. Obstet Gynecol Clin N Am. 2007;34(4):717–37, ix.
30. Ronghe R, Gaudoin M. Women with recurrent postmenopausal bleeding should be re-investigated but are not more likely to have endometrial cancer. Menopause Int. 2010;16(1):9–11.
31. Varughese J, Richman S. Cancer care inequity for women in resource-poor countries. Rev Obstet Gynecol. 2010;3(3):122–32.
32. Brinton LA, Berman ML, Mortel R, et al. Reproductive, menstrual, and medical risk factors for endometrial cancer: results from a case-control study. Am J Obstet Gynecol. 1992;167(5):1317–25.
33. Woodruff JD, Pickar JH. Incidence of endometrial hyperplasia in postmenopausal women taking conjugated estrogens (Premarin) with medroxyprogesterone acetate or conjugated estrogens alone. The Menopause Study Group. Am J Obstet Gynecol. 1994;170(5 Pt 1):1213–23.
34. Schiff I, Sela HK, Cramer D, et al. Endometrial hyperplasia in women on cyclic or continuous estrogen regimens. Fertil Steril. 1982;37(1):79–82.
35. Furness S, Roberts H, Marjoribanks J, et al. Hormone therapy in postmenopausal women and risk of endometrial hyperplasia. Cochrane Database Syst Rev. 2009;(2):CD000402.
36. Iqbal J, Ginsburg OM, Wijeratne TD, et al. Endometrial cancer and venous thromboembolism in women under age 50 who take tamoxifen for prevention of breast cancer: a systematic review. Cancer Treat Rev. 2012;38(4):318–28.
37. Early Breast Cancer Trialists' Collaborative Group, Davies C, Godwin J, et al. Relevance of breast cancer hormone receptors and other factors to the efficacy of adjuvant tamoxifen: patient-level meta-analysis of randomised trials. Lancet. 2011;378(9793):771–84.
38. Siiteri PK. Adipose tissue as a source of hormones. Am J Clin Nutr. 1987;45(1 Suppl):277–82.
39. La Vecchia C, Franceschi S, Decarli A, et al. Risk factors for endometrial cancer at different ages. J Natl Cancer Inst. 1984;73(3):667–71.
40. Hoffman BLSJ, Bradshaw KD, Halvorson LM, Scahffer JI, Corton MM. Williams gynaecology. 3rd ed. New York: McGraw-Hill; 2016.
41. Creasman WT, Morrow CP, Bundy BN, et al. Surgical pathologic spread patterns of endometrial cancer. A Gynaecologic Oncology Group study. Cancer. 1987;60(8 Suppl):2035–41.
42. Mariani A, Dowdy SC, Cliby WA, et al. Prospective assessment of lymphatic dissemination in endometrial cancer: a paradigm shift in surgical staging. Gynecol Oncol. 2008;109(1):11–8.
43. ASTEC Study Group, Kitchener H, Swart AM, et al. Efficacy of systematic pelvic lymphadenectomy in endometrial cancer (MRC ASTEC trial): a randomised study. Lancet. 2009;373(9658):125–36.
44. Resnick KE, Cohn DE, Fowler JM. Role of lymphadenectomy in the staging of endometrial cancer. Nat Rev Clin Oncol. 2009;6(7):382–4.
45. Creutzberg CL, Nout RA, Lybeert ML, et al. Fifteen-year radiotherapy outcomes of the randomised PORTEC-1 trial for endometrial carcinoma. Int J Radiat Oncol Biol Phys. 2011;81(4):e631–8.
46. Keys HM, Roberts JA, Brunetto VL, et al. A phase III trial of surgery with or without adjunctive external pelvic radiation therapy in intermediate risk endometrial adenocarcinoma: a Gynaecologic Oncology Group study. Gynecol Oncol. 2004;92(3):744–51.
47. Nout RA, Smit VT, Putter H, et al. Vaginal brachytherapy versus pelvic external beam radiotherapy for patients with endometrial cancer of high-intermediate risk (PORTEC-2): an open-label, non-inferiority, randomised trial. Lancet. 2010;375(9717):816–23.
48. Randall ME, Filiaci VL, Muss H, et al. Randomised phase III trial of whole-abdominal irradiation versus doxorubicin and cisplatin chemotherapy in advanced endometrial carcinoma: a Gynaecologic Oncology Group study. J Clin Oncol. 2006;24(1):36–44.
49. Susumu N, Sagae S, Udagawa Y, et al. Randomised phase III trial of pelvic radiotherapy versus cisplatin-based combined chemotherapy in patients with intermediate- and high-risk endometrial cancer: a Japanese Gynaecologic Oncology Group study. Gynecol Oncol. 2008;108(1):226–33.
50. Kuoppala T, Maenpaa J, Tomas E, et al. Surgically staged high-risk endometrial cancer: randomised study of adjuvant radiotherapy alone vs. sequential chemo-radiotherapy. Gynecol Oncol. 2008;110(2):190–5.
51. Hogberg T, Signorelli M, de Oliveira CF, et al. Sequential adjuvant chemotherapy and radiotherapy in endometrial cancer--results from two randomised studies. Eur J Cancer. 2010;46(13):2422–31.
52. PORTEC-3 Trial. http://clinicaltrials.gov/ct2/show/NCT00411138.
53. GOG 258. http://clinicaltrials.gov/ct2/show/NCT00942357.

61 Emerging Trends and Best Practices in Hospice and Palliative Care

Joseph A. Balogun

Learning Objectives

After reading this chapter, the reader will be able to discuss the:

- Differences between euthanasia, hospice, and palliative care
- Dynamics of a multidisciplinary and interdisciplinary team in hospice and palliative care
- Roles and responsibilities of the interdisciplinary hospice and palliative care team
- Genesis and transmogrification of hospice and palliative care
- Evolution of hospice and palliative care as a medical speciality
- Global demand and utilisation of hospice and palliative care services
- Hospice and palliative care best practices
- Pharmacological management of pain in the hospice and palliative care setting
- Global epidemiology of opioid-related deaths
- Complementary and alternative treatment approaches in hospice and palliative care
- Guidelines that physicians and burgeoning organisations can leverage to develop a high-quality hospice and palliative program
- Status of hospice and palliative care education in Africa

J. A. Balogun (✉)
Chicago State University, Chicago, IL, USA

University of Medical Sciences, Ondo City, Nigeria

Centre of Excellence in Reproductive Health Innovation, University of Benin, Benin City, Nigeria
e-mail: jbalogun@csu.edu; jbalogun@unimed.edu.ng

61.1 Introduction

Hospice and palliative care (HPC) is not the most enchanting discussion to have, yet it is one that we dare not avoid. It is a morbid topic, but a very critical one because death is a universal experience that we all must face in the future. Despite the inevitability of death, one is never really prepared for its occurrence. Shakespeare said that "death is a necessary end that will come when it will come." Death has been feared for ages as attested by Julius Caesar who said: "Cowards die many times before their death, the valiant never taste of death but once." Most affected by death are the survivors, especially when the deceased is young. Attitudes to death and dying are a profoundly emotional event that is multidimensional in reach and varies across cultures. The "cause no harm" ethical code of medical practice embodied in the Hippocratic Oath reflects the obligation that a healthcare provider has commitments towards the well-being of all patients, including those that are terminally ill. Compared to societies in Africa and Asia, in many European countries, death and dying are phenomena that are accepted more readily. In Africa and Asia, family dynamics and religion play significant roles in shaping the concept of death.

In European culture, the young adult early in life becomes independent of their nuclear family. In the African and Asian cultures, the adolescent is bonded within the nuclear family based on marriage, and they are adversely affected by the demise of a family member [1]. The Yoruba and Igbo ethnic groups in Nigeria have a culture of celebrating life and feel anxious about death, especially if the individual is under 60 years of age. When the inevitable is accepted, the culture prefers a delay of the dying process and wants the terminally ill to be at the native birthplace so the family can make their peace and have an opportunity to say farewell.

Africa occupies 22% of the world's landscape, and both communicable and non-communicable diseases undeniably are currently ravaging the continent. Between 2005 and 2015, about 28 million Africans die of chronic illnesses each

F. Okonofua et al. (eds.), *Contemporary Obstetrics and Gynecology for Developing Countries*,
https://doi.org/10.1007/978-3-030-75385-6_61

year. In 2008 alone, there were 715,000 new cases of cancer and the incidence is expected to double by 2030 [2]. Africa carries 69% of the total global disease burden and, to cite one disease as a case in point, the region is affected disproportionately by HIV/AIDS than the rest of the world [3]. In sub-Saharan Africa, in 2011, 23.5 million people lived with HIV/AIDS, and 1.8 million had new infections that year. People living with HIV/AIDS and cancer are particularly in need of hospice and palliative (pronounced pal-lee-uh-tiv) care because "the burden of issues that cause[s] suffering is acutely high for these patients" [4].

Recognised in 2002 by the World Health Organization (WHO) as a medical speciality, HPC is a treatment approach designed to "improve the quality of life of the people living with a terminal illness and their families through prevention and relief of suffering using early identification and impeccable evaluation and treatment of pain and other problems as physical, psychosocial and spiritual" [5]. Attitude towards HPC in the West has changed considerably; it is a topic that is discussed openly within each family. On the other hand, many Africans and Asians still have a vague and hazy knowledge of HPC. Consequently, they do not like to discuss it, because the cultures do not believe people die naturally (except due to old age) but as a result of some supernatural forces that are unknown to man.

Today, in industrialised countries, HPC is the hallmark of end-of-life care. In these societies health care is well-funded, and healthcare professionals practice their trade guided by the core principles of open disclosure of ailments, autonomy, and participation in decision-making concerning their health [6–9]. Just like attitudes to death and dying, caring for individuals with an advanced terminal illness is something that also varies across cultures. As indicated earlier in this preamble, currently Africa faces a tremendous disease burden that will likely increase in the coming years. Accordingly, in the course of their career, healthcare professionals in the region will provide care for people with advanced life-threatening illnesses. Therefore, these professionals need contemporary training on how to deliver high-quality, culturally competent HPC. Unfortunately, educational opportunities in developing countries, particularly in Africa, about HPC are limited [2, 10].

During their training, medical and health sciences students in many developing countries have no access to resources such as encyclopaedia, books, and journals on HPC. This chapter seeks to fill this void and other unsatisfactory educational and human resource gaps. The chapter comprises 15 sections dealing with various topics related to HPC. The introductory section covered a range of issues, including the differences among euthanasia, hospice, and palliative care, multidisciplinary and interdisciplinary healthcare team in HPC, and the roles and responsibilities of HPC interdisciplinary team. The mid-section traces the genesis and evolution of HPC as a medical speciality, global demand, and utilisation of HPC services. Next is the discussion on HPC best practices and global epidemiology of opioid-related deaths. The concluding section examines the relevance of complementary and alternative medicine and clinical guidelines to foster high-quality palliative care. Overall, the article cited over 100 references that an inquisitive learner seeking to go beyond the presentation here can consult for more in-depth information on any of the various topics covered. Finally, the article incorporates schematic diagrams, bar and pie charts that lend a visual exposition to the presentation and engender needed clarity to the discussions.

61.2 Operational Definitions

In this chapter, the term *industrialised countries* refer to the 34 Organization for Economic Cooperation and Development member nations that include the USA, Canada, the Western European nations, Japan, Australia, New Zealand, and others. In general, the Organization for Economic Cooperation and Development countries is more productive with higher per capita income than the 150 developing countries in Africa, Asia, and Latin America which are economically less advanced with low average per capita income.

61.3 Differences Among Euthanasia, Hospice, and Palliative Care

There are apparent distinctions between euthanasia, hospice, and palliative care. The term palliative care derived from the Latin word "palliare" means "to cloak." Euthanasia, also known as mercy killing, is the act of a third party; usually, a physician humanely terminating a patient life typically by administering large doses of pain-killing drugs. Across the world, controversy still swirls the concept of euthanasia. Because in many cultures, life commences from the time of conception to the last breath, an attempt at truncating this process is viewed as abominable. The Igbos and Yorubas of Nigeria believe that people do not die in the actual sense, but transit to join their ancestors. Therefore, it is a taboo to terminate life even in the state of hopelessness because the ancestors will be angry and visit the community with a plague [11].

There is an ongoing debate in the literature on the best drugs to use to end life in countries where assisted dying is legalised. The drugs commonly used are called barbiturates. Lethal injection of barbiturates, the most common form of execution in the USA, became popular in the late twentieth century in place of less than humane methods like gas inhalation, electrocution, hanging, and firing squad. When used in small therapeutic doses, barbiturates are a proper treatment for insomnia or seizures in emergencies. They are used as anaesthesia during surgery in varying dosages and modes of administration.

A hefty dose of barbiturates will efficiently cause the brain to slow down, and after the effect decreases, the respiratory system is shut down and breathing stops. Usually, three conventional medications when injected in fatal doses induce unconsciousness: anaesthetic, such as Sodium Thiopental or Pentobarbital, causes unconsciousness; Pancuronium Bromide (Pavulon) causes muscle paralysis and respiratory arrest, and Potassium Chloride stops the heart. The relative safety and effectiveness of these medications in triggering a peaceful, swift, and untoward death have made them the drug of choice in Belgium, Switzerland, Netherlands, and USA where euthanasia is legal. In contrast, in Australia, Nembutal and Secobarbital are illegal for use in humans but may be used in animals [12].

Unlike euthanasia, the goal of palliative care is not to cause death but to make the end stage of life as comfortable as possible. Palliative care is instituted for people of any age in the terminal phase of life-threatening disease when cure is not the aim of treatment. Palliative care is appropriate for individuals with a diagnosis of a chronic disease involving the heart, liver, and kidney. Other life-threatening diseases subject to palliative care include many kinds of cancer (breast, colon, ovarian, pancreatic, lung, prostate, head and neck, leukaemia, and lymphoma). It also includes congestive heart failure, chronic obstructive pulmonary disease, pulmonary fibrosis, bone marrow transplant, dementia, eosinophil-associated disease, multiple myeloma, multiple sclerosis, sickle cell anaemia, stroke, dementia, HIV/AIDS, Huntington's disease, arthritis, and diabetes [6–8]. As the individual ages and the disease process progresses, the dilapidating effects of the chronic illness will increase in intensity, frequency, and complexity.

Hospice care comes into play when, from the clinical perspective, individuals with a terminal illness have less than 6 months to live, and the physician decides to stop curative treatment but instead concentrate on improving the quality of life. The patient prognosis may range in spectrum from several months of a vibrant full life or just a few days. In the USA, a distinction is made between palliative care and hospice care. The death prognosis timeline of 6 months and the payment process are used as the eligibility criteria for hospice care [6–8]. Hospice care is funded through the government-run Medicare system or other health insurance providers, and services are delivered in an inpatient facility or at the individual's home. In the other parts of the world, a distinction is often not made between hospice and palliative service as all treatment provided for the people living with a terminal illness is usually referred to as palliative care. In many countries, the term hospice usually refers to a physical building or centre that provides palliative care services, rather than to a stage of care progression.

The general tenets now considers hospice care as a decline in functional status, increase dependence on other people for routine activities of daily living tasks, and deterioration in nutritional status (Table 61.1).

Table 61.1 General screening and diagnostic guidelines to determine eligibility for hospice care

Changes in medical status	Clinical indicators	Common terminal illness diagnoses	Clinical indicators
A decline in functional status in the past 6 months	Multiple falls, increased visits to physician or ER, increased number of hospitalisations	Cancer	Curative treatments are not likely to improve the quality or length of life. Metastasis to multiple sites
Increase dependence on other people for routine activities of daily living tasks	Needs more assistance with bathing, dressing, eating, toileting, transferring/ walking, and incontinence	Heart failure	Chest pain and/or shortness of breath with and without activity. Taking multiple cardiac medications. Heart surgery is not a preferred option
A decline in nutritional status	Loss of appetite and progressive weight loss	Chronic obstructive pulmonary disease	Shortness of breath at rest and with any physical activity. Recurring respiratory infections. Using multiple inhalers with poor response
Presence of other chronic illnesses	Co-morbidities	Dementia	Speaks few intelligible words. Needs assistance to sit up. Needs an assistive device to ambulate
Increase in pain or other illness symptoms	Prolonged sleeping pattern, increasing weakness, fatigue, and lethargy	Stroke	Difficulty swallowing, unable to take in adequate nutrition. No feeding tube
Deteriorating cognitive abilities	Change in mental status (less alert, more confused, etc.)	Liver failure	Ascites despite the use of diuretics. Serum albumin 1.5
Recurrent infections and skin breakdown	Pressure sores, decubitus ulcers	Renal failure	Considering stopping dialysis Serum creatinine >8.0 (>6.0 for diabetics)
		HIV/AIDS	CD4+ count 100,000 Secondary conditions such as Kaposi's sarcoma, pneumocystis pneumonia, fungal infections, etc.

(continued)

Table 61.1 (continued)

Changes in medical status	Clinical indicators	Common terminal illness diagnoses	Clinical indicators
		Amyotrophic lateral sclerosis (ALS)	Barely intelligible speech Significant shortness of breath. Difficulty swallowing accompanied by rapid weight loss. No feeding tube or ventilator

The presence of multiple chronic illnesses, increasing weakness, fatigue, and lethargy, deteriorating cognitive abilities, and recurrent infections and skin breakdown are also determinant factors. In addition, the disease-specific diagnosis for the individual living with a terminal illness must be taken into consideration in determining the eligibility criteria for hospice care [6–8]. Top-tier hospitals in the USA now implement protocols that elicit referrals for HPC based on specific clinical characteristics, such as repeated or prolonged hospitalisation, a decline in cognition or functional status, intolerable pain, or emotional distress.

61.4 Dynamics of Multidisciplinary and Interdisciplinary Teams in Hospice and Palliative Care

Traditionally, healthcare systems operate in multidisciplinary teams, and HPC uniquely fits into this approach given the different phases involved in caring for the physical, social, and psychological needs of the individuals with a terminal illness and their nuclear family. The multidisciplinary team in HPC organisations occurs when healthcare professionals from different disciplines come together to deliver high-quality services to address the physical and mental health needs of the people living with a terminal illness [6–8]. For all its attendant benefits, the major pitfall of the multidisciplinary team approach is the inability of the different professionals to develop a cohesive treatment plan as each discipline tends to create an individual treatment plan which makes service delivery fragmented and prone to medical errors.

Because of these downsides, in contemporary healthcare practice, the concept of the multidisciplinary team is being replaced by the interdisciplinary team approach. The latter model is preferred because team members build on each other's expertise to create commonly shared goals which improve communication among team members and produces better clinical outcomes and improved satisfaction on the part of the individuals with a terminal illness and their families. The beneficial features of a high-quality interdisciplinary team are "open communication, the team concept philosophy, good interpersonal relationships, high team commitment, autonomy and the ability to deal with death and dying" [13]. A recent study revealed that the interdisciplinary team approach fosters improved professional performance, although the evidence on outcomes is mixed. Teams with improved coordination experienced a positive impact on outcomes but limited effects on resource utilisation and cost [14, 15].

61.5 Roles and Responsibilities of the Interdisciplinary Hospice and Palliative Care Team

Provision of high-quality HPC services entails access to healthcare professionals with clinical competence to reduce anxiety and improve the safety and comfort of individuals living with a terminal illness. Typically, the interdisciplinary team of an HPC organisation includes a physician who specialises in palliative medicine, a nurse, social worker, clinical psychologist, clergy, physical-occupational-speech, and music therapists. Aside from the physician, nurse, and the clergy, many of these professionals are in acute shortage and therefore practically non-existent in many developing countries. Thus, the roles and responsibilities of the members of an HPC interdisciplinary team are described below.

The *palliative medicine physician* collaborates with the other members of the interdisciplinary team to provide curative and rehabilitative treatments and referral for additional supportive services. The palliative medicine physician must be astute on the trajectories of the common chronic diseases, and the psychometric tools needed for prognostication. Several of the existing validated psychometric tools that are performance status-based and used in combination with clinical indicators are the Palliative Prognostic Score and Flacker Mortality Score, as well as disease-specific instruments, such as Model for End-Stage Liver Disease, and Charlson Comorbidity Index for End-stage Renal Disease [16–19]. The Patient-Reported Outcome Mortality Prediction Tool is commonly used in older adults to predict the projected six-month mortality period [20]. However, more validation studies are needed for it to gain broader clinical use.

People living with a terminal illness often confront limitations in carrying out routine activities of daily living tasks. Consequently, they need assistance to navigate the anxieties and perception that they are a burden to their nuclear family. The HPC *nurse* assists the individuals with administering their medications, bathing, and dressing. The team *physiotherapist plays* a significant role in maintaining physical function, independence, and rehabilitation after surgery or illness. They also evaluate the patient to determine their level of physical functioning and train them on how to exercise to reduce pain and maintain muscle strength and joint flexibility. As well, when indicated, the physiotherapist provides mobility assistive aid devices, such as wheelchairs, walking frames, and canes. To manage the fatigue that people living with a terminal illness commonly experience, physiotherapist collaborate with the *occupational therapist* to engage them in low-impact aerobic exercise and train them in energy conservation techniques, such as pacing activities, and minimising physical stressors [21].

While the goal of physical and occupational therapy is not the restoration of premorbid functionality, but rather to give the individuals with a terminal illness some degree of independence, to reduce the care burden, and promote improved quality of life. In cases when physical functionality is limited or not possible, such as in instances of neurodegenerative diseases, the individual should be given psychological, emotional, and spiritual care. The occupational therapist works to improve the quality of life of the individuals with a terminal illness through participation in the activities of everyday life by providing training and advice on how to adapt to their current statuses, manage fatigue, and conserve energy by making daily activities more comfortable. The individuals with a terminal illness must be prepared to participate in safety-oriented physical activities, such as bathing, getting in and out of bed, and sitting. For a safer, more easily accessible environment, the occupational therapist often recommend modifications to the home and teach patients on the use of aids to assist with personal care, such as putting on socks and shoes, household tasks [21].

The loss of vocalisation also affects the ability of people living with a terminal illness to adequately express their feelings and concerns. The sensation of food sticking in the oesophagus, discomfort with swallowing tablets, eating, or drinking may cause difficulties with speech. These complications will affect the ability of people living with a terminal illness to make choices. In these instances, the *speech therapist* (speech language pathologist) engages them to reduce the risk of coughing and choking. Treatment focuses on the quality of the speech by tapping into other means of communication that will engender independence and quality of life. The speech therapist also assists the individuals with problems recalling words, speaking, and those who are aphasic and dysarthria, as well as those with voice changes (poor volume or intonation; creaky, whispery, breathy, hoarse qualities). The speech therapist also work with people living with a terminal illness who are unable to verbalise their concerns to use other means of communication, such as gesture, writing, and drawing using computer technology or a keyboard with voice output. Individuals with poor swallowing will require a gastrostomy tube; support for them and their families, and training of the other healthcare providers on the aforementioned skills [6–8, 22].

Music therapists create a safe and secure environment for people living with a terminal illness to use music to express their feelings, instead of words. Music therapy session promotes relaxation, reduces stress, anxiety, and perception of pain. It also reduces the feeling of breathlessness, depression, helplessness, isolation, and withdrawal. And stimulates creativity and provides an opportunity for the individual with a terminal illness to express thoughts and feelings as they assume responsibility and participation in their treatment [22].

Social workers advocate for people living with a terminal illness and assist them to actively participate in their care, as well as make decisions and choices about what is important to them as their priorities and needs change. The team social worker must discuss honestly and non-judgmentally, as the individual experience roller-coaster emotions of fear, anger, anxiety, and sadness, tinged with hope [6–8, 22].

Clinical psychologists address the adjustment to illness, lifestyle changes, and relationships of individuals with a terminal illness with their family and friends. They also manage their anxiety, depression, and loneliness, reactions to loss, as well as helping them to set realistic future goals and living well. The *clergy* is *clergies* are trained to provide culturally appropriate spiritual and emotional support. They offer a calm presence and encourage the individuals with a terminal illness and their families to explore the ultimate meaning of life, as well as an observance of the sacraments and rituals of their faith [6–8, 22].

61.6 Genesis and Transmogrification of Hospice and Palliative Care

The concept of HPC is not new. The practice dates back to 460 BC, when Hippocrates, celebrated as the father of medicine, provided symptomatic relief of pain to his dying patients [23]. Dr. Cicely Mary Strode Saunders, a nurse who later trained as a social worker and physician and worked at the end of her career at St. Thomas' Hospital, London, in the latter part of 1950, conceptualised the modern-day hospice care. After close observation of the loathsome services that the people living with a terminal illness received, she advocated for an interdisciplinary team approach to relieving their pain and that of their family [24].

In the 1960s, Elisabeth Kübler-Ross, a Swiss-American psychiatrist, and instructor at the University of Chicago's Pritzker School of Medicine lampooned the traditional psychiatry practice of treating dying patients. She confronted fierce resistance when she advocated that the people living with a terminal illness be treated with respect, openness, and honest communication. The extensive work she did with individuals with life-threatening disease led her to develop a five-stage model of death and dying now referred to by the acronym "DABDA" —denial, anger, bargaining, depression, and acceptance - the concept used today in grief counselling is an adjustment technique. Kübler-Ross charismatic presentations and classic book on death and dying revolutionised and interjected care with dignity in the treatment of people living with terminal illnesses [25].

In 1974, Dr. Balfour Mount, a surgical oncologist at the Royal Victoria Hospital of McGill University in Montreal, Canada, invented the term "palliative care" in place of "hospice" that had pervasive negative connotations within the French culture. He popularised Dr. Saunders' innovations within the teaching hospitals in Canada by advocating the concept of holistic care for dying individuals and their families—who may also be enduring physical, psychological, social, or spiritual distress [25].

A report commissioned by the U.S. Institute of Medicine in 1977 brought palliative care into the mainstream of the American healthcare system by highlighting the deficiencies in the end-of-life care services. In the same year, the General Medical Council in the United Kingdom prosecuted some physicians for failing to provide care or refer the individuals living with a terminal illness for palliative care [26]. For over two decades, following these inauspicious beginnings, HPC has become the standard service offered to individuals with terminal diseases in industrialised nations. In the last decade, the number of hospitals with palliative care teams in the USA has tripled, but access to services is still limited. For example, only 267 (60%) of California's 448 hospitals surveyed in 2011 by the Centre to Advance Palliative Care had functioning palliative care teams [6–8, 26].

In 2005, the World Health Assembly proclaimed HPC a fundamental human right [27]. Today, many countries have developed policies to translate the World Health Assembly's goal into action. There has been rapid progress in integrating HPC into the healthcare system of many developing countries around the world. As a result, countries such as India, Saudi Arabia, and Pakistani now have robust and functional HPC resources within their healthcare system [28–30]. In West Africa, HPC services are still grossly underdeveloped and not integrated into the healthcare system [31, 32].

Hospice care was first introduced into Nigeria in 1993 by Mrs. Olushola Fatunmbi, and Dr. Anne Merriman, but their efforts did not receive the desired support from the national government [33]. The lack of governmental support led Dr. Merriman to relocate to Kenya and later Uganda. In 2007, Dr. Merriman facilitated the inauguration of the Hospice and Palliative Care Association of Nigeria through funding from the African Palliative Care Association. The University College Hospital, Ibadan, is the leading tertiary hospital and the first to develop a structured HPC services, in 2007. The project started as a partnership between the University College Hospital and the Centre for Palliative Care, a non-profit organisation in Nigeria. The services offered provide both hospital-based palliative care as well as home-based care for those individuals who cannot come to the hospital for various reasons [34–36].

61.7 Evolution of Hospice and Palliative Care as a Medical Speciality

Propelled by modern technology, demographic pressures that pushed death and dying issues in front of the medical, legal, and political agendas, HPC has evolved into a clinical speciality/sub-speciality in many industrialised countries. In the UK, the Royal College of Physicians recognised HPC as a speciality in 1987 when specialization in the discipline commenced [37]. In 1991, the Royal Australasian College of Physicians in Australia and New Zealand created sub-speciality training in HPC [38].

Ireland received speciality status accreditation for HPC in 1995. A year later, five other European countries—Germany, France, Romania, Poland, and Slovakia—recognised HPC as a sub-speciality [39]. Subsequently, the medical association of ten different European countries in Spain, Sweden, Czech Republic, Finland, Denmark, Iceland, Latvia, Malta, Israel, and Norway granted sub-speciality status following full recognition in an established speciality. Across Europe, there is a disparity in the criteria for certification, and wide variability in the rigour of the education provided [39].

After several years of struggle for recognition, in September 2006, the American Board of Medical Specialties granted accreditation to HPC as a sub-speciality in anaesthesiology. The field now has over 3000 members [25]. In 2014, the Royal College of Physicians and Surgeons in Canada officially recognised HPC as a two-year sub-speciality within internal medicine, anaesthesia, neurology, or paediatrics [40].

61.8 Global Demand and Utilisation of Hospice and Palliative Care Services

As a result of the world's ageing population and the increase in the incidence of cancer and other chronic diseases, the need for HPC has grown at a rapid pace. Across the world, over 29 million people died from illnesses that require HPC [41]. Of that number, 94% are adults, 69% were over 60 years old, 25% were 15 to 59 years old, and only 6% were children. The overwhelming majority of adults requiring HPC died from cardiovascular diseases (39%), cancer (34%), chronic respiratory infections (10%), HIV/AIDS (5.7%), and diabetes (4.5%). Those dying from HIV/AIDS are primarily persons in the younger age group, 15 to 59, whereas those with cardiovascular diseases, such as Alzheimer's, diabetes, chronic respiratory diseases, rheumatoid arthritis, Parkinson's, and cancer, are primarily individuals in the older age group [41].

Despite the need for HPC globally, it is still underdeveloped, with the reality that outside North America, Europe, and Australia, access to high-quality service is scarce. In 2011, 58% (136) of the world's 234 countries had at least one HPC service. This number represents a 9% [21] increase from 2006. Africa has the most significant improvement, but only 8.5% [20] of the countries have so far achieved "advanced integration" of HPC into their health system [2].

In the USA, approximately 90 million people live with life-threatening diseases, and with the ageing of the baby boomers (individuals born between 1946 and 1964), the number of people affected is expected to double over the next 25 years. Seven out of every 10 Americans today die from life-threatening illnesses. The number living with at least one chronic fatal illness is expected to surge to 157 million by 2020 [42]. In 2014, about 67,000 accredited HPC organisations - broken down into 30,200 assisted living residential facilities, 15,600 nursing homes, 12,400 home health agencies, 4800 adult day centres, and 4000 hospices - served about nine million Americans [43]. A 2015 national study revealed that, despite the increasing number of hospitals with palliative care services, access to care remains inadequate for people living with life-threatening illnesses [44].

In the UK, philanthropic organisations provide HPC through donations from citizens [45]. In 2015, charitable organisations offered HPC services to approximately 200,000 people with life-threatening illnesses, which represents 44% of the population that need the services. In the same year, hospices provided bereavement support for 41,000 people with life-threatening illnesses, their families, and paid family caregivers. Also in 2015, the UK government spent £868 million on care for people living with a terminal illness, their family caregivers, and families [45].

In Australia, neonatal units, paediatric services, general practices, acute hospitals, residential and community-based care services, and generalist community services are the primary providers of HPC [46]. Between 2014 and 2015, 65,000 hospital admissions in Australia were HPC-related. This number represents a 19% increase when compared with the 2010 and 2011 figures. One in every six public acute hospitals in Australia had an HPC facility. And one of every 1000 general practitioners' practice in an HPC-related setting, and seven in every 1000 medical specialists are a palliative physician. Similarly, one in every 90 nurses had palliative care training. About 46% of all inpatient who died received palliative care and 3% of all residential individuals with a terminal illness required palliative care [46].

In Middle Eastern countries, such as Turkey, Pakistan, Morocco, Palestine, Cyprus, Israel, Lebanon, Iran, and Jordan, HPC is often misconstrued by the health professionals and the general public because of the tradition and religious beliefs of inhabitants of these countries. The result is that of all Middle Eastern countries, only Turkey and Israel have implemented a national HPC policy. The primary barriers to the implementation of HPC and pain treatment are the shortage of opioids and inadequate training of healthcare professionals. In the Middle East, injectable morphine is available only in Israel, Iran, and Turkey. In the three countries, oral morphine is available in tertiary hospitals, but less accessible in rural health centres. Consequently, people with a terminal illness with severe pain attend tertiary hospitals in urban centres. Compared to the urban centres, the cost of pain treatment in rural health centres is more prohibitive [30].

As of 2004, only five of the 53 African countries provide HPC services [30, 31]. By 2011, nearly 50% of African nations, had HPC services, but less than 5% of the population in need of services had access to those services. By 2011, only four countries (Kenya, South Africa, Tanzania, and Uganda) in Africa have integrated HPC into their healthcare system. Rwanda and Swaziland developed a unique standalone national palliative care model [2]. Swaziland followed by South Africa had the lowest indicative ratio of HPC services to the population of 237 and 239, respectively. Swaziland and South Africa ranked numbers one and two out of the 53 African countries. Morocco and Ethiopia with a ranking of 27 and 28 had the highest indicative ratio of 31,993 and 41,412, respectively. Nigeria, the most populous nation on the continent, ranked number 24 out of 28 with an indicative ratio of 22,104 (Table 61.2).

Côte d'Ivoire with a population of 23.1 million was the first nation in West Africa with a credible HPC facility. In contrast, Togo with a population of 7.4 million has no single HPC facility [31]. Between 2006 and 2011, Côte d'Ivoire established 26 HPC facilities (22 government health centres, three mission hospitals, and one private hospital) within their healthcare system and noticed the most significant improvement. Kenya with 44 palliative care centres in 2011 made "much progress" when compared to the number available in 2006.

As of 2013, Nigeria had seven (two private hospices and five federal government-funded tertiary hospitals) HPC facilities, five credentialed palliative physicians and four nurse specialists, but did not improve its overall classification grouping [2]. Despite the increasing occurrence of cancer and other debilitating diseases in Nigeria, HPC still takes the back burner within the healthcare system. However, it is beginning to receive the much-needed federal government attention. In less than a decade, 15 HPC centres were established in five out of the six geopolitical zones across the

Table 61.2 Indicative ratio of hospice and palliative care centres to the population of the countries in Africa as of 2011 [2]

Number of country ratio[a]				
Country	HPC Facility	Population	1:1000	Ranking
Swaziland	5	1,185,000	237	1
South Africa	210	50,110,000	239	2
Botswana	4	1,950,000	490	3
Namibia	3	2,171,000	724	4
Reunion Island	1	800,000	800	5
Côte d'Ivoire	26	21,075,000	811	6
Kenya	44	39,802,000	905	7
Uganda	34	32,710,000	962	8
Zimbabwe	13	12,523,000	963	9
Zambia	13	12,935,000	995	10
Malawi	9	15,263,000	1696	11
Gambia	1	1,705,000	1705	12
Lesotho	1	2,067,000	2067	13
Tanzania	20	43,739,000	2187	14
Congo	1	3,683,000	3683	15
Ghana	5	23,837,000	4767	16
Rwanda	2	9,998,000	4999	17
Tunisia	2	10,272,000	5136	18
Sierra Leone	1	5,696,000	5696	19
Cameroon	3	19,522,000	6507	20
Mali	1	13,010,000	13,010	21
Angola	1	18,498,000	18,498	22
Sudan	2	42,272,000	21,136	23
Nigeria	7	154,729,000	22,104	24
Mozambique	1	22,894,000	22,894	25
Egypt	3	82,999,000	27,666	26
Morocco	1	31,993,000	31,993	27
Ethiopia	2	82,825,000	41,412	28

[a]To normalise for differences in the population across the different countries, an indicative ratio of hospice and palliative care services was computed

country [10, 34–36]. In 2015, approximately 4.6 million Nigerians were estimated to be in need of HPC services [10, 47]. Those in desperate need of services were children, people living with HIV/AIDS, prisoners, soldiers, and rural dwellers [47].

Within the next two decades, there will be a 300% surge in demand for HPC in Africa [31]. People living with HIV/AIDS will need more continued support than the general population. The significant barriers in rendering HPC services in Africa are the local culture and belief systems. The challenge is compounded by the taboo against open discussion of impending death, limited culturally appropriate information about dying, and the "death denial" mentality ingrained in the psyche of the individuals living with a terminal illness, their relatives, and healthcare professionals.

The future development of HPC in Africa lies in increasing the number of people receiving high-quality services while creating dynamic and flexible action plans to address the evolving illness patterns and counter the unprogressive local belief system. Ingenuity in the distribution and use of available resources and employing new technologies, such as mobile phones, while respecting non-harmful cultural practices, has been advocated by health policy technocrats as the best way forward [31]. The demand for HPC will continue to outpace supply and available resources. On a positive note, more African countries have recently adopted a public health system with increased networking. Similarly, the palliative care associations and governments in the continent are beginning to integrate HPC into the healthcare systems [31].

61.8.1 Hospice and Palliative Care Best Practices

In the last two decades, there has been a paradigm shift in the healthcare industry, including the HPC system, away from the theoretical propositions of the basic science towards evidence-based practice (EBP). Professor David Sackett, a Canadian medical epidemiologist and progenitor of EBP, defined it as "the integration of the clinical expertise, patient values, and the best research evidence into the decision-making process to deliver high-quality healthcare." [48] The implementation of EBP relies on the rigour of the experimental design and availability of existing literature that meets pre-defined criteria of quality. The dawn of EBP in HPC is already here, but its application has lagged significantly behind other clinical specialities because of the discordance between the clinical contexts of HPC and the foundational expectations and procedures of EBP [48].

The concept of EBP is still new in many developing nations, and a host of reasons impedes its implementation. Among the reasons are the limited resources and access to the internet, especially in rural communities, and the epileptic electricity supply in the urban centres, leading to the inconsistent internet connectivity needed for literature searches. Presently, in many developing countries, EBP studies on HCP are lacking, an occurrence that makes this void a gold mine for budding scientists.

Many of the available clinical guidelines for different patient populations now incorporate HPC into the standard-of-care treatment. One model that has been found useful in people living with a terminal illness is having the palliative physician clarify prognosis at the first visit and provide well-defined goals at each stage of transition. The physician must contextualise clinical decisions around the care goals; such as to preserve hope and optimism for the individual, and the treatment reoriented towards clearly defined objectives. Palliative care is part of a more extensive continuum of care; therefore, abrupt changes in the medical treatment must be avoided [15].

Hospice care is typically broken down into five stages, bearing in mind that every individual living with a terminal illness has different needs and diverse end-of-life pathways

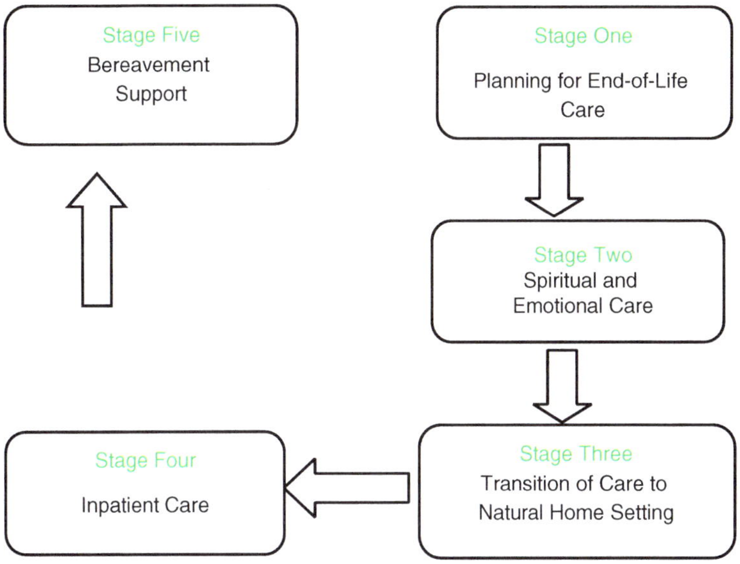

Fig. 61.1 Five phases of hospice care. I have attached pdf and word files for this unacceptable figure.

(Fig. 61.1). The best practice care routinely provided at the end-of-life will be discussed next.

61.8.2 Stage One: Planning for End-of-Life Care

For healthcare professionals, discussing HPC with the individuals living with a terminal illness can be a tricky and unsettling proposition. However, when approached with perspective and preparation, it can be more comfortable for both parties. The best approach is for the interdisciplinary team to discuss HPC and the associated myths as early as possible in the disease process [49]. The best practice for having the initial conversation with people living with a terminal illness is for the team to meet in a quiet room free of distractions, and in relaxed seating. Subsequently, the team can probe the individuals on their health status and then proceed to explain the disease process, allowing adequate time for assimilation of the information. Then the discussion of prognosis and treatment options and goal setting can follow.

In subsequent meetings, the team clinical psychologist, social worker, and clergy must discuss advance directives and coping strategies. At this stage, hospice information-gathering visits must be explored [49]. The cost of care is often a significant source of stress and anxiety for the people living with a terminal illness and their families. Wherever possible, the individual must be empowered to make decisions regarding their care in advance, and opportunities provided for them to clarify what help they will need and from where that support will come. Having their questions answered by knowledgeable professionals can reduce the concerns and allow them to enjoy their remaining days with dignity.

A minimal level of depression and anxiety is associated with severe illness. The interdisciplinary team must communicate prognosis openly and honestly with family members and provide regular updates on treatments. The family member must also actively participate in establishing care goals and focus on the strength of the individual living with the terminal illness. They must be encouraged to keep a daily journal and engage in other activities (exercise, prayer, and listening to music) that can distract from depression and anxiety [6–8]. Severe depression and anxiety must be treated by the physician with medication, in combination with counselling and complementary therapies.

The individuals living with a terminal illness must be encouraged to make their wishes known early through legal healthcare documents called "advance directives." The directive includes a living-will that provides instructions, regarding what type of treatment the patient would or would not like, such as the use of feeding tubes, ventilators (breathing machines), and cardiopulmonary resuscitation. The advance directives also include the medical power of attorney or healthcare proxy (agent) which identifies someone who will make healthcare decisions for the individual when they are no longer capable [6–8]. In many African cultures, implementing advance directives, such as a living-will or healthcare proxy, is despised as a taboo because of the superstition that it hastens the demise of the loved one at the end-of-life stage.

61.8.3 Stage Two: Spiritual and Emotional Care

This phase of the hospice care proceeds in tandem with the other treatments from the beginning to the very end-of-life. During this period, the loved ones and the healthcare providers must use a calm, reassuring tone, devoid of loud noise and night interruptions. The emotional and spiritual needs of the individuals with the terminal illness must be addressed by the team clinical psychologist, social worker, and clergy to prepare them and their families to accept death when the time comes. The healthcare professionals must also be well informed about the concerns of the individuals and their family members. In several African cultures, family support plays a critical role in dealing with death and dying. However, with urbanisation and assimilation of Western education and values, family support is decreasing and changing from extended to nuclear families. Other forms of assistance from caregiver organisations or religious support groups will be needed to fill the void in the decreasing family roles/support [49].

61.8.4 Stage Three: Transition of Care to a Natural Home Setting

People living with a terminal illness often need assistance with their everyday tasks and deserve to be near their nuclear family. In industrialised countries, it is best practice to provide them care in the natural environment that is comfortable, usually in their home [6–8]. The transitioning of HPC services to the home setting will be impractical in many developing countries due to lack of essential amenities in many homes, particularly in the rural areas where most people live. Poverty and health disparity is rife throughout Africa. In countries where these services are available, many people living with a terminal illness cannot afford the cost of HPC services and are often abandoned in the hospital ward. Due to the shortage of human and financial resources, intensive care units are commonly used to provide palliative services in many developing countries [50, 51].

61.8.5 Stage Four: Inpatient Care

Not all the people living with a terminal illness are a good candidate for inpatient care. For those who need it, hospitals or nursing facilities should be made available as a possible option. Some hospices offer inpatient services in hospitals, skilled nursing facilities, hospice facilities, and assisted residential living facilities [6–8]. In the USA, most hospice agencies do not provide full-time family caregivers at home and require an alternative arrangement be made for one.

Given that the primary goal of hospice care is a pain-free death, individuals at the end-of-life stage are prescribed potent opioids. The common side effects of the medications are shortness of breath, sedation, nausea, vomiting, constipation, delirium, anxiety, and loss of appetite, disorientation, and organ failure. These symptoms are best managed medically by the palliative team physician. As with pain control, there are complementary and alternative treatment approaches for managing the symptoms, but healthcare providers often ignore them because of lack of knowledge about their existence.

At the end-of-life stage, people living with a terminal illness will show physical symptoms and signs that both healthcare providers and family members must be alert to and provide appropriate assistance. Upright positioning is ideal at the end-of-life stage, and the physiotherapist can teach the individuals living with terminal illness breathing control techniques to manage shortness of breath. Healthcare providers must identify the triggers that cause the problem and eliminate them. The windows must be opened to allow more air in the room. The use of fan, humidifier, or air conditioning is recommended in hot condition [6–8].

To prevent nausea and vomiting, the people living with a terminal illness must avoid eating foods and odours that precipitate the symptoms. Eating fatty and fried foods must be equally discouraged, but encouraged to suck on hard candy, eat small and frequent meals [6–8]. Certain fruits and vegetables, such as prunes, mangoes, pawpaw or papaya, tamarind (black tumbler), and spinach can help in controlling constipation. They must avoid eating bananas when constipated.

Loss of appetite is typical and does not mean the individual is starving as one can live for an extended period with little food. There are various reasons for loss of appetite, which the physician must manage. The healthcare provider or family member must not force them to eat or drink if they don't want to make them more uncomfortable. Appetite can be improved through careful menu planning and eating small portions and easy-to-swallow foods, such as pudding or pureed food.

The lower and upper extremities may increasingly become cold, and skin colour may become mottled. The individual should be kept warm as they become uncommunicative and unresponsive. The healthcare providers and family members must introduce self by name before speaking and speak clearly, and truthfully. The individual may sleep more and difficult to arouse. The healthcare providers and family members must sit quietly with them, speak in a normal voice and hold their hand assuming they can hear everything said to them.

The urine output may reduce and become tea coloured. The individual may become incontinent. It is essential to keep them clean and comfortable. Due in part to decrease in oxygen, the individual may be feverish, restless, and make repetitive motions such as pulling the bed linen. The healthcare provider or family member should not restrain them but must speak in a low voice, lightly massage their forehead, read to them and play soothing music. If feverish, a cold, moist cloth on their forehead might help to calm them down.

The lungs will be congested, and the individual may produce a loud sound which does not indicate the onset of severe pain. The healthcare provider or family member must gently turn their head to the side to drain secretions and wipe the mouth with a moist cloth. The breathing pattern of the individual may change with shallow breaths interspaced with periods of no breathing for a few seconds to a minute and periods of rapid, shallow panting. The healthcare provider or family member must elevate their head or turn them on their side for comfort, hold their hand and communicate with them gently.

The living-will of the individual with the terminal illness must be shared in advance with the interdisciplinary team. At the end-of-life stage, the road to death can be smooth (tranquil) or chaotic with variations among the individuals (Fig. 61.2).

The smooth path to death is usually short and peaceful, while the chaotic route is prolonged and fraught with many complications before death finally arrives. The family member and healthcare professionals working with the individuals at this delicate end-of-life stage must be alert and look for progressively declining signs such as restiveness, confusion, stupor, quivering, delirium, myoclonic jerks, and seizures that may eventually lead to the comatose state and death. Ideally, the healthcare proxy (agent) of the person with the terminal illness must be around to reaffirm whether cardiopulmonary resuscitation should be instituted or not.

Best clinical practices of using electronic orders, instead of the manual paper-based materials have improved clinical outcomes of hospitalised individuals at the end-of-life [52]. Recent studies have demonstrated that people living with a terminal illness who received HPC have less depression and illness symptom burden, enjoy better control, and can avoid the risks associated with treatment and hospitalisation. Compared to traditional cure-directed care, individuals with a terminal illness who receive HPC have a better quality of life, lower treatment cost due to improved utilisation of healthcare resources, higher satisfaction with the quality of care [52], and improved survival rates when compared to matched controls who received standard treatment [53].

Stage Five: Bereavement support.

The death of the individual with a terminal illness takes an emotional toll on the nuclear family. There are seven phases that the individuals going through grief transcends and the members of the interdisciplinary team must be able to recognise the associated symptoms (Fig. 61.3).

Phase one, denial, reflects the unwillingness of the bereaved to accept the loss. Phase two in the form of annoyance towards the self or the creator for allowing the loved one to die. In the bargaining phase, the bereaved often conclude that it was okay that death came at such time at least to put an end to the loved one's suffering. Phase four, depression, sets in when the survivors get unnecessarily bitter and start to think that the death of the loved one is due to some inadequacies on their part. Next, the panic phase is when the bereaved begin to feel their psychological survival is keeping the loss from occurring. Phase six is when the bereaved start

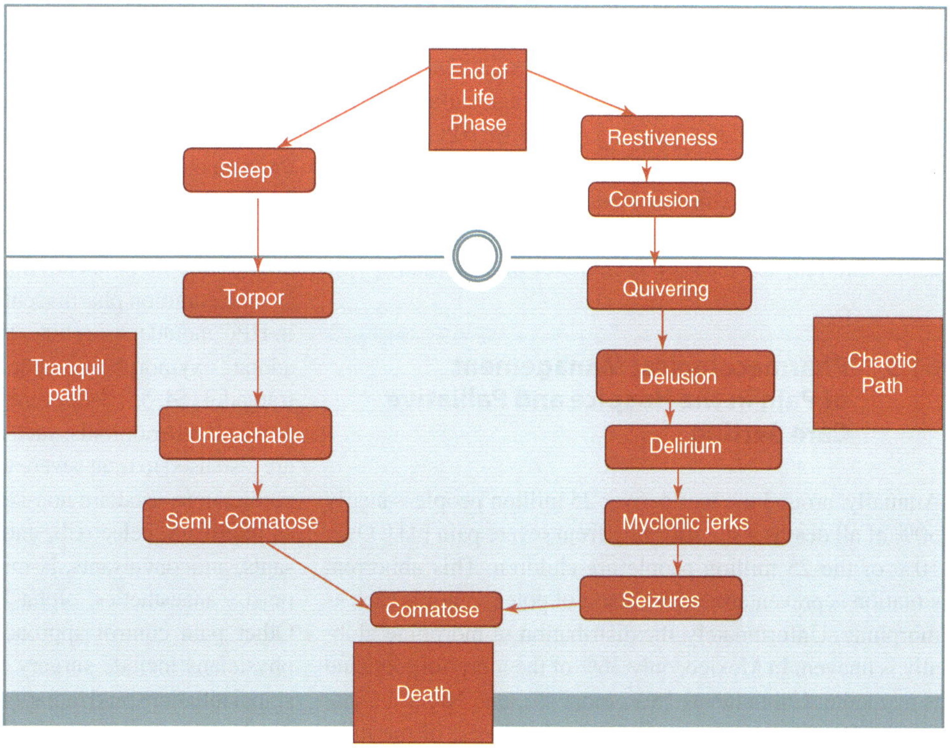

Fig. 61.2 The tranquil and chaotic paths to death

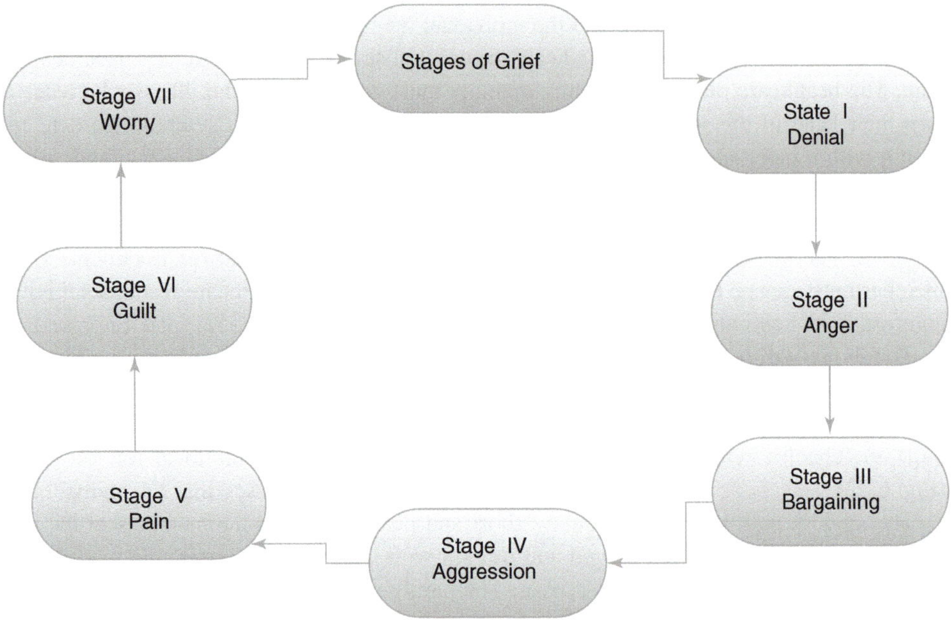

Fig. 61.3 Seven phases of grieving

to blame self for not taking the appropriate measures to forestall the death of the loved one through statements such as "if only I have done something differently." The worry phase is when the bereaved have come to accept the loss and started to think of the future and what life will be like in the absence of the loved one. The seven phases have one theme in common; the feelings are very humane. Grieving may not necessarily occur in the order stated nor did every survivor have to pass through all the phases and the time it takes to move from one stage to another is highly variable. The form and manifestations of these symptoms may vary significantly based on the level of education, personality, and cultural background of the individual grieving. Frontline HPC organisations with best practice culture will routinely provide bereavement support in the form of individual and group counselling and expressive arts bereavement sessions for the adult, children, and teens of the families of the dead [6–8].

61.9 Pharmacological Management of Pain in the Hospice and Palliative Care Setting

Annually, around the world, over 25 million people—nearly 50% of all deaths—die suffering from severe pain [41]. Over 10% of the 25 million people are children. This abhorrent situation is preventable with the use of potent opioids such as morphine. Unfortunately, the distribution of morphine globally is uneven. In Mexico, only 36% of the morphine demand is available; China meets 16%, India 4%, and Nigeria a dismal 0.2% of the needs are available. In several of the most impoverished countries, such as Haiti, Afghanistan, and Africa, the use of oral morphine in HPC is virtually nonexistent. Not only is morphine not readily available in the developing countries, but as of 2017 it is also more expensive; it costs about 16 US cents for 10 milligrams of morphine in developing nations compared to three cents in the industrialised world.

There are many modes of pain relief medication administration available to the palliative physician, including by mouth, via suppositories and patches, or through a tube inserted into the blood vessel or injected under the skin. In many countries around the world, Fentanyl is used for postoperative pain control through intravenous and epidural routes of administration. Transdermal patches are applied in the management of chronic pain, while transmucosal dosage is used to control cancer pain. Opioid medication is routinely administered via a pump that allows the patient to control the dosage of pain medication needed to bring relief [53–56].

The common pharmaceutical opioids used for pain control in HPC include: morphine, buprenorphine, oxycodone, methadone, oxymorphone, codeine, hydrocodone, fentanyl, and tramadol [54, 55]. Morphine is routinely prescribed for severe pain and other opioids, such as oxycodone and oxymorphone, are also used to treat severe to moderate pain. Other painkiller medications used are non-steroidal anti-inflammatories, such as naproxen, celecoxib, and ibuprofen, tricyclic antidepressants, anticonvulsants, N-methyl D-aspartate receptor antagonists, anaesthetics, alpha-2 agonists, and anticholinergics. Other pain control approaches recommended by palliative physicians include surgery in the form of nerve blocks and spinal infusions, and radiation therapy [55]. In the Netherlands, the three most prescribed drugs in hospice care are morphine, midazolam, and haloperidol. At admission, 89% of their patients in hospice care centres received medication orally and 94% subcutaneously on the day of death. Most of the drugs prescribed are unlicensed for their specific application, and guidelines are based on a low level of evidence [54].

A well-known phenomenon across healthcare settings is the variations in practice protocols, and HPC is no exception. The International Narcotics Control Board opined that opioids are underutilised in the management of pain, especially cancer pain [55]. Indisputably, many physicians in developing countries are afraid to prescribe strong opioids [56]. Suboptimal control of pain in HPC settings is attributed partly to physician's inadequate knowledge of the various appropriate drugs as well as their "failure to accept the terminal nature of the illness" [9]. Moreover, the EBP guidelines recommended for pain control in older patients with cancer are often not used in most clinical settings [55].

Although pain control is the primary focus of HPC, across the world, there is no consensus among physicians on the use of opioids for pain management. Best clinical practice guidelines developed for cancer pain control are available from different sources such as the American Pain Society, the National Consensus Project for Palliative Care, and the National Comprehensive Cancer Network. For the older adults, the American Geriatrics Society Persistent Pain Guidelines, the Acute Pain Management in Older Adults, and the Pain in Residential Aged Care Facilities Management Strategies. There is an ongoing debate on the dosage of morphine needed for pain control. Some physician contends that morphine has no standard dose and the ideal treatment is the amount that controls the pain. The WHO ladder protocol is considered the best practice in the management of the pain of people living with a terminal illness [57]. First, the protocol stipulated that morphine be administered in increasing amounts, and applied until the pain ceases without producing an "overdose," together with tolerable side effects; and individuals with a terminal illness must first be on non-opioids (such as Paracetamol), and an adjuvant drug (such as NSAID), if necessary. Second, a moderate opioid (such as Codeine, Tramadol, etc.) can be added. Third, a potent opiate (such as morphine—gold standard) should be used to control the pain. Finally, in clinical settings when morphine is not available, other potent opioids, such as Fentanyl, Buprenorphine, and Pentazocine, can be use as a substitute [57].

The barriers to effective treatment of pain among dying individuals with a terminal illness in Britain and Korea include fear of euthanasia, the physicians' beliefs and prejudices, and inadequate knowledge [58–60]. People living with life-threatening illness on opioids for a prolonged period may experience physical dependence and tolerance, but psychological addiction is infrequent. Therefore, the risk of reliance must not be a consideration in determining whether to use opioids to modulate pain [57].

The distressing side effects of opioids have been one of the reasons many physicians are hesitant to use them for pain control [61]. In many African countries, the phenomenon of "opiophobia" or apprehension by the physician to prescribe opioids is prevalent due to fear of addiction. This misunderstanding has caused some physicians to prescribe limited opioids, causing the people living with a terminal illness unnecessary pain. Physicians in North-eastern Portugal reported several erroneous beliefs about the side effects of morphine, addiction concerns, and legal limitations [61]. In several countries across the world, governments have enacted laws that make the acquisition of opioids difficult because of the fear of abuse. In several European countries, strict regulations surrounding the use of opioids and high cost contributed significantly to effective cancer pain management and abuse of the drug [62]. Indeed, more clinical research is needed on medication use in palliative care [54].

61.10 Global Epidemiology of Opioid-Related Deaths

Worldwide, 250 million people use drugs, and over 29.5 million (11%) use them at a level that requires treatment. Among the drugs used, opioids have the highest negative health impact, but cannabis remains the most popular recreational drug, with a prevalence of 3.8% among adults. Globally, in the past year, about 183 million people (an estimated 128 to 238 million people) have experimented with cannabis [63]. The current drug epidemic in the USA began in the 1990s when over 100 million adults with chronic pain, were encouraged by physicians to consider pain as a serious clinical problem. Unfortunately, the pharmaceutical companies took advantage of the situation, through an aggressive advertisement campaign, encouraging physicians to prescribe OxyContin and Percocet. Although opioids were found to be useful for short-term treatment of acute pain, the empirical evidence related to their efficient use in chronic pain treatment is weak. Moreover, there was substantial evidence that opioids are dangerous when used for prolonged period.

Today, physicians in North America prescribe more painkillers than their colleagues in other parts of the world (Fig. 61.4).

In the last two decades, the prescription of opioids by physicians increased. Regrettably, the drugs landed in the hands of teens foraging through the first-aid kits and medicine cabinets of their parents, and family members. The death toll from this unfortunate development is consequential.

Vis-à-vis other parts of the world, more people die today of a drug overdose in North America. In 2015 alone, 190,900

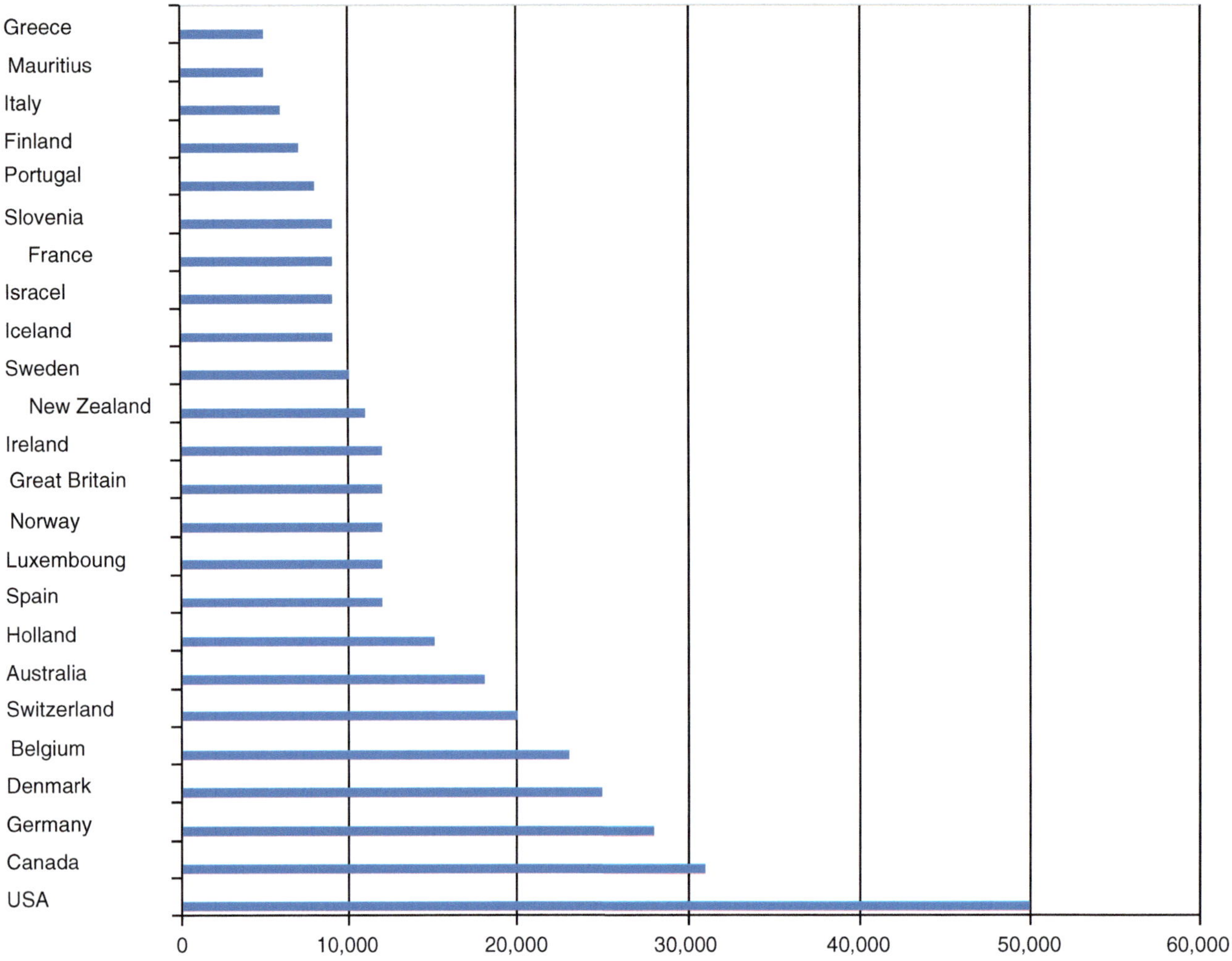

Fig. 61.4 Standard daily opioid dose use by country (for every one million people). (Data Source: United Nations International Narcotics Control Board)

drug-related deaths occurred globally. Of that number, 52,000, accounting for 25% of the total figure, were Americans who died of drug overdoses (Fig. 61.5). Between 1999 and 2015, deaths by overdose more than tripled, most of it from opioids. Between 2012 and 2015, deaths attributed to an overdose of synthetic opioids increased by 265%. From 2014 to 2015, these deaths again increased by 72%, most of it driven by illicit Fentanyl use [63]. Given the surge in deaths by overdose from synthetic opioids, in 2015, life expectancy fell in the United States by 0.1 years from 78.9 to 78.8. The last time such a decline took place was in 1993 when it fell by 0.3 years.

The drug-related mortality rate in North America is more than four times higher than the global average and 2.5 times higher in Oceania (Australia and New Zealand) than the worldwide average. About 35% of the global drug-related deaths occur in Asia, but the mortality rate is below the worldwide average of 39.6 per million persons aged 15–64 years [63] (Fig. 61.6).

Approximately, 60,070 Americans died of drug overdoses in 2016. A retrospective analysis of the data for drug-related death revealed that the figure surpassed the estimated 55,000 deaths that occurred from car crashes at the peak of the epidemic in 1972 and the estimated 40,000 deaths from gun violence at the height of the scourge in 1993. It also surpassed the estimated 43,000 deaths due to HIV/AIDS during that epidemic's peak in 1995; and the 58,220 deaths during the Vietnam War (Fig. 61.7). In a nutshell, the surge in drug-related deaths in the USA is horrifying and a critical lesson that developing countries can learn.

The sociological factors surrounding the misuse of medically prescribed opiates vary in different parts of the world. Easy access to prescribed opioids is not related to abuse and addiction. The contradiction is because some countries which put restrictions on opioid, and maintain a low per-capita medical use, still report high levels of misuse of painkillers [64, 65]. High incidences of opioid abuse are common in Australia and the USA—the two nations with the most per-capita medical use of opioids. In North America, the increase in the abuse of prescription opioids is due to a range of social factors that include the structure of the health

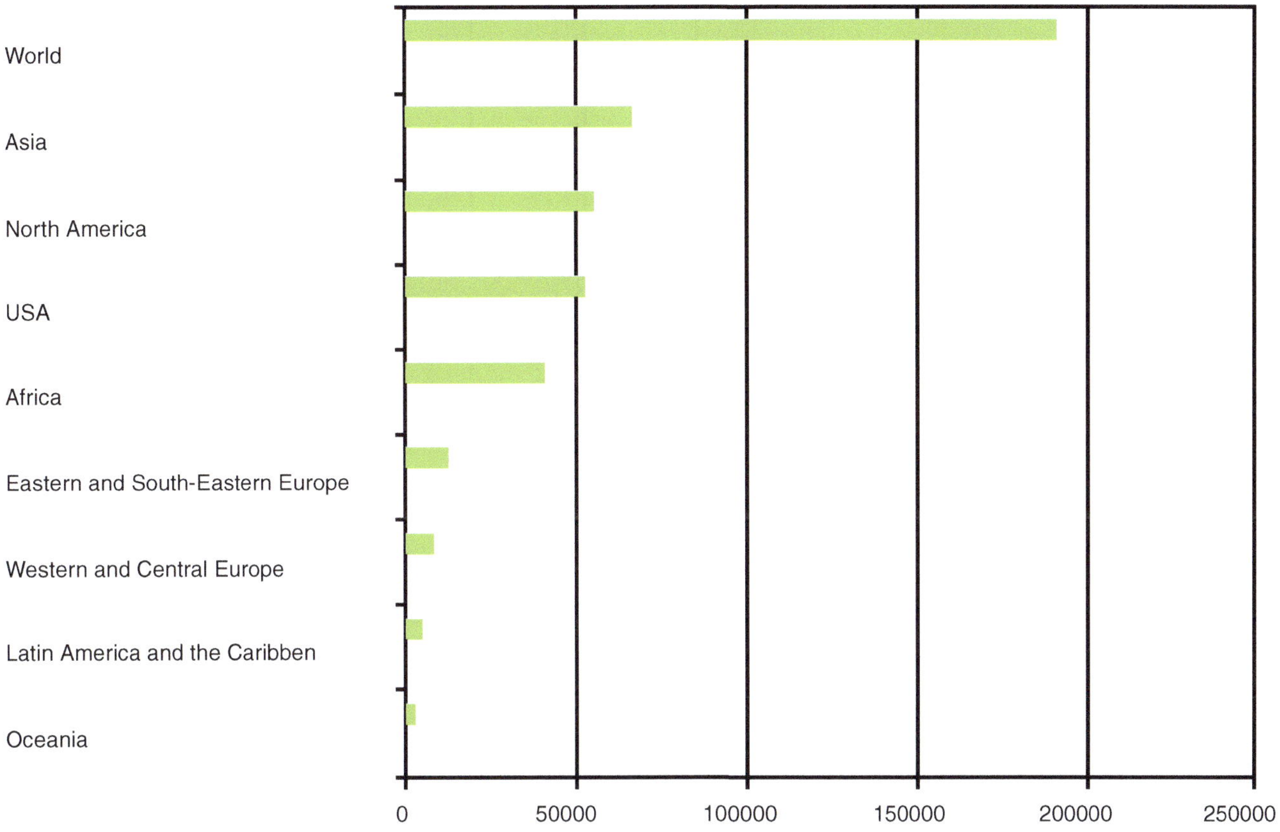

Fig. 61.5 Global drug-related deaths in 2015. (Data Source: United Nations Office on Drugs and Crime)

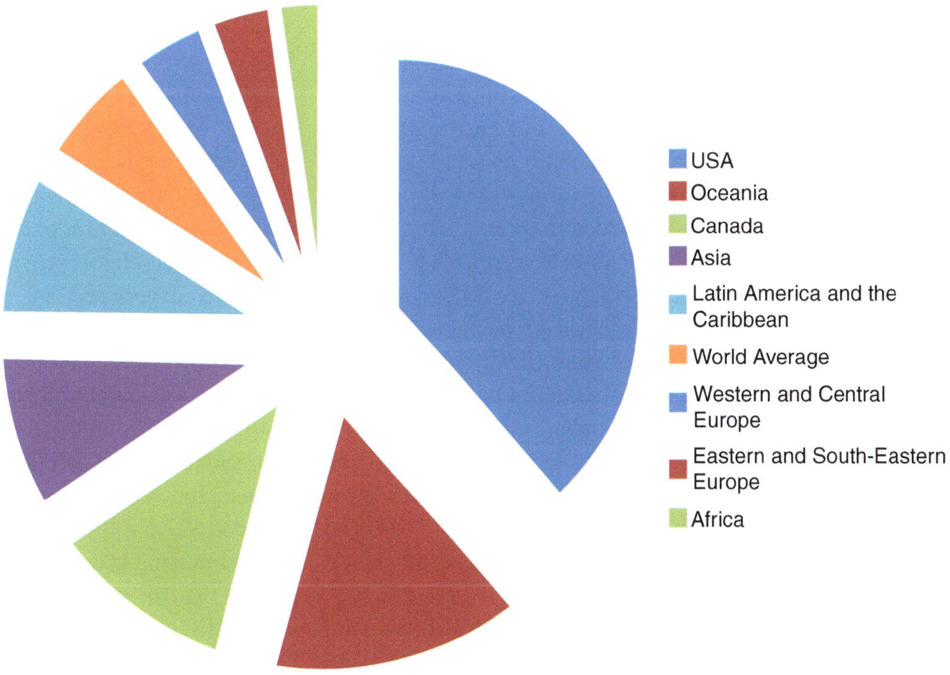

Fig. 61.6 Global drug-death rate in 2015 (mortality rate per million persons ages 15–64). World average is 39.6 mortality rate per million persons aged 15–64 years (Total = 190,900 people). (Data Source: United Nations Office on Drugs and Crime)

system and a medical culture that allows easy access to pain killers. Furthermore, the surge is due to the prescription practices by physicians who write up orders of these drugs for people living with a terminal illness. Many patients, unfortunately, view access to these painkillers as a right [66].

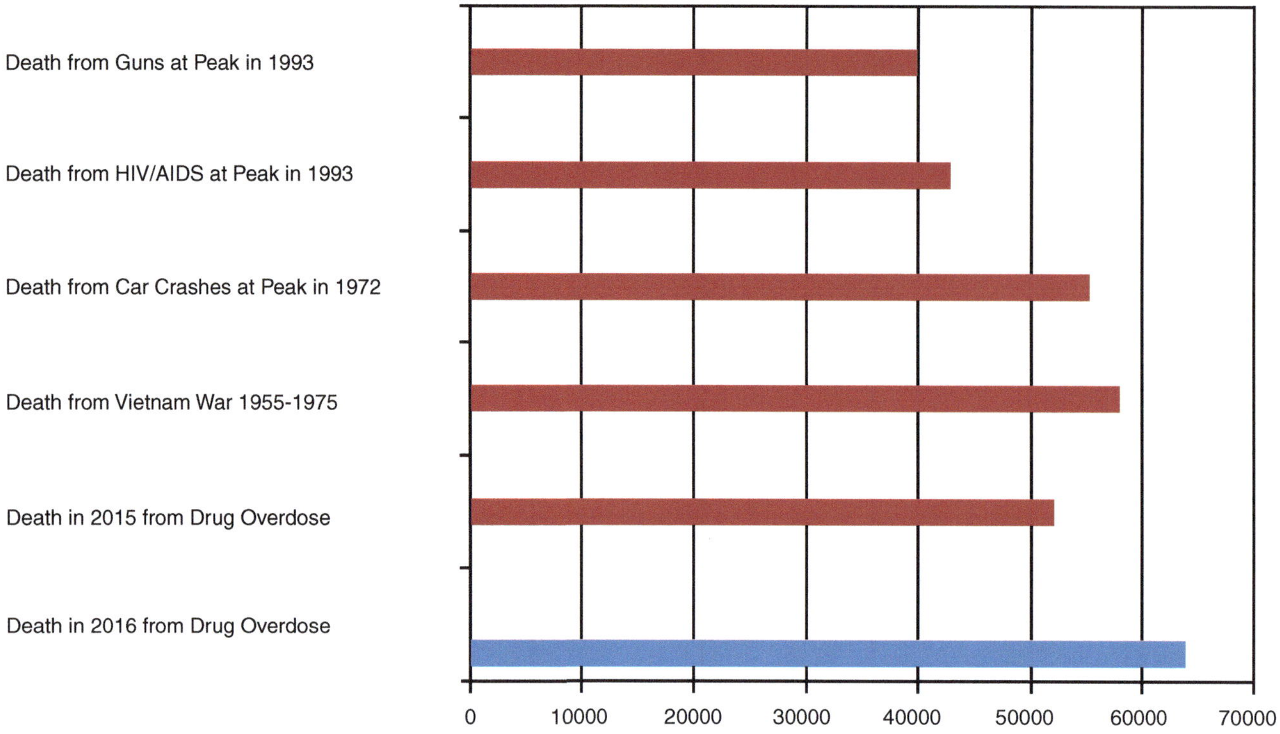

Fig. 61.7 Drug-related death in the USA compared to death from other significant catastrophic events in the nation's recent history

Globally, there is a growing incidence of tramadol misuse among adolescents and young adults, particularly in regions like the United Arab Emirates, Iran, Asia, and Africa. The reasons for the abuse of tramadol is due to its mood-enhancing effect, delayed ejaculation, self-medication for pain and fatigue and a proven treatment option in relieving depression and anxiety. The high levels of misuse of tramadol are due to its widespread availability in pharmacies, its lower cost compared to other illicit drugs, and the perceptions that it is safe and easily hidden [63].

In Nigeria, the Hospital Pain-Free Partnership Project between the American Cancer Society and the Federal Ministry of Health mandated that all healthcare professionals should be trained in the management of pain. Under this innovative program, clinicians at the tertiary health institutions level were empowered to prescribe strong opioids. Consequently, the consumption of opiates escalated. In the view of one analyst, "the previous phobia among hospital staff and patients in the use of the opioid is gradually becoming a cruel past" [10]. The increase in the consumption of opioids must be monitored carefully to ensure that the wrong hands do not have access to the drug and only people living with a terminal illness who need the medication get it. This caution is warranted to prevent the unintended consequences of drug culture and liberal public policy on drugs as in North America. The Federal Ministry of Health is currently the sole importer of opioids, but strict laws must be promulgated to avert misuse.

61.11 Complementary and Alternative Treatment Approaches in Hospice and Palliative Care

The use of complementary and alternative treatment practices continues to grow in popularity around the world. Nearly 40% of Americans annually spend over $34 billion on complementary and alternative medicine (CAM) and more physicians in the USA today are open to the use of CAM than a decade ago. In 1998, 64% and in 2002, 84% of USA medical schools provided CAM-related instruction and clerkship experience in their curriculum. The number declined to 51% in 2015. The most frequently taught contents were traditional medicine, acupuncture, spirituality, herbs, and general information on CAM. The standard instructional methods used were lectures, readings, observation, and receiving CAM treatment. In 1999, the US National Center for Complementary and Alternative Medicine awarded $22.5 million developmental grant to fifteen medical and nursing schools to teach CAM contents. Over 80% (13 of the 16) of the Canadian medical schools in 1999 included CAM contents in their curriculum; the remaining 19% [3] "planned to offer it in the future."

A 2012 study from the UK revealed that 56% of the medical students (N = 450) had not received any education in CAM, but 66% of them already used CAM, and 17% were "currently using it." The most commonly used CAM by the students includes Echinacea, cod liver oil, and aloe vera. Over 50% of the students surveyed were not sure of the efficacy and safety of the CAMs. Notwithstanding, 88% of them reported that they would recommend CAM to others. Only 16% of the students indicated they had informed their physician about their CAM use; 28% expressed interest in receiving instruction in CAM.

Another study from the UK in 2013 revealed that 54% of the medical students surveyed ($N = 95$ representing 25 different medical schools) had received lectures on CAM in their "core course." Approximately, 46% of the students believed the instruction on CAM was "critical," 16% responded as "uncritical," and 39% indicated "discursive."

In 2014, only 47% of the physician in the UK surveyed ($N = 1363$) believed medical schools should teach alternative medicine. To date, medical schools in North America and the UK have not fully integrated CAM-related contents into their medical curriculum. Aside from the training deficit, the role of CAM in HPC is presently not commonly discussed in the literature.

At the end-of-life stage, pain control and patient comfort are the primary focus of treatment. The non-pharmacological complementary methods that have the potential to promote relaxation and pain relief include cognitive-behavioural strategies such as guided imagery, hypnosis, meditation, biofeedback, music, massage, aquatic/hydrotherapy, and acupuncture. Physiotherapy modalities such as mobilisation, manipulation, ergonomically appropriate positioning in bed, exercise, thermotherapy (heat lamps, hot packs and shortwave diathermy), cryotherapy (ice compression wraps, ice packs), and transcutaneous electrical stimulation may be used to reduce the need for potent painkiller drugs and prevent the undesirable side effects.

There are logistical problems associated with the use of heat lamps, hot packs, and shortwave diathermy in the home environment, particularly in developing countries. The equipment needed is bulky and often not readily available. Local adaptations that use low technology should be explored. For example, putting rice grains in socks and microwaving it for 2–4 minutes can be used as a substitute for a heating pad. This treatment option retains heat for a prolonged period. In the tropics where the temperature is typically oppressive, the use of heat for pain modulation may be inappropriate; instead, cryotherapy with crushed ice wrapped in a towel will be a better option for individuals with a terminal illness who can tolerate cold.

In addition to the complementary therapies, other alternative treatment practices outside the realms of conventional orthodox medicine can be utilised to control the pain and illness symptoms of individuals with a terminal illness. Examples of the alternative therapies commonly used in the West are yoga, humour or distraction, therapeutic touch, pet therapy, herbal medicine or phytotherapy, spiritual and Shamanic healing, aromatherapy, naturopathy, and homoeopathy. Unfortunately, randomised controlled studies on the clinical effectiveness of these alternative medicines in HPC settings are presently lacking. The mainstream medical establishments and health insurance companies in many of the industrialised countries do not recognise alternative treatment approaches, and therefore services delivered by their practitioners are not reimbursed. Another drawback of the use of alternative medicine is that at the end phase of life, the dying individuals do not have the financial resources to pay out of pocket for the service.

Alternative medicine informs of traditional healing is used by most of the people around the world. Different societies over the years have employed various forms of indigenous healing practices, which are herbal, spiritual, or faith-based, to ease the pain of dying individuals. Examples are the traditional Chinese medicine, Ayurvedic, and Siddha that is native to India, so is Shamanism in Siberia, Reiki in Japan, Unani or "Greco-Arab" medicine in Greece, ancient Iranian medicine, Iranian (Persian), Islamic medicine, and traditional Korean medicine. In Africa, "Muti" and "Sangoma or Nyanga" are healing practices indigenous to South Africa, so is "Ifá" or "Babalawo" among the Yorubas, "Dibia" among the Igbos, and "Boka" among the Hausa people in Nigeria.

Practitioners of alternative medicine, in the different cultures, claim they treat the terminally ill person holistically by reconnecting their social and emotional equilibrium and bring them back into harmony with their ancestors. In several African communities, religious and local indigenous music with "talking-drums" can be leveraged to calm down and restore transient tranquillity to the people living with a terminal illness. The use of the alternative medicine within the healthcare system is still controversial around the world, even in industrialised countries. Any alternative treatment approach that does not exacerbate the pain or discomfort of a dying individual is worth trying.

61.12 Clinical Guidelines on High-Quality Hospice and Palliative Care

The increasing use of HPC to improve the quality of life of people living with a terminal illness has led to the development of several clinical guideline protocols. Clinical guidelines are carefully crafted statements derived from the systematic review of empirical evidence from the literature considering the pros and cons of all treatment options. Several clinical guidelines developed by HPC organisations and governmental agencies, including the WHO, abound in the literature [67–74]. The salient points drawn from three popular clinical guidelines are summarised below.

In 2009, the National Consensus Project for Quality Palliative Care, based in the USA, published the second edition of a clinical practice guidelines [72]. The monograph pinpointed the following six core competencies. The palliative care physicians must:

- Be compassionate and provide medical care based on EBP in palliative medicine, aimed at optimising the quality of life of people with advanced life-threatening illnesses - the interdisciplinary team must provide care for the patient and their families.
- Be knowledgeable about the established and evolving biomedical, clinical, population science, and social, behavioural sciences relevant to the care of people with advanced life-threatening illnesses and their families and be able to relate the knowledge to HPC practice.
- Be able to evaluate, appraise, and assimilate scientific evidence relevant to HPC and improve his/her clinical practices on caring for people with life-threatening illnesses and their families.
- Have appropriate interpersonal and communication skills necessary for effective relationship-building, information exchange, emotional support, shared decision-making, and bonding with people with advanced life-threatening illnesses and their families.
- Be committed to his/her professional responsibilities, adhere to ethical principles, sensitive to a diverse patient population, with appropriate self-reflection, and devotion to decrease pain and enhance the quality of life of people with advanced life-threatening illnesses and their families.
- Be aware of and responsive to the broader context of healthcare, including hospice and other community-based services for people with life-threatening illnesses and their families.

In 2013, the National Consensus Project for Quality Palliative Care released the third edition of its recommendations relating to people with life-threatening illnesses in all settings, regardless of diagnosis, prognosis, or age [73]. The report was produced through a consensus process among the preeminent HPC organisations in the USA. The recommendations were broken down into eight domains with instructions for each area. The following are their broad prescriptions and benchmark for a high-quality HPC organisation:

Domain 1: Structure and processes of care

- The interdisciplinary team of an HPC organisation must undertake a detailed and timely evaluation of the patient and the family and use the findings to develop a care plan.
- The care plan must be based on the identified and expressed preferences, values, goals, and needs of the patient and family and must be developed with professional guidance and support of the patient's family.
- The services provided by the interdisciplinary team to both the patient and family must be consistent with the care plan.
- The HPC organisations must use trained and supervised volunteers at home as caregivers to the extent feasible.
- The interdisciplinary team must provide support for ongoing quality assurance education, training, and professional development.
- The HPC organisations must be committed to quality evaluation and performance improvement, by implementing a continuous data-driven process that reflects the complexity of the organisation and focuses on clinical outcomes.
- The HPC organisations must recognise the emotional impact of caring for people with life-threatening illnesses on the mental health of the health professionals and caregivers at home.
- HPC organisations must ensure that adequate community resources are available to deliver the highest quality service across the care continuum.
- The physical environment of the HPC organisations must meet the preferences, needs, and circumstances of the people with advanced life-threatening illnesses and their family, to the extent possible.

Domain 2: Physical aspects of care

- The interdisciplinary team must use EBP to evaluate and manage pain and all illness-related symptoms of people with advanced life-threatening illnesses and their family.
- Within the context of the disease progression, the assessment and management of the illness symptoms and medication side effects must be appraised.

Domain 3: Mental health aspects of care

- The interdisciplinary team must use EBP to evaluate and address the psychological and psychiatric aspects of care to optimise the coping capacity and quality of life of people with advanced life-threatening illnesses and their family.
- Based on the desired evaluation, a core component of the HPC must include grief and bereavement services available to the people with advanced life-threatening illnesses and their family.

Domain 4: Social aspects of care

- The interdisciplinary team must use EBP to evaluate and address the social issues of concern to foster patient-family needs and goals and maximise the patient-family strengths and physical well-being.

- A detailed interdisciplinary evaluation must be undertaken to identify the human strengths, needs, and objectives of the individual patient and family.

  Domain 5: Religiosity and existential aspects of care

- The interdisciplinary team must use EBP to evaluate and address the religious, spiritual and existential scope of responsibility.
- Should the need arise, the clinician must conduct a detailed mental evaluation. The assessment should identify spiritual, religious, experiential capacity, preferences, beliefs, ritual practices of the patient and family, bearing in mind the illness symptoms, such as pain, resentment, guilt, hopelessness, despair, and spiritual distress.
- The services provided by the HPC organisation must promote the religious, spiritual, and cultural rituals or practices of the patient and family, even after the passing of the patient.

  Domain 6: Cultural aspects of care

- The professionals who provide HPC must strive to develop appropriate cultural and linguistic competence.
- The HPC organisations must deliver linguistically and culturally sensitive service to individuals with advanced life-threatening conditions and their family.

  Domain 7: Care at the End-of-Life

- The interdisciplinary team must treat the signs and illness symptoms at the end-of-life to meet the physical well-being, psychosocial, spiritual, and cultural needs of people with advanced life-threatening illnesses and their family.
- Working hand in hand with individuals with advanced life-threatening illnesses and their family, the interdisciplinary team must evaluate and undertake a care plan to address preventable and emergency treatment of illness-related symptoms.
- Following the death of the patient, the HPC organisations must provide service in a respectful manner that honours the culture and religious practices of the deceased's family.
- Following the death of the patient, the HPC organisations must develop a bereavement plan that it activates expeditiously.

  Domain 8: Legal and ethical aspects of care

- Applicable state and federal laws and standards of healthcare must inform patient goals, preferences, and decisions.
- Person-centred goals, choices, and decisions must be the basis for the care plan that is developed by the interdisciplinary team.
- The HPC organisations must identify, acknowledge, and address the complex ethical issues that may arise while providing care for people with advanced life-threatening illness.
- The state and federal laws, professional regulations and applicable standards of healthcare must guide the operations of the HPC organisations.

The fourth edition of the National Consensus Project for Quality Palliative Care's guidelines was published in 2018.

For its part, in 2014, the African Palliative Care Association, in collaboration with Global Partners in Care, published a monograph on clinical placement for HPC trainees [74]. The document can be used as a resource by clinicians interested in developing an HPC organisation or for capacity building to train palliative care professionals. It can also be used to build quality clinical placements and improve trainees and supervisors' knowledge about HPC. The report recommended that HPC organisations provide the following operational and workforce resources:

- High-quality end-of-life care for people with life-threatening illness
- Clinical supervision
- Efficient communication operations
- Complementary therapies
- Ethical consideration and respect for human rights
- Grief and bereavement support
- Utilisation of an interdisciplinary healthcare team concept for service delivery
- Timely treatment of opportunistic infections
- Medication management
- Management of pain and illness-related symptoms
- Planning, coordination, and access to HPC
- Financial and legal support for the care providers
- Psychosocial and spiritual support and culturally sensitive care

The report also recommended that HPC organisations implement the following eight steps before admitting people living with life-threatening illness into their facilities:

- Develop an organisational structure for clinical placement and recruit qualified operational staff
- Stipulate the fees and benefits for the trainees
- Define the core knowledge and skills during the clinical internship
- Develop a schedule for clinical placement trainees, including supervisor/mentor
- Develop organisational policies to address legal issues
- Develop a contract that will guide the behaviours of the trainee, supervisor, or mentor
- Implement an orientation session for trainees

- Develop an evaluation protocol and competence guidelines for trainees

The report advocated six steps in developing clinical placements for trainees, including activities before, during, and after the conclusion of deployment.

Before the clinical placement:

- The HPC organisation must assign the trainee a supervisor or mentor.
- The mentor and trainee must discuss the learning objectives and identify specific activities that will enhance the attainment of each learning objective.

During the clinical placement:

- A representative of the HPC organisation must orient the trainee to the program.
- A representative of the HPC organisation and the trainee must meet to discuss and agree on the specificity of each learning objectives, expectations, placement activities, as well as legal and policy issues.
- The supervisor must engage in an ongoing mentoring of the trainee.

After the clinical placement:

- The trainee and supervisor must jointly assess the clinical placement.

The three clinical guidelines showcased above can be used by health professionals, policymakers, and HPC organisations to make informed decisions about the healthcare needs of the people living with a terminal illness. A website now exists that provides up-to-date clinical information on the latest trends on HPC. The site can serve as a reference resource for individuals with terminal illness, health professionals, and HPC organisations [75].

61.13 Status of Hospice and Palliative Care Education in Africa

In industrialised nations, the professional association of allied health disciplines, such as nursing [76], physical therapy [77], occupational therapy [78, 79], music therapy [80], and social work [81], have set clear standards defining their scope of practice in HPC. Furthermore, the current publications emanating from the industrialised nations have articulated the roles and responsibilities of family physicians [82], physical therapists [83], speech therapists [84], music therapists [85], clinical psychologists [86–88], clergies [89–91], and social workers [92, 93], in HPC. An inquisitive reader can consult the relevant citations provided to obtain more advanced information on the related topics.

Around the world, although HPC is now a recognised speciality in medicine, it is still not widely accepted as a speciality in allied health professions. For example, in the USA, HPC is not one of the nine (cardiovascular and pulmonary, clinical electrophysiology, geriatrics, neurology, oncology, orthopaedics, paediatrics, sports, and women's health) recognised specialities in physical therapy [94]. Similarly, HPC is not one of the nine (gerontology, driving and community mobility, mental health, environmental modification, paediatrics, feeding, eating and swallowing, physical rehabilitation, low vision, and school systems) board certification in occupational therapy [95]. Also, HPC is not one of the 11 (ambulatory care, cardiology, critical care, geriatrics, infectious diseases, nuclear, nutrition support, oncology, paediatric, pharmacotherapy, and psychiatric) specialities in pharmacy [96].

Although WHO in 2004 recommended that the curriculum of health workers at all levels include contents in HPC, this goal is still not realised in many developing countries. Africa is currently plagued with a shortage of healthcare professionals, particularly those with expertise in HPC. On the continent, only a few universities in East and South Africa offer degree programs in HPC. None of the universities in West Africa has a degree program in HPC. Nigeria with seven palliative care centres does not field a degree program in HPC. As of June 2021, only two of the 44 medical schools in Nigeria (the University of Ibadan and the University of Ilorin), currently teach elective courses in HPC [10, 97, 98]. In comparison, Congo with only a single palliative care facility (Table 61.2) offers a certificate program in home-based palliative care in Kinshasa. Health establishments in Uganda, South Africa, Kenya, Zambia, Swaziland, and Botswana regularly provides on the job training courses leading to a certificate credential for healthcare workers at all levels [99].

Palliative care is currently integrated into the educational curricula of healthcare professionals in Uganda, Kenya, Namibia, Botswana, Malawi, and Tanzania. This development was made possible by the workforce and funding provided through the Diana Princess of Wales Memorial Foundation in the UK [99]. The Ugandan Ministry of Health has developed a national training manual in HPC for use at all levels of their healthcare system.

The University of Cape Town in South Africa, in partnership with the College of Medicine at the University of Wales (now Cardiff University), developed the first HPC postgraduate diploma and Master of Philosophy degree programs on the African continent in 2011 [99]. Other postgraduate programs in HPC have since been established at Mildmay International (in affiliation with the University of Manchester in UK), the International Medical Technological University in Tanzania, the Institute of Health Sciences in Gaborone, the International University of Management in Namibia, and the College of Medicine and Health Sciences at the University of Rwanda. Nairobi Hospice offers a postgraduate degree program in HPC in collaboration with Oxford Brookes University in the United Kingdom. Also, the Kenya Medical Training College offers an 18-month higher education web-based postgraduate program in HPC for healthcare professionals [99–102].

The Africa Palliative Care Association based in Kampala; Uganda has taken the lead on the continent by developing a training program in community-based HPC for family caregivers. Also, they offer through distance learning, diploma and Bachelor of Science degree programs in HPC. In collaboration with Oxford Brookes University, the Africa Palliative Care Association also offers a diploma in health education and Master of Philosophy degree programs in palliative medicine in partnership with the University of Cape Town in South Africa [101]. The Institute of Hospice and Palliative Care in Africa (Hospice Africa Uganda) in collaboration with Makerere University also offers a diploma and a Bachelor of Science programs in HPC [103].

There are significant challenges associated with the offering of HPC education in Africa. The problems include the shortage of competent educators, clinical placement logistics and inadequate funding of the medical and allied health sciences programs. The training of HPC personnel in Africa should occur at three levels-basic levels aimed at the primary healthcare workers (non-palliative care specialists), intermediate level (technical and auxiliary healthcare workforce), and specialist training of medical and allied health professionals at the university level.

61.14 Summary

Although emotionally draining and stressful, caring for the terminally ill person can be rewarding. Therefore, the needs of the family, friends, and healthcare providers during the arduous and tortuous journey towards death must be carefully considered. All HPC treatments come with burdens and benefits. Medical interventions may help control the illness symptoms of individuals at the end-of-life, but the response may be concomitant with side effects that may be minimal or significantly worsens their quality of life. The interdisciplinary team must weigh the benefits and burdens of the treatment to decide what is right for each patient.

Due to the shortage of human and financial resources, many of the best practices described in this paper are unrealistic in developing countries; presently an academic pipe dream. In developing countries, HPC is still not a recognised medical speciality; many of the physicians in the discipline are not board certified like their counterparts in North America, Europe, and Australia. While taking its root in academic medicine, HPC as a sub-speciality or full speciality enabled physicians to obtain clinical skills and advanced knowledge in the field; other allied health disciplines must strive to develop speciality tracks in HPC.

In the era of EBP, clinicians employed in the HPC setting often find themselves hampered by lack of relevant well-designed randomised controlled studies. Despite the increased use of EBP today, HPC is still not well informed by the level and rigour of evidence found in the other clinical specialities. With tighter regulations and greater scrutiny of outcomes, HPC settings are being challenged to consider the implementation of EBPs. Outcome studies are therefore needed to uncover the efficacy of the traditional and complementary treatment approaches presented in this chapter. The clinical guidelines presented represent best practices and core competencies that palliative physicians and providers are expected to imbibe and internalise. They can be utilised to improve both the quality of care and patient outcomes in HPC settings.

Globally, Nigeria currently lags many other developing nations in the provision of palliative care. The services provided are still not an integral component of health insurance benefits. It is essential that governments at federal and state levels commit to the development of services by expanding the capacity for both in- and out-patient palliative care. Developing nations must adopt culturally appropriate public policies on drugs, to combat the scourge of opioid-related deaths and carefully monitor the implementation of such plans.

References

1. Aniebue UU, Onyeka TC. Ethical, socioeconomic, and cultural considerations in gynaecologic cancer care in developing countries. Int J Palliat Care. 2014: Article ID 141627. Available at https://doi.org/10.1155/2014/141627. Accessed: January 19, 2018.
2. Lynch T, Connor S, Clark D. Mapping levels of palliative care development: a global update. J Pain Sympt Manag. 2013;45(6):1094–106. Available at http://www.jpsmjournal.com/article/S0885-3924(12)00334-X/fulltext. Accessed: March 10, 2018.
3. World Health Organization. The impact of chronic disease in Africa. Geneva: WHO; 2012.
4. Stjernsward J, Foley K, Ferris F. WHO public health approach for palliative care. J Pain Sympt Manag. 2007;33(5):486–93, p. 486.
5. World Health Organization. Cancer pain relief and palliative care. Geneva: WHO; 2002.
6. Palliative Doctors. Available at http://palliativedoctors.org/palliative/care. Accessed: January 19, 2018.
7. Centre for Hospice Care. Available at https://www.hospicesect.org/hospice-and-palliative-care/when-is-it-time-for-hospice. Accessed: January 19, 2018.
8. Get Palliative Care – Available at https://getpalliativecare.org/whatis/disease-types/. Accessed: January 19, 2018.
9. Abbas SQ, Muhammad SR, Mubeen SM, Abbas SZ. Awareness of palliative medicine among Pakistani doctors: a survey. J Pak Med Assoc. 2004;54:195–9.
10. Faith M-P. Palliative care in Africa: an overview. Afr Health. 2011;33(5):19.
11. Chukwuneke FN. Ethics of palliative care in late-stage cancer management and end-of-life issues in a depressed economy. Niger J Clin Pract. 2015: 18(Suppl S1):15–9. Available at: http://www.njcponline.com/text.asp Accessed: January 19, 2018.
12. Chaar B, Isaac S. Euthanasia drugs: what is needed from medications for assisted deaths? 2017. http://www.abc.net.au/news/2017-10-20/assisted-dying-what-is-need-from-drugs-for-voluntary-euthanasia/9069896.

13. Jünger S, Pestinger M, Elsner F, Krumm N, Radbruch L. Criteria for successful multi professional cooperation in palliative care teams. Palliat Med. 2007;21:347–54. Available at https://www.researchgate.net/profile/Lukas_Radbruch/publication/6183248_Criteria_for_successful_multiprofessional_cooperation_in_palliative_care_teams/links/00b49528a446de6a99000000/Criteria-for-successful-multiprofessional-cooperation-in-palliative-care-teams.pdf. Accessed: January 19, 2018.
14. Bosch M, Faber MJ, Cruijsberg J. Effectiveness of patient care teams and the role of clinical expertise and coordination. November 16, 2016;66(Issue 6_suppl), 2009. Available at http://journals.sagepub.com/doi/pdf/ Accessed: January 19, 2018.
15. Mcateer R, Wellbery C. Editorials. Palliative care: benefits, barriers, and best practices. Am Fam Physician. 2013;88(12):807–13. Available at https://www.aafp.org/afp/. Accessed: January 19, 2018.
16. Wilner LS, Arnold R. The palliative prognostic score: fast facts and concepts no. 124. Available at http://www.eperc.mcw.edu/EPERC/FastFactsIndex/ff_124.htm. Accessed: January 27, 2018.
17. Flacker JM, Kiely DK. A practical approach to identifying mortality-related factors in established long-term care residents. J Am Geriatr Soc. 1998;46(8):1012–5.
18. Angermayr B, Cejna M, Karnel F, et al. Child-Pugh versus MELD score in predicting survival in patients undergoing transjugular intrahepatic portosystemic shunt. Gut. 2003;52(6):879–85.
19. Hemmelgarn BR, Manns BJ, Quan H, Ghali WA. Adapting the Charlson co-morbidity index for use in patients with ESRD. Am J Kidney Dis. 2003;42(1):125–32.
20. Han PK, Lee M, Reeve BB, et al. Development of a prognostic model for six-month mortality in older adults with declining health. J Pain Symptom Manag. 2012;43(3):527–39.
21. Onyeka TC, Ezeome ER, Onyeka TC, Amah CC. Ethics of physiotherapy practice in terminally ill patients in a developing country, Nigeria. Niger J Clin Pract. 2015;18:S40–S5.
22. Our Team. Available at http://www.dhhs.tas.gov.au/palliativecare/about/team. Accessed: January 19, 2018.
23. Manual of Cancer Services Standard. London: National Health Services; 2000.
24. Richmond C. Dame Cicely Saunders: The founder of the modern hospice movement dies. 14 July 2005. Available at http://www.bmj.com/content/suppl/2005/07/18/331.7509.DC1. Accessed: January 19, 2018.
25. Loscalzo MJ. Palliative care: an historical perspective. Available at http://asheducationbook.Haematologylibrary.org/content/2008/1/465.full. Accessed: January 19, 2018.
26. Riley J. The general medical council and the right to specialist palliative care. Palliat Med. 1997;11:317–8.
27. World Health Assembly. Available at http://www.who.int/hiv/universalaccess2010/worldsummit.pdf. Accessed: January 19, 2018.
28. Sureshkumar K, Rajgopal M. Palliative care in Kerala. Palliat Med. 1996;10:293–8.
29. Brown S, Black F. Palliative care in the Kingdom of Saudi Arabia. Eur J Palliat Care. 2001;8:196–8.
30. Silverman M, Arnaout M, Daher M, Nestoros S, Pitsillides B, Charalambous H, Gultekin M, Fahmi R, Mostaf KAH, Khleif AD, Manasrah N, Oberman A. Palliative cancer care in Middle Eastern countries: accomplishments and challenges. Ann Oncol. 2012;23(Suppl 3):15–28. https://doi.org/10.1093/annonc/mds084.
31. Grant L, Downing J, Namukwaya E, Leng M, Murra SA. Palliative care in Africa since 2005: good progress, but much further to go. Available at https://doi.org/10.1136/bmjspcare-2011-000057. Accessed: January 19, 2018.
32. Ajayi I, Iken O, Powell R, Soyannwo O, Namisango E, Mwangi-Powell F. Palliative care research in Western Africa. Eur J Palliat Care. 2014;21(1):45–7.
33. Hospice and Palliative Care, UCH Ibadan. Available at http://uch--ibadan.org.ng/hospice_and_palliative_care. Accessed: January 19, 2018.
34. Soyannwo AO. End of Life Care: palliative care initiative in Nigeria. Health life for all Foundation; 20th May 2004. Available at: http://www.hlfonline.org/articles. Accessed: January 14, 2018.
35. Adenipekun A, Onibokun A, Elumelu TN, Soyannwo OA. Knowledge and attitudes of terminally ill patients and their family to palliative care and hospice services in Nigeria. Niger J Clin Pract. 2005;8:19–22.
36. Soyannwo OA. Palliative care and public health, a perspective from Nigeria. J Public Health Policy. 2007;28:56–8.
37. Murie J. Palliative medicine. 2006. Available at http://careers.bmj.com/careers/advice/Palliative_medicine. Accessed: January 19, 2018.
38. Cairns W. A short history of palliative medicine in Australia. Cancer Forum. 2007:31(1). Available at https://cancerforum.org.au/forum/2007/march/a-short-history-of-palliative-medicine-in-australia/. Accessed: January 19, 2018.
39. Centeno C, Noguera A, Thomas Lynch T. Official certification of doctors working in palliative medicine in Europe: data from an EAPC study in 52 European countries Palliative Medicine 2007; 21: 683–7. Available at http://www.eapcnet.eu/LinkClick.aspx?fileticket=sAcHoGky9ZY%3D&tabid=194. Accessed: January 19, 2018.
40. Sullivan P. Specialty status granted to palliative care MDs. 2014. Available at https://www.cma.ca/En/Pages/Specialty-status-granted-palliative-care-MDs-may-aid-recruiting.aspx. Accessed: January 19, 2018.
41. Global atlas of palliative care at the end of life. Worldwide Palliative Care Alliance and the World Health Organization. 2014. Available at http://www.who.int/nmh/Global_Atlas_of_Palliative_Care.pdf. Accessed: January 19, 2018.
42. The Centre to Advance Palliative Care Palliative Care: Facts and Stats. 2014. Available at https://media.capc.org/filer_public/68/bc/68bc93c7-14ad-4741-9830-8691729618d0/capc_press-kit.pdf. Accessed: January 19, 2018.
43. Long-term care providers and services users in the United States: Data from the national study of long-term care providers, 2013–2014. Vital and Health Statistics Series 3, Number 38. Available at https://www.cdc.gov/nchs/data/series/sr_03/sr03_038.pdf Accessed: February 16, 2018.
44. America's care of serious illness: 2015 state-by-state report card. On access to palliative care in our nation's hospitals. Available at https://reportcard.capc.org/ Accessed: January 19, 2018.
45. Hospice care in the UK 2016: Scope, scale and opportunities. 2016. Available at https://www.hospiceuk.org/docs/default-source/What-We-Offer/publications-documents-and-files/hospice-care-in-the-uk-2016.pdf?sfvrsn=0. Accessed: February 16, 2018.
46. Australian Institute of Health and Welfare. Palliative care services. 5/02/2018. Available at https://www.aihw.gov.au/reports--statistics/health-welfare-services/palliative-care-services/overview. Accessed: February 16, 2018.
47. Oyebola FO. Palliative care trends and challenges in Nigeria – the journey so far. J Emerg Intern Med. 2017;1(2):17. Available at http://www.imedpub.com/articles/palliative-care-trends-and-challenges-in-nigeria%2D%2Dthe-journey-so-far.php?aid=21670. Accessed: February 16, 2018.
48. Visser C, Hadley G, Wee B. Reality of evidence-based practice in palliative care. Cancer Biol Med. 2015;12(3):193–200. https://doi.org/10.7497/j.issn.2095-3941.2015.0041. PMCID: PMC4607825.
49. Crossroads hospice and palliative care: approaching the hospice conversation: best practices for physicians. June 20, 2014. Available at https://www.crossroadshospice.com/healthcare-professionals-resources/palliative-care-blog/2014/june/20/

approaching-the-hospice-conversation-best-practices-for-physicians/. Accessed: February 16, 2018.

50. Obinna C. Intensive care units in Nigeria not for palliative care — experts. Vanguard Newspaper. On August 1, 2017. Available at https://www.vanguardngr.com/2017/08/intensive-care-units-nigeria-not-palliative-care-experts/. Accessed: February 16, 2018.
51. Babajo SK. Basic Health: Nigeria lagging behind in providing palliative care — minister – July 20, 2017. Available at http://www.libertytvradio.com/basic-health-nigeria-lagging-behind-providing-palliative-care-minister/. Accessed: February 16, 2018.
52. Beresford L. Home hospice providers offer best practices for end-of-life care. The Hospitalist. 2014(7). Available at https://www.the-hospitalist.org/hospitalist/article/126160/hospice-palliative-medicine/home-hospice-providers-offer-best-practices. Accessed: February 16, 2018.
53. Mcateer R, Wellbery C. Editorials. Palliative care: benefits, barriers, and best practices. Am Fam Physician. 2013;88(12):807–13. Available at https://www.aafp.org/afp/2013/1215/p807.html. Accessed: February 16, 2018.
54. Masman AD, van Dijk M, Tibboel D, Baar FPM, Mathôt RAA. Medication use during end-of-life care in a palliative care centre. Int J Clin Pharm. 2015;37(5):767–75. Available at https://www.ncbi.nlm.nih.gov/pmc/articles/PMC4594093/. Accessed: December 28, 2018.
55. Herr K, Titler M, Fine P, Sanders S, Cavanaugh J, Swegle J, Forcucci C, Tang X. Assessing and treating pain in hospices: current state of evidence-based practices. J Pain Sympt Manag. 2010;39(5):803–19. https://doi.org/10.1016/j.jpainsymman.2009.09.025. Available at https://www.ncbi.nlm.nih.gov/pmc/articles/PMC2884963/. Accessed: February 16, 2018.
56. Onyeka TC. Palliative care in Enugu, Nigeria: Challenges to a new practice. Indian J Palliat Care. 2011;17(2):131–6. https://doi.org/10.4103/0973-1075.84534.
57. World Health Organization. Cancer pain relief: a guide to opioid availability. Available at http://apps.who.int/medicinedocs/documents/s22085en/s22085en.pdf. Accessed: February 23, 2018.
58. Cuttini M, Casotto V, Rodolfo S, Marcello O. Health professionals' beliefs may undermine effective pain relief for dying patients. BMJ. 2003;327:221–2.
59. Chang YJ, Yun YH, Park SM, Lee SW, Park HA, Roy YJ, et al. Nurses' willingness to maximise opioid analgesia for severe cancer pain, and its predictor. Support Care Cancer. 2005;13:743–51. PubMed: 15827729
60. Jeon YS, Kim HK, Cleeland CS, Wang XS. Clinicians' practice and attitudes towards cancer pain management in Korea. Support Care Cancer. 2007;15:463–9. PubMed: 17115200
61. Verloo H, Mpinga EK, Ferreira M, Rapin C, Chastonay P. Morphinofobia: the situation among the general population and health professionals in North-Eastern Portugal. BMC Pall Care. 2010;9:15. PMCID: PMC2900233.
62. Cherny NI, Baselga J, de Conno F, Radbruch L. Formulary availability and regulatory barriers to accessibility of opioids for cancer pain in Europe: A report from the ESMO/EAPC Opioid Policy Initiative. Ann Oncol. 2010;21:615–26. PubMed: 20176694
63. United Nations Office on Drugs and Crime, World Drug Report 2017. ISBN: 978-92-1-148291-1, eISBN: 978-92-1-060623-3, United Nations publication, Sales No. E.17.XI.6.
64. World Drug Report. United Nations Publication, 2014, sales No. E.14.XI.7.
65. Degenhardt L, et al. Benefits and risks of pharmaceutical opioids: essential treatment and diverted medication – a global review of availability, extra-medical use, injection and the association with HIV. Sydney: National Drug and Alcohol Research Centre, University of New South Wales; 2007.
66. Fischer B., et.al. Non-medical use of prescription opioids and prescription opioid-related harms: why so markedly higher in North America compared to the rest of the world? Addiction, 109, 2 (2014), pp. 177-181.
67. Greer JA, Jackson VA, Meier DE, Temel JS. Early integration of palliative care services with standard oncology care for patients with advanced cancer. CA Cancer J Clin. 2013;63(5):349–63. [Medline].
68. Clinical practice guidelines in oncology. Palliative care. Version 1.2016. National Comprehensive Cancer Network. Available at http://www.nccn.org/professionals/physician_gls/pdf/palliative.pdf. Accessed: March 9, 2018.
69. Ferrell BR, Temel JS, Temin S, Alesi ER, Balboni TA, Basch EM, et al. Integration of palliative care into standard oncology care: American Society of Clinical Oncology. Clinical practice guideline update. J Clin Oncol. 2017;35(1):96–112. Available at http://ascopubs.org/doi/full/10.1200/JCO.2016.70.1474.
70. Palliative care fact sheet. Number 402. World Health Organization. Available at http://www.who.int/mediacentre/factsheets/fs402/en/. Accessed: March 9, 2018.
71. Shekelle P, Aronson MD, Melin JA. Overview of clinical practice guidelines Available at https://www.uptodate.com/contents/overview-of-clinical-practice-guidelines. Accessed: March 9, 2018.
72. Hospice and palliative medicine core competencies for quality palliative care. Version 2.3, September 2009, 2nd ed. Available at http://aahpm.org/uploads/education/competencies/Competencies%20v.%202.3.pdf. Accessed: February 16, 2018.
73. The National Consensus Project Clinical Practice Guidelines for Quality Palliative Care, 3rd ed., 2013. Available at https://www.nationalcoalitionhpc.org/ncp-guidelines-2013/. Accessed: March 9, 2018.
74. Guidelines for clinical placement in hospice and palliative care in Africa. Available at http://www.globalpartnersincare.org/sites/default/files/public/gpc/Clinical_Placement.pdf. Accessed: March 9, 2018.
75. https://www.uptodate.com/contents/whats-new-in-palliative-care. Accessed: March 9, 2018.
76. Hospice and Palliative Nurses Association (HPNA). Standards for clinical education of hospice and palliative nurses. July 2015. Available at http://hpna.advancingexpertcare.org/wp-content/uploads/2015/08/HPNA-Clinical-Education-Standards.pdf. Accessed: March 10, 2018.
77. American Physical Therapy Association (APTA). Hospice and palliative care. 2015 Available at http://www.apta.org/PatientCare/HospicePalliativeCare/. Accessed: March 10, 2018.
78. The role of occupational therapy in palliative and hospice care. American Occupational Therapy Association. Copyright © 2015. Available at https://www.aota.org/~/media/Corporate/Files/AboutOT/Professionals/WhatIsOT/PA/Facts/FactSheet_PalliativeCare.pdf. Accessed: March 10, 2018.
79. Occupational therapy in palliative care: a position paper. Occupational Therapy Australia 2015. Available at http://www.otaus.com.au/sitebuilder/advocacy/knowledge/asset/files/21/positionpaper-occupationaltherapyinpalliativecare%5Baugust2015%5D-occupationaltherapyaustralia.pdf. Accessed: March 10, 2018.
80. American Music Therapy Association. Standards of clinical practice. Available at https://www.musictherapy.org/about/standards/. Accessed: March 10, 2018.
81. Social workers in hospice and palliative care: occupational profile. ©2010 National Association of Social Workers. Available at https://www.socialworkers.org/LinkClick.aspx?fileticket=l_dSmnRuGfY%3D&portalid=0. Accessed: March 10, 2018.
82. Ramanayake RPJC, Dilanka GVA, Premasiri LWS. Palliative care: role of family physicians. J Family Med Prim Care. 2016 Apr-Jun; 5(2): 234–237. Available at https://www.ncbi.nlm.nih.gov/pmc/articles/PMC5084539/ Accessed: March 10, 2018.

83. Kumar SP, Jim A. Physical therapy in palliative care: from symptom control to quality of life: a critical review. Indian J Palliat Care. 2010; 16(3):138–46. Available at https://www.ncbi.nlm.nih.gov/pmc/articles/PMC3012236/. Accessed: March 10, 2018.
84. Toner MA, Shadden BB. Foreword: end-of-life care for adults what speech-language pathologists should know. Top Lang Disord. 2012 ;32 (2):107–10. Available at https://journals.lww.com/topicsinlanguagedisorders/Fulltext/2012/04000/Foreword__End_of_Life_Care_for_Adults_What.2.aspx. Accessed: March 10, 2018.
85. Ko L. Music therapy in palliative care. September 01, 2010. Available at https://www.clinicaladvisor.com/commentary/music-therapy-in-palliative-care/article/177883/. Accessed: March 10, 2018.
86. Strachan J, Finucane AM, Spiller J. Clinical psychologists in specialist palliative care: what do we actually do? Available at https://www.palliativecarescotland.org.uk/content/publications/04.-Clinical-Psychologists-in-specialist-palliative-care%2D%2D-what-do-we-actually-do.pdf. Accessed: March 10, 2018.
87. Jünger S, Payne S. Guidance on postgraduate education for psychologists involved in palliative care. Available at http://www.eapcnet.eu/LinkClick.aspx?fileticket=7kOIkiphMt0%3D&tabid=194. Accessed: March 10, 2018.
88. Kasl-Godley JE, King DA, Quill TE. Opportunities for psychologists in palliative care working with patients and families across the disease continuum. Am Psychol. 2014:364–76. Available at https://www.apa.org/pubs/journals/releases/amp-a0036735.pdf. Accessed: March 10, 2018.
89. Balboni MJ, Sullivan A, Enzinger AC, Smith PT, Mitchell C, Peteet JR, Tulsky JA, VanderWeele T, Balboni TA. U.S. Clergy religious values and relationships to end-of-life discussions and care. 2017. J Pain Sympt Manag. Available at https://projects.iq.harvard.edu/files/rshm/files/clergy_jpsm_2017_01.pdf Accessed: March 10, 2018.
90. LeBaron VT, Smith PT, Quinones R, Nibecker C, Sanders JJ, Timms R, Shields AE, Balboni TA, Balboni MJ. How community clergy provide spiritual care: toward a conceptual framework for clergy end-of-life education. J Pain Symptom Manag. 2016;51:4.
91. Holland JC, Chertkov L. Clinical practice guidelines for the management of psychosocial and physical symptoms of cancer. Available at https://www.ncbi.nlm.nih.gov/books/NBK223528/. Accessed: March 10, 2018.
92. Hospice social work: linking policy, practice, and research a report from the March 25, 2010 symposium. Available at http://www.socialworkpolicy.org/wpcontent/uploads/2010/09/SWPIHospice-Report-FINAL.pdf. Accessed: March 10, 2018.
93. LeClaire J. Social workers gets new standards for end-of-life care. Available at https://www.monster.com/career-advice/article/social-workers-end-of-life-care-guidelines Accessed: March 10, 2018.
94. American Physical Therapy Association. Available at http://www.apta.org/Media/Releases/Association/2016/6/. Accessed: March 14, 2018.
95. American Occupational Therapy Association. Available at https://www.aota.org/Education-Careers/Advance-Career/Board-Specialty-Certifications.aspx. Accessed: March 14, 2018.
96. Board of Pharmacy Specialties. Available at https://www.bpsweb.org/bps-specialties/. Accessed: March 14, 2018.
97. Ilori AF. Nigeria needs more hospices, palliative centres, says HPCAN. 2015. Available at https://guardian.ng/features/nigeria--needs-more-hospices-palliative-centres-says-hpcan/. Accessed: March 14, 2018.
98. Onwumere O. Perils of operating palliative care in Nigeria. Modern Ghana Newspaper. Available at https://www.moderngh-ana.com/news/471174/perils-of-operating-palliative-care-in-nigeria.html. Accessed: March 14, 2018.
99. Rawlinson FM, Gwyther L, Kiyange F, Luyirika E, Meiring M, Downing J. The current situation in education and training of health-care professionals across Africa to optimise the delivery of palliative care for cancer patients. Ecancermedicalscience. 2014;8:492. Available at https://www.ncbi.nlm.nih.gov/pmc/articles/PMC4303614/. Accessed: March 14, 2018.
100. Onyeka TC, Velijanashvili M, Abdissa SG, Manase FA, Kordzaia D. Twenty-first century palliative care: a tale of four nations. Eur J Cancer Care. 2013;22(5):597–604. Available at https://onlinelibrary.wiley.com/doi/pdf/10.1111/ecc.12064. Accessed: March 14, 2018.
101. Fraser BA, Powell RA, Mwangi-Powell FN, Namisango E, Hannon B, Zimmermann C, Rodin G. Palliative care development in Africa: lessons from Uganda and Kenya. J Glob Oncol. Available at http://ascopubs.org/journal/jgo. Accessed: March 14, 2018.
102. African Palliative Care Association. Palliative care in education programmes. Available at https://www.africanpalliativecare.org/integration/palliative-care-in-education-programmes/. Accessed: March 14, 2018.
103. Makerere University. Call for applications: bachelor of science in palliative care and diploma in palliative care. Available at https://news.mak.ac.ug/2013/10/call-applications-bachelor-science-palliative-care-and-diploma-palliative-care. Accessed: March 14, 2018.

Part VI

Health Systems Organisation, Research Methodology and Biostatistics

Leadership of Healthcare Teams, Organisations and Systems: Implications for Curriculum Revision in Medical Education

62

Joseph A. Balogun

Learning Objectives

After reading this chapter, the reader will be able to:

- Articulate the differences between management and organisation.
- Discern the different types of healthcare team practice.
- Discuss the current status of healthcare team practice in Nigeria.
- Contextualise the role of leadership within the contemporary healthcare system.
- Discuss the skills needed to lead heath care organisations and healthcare systems.
- Discuss the major leadership theories.
- Describe the five leadership styles that are relevant in contemporary healthcare setting.
- Describe the leadership skills needed to effectively manage conflicts within healthcare teams, organisations and systems.
- Discuss why some of the leadership theories in the West may not be externally valid in developing countries.
- List five core competencies that clinicians, irrespective of discipline, would need to be able to practice in the twenty-first century effectively.
- Discuss the non-clinical related contents needed in the Nigerian medical school curriculum to bring it up to the global standard.

J. A. Balogun (✉)
Chicago State University, Chicago, IL, USA

University of Medical Sciences, Ondo City, Nigeria

Centre of Excellence in Reproductive Health Innovation, University of Benin, Benin City, Nigeria
e-mail: jbalogun@csu.edu; jbalogun@unimed.edu.ng

62.1 Introduction

The modern-day healthcare practice was imported into the region now known as Nigeria over 500 years ago, through the trans-Sahara trade routes by European traders, explorers, colonial military and civilian administrators, and later missionaries. Today, the local, state and federal governments are responsible for healthcare delivery in the country. The federal government is responsible for funding the university teaching hospitals, federal medical centres, and specialist hospitals (tertiary healthcare), while the state government coordinates the general hospitals (secondary healthcare), and the local government operates the health centers and dispensaries (primary healthcare). In recent years, the private sector now plays a vital role in healthcare.

Having effective leaders is essential for healthcare teams, organisations and systems to achieve their primary goal of providing quality and efficient healthcare. To meet this primary goal, clinicians and chief executives of organisations and systems must understand the different organisation and leadership theories. The beginning of the twentieth century witnessed an increased interest in the study of leadership. Between 1940 and 1980 several leadership behavioural theories were postulated. Similarly, between 1950 and 1980 other leadership theories emerged that consider the employee's needs, environment and the task performed. In later years, the "interactional" leadership theory focused on the interaction and relationship of the leader with the followers. Another management approach that emerged from the study of business enterprise was the "supportive" leadership theory that affirmed that employees are happier and more satisfied when the leader is supportive and empathise at a personal level. Studies in the business enterprise have shown that when leaders are inspirational and competent, their followers are motivated and perform at high levels [1–6].

The Nigerian healthcare system is plagued by antiquated equipment, old facilities and incessant industrial actions by health workers agitating for better conditions of

F. Okonofua et al. (eds.), *Contemporary Obstetrics and Gynecology for Developing Countries*,
https://doi.org/10.1007/978-3-030-75385-6_62

service [7–9]. Low morale due to poor remuneration and detestable work condition combined to produce a health system that is inefficient with poor health outcomes [10]. The peril in the health sector has been attributed to the lack of administrative skills and poor management of human and fiscal resources at all levels by chief medical officers, health commissioners and ministers; positions that are occupied predominately by physicians [11–14]. Unfortunately, the educational curriculum of medical schools in Nigeria lacks content in leadership and program administration [12–14].

Good knowledge of medicine and being an astute physician does not often translate into effective leadership in administering the affairs of large organisations or in steering the ship of the nation's healthcare system. Drawing examples from physicians in top administrative positions in Nigeria who have performed less creditably, Ojo and Akinwumi are of the opinion that most physicians in the leadership position are "bad managers" [12]. Thus, Nigeria desperately needs uncompromised visionary leaders with excellent administrative experiences that will address the multi-factorial challenges within the healthcare system.

Interdisciplinary healthcare teams, which are now a sine qua non-practice in developed nations, are universally recommended to promote genuine collaboration among healthcare providers [15–17]. Unfortunately, the practice is still nascent in many developing countries around the world. The health professions in Nigeria are divided and embroiled in territorial professional turf wars [13, 14]. In most clinical settings, there is limited communication or interaction among health professionals. This unacceptable situation is pervasive because interdisciplinary team dynamics, organisation and leadership theories are currently not taught in Nigerian medical schools. These curriculum deficits no doubt affect the ability of medical graduates to lead healthcare teams, large organisations, and systems effectively.

The first medical school in Nigeria was established in 1948 at the University College, Ibadan, as an affiliate campus of the University of London until 1962 when it gained full independent status. From inception, the medical school adopted the University of London medical curriculum, which was later exported to the other newly created medical schools [18]. For over six decades, no concerted effort was made to align the contents of the medical curriculum with global standards, despite appeals from several quarters [11–14, 18]. Meanwhile, the Nigerian healthcare system continues to crumble.

The purpose of this chapter is to contextualise the perceived weaknesses in the non-clinical aspect of the medical curriculum that currently impact graduate's ability to provide effective leadership for healthcare teams, large organisations, and systems.

62.2 Operational Definitions

- In this chapter, the term *leader* refers to the chief executive officer who inspires, motivates and directs the followers to achieve the defined goals of teams, organisations or systems.
- The *follower* is a member of healthcare teams, employee or subordinate in organisations or systems who reports to a leader.
- *Leadership*, also known as headship, is the chief executive officer or an individual in the position of authority who exerts power and influence on the followers.
- *Leadership style* is the behaviour of the chief executive officer or leader responsible for coordinating and administering the activities of teams, organisations or systems.
- *Organisation* is the group of people hired and assembled to accomplish well-defined goals.
- *Healthcare team* is a group of professionals with different clinical expertise working collaboratively to provide service to patients. Examples: cancer team, hospice team or poliomyelitis team. The traditional members of a healthcare team are physician, nurse, physiotherapist, occupational therapist and social worker.
- *Healthcare organisation* is an institution, hospital or centre that provides services to meet the health needs of the target population or community. It may be privately (for-profit) funded or owned by the government or non-government establishments. Examples: state general hospitals, university teaching hospitals, specialist hospitals, religious proprietary hospitals or non-governmental organisations.
- *Health system*, also referred to as the *healthcare system* or simply *system*, is a complex network of delivering healthcare services to citizens at the local, state or federal levels. Examples: local government health department, state ministry of health and the federal ministry of health.
- *Discipline* is the academic domain of knowledge such as medicine, dentistry, pharmacy, physiotherapy, etc.
- *Interdisciplinary* is when two or more disciplines come together to provide service to solve a patient problem or gather clinical information. For example, a child with a diagnosis of autism spectrum disorder and developmental delay in attaining the significant milestones will need a team of a paediatrician, physiotherapist, occupational therapist, speech-language pathologists and dietician to work together to treat the patient.
- *Interprofessional* is when two or more disciplines actively collaborate to learn together.

62.3 Differences Between Management and Administration

The term administration and management are often used in error interchangeably. There is a clear distinction between the two concepts. Management, on the one hand, is the skill of motivating and directing followers to work together in a profit-making business enterprise. On the other hand, administration emphasises the formulation of policies, development and implementation of strategic plan in a government or military establishments, hospitals, religious and educational organisations [6]. Management is under the operational control of an administration. For parsimony of time and space purposes, the significant differences between the two terms are summarised in Table 62.1.

62.4 Types of Healthcare Team Practice

Healthcare practice is a collaborative team effort that is critical to patient care, safety and optimum treatment outcomes. The more the members of a health team work together, the better they can provide the best quality care possible. Each professional in a healthcare team serves a unique role, perspectives and expertise. Some team members diagnose disease, and others are experts who treat illness or care for individuals with physical disabilities and emotional needs.

Over the last half century, healthcare practice all over the world has evolved from the "lone-ranger, I know it all" practitioner to an interdisciplinary team approach; a concept that is alien to the Nigeria healthcare system. Therefore, an opportunity to discuss it further here. The following are the different types of healthcare team practices around the world:

Table 62.1 Differences between administration and management [6]

	Basis of difference	Administration	Management
1	Application	Government or military establishments, hospitals, religious and educational organisations	For profit business enterprise associated with production of goods or delivery of services
2	Scope	Systematic process of administering an organisation by leaders	Managing people and resources
3	Function	Determinative – decisive	Executive
4	Level of authority	Top level	Middle and lower level
5	Focus	Formulation of policy, setting objectives, allocation of budget and effective use of resources	Implementation of policy and putting plans into actions
6	Competence of the leader	Administrative skills	Technical skills

1. The multidisciplinary team consists of a group of professionals from various health disciplines who provide service to the patient, but their care does not overlap. Each professional providing service to the patient has separate treatment plans and rarely communicate or interact with one another. Consequently, multidisciplinary team practices are not coordinated and can therefore not achieve the goal of efficient delivery of health services.
2. The interdisciplinary team consists of healthcare professionals from diverse fields who organise their effort towards a common goal for the patient. Each professional is involved in establishing a treatment plan designed to achieve optimum outcomes. The composition of the team varies depending on the diagnosis, but the patient is always a member of the team. The purpose of the interdisciplinary team approach is to enhance the structure and consistent communication among the various health disciplines and to establish, prioritise and achieve treatment goals. Successful implementation of interdisciplinary care depends on the administrative skill of the team leader and the cooperation of the professionals within the team. Empirical evidence has demonstrated that positive health outcomes and quality services occur through the utilisation of an interdisciplinary team approach to healthcare.
3. The intradisciplinary team consists of a group of professionals who are all from the same profession, such as three physicians from different specialties and expertise collaborating on the same case.
4. The transdisciplinary team is composed of various healtcare professionals cooperating across different fields to improve healthcare through practice and research.
5. Cross-organizational team is an example of a transdisciplinary team in the workplace designed to break down divisional, functional, or departmental lines and cause collaboration in an important project is a cross-organizational team.

A systematic review of the literature by Nancarrow and associates identified ten attributes that are paramount for effective interdisciplinary teamwork. The characteristics are (1) competent and inspirational leader; (2) clear communication structures; (3) personal rewards and capacity building opportunities; (4) clear organisation procedures and adequate resources and (5) appropriate clinical expertise by the members. Also crucial for productive teamwork are (1) conducive work environment; (2) attributes of the individual team member that supports collaborative partnership; (3) unambiguous organisation and team vision statement; (4) high standard of healthcare provided within the organisation and (5) team members' respect for the distinct clinical roles and responsibilities of their peers [15].

Organisation theorists [16] contended that the functioning of the interdisciplinary team will be cohesive and effective when each member of the group understands their expertise and knowledgeable about the clinical goals and treatment outcomes for each patient, including the roles of the other team members. Other organisation theorists affirmed that healthcare teams are more productive when members communicate respectfully and compassionately with one another and support the leader appointed to coordinate the services [17].

62.5 Current Status of Healthcare Team Practice in Nigeria

In Nigeria, there are 44 medical schools as of June 2021, with the majority offering degree programs in medicine, dentistry, pharmacy, physiotherapy, occupational therapy, optometry, radiography, medical laboratory science, environmental and community health, biomedical engineering, prosthesis and orthotics and nursing [18]. Presently, healthcare in Nigeria is primarily a solo (single discipline) practice. In most clinical settings, there is limited communication or interaction among the different professionals providing service for patients. Thus, for the most part, the healthcare service provided is fragmented and inefficient. Besides the lack of productive communication and interaction, the various professions are continually feuding, suspicious of one another, and jostling for supremacy [10–14]. Unfortunately, to the detriment of the individuals that they serve. The hatred and antagonism among the healthcare providers are inimical to effective health outcomes and unequivocally one of the significant banes of the Nigerian healthcare system.

One of the first empirically based study on interdisciplinary healthcare team in Nigeria was conducted in 2015 at the University of Nigeria Teaching Hospital Enugu and the Federal Teaching Hospital Abakaliki, in Ebonyi State [19]. The cross-sectional study investigated the attitudes of obstetricians and gynaecologists towards the team approach to healthcare. Of the 160 obstetricians and gynaecologists employed in both hospitals, 116 of them (73%) completed the survey. The investigation revealed that 74% of the respondents were aware of the interdisciplinary team concept and had a positive attitude towards team approach of delivery of healthcare. Unfortunately, only 29% of the knowledgeable respondents had received formal instruction on the interdisciplinary team during professional development. The authors concluded that the attitudes of the physicians are supportive of interdisciplinary team approach. The findings are encouraging because both attitudes and knowledge can change with appropriate educational intervention. Undoubtedly, the findings underscore the need to urgently revise the curricula of the medical and allied health professions in line with global best practice to include contents on the dynamics of the interdisciplinary team [20]. Additional qualitative and quantitative studies are needed to better understand the status and barriers against interdisciplinary healthcare team practice in Nigeria.

62.6 Leadership of Healthcare Team

Leadership is part and parcel of the interdisciplinary healthcare team, and the discipline that leads the team has historically been a contentious issue in the literature [21]. In the new landscape, physicians, who traditionally assumed the leadership of the healthcare team, are constantly challenged and required to balance changes in the industry along with new demands needed to lead teams effectively. With new laws, regulations and new payment models, healthcare professionals are required to work more collaboratively and adjust to new practice models in treating their patients. The long-established leadership beliefs are changing as physicians and other healthcare professionals are adapting to an interdisciplinary team-based treatment approach to deliver adequate service to their patients.

It is now recognised more widely in developed countries that what makes a physician a great clinician may not necessarily make them a great leader. Dr. Atul Gawande, a physician in the USA, stated it best when he opined that "healthcare is moving towards teams, but that collides with the image of the all-knowing, heroic healer. We've celebrated cowboys, but what we need is more pit crews. There's still a lot of silo mentality in healthcare." The same point of view was echoed by Dr. Thomas Lee, also from the USA, who affirmed that the problem with healthcare is that "people like me – doctors (mostly men) in our fifties and beyond, who learned medicine when it was more art and less finance. The only way to ensure quality was to adopt high personal standards and then meet them. Now at many healthcare institutions and practices, we are in charge. Also, that's a problem because healthcare today needs a fundamentally different approach – and a new breed of leaders" [22].

In the new healthcare landscape, the team leader at any stage naturally emerges during the different phases of the hospitalisation and rehabilitation services provided to the individuals. Typically, the healthcare professional with the unique beneficial clinical skill, interest or knowledge in a particular case will take on the leadership role. For example, during admission and the inpatient (hospitalisation) phases, the physician will assume the leadership role to make a medical diagnosis, but the leadership may change as the treatment plan progresses to the rehabilitation phase. Similarly, a dentist may lead an interdisciplinary team managing a patient with temporomandibular joint pain. In the same vein, a physiotherapist may lead a team caring for individuals with autism or poliomyelitis during the rehabilitation phase.

62.7 Leadership of Healthcare Organisations and Systems

Globally, the healthcare industry is in transition, and new leadership is needed to motivate the employees to deliver efficient and quality care. The leader of the healthcare organisations and systems is now required to have appropriate administrative skills to prevent intra- and interprofessional conflicts and to increase employee productivity and financial solvency.

In developed countries, the leadership of healthcare organisations and systems is no longer the exclusive domain of any particular professional group, but all members of the healthcare team are potential leaders [23]. The existing literature has emphasised the relevance of effective leadership in the delivery of a high-quality healthcare system that provides safe and efficient care consistently. Unfortunately, the administration of healthcare organisations, because of its unique characteristic, is very complex, and some observers claim it faces unique contextual challenges.

The early leadership theories were developed from the study of large organisations in business and later applied to the healthcare system. A recent study by Sfantou and associates [24] found that leadership styles are determinant of the quality of healthcare services delivered. The authors concluded that leadership is a core element needed for an efficient and well-integrated healthcare system, both from the standpoint of the patients and healthcare professionals [24].

In general, healthcare professionals around the world are not well prepared to lead large organisations and systems. In the past decades, professional organisations in developed countries have recognised this problem, and curricula revision has been implemented to address the perceived deficiencies. In the UK, a Medical Leadership Competency Framework was developed to better prepare physicians for leadership roles. The model was widely embraced by the medical establishments, regulatory bodies and educational institutions as the "gold standard" for leadership. Similarly, a Clinical Leadership Competency Framework was formulated from the Medical Leadership Competency Framework to include leadership competencies in the undergraduate, postgraduate and continuing professional education of all regulated health professions [23].

Other countries such as New Zealand and Australia have revised the curricula of their undergraduate health programs to include contents in leadership for physicians, nurses and allied health professionals. Some of these curricula reforms have similar features to the UK's leadership frameworks and its associated strategies [23].

Unfortunately, despite the global recognition of the importance of having competent leaders to achieve efficient and quality healthcare, significant barriers to the management of organisations and systems abound. Such challenges include low morale arising from poor remuneration, lack of interdisciplinary confidence and pervasive cynicism, poor communication and limited administrative preparation for leadership roles. Other barriers include lack of vision by the leaders, the limited commitment by the governing board, poor interdisciplinary collaboration, role conflicts, rejection of the "leader" as unacceptable impost and resistance to change [23]. Although considerable global improvement in power-sharing within healthcare organisations and systems have occurred, there continues to be a significant disconnect between the professional groups and bureaucratic imperatives, and the debate on who is best qualified to lead healthcare teams, organisations and systems continue.

62.8 Organisational Theories

Knowledge of organisation theories is of paramount importance for leaders of healthcare teams, organisations and systems to be successful in discharging their duties. Organisational theories study the effect of the social relationships between the followers and their behaviours on the whole organisation. It also explores the impact of internal and external business environment including political, legal and cultural norms on the organisation. Organisational theories study not only the relationships between the followers but also their overall effect on the performance of the organisation. The administrative structure of the organisation plays a critical role in determining the effectiveness and success of any enterprise. And organisational theorists are positioned to identify the appropriate structure that is efficient to deal with any establishment-specific problems [25]. The six primary organisational theories are presented next.

1. The classical theory is the traditional approach that emphasises the importance of the organisation more than the employees. The theory is built on the accounting model that considers the organisation as a machine and the employees as the different parts of the device. The organisation structure is well integrated, but the authority and control are vested on the central body only. The theory considers employees to be relatively homogeneous, unmodifiable and relatively stable when there is a change

within the organisation. The classical approach is more concerned with productivity levels than the welfare of the employees and focuses on detecting errors within the organisation and correcting them immediately. While some classical theorists emphasised how the organisation can be made more efficient with the use of technology, others stressed the importance of the structural factors and that employees collectively can be more efficient. The classical theory considers the employees as a means of production.

2. The scientific management theory popularised by Fredrick Winslow Taylor, often called the "Taylorism," follows the bottom-up approach and is widely applied in engineering science at the production floor levels. It focuses on improving the production efficiency of the organisation by intensive use of mechanisation and automation rather than the broader behaviour of the employees in the organisation. In the performance of routine tasks, the employees are considered adjuncts to machines. The theory entails the work performed on the production floor which is repetitive and entirely different from the other functions performed within the organisation. The employees on the production floor perform cyclical, repetitive tasks that do not require complex problem-solving activity, but the imposition of standardisation of working condition is needed. The theory recommends that employees should be hired and trained using scientific principles, including time, motion analysis and fatigue studies, to determine the optimum amount of work for each employee.
3. Administrative theory developed by Henri Fayol follows the top-down approach which contends that organisational management is more important than the human and behavioural factors. Thus, the focus is on the departmentalisation of the organisational structure and how well the employees are organised to accomplish the tasks assigned to them. The theory first emphasises how to improve and standardise the effectiveness of the management before the operational-level employees, who are later informed of the changes, and how to implement them in their routine jobs. The administrative theory is contrary to the scientific management theory which emphasises the improvement of the efficiency of the employees at the operational level first which in turn enhances the effectiveness of the management.
4. The bureaucratic theory, developed by Max Weber and regarded as the father of bureaucracy organisation philosophy, emphasises the structure and administrative process of the organisation. The bureaucratic organisation has a hierarchy of authority, specialised workforce, standardised rules, regulations, processes, procedures and patterns that are developed to reduce the complexity of the functioning of the enterprise. Max Weber affirmed that bureaucratic organisation is the most reasonable means to exercise appropriate control over employees. Bureaucratic organisations have a clear hierarchy in the lines of authority, and the employees know the immediate leader to whom they are directly accountable. The evaluation of employees' performance is against specified criteria, and promotion is merit-based. Weber's bureaucratic theory posits that clear organisation structure with unambiguous organisational lines of authority is required to have a productive workplace. This line of reasoning is a significant contribution to the classical organisational theory. A frequent critic is that bureaucratic organisations are detached and impersonal.
5. The neoclassical theory is the refined version of the classical theory which integrated behavioural sciences in management. It espouses the view that the organisation is a social system that its performance is not affected by human actions. The classical theory focusses on physiological and mechanical factors and considers them as the prime determinant of organisational efficiency. Unfortunately, on the evaluation of the organisational effectiveness, despite the positive influence of the physiological and mechanical variables, the anticipated increase in work performance was not evoked. This paradoxical finding led to the formation of the neoclassical theory which primarily focused on the employees in the organisation. This approach is called the "behavioural theory of organisation" or "human relations" approach in organisations. The neoclassical theory asserts that employees are motivated differently based on their specific needs. And excellent communication is a critical yardstick to measure the efficiency of the information conveyed to and from the different levels of the organisation. Teamwork, which can be achieved through a behavioural approach when employees interact with each other, is an essential requisite for the effective functioning of the organisation.
6. The modern theory, developed by scientists from different fields, integrates the valuable concepts of the classical theory with the social and behavioural sciences. The theory asserts that organisation is a dynamic system influenced by changes in both the internal and external climate. The modern approach considers the organisation as an open system which is dynamic and consistently interacts with its environment to sustain and grow the market. Thus, the modern method differs from the classical approach which considers the organisation as a closed system. The contemporary theory affirms that organisation is adaptive and adjusts itself to the changing climate because it is an open system, whose growth and the changes in the environment determine its sustenance. The modern theory covers the multilevel and multidimensional aspects of the organisation. That is, it encompasses both the micro (internal) and macro (external) environment of the organisation. The modern theory considers multiple variables which

could be interrelated or interdependent concurrently. The approach emphasised the importance of excellent communication and integration of the interests of the employees and the establishment as requisites for the smooth operation of the organisation [25].

62.9 Leadership Theories

Leaders exert different types of powers – legitimate power, reward power, coercive power, expert power and referent power. Legitimate power is the authority bestowed on a leader under the position hierarchy. Reward power is the ability of a leader to provide or curb tangible and intangible perquisites and perks. The ability of a leader to penalise and discipline followers is coercive power. Expert power is the specialised knowledge and skills that a leader possesses. Referent power originates from follower's respect, admiration and loyalty towards the leader [26].

Today, many different theories of leadership have emerged [27]. The old arguments focused primarily on the qualities that distinguished leaders from followers, while recent investigations examined other variables such as situational factors and competence. The following 12 theories which mostly evolved from the study of business enterprise have influenced the leadership approaches now commonly applied in healthcare teams, organisations and systems.

1. The "great man" leadership theory is the first leadership theory to be conceptualised, and it assumes that leadership capacity is an inherent male quality, especially concerning military leadership. The theory posited that great leader is born, not made, and portrays them as heroic, mythical and destined to lead when needed.
2. The trait leadership theory is closely aligned with the "great man" theory, and it affirmed that people inherit certain qualities and characteristics that make them better leaders. The approach often identifies some personality or behavioural attributes shared by heroic leaders. Detractors of this theory have argued that if specific traits are critical features of administration, it is difficult to explain why certain people who possess those qualities are not effective leaders. This schism is one of the challenges in using the trait theory to define effective leadership.
3. The behavioural leadership theory, which is rooted in behaviourism, assumes that great leaders are made, not born. The approach focused on the actions of leaders, not on their mental abilities or internal states, and posited that they learn to become effective leaders through teaching, observation, mentoring and shadowing.
4. Transformational leadership theory emphasises the well-held belief that employees work more effectively when the organisation mission and vision statements are communicated in a manner that is exciting, meaningful and empowering with a collective purpose. Transformational leaders can motivate performance beyond expectations through their ability to influence attitudes.
5. The collaborative leadership theory emphasises the importance of communication of information to organisation leaders and employees for them to make appropriate informed decisions. The theory assumes that collaboration is a positive process that occurs when employees work together towards mutual symbiosis benefit. Collaborative communication strategies reduce organisation administrative complexity by promoting dialogue and interaction among multiple stakeholders and sharing of knowledge and experiences. Collaborative leadership fosters a synergistic work environment by encouraging the various parties to work together to implement effective practices and processes that promote understanding of the different cultures within the organisation and facilitate integration and interdependency among numerous stakeholders. Shared visions and values unify employees, and the synergistic working practices achieved can produce outcomes that are better than the sum of the individual efforts. To raise the levels of motivation and nurture interdependency between the different healthcare practitioners, the organisation leaders must first model collaborative behaviours.
6. The shared leadership theory posited that highly qualified autonomous healthcare professionals with direct responsibility for their patients are opposed to authoritarian leadership style but readily embrace the shared leadership style – a team management system that empowers personnel in decision-making by offering an opportunity for employees to manage and develop within the organisation. Numerous studies have shown that shared leadership style is effective in improving the work environment because it fosters employees' job satisfaction. The promotion of effective collaborative relationships through support and task delegation encourages shared governance, continuous workplace learning and the development of productive working relationships. Ideally, shared leadership style fosters greater autonomy and improved healthcare outcomes with employees adopting leadership behaviours. Shared leadership in an organisation presumes a good working relationship between managers and staff and continuous evaluation is required to be responsive to the continually changing healthcare challenges. Barriers to developing shared leadership include a poor team ethos, high workload and staff turnover rates, monotonous work, lack of responsibility and insufficient goal setting.

7. The distributed leadership theory argued that as a result of globalisation, large corporations have come to recognise that trust and initiative are spread widely by becoming less hierarchical and more collaborative in their leadership approach. The goal of the distributed leadership style is to create a system where employees can complement one another's strengths and offset their weakness, with leadership distributed throughout the organisation. The approach requires four interdependent characteristics – sensemaking, relating, visioning and inventing. Sensemaking is the ability to understand the continually changing business environment and interpret the ramifications of changes within an organisation. Relating is the ability to build trusting relationships, balance advocacy with inquiry and cultivate networks of supportive confidants. Visioning is creating credible and compelling images of the desired future that those in the organisation can work towards, and inventing is creating new ways of approaching tasks or overcoming seemingly insurmountable problems. Effective leaders are able to identify their capabilities, strengths and weaknesses.
8. Ethical leadership theory espoused the view that leaders exhibit behaviours that impact the lives of their staff, healthcare outcomes and the fate of an organisation. Such leaders influence their employees by (1) creating enthusiasm for risky strategies; (2) changing underlying beliefs and values and (3) making decisions that favour some at the expense of others. Unfortunately, by practicing such effective leadership behaviours, in some instances, the leader may unintentionally influence employees to engage in crimes and unethical acts. A good leader must have good intentions with sound moral values and behaviours that respect employee's rights.
9. The situational leadership theory embraced the view that no one single leadership style is adaptable to all circumstances. And that leadership style or strategy should be versatile to address the situation at hand. The theory argued that effective leaders often adapt their style to the tasks at hand and continuously explore factors that may impact the realisation of the primary goals of the team, organisation or system [28].
10. The interactional leadership theory which emanated in the 1970s asserted that the work environment, organisational value system and situational complexities influence the emergence of leadership. The theory argues that the way team members or employees interact with one another is of critical importance in setting the climate of the work environment and have a significant impact on morale and productivity. The theory encourages leaders to interact (face-to-face contact) with followers on a regular basis and dedicate time to exploring the interactions among team members or followers and how it could impact the work environment [29, 30].
11. Supportive leadership theory which emanated in the 1990s asserted that leaders do not merely delegate tasks and receive feedback from their followers but must support them until the job is completed. The negative side to supportive theory is that the leader will work with the followers until they are empowered and adequately skilled in handling tasks with minimal supervision. This management approach requires significant time investment by the leader [31]. The primary tenets of supportive leadership theory are that leadership keeps the channels of communication with followers open, accepts corrections, criticisms and recommendations. Furthermore, supportive leaders do not only set rules and regulations, but they listen to complaints from followers and help them cope with stressful events. The leader is empathetic and shows a high degree of sensitivity towards followers' concerns and teach them how to deal with it in the future [31, 32]. Supportive leadership theory encourages leaders to promote teamwork but also make their expectations known and remain committed to the team members and the project at hand. Leadership should foster quality relationships with followers by organising team building events where members can bond. It has been debunked that supportive leadership style may not be applicable in every setting but is suitable for flat organisations [31].
12. Functional results-oriented healthcare leadership theory emphasised the challenges that leaders face in the complex milieu of the modern healthcare organisation which includes different and high staff turnover rate, changing individual needs and expectations and the high cost of healthcare services. This situation requires organisation leaders to consider the needs of the broader patient population and the capacity to deliver high-quality care. The functional results-oriented leadership style emphasised effective and efficient organisation processes. Consequently, the leadership must have specific role and skills necessary to achieve the desired results of the group and in meeting the needs of the organisation in three areas: the employees, team and tasks.

Of the 12 leadership theories reviewed, the situational leadership theory is more practical because the leader can adapt to match the situation at hand and continuously assess the internal and external climate that impacts the functioning of the organisation.

62.10 Contemporary Leadership Styles in the Changing World

In the modern world, five leadership styles are most widely embraced in the healthcare setting – charismatic, transformational, visionary, transactional and servant leadership styles.

They all involve leaders appealing to their followers' commitment to fulfilling challenging missions in a vastly changing healthcare environment [33]. Charismatic leaders have natural ability and charming personality to attract and inspire followers to commit to a cause. Charismatic leaders have a dramatic influence on the behaviours of their followers. There is a positive relationship between charismatic leadership and follower's performance and satisfaction. Visionary leaders have the unique ability to predict the future and inspire the followers to achieve the jointly set goals.

Transactional leaders allocate contractual tasks to followers and expect prompt delivery of results based on the assumption that rewards and punishment are key motivators in the workplace. Servant leaders are not overtly noticeable, but they operate from the background and serve the followers by upholding the "do as I do" principle. They lead democratically through the participatory decision-making process and allow followers to take credit for the organisation effectiveness; a stark departure from the dominant traditional leadership style of telling followers what to do. Transformational leaders have vision and creativity and make positive changes within the organisation to enhance high performance. They motivate and improve morale by acting as role models to their followers.

A systematic review by Sfantou and associates [24] investigated the relationship between the different leadership styles and selected healthcare quality outcomes from 18 relevant articles. The study revealed that leadership style is strongly related to quality healthcare services and associated measures (moderate-severe pain, physical restraint use, high-risk residents having pressure ulcers, the catheter in the bladder). The "resonant" leaders positively influenced the quality of safety measures by decreasing the number of medication errors and 30-day mortality. The "task-oriented" leaders had higher levels of quality care based on the assessment made by relatives and staff. The "formal" leadership style was associated with learning minor and moderate safety events, while "informal" leaders presented no safety effect. Patients are generally more satisfied with "transactional" leaders. The latter finding is discordant with results from previous studies that found no association between leadership style and individual satisfaction [24].

62.11 Studies on Leadership from Nigeria

A dose of caution is warranted when trying to extrapolate the results of studies conducted in the West to developing countries. Due to cultural differences, the findings of studies emanating from the West may not be externally valid in patriarchal societies where the male gender and old age are more revered than the female gender and youth. The moderating correlates of gender, age and leadership effectiveness require investigation in patriarchal societies in Africa and the Middle East.

A plethora of studies on leadership in higher education, government, industry, trade union, small scale and banking sectors in Nigeria have been published [34–44]. On the other hand, no single peer-reviewed study on leadership in the health sector was found after exhaustive literature searches of the PUBMED and the Cumulative Index to Nursing and Allied Health Literature databases using the keywords of Nigeria, leadership, healthcare teams, organisations and systems. Given the absence of any research on leadership in the Nigerian health sector, qualitative and quantitative studies are desperately needed to corroborate or refute the theoretical leadership constructs developed in the West.

In 2013, an ethnographic study investigated the leadership practices of government officers in the Eastern region of Nigeria and found that most of the leaders and policymakers lack effective leadership skills for their position. And the system is riddled with high-level corruption, bad governance, political instability and a cyclical legitimacy crisis that currently make the followers not to have confidence in their political leaders and political system [44].

The effect of cultural norms on leadership effectiveness was investigated in 2014 by Amos and associates [45]. The study found that the Nigerian culture of interdependency, "godfatherism" and nepotism contributes greatly to their leader's corrupt practices. The authors averred that the Nigerian "mind, culture and value system need to be purified" for national development to occur.

Leadership theorists from the West contended that ethical leaders who exhibit empathy, trustworthiness, selfless attitude and focus on collective mission tend to maintain optimal leader-follower relationships. On the contrary, Njoku [43] argued that the mindset of the average Nigerian worker is centred on personal rather than group goals, and followers perceive an empathetic, selfless and considerate attitude of a leader as a weakness and that Nigerian employees generally seek ways to enrich themselves instead of improving their organisation [43]. Indeed, one single leadership style may not be practical to get Nigeria out of its national malaise. A persuasive and charismatic leader capable of changing the political structure and mindset of the people will be the most successful in moving the nation forward.

62.12 Conflict Resolution Strategies

Conflict is a pervasive foe within healthcare teams, organisations and systems. Despite the recognised importance of the need for collaboration, only a small proportion of time in healthcare is devoted to genuine collaborative efforts. The healthcare team leader and administrator of large health organisations and systems must be astute at conflict management. The most common sources of conflict in healthcare teams and organisations are intra- and intergroup misunderstanding, the aberrant behaviours of individual professionals, poor communication and unclear organisational structures. The leader must first be able to identify the source of the disagreement and the major power players at the centre of the dispute to be effective in diffusing a conflict.

Usually, conflict develops from underlying latent issues which often progress to perceived conflict (where the problem becomes apparent) and subsequently manifest the behavioural/action phase), and lastly the aftermath of the battle. The leader can utilise any of the following approaches to creating a positive outcome for all feuding parties – compromise, accommodation, collaboration, bargaining/negotiation, mediation, facilitating communication, seeking consensus and engendering vision to aid the resolution of the conflict at all stages of its development.

There are essential qualities that the leaders of healthcare teams, organisations and systems must possess while managing a crisis-riddled and fast-changing practice landscape. The leader must be (1) be an independent thinker who understands the emerging healthcare market; (2) passionate about meeting the needs of the followers; (3) a change agent for their organisation; (4) able to motivate and inspire the team members; and (5) able to run a lean, high-quality organisation. Most importantly, the leader must be familiar with the following strategies needed to create harmony and to prevent conflicts within a team:

1. Set some ground rules during the first and subsequent meetings to address what process will be taken to resolve disputes and inform the parties involved that their ideas are valid and will not be dismissed outright.
2. Understand destructive conflicts that develop when no resolution is in sight or the issue cannot be resolved. The leader must not slip into the fray but must try to recognise the ongoing team dynamics.
3. Resolve all conflicts as quickly as possible before it festers.
4. Understand the entire story and the perspectives of all parties involved to address differences of opinions and to prevent miscommunication or misunderstanding.
5. Make compromise between parties a goal and must create harmony among followers.
6. Must avoid falling into group thinking mentality that will suppress the views of other members.
7. Must not try to change the unique ideas and forms of expression of the team members as this may lead to resentment.
8. Propose alternatives by listing the benefits of other ideas, but ultimately must accept the fact that followers may disagree with the outcome of the resolution efforts [22, 46–48].

62.13 The Much-Needed Medical Education Reforms, Anticipated Benefits and Barriers

As of June 2020, only 3 of the 44 medical schools in Nigeria have embraced the collaborative philosophy of education. The challenges in the healthcare system highlighted in this chapter underscores the need to reform the medical curriculum [18]. Globally, there are three primary instructional methods used in medical and allied health education – discipline-specific (non-collaborative), multidisciplinary and interprofessional approaches. The terms multidisciplinary and interprofessional education is often used in error interchangeably; therefore, the distinction between them needs clarification here.

Multidisciplinary education combines students from two or more professions in learning a topic or offers the entire course in tandem, but there is no active real-life purposeful, collaborative learning among the students. Interprofessional education is a student-centred dynamic learning approach which brings together students from two or more professions collaborate during the learning process to break down the artificial barriers that exist across disciplines. In 1988, the World Health Organization (WHO) defined interprofessional education as "the process by which a group of students or workers from the health-related occupations with different backgrounds learn together during certain periods of their education, with interaction as the important goal, to collaborate in providing promotive, preventive, curative, rehabilitative, and other health-related services" [49]. Of the three instructional methods, the interprofessional strategy is best suited to deliver efficient healthcare services.

Although the discussion of interprofessional education concept began to take roots during the 1960s in the USA, Canada, Australia, England, Germany, Jamaica and Mexico, its implementation is relatively contemporary [50]. Multiple and complex forces influenced the development of interprofessional education in different countries around the world. Today, the concept is shared globally among international organisations and task forces [50].

In 2001, the Institute of Medicine in the USA in a landmark document titled "To Err is Human: Building a Safer Health System," called for the implementation of interprofessional teams in healthcare to improve quality care and patient safety [51]. Two years later, in another report, the Institute of Medicine echoed the nexus between interprofessional collaboration and healthcare quality and urged medical and allied health educators to adopt interprofessional instructional methods in their institutions [52]. The report proposed five core competencies that all health sciences disciplines should train their entry-level students to be able to

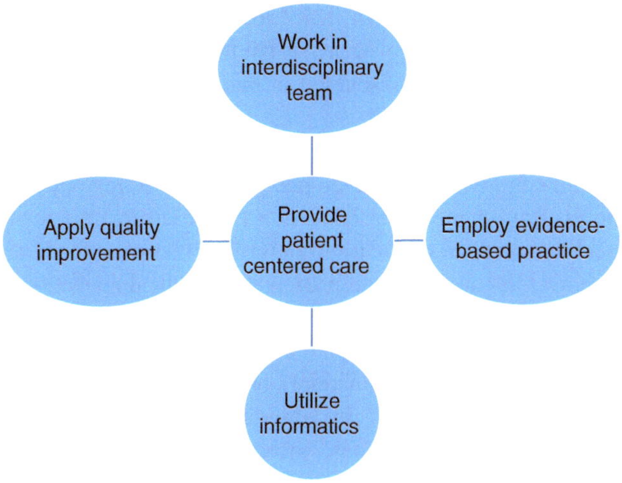

Fig. 62.1 Five core skills needed to practice effectively in the twenty-first-century healthcare system

practice effectively in the twenty-first-century healthcare system. The recommendation calls for revision of the curriculum to ensure all entry-level graduates can work in an interdisciplinary team, provide patient-centred care, employ evidence-based practice, apply quality improvement strategies to mitigate medical errors and utilise informatics to communicate effectively (Fig. 62.1).

In providing patient-centred care, the clinician must always respect and value patients' expressed needs, differences and preferences. They must listen to, communicate with and educate patients, relieve their pain and suffering and share decision-making and management with the other healthcare team members. Also, the clinician must continuously advocate disease prevention and promote wellness, healthy lifestyles, including a focus on community health. And must work in interdisciplinary teams by cooperating, collaborating, communicating, integrating and coordinating care continuously and reliably. At all times, the clinician must utilise evidence-based practice by combining the best research with clinical expertise and considering the patient values for optimum care and engaging in ongoing research activities.

The clinician must apply quality improvement skills to identify medical errors and hazards in the clinical environment and implement safety design principles by standardising and simplifying operations. Understanding and assessing the quality of care in terms of structure, process and outcomes reflect patient and community needs. Must design and test interventions that change processes and systems of care to improve quality. Finally, the clinician must utilise information technology skills to communicate, manage knowledge and prevent medical error. The five core competencies described should be included in all healthcare education programs' accreditation standards without further delay.

Today, these five core competencies are integrated into the accreditation standards of health professions in the USA. In Nigeria, the origin of multidisciplinary medical education started at the University of Ibadan in the early 1970s, later at the University of Ife (now Obafemi Awolowo University) in the 1980s and more recently in 2015 at the University of Medical Sciences, Ondo. In the three medical schools, the curriculum mandates medical, dental, physiotherapy and nursing students take anatomy, physiology and biochemistry courses together [54]. Unfortunately, the multidisciplinary learning experience in the three universities never extended to the clinical courses. Consequently, the full potential of interprofessional education was never realised in the country.

As a means to promote the understanding of the roles and responsibilities of the healthcare team and to facilitate better communication, and ultimately foster the well-being of patients, the implementation of the interprofessional experience must begin early in the curriculum [53]. To engender genuine collaboration early in the medical curriculum, the preclinical courses (anatomy, biochemistry, physiology) should be fashioned into credit units. The interprofessional curriculum approach will allow students from the different health disciplines take some of their classes in tandem as dictated by their curriculum pattern. In the first clinical year, the students should be provided structured case study reviews and taught organisation and leadership theories and program administration [11–14, 18]. The clinical clerkship experience will facilitate interaction among the faculty members and students from the different professions during ward rounds and community outreach events. To effectuate the anticipated benefits, only experienced faculty members who model effective interdisciplinary collaboration should participate in the proposed clinical instructional activities.

The actualisation of interprofessional education in Nigerian medical schools will (1) force the students to consider other viewpoints and develop transferable critical thinking and synthesis skills; (2) enable students to consolidate their learning by synthesising ideas from diverse perspectives and by exploring alternative ways of knowledge acquisition and (3) motivate students to pursue new knowledge outside their discipline. The institutional change will allow students to cover topics in more depth because they will approach the problem utilising their diverse training and life experiences. The experience will also develop the students' research skills with potential for greater creativity. These developments will create a positive learning environment and foster mutual respect between the members of the healthcare team [20, 55]. These anticipated benefits in its totality will produce the competent leaders that Nigeria desperately needs to manage its healthcare organisations and systems.

The proposed seismic change may improve the quality of communication among members of the healthcare team and modulate the disharmony and conflicts among the health professionals. The move will go a long way in sanitising the health sector by decreasing the stereotyping that exists among the different health professions. It will also lead to a more effective healthcare system that will reduce the mortality rates of infants and improve quality of life and life expectancy of Nigerians.

There are six daunting logistical challenges to overcome in the implementation of interprofessional education in Nigeria. First, due to time constraints, adding new information to any curriculum is always a contentious issue among faculty. Second, internal politics and turf protection among the faculty are plausible reasons for inaction. Third, for self-preservation purposes, faculty members who want to maintain the status quo will sabotage any attempt at curriculum reform. Fourth, the paradigm shift may generate unfair competition for discipline identities, values and cultures. Fifth, the introduction of interprofessional education initially might further promote the stereotyping of other professions, with the potential for interdisciplinary conflicts. Finally, given that a few health disciplines have no collaboration experience, bringing these professions along to embrace the new way of doing things will be a challenge to overcome.

The incessant industrial strike by the health workers has been the bane of quality health services in Nigeria. Ineffective leadership, deplorable conditions of service and salary and the failure of the government to implement agreements are the root causes of the strikes [13, 14]. Other critics affirmed that the persistent industrial action is due to disagreements between physicians and the other health occupations over salary levels and pay, the leadership of teaching hospitals and appointment of the Minister of Health. Two commissions have been constituted by the federal government to address the intractable dilemma, but they were both unsuccessful in resolving the disputes [11]. Until both parties come to a mutually acceptable position, the health system will continue to experience disruption of services, and the Nigerian people will continue to suffer from the aftermath.

62.14 Non-clinical Related Curriculum Weaknesses

Given the myriad of problems in the healthcare system, it is astonishing that the 1948 British medical curriculum imported to the country has not undergone any significant content revision despite the repeated appeals from different quarters to reform [11–14, 18]. Clearly, there are other non-clinical related areas of weakness in the medical curriculum beyond those so far discussed in this chapter that must be considered.

Many medical graduates in Nigeria are finding it difficult to find employment and even postgraduate training opportunities. Entrepreneurship education is needed to free newly qualified medical graduates from the shackles of dependency on government jobs. Entrepreneurship medical education is a vehicle for training students about innovations in technology, development of therapeutic tool and conversion of creative ideas into commercial products [56, 57]. The entrepreneurship course in Nigeria should emphasise the business aspects of medicine, including the nuts and bolts of how to start and operate a private practice. If this proposal is implemented, it has the potential to curb unemployment and promote self-actualisation and financial independence of newly qualified medical graduates.

The University of Medical Sciences, Ondo City is the, first and so far, only medical school in Nigeria that has incorporated entrepreneurship contents into all their undergraduate curricula. This feat is commendable because, even in developed countries, the inclusion of entrepreneurship in medical education is relatively new. As of 2016, only 13 of the 175 (141 MD and 34 DO degree-granting) medical schools in the USA (7.4%) have integrated entrepreneurship content in their curriculum. In 2018, the School of Medicine at Case Western Reserve University debuted an innovative entrepreneurship course in the preclinical year that offers biweekly seminar and a mentored project. The Feinberg School of Medicine at Northwestern University also offers a six-month interdisciplinary course that introduces the students to the development of medical technologies. Similarly, the School of Medicine at the University of Michigan develops an entrepreneurship course to teach surgical innovation.

In the USA, the Accreditation Council for Graduate Medical Education has approved the training of residents in quality improvement, but entrepreneurship education is yet to be incorporated fully into the undergraduate and residency curricula [56]. In the UK, about 100 newly qualified medical graduates in 2017 completed a "clinical entrepreneur training program" offered by the National Health System in collaboration with Health Education, England. Today, many of the physicians have transformed their creative ideas into innovative commercial products, apps and services to improve healthcare and promote learning [57, 58].

Clinical practice in Nigeria has evolved in scope over the years, and the roles of physicians have grown from a healthcare provider to research and teaching [12]. However, it is no secret that the standard of instruction in the medical schools is not at par with the norm in other parts of the world. The university system often assumed that being an expert clinician will translate into an effective teacher. This assumption is far from the truth, as most clinicians are ineffective in the classroom. Unfortunately, lecturers employed in medical schools rarely receive formal instruction in the fundamental principles of teaching. This paradox is unacceptable because no one will allow a teacher to perform surgery. So, why let a physician who has no andragogy experience teach students? We need to understand that teaching is a profession and, like the practice of any occupation, requires training to develop expertise and specialisation in andragogy.

Graduating competent and professional physicians is a complicated learning experience that is influenced by both the physical resources and the clinical and instructional expertise of the faculty employed to teach the students. The poor quality of medical education in Nigeria has been attributed to the curriculum deficiencies in teaching. Thus, the justification to develop a course that will teach the following fundamental elements of andragogy: evidence-based teaching, learning domains, Bloom's taxonomy, curriculum mapping, program learning objectives, course and syllabus objectives development, and program assessment.

Most physicians employed in the top administrative position in government establishments in Nigeria have no basic knowledge of the principles of finance. It is therefore not surprising that most large organisations and systems in Nigeria led by physicians are financially challenged. A course in health economics or healthcare financing that covers the fundamental elements of accounting, mobilisation of funds, distribution of financial risks, allocation and utilisation of services, provider payment incentives, costs, pricing, expenditure, essential drugs, supplies and human resource management, will address this apparent management deficit in the medical curriculum.

62.15 Summary

This chapter was written to provide clinicians, irrespective of discipline, the primary leadership and administrative knowledge needed to be a successful leader of healthcare teams, organisations or systems. A curious health professional seeking more advanced knowledge on any of the topics covered in this chapter can consult the appropriate references cited.

Based on the multitudes of problems in the Nigerian healthcare system, an overhauled of the medical curriculum is warranted. The revised curriculum should include contents in the five interprofessional core competencies discussed in this chapter: organisation and leadership theories, program administration, healthcare financing, essential drugs, supplies and human resource management, entrepreneurship and andragogy. Implementation of this recommendation will foster interdisciplinary work and improve the quality of medical education and healthcare delivery. As the first step towards change, both the National Universities Commission and the professional regulatory board should include the above contents in their accreditation standards.

References

1. Van Wagner K. 8 major leadership theories. 2008. Available at http://unpan1.un.org/intradoc/groups/public/documents/APCITY/UNPAN030550.pdf. Accessed 2 Feb 2019.
2. Cherry K. The major leadership theories. 2018. Available at https://www.verywellmind.com/leadership-theories-2795323. Accessed 2 Feb 2019.
3. Sundheim D. The trouble with leadership theories. 2014. Available at https://hbr.org/2014/05/the-trouble-with-leadership-theories. Accessed 2 Feb 2019.
4. Leadership Theories (n.d.). Available at https://www.leadership-central.com/leadership-theories.html. Accessed 2 Feb 2019.
5. Hasan S. Top 10 leadership qualities that make good leaders. 2017. Available at https://blog.taskque.com/characteristics-good-leaders/. Accessed 2 Feb 2019.
6. Surbhi S. Difference between management and administration. 2015. Available at https://keydifferences.com/difference-between-management-and-administration.html#ComparisonChart. Accessed 2 Feb 2019.
7. Adeloye D, David RA, Olaogun AA, Auta A, Adesokan A, Gadanya M, Opele JK, Owagbemi O, Iseolorunkanmi A. Health workforce and governance: the crisis in Nigeria. Human Resources for Health 15:32. 2017. Available at https://human-resources-health.biomedcentral.com/articles/10.1186/s12960-017-0205-4#Bib1. Accessed 16 Jan 2019.
8. Ugah N, Otokpa AR, James C. Strike: FG has not invited us for talks –JOHESU. 2018. Available at https://newtelegraphonline.com/2018/04/strike-fg-has-not-invited-us-for-talks-johesu/. Accessed 16 Jan 2019.
9. Atueyi U. A glorious end to fellowship, PhD controversy for clinical teachers. 2017. Available at https://guardian.ng/features/a--glorious-end-to-fellowship-phd-controversy-for-clinical-teachers/. Accessed 16 Jan 2019.
10. Ihekweazu C. Three reasons strike will continue in Nigeria's health sector. 2015. Available at http://nigeriahealthwatch.com/three-reasons-strikes-will-continue-in-nigerias-health-sector/. Accessed 16 Jan 2019.
11. Alubo O, Hunduh V. Medical dominance and resistance in Nigeria's healthcare system. Int J Health Serv. 2017;47(4):778–94.
12. Ojo TO, Akinwumi AF. Doctors as managers of healthcare resources in Nigeria: Evolving roles and current challenges. Niger Med J. 2015;56(6):375–80. Available at https://www.ncbi.nlm.nih.gov/pmc/articles/PMC4743284/. Accessed 16 Jan 2019.
13. Oleribe OO, Udofia D, Oladipo O, Ishola TA, Taylor-Robinson SD. Healthcare workers' industrial action in Nigeria: a cross-sectional survey of Nigerian physicians. Hum Resour Health. 2018;16(1)
14. Oleribe OO, Ezieme IP, Oladipo O, Akinola EP, Udofia D, Taylor-Robinson SD. Industrial action by healthcare workers in Nigeria in 2013–2015: an inquiry into causes, consequences and control—a cross-sectional descriptive study. Hum Resour Health. 2016;14(1):46.
15. Nancarrow SA, Booth A, Ariss S, Smith T, Enderby P, Roots A. Ten principles of good interdisciplinary teamwork. Hum Resour Health. 2013;11:19. Available at https://www.ncbi.nlm.nih.gov/pmc/articles/PMC3662612/. Accessed 2 Feb 2019.
16. The HRH Global Resource Centre (n.d.) Why is teamwork in healthcare important? Available at https://www.hrhresourcecentre.org/HRH_Info_Teamwork.html. Accessed 2 Feb 2019.

17. Venzin K. 5 things to know when working with an interdisciplinary healthcare team. 2018. Available at https://covalentcareers.com/resources/5-tips-interdisciplinary-healthcare-team/. Accessed 2 Feb 2019.
18. Balogun JA. The case for a paradigm shifts in the education of healthcare professionals in Nigeria. 2016. Available at https://www.researchgate.net/publication/317387397_The_case_for_a_paradigm_shift_in_the_education_of_healthcare_professionals_in_Nigeria. Accessed on June 11, 2021.
19. Iyoke CA, Lawani LO, Ugwu GO, Ajah LO, Ezugwu EC, Onah P, Onwuka CI. Knowledge and attitude toward interdisciplinary team working among obstetricians and gynaecologists in teaching hospitals in South East Nigeria. J Multidiscip Healthcare. 2019;8:237–44. Available at https://www.ncbi.nlm.nih.gov/pmc/articles/PMC4451848/ 2015. Accessed 16 Jan 2019.
20. Gill SV, Vessali M, Pratt JA, Watts S, Pratt JS, Raghavan P, DeSilva JM. The importance of interdisciplinary research training and community dissemination. Clin Transl Sci. 2015;8(5):611–4. Available at https://www.ncbi.nlm.nih.gov/pmc/articles/PMC4625396/. Accessed 2 Feb 2019.
21. Kaini BK. Interprofessional care and role of team leaders. JNMA J Nepal Med Assoc. 2015;53:197–404. Available at https://www.slideshare.net/bachchukaini/interprofessional-care-and-role-of-team-leaders. Accessed 16 Jan 2019.
22. Dodson D. What's the best leadership style for healthcare? 2017. Available at https://nchica.org/whats-the-best-leadership-style-for-healthcare/. Accessed 16 Jan 2019.
23. Daly J, Jackson D, Mannix J, Davidson PM, Hutchinson M. The importance of clinical leadership in the hospital setting. J Healthcare Leadership. 2014;6:75–83. Available at https://www.dovepress.com/the-importance-of-clinical-leadership-in-the-hospital-setting-peer-reviewed-fulltext-article-JHL. Accessed 16 Jan 2019.
24. Sfantou DF, Laliotis A, Patelarou E, Sifaki-Pistolla D, Matalliotakis M, Patelarou E. Importance of leadership style towards quality of care measures in healthcare settings: a systematic review. Healthcare. 2017;5(4):73. Available at https://www.mdpi.com/2227-9032/5/4/73/pdf. Accessed 16 Jan 2019.
25. Organization Theory. Available at https://businessjargons.com/organizational-theory.html. Accessed 16 Jan 2019.
26. Al-Sawai A. Leadership of healthcare professionals: where do we stand? Oman Med J. 2013;28(4):285–7. Available at https://www.ncbi.nlm.nih.gov/pmc/articles/PMC3725246/ 2013. Accessed 2 Feb 2019.
27. Consador K. Definition of leadership theories. 2017. Available at https://bizfluent.com/about-5386863-definition-leadership-theories.html. Accessed 2 Feb 2019.
28. Cherry K. Situational theory of leadership. 2018. Available at https://www.verywellmind.com/what-is-the-situational-theory-of-leadership-2795321. Accessed 2 Feb 2019.
29. Tang K (n.d.). Interactional approach theory in leadership. Available at https://yourbusiness.azcentral.com/interactional-approach-theory-leadership-14743.html. Accessed 2 Feb 2019.
30. Schreinerht E (n.d.). Interactional approach theory in leadership. Available at https://smallbusiness.chron.com/interactional-approach-theory-leadership-36412.html. Accessed 2 Feb 2019.
31. Lacoma T (n.d.). Definition of supportive leadership style. Available at https://smallbusiness.chron.com/definition-supportive-leadership-style-21835.html. Accessed 2 Feb 2019.
32. Corporate Finance Institute (n.d). What is supportive leadership? Available at https://corporatefinanceinstitute.com/resources/careers/soft-skills/supportive-leadership/. Accessed 2 Feb 2019.
33. Olowookere, EI, Elegbeleye AO. (n.d.). Transformational leadership style as a catalyst for change in the Nigeria academia. Available at http://m.covenantuniversity.edu.ng/content/download/34462/236997/file/Article+4+.pdf Accessed 16 Jan 2019.
34. Orji MG, Malachy OD, Boman SA, Emmanuel A. Leadership styles and employee performance in Nigerian higher educational institutions. Am J Environ Resour Econ. 2017;2(1):12–21. Available at http://article.sciencepublishinggroup.com/html/10.11648.j.ajere.20170201.12.html. Accessed 16 Jan 2019.
35. Tugbobo AN. The factors influencing the leadership style of Nigerian small scale business entrepreneur. Eur J Bus Manage. 2014;6(1):78. Available at https://iiste.org/Journals/index.php/EJBM/article/viewFile/10218/10427. Accessed 16 Jan 2019.
36. Adanri AA, Singh RK. Transformational leadership: towards effective governance in Nigeria. Int J Acad Res Bus Soc Sci. 2016;6:11. Available at https://pdfs.semanticscholar.org/7d2b/599c88249ec5f9ab053edbd3de363b87ff9c.pdf. Accessed 16 Jan 2019.
37. Igbaekemen GO, Odivwri JE. Impact of leadership style on organization performance: a critical literature review. Arabian J Bus Manag Review. 2015;5:142. Available at https://www.omicsonline.org/open-access/impact-of-leadership-style-on-organization-performance-a-critical-literature-review-2223-5833-1000142.php?aid=58909. Accessed 16 Jan 2019.
38. Abasilim UA. Transformational leadership style and its relationship with organisational performance in Nigerian work context: A review. 2014. Available at https://www.researchgate.net/publication/280324869_Transformational_Leadership_Style_and_Its_Relationship_with_Organisational_Performance_in_Nigerian_Work_Context_A_Review. Accessed 16 Jan 2019.
39. Ajibade OE, Ajayi TO, Shobowale O. Leadership style and employees' performance in Nigerian Federal Polytechnics: a study of Federal Polytechnic, ILaro, Ogun State. J Public Administration, Finance and Law. 2017; 11 17. Available at http://www.jopafl.com/uploads/issue11/LEADERSHIP_STYLE_AND_EMPLOYEES_PERFORMANCE_IN_NIGERIAN_FEDERAL_POLYECHNICS.pdf. Accessed 16 Jan 2019.
40. Genty IK. Leadership Styles and their Implications for prosperous industrial relations in Nigeria. Eur Sci J. 2014;560(574):1857–7881. Available at https://www.researchgate.net/publication/317003882_Leadership_Styles_and_their_Implications_for_Prosperous_Industrial_Relations_in_Nigeria/. http://m.covenantuniversity.edu.ng/content/download/34462/236997/file/Article+4+.pdf. Accessed 16 Jan 2019.
41. Zirra CTO, Ezie O. Dynamics of leadership styles and the management of small businesses in Nigeria. IOSR J Bus Manage. 2017;19(3). Available at http://www.iosrjournals.org/iosr-jbm/papers/Vol19-issue3/Version-1/T190301116125.pdf. Accessed 16 Jan 2019.
42. Agbato A. Nigerian banking governance, leadership style, and performance during the 2008-2009 financial crisis. Walden Dissertations and Doctoral Studies Collection. 2016. Available at https://scholarworks.waldenu.edu/cgi/viewcontent.cgi?referer=&httpsredir=1&article=4052&context=dissertations. Accessed 16 Jan 2019.
43. Njoku MGC. Leadership strategies for Nigeria. Available at http://www.strategiimanageriale.ro/papers/130405.pdf. Accessed 16 Jan 2019.
44. Ejimabo NO. Understanding the impact of leadership in Nigeria: Its reality, challenges, and perspectives SAGE Open, vol. 3, 2. Available at https://journals.sagepub.com/doi/full/10.1177/2158244013490704 2013. Accessed 16 Jan 2019.
45. Amos NA, Emmanuel O, et al. The influence of "Nigerian Culture" on leadership and its implication on the sustainable development of the nation. Educ Sci J. 2014;4(1). Available at https://www.researchgate.net/publication/309136559_THE_INFLUENCE_OF_NIGERIAN_CULTURE_ON_LEADERSHIP_AND_ITS_IMPLICATION_ON_THE_SUSTAINABLE_DEVELOPMENT_OF_THE_NATION. Accessed 16 Jan 2019.

46. Bunashe J, Broder L. How leaders can best manage conflict within their teams. 2015. Available at https://www.entrepreneur.com/article/247275. Accessed 16 Jan 2019.
47. Reddy K (n.d.). Strategies for conflict resolutions in teams. Available at https://content.wisestep.com/conflict-resolution-in-teams/. Accessed 2 Feb 2019.
48. Woodard R (n.d.). 10 methods of resolving conflict in your project team. Available at https://www.brighthubpm.com/resource-management/95564-ten-ways-to-halt-conflicts-with-project-team-members/. Accessed 2 Feb 2019.
49. World Health Organization WHO. Learning together to work together for health. Report of a WHO study group on multi-professional education of health personnel: The team approach. World Health Organization Technical Report Series, vol. 769. Geneva: World Health Organization; 1988. p. 1–72.
50. Lavin M, Ruebling I, Banks R, Block L, Counte M, Furman GE, Miller P, Reese C, Viehmann V, Holt J. Interdisciplinary health professional education: a historical review. Adv Health Sci Educ. 2001;6:25–47. Available at https://www.researchgate.net/publication/11857303_Interdisciplinary_Health_Professional_Education_A_Historical_Review. Accessed 2 Feb 2019
51. Rouse SM, Delunas LA, Anderson M, Anderson JJ. Interprofessional education: development of an interdisciplinary healthcare team project at a Midwestern U.S. university. Med Sci Educ. 2010;20:2. http://www.iamse.org/mse-article/interprofessional-education-development-of-an-interdisciplinary-health-care-team-project-at-a-midwestern-u-s-university/
52. Institute of Medicine of the National Academies. Educating health professionals in teams: Current reality, barriers, and related actions. Institute of Medicine Report, 2001; 1-10.
53. Institute of Medicine of the National Academies. Health professions education: a bridge to quality. Washington, DC: National Academies Press; 2003.
54. Zwarenstein M, Goldman J, Reeves S, Interprofessional collaboration. Effects of practice-based interventions on professional practice and healthcare outcomes. Cochrane Database Syst Rev. 2009;3
55. Balogun JA, Aka PC, Balogun AO, Obajuluwa VA. A phenomenological investigation of the first two decades of university-based physiotherapy education in Nigeria. Cogent Med. 2017;4(1) https://doi.org/10.1080/2331205X.2017.1301183. Available at https://www.researchgate.net/publication/314878873_A_phenomenological_investigation_of_the_first_two_decades_of_university-based_physiotherapy_education_in_Nigeria_Joseph_A_Balogun_Philip_Aka_Adetutu_O_Balogun_Victor_A_Obajuluwa_Cogent_Medicine_2017_4. Accessed 12 Feb 2019.
56. OpenLearn. What are the benefits of interdisciplinary study? 2015. Available at https://www.open.edu/openlearn/education/what-are-the-benefits-interdisciplinary-study. Accessed 12 Feb 2019.
57. Ju W, Nguyen M. The need for entrepreneurship education in medical school and residency training. Dermatology Times, 2018; 39 Available at https://www.dermatologytimes.com/business/need-entrepreneurship-education-medical-school-and-residency-training. Accessed 12 Feb 2019.
58. Limb M. The rise of medical entrepreneurs – How students are turning their ideas into innovative apps and products. Student BMJ. Available at http://student.bmj.com/student/view-article.html?id=sbmj.j1694 2017. Accessed 12 Feb 2019.

Mobilising Human and Financial Resources for Maternal Health

63

Rotimi A. K. Jaiyesimi, Adegbola Ojo, and Olubukola Adesina Adewole

Learning Objectives

After reading this chapter, the reader will be able to:

- Describe the mobilisation of financial resources within the Nigerian Healthcare System
- Identify foreign and local sources of funding and define the diminishing role of donor agencies
- Discuss the role of emerging technologies in improving efficiency
- Articulate the importance of a well-resourced health system in terms of the human and financial requirements to strengthen and deliver a quality healthcare system

63.1 Introduction

The delivery of quality healthcare depends on the human and financial resources available to meet the demands of consumers. It is for these reasons that a proper understanding of human capacity building, and how to garner adequate funding, is essential [1]. These factors are interconnected and should be at the forefront of any proposals to set up a healthcare system and are described in this chapter.

The successful management of a healthcare facility requires a strategic and visionary leader with excellent human relations skills who understands the complexities of the healthcare system and ready to acquire the emerging technologies in patient care. Healthcare delivery in any country depends on the principal officers of the Ministry of Health and the Health Committees in the legislative arm of government. Resource mobilisation is critical to all healthcare organisation to ensure the delivery of quality service to clients, support institutional sustainability and improvement of the services currently offered [2].

Over 70% of the disease burden in Nigeria and most sub-Saharan countries can be managed at the primary health centre level. Unfortunately, this level of the healthcare system is poorly funded and poorly staffed. The physical structures are non-existent, dilapidated or non-functional. Emerging technologies have provided new opportunities not previously available for use in the healthcare delivery system. The description of the Geographic Information System (GIS) technology covers the gap in the literature, offering capabilities for tracking the spatial distribution of healthcare providers and allocating resources across different health or administrative areas. This chapter emphasises the importance of identifying an efficient framework for the mobilisation of human and financial resources and incorporating new technologies to provide a quality healthcare system in Nigeria.

63.2 Operational Definitions

In this chapter, the term resource mobilisation refers to all activities involved in securing additional resources to augment the services delivered within the organisation. It also consists of making better use of and maximising existing and obtaining new resources from donors by using different mechanisms to implement pre-determined goals. It deals with acquiring needed funds in a timely, cost-effective manner. Advocates of resource mobilisation have the right type

R. A. K. Jaiyesimi (✉)
Mid and South Essex University Hospitals NHS Foundation Trust, Basildon, UK

Faculty of Law, University of Ibadan, Ibadan, Nigeria
e-mail: jaiyesimi@obs-gyn.org

A. Ojo
School of Geography and Lincoln Centre for Water and Planetary Health, University of Lincoln, Lincolnshire, UK

O. A. Adewole
College of Medicine, University of Ibadan, University College Hospital, Ibadan, Nigeria

F. Okonofua et al. (eds.), *Contemporary Obstetrics and Gynecology for Developing Countries*,
https://doi.org/10.1007/978-3-030-75385-6_63

of infrastructures, at the right time, at the right price while making proper use of the acquired resources, thus ensuring optimum utilisation of the same.

The eight Millennium Development Goals (MDGs) described in this chapter were the vision of the United Nations to shape a broad vision to fight poverty in its many dimensions and was the overarching development framework for the world for the past 15 years (2000–2015). The use of the term Sustainable Development Goals in this chapter is consistent with the 17 Global Goals conceptualised in January 2016 by the United Nations Development Programme to end poverty by the year 2030 and ensure that people all over the world protect the planet, enjoy peace and prosperity. The 17 global goals were developed after the successes of the Millennium Development Goals by incorporating new interconnected goals on economic inequality, innovation, climate change, peace and justice and sustainable consumption.

The World Bank assigns the world's economies into four income groups, high, upper-middle, lower-middle and low, based on gross national income (GNI) per capita. While the GNI/capita of high-income countries is more than $12,235, countries with a GNI/capita of $1006–3955 are referred to as lower-middle income countries.

63.3 Human Resource Mobilisation and Training: Human Capacity Building

The Nigerian healthcare system is run at three levels, primary, secondary and tertiary, each level being the responsibility of the local, state and federal governments, respectively. The healthcare centre system is a complex organisation, not dependent alone on the clinicians who have direct contact with patients but includes a myriad of equally important personnel required for the running of the hospital. These include administrators, procurement officers, porters, kitchen staff, business analysts and financial officers, among others. Irrespective of what each employee brings to the workforce, they need ongoing training to attain the competency needed to perform their duties effectively.

Healthcare delivery takes place in a variety of settings and require a variety of personnel with differing expertise, skills, knowledge and performance. These settings could be in rural or urban environments and vary from Health Centres, Primary Healthcare Centres, General Hospitals to Tertiary Healthcare Centres.

Human resource is critical for the successful operation of these services and requires ongoing personnel training and a critical mass of human capacity to provide adequate staffing levels. The skills can be achieved through continuous professional development, mindful of the development of competencies which are relevant to the individual needs and the needs of hospital services. Delivering these capabilities require funding to attend training courses and conferences. These courses are increasingly becoming more expensive for employees to pay out of pocket. Therefore, organisations should in their strategic plan allocate funds for staff training. Of particular importance concerning service delivery in the public sector are human resource shortages. There is an urgent need for the Ministries of Health and the policymakers to develop a long-term human resource strategic plan to formulate ways of recruiting, training and retaining health workers.

63.4 Recruitment and Retention of Healthcare Personnel

The difference in the social infrastructure and quality of life between urban and rural towns affects the recruitment and staffing of health centres. There is a preference by healthcare workers to work in urban centres rather than rural centres [3]. This schism leaves many primary healthcare centres understaffed or poorly staffed. The conditions of service for staff working in rural areas need to be improved to attract and retain experienced healthcare personnel. Failure to do so will no doubt negatively impact the accessibility and quality of services in the rural areas. Human resources should be deployed to the area of need, and the financial resources should be used judiciously to enhance evidence-based clinical practice.

63.5 Financial Resource Mobilisation

Strategy formulation entails the articulation of a mission, a set of long-term objectives to be achieved within the stated purpose and an action plan specifying how to accomplish the stated tasks and goals. In the context of health care, a mission common to governments of most countries is to provide or committed to health care for all citizens of the country. Long-term objectives include an efficient provision of quality health care that is accessible and equitable, in a manner that is socially and ethically acceptable. One of the principal components of an action plan to achieve these objectives is to find ways and means to finance the provision of health care [4].

Globally, healthcare services are financed either directly by consumers or by the government. Direct financing by consumers takes many forms, such as payment at the point of service in public or private facilities, contributions to private or government insurance funds, private donations and purchase of drugs and other medical supplies from pharmacies. Similarly, government financing of health services uses resources generated from various sources, such as through increased allocations from general government revenue, specially targeted public revenue-raising efforts, public sector user fees, social health insurance and foreign assistance [5].

A resource mobilisation strategy comprises the mix of mechanisms that government employs to directly finance its production and delivery of health care in a manner that is efficient, equitable, sustainable, transparent and improves quality of care. The resources available to the government to fund healthcare services are tax revenues, public sector user fees, insurance and donor funding. In most developing countries, the estimation of national health expenditures is still at a preliminary stage. However, recent work has shown that the National Health Account methods use a detailed breakdown of sources, and the expenditure can be used feasibly, affordably and usefully. The National Health Accounts, which describe the expense flows – both public and private – within the health sector of a country, is one avenue to assess health expenditures in a rigorous and timely manner. They represent the sources, uses and flow of funds within the healthcare system and are an essential requirement for optimal management of the allocation and mobilisation of health sector resources [1].

Implementation of disease prevention programmes requires adequate human resources, finance and infrastructure. The two strands to resource mobilisation are to obtain the financial and human resources needed to deliver the services and prioritising the service(s) that require prompt implementation.

Healthcare funding around the world comes from the national government and global partners such as The Global Fund, United States Agency for International Development, President's Emergency Plan for AIDS Relief, United Nations Programme on HIV and AIDS, World Health Organisation, United Nations International Children's Emergency Fund and others. The external partners make substantial contributions towards disease prevention programmes such as immunisation against infectious diseases, malaria, HIV and AIDS.

In April 2001, the African Union countries pledged to set a target of allocating at least 15% of their annual budget to improve the health sector and urged each nation to scale up support. Unfortunately, these goals never materialised and international assistance dropped. Many African Union countries failed to achieve the Millennium Development Goals as a result of inadequate funding [6]. Low- and medium-income countries can no longer rely on international support due to donor fatigue and political changes within the foreign countries. For example, the recent changes in tax laws in the USA under the Trump presidency have seen a slow, long-term drop in the philanthropic donations which in effect jeopardises the work and impact of many of the charities [5].

The problems of financial resource mobilisation are not limited to low- and medium-income countries; United Kingdom, USA and other developed nations also have financial constraints on health expenditure. Providing affordable, high-quality services is a challenge for countries at all income levels, as data from 183 countries in the World Bank Group's 2018 Health Equity and Financial Protection Indicators database indicate. Universal healthcare coverage is about all people having access to the care they need without financial hardship.

63.6 Healthcare Financing

All over the world, the healthcare system is financed differently in different countries. Health insurance, a critical component of financing health, is a social security system that provides health services to persons covered who pay token contributions at regular intervals to a shared pool, usually held by a third party. These funds are then used to pay for the healthcare costs of the members of the pool. Health insurance is risk-averse, and the primary objective is to protect people from the financial risk of seeking medical care when they fall ill. Therefore, the premium and list of medical conditions covered by the insurance scheme must be defined explicitly for the consumers. A contentious area of health insurance coverage is in cancer care because it is exceedingly expensive. Unfortunately, in many countries around the world, consumers with pre-existing medical conditions including cancer and chronic diseases are often unfairly treated because they are made to pay a higher premium for their health insurance coverage. Overall, health insurance has significant implications for revenue generation, sustainability, efficiency, equity and quality of care [7].

In comparison to tax-based revenues and consumers' fees payment mechanisms, insurance policies have more significant potential to contribute to revenue generation because in many developing countries tax avoidance is high. The insurance contributions are an 'earmarked' contribution; they are kept separate and tied to specific benefits. Indeed, consumers of health care often do not have funds readily available at the time of need to pay for charges. Since the ability to pay is low in times of illness, consumers find it easier to make smaller contributions at periodic intervals than substantial contributions when sick [4].

Around the world, health insurance schemes vary from country to country, so is the degree of success. Health insurance in Rwanda is flagged up as one of the success stories with the highest enrolment in sub-Saharan Africa. The community-based health insurance scheme implemented in Rwanda is pivotal in setting the path to universal health coverage, which now covers more than 75% of the population [8]. The commitment to expanding health insurance coverage was made possible by a dominant political settlement, defined as the balance or distribution of power between contending social groups and social classes [9]. Unlike the Rwandan success, Nigeria's National Health Insurance Scheme established in 1999 to improve access to health care at an affordable cost through various prepayment systems has only achieved about 5% coverage. This poor performance is not due to Nigeria's large population but the absence of strong political will and transparency in the operational and financial management of the scheme [10].

As far as the sustainability of the health system is concerned, insurance systems have the potential to improve sustainability because the increased revenue contribution may reduce the government's burden of financing the health system. In addition, management of insurance systems entails a complex system of billing and collection, accounting, bookkeeping, maintaining individual records, keeping detailed accounts of various charges and is likely to lead to the development of a group of trained accountants and professionals, which is expected to lead over time to better management of the health system [11].

Health insurance coverage in developing countries can lead to improvements in economic and social efficiency. Health insurance is risk-averse, and consumers must be willing to pay for the risk associated. Provision of risk coverage, therefore, is an efficient use of scarce resources. Health insurance can potentially improve social welfare by setting in place a mechanism for spreading costs over the unwell and the healthy. Moreover, insurance policies are designed to permit income redistribution in favour of the poor which represents the social efficiency objective. However, the welfare-enhancing potential of insurance is reduced by several risks associated with third-party insurance. For example, the introduction of third-party insurance often leads to an increase in the utilisation of health services. When the unit price of health care is meagre, there will be a tendency among consumers to overuse health care and the potential for increased costs [12].

The introduction of insurance in a healthcare system may lead to an increase in the use of services. In a specific payment system such as in a fee-per-service system, providers are incentivised to oversupply services with the potential to increase costs. Insurance systems can face significant cost overrun risks and have a negative impact on welfare if risks are not spread across broad segments of the population. This situation may happen if only the sick seek insurance (demand side adverse selection) and the sick are not encouraged to participate in the insurance plan (supply side adverse selection). It is debatable whether public or private held or run insurance schemes always translates to the provision of and access to the required quality health care. Tax insurance is often designed in a manner that ensures vertical equity (persons or families of unequal ability to pay and make appropriately dissimilar payments) and horizontal equity (persons or families with the same ability to pay and make the equal contribution).

63.7 International Donors

Low- and medium-income countries receive support in a variety of ways from donor countries and international organisations from the West and more recently from China and other Asian countries. The resources come in the form of monetary donations, loans and technical support. Accountability for the resources can be challenging as payments at times do not get to the recipients directly but made to a group of countries, and under this unique circumstance, funds are spent outside the recipient country [13].

In developing countries, most healthcare programmes to some extent rely upon external support. It is therefore desirable to encourage major donors to participate in a strategic planning process with the recipient organisation at the initial stage of grant approval. The planning process should involve all key stakeholders since donors may have specific concerns or priorities that do not always match national priorities. Their active participation will ensure coherence and maximise the allocation of the resources to priority areas. Besides the various 'communities' mentioned above, the 'key stakeholders' at this stage will include not only international donors but also, hopefully, some new or potential resource partners as identified through need assessments.

Through multilateral or bilateral financial donations from Overseas Development Agencies such as the British Department for International Development, many low- and medium-income countries tackle global health challenges. Similarly, not-for-profit organisations such as the Bill and Melinda Gates Foundation have made significant contribution to the improvement of health care in low- and medium-income countries; prevention of malaria being one of the significant achievements.

One difficulty encountered in appreciating the exact contribution of non-governmental organisations or external donors to health financing is that in many countries they are not required to report their in-country expenditures, or if they are required to submit budgets with proposals at the time they gain permission to work in the country, there is no database where this information is systematically captured nor where actual expenditures are recorded. This also applies to domestic non-governmental organisations and other charitable organisations supporting the health sector, where it is often difficult to track expenditures [13].

Development aid from bilateral donors remain a critical source of healthcare funding in developing countries. In recent years, multilateral support has generally diminished and is now focused more on catalytic action, technical assistance and advocacy, including efforts to leverage additional resources [14].

63.8 Sustainability of Gains

A strong political will is needed to sustain the gains in healthcare development and must not be subject to the whims and caprices of politicians in power. Indeed, human and financial resources needed to deliver quality health service on long term must be made available irrespective of which political party is in power. Short- and long-term strategic plans must be developed to meet the nation's health needs, and successive governments should implement the programmes. Sustainability occurs when an organisation has sufficient funds to cover its activities; however, it is a broader concept. Three critical factors are essential to the survival of any organisation: institutional, financial and programmatic sustainability [2].

Partisan politics should not influence the sustainability of human and financial resources but impacted by the three factors hitherto mentioned. Programmatic sustainability is where the organisation delivers services that meet the needs of the clients, and the success enables expansion of the client base. Institutional sustainability is when the organisation has a strong, flexible structure with accountable and transparent governance practices. The organisation structure and good governance allows it to respond to the shifting priorities of its clients and other stakeholders while creating a favourable work environment for its employees. Funds are required to keep an organisation operational, and financial sustainability of the organisation is obtained from various sources, allowing it to support its ongoing efforts and to undertake new initiatives [1]. Figure 63.1 illustrates how all of these streams of sustainability are interrelated in an organisation.

The strategic plan is the anchor, on which organisation's programmes, structure and systems, as well as financials, are reviewed and new business opportunities identified. These new directions and opportunities are then pursued using a distinct resource mobilisation approach such as grant proposal or business plan development. These instruments are designed to showcase an organisation's programmes, institutional structure and financial health [1].

63.9 Application of Technology in Human Resource Mobilisation

Spatial technologies such as the Geographic Information Systems (GIS) are rapidly gaining popularity within the public health arena. Generally, they are tools used for integrating multiple data sources, visual representations of complex spatial data for facilitating the compilation and tracking of information on the incidence, prevalence and spread of disease [15]. Although disease surveillance and forecasting remain the most dominant health application areas of GIS, the technology also contributes towards the strengthening of health systems in at least two other ways – the mapping and deployment of healthcare personnel and the prudent allocation of financial resources. We will discuss next the applications of GIS in human and financial resource mobilisation in the healthcare system.

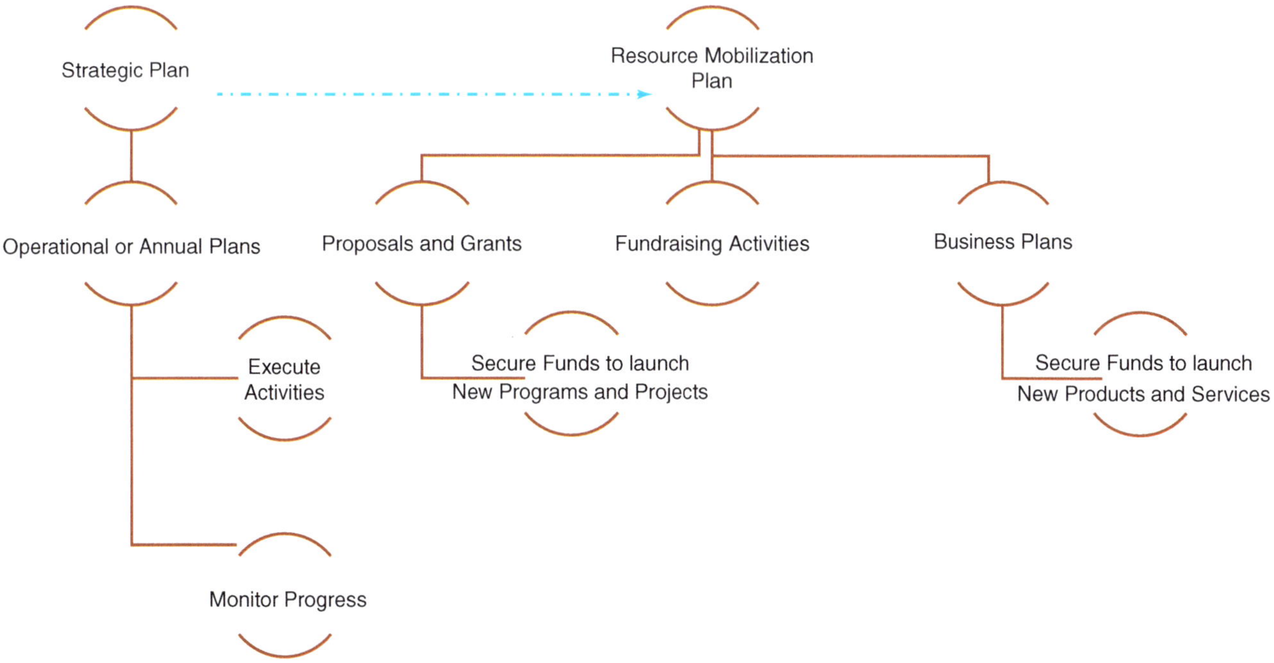

Fig. 63.1 Strategic plan and resource mobilisation. (Source: Judith B. Seltzer (2014) – What is resource mobilisation and why is it so important? This material was made possible by the support of the American people through the United States Agency for International Development (USAID). The Health Communication Capacity Collaborative (HC3) was supported by USAID's Office of Population and Reproductive Health, Bureau for Global Health (2012–2017) and led by the Johns Hopkins Bloomberg School of Public Health's Centre for Communication Programs. Management Sciences for Health)

63.10 Monitoring Human Resources in Public Health Programmes

To track improved patient outcomes, programme managers regularly require the capacity to quickly compare demographic and epidemiologic data with information on service site locations and human resource capacity for disease diagnosis and management. Techniques subsumed within GIS facilitate the analysis and visualisation of the location, distribution and relationships between healthcare providers and those who require care. Results from this type of analysis offer both strategic and operational utility by improving understanding of programmes that are in operation relative to where healthcare personnel is located [16].

To illustrate this application, we draw on the World Health Organization's example from Oromiya, Ethiopia, which focused on helping healthcare programme managers to triangulate and monitor the availability of tuberculosis services, human resources, case distribution and case outcomes [17]. The GIS was used to map current staff against staffing norms at each tuberculosis facility, visualise the availability of health staff based on nearby population, monitor staff caseload as a function of out-patient department patients and also map the proportion of staff trained in tuberculosis management compared with the corresponding caseload.

63.11 Health Equity and Access

Physicians and policymakers in developing countries recognise that systemic differences in the health status of different population groups can have significant adverse effects on individuals and broader society. Health disparities tend to be generally more pervasive among vulnerable segments of the population which include women and children in poorer households [18]. Combating health inequities and improving outcomes for susceptible population groups is at the top of virtually all national health policies, strategies and plans in developing countries.

Different social, structural and economic circumstances combine to influence and exacerbate widespread disparities in health outcomes. In 1991, Dahlgren and Whitehead illustrated a model which is one of the most useful frameworks for researching the determinants of health disparities [19]. They plotted the relationship between the individual, their environment and disease. Individuals are positioned at the centre with a set of fixed genes. Surrounding them are influences on health that can be changed. The first layer in the Dahlgren and Whitehead model [19] is personal behaviour and ways of living that can promote or damage health. This includes behaviours like the choice to smoke or not. The next layer is social and community influences, which provide mutual support for members of the community in unfavourable conditions. These broader community influences can also have a negative effect on health. The third layer includes structural factors: housing, working conditions, access to services and provision of essential facilities.

The Dahlgren and Whitehead framework [19] has helped researchers to construct a range of hypotheses for exploring the relative influence of these determinants on different health outcomes and the interactions between the various factors. One of the health determinants relays access to healthcare and related services. Lopsided access to healthcare services widens inequalities in health. In many developing countries, access to health care is correlated directly with the spatial distribution of healthcare providers. This implies that those areas where there are more physicians relative to the population at risk enjoy greater healthcare access when compared to areas that attract fewer physicians. The density of healthcare providers in developing countries increases with the average income of the geographical areas served, with urban centres often benefiting more than rural areas. This pattern is illustrated further by the fact that healthcare systems depend significantly upon providers of private care who depend upon profit-making to survive. All these factors combine to distort the spatial distribution of healthcare providers in favour of people who can afford their services and further deepen disparities in health outcomes.

The GIS technology offers capabilities for tracking the spatial distribution of healthcare providers and allocating resources across different health or administrative areas. This can be achieved by calibrating spatial indices that relate the number and distribution of varying health physicians to the corresponding at-risk population size and structure with the spatial distribution of healthcare providers. This implies that those areas where there is more physician's relative to the population at risk enjoy greater healthcare access when compared to areas that attract fewer physicians. The density of healthcare providers in developing countries increases with the average income of the geographical areas served, with urban centres often benefiting more than rural areas. This pattern is illustrated further by the fact that healthcare systems depend significantly upon providers of private care who depend upon profit-making to survive. All these factors combine to distort the spatial distribution of healthcare providers in favour of people who can afford their services and further deepen disparities in health outcomes.

The Geographic Information System (GIS) technology offers capabilities for tracking the spatial distribution of healthcare providers and allocating resources across different health or administrative areas. This goal can be achieved by calibrating spatial indices that relate the number and distribution of varying health physicians to the corresponding at-risk population size and structure [20].

63.12 Workforce Demand-Supply Analysis and Forecasting

The task of ensuring impartiality in access to health services is a vital obligation for governments across the world. Stipulations enshrined in the United Nations Universal Declaration of Human Rights make this even more pertinent [21]. The focus of contemporary policy debate is therefore often directed towards the provision of services that meet peoples' needs, provide choice and access and are appropriate to dealing with patient's problems as they present themselves in daily life [22]. One of the challenges that often confront healthcare managers involved in the strategic mobilisation of human resources across different health geographies is the need to meticulously align the needs and priorities of healthcare organisations with those of the workforce and the general public to ensure legislative, regulatory and organisational objectives are met.

Seamlessly achieving these objectives requires a vast amount of data and sophisticated techniques and processing power. Some of these capabilities can be derived when GIS is combined with parallel computing processes and sufficient workforce data [23]. These new methods can help healthcare organisations to better forecast current and future staffing needs about strategic and operational business objectives and then address matters relating to the demand and supply of labour. Typical methods for achieving this might include calibration of reductions in labour costs in favour of workforce deployment and flexibility; spatial identification and response to changing patient's needs; geographic mapping of relevant strategies for focussed people development, inefficiencies and requirements; and forecasting areas with most significant requirements for employee retention based on changing patient social and demographic characteristics.

Furthermore, GIS-based approaches offer a powerful potential for highlighting the nexus between the professional capabilities of care providers and the demand for their skills at granular geographic scales. This approach may provide for identification and forecasting of health inequalities at a local level. By undertaking analysis using this approach, it may be possible to both better identify the scale of inequalities that prevail and support more effective targeting of interventions in the future.

63.13 Tailoring Resource Mobilisation to Patient's Spatial Positioning

Patients are not static, and their dynamic mobility represents one of the most significant processes driving changes in the pattern of epidemiology across much of the developing world. Understanding the flow of patients and diseases within and across health jurisdictions is therefore central to the mobilisation and allocation of resources needed to cater to their corresponding care in emergencies for instance. One of the challenges associated with tailoring health resource mobilisation to disease outbreaks resulting from patient flows is the requirement for timely, accessible and accurate mobility information about at-risk population groups. However, advancements in the capability of GIS platforms and their interoperability with other digital technologies such as the Global Positioning Systems and satellite imageries have made it possible for these technologies to be combined with data from the mobile phones of patients to track movements in real time and channel relevant health resources to meet patient needs [24].

63.14 Emerging Technologies and Supply of Vaccines and Laboratory Chemical Agents

Vaccines are critical resources for every child, yet it is still challenging to get these resources to children in the rural areas where there is no electricity to maintain the temperature-controlled supply chains, also known as cold-chains. Vaccine efficacy is affected by storage temperature, and this makes it essential that the supply of vaccines reaches the patients while still retaining its potency. The terrain in low- and medium-income countries and the transport facilities are obstacles to an efficient supply chain due to the inefficiency of the supply chains that are used to store and distribute these resources. The World Health Organization estimates that more than 50% of vaccines may be wasted globally every year because of temperature control, logistics and shipment-related issues [25].

Supply chain technology allows for the tracking of critical resources from start to finish, and emerging technologies such as Artificial Intelligence, the Internet of Things and Blockchain can be used to track products in the supply chain and gather data about each product. Access to such data helps in preventing failures of distribution, predicting the demand and capacity levels and reducing the cost and wastage of all limited resources. As the vaccines and other laboratory agents go through different segments of the supply chain, the quality and additional vital information such as temperature and location are recorded. The data collected allow for transparency of the movement of the vaccines and other similar goods.

It becomes imperative that economic mobilisation takes into consideration the necessary funding required to obtain data and set up effective vaccines (and food, essential drugs) supply chain. Training in establishing this system would include data collection and validation and the use of this information to drive improvement. This system can be run centrally rather than in silos, thus saving costs and improving efficiency.

Funding for emerging technologies such as telemedicine and teleradiology services should be made available at the primary healthcare level to link local government healthcare personnel to the specialist at state hospitals. The provision of these services will assist staff in primary health centres, or general hospitals in rural areas have access to specialist support and hence improve patient care.

63.15 New Paradigms of Doing Business in Health Care

There is a charitable element to health care, and health care in itself is expensive to deliver. There is no bottomless pit for the finance required to provide health care. The health sector faces a severe crisis of underinvestment. The cost of essential health services globally is put at about US $90 per person per year [26]. In 2015, 71 countries invested less than this in the health of their citizens, and 41 nations, with a combined population of 2.6 billion, spent less than the US $25 per person [26].

Developing countries need to improve the efficiency of their investments in the health sector, to ensure they are getting the best possible outcomes. External assistance for health development and other global partnerships can play a complementary and catalytic role to domestic resources, which form the vast majority of the health investments in many countries around the world.

Quality health care is not dependent on money alone. There is the need to work smarter through central procurement, avoidance of overstaffing, ghost workers and corruption. The central acquisition helps the government to source the best equipment at a negotiated beneficial price. It is more expensive for healthcare facilities to procure product from manufacturers or through intermediaries than through a central unit system. It is for this reason that state and federal governments including healthcare facilities should consider procurement through a central system. The supply chain team plays a critical role in the overall financial health of a healthcare organisation. As non-labour supply expenses continue to rise, mostly due to new product technology, governments and organisations in developing countries must look for ways to control costs and combat pricing variations of up to 300% for the same products, as seen from our comparative analysis [27].

The continuous renegotiation of supply pricing has been the most common weapon of the supply chain team, but the price is just one factor; utilisation is also influencing the cost of healthcare. Identifying and reducing unwanted variation in utilisation practices can have a significant impact on healthcare bottom line. The integration of supply chain system with the electronic patient records system will allow data analysis across both systems to be cost-effective and hopefully deliver efficient procurement system across all levels of the healthcare system. This development will eliminate the variation in the types and costs associated with the delivery of healthcare services such as the cost of prosthesis used in orthopaedics, dentistry and physiotherapy. It will also deter corrupt tendering and trade practices. An integrated system will eliminate variances in practice and help with the proper implementation of the financial mobilisation of the healthcare system. Both public and private sector organisations must be in the business of generating new ways of conducting business to remain in business.

63.16 Political Feasibility and Consensus Building

There are two elements in the assessment of the political feasibility concerning resource mobilisation strategies [4]. The first relates to the viability of the decision processes surrounding the choice and commitment to the various methods of resource mobilisation available to the government. Stakeholders within the government are likely to respond differently to multiple ways of resource mobilisation, insofar as they impinge their organisational and individual interests. For example, organised interests within the government may find it difficult to assume a regulatory role as opposed to a direct service provision role, which may follow a shift to social insurance.

The second relates to the political aspects of popular acceptability of policies relating to making payments for a service largely considered an entitlement. Public reaction to resource mobilisation strategies will likely occur after the effects of the approach are felt. In particular, it may be challenging to implement user fees without concurrent improvements in the quality of health services. Similarly, while it may be easy to introduce social insurance in the formal sector, it will likely require an extra effort to reach the rural, self-employed and poorer sections of society.

The importance of consensus building must not be underestimated. The understanding of stakeholder interests, openness to negotiation and frequent information-sharing are critical to the success of any combination of resource mobilisation methods. Experience worldwide indicates that the best of policies fails without adequate attention to consensus building and public comprehension and reaction to policy reforms [4].

63.17 Long-Term Sustainability of Human and Financial Resources

The development of an effective national framework for mobilising human and financial resources will provide a long-term strategy for achieving an impactful desired goal. To date, many developing countries, including Nigeria, have failed to attain the Millennium Development Goals. Coincidentally, another opportunity now exists to improve the welfare and health of citizens of Nigerians by committing to achieve the Sustainable Development Goals by 2030, the blueprint to achieve a better and more sustainable future for all. These goals address the global challenges we face, including those related to poverty, inequality, climate, environmental degradation, prosperity and peace and justice. The Goals interconnect, and in order to leave no one behind, it is important that we achieve each Goal and target by 2030.

To achieve the SDGs, there will be a need for intersectoral cooperation between the Executive and Legislative arms of government. This cooperation should enable the Ministry of Finance, the Ministry of Economic Planning, Department of Labour, Ministry of Justice and Civil Liberties Organisations work together to deliver a national framework on the SDG goals, to leave no one behind. Furthermore, such a framework should subsume mechanism that allows for adequate budgetary allocations for the mobilisation of human resources needed to operationalise and implement the SDGs at the local government area level.

63.18 Summary

It is essential to pay attention to human and financial resource needs, to enable low- and medium-income countries to deliver quality healthcare to their citizens. By increasing the annual health budget to 15% consistent with the African Union treaty and deployment of competently trained personnel to key positions within the states and federal Ministries of Health, Nigeria will no doubt achieve the 2030 Sustainable Development Goal. Reforms designed to meet the needs of the people should come from within the country, and it should ensure the efficient use of the funds allocated to health care by reducing waste and eliminating corruption.

Personnel is the most critical resource, and due attention is paid to the training and the professionalisation of healthcare providers in the urban and rural settings. The mobilisation of an adequate human and financial resource and staff training would provide the necessary framework needed for the delivery of quality health care. The world is a global village and what affects developing countries can quickly spread to the developed world. Therefore, globally, the provision of adequate human and financial resources and ongoing training should be the responsibility of healthcare organisations and governments.

References

1. Rannan-Eliya R, Berman P. National health accounts in developing countries: improving the foundation. Boston: Harvard School of Public Health; 1993.
2. Seltzer JB. What is resource mobilisation and why is it so important? 2014. Available at: https://healthcommcapacity.org/resource-mobilisation-important/. Accessed 31 Nov 2018.
3. American College of Obstetricians and Gynaecologists. Health disparities in rural women. Obstet Gynaecol. 2014;123(2):384–8.
4. Chawla M, Berman P. Developing and implementing a resource mobilisation strategy. Boston: Harvard School of Public Health; 1996.
5. Berr J. Tax reform is squeezing charitable giving. CBS News, June 5, 2018. Available at: https://www.cbsnews.com/news/trump-tax-reform-is-already-squeezing-charitable-giving/. Accessed 26 Dec 2018.
6. World Health Organization. The Abuja declaration: ten years on. 2011. Available at: https://www.who.int/healthsystems/publications/abuja_report_aug_2011.pdf?ua=1. Accessed 31 Nov 2018.
7. Gilson L. The lessons of user fee experience in Africa. Health Policy Plan. 1997;12(3):273–85.
8. Chemouni B. The political path to universal health coverage: power, ideas and community based health insurance in Rwanda. World Dev. 2018;106:87–98.
9. Di John J, Putzel J. Political settlements. Birmingham: Governance and Social Development Resource Centre; 2009.
10. Okebukola PO, Brieger WR. Providing universal health insurance coverage in Nigeria. Int Q Community Health Educ. 2016;36(4):241–6.
11. Cleverley WO, Cleverley JO. Essentials of healthcare finance. Burlington: Jones and Bartlett Learning; 2018.
12. Nay O, Béjean S, Benamouzig D, Bergeron H, Castel P, Ventelou B. Achieving universal health coverage in France: policy reforms and the challenge of inequalities. Lancet. 2016;387(10034):2236–49.
13. World Health Organisation. Health systems financing. 2010. Available at: https://www.who.int/healthinfo/systems/WHO_MBHSS_2010_section5_web.pdf. Accessed 19 Dec 2018.
14. UNAIDS. Guide to the strategic planning process for a national response to HIV/AIDS, resource mobilisation. Joint United Nations Programme on HIV/AIDS, (UNAIDS) 2000. Available at http://data.unaids.org/publications/irc-pub05/jc431-stratplan4_en.pdf. Accessed 20 Dec 2018.

15. Ostfeld RS, Glass GE, Keesing F. Spatial epidemiology: an emerging (or re-emerging) discipline. Trends Ecol Evol. 2005;20(6):328–36.
16. Rais A, Viana A. Operations research in healthcare: a survey. Int Trans Oper Res. 2010;18(1):1–31.
17. Moise IK, Cunningham M, Inglis A. Geospatial analysis in global health M&E: a process guide to monitoring and evaluation for informed decision making. 2015, Available at https://www.measureevaluation.org/resources/publications/ms-14-98. Accessed 21 Dec 2018.
18. Wilkinson RG. Unhealthy societies: the afflictions of inequality. London: Routledge; 2002.
19. Dahlgren G, Whitehead M. Tackling inequalities in health: what can we Learn from what has been tried? Oxfordshire: King's Fund; 1993.
20. Abbas J, Ojo A, Orange S. Geodemographics – a tool for health intelligence. Public Health. 2009;23(1):35–9.
21. United Nations. Universal declaration of human rights. 1948. Available at: http://www.un.org/en/universal-declaration-human-rights/. Accessed 24 Dec 2018.
22. WHO. WHO global strategy on people-centred and integrated health services. Geneva: World Health Organisation; 2015.
23. Craglia M, Maheswaran R, editors. *GIS in public health practice*. Boca Raton: CRC Press; 2016.
24. World Health Organisation. Monitoring vaccine wastage at country level – Guidelines for programme managers. WHO/V&B/03.18. Rev.1, 2005. Available at: https://apps.who.int/iris/bitstream/handle/10665/68463/WHO_VB_03.18.Rev.1_eng.pdf?sequence=1&isAllowed=y
25. Wesolowski A, Eagle N, Tatem AJ, Smith DL, Noor AM, Snow RW, Buckee CO. Quantifying the impact of human mobility on malaria. Science. 2012;338(6104):267–70.
26. The World Bank. Lack of health care is a waste of human capital: 5 ways to achieve universal health coverage By 2030, December 7, 2018. Available at: http://www.worldbank.org/en/news/immersive-story/2018/12/07/lack-of-health-care-is-a-waste-of-human-capital-5-ways-to-achieve-universal-health-coverage-by-2030?cid=ECR_TT_worldbank_EN_EXT. Accessed 26 Dec 2018.
27. Corban G. Connecting supply chain with clinical practice: a how-to guide. Modern Healthcare, 2018. Available at: https://www.modernhealthcare.com/article/20181026/SPONSORED/181029932. Accessed 4 Jan 2019.

64 The Role of Professional Associations in Obstetrics and Gynaecology

Christopher Odianosen Aimakhu and Olusegun Adeoye

Learning Objectives

At the conclusion of this chapter, the learner will be able to:

- Identify professional associations in Obstetrics and Gynaecology.
- Discuss and articulate the aims and roles of the Obstetrics and Gynaecological professional bodies.
- Know about the Society of Gynaecology and Obstetrics of Nigeria.
- Know some contributions of National Society of Obstetricians and Gynaecologists in other developing countries.
- Write on the role of professional associations in Obstetrics and Gynaecology.

64.1 Introduction

A professional association, also called a professional body, professional organisation, or professional society is usually a non-profit organisation seeking to further the cause of a particular profession, the interests of individuals engaged in that profession and the overall public interest [1]. The members of professional associations are learned individuals with skills in a particular occupation charged with providing oversight for the legitimate practice of that occupation. The professional associations act to safeguard the public and represent the interest of the members and evolve to a status of credibility and influence in the given area of specialty [1].

Obstetrics and gynaecology (commonly abbreviated as OB-GYN, OBG or O&G in United States English, and as OBS and GYNAE in British English) is the medical specialty that encompasses the two subspecialties of obstetrics (covering pregnancy, childbirth, and the post-partum period) and gynaecology (covering the health of the female reproductive systems–vagina, uterus, and ovaries) [2]. Obstetrics and gynaecology is therefore a medical profession that specialises with expert knowledge and skill in the delivery of babies and also in treating diseases of the female genital organs. Postgraduate training programs for both fields are usually combined, preparing the practicing obstetrician–gynaecologist to be adept both at the care of female reproductive organs' health and at the management of pregnancy, although many doctors go on to develop subspecialty interests in one field or the other [2].

The professionals involved in obstetrics and gynaecology practice have over time formed associations that have developed consistently to provide competent representation for the interest of its members and eventually collective interest of their clients. The focus of obstetrics and gynaecology is specifically on women's health [3]. The global professional body is the International Federation of Gynaecology and Obstetrics (FIGO), could be continentally represented like the African Federation of Obstetrics and Gynaecology (AFOG), regionally represented and with country-specific representation like the Royal College of Obstetricians and Gynaecologists (RCOG) in the United Kingdom and the Society of Gynaecology and Obstetrics of Nigeria (SOGON) in Nigeria. The professional associations in Obstetrics and Gynaecology have over time evolved and organised into credible and influential entities to foster the health of the mother and the new-borns.

C. O. Aimakhu
College of Medicine, University of Ibadan and University College Hospital, Ibadan, Nigeria

Society of Gynaecology and Obstetrics of Nigeria (SOGON), Kaura District Abuja, Nigeria

O. Adeoye (✉)
Society of Gynaecology and Obstetrics of Nigeria (SOGON), Kaura District Abuja, Nigeria

F. Okonofua et al. (eds.), *Contemporary Obstetrics and Gynecology for Developing Countries*,
https://doi.org/10.1007/978-3-030-75385-6_64

64.2 Aims and Roles of the Obstetrics and Gynaecological Professional Body

The aim of most professional associations in obstetrics and gynaecology, such as the RCOG and SOGON, is to set standards that will "improve women's health and the clinical practice of obstetrics and gynaecology in the countries they practice and across the world." Their charitable objectives are to "encourage the study, and advance the science and practice of obstetrics and gynaecology." They promote leadership, innovation, caring, inclusiveness, trust, and integrity; and operate with transparency in its work, at all times, to the highest standards. The RCOG Strategic Plan for 2017–20 aims to fulfil their dual ambitions of becoming the "go-to" place in the UK to acquire knowledge in women's health and a global leader for women's health and reproductive healthcare.

Obstetrics and gynaecology professional associations have several common identified roles which include:

1. Advocacy

Advocacy is the willingness to enable groups to voice their opinions and create conditions to be heard. It involves that interest groups participate in both a formal network of institutions and an informal network that serves to form the image of the organisation and create partnerships where active communication is needed [4]. For example, in 2013, the FIGO Leadership in Obstetrics and Gynaecology for Impact and Change (LOGIC) developed an initiative in maternal and new-born health. The effort was based on the assumption that organisational capacity strengthening in eight low-and-middle-income countries would result in the improved ability of its member associations to engage stakeholders in the health sector to discuss evidence and facilitate policy change and clinical practice in maternal and new-born health. This initiative improved the leadership roles of the member associations that were involved in project [4].

2. Research and Scientific Conferences

Professional associations typically hold scientific conferences at consistent periods. For instance, the Annual Scientific Conference and Annual General Meeting of the Society of Gynaecology and Obstetrics of Nigeria (SOGON) [5], which is the Nigeria professional association of Obstetrics and Gynaecology, holds every year while the International Scientific Conference or Congress of the International Federation of Gynaecology and Obstetrics (FIGO) is held every 3 years [4]. These conferences are avenues for dissemination of information about the current practice, best practices, research results and innovative ideas and discoveries in women and new-born health.

3. Setting Standards of Practice

Professional associations play a vital role in ensuring that there is an evidence-based fixed standard of clinical practice and ensures that they are disseminated widely amongst its members in its general conferences, workshops and various channels of information dissemination. This role has influenced the quality of service rendered by the members of the group over time. Members design these practices which may be in the form of guidelines, protocols amongst others with expert opinions in various specialties in the field and reach consensus opinions.

SOGON recently developed and updated in 2018 four clinical guidelines. These are guidelines for the prevention of cervical cancer, management of post-partum haemorrhage, management of severe pre-eclampsia and eclampsia, and the Volunteer Obstetric Scheme (VOS)

4. Capacity Building

Professional associations have over time invested in strengthening the organisational capacity of members associations. An example is the Organizational Capacity Assessment and Organizational Capacity Improvement Framework of the Society of Obstetricians and Gynaecologists of Canada (SOGC) administered on Obstetrics and Gynaecology professional association to strengthen their capacities [6]. This role involved an actively participatory approach, working with key stakeholders within the associations and also senior management and finance staff. A process based on self-examination against standards in repeated cycles of self-assessment, action, and learning. This capacity building also extends to supporting training of skilled birth attendants to improve proficiency and skills when attending to women during delivery. This skill transfer has significantly improved the outcome of child delivery [7]. An example of this is the involvement of Society of Gynaecology and Obstetrics of Nigeria (SOGON) in partnership with Nigeria Primary Healthcare Development Agency in development of curriculum and training of midwives across Nigeria under the Midwifery Life Saving Scheme [5].

5. Intervention Programme Management

Obstetrics and Gynaecology professional associations have gone beyond associations that promote the profession amongst its members only but have also evolved into an organisation that provides intervention projects that impact on the adverse maternal and new-born health mortality. In Nigeria, SOGON has been involved directly in implementing several projects and have developed notably, the Volunteer Obstetrician Scheme where obstetricians are made to volunteer available time in health facilities and communities that are underserved by the services of Specialised Birth Attendants. SOGON has also trained members and health professional with its project on Maternal Perinatal Death Surveillance and Response which it initiated and has been adopted for the whole country by the Federal Ministry of Health.

6. Professional Fellowship Examinations

Some professional Obstetrics and Gynaecology associations such as the Royal College of Obstetricians and Gynaecologists (RCOG) in the United Kingdom are responsible for the training and examinations of trainees and specialists in the field. The RCOG developed the framework and curriculum of postgraduate training in Obstetrics and Gynaecology in the United Kingdom. It conducts two major examinations: The Membership examination (MRCOG) and the Diploma examination (DRCOG). The DRCOG examination is for medical doctors, especially general practitioners, who wish to be credentialed in obstetrics and gynaecology. The MRCOG was first administered in 1931 and is intended for those who want to specialise in Obstetrics and Gynaecology. The examination is in two parts; Part 1 is a written examination designed to evaluate primary and clinical sciences relevant to the subject. Part 2 consists of written and clinical sections administered separately [8]. SOGON is not an examination body, but it has developed a Medical Training Initiative Scheme in collaboration with the RCOG to prepare Obstetricians and Gynaecologists in Nigeria to train in the United Kingdom towards the attainment of the MRCOG.

64.3 The Society of Gynaecology and Obstetrics of Nigeria

The Society of Gynaecology and Obstetrics of Nigeria (SOGON) is the umbrella professional organisation for gynaecologists and obstetricians in Nigeria [5]. It was inaugurated in April 1965 and registered with the Corporate Affairs Commission of Nigeria in 1999 as a Non-Government and non-profit Organisation (RC No. 2156). It is an affiliate member of the International Federation of Gynaecology and Obstetrics (FIGO) and the African Federation of Obstetrics and Gynaecology (AFOG) [9]. It currently has more than 1300 Registered Full Members who have completed their postgraduate training in Obstetrics and Gynaecology. It also has some Associate Members who are residents doctors in training in obstetrics and gynaecology. SOGON collaborates with the Federal Ministry of Health, International Development Partners, and other professional and non-governmental organisations in Nigeria in promoting women's health. Members are from across the 36 states and the Federal Capital Territory of Nigeria, and from outside the country.

SOGON's members are "professionally empowered and committed to the pursuit of the rights of women to achieve the highest possible standards of physical, mental, reproductive and sexual health and wellbeing throughout their lives." In addition, SOGON is "dedicated to the improvement of women's health and rights and the reduction of maternal and newborn, as well as advancing the science and practice of Gynaecology and Obstetrics in Nigeria." The core values [8] of SOGON include:

- Commitment to women-friendly care
- Respect for clients' rights
- Respect for providers' rights and needs
- High ethical standards
- Quality consciousness
- Transparency and accountability
- Professionalism

The rights, benefits, and privileges of members of SOGON include:

1. The reduction in registration fees in SOGON activities including Conferences
2. Eligibility to partake in SOGON meetings including voting and vying for elective office
3. Entitlement to free copies of SOGON publications. These include the Associations Journal which is the Tropical Journal of Obstetrics and Gynaecology and the SOGON News
4. Participation in Continuing Medical Education activities
5. Access to SOGON members-only site in the SOGON website
6. Access to SOGON guidelines and protocols
7. Recommendation and/or selection to attend local and international meetings and conferences
8. Enjoy all other privileges accorded to gynaecologists and obstetricians including discounted hotel rates in some hotels in Abuja, Lagos, and other cities in Nigeria [9]

The focus of the association's 2012–2017 Strategic Development Plan [10] is in the areas of:

- Leadership and Governance
- Human Resources Development
- Service Delivery
- Business and Finance
- Knowledge Management
- Research, Innovation, and Partnership

A new Strategic Development Plan for 2018–2023 has been completed and will be launched soon.

64.4 Global Affiliation and Organisational Structure of SOGON

SOGON is a member of the International Federation of Gynaecology and Obstetrics (FIGO) and the African Federation of Obstetrics and Gynaecology (AFOG). SOGON members have held various positions in the Executive Committees of both FIGO and AFOG [7]. The National Secretariat of SOGON is in Abuja. At the National level, the Executive Officers comprise of the President, First Vice-President, Second Vice-President, Secretary General, Honorary Treasurer, and the Editor of the Tropical Journal of Obstetrics and Gynaecology. The Executive Officers with the support of the Secretariat staffs administer SOGON daily. Due to the increasing size of the society, and the fact that members are distributed widely across the country, SOGON is administratively divided into "sectors." Presently, there are eight sectors. These sectors are the North East, North West, North Central, Lower Middle Belt, Mid-West, Western, Eastern, and Lagos sectors. Each sector has a local administrative committee which includes a Chairman, Secretary, and Treasurer. The position of State Coordinators was recently introduced to enhance effectiveness at the state level, and to oversee SOGON activities in various states and the Federal Capital Territory.

The primary administrative organ of SOGON is the Council. The SOGON Executive Council comprises of the Executive Officers, the Immediate Past President, Immediate Past Secretary General, the Assistant Secretary Generals, and three representatives from each of the sectors. The Council meets at least three times annually to deliberate on critical issues affecting SOGON and to make substantive decisions.

The General Assembly is the apex decision-making organ of the Society. It comprises of all members of the Society and meets once a year as part of the Annual General Conference. Apart from General Meetings, there are statutory committees that make recommendations on various issues for consideration by Council.

The current statutory committees of SOGON include:

- Finance and General Purpose Committee
- Technical Committee
- Ethics and Practice Committee
- Business Development Committee
- Clinical Practice Guidelines Committee
- Continuous Professional Development Committee
- Curriculum Development Committee

As sub-committees of Council, the committees make recommendations for consideration to Council and occasionally implement projects on behalf of SOGON. There is also a Board of Trustees of the Society consisting of senior members of the Society and the public, which ensures SOGON's compliance with their policies and mission.

64.5 Leadership Roles of SOGON

SOGON has been providing leadership roles in the area of maternal health policy administration and management in Nigeria for several years. One of the new functions is the involvement of SOGON in mobilising the government and the maternal health community on the need for even distribution, capacity building of skill birth attendants and the increased uptake of their services during delivery through access [10]. These roles have turned the attention of the government to maternal death audits, capacity building for skill birth attendants and provision of adequate investment for them. Besides, the government is committed to resources and budget implementation and provision of effective leadership to the various networks.

In 2008, FIGO included Nigeria in the list of eight countries to be supported by the LOGIC project to build its capacity and strengthen their leadership capacity to make an impact in the maternal health community. Under that project, the capacity of SOGON was strengthened, and SOGON adapted a programme management approach to making an impact. During the project, a five-year Strategic Development plan was developed and has been the guiding document for SOGON and Ministry of Health activities. Now SOGON has a programme management office and has been involved in implementing several projects including the MacArthur Foundation Maternal Death Review Project, the Jhpiego Maternal and Child Survival Programme Project, Volunteer Obstetrician scheme, Maternal Perinatal Death Surveillance and Response and many others [11].

64.6 Contributions of National Societies of Obstetricians and Gynaecologist in Other Developing Countries

The International Federation of Gynaecology and Obstetrics (FIGO) represents national societies of obstetricians and gynaecologists in 132 counties and territories, with active participation via specialist committees and working groups [12]. Each member society is committed to supporting FIGO's aim for women of the world to achieve the highest possible standards of physical, mental, reproductive and sexual health, and well-being throughout their lives. FIGO's diverse membership, along with its global reach and connections with other world organisations, strengthens its position as the global voice for women's health [12] (Table 64.1).

Various national societies of obstetricians and gynaecologist in many counties focus on certain areas rather than tar-

Table 64.1 National Societies of Obstetricians and Gynaecologist in Developing Countries[a]

Serial number	Country	Name of the society Africa
1.	Algeria	Société Algérienne de Gynécologie-Obstétrique
2.	Benin and Togo	Societe de Gynecologie et d'Obstetrique du Benin et du Togo
3.	Burkina Faso	Société des Gynécologues et Obstétriciens du Burkina
4.	Cameroon	Society of Gynaecologists and Obstetricians of Cameroon
5.	Congo	Société Congololaise de Gynécologie et d'Obstétrique
6.	Egypt	Egyptian Society of Gynaecology and Obstetrics
7.	Eritrea	Eritrean Medical Association
8.	Ethiopia	Ethiopian Society of Obstetricians & Gynaecologists
9.	Gabon	Société Gabonaise de Gynécologie Obstétrique et de la Reproductio
10.	Ghana	Society of Obstetricians and Gynaecologists of Ghana
11.	Guinea	Societe Guineenne de Gynecologie-Obstetrique
12.	Ivory Coast	Societe de Gynecologie et d'Obstetrique de Cote d'Ivoire
13.	Kenya	Kenya Obstetrical & Gynaecological Society
14.	Libya	Libyan Obstetrical & Gynaecological Association
15.	Malawi	Association of Obstetricians and Gynaecologists of Malawi
16.	Mali	Societe Malienne de Gynecologie Obstetrique
17.	Morocco	Societe Royale Marocaine de Gynecologie Obstetrique
18.	Mozambique	Associação Moçambicana de Obstetras e Ginecologistas
19.	Niger	Société de Gynécologie et Obstétrique du Niger
20.	Nigeria	Society of Gynaecology & Obstetrics of Nigeria
21.	Rwanda	Rwanda Society of Obstetricians and Gynaecologists
22.	Senegal	Association Sénégalaise de Gynécologie-Obstétrique
23.	Sierra Leone	Sierra Leone Association of Gynaecologists & Obstetricians
24.	South Africa	South African Society of Obstetrics & Gynaecology
25.	Sudan	Obstetrical & Gynaecological Society of Sudan
26.	Tanzania	Association of Gynaecologists & Obstetricians of Tanzania
27.	Tunisia	Société Tunisienne de Gynécologie-Obstétrique
28.	Uganda	Association of Obstetricians and Gynaecologists of Uganda
29.	Zambia	Zambia Association of Gynaecology and Obstetrics

Table 64.1 (continued)

Serial number	Country	Name of the society Africa
30.	Zimbabwe	Zimbabwe Society of Obstetricians & Gynaecologist
Serial number	Country	Name of society Asia
1.	Afghanistan	Afghan Society of Obstetricians and Gynaecologists
2.	Armenia	Republic of Armenia Association of Obstetrician/Gynaecologists & Neonatologists
3.	Azerbaijan	Supporting the development of Gynaecology and Perinatology
4.	Bangladesh	Obstetrical & Gynaecological Society of Bangladesh
5.	Cambodia	Societe Cambodyenne de Gynaecology et Obstetrique
6.	China	Chinese Society of Obstetrics and Gynaecology
7.	Cyprus	Cyprus Gynaecological & Obstetrics Society
8.	Georgia	Georgian Obstetricians Gynaecologists Association
9.	Hong Kong	Obstetrical & Gynaecological Society of Hong Kon
10.	India	Federation of Obstetrics & Gynaecological Societies of India
11.	Indonesia	Perkumpulan Obstetri Dan Ginekologi Indonesia
12.	Iran	National Association of Iranian Obstetricians & Gynaecologists
13.	Iraq	Iraqi Society of Obstetrics and Gynaecology
14.	Israel	Israel Society of Obstetrics & Gynaecology
15.	Japan	Japan Society of Obstetrics & Gynaecology
16.	Jordan	Jordanian Society of Obstetricians & Gynaecologists
17.	Korea	Korean Society of Obstetrics and Gynaecology
18.	Kuwait	Kuwait Medical Association
19.	Kyrgyzstan	Kyrgyz Association of Obstetricians, Gynaecologists & Neonatologists
20.	Lebanon	Société Libanaise d'Obstétrique et de Gynécologie/Lebanese Society of Obstetrics & Gynaecology
21.	Malaysia	Obstetrical & Gynaecological Society of Malaysia
22.	Mongolia	Mongolian Association Obstetrics, Gynaecology Neonatology
23.	Myanmar	Myanmar Medical Association Obstetrical & Gynaecological Society
24.	Nepal	Nepal Society of Obstetricians and Gynaecologists
25.	Pakistan	Society of Obstetricians & Gynaecologists of Pakistan
26.	Palestine	Society of Palestinian Obstetricians and Gynaecologists

(continued)

Table 64.1 (continued)

Serial number	Country	Name of the society Africa
27.	Philippines	Philippine Obstetrical & Gynaecological Society Inc.
28.	Saudi Arabia	Saudi Obstetric & Gynaecological Society
29.	Singapore	Obstetrical & Gynaecological Society of Singapore
30.	Sri Lanka	Sri Lanka College of Obstetricians & Gynaecologists
31.	Syria	Syrian Society of Obstetricians & Gynaecologists
32.	Taiwan	Taiwan Association of Obstetrics & Gynaecology
33.	Thailand	Royal Thai College of Obstetricians & Gynaecologists
34.	Turkey	Turkish Society of Obstetrics and Gynecolog
35.	United Arab Emirates	Emirates Medical Association Obstetrics & Gynaecology Society
36.	Uzbekistan	Uzbekistan Association of Gynaecology and Obstetrics
37.	Vietnam	Vietnam Gynaecology & Obstetrics Association
Serial number	Country	Name of society south America
1.	Argentina	Federación Argentina de Sociedades de Ginecología y Obstetricia
2.	Bolivia	Sociedad Boliviana de Ginecologia y Obstetricia
3.	Brazil	Federaçao Brasileira das Sociedades de Ginecologia e Obstetrícia
4.	Chile	Sociedad Chilena de Obstetricia y Ginecologia
5.	Colombia	Federación Colombiana de Asociaciones de Obstetricia y Ginecología
6.	Ecuador	Federación Ecuatoriana de Sociedades de Ginecología y Obstetricia
7.	Paraguay	Sociedad Paraguaya de Ginecologia y Obstetricia
8.	Peru	Sociedad Peruana de Obstetricia y Ginecologia
9.	Uruguay	Sociedad Ginecotocologica del Uruguay
10.	Venezuela	Sociedad de Obstetricia y Ginecologia de Venezuela

[a]Full list in https://www.figo.org/our-members

geting too many activities within the country. Many societies in developing countries focus mainly on the burden of maternal mortality, unsafe abortion, and genital cancers. Some of the contributions of societies in some countries are:

1. In West and Central Africa, abortion-related maternal mortality rates are extremely high. The prevalence of modern contraceptive in these countries use is very low, and the unmet need for family planning is also high. The FIGO Initiative for the Prevention of Unsafe Abortion and its Consequences has contributed substantially towards increasing awareness of the problem of abortion, bringing abortion-related issues to the attention of the professional societies, individual gynaecologists and obstetricians, Ministries of Health, healthcare providers, and to the community in general [13].
2. In Ethiopia the major focus of its Obstetrics and Gynaecological association is on intervention including safe motherhood, prevention of mother-to-child transmission of HIV/AIDS, prevention of post-partum haemorrhage, care for survivors of sexual assault, improving access to quality Comprehensive Emergency Obstetric Care services, introducing national standards and guidelines [14].
3. India is the second most populous country of the world and has fast-changing socio-political-demographic patterns that have been drawing global attention in recent years. Approximately one quarter of all pregnancy and delivery-related maternal deaths worldwide occur in India. Strategies to improve coverage of effective interventions during pre-reproductive period by involving doctors and government and other manpower are being used to reduce the incidence of health-related complications or mortality and morbidity in rural India. Early intensive efforts to improve family planning, to control of fertility choices, to provide safe abortion and integrated maternal health services – were the most important interventions to reduce pregnancy-related mortality that is, 150,000 maternal deaths-could be prevented in next 5 years [15].
4. The FIGO LOGIC Toolkit was developed and designed for FIGO member associations and other health professional associations seeking to improve their organisational capacity, including their capacity to influence health policy and improve clinical practice [16]. It is meant to be educational, as to demystify the capacity building process and provide an opportunity for associations to gain greater insight into what makes health professional associations strong and sustainable, but also practical, in order to support concrete and viable capacity building efforts within these associations.

64.7 Summary

The professionals involved in obstetrics and gynaecology practice have over time formed associations that have focused on addressing the health of women in their countries. These groups provide competent representation for the interest of its members and eventually collective interest on women's health. They focus on certain areas rather than targeting too many activities within the country so as to reduce the problems affecting women in their country. In this way their desired impact is achieved.

References

1. Professional association. https://en.wikipedia.org/wiki/Professional_association
2. Obstetrics and gynaecology. https://en.wikipedia.org/wiki/Obstetrics_and_gynaecology
3. British Medical Association (BMA) https://www.bma.org.uk/advice/career/studying-medicine/insiders-guide-to-medical-specialties/nhs-career-choices/obstetrics-and-gynaecology
4. Shaw D. Advocacy: the role of health professional associations. Int J Gynaecol Obstet. 2014;127(Suppl 1):S43–8.
5. Society of Gynaecology and Obstetrics of Nigeria (SOGON). http://www.sogon.org/conference/
6. Bateson DS, Lalonde AB, Perron L, Senikas V. Methodology for assessment and development of organization capacity. J Obstet Gynaecol Can. 2008;30(10):888–95.
7. Obstetric Gynaecology Society of Bangladesh/Ministry of Health/WHO. A report of needs assessment for conducting training of skilled attendant at delivery in Bangladesh, Dhaka. WHO/Bangladesh, Dhaka; 2002.
8. Royal College of Obstetricians and Gynaecologists. MRCOG: a global exam. https://www.rcog.org.uk/en/careers-training/mrcog-exams/
9. Society of Gynaecology and Obstetrics of Nigeria (SOGON). Directory of gynaecologists and obstetricians in Nigeria 2017.
10. Society of gynaecology and obstetrics of Nigeria 2013–2017 strategic plan.
11. FIGO LOGIC initiative https://www.figo.org/figo-logic-initiative
12. FIGO Website. https://www.figo.org/our-members
13. Leke RJI. Contribution of obstetrics and gynaecology societies in West and Central African countries to the prevention of unsafe abortion. Int J Gynaecol Obstet. 2014;126:1,17–9. https://www.sciencedirect.com/science/article/pii/S0020729214001581
14. Website of the Ethiopian society of obstetricians and gynaecologists. http://esog-eth.org/index.php#
15. Strategies to reduce maternal mortality and morbidity in rural India. https://www.fogsi.org/strategies-to-reduce-maternal-mortality-and-morbidit/y-in-rural-india
16. FIGO LOGIC Initiative in Maternal and Newborn Health. Strenghening organisational capacity of health professional associations.Toolkit. http://figo-toolkit.org/wp-content/uploads/2012/08/3.16_Toolkit_AMOGstrategicPlan.pdf

Ethics, Liability, and Risk Management in Obstetrics and Gynaecology

65

Dilly O. C. Anumba

Learning Objectives

At the conclusion of this chapter, the reader will be able to:

- Understand the underpinning principles of ethical clinical practice in Obstetrics and Gynaecology.
- Appreciate the broad areas of the application of ethics in Women's Healthcare.
- Understand the interface and interrelationships between Medical Ethics and Medical Law in Clinical Practice generally and in Obstetrics and Gynaecology in particular.
- Appreciate the legal principles of clinical liability, clinical negligence and clinical litigation.
- Appreciate how clinical risk management principles can enhance clinical error mitigation thereby enhancing patient safety.
- Reason through the unique challenges and approaches to ethical clinical practice and risk reduction in Obstetrics and Gynaecology in Developing Countries and cultures.

65.1 Introduction

Ethics is a branch of philosophy dealing with values pertaining to human conduct, considering the rightness and wrongness of actions and the goodness or badness of the motives and ends of such actions. Professional ethics deals with the systematic rules or principles governing right conduct. Each practitioner, upon entering a profession, is invested with the responsibility to adhere to the standards of ethical practice and conduct set by the profession. Medical ethics encompass the values and guidelines governing decisions in medical practice.

There are few spheres of medicine that pose as many ethical and legal dilemmas as human reproduction. All medical treatments, since the time of Hippocrates, have been predicated on the ethical doctrine of "first do no harm - primum non nocere" (Hippocrates, c.460–400 BC). The physician owes the patient a duty of care to provide treatment whilst avoiding injury or harm to the patient, either in the course of appropriate treatment or as a result of inappropriate treatment. This doctrine is based on the understanding that the patient who is at the centre of the care experience dictates what treatment to accept and judges the treatment so received against their expectation and the relief of their symptoms.

Central to ethical principles governing care for patients is the patient's inherent right to autonomy. Autonomy is firmly established in legal principles since the turn of the twentieth century where in the case of Schloendorff v Society of New York Hospital (1914) [1], it is stated that *"every human being of adult years and sound mind has a right to determine what shall be done with his own body."* Autonomy is defined as the patient's right of self-determination, a right to choose and permit her treatment. The physician is duty bound to respect patient's autonomy, including accepting their right to make their own decisions. Even if the practitioner does not believe that the decision is in a patient's best interests, provided it is reached after full consideration of the available options, and is therefore an informed decision, the patient is entitled to fulfil his/her right to self-determination. On the other hand, as also espoused since Hippocrates, the physician has a "duty of care" to the patient, being skilled to do so by reason of training, knowledge and expertise. The patients, in exercising their autonomy, require to be informed about their treatment choices in the light of the "privileged knowledge" of the physician by reason of their training. However,

D. O. C. Anumba (✉)
Faculty of Medicine, Dentistry and Health, University of Sheffield, Sheffield, UK

The Jessop Wing, Sheffield Teaching Hospitals NHS Foundation Trust, Sheffield, UK
e-mail: d.o.c.anumba@sheffield.ac.uk

F. Okonofua et al. (eds.), *Contemporary Obstetrics and Gynecology for Developing Countries*,
https://doi.org/10.1007/978-3-030-75385-6_65

a brief patient–doctor consultation, during which potentially copious medical information needs to be transmitted to the patients by the physician to inform their treatment choice, may militate against the patient's right to exercise their autonomy as well as the doctor's duty of care to fully inform the patients about their treatment options. The physician may therefore abbreviate the process, at his own behest or as requested by the patient, and direct the patients as to what treatment is best for them given the aphorism that "the physician knows best." Such exercise of the duty of care by the physician "in the patient's best interest" is the ethical principle of paternalism. Thus, on the one hand is physician's paternalism and on the other is the patient's autonomy. Influencing these considerations are the dictates of the law and the norms of the society. These factors are illustrated in Fig. 65.1. The tension that can arise as a consequence of these two ethical principles is often the challenge of practicing medicine ethically free of legal liability, and underpins the principle of shared decision-making which many ethicists now propose.

In the vast majority of consultations, both parties agree on common grounds around which a treatment can proceed and a state of equipoise is achieved. However "ethical clashes" can arise when patient rights versus physician duties may seem at cross-purposes. It is on the basis of seeking to attain some equipoise between patient autonomy and physician's paternalism that the legal and ethical doctrine of informed consent emanates – the physician gives the patient the expert information in comprehensible terms on the basis of which the patient then consents to a treatment, sometimes having to choose one form of treatment over another, or between having one treatment and doing nothing.

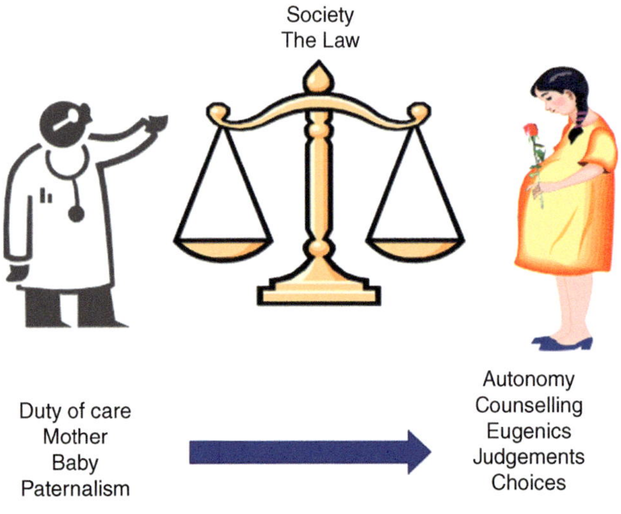

Fig. 65.1 Depiction of the ethical duties of the doctors towards the patient, and the patient's ethical rights. Societal norms and the law govern these ethical relationships

In Obstetrics and Gynaecology, a third factor that is often considered in the ethical equation is the unborn baby and their perceived rights. Does the mother have a right to make decisions based on her autonomy that may be detrimental to the foetus who may be considered to have some "autonomy" even if not able to voice such autonomy? How can these fundamental ethical doctrines influence such aspects of human reproduction as assisted conception with donor gametes or surrogacy? In this chapter, the main ethical principles and dilemmas in Obstetrics and Gynaecology are detailed. Their influences on legal liability and the tort of clinical negligence are then discussed and the clinical risk management principles to circumnavigate the ethical and legal minefields that make Obstetrics and Gynaecology the most litigious specialty worldwide are discussed.

65.2 Ethics in Women's Health

Advances in health technology over the last few decades have highlighted the need for physicians to ask increasingly complex ethical questions in many spheres of Obstetrics and Gynaecology. Such advances that pose complex ethical questions include the use of assisted reproductive technologies, prenatal diagnosis and selective abortion, medical care at the beginning and end of life, and genetics, including preimplantation genetic screening and diagnosis and fetal gender selection. The abortion debate rages worldwide and ethical and legal issues remain in respect of abortions for social reasons and those indicated on medical grounds. Decision-making in all of these spheres requires responsible and thoughtful consideration of the values, interests, goals, rights, and obligations of those involved. Medical ethics, being the science of the morals of human conduct in relation to medicine, helps doctors and other healthcare workers navigate the dilemmas of providing care to the benefit of the patients. It is therefore imperative that doctors are conversant with the ethics of their spheres of practice [2].

65.2.1 Ethical Frameworks and Perspectives

An extensive discussion of current perspectives to ethical frameworks and approaches in Obstetrics and Gynaecology is provided in an opinion paper [2]. Only a brief outline is provided here.

Principle-Based Ethics has dominated medical ethics and is the most frequently practiced [3]. With this approach, four principles are employed to systematically and objectively identify, analyse, and address ethical issues and dilemmas: (1) respect for patient autonomy, (2) beneficence ("doing good, acting for the benefit of others"), (3) non-maleficence (an obligation not to inflict harm intentionally), and (4) justice. Other approaches have been suggested in an attempt to better evaluate clinical problems: virtue-based ethics, an ethic of care, feminist ethics, communitarian ethics, and case-based reasoning, all of which have merits as well as limitations.

Virtue Ethics. This approach can be complimentary to principle-based ethics, and relies on qualities of character, such as trustworthiness, prudence, fairness, fortitude, temperance, integrity, self-effacement, and compassion that dispose health professionals to promote the well-being of patients and respect their autonomous choices. It requires practitioners to ask questions such as: "what would a good, morally virtuous, trustworthy, and compassionate physician do in these circumstances"?

Care-Based Ethics is concerned primarily with responsibilities that arise from attachment, commitment, empathy, compassion, and love to others rather than with impartial principles. This perspective seeks to address the repercussions of decisions on the relationship between the caregiver and the patient.

Feminist Ethics employs feminist theory to examine ethical issues in several ways. First, it indicates how gendered conceptions and human society constrain and restrict women, tends to be male-centred, and woman is viewed as deviant. Thus, feminist ethics can expose androcentric reasoning in the ethics of clinical care and public policy, and questions historically entrenched associations between man and reason, and woman and emotion. It also helps to identify and challenge dominance and oppression not only of women, but also of other groups oppressed because of race, class, or other characteristics. It can also assist in addressing significant health disparities by applying such principles as respect for autonomy and justice to highlight and redress various kinds of domination, oppression, and bias. This ethics approach finds particular application in consideration of women's healthcare given that gender inequities are at the root of several adverse health statistics regarding women – maternal mortality, infant wastage, domestic violence, and rape. Feminist ethics can promote the education and employment of women and Planned Parenthood to address poor health indices.

Communitarian Ethics challenges the primacy often attributed to personal autonomy in contemporary biomedical ethics, by emphasising a community's other shared values, ideals, and goals. It suggests that the needs of the larger community should take precedence over the rights and desires of individuals. Proponents of this ethics, tend to interpret principle-based ethics [4] through the lens of community, stressing benefits and harms to the community as well as the need to override individual autonomy in some cases. This ethic finds utility in public health but still poses questions in a pluralistic society about which community is relevant. Even though there is a broad consensus that communal values and interests sometimes trump personal autonomy, disputes persist about exactly when it is justifiable to override personal autonomy. An illustration is in regard to notifiable diseases where a patient's requirement of privacy and confidentiality needs to be balanced against risks to others. In addressing this contention, the communitarian ethical perspective seeks to ask and answer the question: how probable and serious must the harm be to justify a breach of privacy and confidentiality?

Case-Based Reasoning refers to ethical decision-making that builds on precedents set in specific cases, analogous to the role of case law in jurisprudence. By this approach, a body of influential cases and their interpretation provide moral guidance for the analysis and resolution of current cases. In considering a particular case, someone taking this approach would seek to determine whether there are any relevantly similar cases, either positive or negative that enjoy an ethical consensus.

Justice refers to the ethical principle of rendering to others what is due to them. An underpinning of this ethic is the obligation to ensure that individuals receive equal treatment unless scientific and clinical evidence establishes that they differ from others in ways relevant to the treatments in question. At the societal level, it addresses the criteria for allocating scarce resources, whilst at a more local level, it is relevant to questions such as which patients (and physicians) receive priority for operating room times. This principle can apply to matters such as when to discharge a patient to free up bed space for another sick patient. It often underpins the role of the physician as the patient's advocate and champion when institutional decisions about allocation of resources need to be made.

The conflict between principles of beneficence – nonmaleficence in relation to a patient and respect for that patient's personal autonomy is a universal ethical challenge from which the obstetrician–gynaecologist is not immune. When such conflict arises, the physician's judgement about what is in the patient's best interests could be at odds with the patient's preferences. Acting on the basis of what the physician believes is the better outcome for a patient rather than what the patient judges to be the right course of action – paternalism – has been challenged repeatedly. Similarly, and at the opposite end of the ethical spectrum, the model of following patients' choices, whatever they are, as long as they are informed choices, also has been criticised for reducing the physician to a mere technician. In the final analysis, these ethical perspectives should be employed to address the moral dilemmas and imperatives of providing safe and equitable healthcare in Obstetrics and Gynaecology. Consensus is emerging around the fact that the best care is one whereby the patient and the physician carry themselves along with a course of action to achieve the best outcome for the patient. Other models have been proposed, such as negotiation and shared decision-making.

65.2.2 Common Ethical Issues and Problems in Obstetrics and Gynaecology

Several broad areas of care generate the majority of issues that pose ethical challenges in Women's Health. These are: the role of the obstetrician–gynaecologist in the society at large; the process of voluntary, informed consent; confidentiality; and conflict of interest.

65.3 The Obstetrician–Gynaecologist's Role in Society

Quite apart from their ethical responsibilities in direct patient care, obstetrician–gynaecologists exercise ethical responsibilities related to their involvement in the organisation, administration, and evaluation of healthcare through membership of professional organisations; engagement with community leaders, government officials, and members of the judiciary; expert witness testimony; and education of the public. In the developing countries of the world where healthcare is underfunded and inequitable, obstetrician–gynaecologists should offer their support for institutions, policies, and practices that ensure quality, more equitable access to healthcare, especially for women and children. In this respect, they should exercise the virtues of truthfulness, fidelity, trustworthiness, and integrity.

65.4 Informed Consent

This is defined as "the willing acceptance of a medical intervention by a patient after adequate disclosure by the physician of the nature of the intervention with its risks and benefits, and of the alternatives with their risks and benefits" [5]. Whilst the form simply documents the process and the patient's decision, the primary purpose of the consent process is to protect patient autonomy. The information given by the practitioner should be objective, and as much as possible, free of the informant's bias. The patient's right to accept or refuse recommended medical treatment has legal as well as ethical foundations, and many medical liabilities arise as a consequence of these rights being denied to patients. An important element of informed consent is the patient's capacity to understand the nature of her condition and the benefits and risks of the treatment that is recommended, as well as those of the alternative treatments [6]. Capacity is influenced by the patient's maturity, state of consciousness, mental acuity, education, cultural background, language, the opportunity and willingness to ask questions, and the way in which the information is presented. Critical to the process of informing the patient is the physician's integrity in choosing the information that is given to the patient, as well as respectfully presenting it in a comprehensible way. The patient should be free to choose from treatment alternatives free from coercion, pressure, or undue influence. A key aspect of the consent process is the need to fully document not only the particulars of the consent itself but also the discussions that led up to such consent.

Difficulties arise regarding obtaining informed consent and safeguarding the reproductive rights of women in patriarchal and patrilineal societies such as in many African states. In these societies, the male holds primary power and dominance regarding roles of political leadership, moral authority, social privilege, and control of property. In these settings, women may be disempowered from making choices and decisions about their own bodies and health, relying on the male partner or relative to be dominant and traditionally take decisions for them. In obtaining consent, conflicts can therefore arise where a woman's views and decisions are at variance with that of the dominant male influence in her life or family. Given that the woman has capacity to make the decisions and give informed consent, every effort must be made where possible to empower her by allowing her time to come to that decision herself, give her consent or withhold it, and resolve any conflicting views and decisions with the male partner or relative. This can sometimes mean rescheduling the consultation to give the couple more time to ponder their choices, or recruiting advocates of influence to intercede on her behalf so that her consent can be obtained in a way that respects her autonomy whilst also ensuring that her relationship with the dominant male in her life is not compromised in the process.

Confidentiality is based on the principle of respect for patient autonomy, which includes a patient's right to privacy. Assurance of confidentiality encourages patients to disclose information that may be essential in making an accurate diagnosis and planning appropriate treatment. Confidentiality is seriously threatened by the need to store and transmit medical information about patients. In Obstetrics and Gynaecology, confidentiality is particularly required in dealing with adolescents, especially regarding the diagnosis and treatment of sexually transmitted diseases, contraceptive counselling, and pregnancy. However, rules of confidentiality are not absolute, and legal exceptions to confidentiality in Obstetrics and Gynaecology include the requirements to report certain sexually transmitted diseases or suspected child abuse, and in rare cases to protect others from serious harm.

65.5 Conflict of Interest

Abortion	"Social" abortions (pro-life vs. pro-choice), indicated abortions, rape, late abortions, fetal "rights," multifetal reduction, foeticide
Embryo and stem cell research	Embryo manipulation, pre-implantation embryo selection, use of stem cells from animals and foetuses
Assisted conception	Donor gametes, gender selection, same sex conception, age of potential parents

Table 65.1 Main areas of ethical and legal dilemmas in Obstetrics and Gynaecology

Legal and ethical issues in medical practice	Examples of ethical dilemmas
Mental health law	Capacity, consent for treatment
Clinical research.	Consent and conduct of research, data protection and management, and handling and disposal of human tissue
Organ transplantation	Supply or organs, use of living donors, minors donating, donating to drug and alcohol abusers, and use of organs from animals and foetuses
End of life decisions	Do not resuscitate guidance, withdrawal of life support ("when is dead dead?"), assisted suicide
Legal and ethical issues in reproduction	**Examples of ethical dilemmas**
Surrogacy.	Right of donor vs. surrogate, payment for surrogacy
Prenatal screening	Eugenics, definition of serious handicap, HIV screening and information governance and confidentiality
Refusal of treatment for fetal benefits.	Refusing caesarean section, refusing antiretrovirals therapy to prevent mother-to-child transmission of HIV.

A conflict of interest exists when a primary interest (usually the patient's well-being) is in conflict with a physician's secondary interest (such as financial interest). A conflict of interest is not necessarily wrong, but may create the occasion and temptation for the physician to breach a primary obligation to the patient. These conflicts are rife in obstetrics and gynaecology: a physician recommends products to patients that are sold for profit in his or her office, or refers patients for tests at an entity in which he or she has financial interest. Accepting gifts from a pharmaceutical or medical device company can compromise the ability of a physician to make impartial judgements in relation to care for their patient [7]. Where conflicts exist, they should be declared up front and where the conflict is too great, the physician should withdraw from engaging in that treatment activity. When unavoidable and material to patients' decisions, organisational rules should mandate physicians to disclose conflicts of interest to patients and relevant others.

An exhaustive discussion of ethical and legal challenges in Obstetrics and Gynaecology is outside the scope of this chapter. However, a synopsis with examples is outlined in Table 65.1. Some such dilemmas are general to medical practice whilst others are unique to the practice of Obstetrics, Gynaecology, and Paediatrics.

65.5.1 Making Ethical Decisions in Practice

Given that in medical practice there are often more than one justifiable course of action, it behoves the physician to carefully consider the ethical ramifications of their decisions regarding care to their patients. This is best done by considering a number of logical issues in a step-wise fashion that takes into account all the relevant ethical, legal and clinical issues, employing all the faculties of critical thinking that are required for clinical decision-making. A consistent approach is outlined in Fig. 65.2, adapted from an American College of Obstetricians and Gynecologists. (ACOG) Committee Opinion [2].

The first step is to identify the decision-makers, usually the patient and her family and in patriarchal societies, often the husband or a male relative. This should include determining whether the patient has capacity to make that decision and who may assist her in that process, usually family members or close friends. The next step should involve collecting pertinent information and establishing the facts around which the decision has to be made. An evaluation of all the options according to the relevant ethical values and principles should be undertaken, taking into account ethical conflicts and priorities. In this respect factors that influence ethical decision-making to be taken into account include: personal values, accountability and responsibility for one's actions, religious and cultural beliefs, and individual approaches to problem solving. These steps usually enable the identification of the most justifiable option for selection. Following implementation, re-evaluating the decision should enable improved decision-making should a similar ethical decision need to be made in the future.

65.5.1.1 Providing Counselling to Inform Ethical Decisions

Integral to ethical decision-making is the need for the patient to be provided with the facts and the options to inform her decision-making as she exercises her autonomy. The skills required to provide such counselling are not in the least trivial given that the physician has to deftly balance the inkling to be paternalistic against the need to respect the patient's autonomy. This requires in the main that counselling is non-directive – the patient is presented with the facts of what is known about the condition as well as the options for care, and she makes up her own mind what treatment approach to adopt. There is considerable ethical, medical, and legal debate about the pros and cons of adopting non-directive counselling. For instance, a rigidly applied non-directiveness may not meet the patients' treatment need, if a family does not fully understand the potential implications of the condition that may affect the patient or indeed a future child. On the other hand, withholding information is against autonomy and disables informed decision-making. Indeed, patients often request that the physician adopts a paternalistic approach by deciding for them which treatment option is best given their "superior knowledge." In a developing country such as Nigeria and other resource-poor economies, paternalism holds sway for most clinical decision-making, unlike in high-income economies where women are more

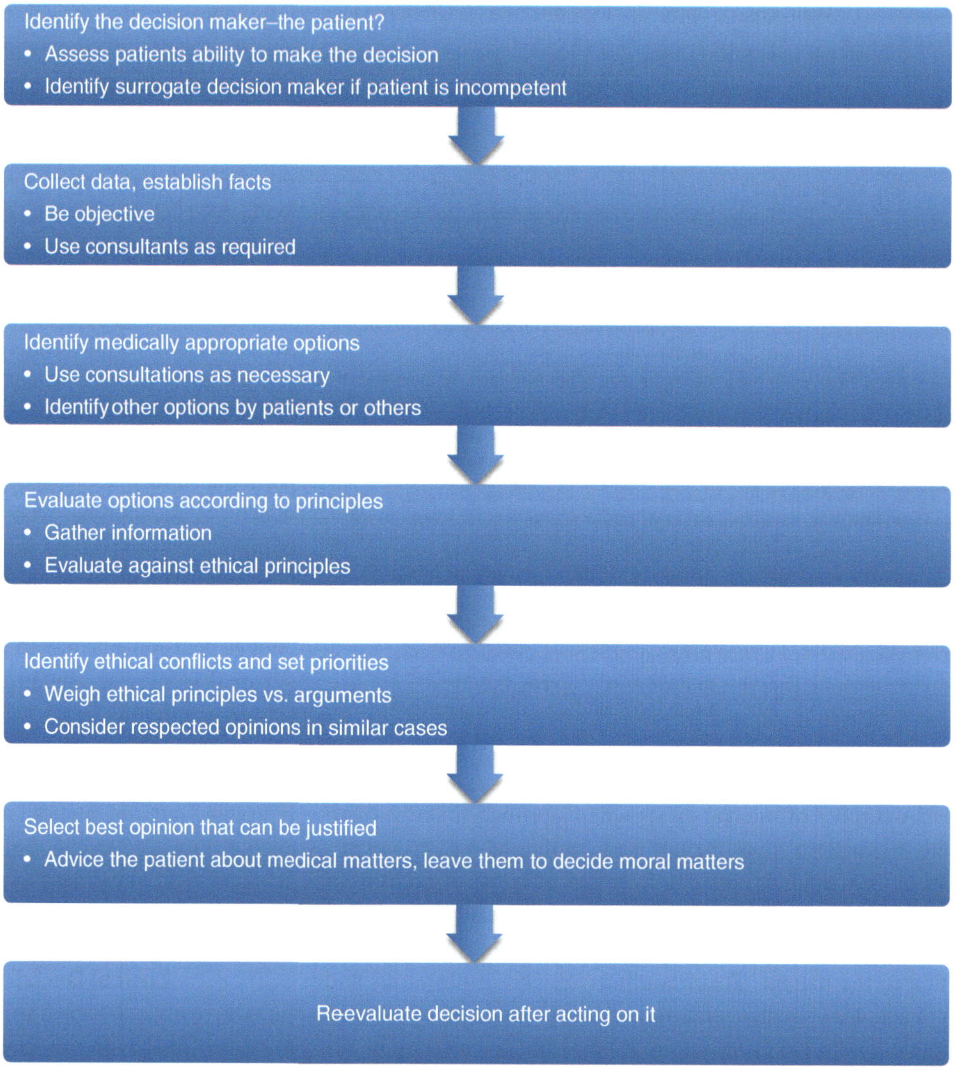

Fig. 65.2 Steps to ethical decision-making

empowered and educated to make their own decisions. Nevertheless, if the goal is to allow women to make informed choices, the duty of health professionals must first be to present the medical and ethical facts to the patients who must have the first option to make their own decisions. However, given that a physician refusing to advice a patient about a treatment choice may impede trust, such advice when given should always be followed by concerted effort to ensure that the patient understands the rationale for such choice and its perceived ethical or clinical advantages over other options. This is ethically justifiable as patient autonomy may include the choice to relinquish the right of determination to another, in this situation the physician.

65.6 Liability in Law and Ethics

Liability in clinical negligence arises and is based on the principle of tort of injury. A tort in common law is defined as a civil wrong that unfairly causes someone else to suffer loss or harm resulting in legal liability for the person who commits the tortious act.

Liability is a comprehensive legal term that describes the condition of being actually or potentially subject to a legal obligation. Clinical negligence is defined as "a breach of duty of care by members of the health care professions employed by a healthcare body or by others consequent on decisions or judgements made by members of those professions acting in their professional capacity in the course of their employment, and which are admitted as negligent by the employer or are determined as such through the legal process." Not only doctors can be liable. The term healthcare professional includes hospital doctors, dentists, nurses, midwives, health visitors, pharmacy practitioners, registered ophthalmic or dispensing opticians (working in a hospital setting), members of professions allied to medicine and dentistry, ambulance personnel, laboratory staff, and relevant technicians.

Two forms of tort are commonly described – intentional and non-intentional tort. An intentional tort is the deliberate interference with a legal right, such as the right to bodily integrity, emotional tranquillity, dominion over property, seclusion from public scrutiny, and freedom from confinement or deception. Violation of these interests results in the intentional torts of assault, battery, trespass, false imprisonment, invasion of privacy, conversion, misrepresentation, and fraud. In these situations, intent is established when the tortfeasor acts with the desire to bring about harmful consequences and is substantially certain that such consequences will follow. Mere reckless behaviour, sometimes called wilful and wanton behaviour, does not rise to the level of an intentional tort. In contrast, unintentional tort, also described as negligence, is the term used to characterise behaviour that creates unreasonable risks of harm to persons and property. A person acts negligently when his behaviour departs from the conduct ordinarily expected of a reasonably prudent person under the circumstances. In general, the law requires the judge or jurors to use their common sense and life experience in determining the proper degree of care and vigilance with which people must lead their lives to avoid imperilling the safety of others.

There can be some overlap of liability between civil and criminal law: tort may be deemed intentional or so negligent as to give rise to criminal rather than civil proceedings. When this is the case, liability can arise in criminal rather than, or as well as, civil law. To constitute a crime, there must be an *"actus reus"* – a guilty act – accompanied by the "*mens rea*" – the mental element of a person's intention to commit a crime; or knowledge that one's action or lack of action would cause a crime to be committed. In the prosecution of result crimes the issue as to whether the accused intended the consequences of the prohibited act has been most problematic in the construction of criminal responsibility. Negligence shows the least level of culpability, intention being the most serious, and recklessness being of intermediate seriousness, overlapping with gross negligence. The distinction between recklessness and criminal negligence lies in the presence or absence of foresight as to the prohibited consequences. Recklessness is usually described as a "malfeasance" where the defendant knowingly exposes another to the risk of injury. The fault lies in being willing to run the risk. With criminal negligence, the fault lies in the failure to foresee, and therefore allowing otherwise avoidable dangers to manifest. In some cases, this failure can rise to the level of wilful blindness, where the individual intentionally avoids adverting to the reality of a situation. The degree of culpability is determined by applying a reasonable-person standard. Criminal negligence becomes "gross" when the failure to foresee involves a "wanton disregard for human life." For instance, a surgeon who undertakes to perform an operation for which they are not trained, and causes the death of a patient from such behaviour, may be at risk of criminal as well as civil proceedings from such undertaking, and could be liable for manslaughter under criminal law.

However, not every medical accident producing injury gives rise to liability for negligence as some medical accidents cannot be avoided even with the exercise of reasonable care. For a plaintiff to succeed in a suit based on a claim of negligence, he or she must prove the following elements: (1) the defendant owed the plaintiff a duty to adhere to a standard of care; (2) the defendant's conduct fell below the standard of care, and the duty was breached; (3) an injury or loss occurred; (4) there was causation in fact, and the breach of duty caused the injury; and (5) the breach of duty was the legal or proximate cause of the injury [8]. No claim in tort may succeed without fulfilling all of these elements. Furthermore, the injury and resulting loss complained about by the person treated must have been reasonably foreseeable as a possible consequence of the breach. Unlike actions for breach of contract, tort actions are not dependent upon an agreement between the parties to a lawsuit. Unlike criminal prosecutions, which are brought by the government, private citizens bring tort actions. Remedies for tortious acts include money damages and injunctions. Tortfeasors are neither subject to fines nor incarceration in the civil court.

Duty of care is a legal obligation imposed on an individual requiring adherence to a standard of reasonable care whilst performing any acts that could foreseeably harm others. Breach of duty relates to discharging such a duty below reasonable standards, as judged by a reasonable body of opinion of people of similar skill and competence in that act or duty. This general test for clinical negligence, the Bolam test, affords a defence to a clinician "if he has acted in accordance with a practice accepted as proper by a responsible body of medical men skilled in that particular art" [9]. However, case law has since evolved such that the courts determined that the quality and credence to be given to such peer professional opinion must remain within the prerogative of the courts to assess. Thus, in the courts summarised that "…in cases of diagnosis and treatment there are cases where, despite a body of professional opinion sanctioning the defendant's conduct, the defendant can properly be held liable for negligence [10] that is because, in some cases, it cannot be demonstrated *to the judge's satisfaction* that the body of opinion relied upon is reasonable or responsible." In this case, the House of Lords modified the Bolam principle by stating that in rare cases, it would be negligent to act in accordance with a professional opinion that "is not capable of withstanding logical analysis." These broad principles apply in law across most developed and developing countries and jurisdictions, cases often being determined on individual merits but informed by legal precedence and expert witness testimony.

Causation is established when it is shown in evidence that a defendant's act of omission was a necessary antecedent to the plaintiff's injury. Courts analyse this issue by determining whether the plaintiff's injury would have occurred "but for" the defendant's conduct. If an injury would have occurred independent of the defendant's conduct, causation would not be established, and no tort would be deemed to have been committed. When multiple factors have led to a particular injury, the plaintiff must demonstrate that the defendant's action played a substantial role in causing the injury. It can therefore be summarised that determining causation is very complicated and is often the primary issue in dispute for most malpractice cases, the reason that malpractice litigation is so expensive.

Claims in tort can generally be brought only during a limited period of time after the alleged injury. Such a period is defined as the limitation period. In England, under the Limitation Act 1980, claims have to be made within 3 years from the date of the injury, or alternatively 3 years from the date that the claimant knew they had suffered an injury. In the case of minors, the limitation period does not start until they reach the age of 18. Persons with a mental disability have unlimited time in which to make a claim.

Personal injury clinical negligence victims would usually seek to recover all their past, present, and future damages cost. Such costs could relate to physical, psychological, and emotional injury, and may include permanent disability, pain and suffering, disfigurement, humiliation, embarrassment, distress, impairment of earning capacity, lost wages or profits, medical costs, and out-of-pocket expenses. Expert witness testimony is often required to assist the courts to determine the quantum of such costs.

The employing authority of the doctor, or the injured patient herself, could also bring action against the doctor before the professional regulatory authorities charged with guarding the professional standards of conduct of the medical practitioner aimed to protect patients. Such action may lead to acquittal, suspension, or withdrawal of the licence to practice, a so-called form of "double jeopardy" of medical malpractice or professional misconduct where a doctor who has been the subject of a trial by a jury or magistrate in the criminal courts may be at risk of a regulatory medical council "prosecution" (in a regulatory/disciplinary sense) for the same alleged misdemeanour, by way of fitness to practice proceedings.

65.7 Who Is Liable for Clinical Negligence?

Clinical liability claims are usually brought against employing hospitals rather than individual doctors or other health professionals. In the UK, the National Health Service (NHS) Hospital Trusts [14] are vicariously liable for claims against their employees. These hospitals take out indemnity insurance against medical malpractice on behalf of their staff and have done so since 1990 under a Clinical Negligence Scheme for Trusts (CNST). The NHS Litigation Authority [14] manages this scheme. General Practitioners (family doctors) are self-employed and may be sued directly, as may hospital doctors undertaking private practice in private health establishments. These self-employed doctors are mandated to take out subscriptions privately to ensure that they are indemnified for claims that may be made against them by patients and their representatives. The CNST incentivises safety by offering subscription discounts to hospital trusts who comply with its prescribed risk management and healthcare quality standards.

Despite these measures, there has been a rise over the last two decades in the rates of claims brought against hospital trusts in England and Wales, the United States and other developed countries of the world. However, it is not yet clear whether this trend has continued in the more recent past. In the UK, in 1978, the Royal Commission on Personal Injury Compensation estimated that there were about 500 claims against doctors, dentists, and pharmacists per year. This increased in the 1980s by approximately 500%, with a corresponding increase in the costs of settling claims: these rose by up to 250% [11]. Between 1978 and 2006, the level of claims increased dramatically by 1200% [12]. By 2010/11, 8655 claims of clinical negligence and 4346 claims of non-clinical negligence against NHS bodies were received by England's NHS Litigation Authority. In terms of financial cost, £863 million was paid in connection with clinical negligence claims during the same period [13].

Maternity claims represent the highest value and second highest number of clinical negligence claims reported to the NHS Litigation Authority (NHSLA) [14]. An analysis of 10 years of maternity claims between first April 2000 and 31st March 2010 revealed that 5087 claims, representing less than 0.1% of all births, were made, with a total value of £3.1 billion. The commonest categories of claim were those relating to management of labour (14%), caesarean section (13%), and cerebral palsy (11%). Cerebral palsy and management of labour, along with cardiotocography (CTG) interpretation, were the most expensive and together accounted for 70% of the total value of all the maternity claims (NHSLA 2012) [14].

The prevalence of liability claims in the United States is reviewed [15]. In 1999, the Institute of Medicine made front-page news by estimating that medical errors kill 44,000–98,000 hospitalised patients annually and injure many more [16]. Fatal injuries are only the tip of the adverse event/medical error iceberg, since over a million people are injured by medical treatments annually in the U.S. One study concluded that medical errors and quality problems in outpatient care resulted in "116 million extra physician visits, 77 million extra prescriptions, 17 million emergency department visits, 8 million hospitalisations, 3 million long-term admissions and 199,000 additional deaths" [17]. However, lack of comprehensive national data makes it difficult to determine whether the number of errors has continued to rise.

There is evidence outside of peer-reviewed journals that the frequency of errors greatly exceeds the number of claims. At the national level, in 2000, there were roughly 87,000 medical malpractice lawsuits filed. At the state level, in 2009, a Florida agency received reports of 4137 injury incidents from medical facilities but the number of new malpractice claims was only 855. A study of 1047 patients at a Chicago hospital found that although 17.7% patients experienced "one or more errors with a serious injury," only 39 (3.7%) requested their medical records, only 5 (<0.5%) sent letters of complaint, and only 13 (1.2%) brought a claim. Similarly, it is unclear whether, and to what extent, legal payouts have skyrocketed in the United States in the last few decades. The assertion of escalating numbers of claims is sometimes based on unrepresentative anecdotes or unpublished data that do not adjust for changes in the mix of injuries. Indeed, some studies suggest a recent decline in liability claims. For example, a report from the Missouri Department of Insurance examined 6694 malpractice claims that closed with payments from 1990 to 2001. Using a time series regression model that controlled for healthcare inflation, real wages, and injury severity, the model showed that Missouri's liability system became stingier over time. They concluded that without increases in healthcare costs and average wages, and if injury severities remained constant, average payments would have decreased fairly significantly during the 1990s [15]. A further assessment in a 2013 report showed that after new claims spiked sharply in 2005, newly opened claims declined substantially in subsequent years up until 2013 [18]. All in all it would seem that rates of claims have plateaued somewhat in the United States, although the costs of litigation for medical malpractice remain prohibitive.

In its 1999 report, the Institute of Medicine estimated that medical errors cost the U.S. between $17 and $29 billion per year. In 2008, the Agency for Health Care Research and Quality estimated that surgical errors cost nearly $1.5 billion per year. In 2006, drug-related errors were estimated to cost as much as $3.5 billion per year. Overall annual costs of all adverse events in the US are estimated at $19.5 billion. When direct and indirect costs including bills for defensive medicine are combined tort reform advocates claim that defensive medicine may cost the US taxpayer between $100 and $300 billion per year. In terms of trends the Missouri report in 2014 showed that after a significant increase in 2007, the number of claimants receiving a recovery subsequently declined. The average award per claimant stood at $275,808 in 2013 [18].

Regarding developing countries of the world such as sub-Saharan Africa, data are sparse but there is some suggestion that liability claims and payouts are on the rise as patient expectation of clinical services quality rises. A survey reported by the Medical Protection Society of South Africa has shown that the cost of reported negligence claims soared by 132% in South Africa between 2008 and 2010. Reliable legal or medical data regarding clinical negligence claims in the majority of West African countries such as Nigeria are not available, sparse data being limited to a handful of cases documented for reports to professional regulatory bodies or in law reports. However, the situation in these countries is likely to be similar to what currently pertains in South Africa where litigation for clinical liability is on the increase with rising patient expectation and awareness.

65.8 Does Litigation for Liability Improve Patient Safety?

The most promising rationale for a connection between tort law and patient safety is that the threat of litigation can deter dangerous practice – the so-called defensive medicine thesis. Nevertheless, there is no clear evidence connecting the threat of civil action with safer healthcare although intuitively it would seem logical to expect that complaints and litigation have substantial influence on medical practice. It has been noted that better note keeping and more detailed consultations were common reactions to the fear of litigation and complaints. The fear of litigation may also play some role in encouraging institutions to take patient safety seriously to prevent financial penalties and the ignominy associated with litigation.

However, the practice of defensive medicine is not necessarily consistent with safety, in that caution and conservatism may be unsafe in certain situations (i.e. not doing something that ought to be done for fear of being sued). There is some suggestion that the inadvertent "name and shame" principle associated with addressing clinical liability by litigation encourages practitioner secrecy rather than the openness and candour that are essential for promoting patient safety. A "safer medicine" thesis is therefore arguably a more appropriate term than "defensive medicine." All in all, literature reviews in both the US and the UK have found no firm evidence suggesting that litigation enhances patient safety from deterrence theory.

65.9 Clinical Governance and Risk Management

The malpractice system deals with medical errors and adverse events after they occur, although it is supposed to create added incentive to avoid such outcomes. Clinical governance and risk management, on the other hand are mainly about preventing such errors and improving patient safety before malpractice occurs.

It is increasingly recognised that the best way to reduce the socioeconomic burden of rising clinical liability is to improve patient safety, and that the rising costs of claims and lawsuits appear to result in part from a lack of clinical safety culture.

To better address the issues that lead to litigation for clinical liability, the principles of risk management and clinical governance were developed and have found widespread adoption globally. Clinical governance has been defined as a framework through which health organisations are accountable for continuously improving the quality of their services and safeguarding high standards of care by creating an environment in which excellence in clinical care will flourish. It encompasses the principles that are required for managing clinical risk. Clinical risk management is defined as a logical and systematic method of establishing the context, identifying, analysing, evaluating, treating, monitoring, and communicating risks associated with any clinical activity, function, or process in a way that will enable organisations to minimise losses and maximise opportunities. Risk management is as much about identifying opportunities as avoiding or mitigating losses. Risk management being an integral part of good management practice is an iterative process consisting of steps, which when undertaken in sequence, enable continual improvement in decision-making.

Risk is defined as exposure to events which may threaten or damage the organisation and its interests. Risk management involves three processes: identification, analysis, and control of risk. Applied to the health sector and for any health service it involves balancing the costs of risks and their consequences against the costs of risk reduction. It includes obtaining and analysing existing data on clinical incidents and quantitative and qualitative analysis of causes and consequences of clinical risks. It also involves measuring and controlling risk by changing systems to minimise the consequences of risk or acting to minimise them through risk transfer. Although initially adopted in healthcare systems to stem the escalating costs of clinical negligence claims to the taxpayer, it has evolved to the potentially cheaper and better principle of enhancing clinical care quality and patient safety.

In the UK, risk management as part of clinical governance has informed recent health quality and safety agendas set by the Department of Health and the National Health Service. It was developed in the UK in the late 1990s, and has been expanded in response sometimes to major widely publicised major adverse incidents and systemic failures. In parallel to these developments, and informed by funding limitations to compensate for clinical service failures under the tort system, the Crown indemnity service was introduced from which emerged the Clinical Negligence Scheme for Trusts (CNST), administered by the NHS Litigation Authority (NHSLA) [14]. In addition to dealing with compensation for clinical liability within the NHS, the NHSLA now also prescribes quality and clinical risk management standards for hospital organisations which subscribe to the CNST for compensating patients who bring liability actions against hospitals. Hospitals are vicariously liable for the clinical mistakes made by their staff. Attaining the standards of risk management prescribed by the NHSLA enables Hospitals to get a discount on their subscriptions.

Risk management principles can be employed to prevent and mitigate risk across several domains: direct and indirect patient care risks, risks relating to health and safety issues, and organisational or corporate risks. Risk management involves integrating several approaches to improve the patient's healthcare quality experience. These include the adoption of clinical and medical audit, and the prescription of care standards through clinical guidelines and protocols. It is useful to mandate clinical governance and risk management by appropriate legislation. For instance, the UK's 1999 Health Act statutorily mandates NHS and Primary Care Trusts to assure and improve the quality of the care that they deliver by a process of implementation of clinical governance. Risk reduction programmes and critical incidence reporting are also key components of clinical governance and risk management. In Obstetrics and Gynaecology, the systematic reporting of Maternal Deaths and serious morbidity has played a key role in risk management and has translated to improving care standards and safer child birth in developed and developing countries.

Clinical governance and risk management strategies are instituted at local hospital or regional levels but need to be underpinned by a co-ordinated national policy of healthcare quality improvement. In the UK an NHS Modernisation agenda has set out clear national standards for services and treatments, through National Service Frameworks and the National Institute for Clinical Excellence (NICE). These national frameworks support and guide local delivery of high-quality healthcare, through clinical governance underpinned by modernised professional self-regulation. Care quality is also improved when there is a statutory requirement for health professionals to engage in lifelong learning and development, and a monitoring framework for assessing clinical performance.

An important component of clinical governance is the involvement of patients and service users in gauging healthcare quality and in capturing their experience of the healthcare service through surveys and membership of relevant service committees and structures. A key benefit of the increasing application of governance to managing clinical risk is in the prevention of serious service failures that lead to much public concern.

65.9.1 Error Classification

Managing clinical risk requires understanding of the sources of human error with potential for harm to patients. Given the

Table 65.2 Classification of error types

Types of errors
Leape et al. [21]
Diagnostic
Error or delay in diagnosis failure to employ indicated tests
Use of outmoded tests or therapy
Failure to act on results of monitoring or testing
Treatment
Error in the performance of an operation, procedure, or test
Error in administering the treatment
Error in the dose or method of using a drug
Avoidable delay in treatment or in responding to an abnormal test
Inappropriate (not indicated) care
Preventive
Failure to provide prophylactic treatment inadequate monitoring or follow-up of treatment
Other
Failure of communication – involving patients and healthcare workers
Equipment failure
Other system failure

diverse nature of error and systemic failures, a system of classification would facilitate interventions to minimise such errors. Several classification approaches have been published. Table 65.2 summarises a classification based on whether they relate to diagnosis, treatment, or prevention of an adverse outcome [21]. This classification also recognises sources of error resulting from failure of communication, equipment failure, or other system failure.

65.9.2 Understanding and Managing Adverse Events

An appreciation of the types of error improves understanding of how adverse events can occur as a consequence of such errors. These are illustrated in Fig. 65.2. Adverse events may arise because management decisions and organisational processes are deficient leading to conditions that are conducive for error or violations of protocols, procedures, or guidelines. For instance staff shortages during night-time shifts could mean that inadequate care is provided to patients leading to errors. Similarly an organisation that does not pay attention to facilitating regular training and up skilling of the staff sets itself up for errors from poor competence. There are usually defence barriers at organisational or individual levels that are created to prevent or mitigate errors and reduce the risk of clinical mishaps so that no adverse event occurs. These barriers are integral to the so-called Swiss Cheese model of error mitigation. The Swiss Cheese model of accident causation is a model used in risk analysis and risk management, including aviation, engineering, and healthcare. It likens human systems to multiple slices of Swiss cheese, stacked side by side, in which the risk of a threat becoming a reality is mitigated by the differing layers and types of defences which are "layered" behind each other [19]. Therefore, in theory, lapses and weaknesses in one defence do not allow a risk to materialise, since other defences also exist, to prevent a single point of weakness. Adverse events only occur when individual or organisational processes and practice generate errors and violations, and when the barriers set up to prevent mishaps are insufficient to prevent a subset of such human or systemic errors (Fig. 65.3).

Risk management is about putting in place mechanisms that seek to improve organisational and individual structures in order to minimise the chance of error. It is also about erecting specific barriers that serve to minimise the chance of an adverse outcome even when an error has been. This often involves taking steps to strengthen a cycle of prevention of error and medical accidents. Aspects of this generic cycle of managing clinical risk are illustrated in Fig. 65.4. This involves putting in place structures that are able to detect substandard care, mechanisms for analysing how such mistakes occurred (often involving a root-cause analysis), and a mechanism for taking corrective action regarding the case in question, as well as elucidating corrective actions that can be sustained within the clinical setting to prevent recurrence of such error in the future.

Managing clinical risk requires an integrated structure of governance that should serve to promote safe delivery of care as well as service improvement. Hospital organisational structures should be established to provide the cardinal pillars of clinical governance, which should include a corporate policy of risk management, as well as effective structures for periodic evaluation of aspects of the clinical service, a strategy for monitoring clinical effectiveness and quality assurance. A framework for clinical research and development as well as policies and support structures to promote staff development are also required to deliver a high-quality clinical service that is safe for the patient. These structures are illustrated in Fig. 65.5.

65.9.3 Clinical Governance and Risk Management in Obstetrics and Gynaecology

Risk management is recognised as an important component of obstetric clinical governance. In the UK for example, a report by the Department of Health, identified maternity care as an area for improvement and outlined strategies for reducing the number of cases of negligent harm in obstetrics and gynaecology.

Every obstetric unit should have a risk management committee. This committee should be tasked with managing the reporting and investigation of incidents within the unit. They should deal with any complaints from patients by investigating them carefully and ensuring that lessons are learnt from

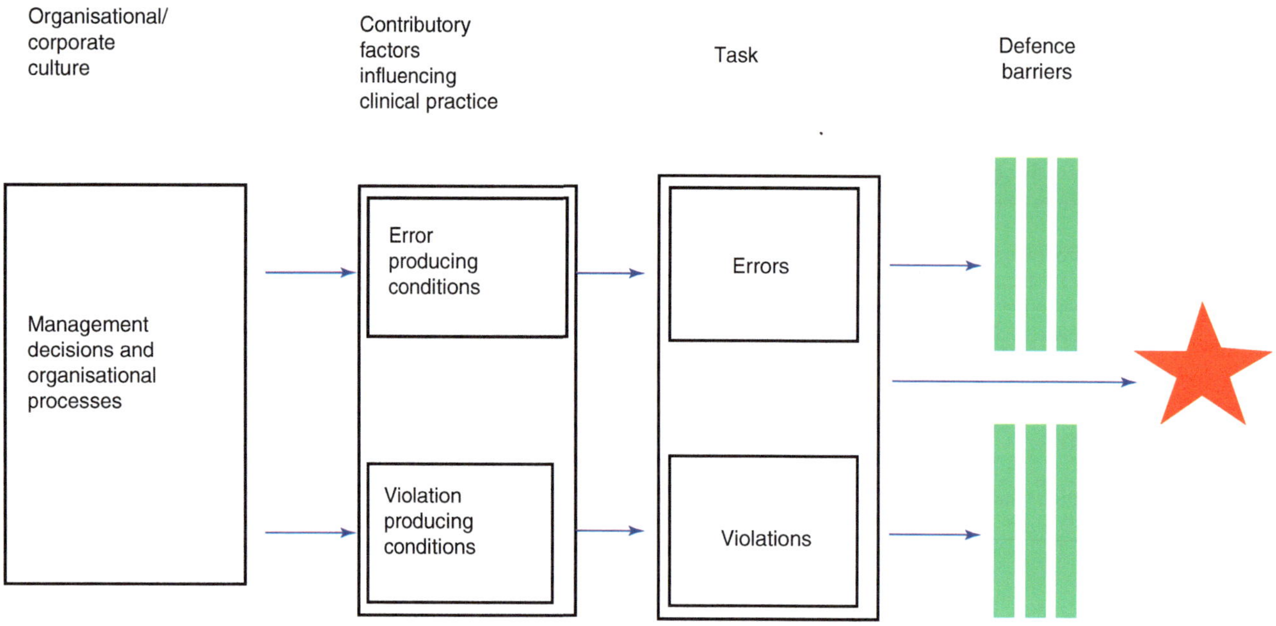

Fig. 65.3 How adverse events occur

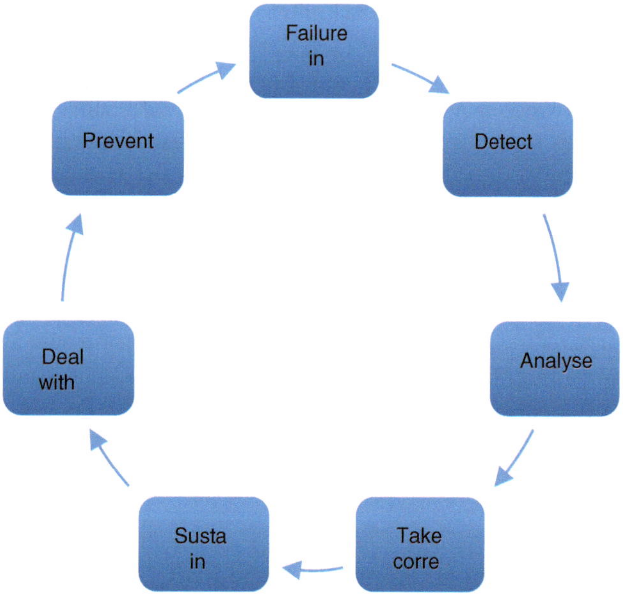

Fig. 65.4 The risk management cycle

any mistakes. They should provide feedback, positive and negative as appropriate, to staff involved with providing the care. They should also highlight and refer potential litigation cases and issues to the legal staff of the hospital. They should also identify and deal with any service failures to ensure that they do not recur. This committee should work closely with the guideline committees to update them regularly to ensure clarity and safe care.

Examples abound in Obstetrics and Gynaecology regarding interventions at an organisational level that can minimise the risk of errors and medical accidents. These relate to equipment, manpower training and capacity, and the inculcation of a culture of cross-disciplinary communication and referral (Table 65.3).

The use of "fire drills" was advocated in the 1999 Confidential Enquiry into Maternal Deaths and Towards Safer Childbirth in the UK in anticipation of obstetric emergencies and has found widespread adoption in effective risk management strategies [20]. In the UK, implementation of these drills is necessary for level 2 accreditation by the Clinical Negligence Scheme for Trusts, which conveys a 20% discount in liability premiums for hospital trusts. Simulation is useful for training both doctors and midwives to manage obstetric crises. Training with high fidelity simulation has been shown to improve the speed with which anaesthetists respond to emergencies and the quality of their care. Simulation can also be used to rate technical skills and behavioural performance during the management of emergencies, suggesting a role for this tool in a risk management strategy. Multidisciplinary drills, or on-site simulations, using both manikins and actors, have been described for major obstetric haemorrhage, shoulder dystocia, and cord prolapse.

A recent review of maternity legal claims in the UK National Health Service identified key risk management themes for which additional action is required to reduce claims and payouts. It highlighted the need to engage with the risk management process at all levels. Particular emphasis was laid to provide suitable learning and training; ensure appropriate supervision and support; have in place up-to-

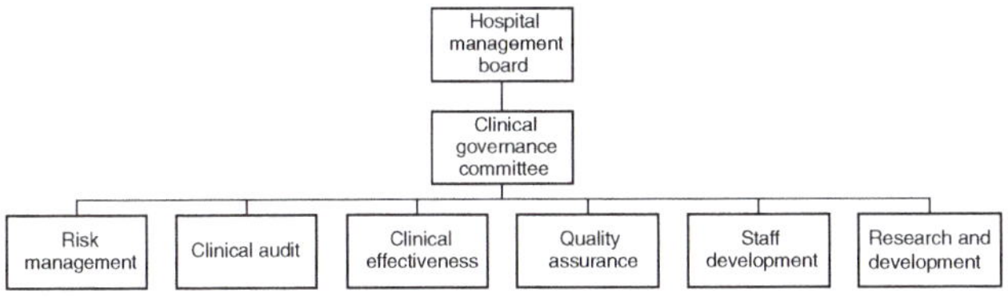

Fig. 65.5 The cardinal "pillars" of hospital clinical governance incorporating risk management

Table 65.3 Examples of risk minimisation approaches in Obstetrics and Gynaecology

Equipment
Ensure no obsolete equipment
Ensure fetal blood gas equipment available
Staffing levels
Minimise use of agency and bank staff
Make time for talking to patients part of work load calculations
Practice "day-time" obstetrics – plan difficult cases electively during the day
Resident doctor training
Ensure mandatory induction at start
Allow protected teaching time
Ensure regular fire drill exercises
Give formal feedback on training
Resident/Consultant doctor work
Write departmental guidelines on routine and emergency practice
Mandate formal hand-overs between shifts
Ensure support from seniors and midwives
Midwives and nurses work
Ensure regular training sessions on fetal monitoring
Have clear definition of roles
Provide direct access to consultant by senior midwife/nurse
Staff communication
Regular delivery suite meetings
Team building social occasions
Clear complaints procedure and feedback from patients' advocates
Notify consultant of problems promptly
Feedback meetings
Surgical safety theatre checklists and team briefs

date protocols and guidance with which staff are familiar; and to learn lessons from claims. The report concludes that the most effective way to reduce the financial and human cost of maternity claims is to continue to improve the management of risks associated with maternity care, focusing on preventing incidents involving the management of women in labour, including the interpretation of CTG traces [14].

65.9.4 Summary Remarks: Clinical Governance and Risk Management in Sub-Saharan Africa

As with issues around clinical liability and litigation, risk management is still rudimentary in many developing countries and frameworks for ethical practice and managing clinical risk are yet to be well-developed. Unlike in developed countries where litigation appears to have driven the patient safety agenda, developing countries have the opportunity to learn from the mistakes of those economies by developing risk management and clinical governance strategies that have the potential to prevent a rise in litigation. More importantly given the poor health indices in these countries, better management of risk will assist to improve patient safety in the developing world and reduce health morbidity and mortality statistics, as well as to improve life expectancy and health-related quality of life, even if claims are seldom brought against practitioners in tort. To err is indeed human but prevention of risk is better than paying damages in tort for harm, injury, and loss of earnings.

References

1. Schloendorff v. Society of New York Hosp., 105 N.E. 92, 93 (N.Y. 1914).
2. ACOG Committee Opinion No. 390. Ethical decision making in obstetrics and gynaecology. American College of Obstetricians and Gynaecologists. Obstet Gynecol. 2007;110:1479–87.
3. Childress JF. Methods in bioethics. In: Steinbock B, editor. The Oxford handbook of bioethics. New York, NY: Oxford University Press; 2007. p. 15–45.
4. Beauchamp TL, Childress JF. Principles of biomedical ethics. 5th ed. New York, NY: Oxford University Press; 2001.
5. Jonsen AR, Siegler M, Winslade WJ. Clinical ethics: a practical approach to ethical decisions in clinical medicine. 6th ed. New York, NY: McGraw-Hill; 2006.
6. American College of Obstetricians and Gynaecologists. Informed consent. In: Ethics in obstetrics and gynaecology. 2nd ed. Washington, DC: ACOG; 2004. p. 9–17.
7. American College of Obstetricians and Gynaecologists. Relationships with industry. In: Ethics in obstetrics and gynaecology. 2nd ed. Washington, DC: ACOG; 2004. p. 107–10.
8. Jerrold L. Understanding foreseeability and causation. Am J Orthod Dentofac Orthop. 2006;130:117–9.
9. Bolam v Friern Hospital Management Committee, 1957; 1 WLR 582.
10. Bolitho v. City and Hackney Health Authority, 1996; 4 All ER 771.
11. Walshe K. Medical accidents in the UK: a wasted opportunity for improvement? In: Rosenthal MM, Mulcahy L, Lloyd-Bostock S, editors. Medical mishaps: pieces of the puzzle. Buckingham: Open University Press; 1999. p. 59–73 at 69.
12. Harpwood V. Medicine, malpractice and misapprehensions. Routledge-Cavendish: Abingdon; 2007.
13. Quick O. Patient safety and the problem and potential of law. Tottels J Prof Neglig. 2012;28(2):81.
14. NHSLA. Ten years of maternity claims, an analysis of NHS litigation authority data. London: NHS Litigation Authority; 2012. p. 1–171.
15. Hyman DA, Silver C. Medical malpractice and compensation in global perspective: how does the U.S. do it, 87 Chi.-Kent. L. Rev. 163. 2012. Available at: http://scholarship.kentlaw.iit.edu/cklawreview/vol87/iss1/8
16. Kohn LT, Corrigan JM, Donaldson MS, Committee on Quality of Health Care in America, Institute of Medicine, editors. To err is human: building a safer health system. Washington, DC: National Academies Press; 2000. p. 1–312.

17. Starfield B. Is US health really the best in the world? JAMA. 2000;284:483–4.
18. Missouri Department of Insurance, Financial Institutions & Professional Registration (DIFP). 2013 Missouri medical professional liability insurance report statistics section. November 2014 available at https://insurance.mo.gov/reports/medmal/documents/2013MissouriMedicalProfessionalLiabilityInsuranceReport.pdf. Accessed 3 Sept 2016.
19. Reason J. Human error: models and management. Br Med J. 2000;320(7237):768–70.
20. Moran NF, Naidoo M, Moodley J. Reducing maternal mortality on a countrywide scale: the role of emergency obstetric training. Best Pract Res Clin Obstet Gynaecol. 2015;29(8):1102–18.
21. Leape L, Lawthers AG, Brennan TA, et al. Preventing medical injury. Qual Rev Bull. 1993;19(5):144–9.

Human Rights and Legal Treaties Relevant to Obstetrics and Gynaecology

66

Oluwadamilola A. Adejumo

Learning Objectives

At the conclusion of this chapter, the reader should be able to:

- Explain the scope, nature and classification of female patient's fundamental human rights which may arise in course of treatment.
- Discuss the rationale for the emergence of women's reproductive rights.
- Recall the human rights treaties and provisions relating to reproductive health.
- Distinguish between effect of treaty provisions and declarations.
- Identify the roles of medical practitioners, especially gynaecologists and obstetricians, in ensuring the protection of reproductive health and rights.

66.1 Introduction

Healthcare professionals including gynaecologists owe patients a duty of care in relating with and in treatment of patients [1]. The breach of the duty of care imposed on them will give rise to a civil claim in negligence under the law of tort, and in more severe cases, a claim may also arise under criminal law.

Implied in the principles of ethics and the duty of care, owed by obstetricians and gynaecologists to patients is the duty to recognise, respect, and give effect to the fundamental human rights and freedoms of patients. Obstetrics is arguably one of the most affected medical specialties in medical liability suits and given its consequences in daily clinical practice [2]. It is thus important to highlight some of the human rights provisions on which the duty of care owed to patients is hinged.

A deep awareness and detailed understanding of these human rights obligations, owed specifically to females, is likely to reduce the situations which give rise to medico-legal issues in the practice of obstetrics and gynaecology, and more importantly, it will result in better and improved care for patients requiring obstetrics and gynaecology care.

The use of a right-based approach to deal with issues in obstetrics and gynaecology care is not to 'play the blame game' or to punish erring individuals but primarily to form a basis for practical accountability on the part of government and healthcare providers in the provision of healthcare services to citizens resulting in safe, functional and effective healthcare systems [3].

66.2 Human Rights: Definitions, Scope, Nature and Classification

The word human has been defined as 'natural to, concerning or belonging to mankind' [4]. The term 'right' has been aptly defined by the learned jurist, Oputa JSC [5] as *'a well-founded claim …enforceable by the power of the State'* [6]. A right has also been defined by the Courts as an interest recognised and protected by the law [7].

Human rights and fundamental freedoms are therefore a set of established claims which are the 'birth right of all human beings' [8]. Accordingly, Cranston [9] defined human rights as *'something of which no one may be deprived without a great affront to justice'*, certain claims which should never be invaded and which are supremely sacred.

In the same vein, the late eminent jurist Kayode Eso, on his part, defined human rights as rights which stand above the ordinary laws of the land and which are in fact antecedent to the political society itself [10].

O. A. Adejumo (✉)
Faculty of Law, Obafemi Awolowo University, Ile-Ife, Ife, Nigeria
e-mail: oaadejumo@oauife.edu.ng

F. Okonofua et al. (eds.), *Contemporary Obstetrics and Gynecology for Developing Countries*,
https://doi.org/10.1007/978-3-030-75385-6_66

Prof. Umozuruike defined human rights as'*... claims, which are invariably supported by ethics and which should be supported by law and such claim can only be legal if legally implemented'* [11].

In all of these definitions, it is crystal clear that human rights are of great importance in every legal order. Human rights are closely linked with ethics, values and morality, and as a result, rights which reflect community values have the most chance of successful implementation [12].

66.3 Classification of Rights

Generally, human rights are classified into three broad categories. The first is civil and political rights, also referred to as the first generation of rights, and they include: the right to life, personal integrity and security, freedom of thought, conscience and religion, freedom of opinion and expression, freedom of peaceful assembly and association, freedom from slavery and servitude, freedom from torture, cruel, inhuman or degrading treatment or punishment. These rights are otherwise known as liberty-oriented rights asserted against the state for protection of the liberty of the individual [13].

The second category consists of economic, social and cultural rights. These are referred to as security-oriented rights. They include: the right to work, the right to a just and favourable condition of work, right to form and join trade unions, right to security, right to protection of and assistance to the family, right to an adequate standard of living, right to education, right to health and the right to take part in cultural life.

The third generation of rights, a more recent category of rights, has been and is still being developed. It is an evolving category and may increase or contract in future [14]. This third category of rights, also referred to as solidarity rights, include the right to development, the right to peace, the right to a healthy and balanced environment, reproductive rights, the right to communication, the right to be different, the right to benefit from the common heritage of mankind, and the right to humanitarian assistance.

These categories of rights, if closely viewed, are rights which are derivatives of other existing rights, particularly socio-economic rights, which seem to have overshadowed them, and hence, the need to have these rights stand, alone as a separate and evolving rights. For instance, the reproductive rights and environmental rights are both derivatives of the right to health and right to adequate standard of living. However, it has become imperative that these rights should naturally evolve and stand alone as core rights which are worthy of recognition and protection.

66.4 General Nature of Human Rights

Despite the categories of rights identified above, one must not lose sight of the very core and inherent nature of human rights. Human rights by their very nature and essence are indivisible and thus they cannot be ranked one above the other on a scale of hierarchy. They form a single package.

The Vienna Conference held in the summer of 1993 supports the view that human rights are universal, indivisible, interdependent and interrelated [15]. This principle was aptly summarised by Catherine Lalumiere [16], who queried as follows:

> *What does the freedom of expression mean to those who have no voice and who live in extreme poverty...what does the right to family life mean to impoverished, divided families whose children are separated from them solely for economic reasons?*

In addition, the United Nations declared at the International Conference held in Teheran [17] that:

> *Since human rights and fundamental freedoms are indivisible, the full realisation of civil and political rights without the enjoyment of economic social and cultural rights is impossible.*

The modern trend which is gaining wide footing is that the classification of rights does not imply divisibility of human rights, and whether first, second, third or emerging generation, they are all one single package.

66.5 Emergence of Women's Reproductive Rights

The neglect of women's reproductive health has been identified as a part of a larger and methodical discrimination against women [18]. Specific laws which protect women's reproductive health are rarely or inadequately implemented under municipal laws.

The principle of non-discrimination and equal enjoyment of fundamental human rights without any form of distinction is at the core of human rights provisions from the United Nations Charter preamble which 're-affirms faith in fundamental human rights ...in the equal rights of men and women...' to other subsequent human rights treaties. Despite the presence of this famous clause in human rights treaties, however, the actualisation of the goal of having equal enjoyment of fundamental rights by both males and females is yet to be a reality.

The plight of women is not restricted only to discrimination, harassment, torture and abuse by their family and non-state organs, but also by State organs in some cases [19]. This plight of women became apparent and gained the attention of the international community with the recognition of the fact that even in developed communities, which are confident of their human rights standards, girls and women are vulnerable members of the society who require more specific and affirmative protection in the society as they are frequently victims of neglect, violence, abuse, poverty and discrimination [20].

As an initial attempt to combat this apparent problem, the United Nations in 1979 adopted the International Convention on the Elimination of all forms of Discrimination Against Women (CEDAW). Despite the adoption of CEDAW which is generally regarded as the International Bill of rights for women, the need to deal with violence and physical abuse by non-state actors and within the family was still apparent.

This may not be far from the reality that violence has a very major and negative impact on women's health, and indeed, the physical and mental health consequences of domestic violence, for instance, represents a serious reproductive health concern among women [21].

It was in recognition of this that the United Nations in 1993 adopted the Declaration on Elimination of Violence Against Women. Also, at the regional level, the Organization of American States adopted the Inter-American Convention on the Prevention, Punishment and Eradication of Violence Against Women in 1994 (ICPPEVAW). The Protocol to the African Charter on Human and Peoples' rights on the Rights of Women in Africa was also adopted by the African Union in 2003 and came into force in 2005 (African Women's Protocol). Similarly, in 2000, the Protocol 12 to the European Convention on Protection of Human Rights and Fundamental Freedoms which guarantees non-discrimination in the enjoyment of any rights set forth by law was adopted to protect women and others who have suffered from various discriminatory norms.

A very crucial aspect of the right to health which has gained notable recognition in recent times particularly in the international community and which aims to step down the tide of discrimination in provision of health services is reproductive health.

The international community has taken recognition of the fact that deaths, which could have been averted, are being recorded amongst pregnant women and that it is fast becoming a huge risk to get pregnant, carry a pregnancy to full term and deliver safely in most rural communities. In Nigeria for instance, a woman's chance of dying from pregnancy and childbirth is reported to be 1 in 13 [22].

Reproductive health is at the core of obstetrics and gynaecology care and will be the core focus of the human rights analysis in this chapter. Reproductive health has been defined as a state of complete physical, mental, social well-being in all matters relating to one's reproductive system, functions and processes [23].

Indeed, the international community [24] recognises that reproductive health includes having a satisfying and safe sex life; having the capacity to reproduce and the freedom to decide if, when and how often to reproduce; being informed of and having access to safe, effective, affordable and acceptable methods of family planning and the right of access to appropriate healthcare services that will enable women to go safely through pregnancy and child birth and provide couples with the best chance of having a healthy infant [25].

All the above indicators of reproductive health find root in and are core principles of reproductive rights which are duly recognised fundamental human rights to which women are entitled and which are enshrined in legal treaties and soft laws.

66.6 Human Rights Provisions Relevant to Obstetrics and Gynaecology

The various human rights provisions and obligations which are of interest to the obstetrician and gynaecologist will be discussed below and an attempt will be made to highlight the key human right provisions of these legal treaties and declarations.

Although the obligations in these treaties are imposed on State parties to the respective treaty, the specific responsibilities to be discharged are to be discharged by individuals and relevant professionals, on behalf of the State, and as such, it is expedient that the key stakeholders should be familiar with and keep the obligations and corresponding rights guaranteed in mind in the discharge of their professional duties.

The discussions will be under two different sub-headings: the first is a consideration of specific treaty provisions which expressly relate to reproductive health and other general human rights provisions; and the second sub-head focuses on declarations and proclamations at international conferences on reproductive and sexual rights.

A. *Specific Treaty Provisions Relating to Reproductive Health*

1. *International Convention on Elimination of All Forms of Discrimination Against Women (CEDAW)*

CEDAW is a core gender-specific treaty and was the culmination of more than 30 years' work of the United Nations Commission on the Status of Women [26]. The Commission's work brought to light most areas in which women are denied equality with men. CEDAW is, in fact, the central and most comprehensive document relating to women's rights by the United Nations [27]. The preamble to CEDAW [28] rightly notes and expresses the concern that despite the various human rights instruments in existence, wide-ranging discrimination against women continues to increase.

The standard of equality required by the CEDAW is not limited to the usual formal equality, but it goes further to also provide the basis for realising women's equal access to opportunities in their political, public and private lives. [29] Specifically, it provides and recognises the need to protect the reproductive rights and health of women. Some notable highlights in the provisions of CEDAW are as follows:

- CEDAW provides an all-encompassing definition of discrimination against women [30] and imposes an express obligation on to adopt all necessary measures to achieve full realisation of rights in the treaty [31] to repeal or modify existing laws, penal provisions, social and cultural patterns, customs and prejudicial practices that aid discrimination against women; to eliminate all forms of prejudice based on idea of inferiority or superiority of the sexes or stereotyped roles and particularly, where necessary to accelerate de facto equality between men and women [32].
- CEDAW recognises the right of women to paid maternity leave, protection of their health and function of reproduction, establishment of child-care facilities to support family obligations and work responsibilities [33].
- It also imposes obligation to eliminate discrimination against women in education and to ensure access to education, educational programmes and information on health, family planning, vocational training to reduce existing gap in education between men and women [34].
- There is a further obligation to eliminate discrimination in health care by providing access to healthcare services, family planning, free services where necessary for pregnancy, post-natal and adequate nutrition during pregnancy and lactation [35].
- Specific attention is to be paid to rural women and their peculiar problems by eliminating discrimination against them and giving them opportunity for participation, access to adequate health care, improved living conditions and social security [36].
- CEDAW in addressing discrimination within the marriage and in family relations imposes obligation on states to ensure that women have freedom to determine freely and responsibly number and spacing of children, right to choose a family name, profession and occupation [37].

2. *African Charter on Human and Peoples' Rights (ACHPR)*

The Charter guarantees the right to health [38] as a fundamental human right of all persons.

The right to life [39] is also guaranteed under the ACHPR. The ACHPR emphasises the inviolability of the human life and the integrity of persons.

The fact that there is an undeniable link between the right to life and health cannot be denied. This is well founded in the principle of interrelatedness and indivisibility of human rights.

In actual fact, a woman who is put at risk of death, as a result of unavailability of health facilities to deal with her reproductive health issues during or after pregnancy, cannot be said to be enjoying in reality, a right to life. It is on this premise that the author of this chapter submits that the right to life cannot be enjoyed or fully realised in situations where adequate provisions are not put in place to guarantee one's health.

The ACHPR also guarantees the right to the dignity inherent in the human person and the right to be free from torture and all forms of inhuman or degrading treatment [40]. This right should be borne in mind by medical practitioners in the treatment of persons to ensure that the dignity of the human person is accorded to females even at their lowest state of well-being. Females should not be taken advantage of or subjected to any form of inhuman treatment (including hostile treatments, spanking or subjection to insults, denial of treatment or neglect at the most critical stages of labour and delivery or even at family planning centres), and cases should be promptly handled professionally in total respect for the inviolability of all persons, dignity and respect for all persons.

3. *The Protocol to the African Charter on the Rights of Women (the African Women's Protocol)*

This Protocol was made pursuant to Article 66 of the ACHPR, which provides for special protocols or agreements when necessary, to supplement the provisions of the African Charter [41]. The Protocol which was adopted in 2003 came into force in 2005 as a direct response to women's needs, setting out specific standards and measures by which women's rights should be recognised [42] and their reproductive health and rights duly protected.

This regional Protocol is more detailed than CEDAW and the ACHPR as it specifically addresses certain practices and issues detrimental to the rights of African women. Some notable provisions under the women's Protocol are highlighted below:

- The Protocol has a definitive section and gives concise and precise definitions of phrases including discrimination against women, harmful practices and violence against women. The definition of women under the Protocol also includes girls. There is an obligation on States to implement the rights guaranteed under their national laws and to adopt all measures for the full realisation of the rights and freedoms guaranteed under the Protocol [43].

- The Protocol imposes an obligation to prohibit execution of death sentences on pregnant and nursing women [44], to ensure respect for and promote the reproductive and sexual health of women particularly, to guarantee the right to control their fertility, determine when to have children and spacing of their children, to family planning education and other health services information, to self-protection and protection from STIs and HIV, to be informed of their health status and their partner's status, to guarantee and provide adequate health facilities and to strengthen pre-natal, delivery and post-natal health and nutritional services for women during pregnancy and while breast feeding and to protect the reproductive rights of women by authorising medical abortion in cases of sexual assault, rape, incest and in circumstances where the continued pregnancy endangers the mental and physical health of the mother or the life of the mother or the foetus [45].
- There are imposed obligations to ensure the protection of women's right to nutritious and adequate food, clean drinking water, sources of domestic fuel, supply and storage to ensure food security [46]; to guarantee the right to a healthy and sustainable environment [47]; to guarantee the right of women to sustainable development by introducing gender perspective in national policies and planning procedures and reducing the adverse effect of globalisation to a minimum for women [48]; to ensure protection of poor women, women in distress, pregnant women, nursing women and women in detention [49]; and to provide appropriate remedies to women whose rights under the Protocol has been violated [50].
- There is an obligation on States to embody principle of equality in national constitutions and legislations, take steps and measures to eliminate and prohibit discrimination and harmful practices which endanger the health and well-being of women; to integrate a gender perspective in policy-making and implementation; to modify the social and cultural patterns of the conduct of women and men with a view to achieving the elimination of harmful cultural and traditional practices and all other practices which are based on the idea of the inferiority or the superiority of either of the sexes or on stereotyped roles for women and men [51]. Additional obligations are imposed on States to prohibit and condemn all forms of harmful practices which negatively affect the human rights of women and which are contrary to recognised international standards including Female Genital Mutilation (FGM); provide health, judicial, psychological and emotional services to victims and to protect those likely to be subjected to such harmful practices, violence and abuse [52].

This is particularly important to the reproductive health of females as most of the consequences of these harmful cultural patterns and traditional practices have severe negative consequences on the reproductive health of females. The negative impact of female genital mutilation, for instance, on the health of females is one that has been a cause of worry in developing countries for quite some time.

4. *Inter-American Convention on Prevention, Punishment and Eradication of Violence Against Women (ICPPEVAW)*

This regional Convention was adopted on 9 June 1994 by the General Assembly of the Organisation of American States and entered into force on 3 March 1995 in recognition of the fact that violence against women constitutes a violation of human rights and fundamental freedoms of women and impairs or nullifies the observance, enjoyment and exercise of their rights and freedoms [53].

As noted earlier, violence has a very negative effect on women's health and thus is a major issue to be addressed in discussions relating to women's health. Some notable highlights of the Convention are:

- The Convention gives an all-encompassing definition of violence and list a number of acts which amounts to sexual and psychological violence whether in domestic unit or in the community [54].
- The Convention recognises the rights: to be free from violence; respect for life, inherent dignity, physical, mental and moral dignity [55].
- The Convention imposes the following duties: to give special consideration to women subjected to violence while pregnant or who are disabled, of minor age, elderly, socio-economically disadvantaged, affected by armed conflict or deprived of their freedom [56].

5. *International Covenant on Economic, Social and Cultural Rights (ICESR) 1966*

The very relevant provision of the ICESR in the context of this chapter is the guarantee of the fundamental right of all persons to the highest attainable standard of health [57]. This right has been well expounded by the United Nations Committee on Economic Social and Cultural Rights to necessarily include freedoms, entitlements and specifically sexual and reproductive freedom to control one's body [58]. Thus, the right to health covers and has a full bearing on sexual and reproductive rights of both men and women but with more emphasis on reproductive freedom of females.

6. *International Covenant on Civil and Political Rights (ICCPR) 1966*

The ICCPR like the ACHPR also recognises the right to life and the right to be free from torture inhuman and degrading treatment [59]. The ICCPR specifically recognises the right of all persons not to be subjected to medical or scientific experimentation, without free consent.

Thus, women are not to be subjected to treatments or medical examinations without their consent and shall be treated with humanity and with respect for the inherent dignity of their person at all times [60].

B. *Conference Declarations and Proclamations on Reproductive Rights*

It is important to start this section by making a clear distinction between declarations and treaties. By their nature, declarations are generally not intended to be legally binding, and they do not possess the force of law that treaties possess. Declarations simply represent international consensus on what should be the ideal standards applicable among nations and sets out common standards of achievement for all peoples [19].

In most cases, declarations may eventually evolve to form part of customary international law, and once they have become notorious enough to be considered customary, they acquire a legally binding nature which makes them enforceable.

Declarations are thus 'soft laws' meant to serve as guidelines to assist States in formulating their domestic laws and setting aims of what it should achieve in realisation of human rights.

Notwithstanding the above, the non-binding nature of conference declarations constitutes a major constraint for implementing and enforcing the women's rights in these documents.

In most cases, a sizeable number of representatives and delegations are sent by State parties to attend these international conferences, promises are often made, but on getting back to their home Countries, nothing is hardly ever done to give effect to realisation of the rights recognised in these declarations, and hence, the obligations emphasised at these conferences often remain largely unimplemented and unenforced; this may be attributed, in part, to the non-binding nature of these obligations.

Some notable declarations, some of which have formed part of Customary International law, are discussed below:

1. *Universal Declaration on Human Rights (UDHR) 1948*

This is the foremost universal and international document relating to fundamental human rights. This declaration was adopted by the United Nations General Assembly Resolution 217A (III) on 10 December 1948. The UDHR firmly enshrines the universal nature of human rights and makes no distinction between the various generations of rights and thus incorporates all the three generations of rights.

It must be noted that the Resolution was not intended to be binding, and specifically, the Chairperson of the Human Rights Commission, Eleanor Roosevelt, rightly noted that the declaration is not and does not purport to be a Statement of law or of legal obligation but that it is a '*common standard of achievement*' [19]. The declaration has, however, over time become notorious enough to be considered as forming part of customary international human rights law.

Notable rights in the declaration relevant to obstetrics and gynaecology practice include:

- The right to a standard of living adequate for the health and well-being including access to medical care and necessary social services [61].
- UDHR specifically recognises that motherhood and childhood are entitled to special care and assistance [62].
- Right to life and liberty [63].
- Right to social security and is entitled to realisation of the economic, social and cultural rights indispensable for his dignity [64]. This necessarily include provision of necessary health care facilities and treatment.
- Freedom from inhuman and degrading treatment [65].

2. *United Nations Declaration 2000 and the Millennium Development Goal 5*

The United Nations General Assembly adopted the Millennium Declaration [66] at its 55th Session on 18 September 2000. Women's reproductive health has been identified clearly as one of the key issues for the development of any society, and hence, the Millennium development goal (MDG) No.5 pursuant to this declaration is to improve maternal health by achieving a three-quarter reduction in maternal mortality ratio between 1990 and 2015 and to achieve universal access to reproductive health by 2015 [67].

The declaration also seeks to strengthen respect for and strive for full protection of human rights; to strengthen capacity of states to realise guaranteed human rights of citizens; to combat all forms of violence against women; and to implement the provisions of CEDAW [67].

3. *United Nations Declaration on Elimination of Violence Against Women*

This declaration [68] was adopted by United Nations General Assembly in 1993 in recognition of the urgent need for the universal application to women of the rights and principles with regard to equality, security, liberty, integrity and dignity and borne out of the concern that violence against women is an obstacle to the achievement of equality, development and peace [69], which was duly recognised at the 1985 Nairobi Conference where forward-looking Strategies for the Advancement of Women were identified [70].

The fact that violence has an adverse effect on women's health has been noted earlier, and as such, the declaration emphasises the protection of the fundamental rights of women [71] and recognises a wide range of practices which fall within the scope of violence and which States are enjoined to prohibit and condemn [72].

These practices include: physical, sexual and psychological violence occurring in the family, including battering, sexual abuse of female children in the household, dowry-related violence, marital rape, female genital mutilation and other traditional practices harmful to women, non-spousal violence and violence related to exploitation; within the general community, including rape, sexual abuse, sexual harassment and intimidation at work, in educational institutions and elsewhere, trafficking in women and forced prostitution [73].

4. *International Conference on Population and Development (ICPD)*

This United Nations Conference was held in Cairo, Egypt from 5 to 13 September 1994. Over 179 countries participated and were represented by delegates at the conference [74]. A resolution was passed at the conference to adopt the detailed Programme of Action (POA) which was drafted at the end of the conference. The relevant parts of the POA which has a bearing on women's reproductive health are:

- Chapter II of the POA emphasises women's ability to control their own fertility. This Chapter specifically declares the right of women, including their reproductive rights as inalienable, integral and indivisible part of fundamental human rights [75]. The right of women to universal access to reproductive health care, family planning and sexual health was also recognised and declared to be a core human right [76].
- Chapter VII also emphasises reproductive rights and health of women including family planning and protection from STIs and HIV [77].
- Chapter VIII, which deals with health, morbidity and mortality, goes further to emphasise corresponding duties and rights relating to women's health and safe motherhood [78].

5. *Fourth World Conference on Women*

This conference took place in Beijing from 4 to 15 September 1995. It was a follow up to the 1975 Mexico Conference which is the first world conference on women, the 1980 Copenhagen Conference which is the second world conference on women and the 1985 Nairobi Conference which is the third world conference on women [79].

Certain declarations were made at the conference, and this is now known as the Beijing Declaration. Some of the rights declared which relate to reproductive health of females include:

- The express and unequivocal declaration of women's rights as human rights [80]
- Recognition and reaffirmation of the right of all women to control all aspects of their health, in particular their fertility [81]
- Obligations to ensure equal access to and equal treatment of women and men in education and health care so as to enhance women's sexual and reproductive health as well as education [82]

A Platform for Action (PFA) was adopted at the conference as an agenda to actualise the attainment of the declarations set out. It is worthy of note that several other conferences have been held as a follow up to review progress made in actualising the Beijing Declaration. Notably are the Beijing+5 in 2000, Beijing +10 in 2005 and the 15-year review in 2010.

66.7 Conclusion

The common thread that undeniably weaves through all the definitions, nature and classification of human rights is the fact that they are claims to which all humans are entitled.

Despite this undeniable fact and the emphasised importance of reproductive health, the actual enjoyment and attainment of reproductive health by women who are largely considered as the most vulnerable members of the society is in doubt in most developing countries.

Specifically, healthcare facilities sufficient to cater for the reproductive needs of women are not readily available and accessible. Also, the healthcare providers are often ignorant of the existence of the basic guaranteed rights to which females are entitled.

Even in the very few cases where facilities exist at all, the existing ones fall below international standards, and this, among other factors, is responsible for the high maternal mortality rate which is recorded in most parts of the developing world today [83]. This is in violation of the express provisions of the right to health which entails a necessary obligation to ensure the provision of access to basic facilities required to promote the health and well-being of all persons.

Also, implicit in the right to the highest attainable standard of health is the right of health professionals to discharge their duties efficiently and without negligence and having the duty of care principle at the back of their minds.

Women's reproductive rights advocates striving to improve women's reproductive health; must engage continuously with political elites and stakeholders in the health sector who shape and implement public health policies through legislation and domestication of international treaties [84].

The miracle of life is fast becoming a nightmare of death in most developing countries. 510 per 100,000 was the maternal mortality rate in sub-Saharan Africa in 2015, and this region was the highest rate in the world [85].

The principle of *pacta sunt servanda* is a well-established principle of international law. The principle is to the effect that agreements generally are meant to be binding on parties to them, and thus, where a State has ratified a or consented to a treaty or declaration, the intention to be bound by such document is necessarily implied and should be taken seriously without need for prompting. As such, States need to put in place measures to implement, enforce and guarantee reproductive health and rights provisions of treaties and international declarations signed by them.

A strong political will on the part of the leaders to commit to the actualisation of these rights and policies is what appears to be lacking.

It is not enough for leaders to pay lip service to the issue of reproductive health by sending delegates to 'warm the benches' and mark attendance at international conferences. They should be equally eager to domesticate treaties ratified and give effect to declarations made at these conferences. This will make the reproductive rights protected under treaties and declarations to be not just dangling carrots which cannot be reached by women in the developing world.

There is an urgent need for leaders and all stakeholders in the health sector to take positive and apparently progressive steps by creating an awareness of the existence of duly guaranteed rights and equipping institutions capable of effectively providing these guaranteed rights to its citizens.

66.8 Summary

The practice of obstetrics and gynaecology is one that is prone to litigation and legal claims. A deep awareness and detailed understanding of the human rights obligations owed specifically to females, and the rationale for these obligations is thus crucial for medical practitioners in the field of obstetrics and gynaecology. Identification and understanding of these rights will help avoid medico-legal issues, suits for breach of duty of care and infringement of fundamental human rights, which may arise in the course of practice. Proper understanding of fundamental human rights obligations will also ultimately result in better and improved care for patients requiring obstetrics and gynaecology care.

References

1. Edozien LC. Medico-legal issues in gynaecology. Obstet Gynaecol Reprod Med. 2009;19(7):187–92.
2. Dominguez AP, Belo A, Moura P, Vieira DN. Medico-legal litigation in Obstetrics: a characterisation analysis of a decade in Portugal. Rev Bras Ginecol Obstet. 2015;37(5):241–6.
3. Freedman LP. Averting maternal death and disability- Human rights, constructive accountability and maternal mortality in the Dominican Republic: a commentary. Int J Gynaecol Obstet. 2003;82(1):111–4.
4. Chambers Universal Learners Dictionary. England: Chambers Harrap Publishers Limited, 1995.
5. Retired Justice of the Nigerian Supreme Court.
6. Oputa JCA. Human Rights in political and Legal Culture of Nigeria, vol. 38. 2nd ed. Idigbe Memorial Lectures; 1989.
7. Afolayan v Ogunrinde and Ors (1990) 1NWLR (Pt. 127) 369 at 391.
8. Vienna Declaration. World Conference on Human Rights on 25 June 1993; Paragraph 1. Available at http://www.unhchr.ch/huridocda/huridoca.nsf/%28symbol%29/a.conf.157.23.en. Accessed on 05 Nov 2016.
9. Cranston M. Human Rights: real and supposed. In: Raphael, editor. Political theories and the rights of man, vol. 52. London: Bloomington Press; 1967.
10. Ransome Kuti V A.G Federation (1975) 2NWLR (Pt 6) 211.
11. Eze O. Human Rights in Africa: selected problems. Lagos: Macmillan; 1984. p. 5.
12. Shaw M. International law. 5th ed. New Delhi: Brijbasi Art Press; 2004. p. 248.
13. Shelby D. Development of the concept of rights. In: Human Rights Law and Practice in Nigeria. CUP, vol. 1; 1987.
14. Vasak K. The 3rd Generation of Human Rights: the rights of Solidarity, vol. 2. Strasbourg: Inaugural Lecture Delivered at the 10th Study Session of the International Law of Human Rights; 1979.
15. Vienna Convention 1993; Part 1, para 5.
16. Lalumiere C. Human Rights at the dawn of the 21st century. Council of Europe; 1993. p. 13.
17. Para 13 of the Proclamation of Teheran, Final Act of the International Conference, Teheran 22nd April to 18th May, 1968.
18. Cook RJ. International Human Rights and Women's Reproductive Health. Stud Family Plan. 1993;24(2):73–86.
19. Rehman J. International Human Rights Law. 2nd ed. England: Pearson Education Limited; 2010. p. 80.
20. ibid.
21. Fikree FF, Bhatti LI. Domestic violence and health of Pakistani women. Int J Gynaecol Obstet. 1999;65(2):195–201.
22. UNICEF. Maternal and Child health available at http://www.unicef.org/nigeria/children_1926.html. Accessed on 13 Oct 2016.
23. Aniekwu NI. A legal perspective on reproductive health and gender-specific human rights in Nigeria. J Med Biomed Res. 2004;3(1):21–9.
24. International Conference on Population and Development (ICPD) Programme of Action (POA); 1994.
25. World Health Organisation (WHO). Reproductive health. Available at www.who.int/.../reproductivehealth/en. Accessed on 13 Oct 2016.
26. This Commission was established by the United Nations in 1946 to monitor the situation of women and to promote women's rights.
27. Division for the Advancement of Women, Convention on Elimination of All Forms of Discrimination
28. Against Women. UN Department of Economic and Social Rights http://www.un.org/womenwatch/daw/cedaw/text/econvention.htm. Accessed on 13 Apr 2013. See paragraph 6 of the Preamble.

29. Aniekwu NI. The Convention on the Elimination of All forms of Discrimination Against Women and the Status of Implementation on the Right to Health in Nigeria. Human Rights Brief. Centre for Human Rights and Humanitarian Law, American University, Washington College of Law available at www.wcl.american.edu/humright/centre.cfm. Accessed on 13 Oct 2016.
30. Article 1 CEDAW.
31. Article 24 CEDAW.
32. Articles 2, 3, 4 and 5 CEDAW.
33. Article 11 CEDAW.
34. Article 10 CEDAW.
35. Article 12 CEDAW.
36. Article 14 CEDAW.
37. Article 16 CEDAW.
38. Article 16.
39. Article 4 ACHPR.
40. Article 5 ACHPR.
41. Specifically, Article 2 which affirms the principle of non-discrimination on grounds of sex and Article 18 which calls on all States Parties to eliminate every discrimination against women and to ensure the protection of the rights of women in international conventions and declarations.
42. Aniekwu NI. The Additional Protocol to the African Charter on Human and Peoples' Rights: Indications of capacity for African Municipal Systems. Available at http://www.saflii.org/za/journals/LDD/2009/12.pdf. Accessed on 14 Apr 2016.
43. Article 26 of the Protocol.
44. Article 4 of the Protocol.
45. Article 14 of the Protocol.
46. Article 15 of the Protocol.
47. Article 18 of the Protocol.
48. Article 19 of the Protocol.
49. Article 23 of the Protocol.
50. Article 24 of the Protocol.
51. Article 2 of the Protocol.
52. Article 5 of the Protocol.
53. Paragraph 2 of the Preamble to the ICPPEVAW.
54. Articles 1 and 2 of the ICPPEVAW; these acts include torture, rape, forced prostitution, sexual abuse, trafficking among others.
55. Articles 3–6 of the ICPPEVAW.
56. Articles 7, 8 and 9 of the ICPPEVAW.
57. Article 12.
58. CESCR General Comment No. 14. The Right to Highest Attainable Standard of Health (11/08/00) E/C.12/200/4. 22nd Session 25th April-12th May 2000.
59. Article 6 and 7 of the ICCPR.
60. Article 10 ICCPR.
61. Article 25 UDHR.
62. ibid.
63. Article 3 UDHR.
64. Article 22 UDHR.
65. Article 5 UDHR.
66. United Nations General Assembly Declaration 2000 A/RES/55/2
67. Articles 19 and 25 United Nations Millennium Development Goals available at http://www.un.org/millenniumgoals/ accessed on 10/03/17
68. United Nations General Assembly Resolution 48/104.
69. Paragraphs 1 and 4 of the Declaration.
70. United Nations. Available at http://www.un.org/womenwatch/daw/beijing/.
71. Article 3 of the Declaration.
72. Article 4 of the Declaration.
73. Article 2 of the Declaration.
74. Aniekwu NI. Reproductive health law: A jurisprudential Analysis of Gender specific Human Rights for the African Region. Benin City: Ambik Press; 2011. p. 3.
75. Programme of Action, Principle 4 at page 12 of the POA available at http://www.unfpa.org/webdav/site/global/shared/documents/publications/2004/icpd_eng.pdf. Accessed on 14 Apr 2016.
76. Id, Principle 8.
77. Id, pages 40–49.
78. Id, pages 57 and 58.
79. The United Nations Entity for Gender Equality and the Empowerment of Women at www.un.org/womenwatch/daw/beijing/index.html. Accessed on 14 Apr 2013.
80. Beijing Declaration, Article 14 available at http://www.un.org/womenwatch/daw/beijing/pdf/BDPfA%20E.pdf. Accessed on 14 Apr 2016.
81. Id, Article 17.
82. Id, Article 30.
83. Adedokun N. Curbing maternal deaths in Nigeria. Premium Times 2013 available at http://www.premiumtimesng.com/opinion/132667-curbing-maternal-deaths-in-nigeria.html. Accessed on 13 Oct 2016.
84. Tarrow SG. Power in movement. Cambridge, MA: Cambridge University Press; 1994.
85. United Nations Development Programme (UNDP). Human Development Report. Oxford: Oxford University Press; 2015.

Evaluation of Clinical Significance in Intervention Research

67

Joseph A. Balogun

Learning Objectives
After reading this chapter, the learner will be able to:

- Discuss the general characteristics of intervention research
- Articulate the differences between statistical significance and clinical difference
- Discern the statistical measures of clinical significance
- Discuss the theoretical underpinnings of Cohen-d effect size
- Manually compute Cohen-d and Eta Square (η^2) estimates for two or more groups and repeated test designs
- Contextualise and interpret Cohen-d and η^2 estimates
- Access and use web-based calculators to compute effect size estimates for simple and complex experimental designs

67.1 Introduction

Intervention research has been an essential part of medicine since the eighteenth century, but its application for the betterment of human conditions that is evidence-based is contemporary, and much remains unknown. The importance of intervention research cannot be overemphasised because it forms the centre piece of one of the three fundamental pillars of evidence-based practice – best research evidence using a sound methodology, clinicians expertise and experience and values, preferences, concerns and expectations of the individuals [1]. Obstetrics and gynaecology (Ob-Gyns) intervention studies are designed to evaluate the effectiveness of physical devices/agents, drugs, healthcare service delivery and to establish the safety, cost-efficacy and acceptability of treatment procedures [2–10].

One critical statistical concept that is increasingly receiving attention in the biomedical and allied health literature is clinical significance; also known as practical significance, social validity or real-world treatment outcomes. Effect size is one of the most critical indicators of clinical significance. Most high impact scientific journals now require authors of intervention studies to assess the clinical relevance of any observed statistically significant difference associated with treatment. Failure to do so has recently been one of the primary reasons for rejection of intervention studies manuscripts submitted for publication.

In writing this chapter, a literature search was conducted on the PUBMED database to identify the frequency of reporting clinical significance estimates in obstetrics and gynaecology research publications. The search used the keyword combinations of "obstetrics and gynaecology," "intervention studies," "clinical significance" and "effect size" (Table 67.1).

The literature search showed that the PUBMED database had indexed 13,958 intervention studies in obstetrics and gynaecology, but only 377 (2.7%) of them mentioned clini-

Table 67.1 PUBMED literature search and number of publications

Steps	Level of literature search	Number of publications
1	Obstetrics and gynaecology	189,839
2	Obstetrics and gynaecology and intervention studies	13,958
3	Obstetrics and gynaecology, intervention studies and clinical significance	377
4	Obstetrics and gynaecology, intervention studies, clinical significance and effect size	13

J. A. Balogun (✉)
Chicago State University, Chicago, IL, USA

University of Medical Sciences, Ondo City, Nigeria

Centre of Excellence in Reproductive Health Innovation, University of Benin, Benin City, Nigeria
e-mail: jbalogun@csu.edu; jbalogun@unimed.edu.ng

F. Okonofua et al. (eds.), *Contemporary Obstetrics and Gynecology for Developing Countries*,
https://doi.org/10.1007/978-3-030-75385-6_67

cal significance in the article. Of the 377 studies, only 13 (3.4%) reported clinically significant measures such as confidence interval (CI), risk and odds ratios or effect size. The literature search implied that clinical significance estimates are reported rarely in obstetrics and gynaecology intervention research. Two recently published studies belly the dimension and scope of the problem [11, 12].

A 2016 retrospective study by Glujovsky and associates investigated the proportion of studies published in top infertility journals that reported effect size estimates and their precision [11]. They found that 38% of the 32 studies indexed by PubMed in 2014 did not indicate in the abstract section of their publication whether the difference observed was statistically or clinically significant, and only 6.3% of the studies reported CI. Similarly, in the result section, only 28% and 16% of the findings reported clinical significance estimates and the CI, respectively. In the methods section, only one study documented the minimal clinically significant difference. The authors found the interpretation of the findings to be misleading in 41% of the studies reviewed. They concluded that clinical significance estimates are under-reported in top infertility journals "with a propensity for misleading interpretation of the findings" and recommended that authors should report clinical significance estimates to improve the quality of information presented [11].

A meta-analysis study by Hay and associates in 2017 found that across a broad spectrum of intervention studies, the authors failed to "narrow the CI of an average estimate or change the statistical significance reported in most cases" [12]. The authors recommended that peer review committees of grant applications should "require formal consideration of optimal effect size based on existing evidence in power calculations" [12].

Journal editors reject articles submitted for publication for a variety of reasons ranging from the mundane errors (such as missing title, author names, institutional affiliations, keywords, references, tables, figures and substandard English) to serious methodological malfeasance such as plagiarism [13–15]. The rejection rates of manuscripts submitted to biomedical and allied health journals vary widely ranging from 30% in publications by *Elsevier* to 87% by the prestigious journal of *Nature* [15]. A rejection outcome is frustrating for the researchers who spend years planning the study, securing funding, collecting and analysing data and writing the article with the hope of getting it published. The high rejection rate is due to the limited knowledge of research methods and biostatistics by most medical scientists and practitioner [16–20].

While research methods and biostatistics are not familiar bedfellows of Ob-Gyns, it is nefarious and unethical to publish a statistically flawed study. Although evaluation of clinical significance is now of paramount importance to journal editors and reviewers, many of the biostatistics books available to medical students and practitioners do not cover the concept. And many of the conventional data analysis software, including the Statistical Package for Social Scientists (SPSS) and Statistical Analysis System (SAS), do not provide effect size estimates.

This chapter explores the clinical significance concept and the web-based calculators that can provide effect size estimates with minimal effort. A basic understanding of biostatistics and familiarity with the SPSS program is necessary to comprehend fully the information presented in this chapter.

67.2 Intervention Research

The genesis of intervention research in the modern sense is credited to Dr. James Lind, a British naval surgeon, who in 1747 experimented with 12 sailors suffering from scurvy. He assigned the 12 sailors into six pairs giving each pair different supplements to their regular diet for 2 weeks. The six supplements were vinegar, elixir vitriol, sea water, cider, two oranges and one lemon and a mixture of nutmeg, garlic, mustard and tamarind in barley water. On the sixth day of the experiment, they had no orange and lemon left but noticed that one of the sailors who received orange and lemon supplement recovered fully and his counterpart improved significantly, almost completely healed. Of the other pairs, only the sailors who received cider supplement showed some improvement. The other four pairs that constitute the control group did not improve. This historic study paved the way for true-experimental (randomised controlled trials, RCT) intervention research as we know it today.

From practical perspectives, intervention research is categorised into therapeutic and preventive components. Therapeutic research is typically clinical or laboratory-based, and the patients are treated to prevent death or improve health. Conversely, preventive intervention research is community-based and focuses on pre-emptying the development of emerging diseases. In the preventive research paradigm, healthy individuals or at-risk groups are usually recruited to test the efficacy of vaccines [21].

There are two main methods for investigating a clinical problem or developmental challenge: through the application of quantitative or qualitative research approaches. The quantitative method uses deductive reasoning in arriving at a hypothesis, collect data and statistically analyse it to assess whether empirical evidence exists to corroborate the stated hypothesis. On the other hand, the qualitative method provides an in-depth understanding of the underlying reasons, perceptions and motivations about the phenomenon being studied thereby helping to advance future ideas for quantitative research [21, 22].

The primary types of quantitative research designs include observational, pre-experimental (case studies), quasi-experimental (non-randomised trials), true-experimental (RCT) models, a systematic review and meta-analysis (Fig. 67.1).

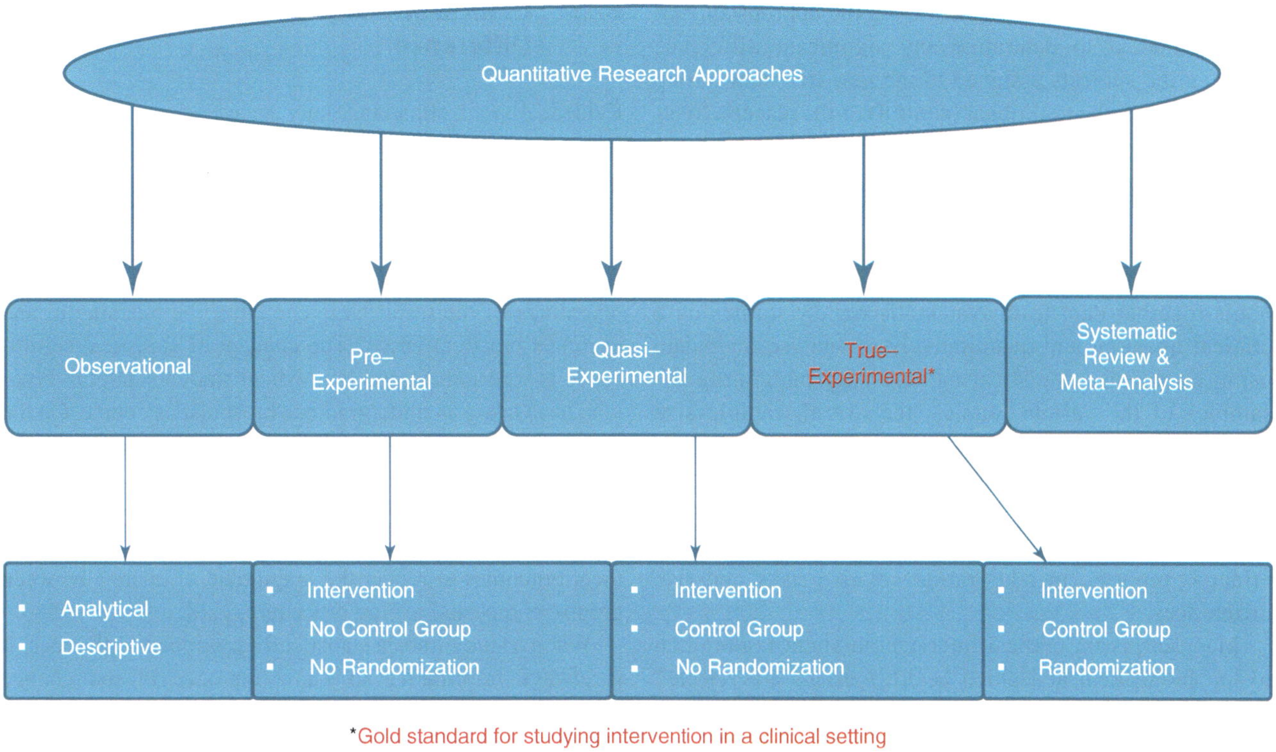

Fig. 67.1 Quantitative research approaches and their major characteristics

Observational design (cohort and case–control studies) investigates the association between disease risk factors, individual characteristics and their likelihood of getting a particular disease [23]. Both observational and qualitative methods do not adequately meet the strict methodological criteria required in intervention studies (i.e. independent groups, randomisation, treatment or intervention and control groups) and also fails to control for the pervasive extraneous factors such as history, repeated testing, maturation, selection bias, experimental mortality, instrumentation and statistical regression [21].

Pre-experimental design is the simplest form of research conducted to understand if further investigation is warranted on the target group. Examples of pre-experimental design are the one-shot case study design, one-group pre- and post-test design and static-group comparison design. In a quasi-experimental design, there is manipulation of independent variables and a control group, but the study participants are not assigned randomly into groups. This design is used typically in field settings where random assignment is either not possible or not required. Examples of quasi-experimental design are the static group comparison design, the non-equivalent control design and the time series design. Although observational, pre-experimental and quasi-experimental designs are useful methods of scientific inquiry, a cause and effect conclusion cannot be inferred from these studies [21].

True-experimental design or RCT, a term commonly used in epidemiological research is the gold standard of clinical research because it eliminates selection and confounding factor biases and a cause and effect conclusion can be drawn from the investigation. Examples of true-experimental design are the post-test-only control group design, the pre- and post-test control group design and the Solomon four-group (multifactorial) design [21]. The overarching goal of true-experimental research is to apply the study outcomes to the general population. In true-experimental research, the study participants are allocated randomly to the experimental (intervention) group receiving the treatment under investigation and a comparison (control) group which gets the traditional treatment or placebo. The groups are then prospectively followed to evaluate the effectiveness of the new treatment compared with the conventional (control) or placebo treatment [21–23]. The random assignment of subjects into groups is to ensure that the treatment and placebo groups are similar in all characteristics before the introduction of the intervention. Indeed, there is no guarantee that the two groups will ever be equal. In rare cases when this occur, the pre-treatment inequalities are adjusted for using the analysis of covariance (ANCOVA) statistical procedure [21].

A double-blind strategy is used in intervention research to safeguard against extraneous variables such as the placebo effect by ensuring neither the researchers taking the measurements nor those following up on treatment protocols know the study participants assigned to the control or the experimental groups until after data collection.

Subsequently, data are analysed using the appropriate statistical method to determine any significant difference between the subjects assigned to the new treatment group compared with the traditional (control) or the placebo treatment group.

A systematic review provides a summary of clinical studies, with conflicting findings, on a clinical question, using specific methods to search, appraise and synthesise the literature critically and systematically. Meta-analysis pools together data from systematic review studies on a clinical question and quantitatively re-analyse their data using established statistical methods. By integrating the samples of the various studies, the overall sample size will increase; thus, improving the statistical power of the analysis and the precision of the treatment effect estimates. Meta-analysis involves the calculation of treatment effect measures for each study at 95% CI. The treatment effect is reported in odds ratios, relative risks and risk differences.

Manuscripts on clinical intervention studies submitted to top biomedical and allied health journals are rejected often for weak research design issues (no control group, no randomisation and inadequate sample size) and invalid statistical analysis methods [11–13]. Through careful planning and use of true-experimental research protocols [22] (Fig. 67.2), the aforementioned methodological pitfalls can be avoided.

67.3 Clinical and Statistically Significant Difference

Evidence-based clinicians daily answer three fundamental questions when comparing the effectiveness of different treatment interventions. First, the clinician would like to know if an observed finding is statistically significant, that is, is it real or could it be due to chance? If it is significant, what is the magnitude of the effect (i.e. effect size)? And is the magnitude of the result large enough to be meaningful and useful in practical terms? The concept of statistical significance is well-understood by medical students and Ob-Gyns who have taken an undergraduate biostatistics course. On the contrary, clinical significance is a less understood entity by researchers in medicine, allied health, social sciences and education [24, 25]. Clinical significance is an adjunct to statistical significance and is used in the interpretation of treatment outcomes to reflect the magnitude of change between groups or repeated testing procedures [26].

When a study finds a statistically significant difference, it is always informative to know the size of the change observed. A statistically significant difference indicates the observed change is authentic and not due to random variation, but we are not sure if the discovery is meaningful in the real world. Incontrovertibly, statistical significance is influenced by sample size, the quality of the data collected and the power of the analytical procedures. With a large sample

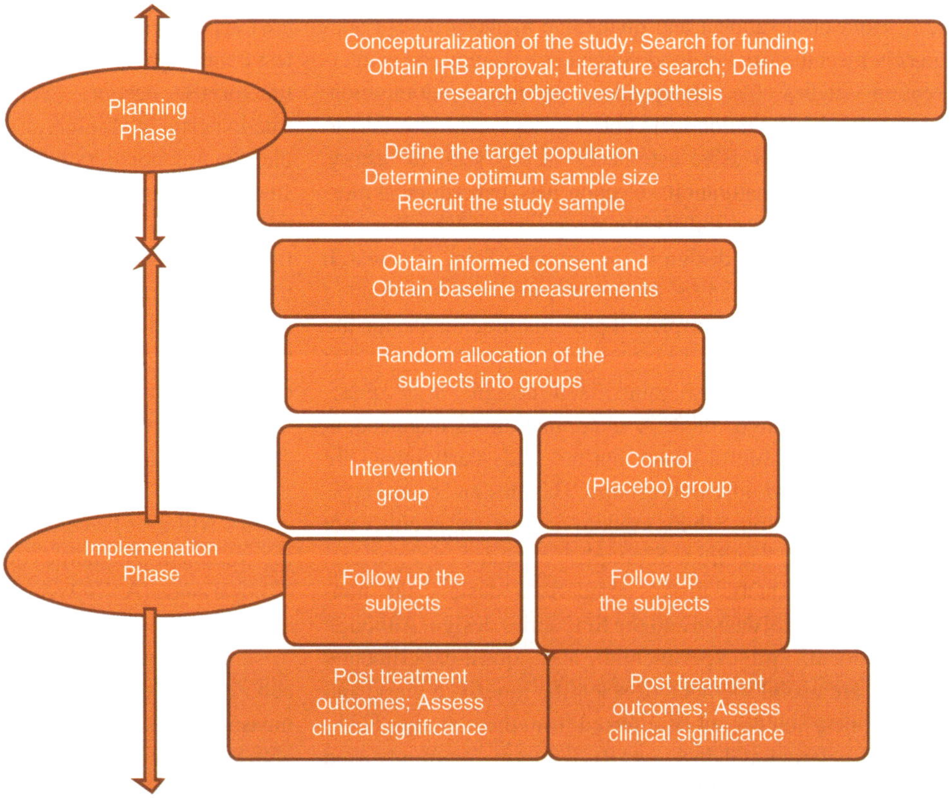

Fig. 67.2 Schematic illustration of the implementation of a true-experimental research

size, as is often the case in epidemiological, laboratory assessment studies, a minimal change in the dependent variables will produce statistical significance [24, 25].

Even though most research publications include information on statistical significance, such information is problematic from a practical standpoint. For example, a statistical significance difference at an alpha level of 0.05 or 0.01 does not tell the readers the size of the observed difference between groups or repeated tests. Under these conditions, the findings cannot be compared easily across different studies [27].

67.4 Measures of Clinical Significance

The following approaches are generally used to translate statistically significant discoveries into the real-life practical situation:

1. Comparison of a Sample to a Reference Group or Norm

By comparing a study mean score to the norm, we can evaluate how well the sample performed relative to the general population. This comparison will allow us to know whether one sample statistic is "small," "intermediate" or "strong" effect when compared to the population [27].

2. Confidence Intervals (CI)

The CI is a range of values that is likely to include the population value with a certain degree of confidence. It is often expressed as a percentage (%) whereby the population means lies between the lower and upper band (interval) interval. Traditionally, they are called "margins of errors." Confidence limits reflect the importance of a finding. A small CI value indicates a high degree of confidence that the study outcome is real. Conversely, if the CI is substantial (wide), it suggests a low degree of confidence and a dose of caution must be exercised in applying the findings from such a study [27].

3. Calculation of Effect Size

When a research finding is statistically significant, the sample size of the study must be "optimum" and not too large. This expectation is because results based on a large sample size may be statistically significant but may not have much practical significance. It is therefore imperative to calculate the size of the change or the effect size of any observed variation. Effect size is a measure of the extent of the impact of the intervention or the magnitude of the differences observed [26]. In practice, we calculate effect size after finding a statistically significant difference between groups or repeated tests. There is no point in estimating the size of intervention if there is no good reason to suppose there is any effect.

67.5 Effect Size Indicators

There are over 50 different indicators of effect size broken down into four major approaches [24, 25, 27].

(i) Correlation indices: Effect sizes based on the percentage of "variance" are explained. This is achieved by evaluating the strength of the relationship between the dependent (Y) and independent (X) variables. Data are analysed by Pearson's product moment correlation coefficient (r) and the multiple correlation coefficient (R^2). Effect size estimates inform that correlation coefficients vary between −1.0 and +1.0 with 0 signifying no effect [25, 27].

(ii) Difference indices: Effect sizes are based on the differences between different groups or repeated measures mean. Examples are Cohen d, Eta-squared (η^2), Glass' Δ and Hedges' g [25].

(iii) Categorical indices: Effect sizes are based on associations among categorical variables using the Chi-squared test. Examples are Phi (related to the point-biserial correlation coefficient), Cramér's V (for variables having more than two levels), Cohen's w and Cohen's h [27].

(iv) Risk potency indices: Effects sizes are based on the calculation of odds and risk ratios, relative risk, risk difference, the number needed to treat (NNT), the experimental event rate, absolute risk reduction and relative risk reduction [28].

In medicine and allied health literature, correlation coefficients (r, R^2), Cohen-d and η^2 estimates are the most commonly reported measures of clinical significance. Epidemiological research usually assesses risk potency indices. Discussion of risk potency is beyond the scope of this article which will focus primarily on the calculation and interpretation of Cohen-d and η^2 effect size estimates. A learner interested in obtaining more in-depth information about risk potency can consult the publications by Jacob and Ganguli [29] and Schnell [30].

67.6 Testing for Statistical Significance in an Independent T-Test Group Design

To calculate effect size estimates, we need to know the arithmetic mean and standard deviation (SD) of the groups or repeated test procedures. We will illustrate our calculations of effect size estimates with a simple posttest-only control group true-experimental design. The hypothetical study sets out to test the null (statistical) hypothesis that a newly discovered hypertensive medication A will not be more effective than the traditional (conventional) medication B in controlling blood pressure.

To test the null hypothesis at an alpha level of 0.05, we recruited 100 patients with hypertension and randomly allocated them to two groups. Group A (newly discovered medication) had 50 patients and those in group B (conventional/standard medication – constitutes the control group) also had 50 patients. We are assuming because the individuals were assigned randomly to the two groups, their baseline (dependent variable) measurements will be the same. Unfortunately, there is no guarantee this assumption will occur. We can improve the design of the study by taking baseline blood pressure measurements at the beginning of the study before taking medication.

Next, the patients in both groups were informed to take their medication for 10 weeks. After 10 weeks, we measured their systolic blood pressure (SBP) and diastolic blood pressures (DBP). In this hypothetical study, we will consider only the SBP for the illustration. The average SBP and SD of the patients' in group A was 140 mmHg with SD of 12.0 and those assigned to group B was 150 mmHg with SD of 13.0.

We can now test for plausible statistically significant difference between the two independent groups – medications A and B. First, we would compute the SD for the SBP measurements and use the independent student (unpaired) t-test formula below to test the hypothesis:

$$t = \frac{\bar{x}_1 - \bar{x}_2}{\sqrt{\frac{s_1^2}{n_1} + \frac{s_2^2}{n_2}}}$$

Where:

$\bar{x}_1$ = Mean SBP value for group A
$\bar{x}_2$ = Mean SBP value for group B
S_1 = SBP SD for patients assigned to group A
S_2 = SBP SD for patients assigned to group B
n_1 = Total number of patients in group A
n_2 = Total number of those in group B

Let us first solve the denominator aspect of the formula:

$$= \sqrt{\frac{(12)^2}{(50)} + \frac{(13)^2}{50}}$$

$$= \sqrt{\frac{(144)}{(50)} + \frac{(169)}{(50)}}$$

$$= 2.5$$

Now that we have calculated the denominator component of the formula, we can now proceed to derive the t-calculated statistic for the two groups:

$$t = \frac{\bar{x}_1 - \bar{x}_2}{\sqrt{\frac{s_1^2}{n_1} + \frac{s_2^2}{n_2}}}$$

t calculated = 140–150/2.50
t calculated = – 4.0
Degree of freedom (DF) = $n_1 + n_2 - 2 = 98$

We now need to derive the t-critical value for the theoretical study from a Standard t-table [31], using a DF of 98 at the stipulated alpha level of 0.05. The derived value from the t-table is 1.984. The t-calculated value of – 4.0 falls outside the normal region/limits of acceptance. Therefore, we would reject the null hypothesis at the 0.05 level and conclude that medication A is better or more effective ($p < 0.05$) than medication B in the management of hypertension.

67.7 Manual Calculation of Cohen-d Estimate for an Independent T-Test Group Design

At this stage, we are still not sure of the magnitude of the observed difference between the two groups. The pertinent question to ask is, how much more effective was medication A better than medication B? We need to calculate Cohen's d effect size estimate to answer this question. Unfortunately, the traditional data analysis software such as SAS and SPSS, do not provide estimates for Cohen's d effect size. However, we can compute it by extracting the relevant information from the SPSS or SAS printout and manually calculate it using the following standard formula:

$$\text{Cohen's d effect size} = \frac{\text{Mean for Group A} - \text{Mean for Group B}}{\text{Pooled Standard Deviation (SD)}}$$

Where pooled SD =

$$SD_{pooled} = \sqrt{\frac{(SD_1^2 + SD_2^2)}{2}}$$

Let us now calculate Cohen's d value for the SBP data from our hypothetical study. To summarise the data collected for the study, the Mean and SD of the SBP for the patients' given medication A at the end of 10 weeks of treatment was 140 mmHg and 12.0, respectively. The SBP for the patients on medication B was 150 mmHg and 13.0, respectively. Again, the formula to calculate Cohen's d effect size is:

$$\text{Cohen's d} = \frac{\text{Mean for Group A} - \text{Mean for Group B}}{\text{Pooled Standard Deviation (SD)}}$$

First, we must calculate the pooled SD component of the formula =

$$SD_{pooled} = \sqrt{\frac{\left(SD_1^2 + SD_2^2\right)}{2}}$$

$$\text{Pooled SD} = \frac{\sqrt{\left(12^2 + 13^2\right)}}{\sqrt{(2)}}$$

$$\text{Pooled SD} = 12.50$$

Second, we can now compute the effect size using the standard formula:

$$\text{Cohen's d} = \frac{\text{Mean for Group A} - \text{Mean for Group B}}{\text{Pooled Standard Deviation (SD)}}$$

$$= \frac{(140 - 150)}{12.50}$$

$$\text{Cohen's d} = -0.80$$

67.8 Interpretation of Cohen's d and Eta Square Estimates

Remember that we have inferred that medication A is statistically more effective ($p < 0.05$) than medication B in the management of hypertension. We can now evaluate the real-life implication of the Cohen's d (−0.80) estimate.

In 1988, Cohen25 proposed the following intervals for the interpretation of effect size estimates:

- 0.1–0.3 = Small practical effect
- 0.3–0.5 = Intermediate practical effect
- >0.5 = Large/Strong practical effect

Applying the above guidelines to the calculated effect size value of – 0.80, we can now affirmatively conclude that the magnitude of the change in SBP at the end of the 10 weeks treatment is of "large" clinical significance.

As stated previously, η^2 is another useful measure of effect size. It is derived typically from the data contained within the analysis of variance (ANOVA) summary table. The interpretation of η^2 is analogous to the description of the coefficient of determination (R^2) in linear and multiple regression analyses. The web-based calculator developed by Psychometrica [32] provides specific guidelines for the interpretation of the magnitude of the correlation. Cohen's-d and η^2 estimates range between 0 and 1 (Table 67.2).

Table 67.2 The interpretation of the magnitude of effect size estimates [32]

Cohen-d	*r* Correlation	$\eta 2$ Eta Square	Interpretation[a] of Cohen-d estimates
<0	<0	–	Adverse effect
0.0	0.00	0.000	No effect
0.1	0.05	0.003	
0.2	0.10	0.010	Small effect
0.3	0.15	0.022	
0.4	0.2	0.039	
0.5	0.24	0.060	Intermediate effect
0.6	0.29	0.083	
0.7	0.33	0.110	
0.8	0.37	0.140	Large effect
0.9	0.41	0.168	
>1.0	0.45	2.000	

[a]Cohen (1988) reports the following intervals for *r*: 0.1–0.3: Small Effect; 0.3–0.5: Intermediate Effect; 0.5>: Strong Effect. The range of the effect size estimates presented in Table 67.2 is consistent with Cohen (1988) guidelines [25]

https://www.psychometrica.de/effect_size.html

67.9 Calculation of Cohen-d Estimate for a Dependent (Repeated Measures) T-Test Design

We will illustrate how to compute Cohen-d effect size estimates for a pre- and post-test repeated measures design with another hypothetical study conducted to evaluate the effects of a customised educational intervention on the knowledge of the fundamental attributes of professionalism by Ob-Gyns. A validated Professionalism Inventory was used to assess the knowledge of professionalism of 47 Ob-Gyns before and after the educational intervention. The customised educational intervention on professionalism consisted of a three-hour classroom lecture and five case study reviews. The SPSS print out for the data collected from the study is presented in Table 67.3.

The result of the paired t-test revealed that post-intervention, the aggregate knowledge of professionalism score improved significantly ($t = 2.34$; $p < 0.05$). We now need to assess the magnitude of the observed change to determine if it is of practical value in the real world.

There are two possible approaches to calculate the effect size. The first approach is to use the following formula to calculate the effect size:

Table 67.3 The SPSS printout from the paired t-test

Paired samples test									
		Paired differences					t	df	Sig. (2-tailed)
		Mean difference	Standard deviation	Standard error mean	95% Confidence interval of the difference				
					Lower	Upper			
Pair 1	Pre-test knowledge score – Post-test knowledge score	−7.4	21.8	3.1	−13.9	−1.0	−2.34	46	0.024

$$\text{Cohen'd} = \frac{\text{Mean difference}}{\text{SD}}$$ (highlighted in red colour in Table 67.3)

Review the SPSS printout closely and look for the "paired samples test" data in Table 67.3.

$$\text{Cohen d} = \frac{7.44681}{21.81624}$$
$$= 0.34$$

Let us now use the second approach with the formula:

$$\text{Cohen d} = \frac{\text{t statistic}}{\sqrt{N}}$$ (highlighted in blue colour on Table 67.3)

$$\text{Cohen d} = \frac{2.340}{\sqrt{47}}$$
$$= \frac{2.340}{6.856}$$
$$= 0.34$$

The same Cohen-d value was obtained using both computational approaches. Based on the calculated Cohen-d value of 0.34, we can conclude that the 3 hours professionalism educational intervention implemented was of small practical significance (Table 67.2).

67.10 Calculation of Eta Square (η^2) Estimate for Three or More Independent Groups Design

The calculation of η^2 estimate from the ANOVA summary table depends on the research design adopted in the study. For example, the calculation of η^2 for experimental designs of three or more groups (due to treatment or intervention ANOVA statistical analysis) will be derived using the following formula:

$$\eta^2 = \frac{\text{Treatment Sum of Squares (SSB)}}{\text{Total Sum of Squares (SST)}}$$

Table 67.4 The one-way ANOVA summary table for the between-groups experimental design

SBP					
	Sum of squares	df	Mean square	F-calculated	Sig.
Between groups	556.6	4	139.1	3.5	0.010
Within groups	3752.8	95	39.5		
Total	4309.4	99			

To illustrate the calculation for η^2, we will consider the SBP data from another fictitious intervention study designed to evaluate the relative effectiveness of four different hypertensive medications and a placebo (sugar-ill) medication. For the study, we will recruit 100 patients with hypertension and randomly assign them into five groups with 25 patients in each group. Table 67.4 presents the one-way ANOVA summary table from the SPSS printout of the study.

- The Treatment Sum of Squares (SSB): Between-groups (556.557) – See the first row (highlighted in red colour)
- The Total Sum of Squares (SST): (4309.390) – See the final row (highlighted in yellow)

$$\eta^2 = \frac{556.557}{4{,}309.390}$$
$$\eta^2 = 0.129$$

The finding revealed that only 13% of the variance in SBP for the five groups was caused by the intervention (treatment). Using Cohen's guidelines in Table 67.2, we can conclude that a η^2 estimate of 0.129 corresponds to a "small" clinical significance.

67.11 Calculation of Eta Square Estimate for Repeated Measures Design

Now let us consider another situation in which we are interested in evaluating the therapeutic effectiveness of a new medication discovered for treating hypertension. Due to limited financial resources and time constraints, we decided to

Table 67.5 The ANOVA summary table for the within-subjects effect

Measure: Test1

Source factor1		Type III sum of squares	df	Mean square	F-calculated	Sig.
	Greenhouse-Geisser	1303.2	1	1303.2	5.5	0.024
	Huynh-Feldt	1303.2	1	1303.2	5.5	0.024
	Lower-bound	1303.2	1	1303.2	5.5	0.024
Error (factor1)	Sphericity assumed	10946.8	46	238.0		
	Greenhouse-Geisser	10946.8	46	238.0		
	Huynh-Feldt	10946.8	46	238.0		
	Lower-bound	10946.8	46	238.0		

Table 67.6 The ANOVA summary table for the between-subjects effect

Measure: Test1

Transformed variable: Average

Source	Type III sum of squares	Df	Mean square	F-calculated	Sig.
Intercept	499175.5	1	499175.5	1631.0	0.001
Error	14074.5	46	306.0		

use a pre- and post-test experimental design. An advantage of the repeated measures testing design is that a smaller number of participants will be required and each study participant will serve as his/her control. We will take the subjects SBP at baseline (pre-test) and again at the end of the 10 weeks (post-test) of taking the new medication. Tables 67.5 and 67.6 presents the repeated measures ANOVA summary table for the hypothetical case. For repeated measures design, the pertinent question to always ask, is the experimental design "between groups" or "within subjects"?

The calculation of η^2 in a pre- and post-test experimental design is slightly more complicated than a group design because we must calculate the Total Sum of Squares for the within-subjects effects using a different formula indicated below:

$$\text{Total Sum of Squares}(\text{SST}) = \text{Treatment Sum of Squares}(\text{SSB}) + \text{Error Sum of Squares} + \text{Error}(\text{Between subjects})\text{Sum of Squares.}$$

Again, the formula for η^2 for ANOVA within-subjects' repeated test design is as follows:

$$\eta^2 = \frac{\text{Treatment Sum of Squares}(\text{SSB})}{\text{Total Sum of Squares for Within Subjects' ANOVA}(\text{SST})}$$

The Total Sum of Squares (SST) is derived as follows: 1303.191 (Table 67.4, Factor1) + 10946.809 (Table 67.4, Error (Factor1) + 14074.468 (Table 67.5, Error) = 26,324.468

Now we can proceed to enter the Total Sum of Squares (SST) in the formula as before:

$$\eta^2 = \frac{1{,}303.191}{26{,}324.468} = 0.0495$$

The computed η^2 revealed that only 4.95% of the variance in the SBP in the fictitious study is because of the effect of the medication. We can now infer that a η^2 of 0.0495 is only of "small" clinical significance (Table 67.2).

67.12 Effect Size Estimation by the Social Science Statistics® Calculator

We have so far presented the step-by-step illustration for the manual computation of Cohen's d and η^2 estimates from the SPSS ANOVA Summary Table. The process is no doubt difficult and time-consuming. To calculate estimates of effect size, we need to know the mean and SD of the groups or repeated test procedures. In practice, the arithmetic mean and SD information will be retrieved from the SPSS print out. Alternatively, we can for a small dataset calculate them efficiently by using a web-based calculator developed by Social Science Statistics® [33].

We will now demonstrate how to use the Social Science Statistics® calculator to derive the Cohen-d estimate for our first hypothetical study designed to test the null hypothesis that medication A will not be more effective than medication B in the management of hypertension. First, let us recap the major points of the study. We randomly assigned 50 patients each to groups A and B and monitored their SBP after they used their medication for 10 weeks. The mean and SD of the SBP for the patients in group A was 140 mmHg and 12.0,

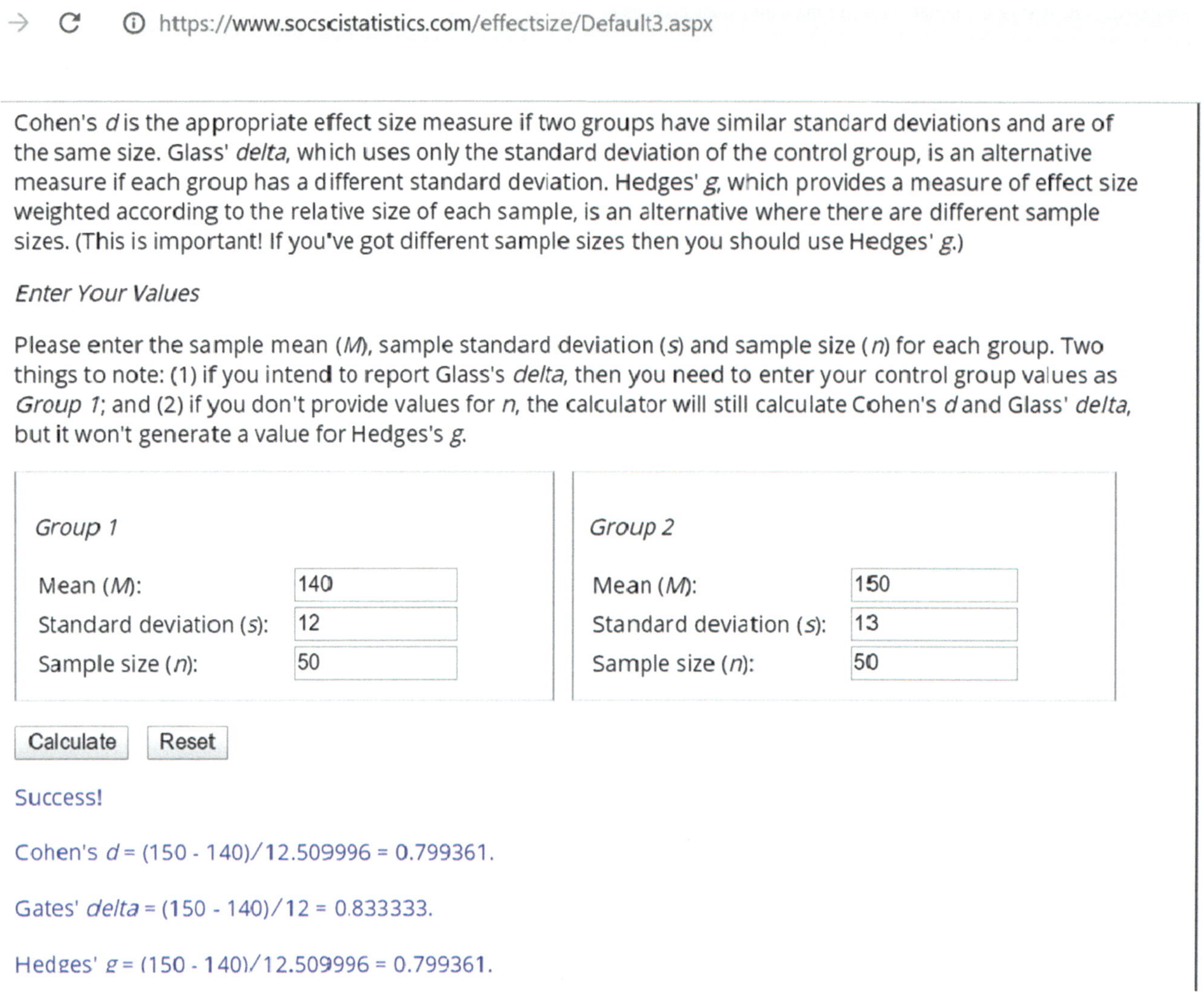

Fig. 67.3 Screenshot image of the output of the Social Science Statistics Calculator [33] after using it to compute a Cohen-d estimate for the first hypothetical study. (http://www.socscistatistics.com/tests)

respectively. The mean SBP for those allocated to group B was 150 mmHg and SD of 13.0.

Proceed to enter the data for the two groups into the Social Science Statistics® calculator [33] and hit the "Calculate" button at the left-hand corner of the template (Fig. 67.3).

A Cohen-d value of 0.799361 was displayed below the "Calculate" button. The value approximates the 0.80 obtained using the manual calculation method illustrated previously. The use of the Social Science Statistics® calculator [33] was effortless as it took less than 2 minutes to accomplish. In addition to calculating Cohen's d effect size for two independent samples, the Social Science Statistics® calculator can be used for a myriad of other statistical analyses listed on their webpage as follows: [33]

- "One-way ANOVA calculator for independent groups design
- One-way ANOVA calculator for repeated measures design
- Binomial test calculator[a]
- Chi-Square calculator for 2 × 2 contingency table[a]
- Chi-Square calculator for 5 × 5 (or less) contingency able[a]
- Chi-Square calculator for the goodness of fit[a]
- Fisher Exact test calculator for 2 × 2 contingency table[a]
- The Friedman test for repeated tests design[a]
- The Kolmogorov–Smirnov test of normality
- Kruskal–Wallis test calculator for independent groups design[a]
- Mann–Whitney U test calculator[a]

- Sign test calculator[a]
- T-test calculator for two independent means
- T-test calculator for two dependent (Paired) means
- T-test calculator for one sample
- Wilcoxon signed-rank test calculator[a]
- Z score calculator for a single raw value
- Z-test calculator for a single sample
- Z-test calculator for two population proportions
- Linear regression calculator
- Multiple regression calculator
- Pearson correlation coefficient calculator
- Spearman's Rho (correlation) calculator[a]
- P-value from Z-score
- P-value from t-score
- P-value from Chi-square score[a]
- P-value from F-ratio score
- P-value from Pearson (r) score
- A single sample confidence interval calculator (t-Statistic)
- A single-sample confidence interval calculator (Z-Statistic)
- An independent samples confidence interval calculator
- Number needed to treat calculator
- Relative risk and odds ratio calculator
- A rank order calculator"[a]

[a]Non-parametric test; remaining tests are parametric

67.13 Estimation of Effect Size with the Psychometrica® Calculator

Another web-based calculator designed to compute effect size is the one developed by Psychometrica [32]. Figure 67.4 is the screenshot image of the Psychometrica® templates for an independent t-test group design.

This platform is flexible, user-friendly and versatile and capable of calculating the effect size for the following experimental designs listed on their webpage: [32]

- "Comparison of groups with equal size (Cohen's d, Glass Δ)
- Comparison of groups with different sample size (Cohen's d, Hedges' g)
- The effect size for pre-post-control studies with the correction of pretest differences

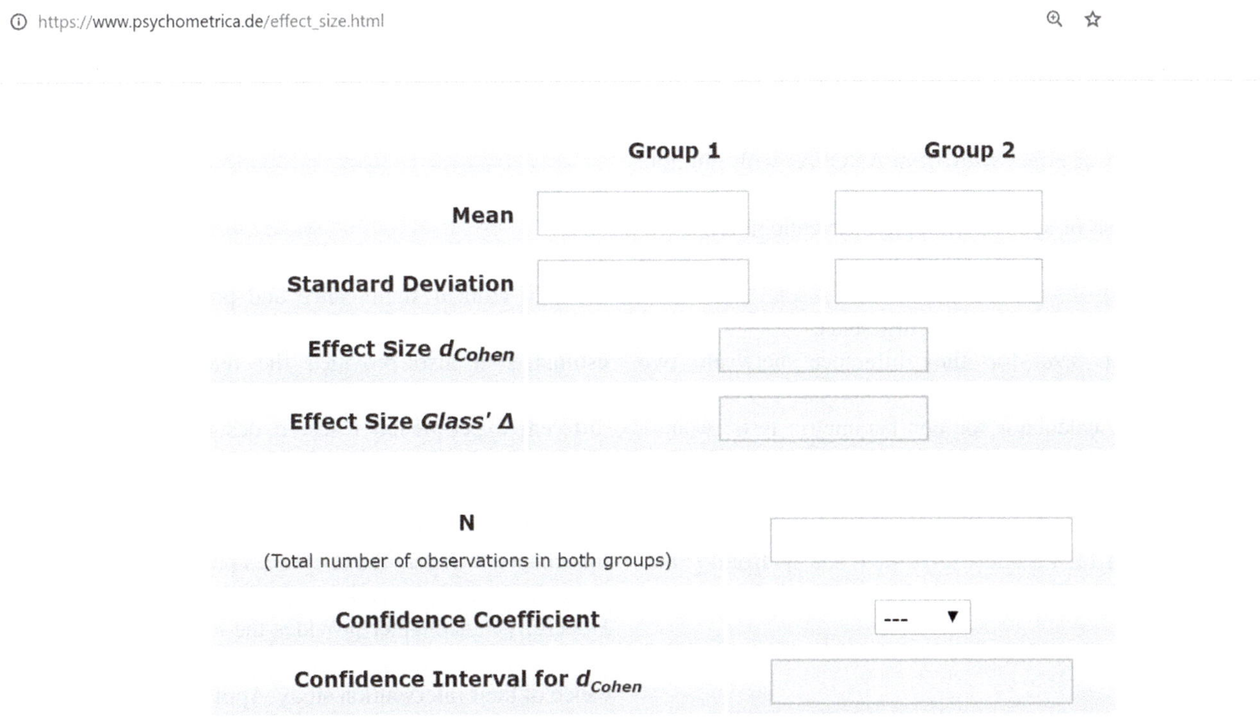

Fig. 67.4 Screenshot image of the output of the estimation of effect size with the Psychometrica® calculator (https://www.psychometrica.de/effect_size.html)

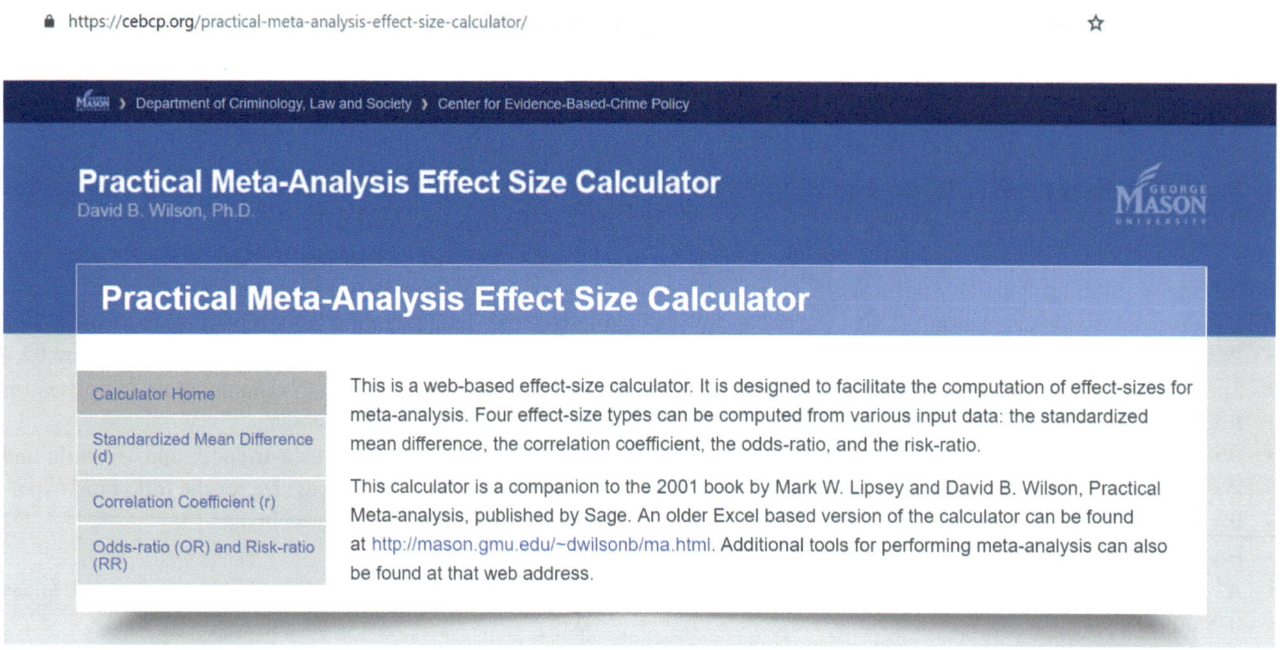

Fig. 67.5 Screenshot image of the output of the practical meta-analysis effect size calculator [34] before using it to compute a Cohen-d estimate for the first hypothetical study. (https://cebcp.org/practical-meta-analysis-effect-size-calculator/)

- Effect size estimates in repeated testing designs
- Calculation of Cohen's d from the test statistics of dependent and independent t-tests
- Computation of Cohen's d from the analysis of variance (ANOVA) F-value
- Calculation of effect sizes from ANOVAs with multiple groups, based on group means
- The increase of success through intervention: The binomial effect size display (BESD) and number needed to treat (NNT)
- Risk ratio, odds ratio and risk difference
- The effect size for the difference between two correlations
- Effect size calculator for non-parametric tests: Mann–Whitney U, Wilcoxon-W and Kruskal–Wallis-H
- Computation of the pooled standard deviation
- Transformation of the effect sizes r, d, f, odds ratio and η^2
- Calculation of the effect sizes d, r and η^2 from χ^2 and Z-test statistics"

67.13.1 Practical Meta-Analysis Effect Size Calculator

The practical meta-analysis effect size calculator [34] is another versatile web-based tool designed to compute effect-sizes of intervention studies (Fig. 67.5).

The practical meta-analysis effect size platform [34] can calculate four types of effect-size from standardised mean difference, correlation coefficient, odds and risk ratios data.

67.14 Summary

This chapter introduces the reader to the fundamental concepts of clinical significance and provides a step-by-step illustration of how to compute and interpret Cohen-d and η^2 estimates. It also provided the reader with web-based resources for calculating clinical significance estimates for different experimental research designs. Additionally, the chapter offer insights on how to assess the underlying assumptions associated with the use of the parametric tests.

A curious learner seeking to go beyond the presentation in this chapter will find the references provided very useful for more in-depth information on any of the topics covered. Hopefully, this chapter provides the learner the knowledge, skills and impetus needed to evaluate the clinical significance of their intervention study. Applying the concepts presented in this chapter will open the floodgate for improved evidence-based intervention studies in medicine and allied health. The more researchers take part in intervention research, the faster we can answer essential clinical questions on how to prevent emerging diseases and find more effective treatments.

References

1. Physiopedia. Evidence-Based Practice (EBP). n.d.. https://www.physio-pedia.com/Evidence_Based_Practice_(EBP). Accessed 12 Dec 2018.
2. Bixo M, Ekberg K, Poromaa IS, Hirschberg AL, Jonasson AF, Andréen L, Timby E, Wulff M, Ehrenborg A, Bäckström T. Treatment of premenstrual dysphoric disorder with the GABAA receptor modulating steroid antagonist Sepranolone (UC1010)-A randomised controlled trial. Psychoneuroendocrinology. 2017;80:46–55.
3. Chakhtoura M, Nassar A, Arabi A, Cooper C, Harvey N, Mahfoud Z, Nabulsi M, El-Hajj FG. Effect of vitamin D replacement on maternal and neonatal outcomes: a randomised controlled trial in pregnant women with hypovitaminosis D. A protocol. BMJ. 2016;6(3):010818.
4. Andersson IM, Benson L, Christensson K, Gemzell-Danielsson K. Paracervical block as pain treatment during second-trimester medical termination of pregnancy: an RCT with bupivacaine versus sodium chloride. Hum Reprod. 2016;31(1):67–74.
5. Whitaker AK, Endres LK, Mistretta SQ, Gilliam ML. Postplacental insertion of the levonorgestrel intrauterine device after cesarean delivery vs. delayed insertion: a randomised controlled trial. Contraception. 2014;89(6):534–9.
6. Monk BJ, Wang J, Stock RJ, Peters WA 3rd, Liu PY, Barrett RJ 2nd, Berek JS, Souhami L, Grigsby PW, Gordon W Jr, Alberts DS. Rethinking the use of radiation and chemotherapy after radical hysterectomy: a clinical-pathologic analysis of a Gynaecologic Oncology Group/Southwest Oncology Group/Radiation Therapy Oncology Group trial. Gynecol Oncol. 2005;96(3):721–8.
7. Polo-Kantola P, Rauhala E, Helenius H, Erkkola R, Irjala K, Polo O. Breathing during sleep in menopause: a randomised, controlled, crossover trial with estrogen therapy. Obstet Gynecol. 2003;102(1):68–75.
8. Entezami M, Heger-Mahn D, Ebert A, Halis G, Lübbert H. Short-term treatment with levonorgestrel does not antagonize the ethinyl estradiol-induced increase of uterine blood flow in postmenopausal women. Contraception. 1997;56(3):181–3.
9. Bofill JA, Rust OA, Devidas M, Roberts WE, Morrison JC, Martin JN Jr. Shoulder dystocia and operative vaginal delivery. J Matern Fetal Med. 1997;6(4):220–4.
10. Hoffman CT 3rd, Guzman ER, Richardson MJ, Vintzileos A, Houlihan C, Benito C. Effects of narcotic and non-narcotic continuous epidural anaesthesia on intrapartum fetal heart rate tracings as measured by computer analysis. J Matern Fetal Med. 1997;6(4):200–5.
11. Höckel M, Vorndran B, Schlenger K, Baussmann E, Knapstein PG. Tumour oxygenation: a new predictive parameter in locally advanced cancer of the uterine cervix. Gynecol Oncol. 1993;51(2):141–9.
12. Glujovsky D, Sueldo CE, Borghi C, Nicotra P, Andreucci S, Ciapponi A. Misleading reporting and interpretation of results in major infertility journals. Fertil Steril. 2016;105(5):1301–6.
13. Hay SC, Kirpalani H, Viner C, Soll R, Dukhovny D, Mao WY, Profit J, DeMauro SB, JAF Z. Do trials reduce uncertainty? Assessing impact through cumulative meta-analysis of neonatal RCTs. J Perinatol. 2017;37(11):1215–9. Available at https://www.ncbi.nlm.nih.gov/pubmed/28880258. Accessed 12 Dec 2018.
14. Thrower P. Eight reasons I rejected your article. 2012. Available at https://www.elsevier.com/connect/8-reasons-i-rejected-your-article. Accessed 12 Dec 2018.
15. Enago Academy. Learning to avoid journal rejection. 2018. Available at https://www.enago.com/academy/learning-to-avoid-journal-rejection/. Accessed 12 Dec 2018.
16. Oosterhaven J. Too many journals? Towards a theory of repeated rejections and ultimate acceptance. Scientometrics. 2015;103(1):261–5. Available at https://www.ncbi.nlm.nih.gov/pmc/articles/PMC4365185/. Accessed 12 Dec 2018.
17. Altman DG, Bland JM. Improving doctors' understanding of statistics. J R Stat Soc A. 1991;154:223–67.
18. Weiss ST, Samet JM. An assessment of physician knowledge of epidemiology and biostatistics. J Med Educ. 1980;55:692–7.
19. Wulff HR, Andersen B, Brandenhoff P, Guttler F. What do doctors know about statistics? Stat Med. 1987;6:3–10.
20. Borak J, Veiullieux S. Errors of intuitive logic among physicians. Soc Sci Med. 1982;16:1939–47.
21. Public Health Action Support Team. Introduction to study designs – intervention studies and randomised controlled trials. 2017. Available at https://www.healthknowledge.org.uk/e-learning/epidemiology/practitioners/introduction-study-design-is-rct. Accessed 22 Dec 2018.
22. Friedman SB, Phillips S. What's the difference? Paediatric residents and their inaccurate concepts regarding statistics. Paediatrics. 1981;68:644–6.
23. Campbell DT, Julian SJ. Experimental and quasi-experimental designs for research. Boston. Available at https://www.amazon.com/Experimental-Quasi-Experimental-Designs-Research-Campbell/dp/0395307872. Accessed 22 Dec 2018.: Hougton Mifflin Company; 1963.
24. Cohen J. Statistical power analysis for the behavioural sciences. Hillsdale, NJ: Erlbaum; 1988.
25. Thompson CJ. What's the difference between statistical significance and clinical significance? 2017. Available at https://nursingeducationexpert.com/difference-statistical-significance-clinical-significance/. Accessed 22 Dec 2018.
26. Cath. Intervention studies. n.d.. Available at http://www.drcath.net/toolkit/intervention-studies. Accessed 22 Dec 2018.
27. Effect size. Available at https://en.m.wikipedia.org/wiki/Effect_size. Accessed 22 Dec 2018.
28. Kraemer HC, Morgan G, Leech NL, Gliner JA, Vaske JJ, Harmon RJ. Measures of clinical significance. J Am Acad Child Adolesc Psychiatry. 2003;42(12):1524–9. Available at https://jaacap.org/article/S0890-8567(09)62138-9/fulltext. Accessed 22 Dec 2018.
29. Jacob ME, M. Ganguli M. Odds ratio: neuroepidemiology. In: Handbook of clinical neurology; 2016.
30. Schnell A. The difference between relative risk and odds ratios. 2008. Available at https://www.sciencedirect.com/topics/medicine-and-dentistry/odds-ratio. Accessed 22 Dec 2018.
31. Statistical Tables. n.d.. Available at https://home.ubalt.edu/ntsbarsh/Business-stat/StatistialTables.pdf. Accessed 22 Dec 2018.
32. Psychometrica. n.d.. Available at https://www.psychometrica.de/effect_size.html. Accessed 22 Dec 2018.
33. Social Science Statistics. n.d.. Available at http://www.socscistatistics.com/tests/. Accessed 22 Dec 2018.
34. The Practical Meta-Analysis Effect Size Calculator. n.d.. Available at https://cebcp.org/practical-meta-analysis-effect-size-calculator/. Accessed 22 Dec 2018.

The Common Statistical Faux Pas in Journal Publications

68

Joseph A. Balogun

Learning Objectives

After reading this chapter, the learner will be able to:

- Describe the critical issues to address during the planning stage of a research study
- Discuss the major statistical tests that are wrongly applied in medical and allied health journals
- Identify the non-parametric equivalence of parametric tests
- Discuss the factors that influence the selection of the appropriate statistical test
- List the underlying assumptions surrounding the use of parametric tests
- Interpret Statistical Package for the Social Sciences (SPSS) printout of tests that evaluate the underlying assumptions of independence of groups, normality, homogeneity of variance, outliers, homoscedasticity and multicollinearity
- Discern the common presentation pitfalls of the study results reported in medical and allied health journals
- Discuss the controversy and recommendations surrounding the precision of reporting measures of central tendency, variability and inferential statistics, such as t, F, χ^2 and confidence interval (CI)

68.1 Introduction

The inappropriate use of statistics in biomedical research was first systematically studied and reported on by Gore and associates in 1977 [1]. The authors of the study evaluated 62 articles in 13 successive editions of the British Medical Journal and found that 52% of the publications had statistical errors; 56% of the mistakes are "fairly serious" in nature. The abstract section of five articles reviewed made some claims that were not supportable by the data presented in the result. Several other investigators around the world have replicated this landmark study with similar results [2, 3]. Regrettably, four decades later the problems identified in 1977 continues till today [2]. Thus, the need to bring renewed attention to this concerting problem.

The misuse and abuse of statistics in biomedical research is attributed to the limited knowledge of statistics by medical and allied health practitioners [2]. A recent study [3] reported that 54% of faculty and medical students found statistics to be "very difficult," 53% could not define correctly the meaning of p-value, 37% incorrectly defined standard deviation (SD) and 51% cannot calculate sample size accurately. Approximately 50% of the articles published in medical journals have one or more statistical mistakes [3]. Thiese, Arnold and Walker opined that the reported percentages above underestimates the dimension of the problem because many journals often omit or conceal data, thus, making a priori analysis difficult [2].

Although most misuses of statistics occur because of ignorance and poor planning, there are cases of abuse that have deliberate intent to achieve the desired outcome. It has been reported that about 34% of researchers confessed to unethical research practices which include embellishing data to improve study outcome, dubious exposition of data, withholding details of methodology or data analysis, exclude data points from statistical analyses because of a "gut feeling that they were inaccurate" and deceptive reporting of the experimental research design and results [3]. As a result of

J. A. Balogun (✉)
Chicago State University, Chicago, IL, USA

University of Medical Sciences, Ondo City, Nigeria

Centre of Excellence in Reproductive Health Innovation, University of Benin, Benin City, Nigeria
e-mail: jbalogun@csu.edu; jbalogun@unimed.edu.ng

F. Okonofua et al. (eds.), *Contemporary Obstetrics and Gynecology for Developing Countries*,
https://doi.org/10.1007/978-3-030-75385-6_68

the appalling practices and dire developments, several medical and allied health journals have adopted new rigorous "*Statistical Analyses and Methods in the Published Literature*" [4] and the "*Strengthening Analytical Thinking for Observational Studies*" [5] guidelines. In addition, many of the journals have expanded the pool of statistical reviewers/consultants on their editorial board to curtail the problems. Despite these reforms, little has changed over the years, with recent reports confirming the persistence of the problems [2, 3, 6].

This chapter discusses the major statistical flaws in published medical and allied health journals with the hope that researchers will avoid making similar errors when conducting and reporting their research findings. To comprehend fully the information presented in this chapter, a basic understanding of statistics and familiarity with the SPSS program is assumed.

68.2 Prevention of Statistical Faux Pas

Two pertinent questions central to this chapter are: why is statistical abuse so pervasive in the published literature? And what can be done to prevent it? Experimental studies that are not carefully planned are prone to major methodological and statistical faux pas. The planning phase of any research is the most crucial to prevent statistical errors; any shortcomings occurring at this stage can have an enormous negative impact on the external validity of the study [6]. That said, it is, therefore, prudent to consult a biostatistician at the planning stage to help formulate the study aims, experimental design, sample size, psychometric properties of the instruments, data collection protocols and outcome measures. Furthermore, the research hypotheses and the statistical analyses methods should be pre-defined and explicitly stated at the planning stage. If no hypothesis is postulated, as in descriptive and qualitative research approaches, it is imperative to clarify the exploratory nature of the study at this stage.

Whenever possible, the experimental design should ensure random sample selection, randomisation of subjects into groups and include double-blind data collection protocol to avoid potential confounding bias. Although this "gold standard" condition is not possible in most cases, the limitations of the experimental study design must be recognised and appropriately stated in the discussion section.

68.3 Sample Size Imperfections

Inadequate sample size is one of the common weaknesses of articles published in major medical journals. This situation usually occurs when a statistical power calculation to determine the optimum sample size is not done before the initiation of the study. Estimation of sample size is a complicated and cumbersome process, particularly when undertaken by manual calculation. Fortunately, several web-based calculators are now available that can perform the task effortlessly at any of the following sites:

- https://clincalc.com/stats/samplesize.aspx
- http://powerandsamplesize.com/Calculators/
- http://psych.wisc.edu/henriques/power.html
- https://www.dssresearch.com/KnowledgeCentre/toolkit-calculators.aspx
- http://www.sample-size.net/
- https://www.ai-therapy.com/psychology-statistics/sample-size-calculator
- https://www.anzmtg.org/stats/PowerCalculator/PowerTtest
- https://www.anzmtg.org/stats/PowerCalculator/PowerANOVA

68.4 Selection of Wrong Statistical Tests

Selection of appropriate statistical test depends on the research question posed, the level of measurement of the variables and whether the data distribution met the underlying assumptions of parametric tests. Statistical errors come in different forms ranging from inappropriate use of parametric and non-parametric tests, failure to apply correction adjustments and inappropriate selection of the correct analysis to mention a few examples. There is presently no consensus among biostatisticians on the best approach for reporting the results from quantitative comparative studies. Some biostatistician advocates the use of confidence intervals [6], instead of the point estimation hypothesis testing method [9]. Strasak and associates [6] argued that probability (p) value alone does not provide meaningful information about the magnitude of the effect size and advocated reporting the p-values precisely as obtained, instead of the hypothesised alpha level of "$p < 0.05$" or "$p > 0.01$" or arbitrary terms such as "p = ns."

Abuse of statistics frequently occurs in comparative studies when authors select the wrong version of the t-test. There are cases in which authors in error inappropriately apply the Student t-test (indicated for comparing two independent groups) instead of paired t-test (for two repeated measures) or vice versa and the one sample t-test (ideally used for examining a sample mean to a norm or previous mean data). Before using the independent Student t-test, many articles often ignore to evaluate whether the two groups have equal variance (homogeneity). The evaluation of group homogeneity is usually done with the Levene's test. Some biostatisticians argue that the equal variance two-sample t-test is not robust to situations when the two groups have unequal variance (heterogeneous) even when the sample sizes are the same. The Welch's t-test, which is a modified form of Student's t-test, is recommended when the two samples have unequal variances (heterogeneity) or unequal sample sizes.

Many published articles, in error, use multiple Student t-tests to evaluate differences between three or more groups instead of the ANOVA followed by a posthoc test when the calculated F-ratio is significant. Multiple comparisons of groups with both t-test and ANOVA may require adjustment; a correction process that is controversial in the literature [6]. Another frequent misuse of statistics occurs when the t-test is used to analyse ordinal data – variables on the ordinal scale cannot approximate a normal distribution and the equivalent nonparametric test is the appropriate analysis for such dataset.

Chi-square non-parametric tests are regularly misused because their underlying assumptions are not evaluated before application and the appropriate corrections are often not applied when the sample size is small. For example, some biostatistician argued that Chi-square techniques should not be employed when the expected number in a cell is less than five because under these circumstances their approximation is no longer reliable. Hence, many biostatisticians recommended that when the Chi-square test assumption is violated or when the number of subjects in a cell is less than five, Fisher's exact test should be used. When the number in a cell is less than 10, the Yates-continuity correction is indicated [6].

68.5 Evaluation of the Underlying Assumptions for Using Parametric Tests

Most medical and allied health professionals who use statistics are more familiar with parametric tests than the non-parametric analyses which are the distribution-free tests that do not assume a normal distribution [7, 8]. A common dogma taught to undergraduate medical and health sciences students is to use non-parametric tests when the assumption about normally distributed data is violated. While the prescription is simplistic and straightforward, unfortunately, the issue is more complex because there are additional assumptions to be evaluated. Often authors use parametric tests without determining whether their data violate the underlying assumptions by testing for the independence of group observations, normality, homogeneity of variance, outliers, homoscedasticity and multicollinearity [9].

Due to the lack of in-depth knowledge of biostatistics, there is a general preference by neophyte scientists to select parametric tests over non-parametric tests. Many authors have expressed the opinion that parametric tests are overused in medical research because practitioners are often unfamiliar with the assumptions associated with the different parametric tests [2, 6]. It has been documented that over 90% of articles published in medical journals lacked discussion of the underlying statistical assumptions for parametric statistics [2]. Although this finding has been reported for some time, none of the previous reviews [1, 2, 6–8] addressed the problem.

The assumptions surrounding the use of parametric tests can be conducted efficiently using the SPSS statistical software which is typically subscribed by most institutions of higher learning around the world. The violation of the assumptions of the parametric test often leads to overestimations of significant effects, inappropriate interpretations of experimental findings which may impact the ability of other authors to replicate the results reported, with potential for misdiagnosis and medical treatment errors [10, 11].

In this chapter, I will use the data from a cross-sectional study to illustrate how to test for the underlying assumptions of parametric test. The aforementioned cross-sectional study measured the anthropometric indices, blood glucose and serum cholesterol levels of 100 rural dwellers of various physical activity levels. First, we would like to determine, using the Levene's test, if the blood glucose level of the study participants who are sedentary (n = 50) and those who are moderately active (n = 50) have equal variance. It is relevant to note that blood glucose in SI unit is measured in millimoles per litre (mmol/L). In the USA and Germany, it is usually measured in milligrams per decilitre (mg/dL). To convert blood glucose levels to mg/dl, multiply mmol/L by 18. The SPSS printout of the Levene's test from the cross-sectional study is presented in Table 68.1.

The p-value for the blood glucose data (0.971) is higher than the 0.05 alpha level adopted at the planning phase of the study. Therefore, the null hypothesis is accepted and we conclude that the assumption of homogeneity is not violated. That is, the variance of both groups is equal.

Based on this finding and the fact that subjects in both groups are equal and blood glucose is on the ratio scale, we can now proceed to use the independent Student t-test to evaluate the plausible difference in blood glucose level.

Table 68.1 The SPSS print out of Levene's test for homogeneity of variance

Test of homogeneity of variances[a]					
		Levene statistic	df1	df2	Sig.
Blood glucose	Based on mean	0.001	1	98	0.971
	Based on median	0.027	1	98	0.869
	Based on median and with adjusted df	0.027	1	73	0.869
	Based on trimmed mean	0.027	1	98	0.871

[a]Analysis obtained from SPSS via the One-way analysis of variance (ANOVA)

Using the same dataset, we can now proceed to test for normality of the blood glucose level. Recall that the number of subjects in the study is 100. The Shapiro–Wilk test is the appropriate test for normality assessement when the sample size is small, between 50 and 2000. When the sample size is more than 2000, the Kolmogorov–Smirnov will be the appropriate test to select. Table 68.2 displayed the SPSS printout of the Shapiro–Wilk test.

The result revealed that the blood glucose level of the sedentary subjects ($p = 0.252$) is normally distributed ($p > 0.05$). Conversely, the blood glucose of the subjects who are engaged in a moderate level of physical activity ($p = 0.001$) did not meet the assumption of homogeneity ($p < 0.001$). Generally, there is no consensus which tests to use when the assumption of normality is not met. The t-test is deemed by some biostatisticians to be "reasonably robust" when the distributions of the samples depart from normality we can use the parametric test. Others disagreed and argued that the question of robustness is challenging to answer because the assumptions can be violated in different degrees in many ways. Given the discord among biostatisticians, it is prudent to run both the parametric (Student t-test) and non-parametric (Mann–Whitney U-test) tests and report both results for the readers to decide.

For the same study presented above, we decided to derive a prediction equation for blood glucose level from anthropometric indices of weight, height and body-mass index (BMI). For the prediction research, we would use the multiple regression model because the three anthropometric measures (weight, height and BMI) are on the ratio scale.

The unstandardised coefficient for BMI, weight and height is 2.542, – 0.289 and – 0.952, respectively. The unstandardised coefficient value for each predictor variable is used to generate the multiple regression equation as follows:

Serum cholesterol = 261.818 – 2.542 (BMI) – 0.289 (Weight), – 0.952 (Height)

To compare the relative importance of each predictor variable in a multiple regression model, use the data in the standardised beta coefficient column. The standardised beta coefficient for BMI, weight and height is 0.140, −0.045 and −0.115, respectively. That means for every 1 (SD) increase in serum cholesterol, the patient BMI (SD) will increase by 0.140. This relationship is true, assuming the other variables (weight and height) are held constant.

To determine the presence or absence of homoscedasticity, proceed to review the "Coefficients" data from the SPSS printout regression analysis. First, determine if the independent (predictor) variables (weight, height and BMI) met the underlying assumptions of homoscedasticity and multicollinearity (Table 68.3).

In (Table 68.3), look for the significant level of the independent variables (for clarity purposes, they are highlighted in red colour). The p values for the three predictor variables ($p = 0.579$, 0.858 and 0.391) are higher than 0.05 ($p > 0.05$).

Table 68.2 The SPSS print out for the normality assumption test

Tests of normality[a]							
	Physical activity	Kolmogorov–Smirnov[b]			Shapiro–Wilk		
		Statistic	df	Sig.	Statistic	df	Sig.
Blood glucose	Mostly sitting down	0.083	49	0.200[c]	0.970	49	0.252
	Moderate level of physical activity	0.189	51	0.001	0.789	51	0.001

[a]Analysis obtained from SPSS via Explore
[b]Lilliefors Significance Correction
[c]This is a lower bound of the true significance

Table 68.3 The SPSS printout of the multiple regression analysis depicting the coefficients data[a]

Coefficients[a]									
		Unstandardised Coefficients		Standardised Coefficients			Collinearity Statistics	
Model[b]		B	Std. Error	Beta	t	Sig.	Tolerance	VIF
1	(Constant)	261.818	188.386		1.390	.168	Tolerance	VIF
	BMI	2.542	4.566	.140	.557	.579	.160	6.367
	Weight	-.289	1.612	-.045	-.179	.858	.157	6.353
	Height	-.952	1.105	-.115	-.862	.391	.570	1.756

[a]Analysis obtained from SPSS via regression; univariate model
[b]Dependent variable: blood glucose

Table 68.4 The SPSS printout of Pearson's product moment correlation coefficient (r) matrix

Coefficients*				
Blood Glucose	1	.05	-.15	.21*
Weight		1	.19	-.22*
Height			1	-.18
Age				1

*Correlation is significant at the 0.05 level (two-tailed)

Table 68.5 The SPSS printout of the ANOVA model summary showing Durbin–Watson values for testing for the independence of observation

Model summary[b]

					Change statistics					
Model	R	R square	Adjusted R square	Std. error of the estimate	R square change	F change	df1	df2	Sig. F change	Dubin-Waston
1	0.176[a]	0.031	0.001	54.7	0.031	1.027	3	96	0.384	1.777

[a]Predictors: (Constant), BMI, Height, Weight
[b]Dependent Variable: Bloodglucose

Therefore, we accept the null hypothesis and conclude that there is no heteroscedasticity problem. That is, the assumption of homogeneity in our model is not violated.

As a rule of thumb, multicollinearity becomes a problem in a regression model when the coefficients of determination (R^2) between the independent variables are higher than 0.75 and a serious problem when the R^2 reach 0.90. The correlation matrix depicting the relationship (r) between the independent variables is highlighted in red colour (Table 68.4). None of the R^2 value is anywhere close to the 0.75 threshold value. Thus, suggesting that multicollinearity is not a problem in the prediction model.

We can confirm whether the assumption of multicollinearity is met by reviewing the numerical value of the data in the Tolerance (highlighted in blue) and the Variance Inflation Factor (VIF) column (highlighted in purple) presented within the Collinearity Statistics in Table 68.3. Biostatisticians agree that multicollinearity is ruled out (i.e. the assumption is met) when the Tolerance value is greater than 0.1 and the VIF (calculated as a reciprocal of Tolerance) value is less than 10 for all variables. From the numerical values of the Tolerance and VIF data in Table 68.3, we conclude that no significant multicollinearity exists among the three predictor variables.

One of the primary assumptions of linear and multiple regression analyses is that the observations are independent. When different observations are made over time, it is most likely that consecutive observations will be related. If there is no autocorrelation (subsequent observations are related), then the Durbin–Watson statistic should be between 1.5 and 2.5. The Durbin–Watson statistic value in the cross-sectional study illustrated in this chapter is 1.777 (Table 68.5) which falls between 1.5 and 2.5. Therefore, we conclude that the data are not autocorrelated, that is, the observations are independent of one another.

Another primary assumption of linear and multiple regression analyses is that there are no significant outliers in the dataset. Outliers are identified by plotting scatterplot and boxplot as shown in Figs. 68.1 and 68.2, respectively.

The scatterplots (Fig. 68.1) showed linear relationships between blood glucose and the anthropometric variables. The boxplot (Fig. 68.2) is typically used to diagnose the presence of outliers

Outliers represent cases that fall more than 1.5 box lengths from the lower or upper hinge of the boxplot and represented by a circle. Extreme outliers have values greater than three box length from either hinge or are represented on the boxplot with the asterisk. As shown in the boxplots in Fig. 68.2, no single outlier is seen in the blood glucose data for the subjects who are sedentary. Conversely, outliers are evident in the moderately active group; particularly noticeable for study participants with identification number 13, 92, 95 and 32. Although the plots are suggestive of outliers in the blood glucose data, there are specific statistical tests to confirm if the outliers are statistically significant [12].

There is no consensus among biostatisticians on how to report significant outliers. While some biostatisticians recommend excluding the outliers from the dataset because they may unduly impact the statistical model,

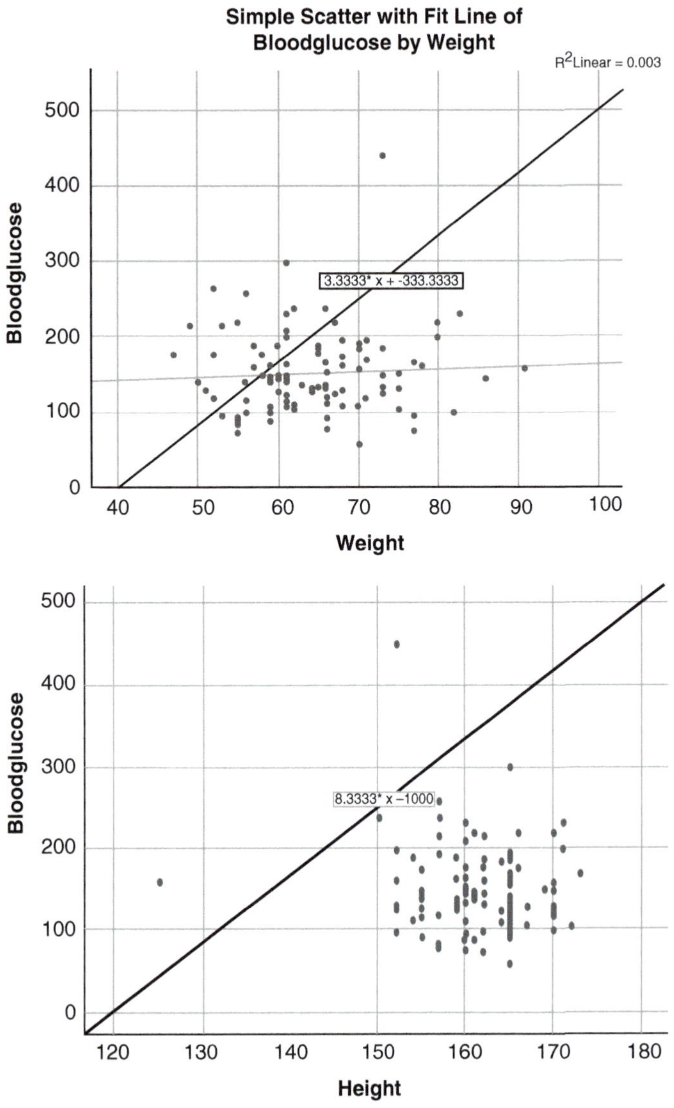

Fig. 68.1 Scatterplots of blood glucose against weight, BMI and height

Fig. 68.2 Box plot of blood glucose for the subjects who are sedentary and those who are moderately active

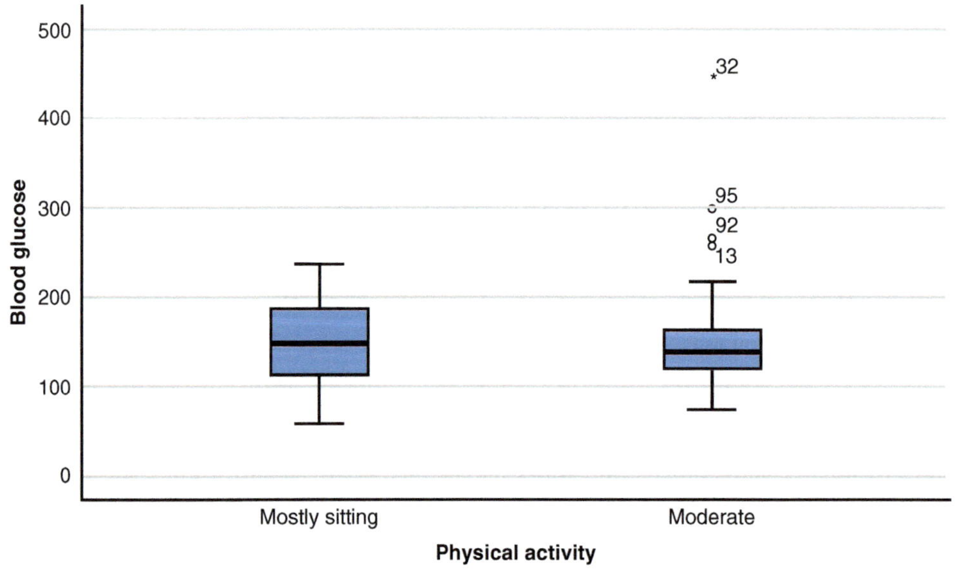

especially when the sample size is small, other biostatisticians worry that omission of outliers from the dataset may exclude valid data that don't fit a pre-defined pattern or hypothesis. Thus, committing an error that may have minimal impact on the results. On the other hand, the error may be fatal and may completely invalidate the study outcomes. The reasonable approach is to analyse the data with the outliers included and rerun the test with the outliers excluded from the dataset. In the spirit of full disclosure and transparency, it is judicious to present the results of both analyses and allow the readers to arrive at their own conclusions regarding the impacts of the outliers on the study outcome [2].

68.6 Levels of Measurements

In research studies, variables are quantified generally on a nominal (categorical), ordinal, interval or ratio (continuous) scales. An in-depth understanding of the levels of measurements and its implications for the type of data analysis to employ is critically important. It is common in published articles where ordinal data, such as level of pain ratings, the stages of cancer ratings and the Appearance, Pulse, Grimace, Activity and Respiration (APGAR) scores of babies postpartum, are analysed in error with parametric tests.

Typically, subjective ratings on questionnaires and clinical variables derived from Likert scales are ordinal. However, in practice, most researchers think of such data as interval or ratio level scales. Some biostatisticians argue that treating ordinal scales as interval or ratio scales violate a technical canon, and in many cases, the outcome has a demonstrable application [9]. Also, variables derived by adding some ordinal variables together are still regarded as ordinal data. The cardinal rule is that non-parametric tests should be used to analyse nominal and ordinal scale data and parametric tests used for interval and ratio scale data [9].

In general, the level of measurement of the dependent variables in survey research is on nominal and ordinal scales. Therefore, they will typically violate the underlying assumptions of parametric tests which are used for variables on interval and ratio scales. Such analysis, when used to analyse survey research data, will produce a Type I error (inferring a significant difference, when in reality no such distinction exists).

68.7 Parametric and Non-parametric Equivalent Tests

When the assumptions of parametric tests are not met, the non-parametric equivalent of the test should be selected. Many novice scientists are inept on the appropriate non-parametric test to choose when the assumptions for the parametric analysis is violated. Table 68.6 can be used as a guide to discern the non-parametric equivalent tests to use when the underlying assumptions of the parametric tests are not met.

Table 68.6 must be used with a dose of caution because there are differing opinions on the level of measurement of variables derived from questionnaire scales [19]. The schism is because many of the scales have arbitrary zero points as determined by the creator of the instrument and they have no standard unit of measurement comparable to standard measures such as cm and kg. As a general principle, the non-parametric tests listed in Table 68.6 should be the statistical methods of choice to select in analysing survey research data. For example, Spearman rank rho or Phi correlation should be used to evaluate the association between two variables that violate the assumptions of correlation and linear regression parametric tests. Chi-Square test is indicated for two group comparisons that break the assumptions of t-test parametric tests. The binary logistic regression should be used for dichotomous dependent variables instead of linear or multiple regression analyses.

68.8 Presentation of Study Outcomes

Sloppy and inaccurate presentation of the statistical analysis methods and results are weaknesses of many articles published in medical and allied health journals. Specifically, all statistical methods employed and the reasons for using them should be stated explicitly. Unfortunately, many published articles, particularly in low impact peer-reviewed journals, often state "we used appropriate statistical tests" without specifying the type of analysis. The statistical methods used should be specified with enough details that will enable anyone with access to the raw data, to recalculate all results. In cases when more than one statistical analysis is used, as it is often the case, it is essential to specify the test performed on each dataset [6].

When presenting the study findings, it is essential to specify the appropriate statistical measures of central tendency and variability. Arithmetic means and SD should be used only when data are distributed normally and not skewed. When the dataset is skewed, it is appropriate to use median, ranges or interquartile ranges. It is preferred to report SD in parentheses [i.e. Mean (SD)] instead of using Mean ± SD expressions because most readers tend to confuse the ± specification with a 95% confidence interval.

Instead of the SD, quite often, the standard error of the mean (SEM) is erroneously applied to report the variability of normally distributed data. The SEM is not a descriptive statistic, but an inferential index used for statistical estimation. The error associated with the use of SEM is perhaps common because it makes the data seem less variable. It is

Table 68.6 Parametric and non-parametric equivalent tests

	Study design	Parametric test (Interval/ratio data; test on means)	Non-parametric test (Norminal/ordinal data; test on median)
1	Correlation (measuring association between two variables)	Pearson's product moment correlation (interval/ratio scales, data are normally distributed, no outliers)	Spearman rho rank (both variables are on the ordinal scale, data are not normally distributed)
			Phi (both variables are dichotomous nominal scale)
			Kendall's Tau (both variables are ordinal scale)
			Point biserial: (one variable is dichotomous and the other variable is on ratio scale)
		Intra-class correlation (>2 repeated measurements/tests)	SPSS Generalised Estimating Equations
	Agreement (association of scores between 2 raters)	Pearson's product moment correlation (interval/ratio scales, data are normally distributed, no outliers)	Kappa when variables are on nominal scale Kendall's Tau for 2 raters on ordinal scale Kendall's W for > 2 raters on ordinal scale
2	One sample compared to a norm group	One sample t-test	The one sample Sign test is based on the median data from a non-symmetrical distribution The one sample Wilcoxon test is based on the median data from a symmetrical distribution
3	Two independent groups design	Student t-test	Chi-Square (χ^2) test used for nominal/ordinal scale (frequency) data with adequate sample size Fisher's exact test is recommended when χ^2 assumption is violated and when N is less than five/cell). Yates correction is used when N is less than 10/cell The Mann–Whitney U test is used for variables on the interval/ratio scale The Welch's t-test, which is a modified form of Student's t-test, is recommended when the two samples have unequal variances (heterogeneity) or unequal sample sizes
4	Dependent repeated measures design	Paired t-test	The McNemar's test is used for variables on the nominal scale or matched groups or twins. The Wilcoxon signed-rank test is used to compare the difference between two paired samples when the dependent variable is an ordinal scale. It is also used for variables on interval/ratio scale when the population cannot be assumed to be normally distributed
5	Three or more groups design	One-way analysis of variance	χ^2 test is used for variables on a nominal/ordinal scale (frequency data) with adequate sample size and k independent groups Kruskal-Wallis H – The test is based on the equality of medians from two or more populations. It is more powerful than the Mood's Median test, but it is less robust to outliers Mood's Median – The test is based on the equality of medians from two or more populations and it is more robust to outliers than the Kruskal–Wallis test, but it is less powerful
6	Three or more repeated measures design	Repeated measures ANOVA	Friedman's test is based on (ordinal) median data when samples are taken from the same people for nominal scale, using a randomised block design. Use the SPSS linear mixed effects model Cochran's Q when samples are taken from the same people for nominal scale Kruskal–Wallis H for ordinal data when samples are not taken from the same people for nominal scale Chi-square when samples are not taken from the same people for nominal scale
7	Two factors – group/time design	Mixed ANOVA design	Noguchi et. al. [15] Zuur et al. [16] Saste, Sananse and Sonar test Simpson SH

Table 68.6 (continued)

	Study design	Parametric test (Interval/ratio data; test on means)	Non-parametric test (Norminal/ordinal data; test on median)
8	Prediction studies	Linear/multiple regression	Binary logistic regression analysis

[13] https://www.youtube.com/watch?v=RtsdTydUiGw
[14] https://www.r-bloggers.com/beware-the-friedman-test/amp/
[15] https://www.researchgate.net/publication/267559451_nparLD_An_R_Software_Package_for_the_Nonparametric_Analysis_of_Longitudinal_Data_in_Factorial_Experiments
[16] https://www.r-bloggers.com/beware-the-friedman-test/
[17] http://www.allresearchjournal.com/archives/2016/vol2issue7/PartJ/2-6-122-317.pdf
[18] https://www.ncbi.nlm.nih.gov/pmc/articles/PMC4483789/
[19] https://www.cjhp-online.ca/index.php/cjhp/article/view/1471/2168 Accessed 7 June 2021

not appropriate to publish Mean and SEM data as a measure of dispersion [Mean (SEM)]. Similarly, it is essential that any "±" specification within the article and tables is specified as SD when it first appears, and in graphical illustrations, the meaning of the error bar (SD) specified. Another common appalling gaffe in many journal publications is the drawing of line and bar charts illustrating group mean data without error bars. Plots without a measure of variability (SD) are not instructive and should be avoided in scientific publications.

Conceptually, parametric tests are associated with arithmetic means and SD while non-parametric tests use median, range or interquartile range for comparing differences between groups. Unfortunately, many articles published in peer journals conflate this basic statistical concept.

Quite often numeric data are misreported in published studies with a level of precision with too many digits than what is possible with the instrument used to collect the data [6]. It is crucial that numeric data be reported to conform realistically with the level of precision/sensitivity of the instrument that took the measurement. The precision of a numeric data relates to the number of figures to the right of the decimal point. Another common doctrine taught to undergraduate medical and health sciences students is that "numeric research data should be rounded up appropriately and not too much and not too little" with the "numbers given in 2–3 effective digits" [18]. Clearly, these off-the-cuff statistical canon prescriptions are simplistic and confusing. There is currently no unanimity in the literature on the number of digits that numeric and inferential data should be presented.

There are confusing numeric reporting rules recommended in the literature such as rounding numbers to two decimal places, rounding numbers to significant digits and a mixture of the two rules (e.g. specifying the number of decimal places to ensure two significant figures for the SD). In a 2015 publication, after an extensive review of the emerging controversies in the literature, Cole offers the following general recommendations for reporting measures of central tendency, variability and inferential statistic measures [18].

1. Arithmetic Means: The rule of thumb is to report the value to conform to the level of precision of the instrument used in taking the measurement. For example, mechanical bathroom scales measure weight only to the nearest whole number (integer), for example, 70 kg. Thus, the means for weight should be reported to the nearest whole number consistent with the sensitivity of the weighing scale used, for example, M (SD) as 4430 (9.23) g or 4.43 (9.23) kg.
2. Standard Deviation: Report it to two significant digits for values under 10, for example, 0.83 kg.
3. Standard Error: Report it to one significant digit, for example, 3.6 kg.
4. Percentage: Use whole numbers or integers for values under 10% and one decimal place for values of 90% if their complement is informative. When the range of values is less than 0.1%, use two or more decimal places, for example, 0.2%, 6.4%, 25%, 88% and 99.7%.
5. Inferential test statistics such as t, F and χ^2: Report it up to one decimal place and up to two significant digits. When the calculated statistic value is significant, reporting t = 30 will be appropriate for a one decimal place t-value of 30.01, as it is so highly significant. Similarly, specifying two significant digits for t = −0.11 is unnecessary. Again, the extra precision is irrelevant as it is far from significant. It will be appropriate to report it as t = − 0.1. Report it to one decimal place and up to two significant digits. Examples t = −15, F = 11 and $\chi^2 = 4.1$.
6. p-values: Round it up to one significant digit, within the limits of the examples provided. The lower limit may be less than 0.001, but not greater than 0.000, for example, 0.3, 0.1, 0.07, 0.04 and 0.002, $p < 0.001$.

7. CI and effect size (for mean, percentage, mean difference, regression coefficient and correlation coefficient or risk ratio): Report them to one less significant digit, for example, the present risk ratio of 0.030 as 0.299. Consequently, 33.68, will be reported as 33.7 (95% CI: 7.5 to 74) or as 23 (95% CI: 8 to 70). Report it to two or three significant digits for effect sizes and two significant digits for measures of variability.
8. Mean difference and regression coefficients: Report the SE to one or two significant digits and the standardised mean difference to one or two decimal places.
9. Correlation coefficient: Report it to one or two decimal places or more when they are very close to ±1, for example, 0.02, − 0.6, 0.89 and 0.999.
10. Risk ratio: Report the data to two significant digits when the leading non-zero digit is four or more, otherwise round to three. Alternatively, use one/two significant digits rather than two or three. For odd ratios (ORs) when using logistic regression with ratio scale independent variable, report it to three decimal places. Alternatively, report the data as log OR×100 as the percentage odds to one decimal place. Examples are: 0.0321, 0.062, 0.76, 1.05, 4.2, 11.3, 55 and 1.042 [18].

68.9 Summary

This chapter discussed the sources and common statistical faux pas in articles published in medical and allied health journals. Undoubtedly, the errors highlighted in this chapter underscore the need for global reforms in medical and health sciences education by increasing the emphasis and time allocated in the curriculum to research methods, biostatistics and ethical issues in research. With adequate knowledge of the matters discussed and careful planning before the initiation of the study, the statistical flaws can be prevented easily.

Hopefully, the readers of this chapter will apply the knowledge gained to avoid the statistical mistakes highlighted and thus improve the quality and rigour of the statistics used in evidence-based research in medicine and allied health.

References

1. Gore SM, Jones IG, Rytter EC. Misuse of statistical methods: critical assessment of articles in BMJ from January to March. BMJ. 1977;1:85–7. Available at https://www.ncbi.nlm.nih.gov/pmc/articles/PMC1604073/. Accessed 27 Dec 2018.
2. Thiese MS, Arnold ZC, Walker SD. The misuse and abuse of statistics in biomedical research. Biochem Med. 2015, 25;(1):5–11. Available at https://www.ncbi.nlm.nih.gov/pmc/articles/PMC4401313/. Accessed 27 Dec 2018.
3. Fanelli D. How many scientists fabricate and falsify research?. A systematic review and meta-analysis of survey data. PLoS ONE. 2009;4:e5738. https://doi.org/10.1371/journal.pone.0005738.
4. Sauerbrei W, Abrahamowicz M, Altman DG, Cessie S, Carpenter J. Strengthening analytical thinking for observational studies: the STRATOS initiative. Stat Med. 2014; https://doi.org/10.1002/sim.6265.
5. Lang TA, Altman DG. Basic statistical reporting for articles published in biomedical journals: the "statistical analyses and methods in the published literature" or the SAMPL guidelines." Science editors' handbook, European Association of Science Editors. 2013.
6. Strasak AM, Zaman Q, Pfeiffer KP, Göbel G. Statistical errors in medical research--a review of common pitfalls. Swiss Med Wkly. 2007;137(3–4):44–9. Available at https://pdfs.semanticscholar.org/f209/5ccffd99ff9457f782d283dc2b990cfdb7ba.pdf?_ga=2.21952571.1036601531.1545322665-1476164196.1545322665. Accessed 27 Dec 2018.
7. Ogee A, Ellis M, Scibilia B, Pammer C, Steele C, Keller D. Choosing between a nonparametric test and a parametric test. Available at http://blog.minitab.com/blog/adventures-in-statistics-2/choosing-between-a-nonparametric-test-and-a-parametric-test 2015. Accessed 27 Dec 2018.
8. Wayne W, LaMorte. When to use a nonparametric test. Available at http://sphweb.bumc.bu.edu/otlt/MPH-Modules/BS/BS704_Nonparametric/BS704_Nonparametric2.html. 2017. Accessed 27 Dec 2018.
9. Kellar SP, Kelvin EA. Munro's statistical methods for healthcare research. 6th ed. Lippincott Williams & Wilkins; 2013.
10. Berger VW, Lunneborg CE, Ernst MD, Levin JG. Parametric analyses in randomised clinical trials. J Modern Appl Stat Methods. 2002;1(1):11, 74–82.
11. Burke DA, Whittemore SR, Magnuson DSK. Consequences of common data analysis inaccuracies in CNS trauma injury basic research. J Neurotrauma. 2013;30(10):797–805. Available at https://www.ncbi.nlm.nih.gov/pmc/articles/PMC3660075/. Accessed 22 Dec 2018.
12. Steiger JH. Outliers, leverage, and influence. n.d.. Available at http://www.statpower.net/Content/313/Lecture%20Notes/Outliers.pdf Accessed 22 Dec 2018.
13. Raj J. Mood's median test. n.d. Available at https://www.youtube.com/watch?v=9Vu5aJblYpY. Accessed 22 Dec 2018.
14. SPSS Linear mixed effects model. Available at https://www.r--bloggers.com/beware-the-friedman-test/amp/. Accessed 22 Dec 2018.
15. Noguchi, et al. An R software package for the nonparametric analysis of longitudinal data in factorial experiments. J Stat Soft. 2012;50(12). Available at https://www.researchgate.net/publication/267559451_nparLD_An_R_Software_Package_for_the_Nonparametric_Analysis_of_Longitudinal_Data_in_Factorial_Experiments. Accessed 22 Dec 2018.
16. Zuur et al. Mixed effects models and extensions in ecology. Available at https://www.jstatsoft.org/article/view/v032b01/v32b01.pdf. Accessed 27 Dec 2018.
17. Saste SV, Sananse SL, Sonar CD. On parametric and nonparametric analysis of two-factor factorial experiment. Int J Appl Res. 2016;(2, 7):653–6. Available at http://www.allresearchjournal.com/archives/2016/vol2issue7/PartJ/2-6-122-317.pdf. Accessed 27 Dec 2018.
18. Cole TJ. Too many digits: the presentation of numerical data. Arch Dis Child. 2015;100(7):608–9. Available at https://www.ncbi.nlm.nih.gov/pmc/articles/PMC4483789/. Accessed 22 Dec 2018.
19. Simpson SH. Creating a data analysis plan: what to consider when choosing statistics for a study. CJHP. 2015;68(4):311–7. Available at https://www.cjhp-online.ca/index.php/cjhp/article/view/1471/2168. Accessed 7 June 2021.

Survey Research Major Methodological Flaws: Caveat Lector

69

Joseph A. Balogun

Learning Objectives

After reading this chapter, the learner will be able to:

- Discuss the primary reasons for rejection of survey research manuscripts submitted for publication in top medical journals.
- Describe how to achieve a cross-cultural and conceptual equivalence of an adapted questionnaire.
- Discuss how to determine and interpret the readability of a questionnaire.
- Describe the different methods for calculating the optimum sample size for a survey study.
- Use web-based calculators to compute sample size and power for survey and intervention studies.

69.1 Introduction

Survey research is a structured and systematic (non-experimental) descriptive method of scientific inquiry frequently utilised by obstetricians and gynaecologists (Ob-Gyns) to gauge patients' and practitioners' knowledge, perceptions and attitudes on professional, health and social issues, and to determine the prevalence of diseases and primary risk factors that cause them [1–12]. For the findings from a survey study to be externally valid, it is essential that the sample selected to participate in the investigation adequately represents the target population [13]. Selection of the optimum sample size from the general population is an important statistical issue that must be addressed at the planning stage of any research [14, 15]. Unfortunately, the problem is generally overlooked because of the rigour and the computational complexities involved. Luckily, there are now web-based calculators that make this process less burdensome, but many clinicians are presently not familiar with these practical and pragmatic resources.

Many novice clinicians and scientists assumed that they could directly adopt a questionnaire developed in another country without obtaining the cross-cultural and conceptual equivalence of the instrument. Besides, inexperienced researchers often translate the questionnaire from another language and proceed to use them. These gaffes are misguided and a primary reason for rejection of survey research manuscripts submitted for publication in top medical and allied health journals [14, 15]. The aforementioned methodological flaws have been attributed to ignorance and poor planning compounded with limited access to relevant data analysis resources and textbooks [16]. With adequate knowledge of survey research methods and careful planning before the initiation of the study, these methodological pitfalls can be prevented easily.

This chapter seeks to fill the perceived knowledge and skills gaps by addressing the major methodological problems in survey research. The issues presented in this chapter, if taken to heart, will assist researchers engaged in survey study avoid the pervasive methodological flaws.

69.2 Operational Definitions

The terms "*questionnaire*," "*survey*," and *psychometric instrument* are often interchangeably used in the medical and allied health literature. This error is disconcerting because the three terms are separate concepts. A *questionnaire* is composed of a series of structured questions administered to the study participants. While the paper and pencil method that requires participants to write their answers is the most popular technique of conducting a questionnaire,

J. A. Balogun (✉)
Chicago State University, Chicago, IL, USA

University of Medical Sciences, Ondo City, Nigeria

Centre of Excellence in Reproductive Health Innovation, University of Benin, Benin City, Nigeria
e-mail: jbalogun@csu.edu; jbalogun@unimed.edu.ng

F. Okonofua et al. (eds.), *Contemporary Obstetrics and Gynecology for Developing Countries*,
https://doi.org/10.1007/978-3-030-75385-6_69

face to face interview, telephone, and the social media via the internet are also the common medium of administering questionnaires.

A *survey* consists of a questionnaire and the methods of collecting and aggregating the data, and statistically analyse the responses from those questions. That is to say, "questionnaire" describes the content, while "survey" describes the content, method, and data analysis [17]. Medical and allied health survey studies are routinely implemented to assess the knowledge, attitudes, and perceptions of patients, clinicians, lay persons or the public at large on health and social issues. Examples of survey studies in obstetrics and gynaecology are presented in the Appendix.

Psychometric instruments are standardised paper and pencil tests used in clinical practice and research for measuring the mental capacities and behaviours of patients. A few examples of psychometric tools used in obstetrics and gynaecology research and clinical practice includes the Contraceptive Knowledge Assessment [18], the International Index of Erectile Function Instrument [19], Pelvic Organ Prolapse Questionnaire [20], the International Consultation on Incontinence Questionnaire (ICIQ) [21], Obstetric Communication Assessment [22], the System for Evaluation of Teaching Qualities Tool [23], and the Delayed Child Bearing Questionnaire [24].

69.3 Survey Research Process

Conducting survey research entails a rigorous and complex process that requires knowledge of research design, questionnaire development, sample size estimation, data collection protocols, and statistical analysis [13]. The planning phase of survey research is the most critical, as errors and shortcomings that can negatively impact the study outcomes can be identified before proceeding to the subsequent steps of the investigation. At the planning stage, the study objectives, research design, questionnaire, and data collection protocols must be meticulously formulated.

Compared to the other descriptive (observational) research methodologies, the medium of administration of survey research is flexible and relatively inexpensive to implement. The anonymity associated with survey research allows the respondents to be honest and provide unambiguous responses. A well-developed questionnaire will have a clear purpose, easy to complete and not unnecessarily burdensome to the respondents. The major steps in the implementation of survey research are summarised in Fig. 69.1.

A frequent concern expressed by journal editors and reviewers on survey research manuscripts submitted for publication is the limited information presented in the methodology section [14, 15]. Many authors usually fail to discuss where the items in their questionnaire were adapted. Although very vital in understanding the core of any survey study, quite often, many authors do not address the following critical methodological issues:

- The different components of the questionnaire
- The number of open and closed-ended questions
- The format and scaling of the questions asked including the semantic differential terms used and the continuum of the ratings
- Methods of scoring the questionnaire
- The minimum and maximum possible scores
- The meaning and implication of the overall (cumulative) score
- The data analysis methods

Failure to address these issues comprehensively will make the replication of the survey study impossible.

The most concerning methodological faux pas is that many published survey research articles often lack information on the psychometric properties of the questionnaire used. Pertinent data on the readability, reliability, and validity of the questionnaire used in survey research will be needed for the findings of the study to be credible. The process for evaluating the reliability and validity of questionnaires are usually comprehensively covered in most research methods books and will not be repeated here. Unfortunately, the similar information about readability is less commonly available in medical and allied health journals and books, and therefore, is one of the primary topics covered in this chapter.

69.4 Translation and Adaptation of Questionnaires Published in Languages Other than English

The development and testing of the psychometric properties of a questionnaire require a high degree of diligence and effort. Similarly, the adaptation of questionnaires published in another language possesses a unique challenge in medical and allied health research. For example, an Ob-Gyns interested in evaluating the symptoms and impact of urinary incontinence among university students in Nigeria can adapt the Chinese version of the ICIQ [25]. However, the Ob-Gyns cannot translate the ICIQ to English language and then proceed to use the instrument directly. This practice is a common mistake made by inexperienced researchers and clinicians. The first goal of the Ob-Gyns should be to achieve a cross-cultural and conceptual equivalence, not semantic/literacy equality of the ICIQ instrument so that it is natural and acceptable among Nigerian university students. The use of the term "equivalency" here is the degree to which differ-

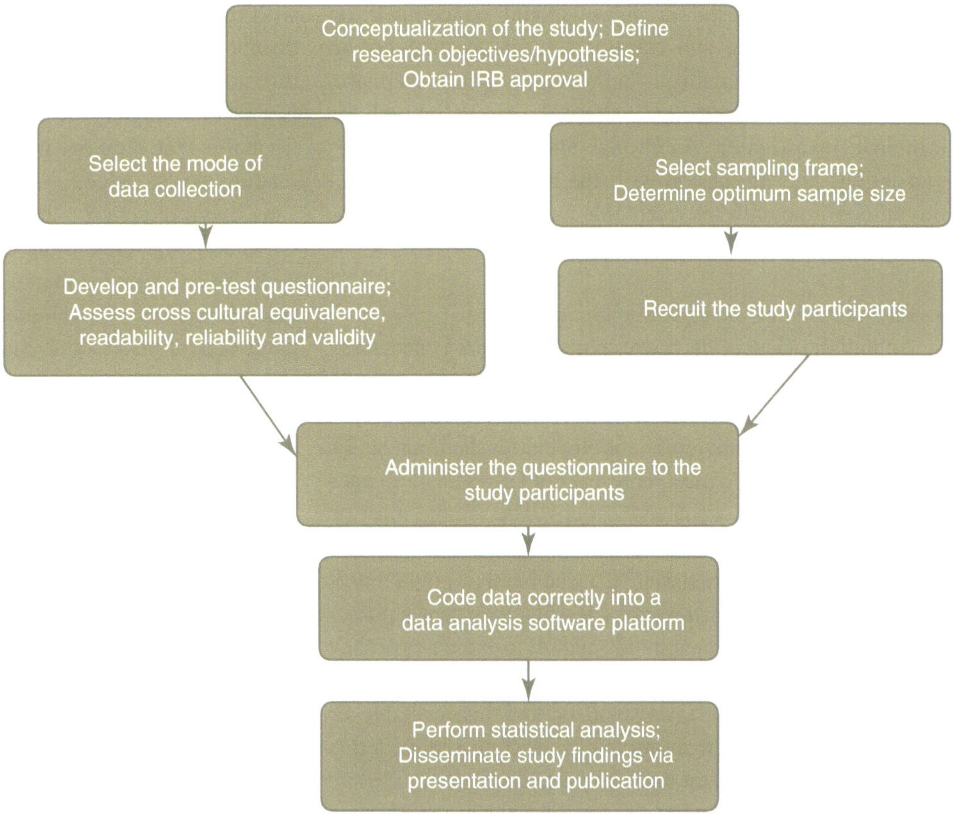

Fig. 69.1 The survey research process framework

ent forms of the same instrument yield similar results. The best strategy to achieve cross-cultural and conceptual equivalence of the ICIQ is to employ the forward and backward translations method proposed by the World Health Organization [26]. A summary of the protocol is provided below to aid the understanding of the strategy.

1. Forward Translation

A health professional with interview skills, fluent in the English language, and whose mother tongue is the primary language of the adapted questionnaire should be appointed as the translator. He/she should understand the contents and terminologies used in the questionnaire and should be given the following specific instructions:

- Focus on the conceptual equivalent of the word or phrase in the questionnaire, and not the word-for-word translation.
- Use simple, concise, and unambiguous terms when formulating a question. Fewer words are preferred.
- Prevent the use of technical terms, jargon, colloquialism, idioms, or vernacular phrases.
- Consider the gender and age of a typical person to whom the questionnaire will be administered and avoid using words that might be offensive to the target population.

2. Bilingual Expert Committee

The principal investigator should constitute a Bilingual Committee of experts fluent in English and the language of the adapted instrument to review the questionnaire and critic the words or expressions used and suggest alternatives and resolve any inadequate expressions or concepts and discrepancies between the forward translation and any previous versions of the research instrument if any. The Bilingual Committee should be provided with all the documents that will make them consistent with the interpretation of the questionnaire. The number of experts in the Bilingual Committee can vary, but it must include the original translator, local health experts, and individuals with questionnaire development, and translation experience. The outcome of this effort should produce a complete translated version of the questionnaire.

3. Back Translation

By using the same approach outlined in the first step, the questionnaire should now be converted back to the English language by another translator, whose mother tongue is the English language and who is not familiar with the questionnaire. This phase of the instrument development should concentrate on selected items on the questionnaire that are sensitive to translation problems across cultures. The emphasis in the back-translation phase should concentrate on achieving conceptual and cultural equivalence and not so much on linguistic equality as in the initial translation phase. At this stage, any inconsistency should be discussed with the Principal Investigator. Additional attempts at forwarding translations and discussion with the bilingual expert panel should continue until an acceptable version of the questionnaire emerged.

4. Pilot Review of the Research Questionnaire

An initial review of the research questionnaire is necessary to ascertain its face and content validity. The researcher should undertake the assessment on a cohort of the study target population – preferably individuals not eligible for the main study. The pilot study sample must represent both genders of all ages and the different socioeconomic groups. The sample must be debriefed systematically and asked (1) what they think each item of the questionnaire meant? (2) whether they could repeat the questions in their own words, (3) when they hear a phrase or term, what comes to their mind? and (4) to explain how they select their answers? They should be asked if there are expressions that they did not understand or find unacceptable or offensive. And should be instructed to select alternative terms that conform better to their usual language.

To gauge the evolving instrument consistency, the answers to each question provided by the pilot study sample should be contrasted with the translator's response to the questionnaire. In-depth personal interviews or focus group discussions must be used to accomplish the pilot testing and cognitive interviewing objectives. The examination must be undertaken under the supervision of an experienced facilitator. A comprehensive report from the recordings of the focus group discussions or interviews should be prepared. The final version of the questionnaire should address the methodological issues described below.

69.5 Readability Defined

Evaluation of the readability of a questionnaire written in English will be necessary to ascertain whether the respondents, can read it and comprehend its contents. A readability score is a computer-generated index which reflects the level of education that study respondents must have in order to understand the questionnaire. The score depends on the complexity of the vocabulary, word semantics, sentence syntactic, and text legibility [27]. Other factors include the reading skills and motivation of the study participants, cultural and social appropriateness, and linguistics.

Word difficulty and sentence length have been found to be the best predictor of questionnaire readability. The overall (mean) readability score of a questionnaire used for persons with limited reading skills may be misleading because they do not reflect the variation in item readability scores. It is difficult for an average person in most countries were English is a second language to comprehend and respond to a questionnaire that requires more than seventh- to eighth-grade reading skills. Indeed, vulnerable populations, such as persons living in poverty, the homeless, and persons older than 65 years of age are among those with limited reading skills.

From a design perspective, it is perilous to use a high literacy (readability) level questionnaire that the study participants cannot understand. Such a questionnaire will be prone to a high item and overall non-response rates. Findings from using such a questionnaire will not be valid and will constitute a waste of time, effort, and resources.

69.6 Determination of the Readability of a Research Questionnaire

There are several web-based platforms available to easily evaluate the readability of a questionnaire [28–31]. Many of the platforms provide easy access without subscription fees. One of them is the *Readable.io*® platform [31] used in this article to determine the readability of the *Autism Spectrum Disorder Questionnaire*. First, type the *Readable.io*® web address into any web browser and acclimatise to the platform by reading the provided instructions. Second, go back, cut the *Autism Spectrum Disorder Questionnaire,* and paste it inside the rectangular space on the left side of the computer screen and follow the direction provided. Several readability indices will be displayed immediately on the right-hand side of the screen (Fig. 69.2). The interpretation of the key indices is provided in this chapter.

Following evaluation of the readability of a questionnaire, if the score is higher than the grade level of the study participants, the following strategies can lower the score.

- Edit the text to shorten the length of the sentences and decrease the use of long words.
- Make reading the questionnaire friendly. Do not put too much information into a single paragraph. Split it up into meaningful chunks and avoid grammatical and syntax errors.
- Frame and tailor the contents of the questionnaire to match the intellectual capacity of the respondents. If the questionnaire is for the general public, then avoid the use of technical jargons or acronyms, and provide a glossary of operational definitions to explain the technical terms.
- The rule of thumb used in the USA is that questionnaires designed for the general public is at the grade level score of 8.

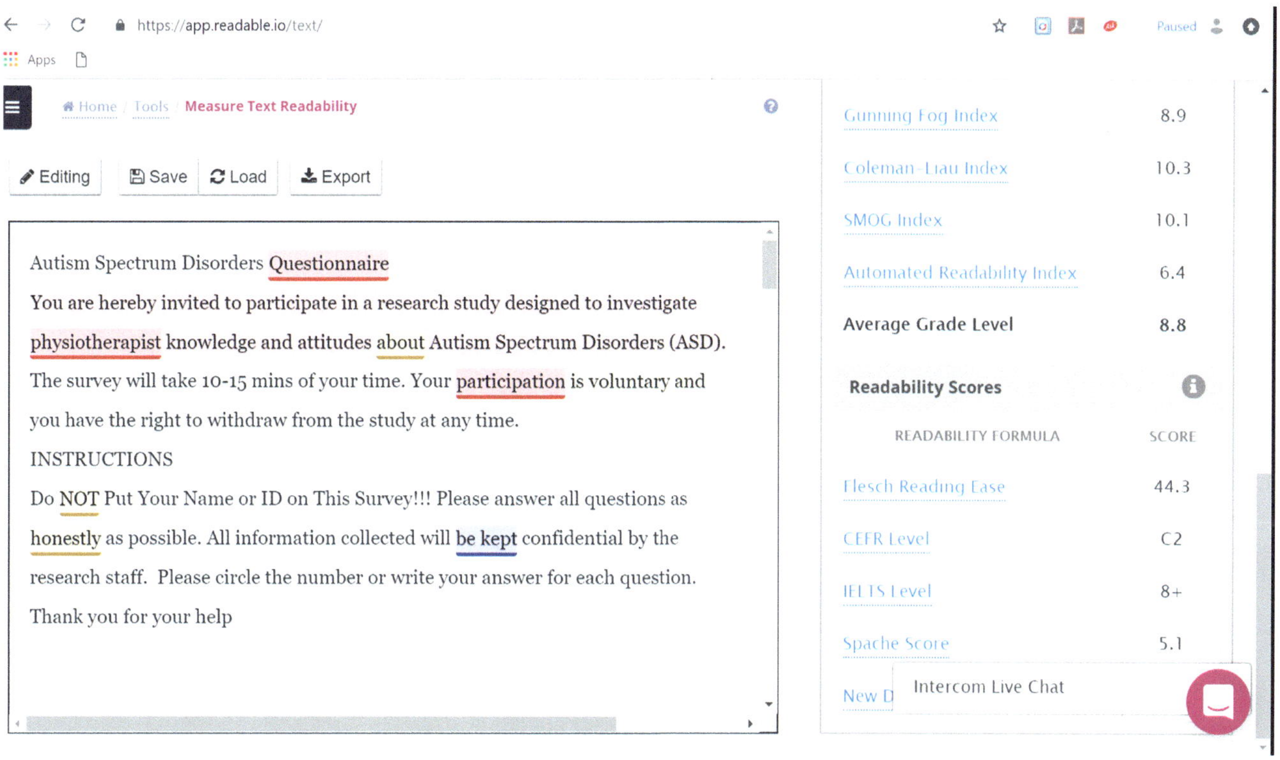

Fig. 69.2 Screenshot image of the *Readable.io*® software [31] after using it to determine the readability of the *Autism Spectrum Disorder Questionnaire*

69.7 Interpretation of the Readability Indices

The two widely used indicator of readability is the Flesch Reading Ease and the Flesch–Kincaid Grade Level scores. Although they both reflect the same core measures (word length and sentence length), they bear different weighting factors. The results of both tests are inversely related. That is, a text with high Flesch Reading Ease test score will have a low-grade level test score. Flesch Reading Ease score ranges between 0 and 100, and a high score indicates that the text is easy to understand. A high Flesch Reading Ease score indicates that the questionnaire is easy to read; a low score suggests that it is difficult to understand. The Flesch–Kincaid Grade Level score corresponds to the US educational grade level or year of education.

The discussion of the other readability indices such as Gunning-Fog Score, Coleman-Liau Index, SMOG Index, and Automated Readability Index indicated on the right-hand corner of the *Readable.io*®, displayed in Fig. 69.2, is beyond the scope of this article. The interpretation of the Flesch Reading Ease score is presented in Table 69.1.

The Flesch Reading Ease and Flesch-Kincaid scores for the *Autism Spectrum Disorder Questionnaire* discussed previously were 44.3 and 8.8, respectively. Both counts are a measure of the literacy difficulty level of the instrument. A Flesch-Kincaid score of 8.8 indicates that a ninth-grade (high school) reading level is needed to be able to comprehend the contents of the questionnaire fully. A Flesch Reading Ease score of 44.3 as indicated in Table 69.1 suggests that the test is relatively easy to understand by 13–15 years of age.

Table 69.1 Guidelines for the interpretation of the Flesch Reading Ease test scores [31]

	Score	Interpretation/Meaning
1	90 – 100	"Easily understood by an average 11-year old student"
2	60 – 70	"Easily understood by 13 to 15-year old students"
3	30	"Best understood by university graduates"

A high score indicates that the questionnaire is easier to read, while a low score reflects that the questionnaire is challenging to read

As indicated in Table 69.2, the ninth-grade (high school) education in the USA corresponds to "Form 3" in Hong Kong and "Year 10" in the British educational system at the age of 14 [32]. Table 69.2 has the potential for use in Nigeria to identify the education grade equivalence level in the USA, Hong Kong, and the UK. As a British colony, after independence, the Nigerian government patterned the educational system after the British, but the system has evolved differently over the years.

Table 69.2 The grade equivalent level in the USA, Hong Kong, and the UK [32]

Education Grade Guide				
Division	US Grade	Hong Kong Grade	UK Grade	Age
Elementary School	Early Childhood 1	Kindergarten 1 (K1)	–	3
–	Early Childhood 2	Kindergarten 2 (K2)	Reception	4
–	Grade 1 Junior	Kindergarten 3 (K3)	Year 1	5
–	Grade 1	Primary 1	Year 2	6
–	Grade 2	Primary 2	Year 3	7
–	Grade 3	Primary 3	Year 4	8
	Grade 4	Primary 4	Year 5	9
Middle School	Grade 5	Primary 5	Year 6	10
–	Grade 6	Primary 6	Year 7	11
–	Grade 7	Form 1	Year 8	12
–	Grade 8	Form 2	Year 9	13
High School	Grade 9	Form 3	Year 10	14
–	Grade 10	Form 4	Year 11	15
–	Grade 11	Form 5	Year 12	16
–	Grade 12	Form 6	Year 13	17

69.8 Manual Calculation of Sample Size

The goal of any survey study is to utilise an optimum sample size needed to produce an externally valid investigation. Small sample size generally produce a questionable outcome, while on the other hand, too large sample size will be a waste of money and time. Except for predictive studies, no precise rule of thumb recommendation exists to determine the sample size. Some biostatisticians posited that at least 10 observations per variable are needed. Using this rule of the thumb recommendation, a hypothetical predictive study containing four independent variables will need a minimum sample size of 40 subjects. This approach is an estimate and not very reliable.

The sample size in predictive studies can be estimated more accurately by using the equation:

Sample size = 50 + 8K. Where K is the number of independent (predictor) variables.

Applying the equation to the previous example:

$$\begin{aligned}\text{Sample size} &= 50+8(4)\\ &= 50+32\\ &= 82\end{aligned}$$

For intervention and survey studies, no such rule of thumb recommendation exists. As a result, researchers will need to compute the optimum sample size or use standard indicative tables.

As stated previously, the estimation of the optimum sample size is an important issue usually addressed at the planning stage of a study. In survey research, the sample size is the total number of completed responses to the questionnaire. Conversely, in clinical trials and laboratory experimental research, the sample size is the number of participants who fully completed all the testing conditions.

Table 69.3 Z-score values at different confidence levels [33]

	Desired confidence level (%)	Z-score
1	80	1.28
2	85	1.44
3	90	1.65
4	95	1.96
5	99	2.58

Typically, the calculation of sample size for survey studies is a complicated and challenging process. The traditional formula used is as follows:

$$\frac{\dfrac{z^2 \times p(1-p)}{e^2}}{1+\left(\dfrac{z^2 \times p(1-p)}{e^2 N}\right)}$$

Where

N = Population size

e = Margin of error (percentage in decimal form)

z = z-score

p = alpha level

Z-score = the number of standard deviations a given proportion is away from the mean, and it can be derived from Table 69.3.

In the above equation, population size represent the number of people living in a state or territory, number of employees in a company, number of students enrolled in a university, or the number of beds in a hospital. The margin of error is the percentage of the respondents who indicate how much the survey results will capture the views of the overall population. The smaller the margin of error, the closer to having the exact answer at a given confidence level. A typical survey will stipulate a confidence level of 95% and a margin of error of 5%. The confidence level reflects how confident the researcher can be about the accuracy of the anticipated study results [33].

69.9 Estimation of Sample Size from a Standard Indicative Table

A less laborious method used in survey research to estimate the optimum sample size and does not require mathematical computation, is the indicative table (Table 69.4).

To use the indicative table [34] successfully, during the planning stage of the study, the researcher must know the number of people in the general population and come to terms with the margin of error and the confidence level. Let

Table 69.4 An indicative table for estimating the sample size in survey studies [34]

Population size	Confidence level = 95%			Confidence level = 99%		
	Margin of error			Margin of error		
	5%	2.5%	1%	5%	2.5%	1%
10	10	10	10	10	10	10
20	19	20	20	19	20	20
30	28	29	30	29	30	30
50	44	48	50	47	49	50
75	63	72	74	67	73	75
100	80	94	99	87	96	99
250	152	215	244	182	229	246
500	217	377	475	285	421	485
700	248	481	653	341	554	672
1000	278	606	906	399	727	943
7500	365	1275	4211	610	160	5165
10,000	370	1332	4899	622	2098	6239
100,000	383	1513	8762	659	2585	14,227
500,000	384	1532	9423	663	2640	16,055
1,000,000	384	1534	9512	663	2647	16,317
2,500,000	384	1536	9567	663	2551	16,478
10,000,000	384	1536	9567	663	2651	16,560
100,000,000	384	1537	9603	663	2651	1,6584
200,000,000	384	1537	9603	663	2654	1,6585
300,000,000	384	1537	9603	663	2654	1,6586

say, we are interested in conducting a nationwide poll to assess the attitudes of Nigerians towards mandatory premarital HIV testing. First, we will need to determine the optimum sample size required for the study. The estimated population of Nigeria as of June 12, 2020 is over 205.89 million [35]. That population size is closer to the 200,000,000, highlighted in red on the left-hand side of the indicative Table 69.4 [34]. At the 5% margin of error and a 95% confidence level, reading off the chart, we would need for the study 384 subjects randomly selected from a sampling frame list of Nigerians.

69.10 Calculation of Sample Size from Effect Size Estimates

Table 69.5 is another less difficult method for obtaining sample size that does not require mathematical computation when the effect size for the study is known [36].

The pertinent question is, how can we know before conducting the study the effect size? One strategy is to perform a small pilot study to obtain a rough estimate or use the results from previously published related research. Another approach is to use clinical judgment to specify the smallest effect size that will be practically relevant.

Assuming for the hypothetical research study, we expect to detect a "small" effect size of the magnitude of 0.52 at an alpha level of 0.05. By reading off the Table 69.5, we would need 200 subjects for the study. The only caution in using the

Table 69.5 Estimation of a sample size from varying effect size values [36]

Sample size	Alpha (α) = 0.05		Alpha (α) = 0.01	
	Effect size (ES)		Effect size (ES)	
	Small (0.2)	Moderate (0.5)	Small (0.2)	Moderate (0.5)
20	0.10	0.34	0.03	0.14
40	0.14	0.60	0.05	0.35
60	0.19	0.78	0.07	0.55
80	0.24	0.88	0.09	0.71
100	0.29	0.94	0.12	0.82
150	0.41	0.99	0.20	0.96
200	0.52	1.00	0.28	0.99

table is the likelihood of overestimating the anticipated effect size. If we overstate the expected effect size, the sample size will be underestimated, and the study will be underpowered. And above all, there will be a lower probability of obtaining a statistically significant result.

69.11 Use of the *Check Market* ® Calculator for Computing Optimum Sample Size

The sample size data that we obtained from Table 69.4 is an estimate that is not accurate. Propitiously, precise computation of the sample size of a survey study can be accomplished easily by using the *Check Market®* calculator [37]. For another survey study, let us assume that we are interested in investigating the knowledge and attitudes of Nigerian Ob-Gyns about Hepatitis C virus (HCV) screening and counselling practice. First, we would need the total number of practicing Ob-Gyns in Nigeria. A previous national survey had reported that there are only 968 Ob-Gyns in the country, with the highest number of practitioners (19%) practice in Lagos State while Yobe and Jigawa State had just 0.2% and 0.1% of the Ob-Gyns, respectively. The South West at 33% had the highest, and North East geopolitical region had the lowest number (at 4.6%) of Ob-Gyns, respectively [38].

The same information needed for using the Indicative Table [34] will also be required for the *Check Market®* calculator. After accessing the platform, enter the number of Ob-Gyns, the 5% margin of error and confidence level of 95%. After plugging the three numbers into the calculator shells, 276 will be displayed on the lower left-hand side of the screen (Fig. 69.3).

For our theoretical survey study, we would need a sample size of 276 people to participate. At 20% projected response rate, we would need to invite 1,380 people. Undoubtedly, the response rate in survey research varies greatly depending on several factors such as the communication and distribution (e-mail, paper, telephone) methods used, the quality of the invitation, and the use of incentives.

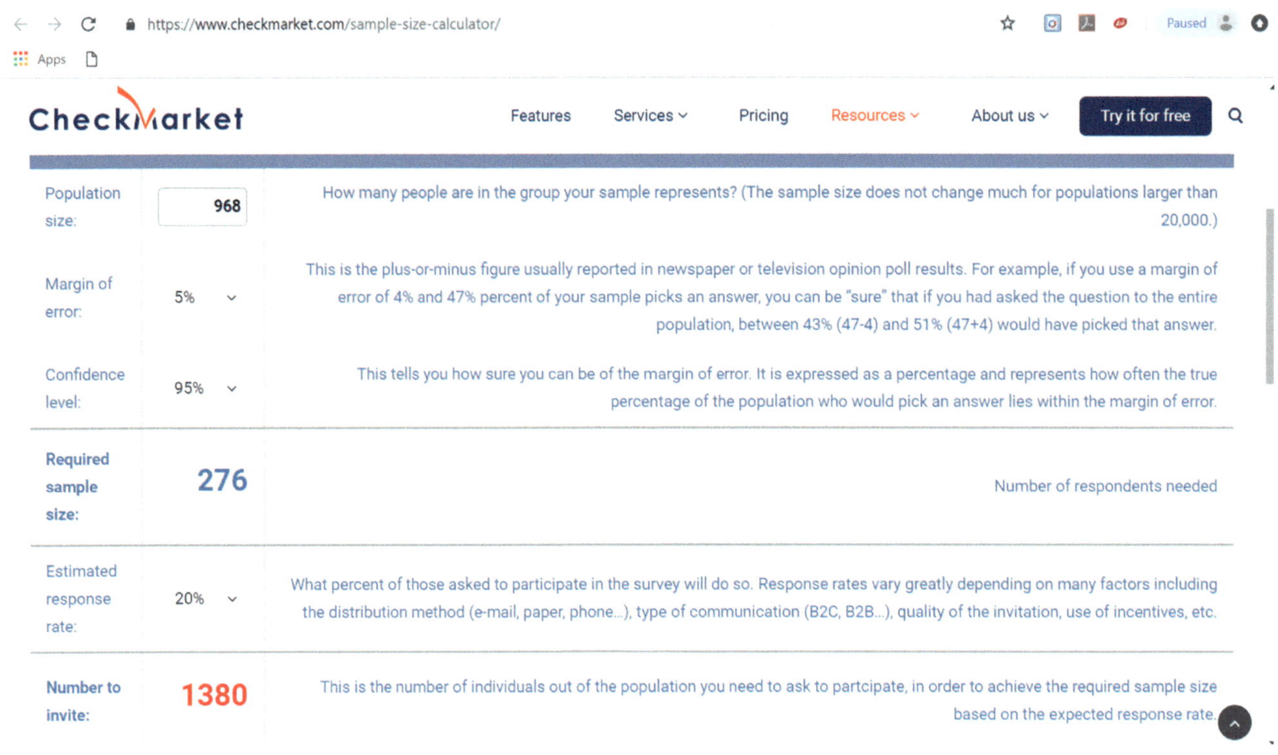

Fig. 69.3 Screenshot image of the Check Market® calculator [37] after using it to compute the sample size

69.12 Determination of Optimum Sample Size with the UCSF Calculator

The University of California at San Francisco (UCSF) developed a web-based calculator to compute the sample size of a study based on simple power/sample size calculations. In other words, the platform can be used to calculate the power of a test for specified sample size and vice versa [39].

To illustrate the application of the UCSF calculator, we will consider a hypothetical one sample study designed to uncover the effectiveness of a new cholesterol-lowering drug. At the planning phase of the study, we posited a null hypothesis (two-sided test) at an alpha level of 0.05 and a power of 0.80. To determine the sample size, we need to first conduct a pilot study to establish the baseline mean total serum cholesterol in the local community where the clinical trial will be implemented. Let us assume that we found the baseline mean total serum cholesterol in the pilot study to be 217.1 and sigma standard deviation value of 38.9 mg/dL (corresponds to mu0 on the UCSF calculator). Next, we need to obtain the normative population value for serum total cholesterol level (indicated as mu1 on the UCSF calculator). We will assume the normal value is 191 mg/dL [40].

Type the web address of the UCSF platform into a browser to access the website and proceed to enter the data mentioned above into the appropriate shells of the UCSF calculator [39]. And, hit the "Calculate" button at the left-hand corner of the calculator (Fig. 69.4).

The numeric value of 18 was displayed, which suggests that we will need 18 subjects for the clinical trial.

In addition to the one sample experimental design illustrated above, the UCSF calculator can also estimate sample size when comparing means or proportions for two independent samples and unmatched case-control study designs.

69.13 Calculation of Sample Size for Correlational Study

The correlational design is a prevalent method used in survey research, to establish a relationship between two variables X and Y. At the planning stage of the study, the investigator must conduct a power analysis to determine the number of participants needed. The web-based calculator developed by *Al-Therapy Statistics* [41] is ideal to decide the minimum number of subjects required to obtain the desired correlation coefficient. The goal of such a study is to ensure that the experiment has enough statistical power. That is, we want some confidence in obtaining the effect size anticipated. In practice, 0.80 or higher is the power value commonly used. The statistical power of 0.80 means the test has an 80% chance of discovering a statistically significant difference if

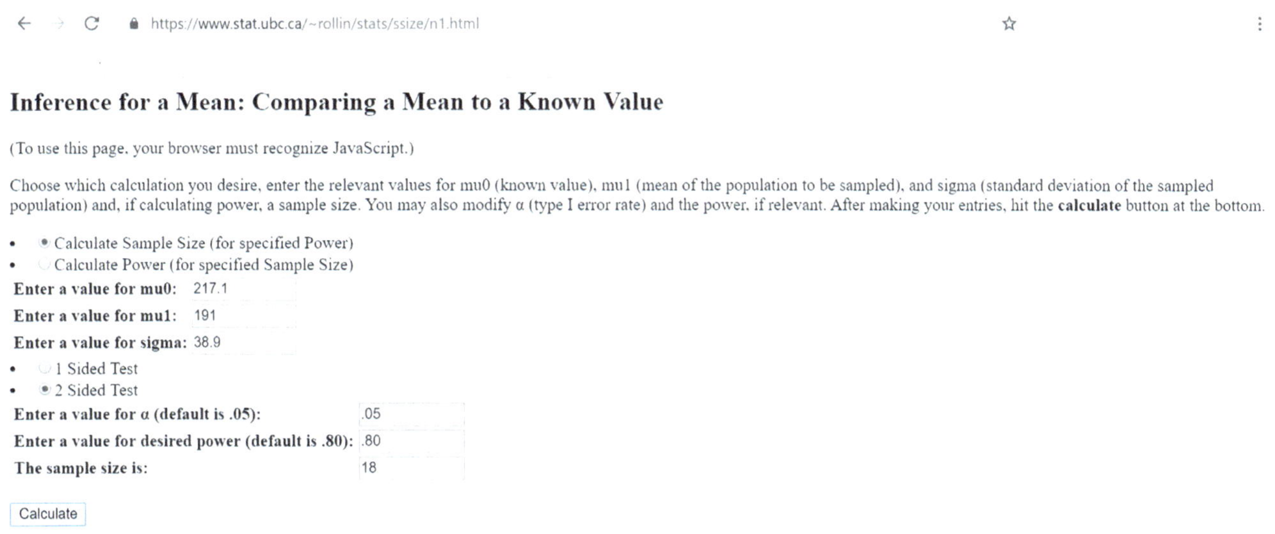

Fig. 69.4 Screenshot image of the UCSF calculator [39] after using it to compute the sample size

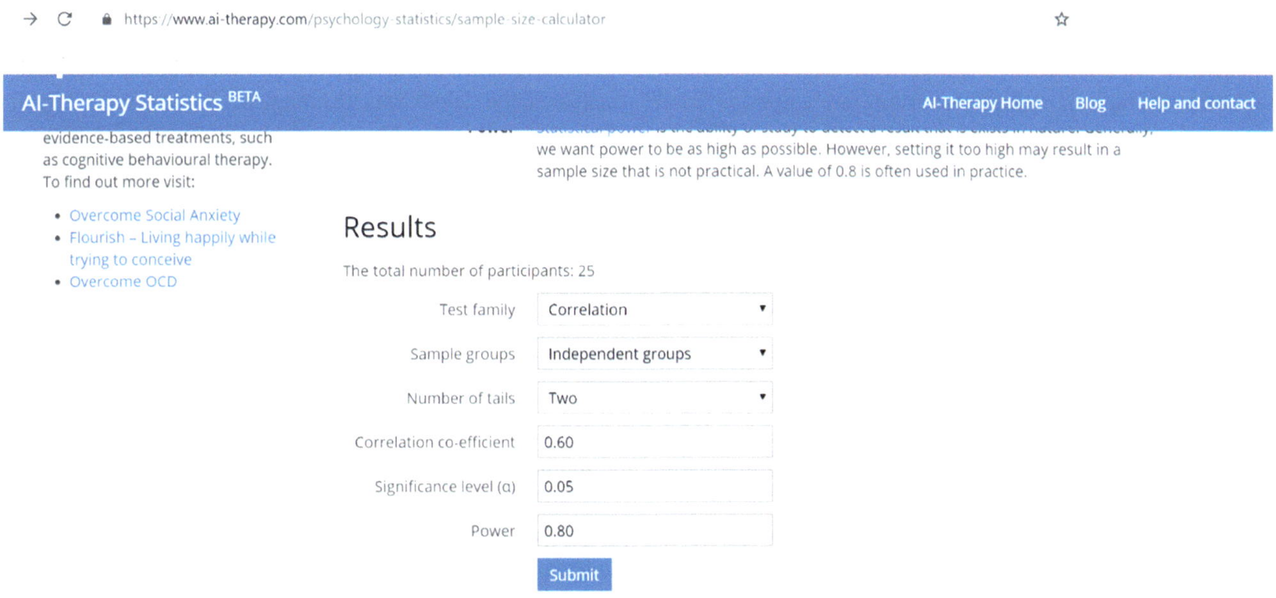

Fig. 69.5 Screenshot image of the *AI-Therapy Statistics* [41] calculator after using it to compute the sample size

one is present. In the theoretical study described above, let us say, we expected a correlation coefficient (r) of 0.60 and adopted a two-tailed test at an alpha level of 0.05 and a power of 0.80.

Type the web address of the *AI-Therapy Statistics*[41] into a browser to access the calculator and enter the desired power analysis information into the platform (Fig. 69.5).

Proceed to hit the "Submit," button at the bottom of the left-hand corner of the screen. In response, the software indicated that we would need 25 participants.

69.14 Conversion of Survey Research Clinical Data

Survey studies are the most efficient and reliable method to obtain authentic feedback from a small representative sample with the goal of using the results to address critical problems affecting the general population [13]. The findings from the sample are used to establish the norms for the population. Normative data describe rather than explain the phenomena of interest that represents the characteristics of a defined population at a specific time. Normative data are of vital importance to clinicians for (1) defining the genesis of clinical conditions in the community; (2) identifying the baseline against which to compare subsequently collected data; (3) making clinical decisions about the normality of a patient's status relative to the population; (4) developing standards of care, and (5) establishing the systematic classification and knowledge of the disease [42].

Many clinicians have in error come to associate survey research exclusively to the use of a questionnaire to investigate perception and attitudes about health and social issues. Indeed, survey research extends beyond that as it is applied in establishing a diagnosis or determining the prevalence of diseases. Physicians are daily challenged to provide relevant medical information to their patients or make an accurate diagnosis. Similarly, physicians compare their patients' laboratory information with the population normative data to arrive at a diagnosis. Such clinical decisions often involve converting laboratory data from one unit to another and determining whether the value obtained is within normal limits.

Situations of this nature occur frequently in developing countries because the major instruments used in the hospitals and institutions of higher learning are imported from abroad. For example, hospitals and universities in Nigeria purchase their primary equipment from all over the world. The Hitachi 704/917 analyser commonly used in Nigerian hospitals and research centres to determine the concentration of substances in the blood is produced by Roche Diagnostics (formerly Boehringer-Mannheim) Indianapolis. The instrumentation when manufactured in the USA provide the level of materials in the blood in mg/dL, but a similar device produced in Canada and Europe offer measurements in SI unit of millimoles per litre (mmol/L). The published normative data in Nigeria for cholesterol levels are reported usually in mmol/L, but many hospitals use the Hitachi 917 analyser manufactured in the USA that provides the level of materials in the blood in mg/dL. The golden rule to convert total serum level from milligrams per decilitre (mg/dL) to the standard SI unit of millimoles per litre (mmol/L) is to multiply by 0.02586. And to convert from millimoles per litre (mmol/L) to milligrams per decilitre (mg/dL) is to multiply by 38.67.

Converting laboratory data from one unit (such as mg/dL) to another (mmol/L) at the bedside clinical situations can be overwhelming and confusing to most clinicians. Interestingly, there are now web-based calculators that convert physical, anthropometric, and biochemical measures such as cholesterol level from mg/dL to mmol/L with minimal effort. An example of such web-based calculator is the Omni® health platform used in obstetrics and gynaecology to calculate the following clinical, anthropometric, and biochemical measures [42]:

- Period
- Ovulation
- Pregnancy due date
- Post-partum appearance, pulse, grimace, activity, and respiration (APGAR) score for new-born
- Pregnancy weight gain
- Human chorionic gonadotropin (hCG) levels
- Progesterone to oestrogen ratio
- Testosterone to oestradiol ratio

69.15 Application of Health Calculator in Clinical Diagnosis

The application of the Omni® health calculator in the conversion of clinical data allows the Ob-Gyns to make a correct diagnosis or to track treatment outcomes [43]. Following the conversion of data from one unit to another, if the patients' laboratory values are outside the normative population range, the diagnosis of a disease/disorder is made, and appropriate therapeutic intervention (surgical or medical) instituted.

In addition to the computation of fertility and pregnancy measures, the Omni® health calculator is versatile and applicable in other clinical scenarios to derive the following anthropometric, clinical, and biochemical measures listed on their website at https://www.omnicalculator.com/health#s-31 [43]:

1. "General health assessment of medication dosage, Glasgow coma scale, opioid conversion, addiction, Alvarado score, blood alcohol content, body surface area, caffeine, free and bioavailable testosterone, medical radiation, noise pollution-maximal exposure time, revised trauma score, sleep, and water intake.
2. The body measurement such as body mass index, body fat, body adiposity index, ideal weight, waist to hip ratio, lean body mass, basal metabolic rate, body shape, Harris-Benedict, Katch-McArdle, ponderal index, waist to height ratio, and army/navy body fat.
3. The metabolic disorders such as end-stage liver disease, blood sugar, protein and resting metabolic rate, total calorie/meal calorie, carbohydrates/fat intake, cholesterol units and ratio, and LDL.
4. Heart indices such as cardiac output, stroke volume, mean arterial pressure, and ECG heart rate.
5. The electrolytes and fluids for creatinine clearance, glomerular filtration rate, corrected calcium, fractional excretion of sodium, sodium correction, Anion gap, arterial blood pH, corrected magnesium, drip rate, free water deficit, sodium correction rate for hypo-and hypernatremia, sodium deficit, total body water, urine anion gap, and venous blood pH.

6. Haematology indices, such as absolute neutrophil count, blood volume, blood donor, blood type, allowable blood loss, eosinophil count, lymphocyte count, reticulocyte count, corrected reticulocyte count, hematocrit /haemoglobin ratio, plasma volume, serum-ascites albumin gradient, and transferrin saturation.
7. Paediatric clinical measures, such as paracetamol/ Ibuprofen dosage, glomerular filtration rate, APGAR score, blood volume, height, and blood transfusion volume.
8. Pulmonary indices such as lung/vital capacity, lung cancer risk, smoking recovery, and endotracheal tube size" [43].

69.16 Summary

This chapter is "a must-read" for Ob-Gyns planning a survey study or contemplating applying the finding from a survey study in clinical practice. More specifically, the chapter provides details on how to achieve cross-cultural and conceptual equivalence of questionnaires translated from another language, ascertain the instrument's readability, and the web-based resources available to calculate optimum sample size in survey research. The judicious application of the information contained in this chapter will improve the standard of survey research published in medical and allied health journals.

References

1. Hankins GD, Erickson K, Zinberg S, Schulkin J. Neonatal encephalopathy, and cerebral palsy: a knowledge survey of fellows of the American College of Obstetricians and Gynaecologists. Obstet Gynaecol. 2003;101(1):11–7.
2. Jones JL, Ogunmodede F, Scheftel J, Kirkland E, Lopez A, Schulkin J, Lynfield R. Toxoplasmosis-related knowledge and practices among pregnant women in the United States. Inf Dis Obstet Gynaecol. 2003;11(3):139–45.
3. Schrag SJ, Fiore AE, Gonik B, Malik T, Reef S, Singleton JA, Schuchat A, Schulkin J. Vaccination and perinatal infection prevention practices among obstetrician-gynaecologists. Obstet Gynaecol. 2003;101(4):704–10.
4. Spong CY, Erickson K, Willinger M, Hankins GD, Schulkin J. Stillbirth in obstetric practice: report of survey findings. J Mater Fetal Neonat Med. 2003;14(1):39–44.
5. Dietrich AJ, Williams JW Jr, Ciotti MC, Schulkin J, Stotland N, Rost K, Baram D, Cornell J. Depression care attitudes and practices of newer obstetrician-gynaecologists: a national survey. Am J Obstet Gynaecol. 2003;189(1):267–73.
6. Boaz K, Fiore AE, Schrag SJ, Gonik B, Schulkin J. Screening and counselling practices reported by obstetrician-Gynaecologists for patients with hepatitis C virus infection. Inf Dis Obstet Gynaecol. 2003;11(1):39–44.
7. Noller KL, Bettes B, Zinberg S, Schulkin J. Cervical cytology screening practices among Obstetrician–Gynaecologists. Obstet Gynaecol. 2003;102:259–65.
8. Margwe JA, Lupindu AM. Knowledge and attitude of pregnant women in rural Tanzania on prevention of anaemia. Afr J Reprod Health. 2018;22(3):71–9.
9. Ramathuba DU, Ngambi D. Knowledge and attitudes of women towards human papilloma virus and HPV vaccine in Thulamela municipality of Vhembe district in Limpopo Province, South Africa. Afr J Reprod Health. 2018;22(3):111–9.
10. Arulogun OS, Adefioye OA. Attitude towards mandatory premarital HIV testing among unmarried youths in Ibadan northwest local government area, Nigeria. Afr J Reprod Health. 2010;14(1):83–94.
11. Nnodu O, et al. Knowledge and attitudes towards cervical cancer and human papillomavirus: a Nigerian pilot study. Afr J Reprod Health. 2010;14(1):95–108.
12. Yotsumoto J, Sekizawa A, Suzumori N, Yamada T, Samura O, Nishiyama M, Miura K, Sawai H, Murotsuki J, Kitagawa M, Kamei Y, Masuzaki H, Hirahara F, Endo T, Fukushima A, Namba A, Osada H, Kasai Y, Watanabe A, Katagiri Y, Takeshita N, Ogawa M, Okai T, Izumi S, Hamanoue H, Inuzuka M, Haino K, Hamajima N, Nishizawa H, Okamoto Y, Nakamura H, Kanegawa T, Yoshimatsu J, Tairaku S, Naruse K, Masuyama H, Hyodo M, Kaji T, Maeda K, Matsubara K, Ogawa M, Yoshizato T, Ohba T, Kawano Y, Sago H, Japan NIPT Consortium. A survey on awareness of genetic counselling for non-invasive prenatal testing: the first-year experience in Japan. J Hum Genet. 2016;61(12):995–1001.
13. Groves, et al. Survey methodology. Hoboken, NJ: Wiley; 2009.
14. Thrower P. Eight reasons I rejected your article. 2012. Available at https://www.elsevier.com/connect/8-reasons-i-rejected-your-article. Accessed 15 Dec 2018.
15. Enago Academy. Learning to Avoid Journal Rejection. 2018. Available at https://www.enago.com/academy/learning-to-avoid-journal-rejection/. Accessed 15 Dec 2018.
16. Thiese MS, Arnold ZC, Walker SD. The misuse and abuse of statistics in biomedical research. Biochem Med. 2015;25(1):5–11. Available at https://www.ncbi.nlm.nih.gov/pmc/articles/PMC4401313/. Accessed 15 Dec 2018.
17. SurveyMonkey. Survey vs questionnaire: what's the difference?. 2018. Available at https://www.surveymonkey.com/mp/survey-vs-questionnaire/. Accessed 15 Dec 2018.
18. Haynes MC, Ryan N, Saleh M, Winkel AF, Ades V. Contraceptive knowledge assessment: validity and reliability of a novel contraceptive research tool. Contraception. 2017;95(2):190–7.
19. Utomo E, Blok BF, Pastoor H, Bangma CH, Korfage IJ. The measurement properties of the five-item International Index of Erectile Function (IIEF-5): a Dutch validation study. Andrology. 2015;3(6):1154–9.
20. Lowder JL, Ghetti C, Oliphant SS, Skoczylas LC, Swift S, Switzer GE. Body image in the Pelvic Organ Prolapse Questionnaire: development and validation. Am J Obstet Gynecol. 2014;211(2):174.e1–9.
21. Athanasiou S, Grigoriadis T, Kyriakidou N, Giannoulis G, Antsaklis A. The validation of international consultation on incontinence questionnaires in the Greek language. Neurourol Urodyn. 2012;31(7):1141–4.
22. Rodriguez AN, DeWitt P, Fisher J, Broadfoot K, Hurt J. Psychometric characterisation of the obstetric communication assessment tool for medical education: a pilot study. Int J Med Educ. 2016;7:168–79. Available at https://www.ncbi.nlm.nih.gov/pmc/articles/PMC4912696/. Accessed 15 Dec 2018.
23. van der Leeuw R, Lombarts K, Heineman MJ, Arah O. Systematic evaluation of the teaching qualities of obstetrics and gynaecology faculty: reliability and validity of the SETQ tools. 2011. Available

at https://journals.plos.org/plosone/article?id=10.1371/journal.pone.0019142. Accessed 15 Dec 2018.
24. Behboudi-Gandevani S, Ziaei S, Kazemnejad A, Khalajabadi F, Farahani FK, Vaismoradi M. Development and psychometric properties of the delayed childbearing questionnaire (DCBQ-55). Healthcare. 2018;6:120. https://doi.org/10.3390/healthcare6040120. Available at www.mdpi.com/journal/healthcare. Accessed 15 Dec 2018.
25. Huang L, Zhang SW, Wu SL, Ma L, Deng XH. The Chinese version of ICIQ: a useful tool in clinical practice and research on urinary incontinence. Neurourol Urodyn. 2008;27(6):522–4. Available at https://onlinelibrary.wiley.com/doi/abs/10.1002/nau.20546. Accessed 15 Dec 2018.
26. World Health Organization (WHO, n.d.). Process of translation and adaptation of instruments. Available at http://www.who.int/substance_abuse/research_tools/translation/en/. Accessed 27 Dec 2018.
27. Available at https://en.wikipedia.org/wiki/Readability. Accessed 27 Dec 2018.
28. Available at https://www.webpagefx.com/tools/read-able/. Accessed 27 Dece 2018.
29. Available at https://readability-score.com/. Accessed 27 Dec 2018.
30. Available at http://www.readabilityformulas.com/free-readability-formula-tests.php. Accessed 27 Dec 2018.
31. Available at https://readable.io/. Accessed 27 Dec 2018.
32. America International School. 2018. Available at https://www.ais.edu.hk/age-grade-guide. Accessed 27 Dec 2018.
33. Survey Monkey: Sample size calculation. n.d.. Available at https://www.surveymonkey.com/mp/lp/sample-size-calculator/?utm_expid=.cOMQLyyUQhqbVct5bsJlAA.1&utm_referrer=. Accessed 27 Dec 2018.
34. Sample size table from the research advisors. Available at https://www.research-advisors.com/tools/SampleSize.htm. Accessed 27 Dec 2018.
35. Worldometer. Nigeria population live. Available at https://www.worldometers.info/world-population/nigeria-population/. Accessed 12 Jun 2020.
36. Complete dissertation by statistics solutions. n.d. Available at https://www.statisticssolutions.com/sample-size-formula/. Accessed 27 Dec 2018.
37. Check Market®. n.d. Available at https://www.checkmarket.com/sample-size-calculator/. Accessed 27 Dec 2018.
38. Agboghoroma CO, Gharorob EP. Coverage and distribution of obstetricians and gynaecologists in Nigeria. Int J Gynaecol Obstetics. 2015;129(1):50–3. Available at https://obgyn.onlinelibrary.wiley.com/doi/abs/10.1016/j.ijgo.2014.09.034. Accessed 27 Dec 2018.
39. UCSF Biostatistics: Power and sample size programs. n.d. Sample size table from the research advisors. Available at http://www.stat.ubc.ca/~rollin/stats/ssize/. Accessed 27 Dec 2018.
40. Centres for Disease Control and Prevention. Serum cholesterol level. 2013. Available at https://www.cdc.gov/nchs/fastats/cholesterol.htm. Accessed 27 Dec 2018.
41. Al-Therapy Statistics. Sample size calculator. 2019. Available at https://www.ai-therapy.com/psychology-statistics/sample-size-calculator. Accessed 27 Dec 2018.
42. O'Connor. Normative data: their definition, interpretation, and importance for primary care physicians. Fam Med. 1990;22(4):307–11. https://www.ncbi.nlm.nih.gov/pubmed/2200734.
43. Omni Calculators. Health Calculators. n.d.. Available at https://www.omnicalculator.com/health#s-31. Accessed 27 Dec 2018.

Appendix

Examples of Survey Research in Obstetrics and Gynaecology

- Assess the knowledge of Ob-Gyns on the aetiology and pathophysiology of neonatal encephalopathy and its relationship to cerebral palsy.[1]
- Determine pregnant women's knowledge about toxoplasmosis and practices to prevent the infection.[2]
- Determine the vaccination and perinatal infection prevention practices among Ob-Gyns.[3]
- Determine the practice patterns of Ob-Gyns in the management of stillbirth.[4]
- Assess the attitudes and behaviour of Ob-Gyns towards depression care.[5]
- Determine the knowledge of Ob-Gyns on the aetiology and pathophysiology of neonatal encephalopathy and its relationship to cerebral palsy.[6]
- Investigate the current cervical cytology screening practices of Ob-Gyns Fellows, to establish a baseline for tracking future changes in practice.[7]
- Determine the knowledge and attitudes of pregnant women about anaemia.[8]
- Determine rural women's knowledge of human papillomavirus and the HPV vaccine.[9]
- Investigate the attitude of unmarried youths towards mandatory premarital HIV testing.[10]
- Assess the knowledge and attitudes of urban and rural women towards cervical cancer and HPV.[11]
- Determine the knowledge and attitudes of Ob-Gyns about HCV screening and counselling practices.[12]

F. Okonofua et al. (eds.), *Contemporary Obstetrics and Gynecology for Developing Countries*,
https://doi.org/10.1007/978-3-030-75385-6

Index

F. Okonofua et al. (eds.), *Contemporary Obstetrics and Gynecology for Developing Countries*,
https://doi.org/10.1007/978-3-030-75385-6

F

I

J

K

L

T

GPSR Compliance

The European Union's (EU) General Product Safety Regulation (GPSR) is a set of rules that requires consumer products to be safe and our obligations to ensure this.

If you have any concerns about our products, you can contact us on ProductSafety@springernature.com

In case Publisher is established outside the EU, the EU authorized representative is:

Springer Nature Customer Service Center GmbH
Europaplatz 3
69115 Heidelberg, Germany

Batch number: 10731665

Printed by Printforce, the Netherlands